CARDIAC AND PULMONARY MANAGEMENT

CARDIAC AND PULMONARY MANAGEMENT

M. GABRIEL KHAN

MB BCh, MD, FRCP(London), FRCP(C), FACP
Associate Professor of Medicine, University of Ottawa
Consultant Cardiologist, Ottawa General Hospital
Ottawa, Canada

Foreword by
HENRY J.L. MARRIOTT

MD, FACP, FACC
Director of Clinical Research
Rogers Heart Foundation
St. Petersburg, Florida
Clinical Professor of Cardiology
Emory School of Medicine
Atlanta, Georgia

LEA & FEBIGER
Philadelphia, London
1993

Lea & Febiger
Box 3024
200 Chester Field Parkway
Malvern, Pennsylvania 19355-9725
U.S.A.
(215) 251-2230

Executive Editor—R. Kenneth Bussy
Manuscript Editor—Denise Wilson
Production Manager—Samuel A. Rondinelli
Developmental Editor—Tanya Lazar

Library of Congress Cataloging-in-Publication Data

Khan, M. Gabriel.
    Cardiac and pulmonary management / M. Gabriel Khan; foreword
by Henry J.L. Marriott.
        p.   cm.
    Includes index.
    ISBN 0-8121-1494-9
    1. Cardiopulmonary system—Diseases.   I. Title.
    [DNLM: 1. Heart Diseases—diagnosis.   2. Heart Diseases—therapy.
    3. Lung Diseases—diagnosis.   4. Lung Diseases—therapy. WG 200
    K45c]
    RC702.K53   1992
    616.1'2—dc20
    DNLM/DLC
    for Library of Congress   92-11602
                                                                               CIP

NOTICE

The author and the publisher have made every effort to ensure that dosage recommendations are accurate and in agreement with accepted standards at the time of publication. Readers must be aware, however, that dosage schedules of newer pharmaceutical agents may change and the possibility of human error always exists. It is advisable, therefore, that you check the product monograph and the recommended dosage if the drug to be administered is one that you use infrequently or have not used recently.

Reprints of chapters may be purchased from Lea & Febiger in quantities of 100 or more. Contact Sally Grande in the Sales Department.

PRINTED IN THE UNITED STATES OF AMERICA

Print number: 5   4   3   2   1

FOREWORD

It is astonishing how many substantial books lack a foreword, the purposes of which can be so useful and diverse. One may contain elements of a book review and provide the opportunity for someone who has already digested the text to take the reader by the hand and lead him to its strengths and, if necessary, its weaknesses. The foreword should, if possible, get the prospective reader into the frame of mind where he can't wait to tackle the pages that follow. It may reemphasize, with the writer's personal slant or bias from his familiarity as a detached but interested reader, what the author has said in his preface about how to use and get the most out of the text; and it may stress virtues that the author is too modest to claim. It may also, if the writer's knowledge and experience permits, add a useful, personal supplement to the text.

In medicine, the two most commonly affected organ systems are the cardiovascular and the respiratory systems. Moreover, there are overlaps and parallels in the symptomatology and therapy of the two; many of the same symptoms can be caused by both heart and lung disease, and disease of the one may be intimately reflected in a response by the other. The two combine to form a natural therapeutic marriage that is consummated in this book.

Dr. M. Gabriel Khan has the unique capacity to combine his encyclopedic knowledge with an ability to condense it and yet keep it readable. He is the author of previous well known and popular handbooks and he has outdone himself with this one. He himself handles all of the cardiologic therapy, except for the nonpharmacologic methods of treating arrhythmias; to deal with respiratory problems, he has assembled a team of outstanding pulmonary and infectious disease experts.

The resulting book is a masterpiece. It is up-to-date, thorough, meticulously detailed and accurate. It is emphatically a text designed for quick and easy reference and not for steady reading. Virtually all aspects of the management of cardiac and pulmonary diseases are covered in concise detail. But there is much more than mere management here: to provide intelligent background for therapy, the pathophysiology, symptomatology, and diagnosis are all summarized, so that the book becomes a veritable textbook of cardiopulmonary medicine.

In the technological age in which we live and work, among the welter of "state-of-the-art" information, it is easy to overlook the simpler measures. And even in this extraordinarily comprehensive text, there are one or two simple but effective emergency measures that are not accorded space. In medicine, the very simplest of mechanical measures is sometimes remarkably effective; consider, for instance, the exquisite simplicity and undisputed efficacy of the Heimlich maneuver—what could be simpler than the concept of using the diaphragm as a piston? A somewhat analogous situation prevails in asthma, in which the patient's difficulty is in getting the trapped air *out of* the lungs. Most therapies are, appropriately enough, directed at relaxing the bronchioles. But in the child with a small and pliable chest, a lot can be done to relieve the acute situation within a few seconds with just a pair of capable adult hands. One can provide prompt and dramatic relief with one hand embracing each hemithorax and reinforcing the child's labored exhalations by rhythmically—synchronous with each expiratory effort—compressing the small chest. The relief can be remarkable, and it is easy enough to keep this up for several minutes—much easier than external cardiac massage in the adult!—while waiting for the bronchodilator to take effect.

And again, in pulmonary edema, the most important single step in treatment is simplicity itself: sit the patient up *with feet on the ground*— not "half-up" in bed, which is awkward and far less efficacious. This alone will bring many patients out of pulmonary edema. The ideal posture, readily obtained if a straight chair is at hand, is to have the patient straddle the seat and face the back; the chair back affords a prop for him to lean on, keeps him upright with legs and feet dependent (which has the same effect as tourniquets—a bloodless venesection), and presents his back to his attendants for serial auscultation as required.

A copy of this remarkably useful and comprehensive book should be available in every emergency room, every coronary care unit, every intensive care unit, and every doctor's office. Appropriately used, and with Dr. Khan's international reputation, it will make a significant contribution to the improvement of urgent patient care in this country and abroad.

Henry J. L. Marriott, M.D.

PREFACE

Diseases of the heart and lung comprise over 70% of medical admissions in an approximate 70:30 ratio.

A cardiologist-in-training must be exposed to all aspects of pulmonary medicine, and the respirologist requires a good cardiologic background to resolve a constellation of symptoms and signs: shortness of breath, chest pain, cough, fatigue, pleural effusion, wheeze, or crackles may be a result of cardiac or pulmonary disease; shortness of breath with crackles and wheeze in conjunction with an abnormal chest radiograph may be caused by heart failure, pulmonary embolism, adult respiratory distress syndrome, or lung carcinoma complicated by infection and lymphangitic carcinomatosis.

Trainees and consultants are often called upon to manage these problems, which must be handled efficiently and rapidly. Knowledge is advancing by leaps and bounds in both areas and it is difficult for consultants, far less the trainee, to keep abreast of new drug or interventional therapies. Therefore, I believe a need exists for an up-to-date text on management of the two most common medical problems encountered in medical wards.

This text is aimed at cardiologists, respirologists, internists, and generalists. The terse format allows the text to accommodate a wealth of practical clinical information, especially in the area of decision-making and application of appropriate therapy, that should appeal to trainees, house staff, and all who care for cardiac and pulmonary patients.

Cardiac and Pulmonary Management should find a place in coronary care units, ICUs, the hands of internists, and importantly, in nursing stations of all medical units where it can serve as a vade mecum for house staff and nurses who administer to cardio-pulmonary patients. Also, professors will be able to quickly retrieve material suitable for seminars in internal medicine, cardiology, and pulmonary medicine. Of necessity, 70% of the text covers cardiologic, and 30%, pulmonary problems, and includes the material considered to be core knowledge for board examinations in cardiology, respirology, and internal medicine.

Experts in their fields were chosen to produce an in-depth text based on careful and critical reviews of current scientific literature; the result is a comprehensive look at "state-of-the-art" management of cardio-pulmonary problems. Cardiac patients may succumb to pulmonary infections, and cardiologists, respirologists, and/or infectious disease specialists are often drawn together to care for critically ill patients. Thus, the chapters on pneumonia and other pulmonary infections, written by Patrick Lynch and Galen Toews of the Pulmonary and Critical Care Division, University of Michigan Medical Center, cover what respirologists and cardiologists need to know about antimicrobial agents and infectious diseases in the critical care setting. Richard Light, Paul Marino, Sanjeev Saksena, and Thomas Shields have enhanced the text by the inclusion of relevant material from their well-received books, *Pleural Diseases, The ICU Book, Electrical Therapy for Cardiac Arrhythmias,* and *General Thoracic Surgery.*

In the preparation of the text, I insisted that discussion of appropriate therapy be based on sound pathophysiologic principles to further strengthen the physician's ability to formulate a reasonable plan of management. Appropriate management or decision-making strategies require integration and orchestration of the following

- accurate diagnosis
- pathophysiologic implications
- prediction of outcome or risk stratification
- knowledge of the action of pharmacologic agents and their correct indications
- advantages and disadvantages of interventional therapy

To cover this wealth of clinical information, we prepared a tersely written text, highlighted by bullets to allow rapid retrieval of vital information on patient management.

The reader will find some material duplicated in several chapters; this has been done purposely to save the busy clinician the difficulty of having to turn from the chapter consulted to another chapter in order to retrieve vital information, especially dosages and adverse effects of drugs. Indeed, both teaching and learning call for different emphases with reinforcement that necessitates some duplication.

The cardiology section gives guidelines for management that are in accordance with the most recent task force reports of the American College of Cardiology and the American Heart Association. Similarly, the pulmonary section reflects a national consensus. The reports of many well-designed clinical trials and information from review articles have been used to create a text that should represent a consensus of medical practice in the United States and Canada. I feel confident that the text is written for a global audience, however, and should succeed on both sides of the Atlantic. Appropriate therapy should essentially be the same worldwide, with subtle differences enforced mainly because of economic differences.

I trust that clinicians will find this information-packed text useful in the day-to-day management of patients with cardio-pulmonary problems, and that strategies and guidelines given will serve to prolong life, alleviate suffering, and improve quality of life for all patients who come in contact with the healing hands.

Ottawa, Canada   M. Gabriel Khan

ACKNOWLEDGMENTS

I gratefully acknowledge permission granted from W.B. Saunders to reproduce tables and illustrations from the 3rd Edition of our book, *Cardiac Drug Therapy*. My trusted colleague, Doctor John S. Geddes, Cardiologist, Royal Victoria Hospital, Belfast and presently Associate Professor of Cardiology, University of Manitoba, Director of Electrophysiology and Pacemaker Clinic, Health Sciences Centre, Winnipeg, reviewed most of the cardiology chapters, and for his criticisms and suggestions I am indebted.

It has been a pleasure for me to deal with Lea & Febiger: my Executive Editor, R. Kenneth Bussy, and John F. Spahr, Jr., President and Chief Executive Officer, have been particularly helpful, as have the effective members of their Editorial/Design/Production team—Tanya Lazar, Developmental Editor; Samuel A. Rondinelli, Production Manager; and Denise Wilson, Manuscript Editor.

My publishing assistant, Hazel Luce, deserves my gratitude for her untiring effort and patience. On a personal note, my wife Brigid and our six children provided understanding support and, most importantly, allowed me the time and freedom to devote myself to this enormous but fortunately pleasurable task.

M.G.K.

CONTRIBUTORS

Diana S. Dark, MD
Associate Professor of Medicine
Division of Pulmonary and Critical
Care Medicine
University of Kansas Medical Center
Kansas City, KS

Randy G. Dotson, MD
Fellow
Division of Pulmonary and Critical
Care Medicine
University of Kansas Medical Center
Kansas City, KS

**John F. Goodwin, MD, FRCP(Lond),
FACC**
Professor Emeritus of Cardiology
Postgraduate Medical School
London, UK

Gerald R. Kerby, MD
Professor of Medicine
Division of Pulmonary and Critical
Care Medicine
University of Kansas Medical Center
Kansas City, KS

**M. Gabriel Khan, MB BCh, MD,
FRCP(Lond), FRCP(C), FACP**
Associate Professor of Medicine
University of Ottawa;
Consultant Cardiologist
Ottawa General Hospital
Ottawa, Canada

Richard W. Light, MD
Professor of Medicine
University of California at Irvine
Irvine, CA;
Associate Chief of Staff for
Research and Development
Veterans Administration Medical
Center
Long Beach, CA

Joseph P. Lynch, III, MD
Associate Professor of Internal
Medicine
Division of Pulmonary and Critical
Care Medicine
University of Michigan Medical
Center
Ann Arbor, MI

Paul L. Marino, MD, PhD, FCCM
Director of Critical Care
Director of Nutrition Support
Service
Presbyterian Medical Center of
Philadelphia;
Clinical Associate Professor
Department of Medicine and
Surgery
University of Pennsylvania School
of Medicine and Surgery
Philadelphia, PA

Davendra Mehta, MD, MRCP(UK), PhD
Clinical and Research Associate
Cardiac Medicine and
Electrophysiology
Eastern Heart Institute
Passaic, NJ;
UMDNJ-Medical School
Newark, NJ

David R. Moller, MD
Assistant Professor of Medicine
Division of Pulmonary and Critical
Care Medicine
The Johns Hopkins University,
School of Medicine
Baltimore, MD

Michael E. Nelson, MD
Fellow
Division of Pulmonary and Critical
Care Medicine
University of Kansas Medical Center
Kansas City, KS

David M. Nierman, MD, FCCP
Assistant Professor of Medicine
Associate Director, Medical ICU
The Mount Sinai Medical Center
New York, NY

Amy O'Brien-Ladner, MD
Assistant Professor of Medicine
Division of Pulmonary and Critical
Care Medicine
University of Kansas Medical Center
Kansas City, KS

Lucy B. Palmer, MD
Assistant Professor
Department of Medicine
Pulmonary and Critical Care
Division
State University of New York at
Stony Brook
Stony Brook, NY

Susan K. Pingleton, MD
Professor of Medicine
Director, Pulmonary and Critical
Care Medicine
University of Kansas Medical Center
Kansas City, KS

Sanjeev Saksena, MD, FACC
Clinical Associate, Professor of
Medicine
UMDNJ-New Jersey Medical School
Newark, NJ;
Director, Arrhythmia and
Pacemaker Service
Eastern Heart Institute
Passaic, NJ

Thomas W. Shields, MD
Professor of Surgery
Northwestern University Medical
School
Chicago, IL

Steven W. Stites, MD
Fellow
Pulmonary and Critical Care
Medicine
University of Kansas Medical Center
Kansas City, KS

Galen B. Toews, MD
Professor of Internal Medicine
Chief, Division of Pulmonary and
Critical Care Medicine
University of Michigan Medical
Center
Ann Arbor, MI

Lewis Wesselius, MD
Associate Professor of Medicine
Pulmonary and Critical Care
Medicine
University of Kansas Medical Center
Kansas City, KS

CONTENTS

Part I
Cardiovascular System

1

HYPERTENSION

M. Gabriel Khan

Hypertension is designated as mild, moderate, or severe based on the height of diastolic blood pressure

- Mild, 90 to 104 mm Hg
- Moderate, 105 to 114 mm Hg
- Severe, 115 mm Hg or higher

No guidelines yet exist for grading the severity of systolic hypertension based on the level of systolic blood pressure. Nonetheless, systolic hypertension is as important as diastolic hypertension in the causation of cerebrovascular and cardiac morbidity and mortality.

Systolic blood pressure constantly above 140 mm Hg or more in patients under age 65 and 165 mm Hg or more in patients over age 65 is significant and requires aggressive control, especially in patients with coronary heart disease (CHD), heart failure, cardiomegaly, renal dysfunction, diabetes, or a strong family history of cardiovascular events. Guidelines for the management of isolated systolic hypertension in patients aged 65 to 85 have been clarified by the results of the Systolic Hypertension in the Elderly Program (SHEP). The SHEP indicates a threefold and twofold increase in the risk of stroke and CHD in elderly hypertensive patients with systolic blood pressures greater than 180 mm Hg. The treated patients in the SHEP showed a 36% reduction in the risk of stroke (p = 0.0003) and a 27% decrease in CHD event rates. A 54% decrease in the risk of left ventricular failure was observed. These beneficial results of antihypertensive therapy should provoke urgent application, which should result in a considerable decrease in mortality, morbidity, and financial burden to patients and to society. The SHEP results indicate that it is advisable to treat all patients aged 65 to 85 who have isolated systolic hypertension constantly greater than 180 mm Hg. In patients with systolic blood pressure in the range from 180 to 240 mm Hg, a 20 to maximum 25% reduction in systolic pressure is recommended, based on the results of the SHEP.

The diagnosis of hypertension is readily made on the basis of two markedly elevated blood pressure readings taken minutes or hours apart. The diagnosis of mild hypertension requires care to avoid unnecessary overtreatment with costly medications that have potential side effects; at least three readings in the hypertensive range obtained on separate days are necessary to confirm the diagnosis. Importantly, blood pressure measured in the office tends to be higher than that observed in the patient's home or at work. Thus, in mild hypertension, it may be necessary to wait 6 months to establish the diagnosis before beginning drug therapy. In some individuals, ambulatory blood pressure readings or estimations at work or during exercise stress testing may prove helpful.

PRIMARY (ESSENTIAL) HYPERTENSION

In about 95% of hypertensive adults aged 20 to 65, no identifiable cause can be determined. Their hypertension should be defined as primary, idiopathic, or essential. In approximately 5% of cases, a secondary cause for hypertension is present. Secondary hypertension will be considered after discussion of primary hypertension.

EVALUATION

Information obtained from the patient's history, physical examination, response to previous drug therapy, complete blood count, urinalysis, serum creatinine, blood urea or blood urea nitrogen, electrolytes, total and high density lipoprotein (HDL) cholesterol, ECG, and chest x-ray should give clues that might initiate further investigation to identify the presence of secondary hypertension. In patients with primary hypertension, data obtained from the evaluation serve as a baseline and may influence the selection of an appropriate antihypertensive drug.

NON-DRUG THERAPY

Non-drug therapy should be rigorously tried in all patients with mild hypertension prior to drug therapy

- Weight reduction
- Low sodium diet
- Cessation of smoking
- Avoidance of alcohol or reduction in alcohol intake
- Removal of stress and/or learning to deal with stress
- Relaxation and exercise

These measures may result in adequate control of hypertension in up to 40% of patients with mild hypertension.

The Joint National Committee on the Detection, Evaluation and Treatment of Hypertension recommends that patients with diastolic pressures of 90 to 94 mm Hg receive a trial of non-drug therapy for about 6 months, followed by drug therapy if pressures remain elevated. Also, systolic hypertension requires aggressive control; the rationale for this recommendation has been discussed earlier.

WEIGHT REDUCTION

Weight loss nearly always results in a lowering of blood pressure. In overweight hypertensive individuals, each kilogram of weight loss is expected to result in a decrease in blood pressure of 2/1 mm Hg and, importantly, a regression of left ventricular hypertrophy may be achieved. More than 25% of North Americans are overweight and the incidence is much higher in black women. Physician dietary advice is necessary but weight reduction is seldom achieved. Small group sessions organized by weight loss clinics have the greatest success.

LOW-SODIUM DIET

There is little doubt that increased salt intake causes mild but significant elevations of blood pressure in "salt-sensitive" individuals and dietary restriction is worth a trial prior to drug therapy. A 2-gram sodium diet is sufficient and compliance is feasible. In "salt-sensitive" individuals, a reduction in blood pressure of about 5 mm Hg diastolic and 15 mm Hg systolic is expected. Patients often fail to achieve a 2-gram daily sodium diet since they relate salt intake mainly to the amount used from the salt shaker. Table 1–1 indicates that three pieces of fried chicken or a large hamburger from a fast food restaurant contains much more than the daily requirement. The patient should understand that 250 ml of canned soup or products such as meat tenderizer, garlic salt, and similar additives contain much more than 0.5 tsp of salt.

If needed, compliance can be assessed; an overnight urine collection should show more than a 30% reduction in urinary sodium content. If the patient is compliant, the urine shows more than 30% reduction in sodium, and there is no appreciable fall in blood pressure over a 3-month period, salt restriction should not be enforced.

ALCOHOL INTAKE REDUCTION

Consumption of one to a maximum of two alcoholic drinks daily appears to produce a mild increase in HDL cholesterol. However, this salutary effect is lost if three or more alcoholic drinks are consumed daily, because this quantity of alcohol may cause a significant increase in blood pressure in sensitive individuals; also, hepatic dysfunction may ensue. Alcohol intake is an important cause of secondary hypertension. Reduction of alcohol consumption in patients with hypertension usually causes a significant lowering of blood pressure.

SMOKING CESSATION

In addition to causing pulmonary complications, cigarette smoking is implicated in the pathogenesis of atherosclerosis, coronary artery vasoconstriction, and sudden cardiac death. Cigarette smoking inhibits the salutary effects of antihypertensive drugs such as propranolol and calcium antagonists. Importantly, the cardioprotective effects of hepatic-metabolized beta blockers are blunted by cigarette smoking.

DRUG THERAPY

Strive for monotherapy in the treatment of systolic or diastolic hypertension whenever possible. The ideal choice is a drug that is effective for 24 hours when given once daily and that produces few or no adverse effects.

TABLE 1–1. LIST OF FOODS WITH COMPARATIVE SODIUM (Na) CONTENT

FOOD	PORTION	MG SODIUM
Bouillon	1 cube	900
Bacon back	1 slice	500
Bacon side (fried crisp)	1 slice	75
Beef (lean, cooked)	3 oz (90 g)	60
Garlic salt	1 teaspoon (15 ml)	2000
Garlic powder	1 teaspoon	2
Ham cured	3 oz (90 g)	1000
Ham fresh cooked	3 oz	100
Ketchup	1 tablespoon	150
Milk pudding instant whole	1 cup (250 ml)	1000
Meat tenderized regular	1 teaspoon	2000
Meat tenderized low Na	1 teaspoon	2
Olive green	1	100
Pickle dill	Large (10 × 4½ cm)	1900
Peanuts dry roasted	1 cup	1000
Peanuts dry roasted (unsalted)	1 cup	10
Wieners	1 (50 g)	500
CANNED FOODS		
Carrots	4 oz	400
(Carrots raw)		40
Corn whole kernel	1 cup	400
(Corn frozen)	1 cup	10
Corn beef cooked	4 oz	1000
Crab	3 oz	900
Peas cooked green	1 cup	5
Shrimp	3 oz	2000
Salmon salt added	3 oz	500
Salmon no salt added	3 oz	50
Soups (majority)	1 cup (250 ml)	1000
Sauerkraut	1 cup (250 ml)	1800
SALAD DRESSING		
Blue cheese	15 ml	160
French regular	15 ml	200
Italian	15 ml	110
Oil and Vinegar	15 ml	1
Thousand Island	15 ml	90
FAST FOOD		
Chopped steak	one portion	1000
Fried chicken	3 piece dinner	2000
Fish & chips	one portion	1000
Hamburger	double	1000
Roast beef sandwich	one	1000
Pizza	one medium	1000

Normal diet contains 1000 to 3000 mg sodium.
Modified from: Khan, M. Gabriel: Heart Attacks, Hypertension & Heart Drugs. 2nd Ed. Toronto, McClelland-Bantam Inc., 1990.

In 1988, the Joint National Committee on Detection, Evaluation and Treatment of High Blood Pressure recommended the use of a beta blocker, small dose diuretic, angiotensin converting enzyme (ACE) inhibitor, or calcium antagonist as the initial drug for the treatment of mild to moderate (diastolic) hypertension. Both systolic and diastolic hypertension, however, require the same attention and measure of control, and identical recommendations apply. One of the four drugs stipulated above is chosen based on characteristics of the individual, such as age, race, and concomitant disease, to manage systolic and/or diastolic hypertension.

Each of the four classes of first-step drugs have unique pharmacologic properties that can be tailored to the hemodynamic, neurohormonal, volume-related factors and concomitant diseases that may exist in certain subsets of hypertensive patients

- Patients under age 65 respond best to beta blockers or ACE inhibitors, but beta blockers have the advantage of providing some cardioprotection depending on the beta blocker used and the presence or absence of smoking (see Chapter 2). The "Quality of Life Study" indicated ACE inhibitors to be superior to propranolol, a beta blocker with maximal central adverse effects
- Patients over age 65 and blacks with low-renin essential hypertension respond best to diuretics or calcium antagonists, but beta blockers are effective in over 50% of blacks and the elderly and are advisable in these patients
- Calcium antagonists are effective at all ages and in all grades of primary and secondary hypertension but provide less cardioprotection than beta blockers
- In females with a high risk for osteoporosis, diuretics are first choice as they are the only antihypertensive agents that increase bone mass. The SHEP has confirmed a salutary effect of low-dose diuretics with or without added beta blocker therapy on cardiovascular and cerebrovascular mortality in patients aged 65 to 86 who have isolated hypertension
- In refractory smokers, hepatic-metabolized lipophilic beta blockers such as propranolol are not advisable because their salutary effects are blunted, whereas timolol, acebutolol, atenolol, nadolol, and metoprolol retain protective effects

Table 1–2 summarizes individual patient characteristics and suggests a rational approach to the choice of an initial antihypertensive drug. This choice is important, considering that more than 60 million Americans have mild to moderate essential hypertension and another 40 million individuals have systolic hypertension. The cost of drug therapy, medical supervision, and laboratory monitoring for adverse effects is also an important consideration. Knowledge of the response and side effects of previous drug therapy aids in the selection of an appropriate drug. Figure 1–1 gives suggested steps in how to manage patients with mild and moderate hypertension. When combination drug therapy is necessary, rational therapy constitutes the combination of two first-choice agents or a first choice combined with a second-choice agent, as indicated in Table 1–2. The following combi-

TABLE 1-2. WHICH DRUG TO CHOOSE AS INITIAL OR MONOTHERAPY FOR MILD HYPERTENSION BASED ON PATIENT CHARACTERISTICS

PATIENT TYPE	BETA BLOCKER	DIURETIC	ACE-I	C	CA	ALPHA₁-BLOCKER	ALPHA₁, BETA-BLOCKER
Age >65	1	1	2	4	1	4	4
Age <65, relatively healthy	1	2	2	4	2	4	4
Blacks	1	1	3	4	2	4	4
Any age group:							
Ischemic heart	1	3	3	4	2	RCI	4
LVH	1	3	2	3	2	RCI	4
Aneurysms	1	3	2	3	2	RCI	3
Cerebral ischemia	1	3	2	3	2	4	4
Heart failure	CI	1	1	RCI	RCI	4	CI
Diabetes:							
Insulin-dependent	RCI	3	1	3	1	3	3
Prone to hypoglycemia	CI	3	1	3	1	3	3
Hyperlipidemia:							
Mild	1	3	3	4	2	3	4
Moderate	1*	4	2	4	1	3	4
Smokers: won't quit	1*	2	3	4	2	4	4
Osteoporosis	1	1**	3	4	2	4	4
Women age >45	1	1	1	4	1	4	4
Chronic lung	CI	1	1	2+	4+	CI	CI
***	2+	1+	4+	2+	4+	2+	3+
†	Yes	Yes	Yes	No	Yes (‡)	No	No

ACE-1 = Angiotensin-converting enzyme inhibitor
C = Centrally acting adrenergic inhibitor
CA = Calcium antagonist
CI = Contraindicated

RCI = Relative contraindication
LVH = Left ventricular hypertrophy
* = Use a non-hepatic-metabolized beta-blocker
** = Increases bone mineral density

*** = Cost: 4+ = expensive, 1+ = low cost
† = proven effective, given alone, once daily
‡ = Preferably nifedipine extended release
1 = first choice; 4 = poor choice

Modified from: Khan, M. Gabriel: Cardiac Drug Therapy. 3rd Ed. London, W.B. Saunders, 1992.

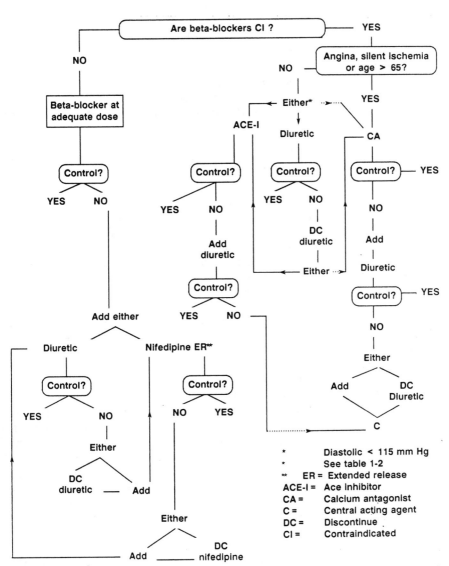

FIG. 1–1. Suggested steps in how to treat mild to moderate (diastolic < 115 mm Hg) essential hypertension. From: Khan, M Gabriel: Cardiac Drug Therapy. 3rd Ed. London, W.B. Saunders, 1992.

nations are suggested, depending on patient characteristics listed in Table 1–2.

- Age less than 65 or in the elderly: A beta blocker plus nifedipine extended release or a beta blocker plus a small dose of a thiazide diuretic. If the latter agent is used and hypokalemia is observed, the thiazide should be switched to a potassium-sparing diuretic, preferably thiazide plus amiloride (Moduretic; Moduret); spironolactone should be avoided, and triamterene may cause renal calculi. Importantly, amiloride is the only diuretic agent that has salutary antiarrhythmic properties (see Chapter 6). Thus, a rational drug combination is: a beta blocker and Moduretic, one tablet each morning. If the diuretic causes adverse effects, switch this agent to nifedipine extended release (Fig. 1–1)

- Blacks: Although it is often stated that diuretics are more effective than beta blockers in these patients, the efficacy difference is small; beta blockers are effective in up to 50% of non-whites, whereas diuretics are effective in approximately 65%. Most importantly, beta blockers may decrease CHD events, whereas diuretics have not been shown to do so in individuals less than age 65. Thus, blacks should be given the same combination recommended above for the elderly

- CHD: In patients with CHD or in those who are at high risk for CHD events, a beta blocker plus nifedipine extended release is a natural choice. The reader is advised to consult Chapter 2 for the appropriate selection of a calcium antagonist. It must be emphasized that ACE inhibitors and alpha$_1$ blockers may cause an increase in angina and are relatively contraindicated in patients with CHD manifested by angina (see later discussion of these agents)

- Hyperlipidemia presents a difficult decision-making scenario. Most beta blockers cause approximately 1 to 10% decrease in HDL cholesterol levels in up to 20% of patients treated; a 6% decrease in HDL cholesterol was observed in the Beta Blocker Heart Attack Trial (BHAT). Acebutolol, however, has been shown to cause no significant change in HDL cholesterol levels in patients treated for over 1 year (Chapter 8). These agents do not increase low density lipoprotein (LDL) cholesterol. In addition, hypertensive patients who have hyperlipidemia are at high risk for CHD events and beta blocking drugs afford cardioprotection, albeit modest. Thus, a logical therapeutic combination is acebutolol plus nifedipine extended release, along with control of hyperlipidemia with diet and/or drug therapy where indicated (see Chapter 8). Although alpha$_1$ blockers do not cause lipid derangements, they may cause deleterious effects on the cardiovascular system and are thus graded as a poor choice for most hypertensive scenarios (see later discussion and Table 1–2). Figure 1–1 gives suggested steps in how to treat mild to moderate hypertension with monotherapy and with appropriate combinations. Table 1–3 gives the dosage and Table 1–4 indicates the more common adverse effects of antihypertensive drugs

BETA BLOCKERS

Beta blockers are considered first-choice therapy for the management of hypertension in several subsets of patients in whom no contraindications to beta blockade exist. When they are contraindicated or produce adverse effects, a calcium antagonist, an ACE inhibitor, or a diuretic can be chosen as first-line therapy (see Table 1–2), based on patients' characteristics.

TABLE 1-3. DAILY DOSAGE OF ANTIHYPERTENSIVE DRUGS

	DOSE (mg)		
	Initial	Usual Maintenance	Maximum*
ACE INHIBITORS†			
Captopril (Capoten)	12.5–25	50–100	150
Enalapril (Vasotec)	2.5–5	10–20	40
Lisinopril (Prinivil, Zestril)	2.5–5	10–20	40
Benazepril (Lotensin)	5	5–30	40
Fosinopril (Monopril) 10 mg	5–10	10–30	40
Perindopril	1–2	2–6	8
Quinapril (Accupril)	2.5–5	5–30	40
Ramipril (Altace)	1.25–2.5	2.5–5	20
ALPHA-ADRENERGIC BLOCKERS			
Prazosin (Minipress)	1 (0.5, UK)	5–15	20
Terazosin (Hytrin)	1	2–10	15
CALCIUM ANTAGONISTS			
Diltiazem ‡60, 90, 120 mg	90	180–240	360
Cardizem CD	180	180–240	300
Cardizem SR 90, 120 mg	90	180–360	360
Adizem SR (UK) 120 mg	120	120–360	360
Nifedipine			
Nifedipine Extended Release:			
Procardia XL, Adalat XL(C) 30, 60, 90 mg	30	60–90	120
Adalat PA 10 mg (C)			
Adalat PA 20 mg (C)	20–40	40–80	120
Adalat Retard 10 mg (UK)			
Adalat Retard 20 mg (UK)	20–40	60–80	80
Verapamil 80, 120 mg, 40, 80, 120, 160 mg (UK)	160	160–360	480
Calan SR 120, 180, 240 mg	120	120–360	480
Isoptin SR 120, 180, 240 mg	120	120–360	480
Verelan 120, 240 mg			
Nicardipine 20, 30 mg	40	40–60	90
Cardene			
Nitrendipine	5	5–20	40
Baypress			
Felodipine			
Plendil 5, 10 mg	5	5–10	15
Isradipine 2.5, 5 mg	2.5–5	5–10	30
DynaCirc			
CENTRAL ACTING			
Clonidine (Catapress)	0.1	0.2–0.8	1
Guanabenz (Wytensin)	4	8	16
Guanfacine (Tenex)	1	1	3
Methyldopa (Aldomet)	250–500	500–1000	1500

TABLE 1–3. (*continued*)

	DOSE (mg)		
	Initial	Usual Maintenance	Maximum*
BETA BLOCKERS			
Acebutolol (Sectral, Monitan)	200–400	400–800	1000
Atenolol (Tenormin)	25–50	50–100	100
Labetalol (Trandate, Normodyne)	100–400	500–1000	1200
Metoprolol (Toprol XL, Lopressor, Betaloc)	50	50–200	300
Nadolol (Corgard)	40–80	40–160	160
Penbutolol (Levatol)	20	20–40	80
Pindolol (Visken)	7.5–15	10–15	30
Propranolol (Inderal)	40–120	160–240	240
Inderal LA	80	80–240	240
Sotalol (Sotacor, C, UK)	80	160	240
Timolol (Blocadren)	5–10	10–20	40
DIURETICS			
Bendroflumethiazide	2.5	2.5	5
Bendrofluazide (UK)	2.5	2.5–5	5
Benzthiazide	12.5	2.5	50
Chlorothiazide	125	250	500
Chlorthalidone	12.5	25	50
Hydrochlorothiazide	12.5–25	25–50	50
Hydroflumethiazide	12.5–25	25–50	50
Indapamide	2.5	2.5	2.5
Methyclothiazide	2.5	2.5	5
Metolazone	1.25	2.5	10
Polythiazide	2	2	4
Quinethazone	25	25	50
Trichlormethiazide	1	2	4
Bumetanide	0.5	1–5	10
Furosemide (Frusemide, UK)	40	40–160	240

* In clinical practice, a dose less than the manufacturer's maximum is advised and reduces the incidence of adverse effects.
† See Table 1–6
‡ Not appropriate for the elderly or those with renal or hepatic impairment (British National Formulary, 1992)
C = Canada
UK = United Kingdom
Note: All drugs are available in the United States, except where labeled "C" or "UK."

Indications

- Patients under age 65, in whom high renin essential hypertension is more prevalent than in the elderly; high-renin essential hypertension is more common in whites than in blacks; these agents are effective, however, in more than 50% of black or elderly hypertensives and should be given a trial. They are indicated in elderly patients with hypertensive, hypertrophic "cardiomyopathy" with impaired ventricular relaxation because diuretics and ACE inhibitors are contraindicated in these patients

TABLE 1–4. ADVERSE EFFECTS OF ANTIHYPERTENSIVE DRUGS	
DRUG TYPE	**ADVERSE EFFECTS**
Beta Blockers	Bronchospasm, exacerbation heart failure, bradycardia, fatigue, dizziness, masking and worsening of hypoglycemia, rarely impotence, nightmares, depression
Thiazide Diuretics	Hypokalemia, hyponatremia, dehydration, postural hypotension, gout, glucose intolerance, impotence, muscle cramps, postural hypotension
Nifedipine Extended Release	Headache, flushing, edema, dizziness, jitteriness, heartburn
Verapamil and Diltiazem	Above, plus bradycardia, rarely sinus arrest, heart block, precipitation of heart failure, constipation, hepatic dysfunction
ACE Inhibitors	First-dose syncope, hypotension, angioneurotic edema, pruritic rash, cough, wheeze, hyperkalemia, worsening of renal failure, loss of taste, mouth ulcers, cerebral circulatory insufficiency, rare: neutropenia, agranulocytosis, proteinuria, membranous glomerulopathy, impotence, pemphigus, hepatitis, +ve ANA.
Centrally acting (methyldopa, clonidine, guanfacine, guanabenz)	Postural hypotension, drowsiness, dry mouth, parotitis, depression, lethargy, impotence, rebound hypertension
Alpha$_1$ blockers	First-dose syncope, postural hypotension, palpitations, precipitation of angina, impotence, retrograde ejaculation, progression of aneurysmal dilatation
Labetalol and other alpha$_1$-beta blockers	No first-dose syncope, otherwise similar to effects given under alpha$_1$ blockers and beta blockers plus +ve ANA, rare lupus-like syndrome, hepatic necrosis

- Beta blockers are first choice in patients with CHD manifested by angina and silent ischemia, and following myocardial infarction, and in individuals at high risk for the occurrence or complications of CHD
- First choice in patients with supraventricular or ventricular arrhythmias
- Patients with left ventricular hypertrophy are at high risk for sudden death; beta blockers are the only antihypertensive agents that have the potential to prevent sudden death in this subset of patients
- They are of particular value in patients with increased adrenergic activity, including the younger age group, who often have high plasma norepinephrine levels, and in patients with hyperkinetic heart syndrome, alcohol withdrawal hypertension, or the hyperdynamic beta-adrenergic circulatory state, with labile or elevated blood pressure and palpitations
- Patients with migraine and hypertension
- Orthostatic hypertension, exaggerated increase in diastolic pressure on standing, usually indicates increased adrenergic tone, and beta blockers produce a salutary effect in these patients

- Patients prone to postural hypotension may benefit since these agents, unlike all other antihypertensives, do not usually decrease systemic vascular resistance
- First choice for patients with aneurysms
- In females over age 55, beta blockers are a rational choice because the incidence of myocardial rupture is high in hypertensive women who sustain a first infarction. Beta blockers protect sufficiently from myocardial rupture to warrant their use in patients considered at risk. The combination of a beta blocking agent and low-dose diuretics is advisable if prevention of osteoporosis also requires therapeutic consideration

There is still no clear consensus regarding the mechanisms by which beta blocking drugs cause a reduction in blood pressure. An interplay of mechanisms appears to be responsible. Negative chronotropic and inotropic effects lead to a reduction in cardiac output and some reduction in blood pressure. Antagonism of sympathetically mediated renin release and reduction in plasma renin have a role, but involvement of renin remains controversial. Added mechanisms include central nervous system effects, reduction in norepinephrine release, reduction in plasma volume and venomotor tone, resetting of baroreceptor levels, as well as inhibition of the catecholamine pressor response to stress.

Dosage

See Table 1–3. It is advisable to use a small dose initially, then titrate to a moderate dose that is within the "cardioprotective" range. If blood pressure is not adequately controlled, it is advisable to add another agent rather than using the manufacturer's suggested maximum dose of beta blocker. At very high doses of a beta blocking drug, cardioprotective properties are lost. Importantly, a 20-mg daily dose of timolol produced significant reduction in mortality in the Norwegian Post Myocardial Infarction Trial. In the BHAT, 160 to 240 mg propranolol achieved a reduction in mortality, and acebutolol (400 mg daily) caused a 48% reduction in cardiovascular mortality. The effect on mortality at lower doses is unknown, and animal experiments using larger doses indicate increased mortality. Therefore, Table 1–3 gives 40 mg as the maximum dose for timolol and 240 mg for propranolol and not 80 mg and 480 mg, respectively, as quoted by other sources. In the management of hypertension, it is advisable not to exceed the 30-mg dose for timolol, 600 mg for acebutolol, 240 mg for propranolol, and 200 mg for metoprolol extended release.

Advantages

Beta blockers decrease cardiac mortality in post myocardial infarction patients. Sudden deaths were decreased some 67% by timolol in the Norwegian Post Myocardial Infarction Trial. Except for aspirin, no oral cardiac medication has shown favorable effects on mortality in any subgroup of cardiac patients and beta blockers are the only agents that have been proven to prevent sudden death. Hypertensives with concomitant CHD or at risk for CHD events deserve therapy with beta blockers even though the protection afforded has been judged by some to be modest (see Chapter 4). Beta blockers reduce the rate-pressure product that determines cardiac workload and myocardial oxygen consumption. Reduction in pulsatile force and decrease in peak velocity, multiplied by the heart rate, decreases hemodynamic stress on the arterial tree, especially at areas just beyond the branching of arteries. Beta blockers protect from the development of aneurysms. It is not surprising that beta blockers play a vital and protective role in the management of dissecting aneurysms in patients, even when blood pressures are in the low normal range (see Chapter 10). Beta blockers are first-line therapy in hypertensive with ventricular ectopy and other arrhythmias. Salutary effects observed in hypertensive patients treated with beta blockers are not obtained with diuretics and/or vasodilators that include hydralazine, prazosin, or centrally acting drugs. Beta blockers prevent left ventricular hypertrophy and cause regression. This finding is not consistently observed with diuretics, some calcium antagonists, or vasodilators that increase sympathetic activity and produce an increase in heart rate.

Unlike the majority of other antihypertensive agents, beta blockers do not usually cause orthostatic hypotension and are a reasonable choice for patients with strokes, cerebral circulatory insufficiency, and neurocardiogenic syncope (see Chapter 15). However, labetalol, which has alpha-blocking properties, can cause orthostatic hypotension. Beta blocking agents have a role in elderly patients with hypertensive hypertrophic "cardiomyopathy" with ventricular diastolic dysfunction in whom ACE inhibitors and diuretics are contraindicated.

Disadvantages

Beta blockers may cause a decrease in HDL cholesterol of approximately 6%; this finding is variable and appears to occur only in susceptible individuals. Several studies have shown no significant fall in HDL with long-term use of beta blockers. An increase in serum triglycerides from 5 to 24% may be observed but occurs in only a few individuals treated over 1 year. Triglycerides are a weak and unproven link in the pathogenesis and manifestations of CHD. A minimal lowering of HDL, 6% in the BHAT, and variable modest increases in triglycerides in a very small percentage of patients treated with beta blockers for prolonged periods should not be regarded as sufficient evidence to disqualify these agents as the mainstay of therapy, considering their aforementioned protective advantages. It must be reemphasized that acebutolol causes no significant lipid derangements during longterm administration. Some antihypertensives, including atenolol, have been shown to decrease blood pressure throughout 24 hours but with less activity between 7 a.m. and 9 a.m. It is important to cover these hours of peak activity and it is advisable in these individuals to give the dose of atenolol or acebutolol every 12 hours or to use timolol twice daily or a longer acting beta blocker, such as nadolol, once daily.

TABLE 1–5. PHARMACOLOGIC FEATURES OF BETA BLOCKERS

	ATENOLOL	ACEBUTOLOL	METOPROLOL	NADOLOL
Cardio selectivity β1	+ + +	+	+ + +	none
Intrinsic sympathomimetic activity (ISA) (partial agonist)	–	+	–	–
Hydrophilic	+ + + +	+	–	+ + + +
Lipophilic*	–	+ + +	+ + +	–
Hepatic metabolized	–	+ + +	+ + + +	–
Renal Excretion	Yes	Partial	None	Yes
Alpha₁ blocker	–	–	–	–

+ = mild
+ + + + = maximum
* Increase concentration in brain

Pharmacologic Features and Subtle Differences

The pharmacologic features of beta blockers are given in Table 1–5. There are important subtle differences. The usual classification into cardioselective and nonselective is an oversimplification. Atenolol and metoprolol are cardioselective beta₁ adrenergic blockers. At high doses, however, these agents can produce bronchospasm, because a small quantity of beta₁ receptors is present in the lungs.

The lipophilic agents are metabolized in the liver and obtain high brain concentration, which may confer some adverse effects. It is possible, however, that increased brain concentration and elevation of central vagal tone may confer greater cardiac protection provided that salutary effects are not nullified by cigarette smoking.

Abald, et al., in a rabbit model, showed that while both metoprolol (lipophilic) and atenolol (hydrophilic) caused equal beta blockade, only metoprolol caused a reduction in sudden cardiac death. Metoprolol, but not atenolol, caused a significant increase in RR interval variation that indicates an increase in parasympathetic tone. Only the beta blockers with lipophilic properties (acebutolol, metoprolol, propranolol, and timolol) have been shown in clinical trials to prevent sudden cardiac death. It is now important for the physician to select an appropriate beta blocker with the understanding that all beta blockers are not alike.

Statements in editorials, such as "Beta blockers do not reduce cardiac mortality in hypertensives," must be considered erroneous because beta blockers possess subtle differences that are clinically important. It is not surprising that cardiac mortality was not reduced by propranolol in smokers in the large hypertension clinical trials of the 1980s. The protective cardiovascular effects of hepatic metabolized beta blockers such as propranolol, oxprenolol, and penbutolol are blunted by cigarette smoking. Thus, in smokers, totally hepatic-metabolized beta blockers and diuretics have about equal beneficial effects in the prevention of cardiovascular events. In hypertensive patients, decrease in cardiac mortality may be sig-

TABLE 1–5. (*continued*)

PENBUTOLOL	PROPRANOLOL	PINDOLOL	TIMOLOL	SOTALOL	LABETALOL
none	none	none	none	none	none
+	−	+ + +	−	−	+
	−	+	+	+ + + +	
+ + + +	+ + + +	+ +	+ +	−	+ + +
+ + +	+ + + +	+ +	+ +	−	+ +
Partial	None	Partial	Partial	Yes	No
−	−	−	−	−	+

nificant with the use of partially metabolized beta blockers that attain high brain concentration, such as metoprolol, timolol, and acebutolol, but studies have not adequately tested this hypothesis. Only timolol, metoprolol, and acebutolol have been shown to be effective in preventing cardiac deaths in smokers and nonsmokers. Insisting that the patient stop smoking is important in preventing cardiovascular events and allows salutary effects of medication to emerge. However, patients who insist on smoking increase their risk of sudden death and other CHD events, and in these patients, the choice of a beta blocker is important.

Thus, until the results of randomized trials are available in smokers, it is advisable to use timolol, metoprolol, or acebutolol for the management of hypertension with the hope that cardiac mortality might be reduced. This advice has not been manifest in the current medical literature and has not been addressed by the Joint National Committee on Detection, Evaluation and Treatment of High Blood Pressure.

Beta blockers with more than moderate intrinsic sympathomimetic activity (ISA) are not recommended because they may blunt the cardioprotective lifesaving potential. Acebutolol has mild ISA activity, has been shown to decrease cardiovascular mortality. Acebutolol is the beta blocking agent of choice in hypertensive patients with hyperlipidemia and/or if other beta blockers cause symptomatic bradycardia (see Chapter 8).

Contraindications

- Heart failure
- Asthma, severe chronic obstructive pulmonary disease (COPD), allergic rhinitis
- Severe peripheral vascular disease
- Heart block, sick sinus syndrome
- Diabetes in patients prone to hypoglycemia

In patients with stable or mild diabetes, however, if beta blocker therapy is needed, a cardioselective agent such as metoprolol is preferred, provided that a low dose of the drug (up to 150 mg daily) is utilized.

Adverse Effects

These include precipitation of heart failure in patients with compromised systolic function. Symptomatic bradycardia is bothersome in less than 10% of treated patients, bronchospasm may be precipitated in asthmatics and patients with chronic obstructive lung disease. Dizziness, weakness, fatigue, vivid dreams, rarely depression, and very rarely psychosis and loss of hearing may occur. Lipophilic beta blockers (propranolol, oxprenolol, penbutolol) have a higher incidence of central nervous system adverse effects than hydrophilic agents (atenolol and nadolol).

Impotence occurs in less than 2% of patients. Based on studies utilizing over 39,000 patients, 0.4% reported impotence. The incidence is much less than observed with the use of diuretics and is not higher than reported with ACE inhibitors or calcium antagonists. Raynaud's phenomenon and worsening of intermittent claudication are bothersome features of beta blocker therapy. A few cases of exacerbation of psoriasis have been reported. Also, rare reports of retroperitoneal fibrosis have been observed with most beta blockers and a lupus-like syndrome has been reported for labetalol. The latter agent is a beta blocker with alpha activity and has two major adverse effects not observed with pure beta blocking agents: postural hypotension is not uncommon, and life-threatening hepatic necrosis has been observed.

Cautions

Avoid abrupt cessation of beta blocker therapy in patients with CHD, because angina may worsen. If necessary, discontinue beta blockers gradually over 2 to 3 weeks and instruct the patient to refrain from moderate exertion. In patients with angina, nitrates or calcium antagonists should be given as beta blocker therapy is withdrawn. Rarely, rebound hypertension is precipitated. Interactions with hepatic-metabolized beta blockers are observed when drugs such as cimetidine or chlorpheniramine, which decrease hepatic blood flow, are used concomitantly. Hypertensive crisis can occur with cough and cold remedies containing phenylpropranolamine. Also, an increased risk for anaphylactoid reaction from contrast media and immunotherapy in patients on beta blockers has been reported, albeit rarely.

Choosing a Beta Blocker

The beta blocking drugs have important subtle differences in pharmacologic and adverse effect profile that may dictate which beta blocker is best for a given clinical situation. Also, switching from one beta blocking agent to another may result in the disappearance of adverse effects and/or improvement of salutary effects.

The following guidelines are suggested

- Depression with propranolol: switch to metoprolol, acebutolol, atenolol, or timolol

- Mild memory impairment on propranolol: switch to metoprolol, acebutolol, or timolol
- Insomnia with propranolol or pindolol: switch to atenolol or timolol.
- Refractory smoker: switch from propranolol to metoprolol, acebutolol, or timolol, to ensure salutary effects including prolongation of life
- Vivid dreams with lipophilic beta blocker: switch to timolol, acebutolol, or hydrophilic agent (see Table 1–5)
- Decreased performance for complex tasks with atenolol: switch to metoprolol
- Marked fatigue with atenolol or sotalol: switch to acebutolol, metoprolol, or timolol
- Sedation with atenolol: change to metoprolol or timolol
- Symptomatic sinus bradycardia with propranolol or other: switch to acebutolol
- Moderate or severe hyperlipidemia, total cholesterol greater than 240 mg/dl (6.2 mmol/l), HDL less than 35/mg dl (0.9 mmol/l): avoid propranolol, switch to acebutolol plus drug therapy for hypercholesterolemia (see Chapter 8)
- Renal failure, serum creatinine greater than 2.3 mg/dl (203 μmol/l): extend the dosing interval of hydrophilic renal excreted agents, atenolol, nadolol, sotalol to alternate day or change to acebutolol, timolol, or metoprolol
- Bronchospasm in a patient with mild COPD: switch from beta$_1$, beta$_2$ agent to beta$_1$ selective metoprolol or atenolol (small dose)
- Postural hypotension with alpha-beta blocker, labetalol: switch to a pure beta blocker

The aforementioned points indicate that the use of metoprolol, acebutolol, or timolol carries major advantages over other agents.

DIURETICS

Diuretics are economical, one-a-day drugs that can still be recommended as first line in selected patients with high blood pressure. Table 1–2 indicates the rationale for the choice of diuretics in many subsets of hypertensives. The SHEP confirms the salutary effects of low-dose diuretic therapy. In the SHEP, chlorthalidone, 12.5 to 25 mg alone or in combination with atenolol, resulted in a significant reduction in the risk of stroke, myocardial infarction, and left ventricular failure. The exact mechanism of action by which diuretics produce a reduction in blood pressure is unknown. A decrease in vascular volume, negative sodium balance, and longterm arteriolar dilatation occurs.

Indications

Small-dose diuretic therapy is particularly useful in the following category of patients:

- Those over age 65

- Blacks, who usually have low-renin hypertension, if a low dose of beta blocking drug fails to control blood pressure
- Those with concomitant heart failure or renal dysfunction
- Those with osteoporosis and particularly females over age 45, who may be at risk for osteoporosis. Diuretics are the only antihypertensive drugs that have been shown to increase bone mineral density and to decrease the risk of hip fractures in both women and men
- Those who require a second-line agent to enhance the blood pressure lowering effect of beta blockers, ACE inhibitors, vasodilators, and/or centrally acting drugs

Disadvantages

Hypokalemia occurs in less than 25% of patients treated with 25 to 50 mg of hydrochlorothiazide or an equivalent dose of another thiazide daily. This occurrence is dose related. A 25- or 50-mg dose of hydrochlorothiazide is expected to cause a reduction in serum potassium of about 0.3 to 0.6 mEq/l, respectively, in susceptible individuals. Patients given a thiazide should be screened in 2 months and then every 6 months for the occurrence of hypokalemia. If hypokalemia develops, it is advisable to change to a potassium-sparing diuretic (Moduretic or Dyazide) after correction of the potassium depletion. However, care is necessary because a few patients may become mildly hypokalemic when taking potassium-sparing diuretics, and at the other extreme, hyperkalemia may occur if renal failure is present.

A diuretic plus a potassium supplement is a cumbersome combination: liquid preparations are often rejected by patients because of unpleasant taste and gastric irritation. Tablets or capsules are large and contain only a low dose of potassium chloride. Thus, several capsules must be taken along with concomitant medications. Each capsule or tablet contains 8, 10, or 20 mEq of potassium. A dose of 60 mEq potassium chloride daily is expected to increase serum potassium levels by 0.3 mEq/l. Patients who show hypokalemia despite potassium supplements or potassium-sparing diuretics are best treated by replacing the diuretic with an ACE inhibitor. Hypokalemia contributes to ventricular ectopy and decreases the ventricular fibrillation threshold, which might be implicated in increased cardiovascular mortality.

Diuretics have not been shown to consistently prevent the development of left ventricular hypertrophy or to produce regression of hypertrophy. Left ventricular hypertrophy is an independent risk factor for ventricular ectopy, ventricular tachycardia, and sudden death. Diuretics, by producing hypokalemia and allowing left ventricular hypertrophy to progress, might increase the risk of cardiac death. Diuretics should be avoided in hypertensive patients with CHD or left ventricular hypertrophy, unless indicated for the management of heart failure. However, in the SHEP, chlorthalidone showed salutary effects on cardiovascular morbidity and mortality.

Hypertensive patients treated with diuretics and followed for over 14 years showed a major increase in the incidence of glucose intolerance; discontinuation of diuretics promptly reversed the hyperglycemic response. The mechanism for the development of diuretic-induced glucose intolerance appears to be the result of a suppressive effect of hypokalemia on insulin secretion. If hyperglycemia develops during diuretic use, the drug should be discontinued and the patient should be assessed for glucose intolerance. If hyperglycemia persists, the patient should be considered diabetic until proven otherwise.

Short-term studies have indicated that diuretics cause minor elevations in serum cholesterol and decreases in HDL. However, longterm trials with large numbers of patients, such as the Medical Research Council Hypertension Trial, showed no significant difference in total serum cholesterol before and after 3 years of treatment with diuretics. Total cholesterol levels and HDL cholesterol levels did not change after 4 to 5 years of therapy with chlorthalidone in the SHEP.

Dosage: Dosages of diuretics are listed in Table 1–3.

Adverse Effects

These include impotence, weakness, and fatigue. The incidence of impotence is higher than that observed with the use of beta blockers. Although rare, hyponatremia may develop over a period of weeks or years in some susceptible individuals. Electrolyte imbalance and hypomagnesemia are well recognized complications. Gout occurs and the prevalence is increased in patients with combined hyperlipidemia. Rarely, thrombocytopenia, agranulocytosis, and pancreatitis occur. Thiazide appears in breast milk, crosses the placental barrier, and can cause decreased placental perfusion, fetal or neonatal thrombocytopenia, jaundice, and acute pancreatitis. Avoid during pregnancy and lactation.

Interactions

- Oral anticoagulants
- Steroids
- An increase in serum lithium levels may occur
- Non-steroidal anti-inflammatory drugs (NSAIDS), including aspirin, interfere with the diuretic effect of furosemide

Bendrofluazide
(Aprinox, Berkozide, Centyl, Neo-NaClex, Urizide)

Supplied: tablets; 2.5, 5 mg

Dosage: 2.5 to 5 mg daily

Hydrochlorothiazide
(Hydrodiuril, Esidrex, Oretic, Hydrosaluric, Direma)

Supplied: tablets; 25, 50, 100 mg

Dosage: Commence with 12.5 mg, then if needed, usual maintenance (25 mg; maximum 50 mg) once daily. Alternate day therapy may suffice in some patients with mild hypertension.

Potassium-Sparing Diuretics

These agents are very useful in the management of hypertension; they also conserve magnesium. They usually are used in combination with other diuretics.

Dyazide
[Hydrochlorothiazide 25 mg and triamterene 50 mg, a potassium-sparing diuretic]

Dosage: 1 tablet each morning

Moduretic; Moduret (UK and Canada)
(Hydrochlorothiazide 50 mg and amiloride 5 mg, a potassium-sparing diuretic)

Moduret 25 or mini-Moduretic (hydrochlorothiazide 25 mg and amiloride 2.5 mg, UK and Europe) is a useful combination.

Contraindications to the use of potassium-sparing diuretics include:

• Renal failure
• Concomitant use of ACE inhibitors and/or K supplements
• Renal calculi, avoid triamterene

Other Diuretics

Indapamide
(Lozol; Lozide, Canada; Natrilix, UK)

Indapamide is chemically related to chlorthalidone but has an added mild vasodilator effect that is not related to diuretic action. The incidence of hypokalemia is similar to that of thiazides, but indapamide produced no disturbances in blood lipid, blood glucose, or insulin levels in hypertensive patients administered 2.5 mg daily for 1 year. Caution: The usual contraindications and cautions to the use of thiazides apply, including avoidance in patients with hypersensitivity to sulfonamides. Because approximately 60% of indapamide is excreted by the kidney, the drug should not be administered to patients with moderate or severe renal failure. Indapamide can be used in patients with mild renal dysfunction; dosing interval does not require adjustment, but periodic evaluation of serum potassium and creatinine is advised.

Supplied: tablets; 2.5 mg

Dosage: 1 tablet each morning. A dose in excess of 2.5 mg daily is not advisable. In some patients with mild hypertension, alternate day therapy may be effective.

Furosemide
(Frusemide, UK)

This powerful loop diuretic is less effective than thiazides in mild hypertension. However, thiazides, with the exception of metolazone, lose their natriuretic effect when the glomerular filtration rate falls below 25 ml/hour but loop diuretics retain their effectiveness. Furosemide is therefore not advised for the treatment of hypertension, except when there is concomitant heart failure or severe renal dysfunction.

Timolide
(Timolol 20 mg and hydrochlorothiazide 25 mg)

Dosage: 1 tablet daily. The disadvantage of 2 tablets daily is excessive dose of thiazide.

Kalten
(Atenolol 50 mg, hydrochlorothiazide 25 mg, and amiloride 2.5 mg)

Kalten is available in Europe and has the advantage of being potassium sparing.

Dosage: 1 tablet daily.

ANGIOTENSIN CONVERTING ENZYME (ACE) INHIBITORS

ACE inhibitors have provided a major advance in the management of hypertension. They are useful first-line agents in some subsets of hypertensive patients (see Table 1–2). These inhibitors of angiotensin converting enzyme prevent the conversion of angiotensin I to the potent vasoconstrictor, angiotensin II. This action causes arteriolar dilatation and a fall in total systemic vascular resistance; diminished sympathetic activity causing vasodilatation (but heart rate does not increase as with other vasodilators); reduction in aldosterone secretion promoting sodium excretion and potassium retention.

The pharmacologic profile of ACE inhibitors is given in Table 1–6, for dosages see Table 1–3.

Indications

- ACE inhibitors are most effective in patients with high renin hypertension and especially in Caucasians under age 65
- Hypertensives with left ventricular dysfunction or heart failure
- Diabetics with hypertension of all grades. Importantly, mild hypertension (systolic 140 to 160 mm Hg, diastolic 90 to 95 mm Hg) in diabetics must be aggressively treated, preferably with an ACE inhibitor

TABLE 1–6. THE PHARMACOLOGIC PROFILE AND DOSAGES OF ACE INHIBITORS

	CAPTOPRIL	ENALAPRIL	LISINOPRIL	RAMIPRIL
USA and Canada	Capoten	Vasotec	Prinivil, Zestril	Altace
UK	Capoten	Innovace	Carace, Zestril	Tritace
Europe	Lopril, Lopirin	Xanef, Renitec	Carace, Zestril	Tritace
Pro-drug	No	Yes	No	Partial
Action				
apparent (hours)	½	2–4	2–4	3–6
peak effect (hours)	1–2	5	4–8	3–6
duration (hours)	8–12	12–24	24–30	24–48
Half life (hours)	2–3	11	13	14–30
Metabolism	Partly hepatic	Hepatic	None	Partial
Elimination	Renal	Renal	Renal	Renal
SH group	Yes	No	No	No
Approved use USA**	Hypertension	Hypertension	Hypertension	Hypertension
Heart failure	Yes	Yes	No	No
Equivalent dose	100 mg	20 mg	20 mg	10 mg
Initial dose	12.5 mg	2.5mg	2.5 mg	1.25–2.5 mg
Total daily dose				
hypertension	50–150 mg	5–40 mg	5–40 mg	2.5–20 mg
heart failure	25–100 mg	5–20 mg		
Dose frequency*	2–3 daily	1–2 daily	1 daily	1 daily
Supplied	12.5, 25, 50, 100 mg	2.5, 5, 10, 20 mg	5, 10, 20, 40 mg; 2.5 UK: 5, 10, 20, 40 mg	1.25, 2.5, 5, 10 mg

* increase dosing interval with renal failure
** Also approved for hypertension: Benazepril (Lotensin) Fosinopril (Monopril); Quinapril (Accupril): see Table 1–3 and text

- The 1992 British National Formulary indicates ACE inhibitors for hypertension only when beta blockers and thiazides are contraindicated, not tolerated, or fail to control blood pressure.

Advantages

ACE inhibitors are most effective in patients with high renin hypertension, especially in Caucasians under age 65. ACE inhibitors have been shown to cause regression and prevention of left ventricular hypertrophy. Other vasodilators may not prevent the development of hypertrophy, presumably because they cause sympathetic stimulation, which results in an increase in heart rate and increased myocardial oxygen requirement.

Unlike ACE inhibitors, other vasodilators, particularly alpha$_1$ blockers, hydralazine, and minoxidil, cause sodium and water retention, and diuretics are usually required to achieve successful antihypertensive effects. The blood pressure lowering response to various doses of captopril flattens after about 75 mg or equivalent ACE inhibitor dosages. A captopril dose higher than 100 mg produces little further reduction in blood pressure. However, addition of a diuretic stimulates the renin angiotensin system and enhances the blood pressure lowering effect of ACE inhibitors. When diuretics are added, blood pressure reduction is similar in white and black hypertensive patients. These agents have been shown to reduce mortality in patients with New York Heart Association (NYHA) Class II, III, and IV heart failure and they are first choice, along with diuretics, in the management of hypertensive patients who have heart failure or left ventricular systolic dysfunction (see Chapter 5). In addition, they blunt diuretic-induced hypokalemia.

ACE inhibitors do not alter lipid levels or cause glucose intolerance. Thus, they are advisable in patients with hyperlipidemia and/or diabetes mellitus. They decrease diabetic proteinuria and appear to preserve nephron life in diabetics. However, hyperkalemia may occur in patients with renal failure and in diabetic patients with hyporeninemic hypoaldosteronism, and caution is necessary. ACE inhibitors increase uric acid excretion and may have a salutary effect in some hypertensive patients with gout. Impotence, weakness, and lethargy observed with methyldopa and diuretics are rarely observed with the use of ACE inhibitors.

Disadvantages

ACE inhibitors are generally well tolerated by patients with mild hypertension. In this group, renovascular hypertension is rare. Caution is necessary therefore, in patients with renovascular hypertension who may have tight renal artery stenosis or stenosis in a solitary kidney since acute renal failure may be precipitated. In patients with severe bilateral renal artery stenosis or stenosis of a solitary kidney, renal circulation depends critically on high levels of angiotensin II. ACE inhibitors markedly decrease angiotensin II and renal blood flow. Renal failure with a sudden elevation in serum creatinine signals this dangerous situation, which should be anticipated and avoided. Patients receiving ACE inhibitors may develop severe hyperkalemia if they have renal failure or diabetes with hyporeni-nemic hypoaldosteronism, or if they are given potassium-sparing diuretics, potassium supplements, or salt substitutes. In addition, ACE inhibitors cause rare but life-threatening angioedema.

Contraindications

- Renal artery stenosis of a solitary kidney or severe bilateral renal artery stenosis
- Severe anemia
- Aortic stenosis
- Hypertrophic and restrictive cardiomyopathy
- Hypertensive, hypertrophic "cardiomyopathy" of the elderly with im-paired ventricular relaxation
- Severe carotid artery stenosis
- Hypertensive patients with concomitant angina
- Uric acid renal calculi
- Pregnancy and breastfeeding
- Porphyria
- Relative contraindications include patients with collagen vascular dis-eases or concomitant use of immunosuppressives, since neutropenia and rare agranulocytosis observed with ACE inhibitors appear to occur mainly in this subset of patients

Adverse Effects

These include hyperkalemia in patients with renal failure, pruritus and rash in about 10% of patients, and loss of taste in approximately 7% of patients. A rare but important adverse effect is angioedema of the face, mouth, or larynx, which may occur in approximately 0.2% of treated pa-tients and can be fatal. Rarely, mouth ulcers, neurologic dysfunction, gas-trointestinal (GI) disturbances, and proteinuria occur in about 1% of pa-tients with pre-existing renal disease; neutropenia and agranulocytosis are rare and occur mainly in patients with serious intercurrent illness, partic-ularly immunologic disturbances, altered immune response, or collagen vascular disease. Cough occurs in about 10% of treated patients and wheez-ing, myalgia, muscle cramps, hair loss, impotence or decreased libido, hepatitis or occurrence of antinuclear antibodies, and phemphigus occa-sionally occur.

Interactions

- Allopurinol
- Acebutolol
- Hydralazine
- NSAIDS
- Procainamide
- Pindolol

- Steroids
- Tocanide
- Immunosuppresives and other drugs that alter immune response
- Drugs that increase serum potassium levels have been emphasized

Captopril
(Capoten)

Supplied: tablets; 12.5, 25, 50, 100 mg

Dosage: Commence with 12.5 mg twice daily, one-half hour before meals, increase gradually to 50 to 100 mg daily, which is the dose required by the majority of patients. The maximum suggested dose is 150mg daily in severe hypertension. Serious side effects are more common in patients given a daily dose of 200 mg or more. Increase the dose interval in renal failure. Decrease the initial dose to 6.25 mg in the elderly or if a diuretic is used concomitantly.

Captopril 100 mg = approximately 20 mg enalapril, 20 mg lisinopril, 20 mg ramipril, 50 mg alecepril, 750 mg pentopril.

Enalapril
(Vasotec; Innovace, UK)

Supplied: tablets; 2.5, 5, 10, 20 mg

Dosage: 2.5 to 5 mg daily, increase over days to months to 10 to 30 mg daily in one or two divided doses with or without food. Maximum 40 mg daily or less often in renal failure. In elderly patients or in those receiving a diuretic, begin with a dose of 2.5 mg daily.

Lisinopril
(Prinivil, Zestril)

Supplied: tablets; 2.5 (UK), 5, 10, 20, 40 mg

Dosage: 2.5 mg once daily, increase to 10 to 30 mg; maximum 40 mg daily or less often in renal failure. Discontinue diuretic for 2 to 3 days prior to commencing lisinopril and resume later if required.

Benazepril
(Lotensin)

Supplied: 5, 10, 20, 40 mg

Dosage: 5 mg, increase as needed to usual maintenance 5 to 30 mg; maximum suggested, 40 mg. Commence with 2.5 mg in the elderly or if a diuretic is given concomitantly.

Fosinopril
(Monopril)

Supplied: tablets; 10, 20 mg

Dosage: 5 to 10 mg once daily, increase slowly, if required, to 20 mg and with assessment of renal function; maximum 40 mg daily with or without food. Initial dose 2.5 mg in the elderly patients or those receiving a diuretic.

Perindopril
(Conversyl, UK)

Supplied: tablets; 2, 4 mg

Dosage: 2 mg daily, increase if required after monitoring of blood pressure to 4 to 8 mg daily. Discontinue diuretic 3 days prior and resume later if needed.

Quinapril
(Accupril; Accupro, UK)

Supplied: tablets; 5 mg (UK), 10, 20, 40 mg

Dosage: 5 mg once daily; usual maintenance 10 to 40 mg daily. Reduce the initial dose to 2.5 mg daily in elderly patients, renal dysfunction, or with diuretic use.

Ramipril
(Altace; Tritace, UK)

Supplied: capsules; 1.25, 2.5, 5, 10 mg

Dosage: 1.25 mg once daily, increase, if needed, to 2.5 to 5 mg and with assessment of renal function; maximum 20 mg daily.

Capozide

Supplied: Contains 15 mg captopril and 30 mg hydrochlorothiazide (HCTZ); in the UK, 50 mg captopril and 25 mg HCTZ. Combinations should be used preferably only after blood pressure is stabilized on two drugs given separately.

Dosage: ½ to 1 tablet daily; maximum 2 tablets daily.

Vaseretic

Supplied: Contains 10 mg enalapril with 25 mg HCTZ.

Dosage: ½ to 1 tablet daily; maximum 2 tablets daily.

TABLE 1-7. PHARMACOLOGIC AND CLINICAL EFFECTS OF CALCIUM ANTAGONISTS

	NIFEDIPINE	DILTIAZEM	VERAPAMIL
Decrease systemic vascular resistance	Marked	Mild	Moderate
Blood pressure	Marked reduction	Mild reduction	Moderate reduction
Coronary dilation	Mild	Mild	Mild
Cardiac output	Mild increase	No change	No change or mild decrease
Heart rate	No change or very slight increase	No change	Mild decrease
Negative inotropic	Very mild	Mild	Moderate
Sinus node depression	None	Moderate	Moderate
AV Conduction	No change	Mild reduction	Moderate reduction
Antihypertensive effect	Excellent	Mild	Good
Antianginal effect	Good	Good	Excellent
Precipitates heart failure	Rarely*	Yes, if EF <40%	Yes, if EF <40%**
Combination with beta blocker	Relatively safe	Caution***	Relative contraindication†

* In patients with severe left ventricular dysfunction
** Contraindicated in all patients with left ventricular dysfunction
† May cause severe bradycardia, sinus arrest

CALCIUM ANTAGONISTS

The blood pressure lowering effects of calcium antagonists are due to peripheral arteriolar dilatation. Normally, calcium enters the cells through slow calcium channels and binds to the regulatory protein troponin, removing the inhibitory action of tropomyosin, which, in the presence of adenosine triphosphate, allows interaction between myosin and actin, resulting in contraction of the muscle cell. Calcium antagonists inhibit calcium entry into cells by blocking voltage-dependent calcium channels, thereby inhibiting contractility of vascular smooth muscle, thus producing vasodilatation.

Table 1-7 gives the pharmacologic and clinical effects of calcium antagonists. The dihydropyridine calcium antagonists, nifedipine, felodipine, nicardipine, and nitrendipine, are more potent vasodilators and more effective antihypertensive agents than verapamil; diltiazem has modest vasodilator properties and high doses are usually required to achieve adequate lowering of blood pressure. In addition, verapamil and diltiazem have added electrophysiologic effects on the sinoatrial and atrioventricular (AV) nodes and can produce bradycardia, sinus arrest, and AV block in susceptible individuals with disease of the sinus and AV nodes.

Indications

- Hypertension of all grades in whites and nonwhites of all ages
- Nifedipine extended release is particularly useful in elderly hypertensive patients because beta blockers and ACE inhibitors are less effective in this subset of patients
- Hypertensives with angina
- Patients with peripheral vascular disease may feel more comfort, although intermittent claudication is not expected to be ameliorated by these agents

Advantages

Fortunately, calcium antagonists do not usually lower the blood pressure of normotensive individuals. They can be used without a diuretic since they have a mild natriuretic effect; their effectiveness may or may not be enhanced by adding a diuretic. Calcium antagonists are useful in hypertensive patients with coexisting angina and peripheral vascular disease or when beta blockers produce adverse effects or are contraindicated. They do not cause abnormalities of lipid or glucose metabolism nor influence potassium and uric acid excretion and have advantages over diuretics in this subset of patients. Nifedipine has shown modest but significant regression and inhibition of progression of atheromatous obstruction of coronary arteries in patients with coronary artery disease. Most calcium antagonists prevent left ventricular hypertrophy and cause regression, although some reports show a lack of salutary effects.

Calcium antagonists, particularly nifedipine, cause no serious adverse effects and their use requires virtually no laboratory monitoring when compared with diuretics and ACE inhibitors. Individual calcium antagonists have advantages that are important in terms of their adverse effects. Nifedipine has less potential than verapamil and diltiazem to cause serious adverse effects. Nifedipine has no electrophysiologic effects and, although uncommon, verapamil and diltiazem can produce bradycardia, sinus arrest, and AV block in susceptible individuals. Verapamil has significant negative inotropic activity and can precipitate heart failure. Diltiazem has mild negative inotropic activity. Nifedipine's mild negative inotropism is relatively balanced by modest reflex stimulation. Indeed, nifedipine extended release can be used with greater safety in the elderly and where the aforementioned concomitant diseases exist (Fig. 1–1). In addition, it is relatively safe to combine nifedipine with a beta blocker in the management of hypertension and when associated with angina. Verapamil must not be added to a beta blocker and diltiazem must be used with great caution. Nifedipine does not alter digoxin levels; however, verapamil and diltiazem cause about a 47% increase in digoxin level and may rarely precipitate bradycardia and AV block. Verapamil and diltiazem cannot be combined with amiodarone or quinidine, but nifedipine is not affected; nifedipine produces much less constipation than verapamil and thus has greater acceptance than verapamil or diltiazem SR in the elderly. Other dihydropiridines are expected to show the same benefit as nifedipine but cause a higher incidence of minor adverse effects when compared with the extended release nifedipine formulation.

Calcium antagonists have few disadvantages when compared with other antihypertensive agents.

Adverse Effects

The approved long-acting preparations for hypertension—nifedepine extended release (Procardia XL, Adalat XL, Adalat PA, Adalat Retard), diltiazem (Cardizem SR), and verapamil SR—produce pedal edema, mild facial flushing, dizziness, headaches, leg cramps, gastroesophageal reflux, and rarely sexual dysfunction in much the same frequency. Minor side effects include gingival hypertrophy, blurring of vision, muscle cramps, and burning in the gums. Rare side effects include depression and psychosis; worsening of renal failure may occur. A case of acute renal failure precipitated by diltiazem has been reported.

Diltiazem may cause mild elevation in liver function tests and rarely acute hepatic injury. The incidence of adverse reactions with Cardizem SR is reported as approximately 13% higher in the elderly and caution is necessary to titrate the dosage. Care is required in patients with severe hepatic dysfunction, and dosage, especially of diltiazem and verapamil, must be reduced to avoid toxicity.

Calcium antagonists should be avoided in pregnancy and by lactating mothers. However, nifedipine has been used during the last trimester of pregnancy as short-term therapy for the control of accelerated hypertension of pre-eclampsia with salutary effects. Further studies are required, however, to document safety of longterm therapy.

Contraindications

- Moderate or severe aortic stenosis
- Diltiazem and verapamil are contraindicated with sick sinus syndrome, arrhythmia, bradycardia, heart block, left ventricular dysfunction, or ejection fraction less than 40%

Interactions

Diltiazem and verapamil may interact with digoxin, amiodarone, quinidine, beta blockers, tranquilizers, oral anticoagulants, and disopyramide (Table 1–8).

Diltiazem
(Cardizem, Cardizem SR, Cardizem CD, Anginyl, Adizem-SR, Britiazim, Calcicard, Herbesser, Tildiem, Tilazem)

Supplied: tablets; 60, 90, 120 mg; Cardizem SR 90, 120 mg (UK, Adizem SR 120 mg); capsules; Cardizem CD 180, 240, 300 mg

Dosage: 60 mg twice daily, increase if needed to 240 to 360 mg daily. The SR preparation given twice daily has a side effect profile similar to

TABLE 1–8. CALCIUM ANTAGONISTS—DRUG INTERACTIONS				
	DIGOXIN LEVEL	QUINIDINE	AMIODARONE	BETA BLOCKER
Nifedipine	No change	No change or ↓	No change	Safe
Diltiazem	40% ↑	↑	Sinus arrest	Caution*
Verapamil	50–75% ↑	↑	Contraindicated	Contraindicated*

* See text.

nifedipine extended release (see Table 2–5). Cardizem CD, 180 to 240 mg daily, maximum 300 mg.

Nifedipine
Extended Release (Procardia XL; in Canada Adalat XL 30, 60, 90 mg; Adalat PA 10, 20 mg tablets; UK, Adalat Retard 10, 20 mg)

Dosage: Nifedipine extended release: Procardia XL or Adalat XL 30 mg once daily, increase if needed to 90 mg once daily; or Adalat PA or Retard, 10 to 40 mg twice daily (given with or after food); maximum 120 mg daily. For pharmacokinetics, see Chapter 2.

Nifedipine combined with a beta blocker is effective in severe hypertension. Nifedipine has virtually replaced hydralazine in triple therapy. The combination of a beta blocker, diuretic, and nifedipine is widely used for moderate to severe hypertension (Fig. 1–1).

Nitrendipine
(Baypress)

Supplied: tablets; 10mg

Dosage: 5 to 10 mg once or twice daily, increase as needed to 20 mg once or twice daily.

Nicardipine
(Cardene)

Supplied: capsules; 20, 30, mg

Dosage: 20 mg tid; maximum 30 mg tid
Vasoselectivity has been claimed, but this agent can cause heart failure and caution is required in patients with left ventricular dysfunction.

Felodipine
(Plendil; Renedil, Canada)

Supplied: tablets; 5, 10 mg

Dosage: 5 mg once daily; maximum 15 mg. In the elderly patients or those with liver dysfunction, blood pressure should be carefully monitored because high plasma concentrations of felodipine may occur and caution is needed in dosing. The 5-mg dose should suffice in the elderly or in patients with impaired liver function; the maximum dose in these patients should not exceed 10 mg daily. Felodipine causes a mild increase in digoxin levels.

This agent exhibits marked vascular selectivity and has not precipitated heart failure in small group studies of patients with left ventricular dysfunction. The results of large clinical trials in patients with compensated heart failure should clarify the safety of felodipine in patients with hypertension and significant left ventricular dysfunction.

Isradipine
(DynaCirc; Prescal, UK)

Supplied: tablets; 2.5, 5 mg

Dosage: 1.25 mg, increase to 2.5 mg twice daily; maintenance 2.5 to 5 mg twice daily, maximum 10 mg twice daily. Elderly: 1.25 to 2.5 mg daily.

Verapamil
(Isoptin, Calan, Cordilox; see Table 1–3)

Supplied: tablets; 80, 120 mg; SR 120, 180, 240 mg

Dosage: 80 mg three times daily, increase to 120 to 160 mg three times daily or preferably 120 mg SR, once or twice daily. The maximum dose, 1.5 tablets of the 240 mg sustained release, should be used with caution; constipation may limit the dosage.

Cautions. Combination with a beta blocker may cause severe bradycardia or sinus arrest because of similar electrophysiologic effects. Verapamil may produce bothersome constipation, especially in the elderly. Serum digoxin levels may be increased 50 to 75% by verapamil and about 45% by diltiazem; nifedipine has little or no effect on digoxin levels (see Table 1–8). Verapamil increases quinidine plasma levels as well as anticoagulant effects, and an interaction occurs with amiodarone.

VASODILATORS

Alpha$_1$ blockers and hydralazine have a small role in the management of hypertension not controlled by first-line agents or their combinations. Combination with a diuretic or a beta blocking drug or centrally acting agent is appropriate in selected patients.

Indications

- Advisable only when beta blockers, diuretics, ACE inhibitors, or calcium antagonists are contraindicated or cause adverse effects
- Combination therapy with beta blockers in selected patients

Advantages

This group of antihypertensive drugs does not cause derangement of lipid or glucose metabolism or alter potassium or uric acid levels. The evidence suggesting that some of these agents cause mild increases in HDL cholesterol is controversial.

Disadvantages

Alpha$_1$ blockers cause an increase in heart rate and in peak velocity multiplied by heart rate. Thus, these agents increase cardiac work and are contraindicated in patients with CHD; also, they may increase the propensity to develop aneurysms. They cause an increase in circulating norepinephrine and activate the renin angiotensin system, causing sodium and water retention; thus, diuretics are often required to potentiate their blood pressure lowering action. The combination with diuretics causes a further increase in cardiac ejection velocity. These agents do not prevent left ventricular hypertrophy or cause regression. Evidence to support the notion that some alpha$_1$ blockers significantly and consistently prevent hypertrophy or cause regression is controversial. Because of these disadvantages, an alpha-blocking agent is considered a poor choice for initial or second line therapy for mild or moderate hypertension and is so indicated in Table 1–2 and Figure 1–1.

Contraindications

- Patients with aneurysms. Undoubtedly, aneurysms may remain occult for several years
- Severe anemia
- Moderate or severe aortic stenosis
- Hypertrophic cardiomyopathy
- Angina, including silent ischemia

Dosage: Dosage of prazosin and terazosin are given in Table 1–3.

Adverse Effects

These include orthostatic hypotension, first-dose syncope, dizziness, impotence, retrograde ejaculation, confusion, rarely paranoid behavior, and psychosis.

Prazosin
(Minipress)

Supplied: capsules; 1, 2, 5 mg; tablets; 1, 2, 5 mg (Canada, UK)

Dosage: Withhold diuretics 1 to 2 days. Give 0.5 to 1 mg test dose at bedtime, then 1 mg twice daily, increase to 5 mg two or three times daily.

As with the use of other vasodilators, after several months of therapy, a diuretic may be required to prevent sodium and water retention and to improve antihypertensive effects. At doses of prazosin greater than 6 mg daily, the addition of a beta blocker is often required to prevent an increase in heart rate and improve blood pressure control. A dose of 10 mg or more is not advisable without concomitant use of a beta blocker or centrally acting agent (see Fig. 1–1).

Terazosin
(Hytrin)

Supplied: tablets; 1, 2, 5 mg

Dosage: 1 mg at bedtime, increase slowly if needed to 5 mg once daily; occasionally twice daily dosing is necessary. Maintenance 2 to 10 mg, maximum 15 mg daily. The drug has action and effects similar to prazosin, but a 12- to 24-hour duration of action and better bioavailability. Terazosin 5 mg = approximately 10 mg prazosin.

Hydralazine

Supplied: tablets; 10, 25, 50 mg

Dosage: 25 to 50 mg three times daily; maximum 200 mg daily. IV 10 to 20 mg/hour; maintenance 5 to 10 mg/hour.

CENTRALLY ACTING AGENTS

Commonly used centrally acting agents include methyldopa, guanabenz, guanfacine, and clonidine.

Indications

- Patients who fail to respond to first-line drugs
- Combination with diuretics and with vasodilators, including calcium antagonists and ACE inhibitors, especially in patients with severe and/or resistant hypertension

Disadvantages

These drugs cause postural hypotension, rebound hypertension, and some sedation. Dry mouth is typical for clonidine, guanabenz, and guanfacine. Impotence and depression are not uncommon. Methyldopa is contraindicated in active liver disease; hepatitis, fatal necrosis, as well as a rare myocarditis have been reported; Coombs' positive hemolytic anemia may occur with this agent.

Clonidine

Supplied: tablets; 0.1, 0.2 mg

Dosage: 0.1 mg at bedtime, then twice daily; maintenance 0.2 to 0.8 mg, maximum 1 mg daily.

Guanfacine

Supplied: tablets; 1 mg

Dosage: 1 mg at bedtime, increase to 2 mg over several weeks; 1 mg twice daily may be necessary with or without a diuretic. The maximum 3 mg dose commonly produces adverse effects.

Guanabenz

Supplied: tablets; 4, 8 mg

Dosage: 4 mg twice daily; maximum 10 mg daily.

Methyldopa

Supplied: tablets; 125, 250, 500 mg

Dosage: 250 mg twice daily, increase if needed to 500 mg two or three times daily; maximum 2 g daily. IV 250 mg over 60 minutes, every 4 to 6 hours.

Contraindications include active liver disease, depressive states, and pheochromocytoma.

ACCELERATED, RESISTANT, OR MALIGNANT HYPERTENSION

In patients with moderate or severe essential or secondary hypertension treated with antihypertensive agents, acceleration and refractoriness of hypertension may occur because of

- Poor compliance
- Increased salt intake in salt-sensitive individuals
- Rebound from discontinuation of centrally acting drugs, clonidine, guanfacine, methyldopa, and rarely, beta blockers or calcium antagonists
- Drug interactions: Phenylpropranolamine combined with beta blockers. NSAIDS decrease the natriuretic action of diuretics and the blood pressure lowering effect of ACE inhibitors and beta blockers; acetylsalicylic acid or other NSAIDS may interfere with the diuretic effect of loop diuretics
- Renal failure: In this situation, thiazides are rendered ineffective and blood pressure may increase

Treated or untreated patients may present with severe hypertension that is difficult to control, including the rare presentation with malignant hypertension and diastolic blood pressures greater than 140 mm Hg with or without end-organ damage. The presence of papilledema is not essential for the diagnosis of malignant hypertension.

In about 15% of cases with severe resistant hypertension, a secondary cause is present. Renal artery stenosis is an important cause in both young and older patients. Atherosclerotic occlusion of the renal artery may suddenly become worse, thus causing accelerated hypertension.

Pheochromocytoma and other causes of secondary hypertension must be excluded. See discussion of secondary hypertension.

THERAPY

In most cases of severe hypertension with diastolic blood pressures greater than 115 mmHg, combination drug therapy is necessary. Renal failure causes resistance to thiazide diuretics and high doses of furosemide combined with other agents may be required. Figure 1–1 gives suggested steps in managing more severe hypertension with combinations of drugs. Provided that heart failure or another contraindication to beta blockade is absent, beta blockers are useful in the majority of patients who have severe hypertension regardless of the underlying cause. All antihypertensive agents, with the exception of beta blockers, cause a decrease in systemic vascular resistance and fortunately have different sites of action. Therefore, they may be combined in these difficult scenarios.

Additional drug therapy is selected to affect each regulatory system

- Diuretics to control renal and other volume-dependent hypertension
- ACE inhibitors or calcium antagonists, particularly nifedipine, to reduce peripheral vascular resistance
- Centrally and peripherally acting drugs that interfere with alpha-mediated vasoconstriction, e.g., methyldopa, clonidine, or guanfacine and alpha$_1$ blockers, prazosin, or terazosin

If edema or severe renal failure is present, 160 to 320 mg furosemide may be required. If the diuretic and blood pressure lowering effects are inadequate, metolazone, 5 to 10 mg, added to furosemide or bumetanide often produces a salutary response; however, hypokalemia may ensue with this potent but useful diuretic combination.

SUGGESTED COMBINATION THERAPY

Combination 1. Beta blocker plus diuretic plus nifedipine at adequate doses; e.g., propranolol 240 mg or atenolol 100 mg plus diuretic plus nifedipine extended release 90 to 120 mg daily (other calcium antagonists if adverse effects occur with nifedipine). Then, if needed, add centrally acting methyldopa or clonidine; then, if needed, an alpha$_1$ blocker is cautiously added to maximize the vasodilator effect of nifedipine. However, the latter combination can cause severe hypotension and caution is required.

Combination 2. Where there is no suspicion of tight renal artery stenosis or a solitary kidney: ACE inhibitor plus diuretic plus a centrally acting agent. Then, if needed, add a beta blocker, plus or minus alpha$_1$, prazosin, or terazosin.

ACE inhibitors in combination with diuretics are particularly useful with accelerated or malignant hypertension in the absence of tight renal artery stenosis, but the latter diagnosis is usually difficult to exclude during the first 48 hours, when urgent antihypertensive therapy is required.

The dose of centrally acting agents and vasodilating alpha blockers may be increased if orthostatic hypertension is not controlled, and the dose of these agents should be decreased if orthostatic hypotension is present.

For hypertension resistant to combination drug therapy, as outlined, minoxidil 2.5 to 10 mg combined with diuretics and beta blockade plus or minus nifedipine may be considered, but baseline echocardiogram and electrocardiogram are advisable. The occurrence of serosanguineous pericardial effusion with tamponade is an undesirable effect of minoxidil therapy, which is rarely required.

Caution is necessary, however, because if maximum doses of drugs are used, careful clinical and laboratory monitoring is necessary to avoid serious adverse effects of combination therapy. Fortunately, interactions producing deleterious effects are rare with antihypertensive drug combinations in patients with accelerated or malignant hypertension. Although uncommon, calcium antagonists plus alpha$_1$ blockade may produce severe hypotension.

Hypertension with diastolic blood pressures exceeding 140 mmHg without end-organ damage, classified as urgent hypertensive crisis, is not an indication for parenteral therapy. Oral medications, especially with oral nifedipine capsules, usually result in a sufficient fall in blood pressure over 1 to 2 hours, then further control is achieved over the following few days.

HYPERTENSIVE EMERGENCIES

Diastolic blood pressure consistently in excess of 140 mm Hg with evidence of target organ damage, e.g., retinal hemorrhages, papilledema, acute pulmonary edema, decreased renal function, cerebrovascular accident, or hypertensive encephalopathy requires immediate but carefully monitored, modest reduction of blood pressure. A 20 to 25% reduction from baseline diastolic and/or systolic blood pressure avoids relative hypotension and is sufficient to produce salutary effects.

Patients with consistently elevated diastolic blood pressure in excess of 130 mm Hg in the absence of end-organ damage designated as having urgent hypertensive crisis are adequately managed with oral nifedipine in combination with other orally acting antihypertensive agents, as discussed earlier.

Hypertensive emergencies are often associated with a malignant phase of essential hypertension, renal failure, cerebrovascular accidents, hypertensive encephalopathy, and rarely pheochromocytoma. In dissecting aneurysm, blood pressure may be markedly elevated or remain modestly elevated in the range of 160 to 190 mm Hg systolic, diastolic 90 to 100 mm

Hg, and is considered a special hypertensive emergency, as blood pressure must be promptly lowered within minutes. This is usually achieved by using nitroprusside; also, a beta blocker is necessary to decrease the rate of rise of aortic pressure, to prevent further dissection (see Chapter 10).

Table 1–9 gives guidelines and choices of drug therapy for the management of hypertensive emergencies associated with various conditions and complications.

In patients with cerebrovascular accident, caution is required because elevations in blood pressure may fluctuate, being triggered by cerebral irritation, and it is essential to carefully monitor the blood pressure for a few hours to confirm that the diastolic pressure is constantly elevated. The need for lowering the blood pressure should be carefully considered and if deemed necessary, the slow controlled titrated lowering of blood pressure with the use of either nitroprusside or labetalol is used, depending on the cause of hypertension, underlying disease process, and complications. There is some evidence that nitroprusside increases intracranial pressure, but clinically the drug is effective. Labetalol is a reasonable alternative, provided that precautions for the use of a beta blocking drug are enforced. Labetalol causes postural hypotension and the patient must remain in bed. Also, the blood pressure lowering effect may occasionally last from 1 to 12 hours, whereas the hypotensive effect of nitroprusside dissipates within minutes of cessation of the infusion.

Pulmonary edema due to severe hypertension can be controlled with oral nifedipine and furosemide. If myocardial ischemia is suspected, nifedipine is contraindicated and nitroglycerin intravenous (IV) infusion is advisable (see Table 1–9). The combination of IV nitroglycerin and furosemide should suffice, but if pressure remains markedly elevated, nitroprusside is indicated. Labetalol is contraindicated with heart failure and captopril could be used in this situation.

Renal failure is usually associated with volume overload, and furosemide 80 to 160 mg IV should be administered. Oral nifedipine also has a role, and in this subset, sublingual nifedipine has been used widely and successfully. The oral preparation, however, lowers blood pressure as quickly as sublingual administration and is the preferred route. Failure of nifedipine therapy should prompt the use of labetalol IV infusion as well as continuation of oral nifedipine capsules to wean the patient off labetalol as quickly as possible.

DRUG THERAPY

NITROPRUSSIDE

Nitroprusside infusion reduces blood pressure to any desired level in almost 100% of patients and is the treatment of choice for most hypertensive emergencies that require the lowering of blood pressure, except when nitroprusside is contraindicated. Caution is needed in patients with inadequate cerebral circulation.

Dosage: 50 mg sodium nitroprusside in 100 ml 5% dextrose water is a convenient solution for use with a nitroprusside infusion pump. See Table

TABLE 1–9. TREATMENT OF HYPERTENSIVE EMERGENCIES ASSOCIATED WITH COMPLICATIONS

AGENT	HEART FAILURE	ENCEPHALOPATHY	CEREBRAL HEMORRHAGE	OTHER CVA	RENAL FAILURE	PHEO	DISSECTING ANEURYSM	PRE-ECLAMPSIA
Nitroprusside	1	1	1	1	CI	2	1	CI
Nitroglycerin	1 or 2	—	—	—	—	—	—	—
Nifedipine	*2†	3*	CI	CI	1 or 2	3	CI	2 or 3+
Diazoxide	CI	2	CI	3	1	CI	CI	CI
Labetalol	CI	2 or 3	1* or 2	1* or 2	1 or 2	AT	2*	2 or 3+
Propranolol**	CI	4 or AT	4 or AT	4 or AT	2 or AT	AT***	1 AT	3 or AT
Trimethaphan	CI	—	—	—	—	—	2	CI
Hydralazine	CI	CI	4	4	2 or AT	CI	CI	1
Furosemide	AT always	4 or AT	—	—	AT always	CI	CI	CI
Methyldopa	4	4 or AT	4	4	3	CI	—	1 or 2
Captopril	1, 2 or AT	—	—	—	—	—	CI	CI
Phentolamine	—	—	—	—	—	1†	—	CI

1 = first choice
2 & 3 = second or third choice
4 = rare use or if other drugs unavailable
AT = added therapy, provides reduction in dosages of combined drugs reduces adverse effects, ensures oral agent commenced early
CI = contraindicated
* = if nitroprusside unavailable, give oral 10 mg nifedipine capsule see dagger
** = or other beta blocker
*** = atenolol or other $beta_1$ selective drug used if severe tachyarrhythmia
— = not recommended
Caution: The goal is to produce an immediate but only modest and preferably titrated reduction in blood pressure.

† = CI in myocardial ischemia
+ = Not approved by the FDA

TABLE 1–10. NITROPRUSSIDE INFUSION PUMP CHART [NITROPRUSSIDE 50 MG (1 VIAL) IN 100 ML (500 MG/L)]

WEIGHT (kg)	40	50	60	70	80	90	100
Dosage (μg/kg/min)				Rate (ml/hr)			
0.2	1	1	1	2	2	2	2
0.5	2	3	4	4	5	5	6
0.8	4	5	6	7	8	9	10
1.0	5	6	7	8	10	11	12
1.2	6	7	9	10	12	13	14
1.5	7	9	11	13	14	16	18
1.8	9	11	13	15	17	19	22
2.0	10	12	14	17	19	22	24
2.2	11	13	16	18	21	24	26
2.5	12	15	18	21	24	27	30
2.8	13	17	20	23	27	30	34
3.0	14	18	22	25	29	32	36
3.2	15	19	23	27	31	35	38
3.5	17	21	25	29	34	38	42
3.8	18	23	27	32	36	41	46
4.0	19	24	29	34	38	43	48
4.5	22	27	32	38	43	49	54
5.0	24	30	36	42	48	54	60
6.0	29	36	43	50	58	65	72

The above rates apply only for a 500 mg/l concentration of nitroprusside. If a different concentration must be used, appropriate adjustments in rates should be made. Start at 0.2 μg/kg/min. Increase slowly. Average dose 3 μg/kg/min. Usual dose range 0.5–5.0 μg/kg/min.
From: Khan, M. Gabriel: Hypertension. In Cardiac Drug Therapy. 3rd Ed. London, W.B. Saunders, 1992.

1–10 for the appropriate rate of infusion based on the weight of the patient. Wrap the infusion bottle in aluminum foil or other opaque material to protect it from light. The solution must be used within 4 hours. Start the infusion at 0.5 μg/kg/min and increase by 0.2 μg/kg/min every 5 minutes until the desired blood pressure is obtained. Dosage range: 0.5 to 6 μg/kg/min. It is important to begin oral antihypertensive agents as soon as possible so that the patient can be weaned off nitroprusside.

Contraindications

- Pregnancy
- Severe anemia
- Severe hepatic dysfunction because cyanide poisoning may occur; if renal disease is present and the use of nitroprusside is extended for more than 2 days, thiocyanate may accumulate.

NIFEDIPINE

Nifedipine administered as capsules is a most useful agent in the management of hypertensive emergencies and is of special value in patients with hypertensive encephalopathy and renal failure when nitroprusside is relatively contraindicated. Nifedipine may be used in patients with heart failure precipitated by severe hypertension, provided that CHD is not present. Nifedipine is contraindicated in the management of cerebrovascular accidents, including hemorrhage, and in patients with CHD, because in these situations, slow, careful titration is needed to avoid a rapid fall in blood pressure, which may precipitate cerebral or myocardial ischemia.

Dosage: 10 mg capsule every 2 to 4 hours for four to eight doses, along with furosemide if volume hypertension or renal failure is present. Then nifedipine dosage is structured four times daily. When blood pressure is under control, a long-acting preparation, e.g., nifedipine extended release (Procardia XL or Adalat XL) 60 to 90 mg once daily is advisable for maintenance therapy. An alternative initial schedule is the administration of sublingual nifedipine. A 5 mg nifedipine capsule is available, or a 10 mg capsule is perforated, squeezed, and the liquid kept sublingually for a few minutes. Alternatively, the patient is instructed to bite the capsule and then swallow it. This technique has been used extensively since 1982 with good results.

Although sublingual nifedipine has gained widespread use, caution is needed because the route has not been approved by the Food and Drug Administration (FDA) and is not warranted by the manufacturer. Sublingual nifedipine is safe in many situations, but occasionally cerebral infarction, myocardial ischemia, and myocardial infarction have been precipitated. This scenario is common to all potent antihypertensive agents that have the potential to cause a marked uncontrolled lowering of blood pressure. Importantly, nifedipine 10 mg capsule, used orally, causes blood pressure lowering that is of the same magnitude and acts as rapidly as the sublingual approach. Thus, oral administration is the method of choice. The higher the blood pressure, the greater the reduction observed with nifedipine use.

Contraindications

- Myocardial ischemia: Abrupt, uncontrolled fall in blood pressure may lead to ischemia and infarction

LABETALOL

This alpha and beta blocker is indicated for the management of hypertensive emergencies caused by renal failure, clonidine withdrawal, and dissecting aneurysm, although in the latter situation, a combination of nitroprusside and a beta blocker is preferable.

Dosage: IV infusion of 2 mg/min, 20 to 160 mg/hour, under close and continuous supervision. The patient must be recumbent during and for 4 hours following the infusion. Hypotensive effects may last from 1 to 12 hours after cessation of the infusion. Alternatively, bolus injections 20 mg over 1 minute, repeated after 5 minutes, if necessary to a maximum of 200 mg. Excessive bradycardia can be controlled with IV atropine, 0.6 to 2 mg, in divided doses.

DIAZOXIDE

Diazoxide has been virtually replaced by nitroprusside, labetalol, and nifedipine. The drug is used when other medications are not available or when renal failure is present and there is concern for nitroprusside toxicity. The drug is of value in malignant hypertension and is used in hypertensive emergencies associated with renal failure and hypertensive encephalopathy.

Dosage: 150 mg IV bolus injected undiluted and within 30 seconds directly into a peripheral vein. The 300 mg dose is not recommended because it causes too great a reduction in blood pressure, is often unpredictable, and has caused cerebral and myocardial infarctions. Diazoxide has sodium-retaining effects and must not be used in patients with heart failure. Furosemide 40 to 80 mg IV should be given following a bolus of diazoxide. Alternative dosage regimen: a slow infusion of diazoxide 5 mg/kg, given at the rate of 15 mg/min over 20 to 30 minutes to a total dose of 300 to 450 mg, is safer than bolus therapy.

Contraindications

• Cerebral hemorrhage
• Cerebrovascular accidents
Controlled blood pressure reduction is necessary in these situations when cerebral circulation is compromised.

HYDRALAZINE

This vasodilator has a role when nitroprusside, nifedipine, and labetalol are not available. The drug is particularly useful for hypertensive emergencies associated with renal failure and in pregnancy.

Dosage: A 10 mg test dose is followed in 30 minutes by IV infusion of 10 to 20 mg/hour; maintenance dose is 5 to 10 mg/hour. The addition of furosemide and a beta blocker to hydralazine greatly enhances antihypertensive effects, and the latter agent prevents hydralazine-induced tachycardia.

TRIMETHAPHAN

This drug is indicated only for the management of dissecting aortic aneurysms when nitroprusside and labetalol are not available (see Chapter 10).

Dosage: 50 mg trimethaphan in 500 ml 5% dextrose and water is given at 1 to 2 mg/min and increased, if needed, to 2 to 4 mg/min via an infusion pump. The head of the patient's bed should be elevated 45° to enhance the drug's orthostatic effect. An IV beta blocker such as atenolol or propranolol is given to reduce ejection velocity and pulsatile flow of blood, which causes further dissection of the aneurysm. Propranolol and other beta blockers used intravenously play a vital role in the management of dissecting aneurysm of the aorta. IV dosages of beta blockers are shown in Table 2–8.

METHYLDOPA

Methyldopa is useful in heart failure, hypertensive encephalopathy, and renal failure. It is not the drug of choice in cerebrovascular accidents because of its sedative properties and slow onset of action but is considered useful if other agents are not available and reduction of blood pressure is not required within the hour.

Dosage: 250 to 500 mg IV every 4 to 6 hours.

NITROGLYCERIN

Nitroglycerin is useful in hypertensive states associated with myocardial ischemia, heart failure, myocardial infarction, and following coronary artery bypass or other vascular reconstructive surgery and during cardiac catheterization.

Dosage: See Infusion Pump Chart, Table 2–9.

HYPERTENSION IN PREGNANCY

Hypertension in pregnancy is present if the blood pressure taken at least 6 hours apart exceeds 140/90 mm Hg or if there is an increase above the baseline of 30 mm Hg systolic or 15 mm Hg diastolic. A mean arterial pressure greater than 90 mm Hg (systolic pressure plus twice the diastolic divided by 3) causes a twofold increase in perinatal mortality.

Blood pressure should be estimated with the patient sitting or semireclined, since the blood pressure may be lower in the recumbent position.

Beta blockers, methyldopa, and hydralazine have all been successfully used in the management of hypertension from the 16th week to delivery and for hypertensive complications during pregnancy. Reduced birth weight, neonatal bradycardia, and hypoglycemia have been reported with beta blockers. However, recent results using beta blockers have shown better control of blood pressure and less effect on the fetus than observed with methyldopa or hydralazine. A combination of pindolol and hydralazine has been used successfully in randomized studies. Atenolol 25 to 75 mg daily has had favorable short- and longterm comparison with methyldopa. Combination therapy lowers the dose of individual drugs and reduces adverse effects.

Caution is necessary to avoid using antihypertensive agents during the first and early half of the second trimester of pregnancy to prevent the rare possibility of inducing congenital malformations. Early pregnancy is fortunately associated with vasodilation, which protects from hypertension. Antihypertensive agents considered relatively safe for chronic use from the 16th week to delivery are

- Beta blockers
- Methyldopa
- Hydralazine

Agents suitable for short-term use during the third trimester if no alternative exists include

- Thiazide diuretics at low dosages, see later discussion
- Nifedipine 10 to 20 mg twice daily for hypertensive emergencies during the last trimester, if other agents are not effective, are contraindicated, or cause serious adverse effects. Nifedipine should be avoided during labor because calcium antagonists may cause cessation of uterine contractions. Diltiazem and verapamil are contraindicated in pregnancy and during lactation. These agents should not be used concomitantly with magnesium sulfate because severe hypotension may occur.

Drugs that are contraindicated are

- Nitroprusside. There is a risk of cyanide toxicity and fetal death
- ACE inhibitors. These agents may cause skull defects and oligohydramnios or may disturb fetal and neonatal renal function and blood pressure control

ATENOLOL

Dosage: 25 mg once daily, increase to 50 mg daily only after several determinations of blood pressure, preferably made during two office or clinic visits. Maintenance up to 50 mg in the morning, 25 mg at night; maximum 50 mg twice daily. Longterm results are similar to those observed with methyldopa. Atenolol should not be used during lactation because the concentration in breast milk is high and adverse effects to infants have been reported.

PROPRANOLOL

Dosage: 20 to 40 mg three times daily, increase if needed to a maximum 80 mg twice daily. The drug is well tried, but atenolol is the preferred agent. Propranolol is the only beta blocker advised during lactation, however, because concentration in breast milk is lower than that of other beta blockers.

LABETALOL

Dosage: 100 to 200 mg twice daily; maximum 800 mg daily is effective but may be implicated in causing retroplacental hemorrhage. Postural hypotension, perioral numbness, itching of the scalp, positive antinuclear antibody (ANA) and Lupus-like syndrome have been observed. Importantly, acute hepatic necrosis is a rare but life-threatening complication. Thus, labetalol must not be considered as just another beta blocking drug.

METHYLDOPA

Dosage: 125 to 250 mg twice daily, increase the dose only after several reassessments over two or three visits; maximum suggested 500 mg twice daily.

In a study of 117 methyldopa-treated women one (0.9%) fetal death occurred; nine (7.2%) fetal deaths occurred in the control group of 125 women. No significant differences were noted at 7-year follow-up of children born to these mothers in both groups.

In blood pressure control is urgently needed prior to delivery, methyldopa is preferred to beta-adrenergic blockers. The addition of hydralazine may be required if methyldopa is not sufficiently effective.

HYDRALAZINE

This pure arterial vasodilator may be used during the last trimester if blood pressure is not adequately controlled with atenolol, pindolol, labetalol or methyldopa. The drug is teratogenic in animals.

Sodium and water retention may occur, requiring the unwarranted use of a thiazide and sinus tachycardia may be troublesome, necessitating beta blockade. Fetal thrombocytopenia has been reported. Thus, this agent is best reserved for a short period of therapy, 1 to 2 weeks, in the last trimester, along with a small dose of methyldopa or atenolol.

Dosage: IV: 5 mg bolus over 1 to 2 minutes, repeated in 20 minutes; then, if needed, infusion 5 mg to maximum of 15 mg/hour, with constant fetal monitoring of heart rate and maternal blood pressure. Oral: 25 mg three times daily for a few weeks.

THIAZIDES

Thiazide diuretics are relatively contraindicated since they decrease placental blood flow causing low birth weight. Thrombocytopenia, neonatal jaundice and occasionally, pancreatitis may occur.

Pre-eclampsia is associated with reduced plasma volume and thiazides are not recommended. Although several studies have indicated freedom from serious adverse effects, the results are questioned and the use of thiazides is restricted. Low-dose thiazide therapy may be considered in the third trimester if other agents are contraindicated or unavailable, particularly in the following category of patients

- Those whose hypertension predated conception or manifested prior to mid pregnancy
- Hypertension causing heart failure associated with volume overload

Dosage: Hydrochlorothiazide 12.5 mg daily (maximum 25 mg) or bendrofluazide 1.25 to 2.5 mg daily for a period of 1 to 6 weeks. After 6 weeks, alternative therapy should be considered.

HYPERTENSIVE CRISIS OF PREGNANCY

Severe hypertension of pregnancy, especially near term or during labor, associated with diastolic pressures greater than 105 mm Hg may require urgent treatment with the following agents and/or combinations.

HYDRALAZINE

Dosage: 5 mg IV over 10 to 20 minutes, and then 5 to 10 mg every 20 to 30 minutes; or, after the first bolus, give by IV infusion 5 mg/h, increase to 10 mg (maximum 15 mg/h) with continuous evaluation of heart rate and blood pressure and fetal monitoring. Fetal distress may occur. In the UK, the drug is given by the above method or by IV infusion initially (200 to 300 μg/min; maintenance 50 to 150 μg/min).

METHYLDOPA

Dosage: 500 mg orally causes blood pressure reduction within 6 hours. IV 250 mg in 100 ml 5% dextrose in water, over 30 minutes to 1 hour, repeated every 6 hours.

LABETALOL

Dosage: IV bolus 10 to 60 mg given every 20 minutes is effective and appears to cause less fetal distress than hydralazine. Clinical trials are necessary to compare efficacy and safety over hydralazine, the preferred drug. Practitioners should ascertain if labetalol is approved for IV use in their areas of practice prior to use. The IV use in pregnancy is not FDA approved.

MAGNESIUM SULFATE

This drug is useful in patients with pre-eclampsia to prevent convulsions and may cause mild transient lowering of blood pressure.

Dosage: 4 g diluted in 100 to 200 ml IV solution infused over 20 minutes, then 2 g/hour with careful monitoring of blood pressure and urinary output. The drug is continued during labor and for at least 24 hours post partum. Combination therapy utilizing the vasodilator action of hydralazine, the central action of methyldopa, and enhancement by magnesium sulfate usually produces salutary effects with less adverse effects than observed with high doses of a single agent. Magnesium sulfate has only mild antihypertensive effects and is not considered an antihypertensive agent, the major benefit of this drug is to prevent seizures associated with pre-eclampsia.

Caution. Magnesium sulfate must not be used concomitantly with nifedipine because severe hypotension may be precipitated; magnesium sulfate should be avoided in patients with renal failure.

SECONDARY HYPERTENSION

Causes of secondary hypertension and their approximate incidence include

- Renal parenchymal disease (3%)
- Renovascular disease (1%)
- Cushing's syndrome (0.1%)
- Pheochromocytoma (0.1%)
- Primary hyperaldosteronism (0.1%)
- Coarctation (0.1%)
- Estrogens (0.4%)
- Alcohol (0.2% or more)

RENAL PARENCHYMAL DISEASE

The history, physical, and laboratory screenings give clues to the type and duration of the underlying disease.
Screening includes assessment for

- The presence and type of urinary casts
- The degree of proteinuria and anemia
- The level of serum creatinine, urea or blood urea nitrogen, serum calcium, phosphate, and albumin

The most common underlying diseases are

- Chronic glomerulonephritis
- Diabetic nephropathy
- Collagen vascular disease
- Polycystic kidney
- Chronic pyelonephritis
- Interstitial renal disease

An increase in total peripheral resistance, hypervolemia, increased total body sodium stores, and a high cardiac output are prominent features that give rise to the hypertension of renal failure.

THERAPY

Furosemide

As emphasized under the section on diuretics, thiazides lose their natriuretic effect in patients with glomerular filtration rates less than 25 ml/hour or serum creatinine greater than 2.3 mg/dl (203 μmol/l).

Dosage: Furosemide 80 to 240 mg daily or bumetanide 5 to 10 mg daily may be expected to produce sufficient natriuresis, which is best reflected in the degree of weight loss. Rarely, up to 500 mg furosemide or 240 mg plus 5 mg metolazone may be required.

Beta Blockers

Beta blockers combined with diuretics are effective in reducing blood pressure in patients with chronic renal failure. Atenolol, nadolol, and sotalol are excreted by the kidney; their dosing interval should be increased, and the total daily dose may have to be reduced in chronic renal failure if exaggerated beta blockade is manifest. Propranolol and metoprolol are actively metabolized, do not require dose adjustment, and are preferred for the management of hypertension with severe renal failure. Timolol and pindolol are partially excreted by the kidney but usually require little or no adjustment in dosage (see Table 1–3 for dosages of antihypertensive agents).

Calcium Antagonists

Calcium antagonists, particularly nifedipine, have had extensive trials and have proven effective in reducing total peripheral resistance, which is usually markedly increased in patients with chronic renal failure. Nifedipine and diltiazem are metabolized and dosages may not require alteration. However, a few patients with renal failure reportedly showed deterioration with nifedipine and diltiazem. Recovery of function occurs upon discontinuing the calcium antagonist. Verapamil may accumulate with renal failure and is not advisable. Nifedipine has commonly replaced hydralazine in the combination beta blocker plus diuretic plus vasodilator, but hydralazine may be added to the combination because the mechanism of vasodilation is different and the effect is additive.

Hydralazine

When calcium antagonists are contraindicated or produce adverse effects, hydralazine has a role in lowering total peripheral resistance and blood pressure and has proven effective in patients with severe hypertension associated with renal failure.

Dosage: 25 to 100 mg twice daily. The dosage interval for hydralazine should be increased with chronic renal failure, with creatinine clearance less than 25 ml/min.

Central Acting Agents

Centrally acting drugs such as methyldopa, clonidine, and guanfacine are useful in combination with furosemide and nifedipine or appropriate agents in managing resistant renal hypertension, including patients on dialysis. Dosing should be reduced to once daily, preferably at bedtime.

RENOVASCULAR HYPERTENSION

Diagnostic considerations in renovascular hypertension include

- Age of onset (before age 30 or after age 50)
- The sudden onset of malignant, accelerated, or resistant hypertension accompanied by a renal bruit

- A sharp rise in serum creatinine after the use of an ACE inhibitor is indicative of significant renal artery stenosis

In such circumstances, the incidence of significant renovascular hypertension ranges from 20 to 33%. Increased diagnostic suspicion is obtained from observation of the IV pyelogram or renal scan. Where available, digital subtraction angiography is preferred to renal arteriography. A difference between the two renal veins from the abnormal and suppressed contralateral kidney giving a renal vein renin ratio greater than 1.5 strongly suggests significant renal artery stenosis, but results are often insufficient to justify the investigation.

THERAPY

Drug therapy includes the judicious use of combination therapy, beta blocker, thiazide (furosemide if renal failure is present), and amiloride, to conserve potassium. Other combinations are suggested in Figure 1–1. ACE inhibitors are contraindicated in patients with severe bilateral renal artery stenosis or stenosis of a solitary kidney since in these patients, renal circulation is dependent on high levels of angiotensin II. Thus, a sharp fall in renal blood flow may occur and renal failure may ensue with the loss of a solitary kidney.

Angioplasty and surgery are equally effective and superior to drug therapy in patients in whom renal artery stenosis is due to fibrous dysplasia and hypertension is present for less than 3 years with normal renal function. Angioplasty has a role in patients who are poor surgical candidates. Restenosis post angioplasty frequently occurs, but a second dilatation may be rewarding. In patients with unilateral renal artery stenosis, elevation of serum creatinine indicates that nephrosclerosis is present in the contralateral kidney, and a salutary effect of angioplasty or revascularization is unlikely.

Surgery appears to be somewhat more effective than angioplasty for atherosclerotic renovascular disease. Either therapy is advisable for atherosclerotic occlusion in younger patients with unilateral renal artery disease, especially when hypertension is difficult to control with antihypertensive agents. A serum creatinine level greater than 1.4 mg/dl (124 μmol/l) and the presence of CHD increase the surgical mortality rate.

PHEOCHROMOCYTOMA

Less than 0.1% of patients with moderate to severe diastolic hypertension are expected to have a pheochromocytoma

- Approximately 10% of these tumors of the adrenal medulla are bilateral
- 10% are malignant
- 10% are outside the adrenals
- 10% are familial

Patients with familial or bilateral pheochromocytomas may be part of the Type II Multiple Endocrine Neoplasia syndrome and should

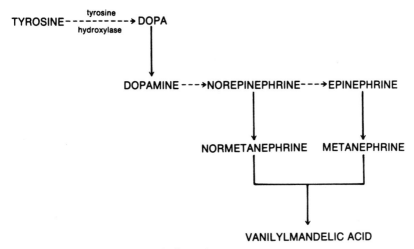

FIG. 1–2. Catecholamine metabolic pathway.

be screened for medullary carcinoma of the thyroid and hyperparathyroidism.

CLINICAL HALLMARKS

These include

- Severe headaches and profuse sweating
- Palpitations and tremor
- Pallor due to vasoconstriction
- Paroxysmal or diastolic hypertension, severe increase of blood pressure with induction of anesthesia, surgery, or use of histamine, phenothiazines, or tricyclic antidepressants
- Postural hypotension
- Weight loss

The catecholamine metabolic pathway involves conversion of tyrosine to normetanephrine and metanephrine (see Fig. 1–2).

DIAGNOSTIC EVALUATION

The following investigations are usually diagnostic

- Elevated 24-hour urine total metanephrine is the most reliable urinary screening test
- Free catecholamines and vanilylmandelic acid (VMA) are often elevated, but interference with urinary screening occurs with phenothiazines, chloral hydrate, and other drugs. Beta blockers, thiazides, calcium antagonists, and ACE inhibitors, however, cause no interference. A special

diet and avoidance of several drugs for at least 3 days are necessary for accurate VMA results.

- An increase in plasma catecholamines: An assessment is carried out with a heparin lock in an arm vein; the patient is sedated with 1 mg of sublingual lorazepam (Ativan) and is allowed to lie quietly for 20 minutes. Blood is then drawn for epinephrine and norepinephrine levels.
- Elevated dopamine serum level is estimated on the same blood sample taken for epinephrine because dopamine may be the only chemical produced by some malignant pheochromocytomas. Plasma catecholamines may be mildly elevated with stress and essential hypertension, diuretics, prazosin, and other alpha$_1$ blockers, hydralazine, labetalol, and calcium antagonists. A computerized tomographic (CT) scan may reveal a tumor. I^{131} meta-iodo-benzyl-guanidine (MIBG) enters chromaffin tissue and an MIBG scan helps identify extra adrenal tumors

THERAPY

Phentolamine
(Regitine; Rogitine, Canada and UK)

Hypertensive crisis may require the use of phentolamine prior to the administration of phenoxybenzamine.

Dosage: 5 to 10 mg IV bolus given over 5 minutes repeated if necessary, or an infusion of 10 to 20 μg/kg/min or 5 to 60 mg over 10 to 30 minutes at a rate of 0.1 to 2 mg/min. The drug has a rapid onset of action and lasts only 10 to 20 minutes.

Caution. Deaths due to arrhythmia and acute myocardial infarction have been reported and beta blockade may be required. If beta blockers are used, care is required in patients who are considered at high risk for precipitation of heart failure.

Nitroprusside

Nitroprusside should be used to lower blood pressure during a crisis and is effective, but complicating tachyarrhythmias may cause problems with management and beta blockade should not be used without adequate alpha blockade (see infusion pump chart, Table 1–10).

Phenoxybenzamine
(Dibenzyline)

Oral therapy with this nonselective alpha blocker is commenced once the blood pressure is under control or if the blood pressure is not severely elevated after control with phentolamine or other agent.

Dosage: 1 to 2 mg/kg daily in two or three divided doses; usually 10 mg every 8 to 12 hours, increase every 3 or 4 days by 10 mg to a maximum

50 mg three times daily. Phenoxybenzamine therapy is usually required for control of blood pressure over a period of 1 to 2 weeks prior to surgery. The drug is contraindicated in heart failure.

Patients with pheochromocytoma are hypovolemic and alpha blockade causes vasodilation. Thus, a marked fall in blood pressure may occur, causing severe postural hypotension. Increase in salt intake and vigorous saline infusion are usually required during the one to two weeks prior to surgery to prevent severe postural hypotension, but careful monitoring is required to prevent the precipitation of heart failure. Postoperative hypotension may be avoided by discontinuing phenoxybenzamine several days prior to surgery.

Nifedipine

This agent, used universally for the management of all grades of hypertension, may be used in the emergency setting with temporary beneficial results expected in some patients and may occasionally avoid the use of nitroprusside (see Table 1–9).

Beta Blockers

Beta blockers must not be used prior to adequate alpha blockade because unopposed stimulation of alpha receptors can cause a severe increase in blood pressure. Beta blockade may be required after 1 week of alpha blockade if catecholamine-induced arrhythmias require control. A beta$_1$ selective drug such as atenolol is preferable to propranolol.

Metyrosine
(Metirosine, UK) (alpha-methyl-L-tyrosine) (Demser)

This agent is an inhibitor of tyrosine hydroxylase (see Fig. 1–2) and, hence, the synthesis of catecholamines. Metyrosine reduces catecholamine production by about 70% and has a role in the preoperative management of pheochromocytomas as an alternative to phenoxybenzamine. The drug is particularly useful for the management of inoperable tumors.

Dosage: 250 mg four times daily, increase daily by 250 mg to reach a maximum of 4 g daily.

Adverse effects. Severe diarrhea, sedation, extra pyramidal symptoms, and hypersensitive reactions may occur.

SURGERY

A transabdominal incision is advisable to allow a search of all abdominal chromafin tissue. Enflurane is considered the safest anesthetic agent, as it does not stimulate catecholamine release or sensitize the myocardium to catecholamines. Management of fluid blood volumes necessitates the use of a Swan-Ganz catheter. Elevated blood pressure is controlled with nitroprusside or nitroglycerin, especially in patients where the occurrence of heart failure is predictable. Postoperative hypotension and heart failure present a greater hazard with the use of alpha blockers and beta blockade than with the use of nitroprusside or nitroglycerin.

A surgical cure is expected in 80% of patients. Approximately 10% of patients have a recurrence, and patients should be screened annually for 5 years. The 5-year survival is about 95% for patients with benign tumors and 45% for patients with malignant tumors.

COARCTATION OF THE AORTA

Hypertension in the arms with weak, absent, or delayed femoral pulses is a hallmark. After the age of 10, chest x-ray shows notching of the fourth to eighth ribs bilaterally or unilaterally and right sided if the coarctation is proximal to the left subclavian.

THERAPY

Drug therapy is often required in the adult prior to surgical correction. Coarctation of the aorta causes activation of the renin angiotensin aldosterone system; thus, ACE inhibitors are first-line agents. All patients should be screened for septal defects, polycystic kidneys, and berry aneurysms; the latter not uncommonly causes the patient's demise.

Surgical repair may not be curative. Postoperative hypertension may be a problem requiring antihypertensive therapy. Aortic dissection may occur distal or proximal to the site of surgical repair. Also, restenosis may require balloon angioplasty, and close follow-up is essential.

Two risk factors have been identified for premature death after surgery

- Age at the time of surgical correction: The younger the patient, the better the outcome
- Hypertension, both preoperative and postoperative, carries a guarded prognosis

BIBLIOGRAPHY

Anastos K, Charney P, Charon RA, et al.: Hypertension in women: What is really known? The women's caucus, working group on women's health of the Society of General Internal Medicine. Ann Intern Med, *1151*:287, 1991.

Calhoun DA, Oparil S: Treatment of hypertensive crisis. N Eng J Med, *323*:1177, 1991.

Cameron DI: Near fatal angioedema associated with captopril. Can J Cardiol, *6*:265, 1990.

Cody RJ: Regression of left ventricular hypertrophy in resistant hypertension. J Am Coll Cardiol, *16*:143, 1990.

Cunningham FG, Lindheimer MD: Current concepts: Hypertension in Pregnancy. N Eng J Med, *326*:927, 1992.

Dabaghi S: ACE inhibitors and pancreatitis. Ann Intern Med, *115*:331, 1991.

Dunn FG, Burns JMA, Hornung RS: Left ventricular hypertrophy in hypertension. Am Heart J, *122*:312, 1991.

Edelson JF, Weinstein MC, Tosteson ANA, et al.: Long-term cost-effectiveness of various initial monotherapies for mild to moderate hypertension. JAMA, *263*:408, 1990.

Felson DT, Sloutskis D, Anderson JJ, et al.: Thiazide diuretics and the risk of hip fracture. Results from the Framingham Study. JAMA, *265*:370, 1991.

Frohlich ED: Left ventricular hypertrophy: Further evidence of risk. J Am Coll Cardiol, *15*: 1295, 1991.

Giannoccaro PJ, Wallace GJ, Higginson LAJ, et al.: Fatal angioedema associated with enalapril. Can J Cardiol, *5*:335, 1989.

Gradman AH: Hemodynamic effects of the vascular selective calcium antagonist felodipine in patients with impaired left ventricular function. Am Heart J, *123*:273, 1992.

Hanson MW, Feldman JM, Beam CA, et al.: Iodine 131-labeled metaiodobenzylguanidine scintigraphy and biochemical analyses in suspected pheochromocytoma. Arch Intern Med, *151*:1397, 1991.

Julien J, Dufloux MA, Prasquier R, et al.: Effects of captopril and minoxidil on left ventricular hypertrophy in resistant hypertensive patients: A 6 month double-blind comparison. J Am Coll Cardiol, *16*:137, 1990.

Khan, M Gabriel: Hypertension. *In* Cardiac Drug Therapy. 3rd Ed. London, W.B. Saunders, 1992.

Kostis JB: Angiotensin converting enzyme inhibitors. I. Pharmacology. Am Heart J, *116*:1580, 1988.

Kostis JB: Angiotensin converting enzyme inhibitors. II. Clinical use. Am Heart J, *116*:1591, 1988.

Kowey PR, Friehling RD, Sewter J, et al.: Electrophysiological effects of left ventricular hypertrophy. Circulation, *83*:2067, 1991.

LaCroix AZ, Wienpahl J, White LR, et al.: Thiazide diuretic agents and the incidence of hip fracture. N Engl J Med, *322*:286, 1990.

National High Blood Pressure Education Program: National high blood pressure education program working group report on hypertension and chronic renal failure. Arch Intern Med, *151*:1280, 1991.

Neutel JM, Schnaper H, Cheug DG, et al.: Antihypertensive effects of β-blockers administered once daily: 24-hour measurements. Am Heart J, *120*:166, 1990.

Oren S, Messerli FH, Grossman E, et al.: Immediate and short-term cardiovascular effects of fosinopril, a new angiotensin-converting enzyme inhibitor, in patients with essential hypertension. J Am Coll Cardiol, *17*:1183, 1991.

Pearson AC, Pasierski T, Labovitz AJ: Left ventricular hypertrophy: Diagnosis, prognosis and management. Am Heart J, *121*:148, 1991.

Phillips RA: Significance of increased left ventricular mass in isolated systolic hypertension of the elderly. J Am Coll Cardiol, *17*:431, 1991.

SHEP Cooperative Study Group: Prevention of stroke by antihypertensive drug treatment in older persons with isolated systolic hypertension: Final results of the Systolic Hypertension in the Elderly Programs (SHEP). JAMA, *265*:3255, 1991.

Slater EE, Merrill DD, Guess HA, et al.: Clinical profile of angioedema associated with angiotensin converting enzyme inhibition. JAMA, *260*:967, 1988.

Szlachcic J, Tubau JF, O'Kelly B, et al.: What is the role of silent coronary artery disease and left ventricular hypertrophy in the genesis of ventricular arrhythmias in men with essential hypertension? J Am Coll Cardiol, *19*:803, 1992.

The Treatment of Mild Hypertension Research Group: The treatment of mild hypertension study. A randomized, placebo-controlled trial of a nutritional-hygienic regimen along with various drug monotherapies. Arch Intern Med, *151*:1413, 1991.

Wassertheil-Smoller S, Blaufox D, Oberman A, et al.: Effect of anti-hypertensives on sexual function and quality of life: The TAIM Study. Ann Intern Med, *114*:613, 1991.

Wilkstrand J, Warnold I, Tuomilhto J, et al.: Metoprolol versus thiazide diuretics in hypertension. Morbidity results from the MAPHY Study. Hypertension, *17*:579, 1991.

Wood SM, Mann RD, Rawlins MD: Angioedema and urticaria associated with angiotensin converting enzyme inhibitors. Br Med J, *294*:91, 1987.

2

ANGINA
M. Gabriel Khan

CLASSIFICATION

- *Stable angina*: No change in the past 60 days in frequency, duration, or precipitating causes. Pain duration less than 10 minutes. In more than 90% of patients, stable angina is caused by a greater than 70% obstruction in at least one coronary artery. In less than 10% of individuals, a lesser degree of atheromatous obstruction, coronary artery spasm, or small vessel disease is present
- *Unstable angina*: There is a change in pattern, increasing frequency, severity, and/or duration of pain, and a lesser degree of known precipitating factors

   Subset I: Changing pattern, i.e., progressive or crescendo angina, worsening of previously stable angina. Pain mainly
   - on exertion
   - at rest

   Subset II: New onset angina present less than 60 days
   - on exertion
   - mainly at rest
   - *Prinzmetal's (variant) angina*: This condition is a rare cause of stable angina. When it does occur, there are often dynamic changes in arterial radius at a point where there is already eccentric organic stenosis

   The Canadian cardiovascular classification grading of angina is widely used to differentiate mild, moderate, or severe stable angina

- Class 1 Angina: Pain is precipitated only by severe and usually prolonged exertion
- Class 2 Angina: Pain on moderate effort, e.g., precipitated by walking uphill or by walking briskly for more than three blocks on the level in the cold, against a wind, or provoked by emotional stress. There is "slight limitation of ordinary activity"
- Class 3 Angina: Marked limitation of ordinary activity; pain occurs on mild exertion, usually restricting daily chores. Unable to walk two blocks on the level at comfortable temperatures and at a normal pace
- Class 4 Angina: Chest discomfort on almost any physical activity, e.g., dressing, shaving, walking less than 100 feet indoors. Pain may be present at rest

STABLE ANGINA

PATHOPHYSIOLOGY

Myocardial ischemia is a dynamic process. It is now clear that three, not two, determinants play a major role in the pathogenesis of myocardial ischemia, which may manifest as the chest pain of angina or remain painless as with silent ischemia.

The three determinants of myocardial ischemia are

- Concentric or eccentric coronary atheroma causing greater than about 70% stenosis; concentric plaques are observed mainly with stable angina and there is a tendency for them to be eccentric in patients with frequent rest pain and in those with unstable angina
- Increased myocardial oxygen demand
- Release of catecholamines occurring at the onset of angina and during the episode in the vast majority of patients with stable angina. Release of catecholamines may actually initiate ischemia, which stimulates further catecholamine release, and a vicious circle perpetuates the oxygen lack (Fig. 2–1)

When angina is manifest, at least one coronary artery is expected to show a greater than 70% stenosis on angiography. The obstructive plaque of atheroma is often focal and usually occurs in the proximal portion of a coronary artery; this combination of proximal and focal lesions dictates the success of angioplasty and bypass surgery. In less than 10% of individuals, and especially in diabetics, multifocal longer segmental or diffuse disease exists in the distal coronary tree.

Figure 2–2 shows coronary angiographic anatomy. An obstructive lesion in the left anterior descending (LAD) artery prior to the septal or first diagonal branch is considered proximal and highly significant because it can jeopardize more than 50% of the left ventricular myocardium. LAD lesions after the first diagonal affect only about 20% of the myocardium. In approximately 85 and 15% of individuals, the right coronary or left circumflex artery supplies the posterior diaphragmatic portion of the interventricular septum and the diaphragmatic surface of the left ventricle, respectively, and is referred to as the dominant artery. The term "dominant" does not imply a more important artery but does have some clinical bearing on decision-making in the management of angina.

A 25% decrease in the outer radius of a normal coronary artery results in about a 60% decrease in a cross-sectional area. However, in an artery with 75% stenosis, a 10% decrease in the outer radius would produce a complete occlusion.

During periods of exercise or exertion, catecholamine release causes an increase in heart rate, an increase in the velocity and force of myocardial contraction producing an elevation in blood pressure, and an increase in myocardial oxygen demand. In the presence of significant coronary artery stenosis, an oxygen deficit may occur. Myocardial ischemia increases catecholamine release, resulting in an additional increase in heart rate and blood pressure, with further oxygen lack, and the vicious circle ensues.

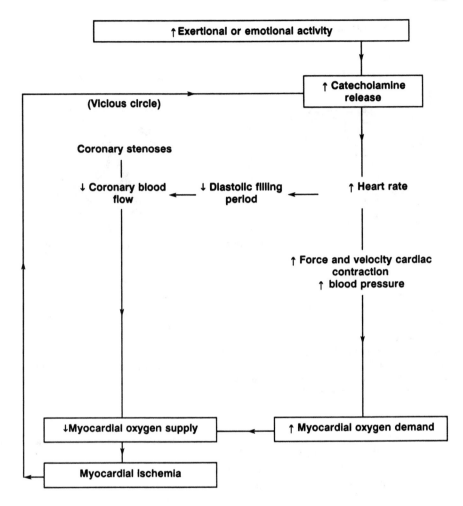

↑ = Increase
↓ = Decrease

FIG. 2–1. Pathophysiology of angina.

Importantly, the coronaries fill during the diastolic period, which is shortened during tachycardia.

Pharmacologic agents that inhibit the initiation or interrupt the dynamic process described above provide rational therapy for myocardial ischemia. It is, therefore, not surprising that beta-adrenergic blocking drugs produce salutary effects in the majority of patients with stable angina and represent first-choice oral medications for the management of angina.

In contrast to the beta blocking drugs, dihydropyridine calcium antagonists, when used alone, tend to increase heart rate and, along with other

CORONARY ANGIOGRAPHIC ANATOMY: REPRESENTATION IN STANDARD PROJECTIONS

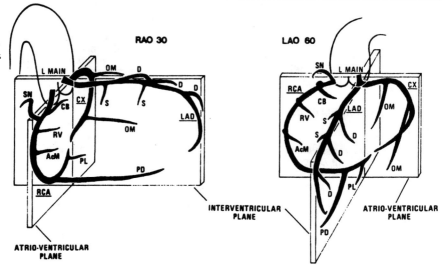

FIG. 2–2. Representation of coronary anatomy relative to the interventricular and atrioventricular valve planes. Coronary branches are as indicated—L Main (left main), LAD (left anterior descending), D (diagonal), S (septal), CX (circumflex), OM (obtuse marginal), RCA (right coronary), CB (conus branch), SN (sinus node), RV (right ventricular), AcM (acute marginal), PD (posterior descending), PL (posterolateral left ventricular). From: Grossman W, Baim DS: Cardiac Catheterization, Angiography and Intervention. 4th Ed. Philadelphia, Lea & Febiger, 1992, p 200.

calcium antagonists, do not inhibit the cardiovascular actions of catecholamines. Nitrates also increase heart rate.

An important consideration in relation to coronary artery spasm is that ischemia from this cause also triggers catecholamine release and worsening of angina. However, coronary artery spasm is a rare cause of myocardial ischemia manifest as stable angina.

DIAGNOSIS

Diagnosis is based on a careful relevant history. The pain of angina is typically a retrosternal discomfort precipitated by a particular activity, especially walking quickly up an incline or against the wind. Pain or discomfort disappears within seconds to minutes of stopping the precipitating activity, in keeping with the concept of oxygen supply versus myocardial demand. Discomfort may start in the lower, middle, or upper substernal area, the lower jaw, or the arm. Typically, the discomfort is a tightness, constriction, squeezing, heaviness, pressure, strangulation, burning, nausea, or an indigestion-like feeling of gradual onset that disappears at rest, except with unstable anginal syndromes. Occasionally, the pain is described as sharp, and at times, discomfort is replaced by shortness of breath on exertion.

The area of pain is usually at least the size of a clenched fist, often occupying most of the central chest area. The patient uses two or more fingers, the entire palm of the hand, or the fist to indicate the pain site. A pencil point area of pain is rarely caused by myocardial ischemia.

Relief of pain in an individual with stable angina always occurs within minutes of cessation of the precipitating exertional or emotional activity. Relief with sublingual nitroglycerin occurs promptly with 1 to 2 minutes.

INVESTIGATIVE EVALUATION

Patients with the same clinical symptoms may have very different prognoses depending on coronary anatomy; one, two, three vessel or left main stenoses; and on left ventricular function.

The failure to predict outcomes based on the clinical presentation often necessitates evaluation with exercise stress testing and echocardiography. Thallium scintigraphy is required in some. It is necessary to evaluate the coronary reserve and degree of proximal stenosis. The goal of initial investigations is to stratify the risk so that those at higher risk can progress to angiography early.

BLOOD WORK

- Lipid levels: Total serum cholesterol is not affected by daily food intake. It is best to request the total cholesterol with the patient in a nonfasting state at the same time as the office visit, as this routine saves patient's time and money. If the total cholesterol exceeds 240 mg/dl (6.2 mmol/l) then request total cholesterol, HDL, LDL, and triglycerides with the patient fasting 14 hours (see Chapter 8)
- The hemoglobin is necessary to exclude the rare occurrence of angina precipitated by anemia in patients with atheromatous coronary stenosis. Renal function, approximately assessed by the serum creatinine, is relevant to the choice and dosage of medications

ELECTROCARDIOGRAM

The ECG is expected to be normal in over 70% of patients with stable angina, except in individuals with previous myocardial infarction or concomitant hypertension. However, even a normal record makes a valuable baseline with which to compare future tracings.

EXERCISE STRESS TEST

Exercise stress testing is important in assessing the coronary reserve and in formulating strategies for other therapeutic interventions, especially in patients with Class 1 and 2 angina. It is also useful in assessing the effect of medical therapy. However, the test is not useful in evaluating atypical chest pain, especially in women. The test is contraindicated in patients with unstable angina, aortic stenosis, and obstructive cardiomyopathy.

Patients under age 60 with angina who can complete more than 6 minutes of a Bruce protocol treadmill exercise test, achieving more than 85% of maximal heart rate without chest pain or ischemia changes, can usually be managed with medical therapy. Patients who can tolerate more than 9 minutes of a Bruce protocol appear to have a good prognosis. In this subset, if medical therapy is judged by physician and patient to be yielding adequate control of symptoms, coronary angiography is usually not required. A positive exercise stress test is indicated by

• Greater than or equal to 1 mm flat or down-sloping ST segment depression, 80 millisecond after the J point occurring in three consecutive beats

A strongly positive test is indicated by

• ST segment depression within the first 3 minutes of exercise, down-sloping ST segment depression of 2 mm or greater, persisting for more than 4 minutes on cessation of exercise or occurring at low work load: heart rate less than 120 per minute, systolic pressure less than 130 mm Hg, i.e., a low rate pressure product. Patients in this category have a poor prognosis and are expected to have a large area of myocardium involved by the ischemic process. Patients with strongly positive tests, ischemia occurring prior to six minutes, and/or hypotension during exercise have a high probability of having multi-vessel or left mainstem disease and are, therefore, at significant risk. Coronary angiography is warranted with consideration for coronary angioplasty or coronary artery bypass surgery (CABS) in such patients.

Figure 2–3 indicates the scatter plot of coronary flow reserve (peak resting blood flow velocity) in vessels of patients with a normal (less than 0.1 mV ST segment depression) exercise test and an abnormal (0.1 mV or greater ST segment depression) test. Table 2–1 shows the relation of coronary flow reserve to exercise electrocardiography and arteriographic stenosis geometry.

Patients with Class 2 angina who are unable to exercise because of arthritis or peripheral vascular disease should undergo dipyridamole-thallium scintigraphy (see Chapter 17). Patients with stable angina Class 3 or unquestionable unstable angina do not require stress testing. Stress testing is particularly hazardous in this last group and coronary angiography is indicated in either situation.

THALLIUM SCINTIGRAPHY

Thallium 201 perfusing the myocardium is removed by myocardial cells. A positive test, a cold spot on the scan, absent thallium uptake with filling in later views, indicates ischemic myocardium. The test is generally performed in conjunction with an exercise test and is useful in patients with left ventricular hypertrophy and atypical chest pain in which conventional exercise stress testing gives a high rate of false positives. The validity of the test depends on a reasonably high rate pressure product being achieved during the preliminary stress period. Thallium scintigraphy has several limitations

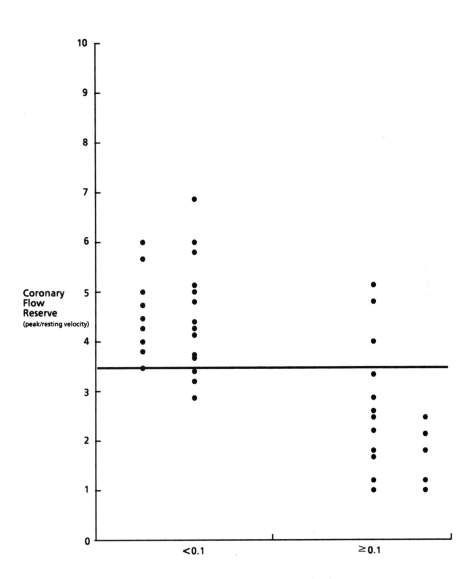

FIG. 2–3. Scatterplot of coronary flow reserve (peak/resting blood flow velocity) in vessels of patients with normal (less than 0.1 mV ST segment depression) exercise test and an abnormal (0.1 mV or greater ST segment depression) test. Sensitivity and specificity of the exercise test in detecting vessels with reduced coronary flow reserve (less than 3.5 peak/resting velocity) were 0.82 and 0.87, respectively. From: Wilson RF, et al.: Accuracy of exercise electrocardiography in detecting physiologically significant coronary arterial lesions. Circulation, *83*:412, 1991.

TABLE 2-1. ACCURACY OF EXERCISE ELECTROCARDIOGRAPHY IN PREDICTING PHYSIOLOGICAL AND ARTERIOGRAPHIC MEASUREMENTS OF STENOSIS SEVERITY

GOLD STANDARD	SENSITIVITY	95% CI	SPECIFICITY	95% CI	OVERALL ACCURACY	95% CI
Coronary flow reserve						
<3.5*	0.82	(0.70–0.94)	0.87	(0.77–0.97)	0.85	(0.74–0.96)
Diameter stenosis (%)						
>50	0.50	(0.35–0.65)	0.71	(0.57–0.85)	0.58	(0.43–0.73)
>60	0.61	(0.46–0.76)	0.73	(0.60–0.86)	0.63	(0.48–0.78)
Area stenosis (%)						
>70	0.57	(0.42–0.72)	0.76	(0.63–0.89)	0.65	(0.50–0.80)
>75	0.80	(0.68–0.92)	0.80	(0.68–0.92)	0.80	(0.68–0.92)

CI, confidence interval
* Peak divided by resting velocity
From: Wilson RF, et al.: Accuracy of exercise electrocardiography in detecting physiologically significant coronary arterial lesions. Circulation, 83:412, 1991.

- Proper methodology is necessary
- Image artifacts are common and can lead to false positive interpretation
- False positive results may occur because of overlying breast shadows; right ventricular blood pool may attenuate inferoposterior myocardial activity
- Myocardial apical thinning causes a local decrease in thallium activity that can be mistaken for ischemic disease
- Left bundle branch block may produce a false positive scan

Most of these difficulties are of importance in relation to fixed defects, reversibility being a strong indicator of myocardium at risk.

Thallium scintigraphy can give a reasonably reliable estimate of the area of myocardium at risk but does not measure myocardial blood flow in ml/g of myocardium. Negative scans may occur with significant lesions in the circumflex or diagonal branches of the left anterior descending artery. Widespread disease with global reduction in uptake will also, paradoxically, yield a negative result. Accumulation of the thallium in the lungs is a sign of left ventricular dysfunction that should be followed up with echocardiography with consideration of angiography.

Dipyridamole thallium scintigraphy is a useful investigation in patients with Class 2 angina with the absence of pain at rest who are unable to exercise because of arthritis or peripheral vascular disease (see Chapter 17). Patients with Class 3 angina require coronary angiographic assessment. Dipyridamole thallium scintigraphy is contraindicated in patients with unstable angina, post infarction angina, and non Q wave infarction; within 3 months of infarction, these patients require coronary angiography. Also, dipyridamole scintigraphy is contraindicated in patients with asthma and chronic obstructive pulmonary disease (COPD).

ECHOCARDIOGRAPHY

Echocardiography is not routinely done but is helpful in some patients with angina to assess.

- Contractility and left ventricular systolic function in anginal patients with previous infarction. Reduction of ejection fraction (EF) may indicate the need for coronary angiography with a view to angioplasty or CABS
- Left ventricular dysfunction, EF less than 40%, would be a relative indication for intervention and would necessitate caution in the use of a beta blocking drug. Verapamil and diltiazem are contraindicated in patients with EF less than 40%, and these agents are now recognized to influence adversely the prognosis when left ventricular function is compromised. Beta blocking agents are used cautiously in patients with EF less than 30 to 40% and are usually contraindicated in patients with EF less than 30%. Exception to this relative contraindication is discussed later in this chapter. The aforementioned points indicate that patients with angina with previous heart failure or suspected left ventricular dysfunction benefit from echocardiographic assessment
- Shortness of breath on exertion in patients in whom mitral regurgitation is suspected with physical signs masked by a thick chest wall or chronic

lung disease. Such patients with significant mitral regurgitation would benefit particularly from ACE inhibitors plus or minus valve surgery

HOLTER MONITOR

Painless ischemia appears to occur more commonly than painful ischemia. However, Holter monitoring can be difficult to interpret and is not cost effective in the assessment of stable angina Class 1 and 2. Patients with unstable angina and those with Class 3 angina have a high incidence of silent ischemia. However, these patients require coronary angiography and Holter monitoring is not indicated unless bothersome or symptomatic arrhythmias are suspected.

CORONARY ANGIOGRAPHY

Indications include the following

- Patients who require coronary angioplasty or CABS. See indications for these interventions
- Ideally, all patients with angina in good general health and with absence of severe concomitant disease that would contraindicate CABS
- Patients with painless ischemia have the same risks as patients with angina and must be evaluated and given consideration for angioplasty or CABS if severe obstructive disease is discovered
- Purely diagnostic to prevent an incorrect label of ischemic heart disease in patients in whom symptoms persist and the diagnosis remains in doubt after careful evaluation, history, and other noninvasive investigations of the heart, lungs, GI tract, and chest wall

THERAPY

General control of risk factors is the necessary first step: weight reduction, cessation of smoking, removal or avoidance of stress, control of hypertension with suitable agents, maintenance of a serum cholesterol less than 200 mg/dl (5.2 mmol/l), LDL less than 160 mg/dl (4 mmol/l) (see Chapter 8).

Suggested steps in therapy for stable angina are given in Figure 2–4. Figures 2–5 and 2–6 give decision-making steps in the management of varying grades of stable angina formulated on knowledge derived from

- The assessment of the patient according to the Canadian Cardiovascular Society functional or similar classification (or similar assessment of clinical severity of angina)
- The exercise stress test
- The anatomic site of atheromatous coronary obstruction, degree of stenosis as determined by coronary angiography, and number of involved vessels
- The presence or absence of lesions angiographically acceptable for balloon angioplasty (Type A) or probably acceptable lesions for balloon angioplasty

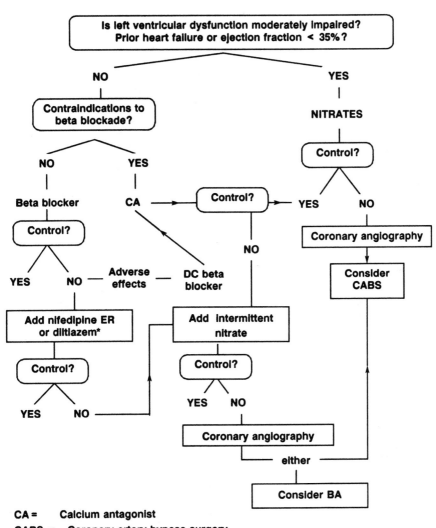

CA =   Calcium antagonist
CABS = Coronary artery bypass surgery
DC =   Discontinue
* Caution with beta blocker combination; avoid if ejection fraction < 40%
BA =   Balloon angioplasty
ER =   Extended Release

FIG. 2–4. Suggested steps in medical therapy for stable angina.

- Radionuclide or echocardiographic assessment of left ventricular function. Patients with significant proximal coronary stenosis affecting three major vessels or two vessels including the left anterior descending and moderate or severe left ventricular dysfunction, EF less than 40% (greater than 20%), show greater benefits from surgery as opposed to medical therapy; surgery is considered to have advantages over angio-

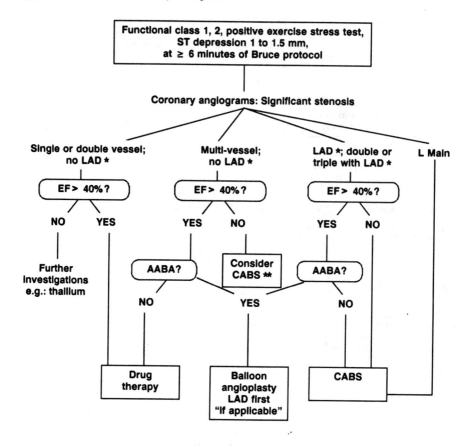

*   **LAD = Left anterior descending severe proximal stenosis**
    EF = Ejection fraction
    AABA = Angiographically acceptable for balloon angioplasty
**   **CABS = Coronary artery bypass surgery**

FIG. 2–5. Decision-making in the management of angina (class 1, 2).

plasty in these patients. However, patients with severe left ventricular dysfunction without reversible ischemia do not benefit from bypass surgery

• The patient's age: Patients aged 35 to 60 are managed preferably by balloon angioplasty if the lesions are considered angiographically acceptable. Thus, surgery is deferred as long as possible to avoid the high risk of vein graft occlusion 10 years later (Table 2–2). The American College of Cardiology (ACC)/American Heart Association (AHA) Task Force Report (1991) strongly advises a left internal mammary artery anastomosis to the left anterior descending. The artery remains attached at its origin from the left subclavian. This is the surgical procedure of choice for all patients, but especially for the relatively young; the 10-year oc-

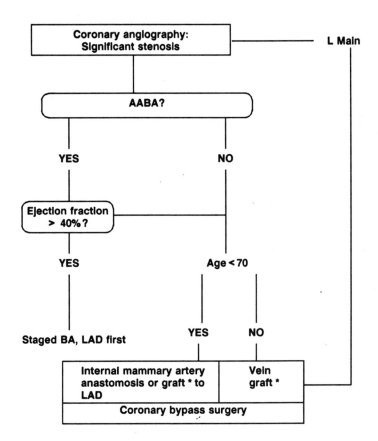

AABA = Angiographically acceptable for BA
BA = Balloon angioplasty
LAD = Left anterior descending
* ACC / AHA Task Force Report; J Am Coll Cardiol 17: 543, 1991
FIG. 2–6. Decision-making in the management of severe angina (class 3, 4, or class 2 with a strongly positive exercise test).

clusion rate is 5%, as opposed to 15% for internal mammary graft and 50% for vein graft (Table 2–2). Even so, internal mammary graft or anastomosis is deferred, if possible, by angioplasty in the younger patient

The algorithms in Figures 2–4, 2–5, and 2–6 give therapeutic guidelines and cannot include all clinical situations.

Although bypass surgery is superior to drug therapy when severe proximal stenosis of the left anterior descending artery is present, there is no evidence indicating that the procedure is superior to angioplasty in patients with good left ventricular function (EF greater than 50%) where the lesion

TABLE 2–2. RESULTS AND COMPLICATIONS OF CORONARY ARTERY BYPASS SURGERY

OCCURRENCE	1 WEEK (%)	1 YEAR (%)	5 YEARS (%)	10 YEARS (%)	15 YEARS (%)
Survival	99	95	87	76	60*
Perioperative myocardial infarction (MI)	2–5				
MI fatal, nonfatal			5	15	35
Reoperation for bleeding	1–4				
Occlusion					
vein graft occlusion	6–10*	12–20*	20	40–50	60
vein graft to LAD				25–30	30–40**
vein graft to other vessels				30–50	60
internal mammary graft				10	
internal mammary anastomosis***				5**	
Symptomatic improvement	90	70			
Asymptomatic angina free	80		50		
Sudden cardiac death				5	10

* = Aspirin 1 hour postoperative = 1.6 and 5.8% (see Table 2–13)
** = ACC/AHA Task Force Report, J Am Coll Cardiol, *17*:543, 1991
*** = Preferred technique
LAD = Left anterior descending

is suitable for angioplasty. Therefore, young patients in this group with relatively good left ventricular function, EF greater than 40%, should be given a trial of angioplasty. Bypass is reserved for later use, utilizing left internal mammary artery anastomosis.

Patients suitable for medical management usually have the following characteristics

• Stable angina functional Class 1 to 2
• Good effort tolerance, negative or weakly positive treadmill exercise test, e.g., beyond 6 minutes of the Bruce protocol. Patients who are unable to exercise because of intermittent claudication or arthritis cannot be graded as Class 1 and 2
• Good ventricular function, radionuclide EF, or estimate from echocardiogram greater than 40%
• Absence of left main disease
• Presence of triple or double vessel disease in the absence of severe proximal stenosis of the left anterior descending artery (Fig. 2–5)
• Concomitant disease and contraindications to bypass surgery
• Age over 75 and not in good general health
• Lesions not ideal for intervention

TABLE 2–3. BETA BLOCKER: FIRST-LINE ORAL DRUG TREATMENT IN ANGINA PECTORIS

EFFECT ON	BETA BLOCKER	CALCIUM ANTAGONIST	ORAL NITRATE
Heart rate	↓	╪	↑
Diastolic filling of coronary arteries	↑	—	—
Blood pressure	↓ ↓	↓ ↓	—
Rate pressure product	↓	—*	—
Relief of angina	Yes	Yes	Variable
Blood flow (subendocardial ischemic area)†	↑	↓	Variable
First-line treatment for angina pectoris	Yes	No	No
Prevention of recurrent ventricular fibrillation	Proven	No	No
Prevention of cardiac death	Proven	No	No effect
Prevention of pain due to CAS	No	Yes	Variable
Prevention of death in patient with CAS	No	No	No

* RPP variable decrease on exercise, but not significant at rest or on maximal exercise
† Distal to organic obstruction
CAS = coronary artery spasm
From: Khan, M. Gabriel: Beta-adrenoceptor blockers. *In* Cardiac Drug Therapy. 3rd Ed. London, W.B. Saunders, 1992.

TABLE 2–4. DOSAGE OF BETA BLOCKERS FOR ANGINA

BETA BLOCKER	INITIAL DOSE* (mg daily)	MAINTENANCE (mg daily)
Atenolol	25–50	50–100
Acebutolol	100–400	400–1000
Metoprolol	50–100	100–300
Toprol XL**	50–100	100–300
Nadolol**	40	80–160
Propranolol	80–120	120–240
Inderal LA**	80	120–240
Timolol	10	10–30

* Elderly: halve initial dose
** Given once daily, all others preferably two divided doses to cover early morning catecholamine surge

Most patients with stable angina Class 1 and 2 are managed with sublingual nitroglycerin and a one-a-day beta blocker. The rationale for a beta blocking drug as a first-choice oral agent is discussed shortly (Table 2–3).

Failure to achieve about a 75% symptomatic relief with an adequate dose of a beta blocker (Table 2–4) might result in the addition of a second agent or the patient may learn to cope with mild angina that quickly disappears on cessation of a precipitating activity. Either a calcium antagonist or a

TABLE 2–5. ORAL AND TRANSDERMAL NITRATE PREPARATIONS AND DOSAGE

NITRATE	DOSAGE	
Isosorbide dinitrate	Initial	15 mg at 700, 1200, 1700 hours
	Maintenance	30 mg at 700, 1200, 1700 hours
Isosorbide dinitrate sustained	Initial	40 mg at 700 hours
release	Maintenance	40 mg at 700, 1500 hours
Isosorbide mononitrate	Initial	10 mg at 700, 1500 hours
	Maintenance	20 mg at 700, 1500 hours
Isosorbide mononitrate	Initial	20–30 mg at 700 hours
sustained release supplied	Maintenance	40–60 mg at 700 hours
as 20, 40, 50 or 60 mg		
Nitroglycerin (*oral* tabs)	Initial	1.3 mg at 700, 1500 hours
(glyceryltrinitrate oral tablets	Maintenance	2.6 mg at 700, 1500 hours
in UK)		
Nitroglycerin (*buccal* tablets)	Initial	1 mg
	Maintenance	1, 2, or 3 mg at 700, 1500 hours
Nitroglycerin (transdermal)	1–2 inches	700, 1300 hours
(glyceryltrinitrate) Ointment		
(paste) 1 in. = approx. 16		
mg		
Phasic-release nitroglycerin	1 patch	700 Remove at 1900 hours
patch: e.g., Transderm-nitro		
0.4, 0.6 mg/hour		

nitrate is considered second choice (Fig. 2–4). If a beta blocker is being used, then nifedipine extended release 30 to 90 mg daily is advisable. If a beta blocker is contraindicated but verapamil is not, then verapamil should be used as the drug of first choice. The rationale for this approach is discussed under calcium antagonists and combination therapy. If a nitrate is selected as second line, a sustained release preparation is selected and given once daily or, at most, twice daily. Preparations and suggested timing of dosing of nitrates are shown in Table 2–5.

If symptoms remain bothersome, triple therapy with beta blockers, calcium antagonists, and nitrates is warranted, but this action should prompt consideration for coronary angiography and interventional therapy.

BETA BLOCKERS

Release of catecholamines plays a major role in the initiation and perpetuation of myocardial ischemia in patients with atheromatous coronary stenosis (Fig. 2–1). Beta blockers can inhibit the initiation of ischemia, interrupt the dynamic process, and provide rational and effective therapy as well as prolong life (Fig. 2–7).

Beta blockers are competitive inhibitors of catecholamines (which they structurally resemble) at beta-adrenergic receptors. Their action depends on the ratio of drug to catecholamine concentration at beta adrenoceptor sites. Beta receptors are part of the adenylcyclase system situated in the cell membrane. The ventricle contains $beta_1$ and $beta_2$ adrenergic receptors in the proportion 70–30. $Beta_2$ predominate in the lung. Adenylcyclase in

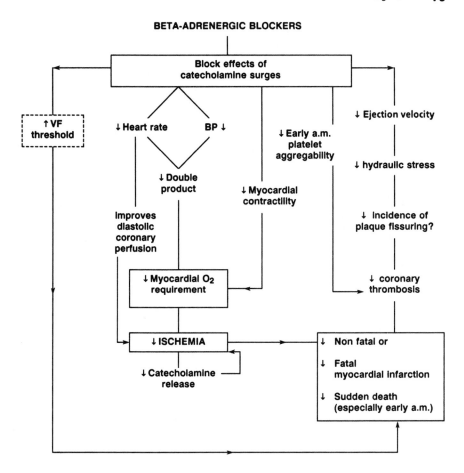

† Increase
↓ Decrease

FIG. 2–7. Salutary effects of beta-adrenergic blockade.

the presence of the stimulatory form of the G protein converts adenosine triphosphate to cyclic adenosine monophosphate (cyclic AMP), the intracellular messenger of beta stimulation.

Beta stimulation causes

- Calcium influx into cells via receptor operated channels, resulting in a positive inotropic effect
- An increase in the pacemaker current in the sinus node resulting in an increase in heart rate
- Increased conduction velocity through the AV node
- Increased phase 4 diastolic depolarization results in increased automaticity (Chapter 6)

Beta blockade results in

- Decrease in heart rate. Cardiac work is reduced and the increased diastolic interval allows for improved diastolic coronary perfusion especially during exercise
- Decrease in velocity of cardiac contraction further reduces myocardial oxygen demand, which is particularly important during exertional activities
- Decrease in cardiac output results in a fall in systolic blood pressure and causes a decrease in the rate-pressure product and a reduction in myocardial oxygen requirement (Table 2–3). The salutary effects of beta-adrenergic blockade are shown in Figure 2–7. These effects are not observed with other antianginal agents
- A decrease in ejection velocity reduces hyperdynamic shearing forces imposed on the arterial wall; this might be important at the site of atheroma. Thus, it is possible that beta blockers may reduce the incidence of plaque rupture and thus protect from fatal or nonfatal myocardial infarction. These agents decrease the incidence of myocardial rupture
- Partial inhibition of exercise-related catecholamines that might initiate vasoconstriction in segments of coronary arteries where atheroma impairs the relaxing effect of the endothelium
- Increase in ventricular fibrillation (VF) threshold and, thus, a decrease in the incidence of VF, which may be responsible for the high mortality during the early hours of acute myocardial infarction and also in VF occurring in other ischemic situations. Beta blockers are of proven value in the prevention of sudden death in the post infarction patient
- A decrease in early morning platelet aggregation and other salutary effects induced by a decrease in catecholamine surges may eliminate the early morning peak of transient ischemic periods and decrease the incidence of early morning mortality and sudden death from myocardial infarction. Beta blockers have been shown to decrease the incidence of sudden death in cardiac patients. This observation has not been documented for any other cardiac medication, including aspirin
- A decrease in phase 4 diastolic depolarization is important in suppressing arrhythmias induced by catecholamines, which increase diastolic depolarization. This action is opposite to that of digoxin. Thus, beta blockers are useful in the management of digoxin toxicity.
- Decrease impulse traffic through the AV node results in slowing of the ventricular response in atrial fibrillation or in the termination of paroxysmal supraventricular tachycardia (PSVT)
- Direct blood flow from the epicardial vessels to subendocardial ischemic areas. In contrast, dipyridamole, a vasodilator used in the management of angina in the early 1960s, is now used to dilate epicardial vessels and produce a "steal." Experimental evidence suggests that some calcium antagonists may also direct coronary blood flow from the subendocardium to dilated epicardial vessels. Nitrates appear to have an effect similar to calcium antagonists

The above-mentioned points have established beta blocking drugs as first-line oral agents in the management of stable angina and indicate the rationale for the algorithmic approach to drug therapy for stable angina given in Figure 2–4.

Dosage

Dosages of available beta blockers are given in Table 2–4. Important dosing considerations include

- In the management of stable angina, titrate the dosage over weeks. Some ethnic groups derive beta blockade at lower than conventional doses
- A concerted effort should be made to get the beta blocker dosage into the important cardioprotective range. Beta blockers protect from fatal and nonfatal myocardial infarction but may do so only at the correct dose range. Coronary studies in animals have convincingly demonstrated that too large a dose of beta blocker is nonprotective and increases mortality, whereas at a well defined smaller dose range, fatal and nonfatal infarctions and ventricular fibrillation are prevented by pretreatment with beta blocking drugs. In the BHAT, a propranolol dose, 180 or 240 mg, conferred protection. In the timolol Norwegian study, 10 to 20 mg timolol offered protection. Acebutolol (400 mg) caused a reduction in cardiac events. Smaller or larger doses of these agents have not been studied in clinical trials. It may be argued that the patients in the quoted studies were post myocardial infarction and the same rules may not apply to patients with angina. The patient with angina or post myocardial infarction is at risk for sudden death. Timolol caused a 67% reduction in sudden death in post myocardial infarction patients and it is quite conceivable that beta blockers would decrease sudden death in patients with angina

Choice

- Beta blockers with partial agonist activity, such as pindolol, should be avoided in patients with ischemic heart disease since cardioprotection is not achieved; acebutolol has only weak agonist activity and one study has shown a beneficial effect
- Do not use hepatic-metabolized beta blockers, propranolol, or oxprenolol in smokers who won't quit, as the salutary effects of these agents are blunted by cigarette smoking (Chapter 1)
- Maximum protection appears to occur with proven agents: timolol and metoprolol in smokers and in nonsmokers, propranolol in nonsmokers

The subtle differences in beta blockers may provide the solution for the apparent lack of protection of some beta blockers. Lipophilic agents that achieve brain concentration may actuate more effective protection from the brain–heart interaction that appears to be involved in the genesis of sudden death in some subsets. This hypothesis must be tested in clinical trials, but predominantly hepatic-metabolized beta blockers should not be given to smokers if all the benefits of beta blockade are to be derived (see Chapter 1).

Atenolol
(Tenormin)

Supplied: tablets; 50, 100 mg

Dosage: 25 to 50 mg for 1 to 4 weeks, then 50 to 100 mg once daily. Observations have confirmed that in some patients, a once daily dose of atenolol may not completely cover the 24-hour period and the patient may be at risk between 6 and 8 a.m. during the early morning period of catecholamine surge. Holter monitoring of patients has documented early morning ischemia in some patients administered atenolol once daily. Thus, it is advisable to give half the dose at 7 a.m. and half at bedtime. Elderly and nonwhite patients usually require a reduced dose to achieve beta blockade. Reduce the dose and increase the dosing interval in renal failure.

Atenolol is a cardioselective agent. The pharmacologic properties of beta blockers are given in Table 1–5.

Acebutolol
(Monitan, Sectral)

Supplied: 200, 400 mg

Dosage: 400 mg once or twice daily, to a maximum of 1,000 mg daily. Acebutolol is mildly cardioselective, possesses mild partial agonist activity, and causes no significant decrease in HDL cholesterol levels during longterm administration (see Chapter 8).

Nadolol
(Corgard)

Supplied: tablets; 40, 80, 120, 160 mg

Dosage: 40 mg once daily for 1 to 2 weeks, then maintenance 40 to 160 mg daily. Clinical practice has documented that the maximum dose of nadolol is much less than that recommended by the manufacturer, and the above dosage is less than that given in the package insert. The drug is nonselective and hydrophilic, has a prolonged action beyond 24 hours, and covers the risk periods when given once daily. As with other beta blockers, adverse effects occur beyond a certain dose range. The drug is eliminated by the kidney, and the dose must be decreased with renal dysfunction.

Metoprolol
(Toprol XL, Lopressor, Betaloc)

Supplied: tablets; 50, 100 mg (Toprol XL 50, 100, 200 mg; Betaloc-SA: 200 mg; Lopressor-SA: 200 mg)

Dosage: Metoprolol 50 to 100 mg twice daily; maximum 300 mg daily. Metoprolol is a cardioselective beta blocker, but this effect is maintained up to a dose of 200 mg daily. A metoprolol dose beyond this dosage or atenolol above 50 mg daily can precipitate bronchospasm. However, when cardioselective drugs are given, bronchospasm is more easily reversed with albuterol (salbutamol) or other beta agonists than when $beta_1$ and $beta_2$ nonselective beta blockers are used. Toprol XL (metoprolol succinate) extended release tablets are effective when administered once daily, 100 to 300 mg daily.

Propranolol
(Inderal; Angilol, Berkolol, UK)

Supplied: tablets; 10, 40, 80, and 120 mg. capsules; Inderal-LA (80, 120, 160 mg)

Dosage: 20 to 40 mg three times daily for several weeks, increase if needed to 160 to 240 mg daily or Inderal-LA, 120 to 240 mg once daily. The drug is noncardioselective, lipophilic, and hepatic-metabolized.

Timolol
(Blocadren; Betim, UK)

Supplied: tablets; 5, 10 mg. Timolol is a noncardioselective $beta_1$, $beta_2$ adrenergic blocking agent that is partially lipophilic and hydrophilic. Thus, the drug causes less central nervous system side effects than metoprolol or propranolol. If vivid dreams occur with metoprolol or propranolol, a switch to timolol or nadolol is advisable. Because the drug is only partially metabolized in the liver, it is effective in smokers and nonsmokers. (See Beta Blocker, Subtle Differences, Chapter 1.)

Dosage: 5 mg twice daily for 1 to 2 weeks, then 10 to 15 mg twice daily. This dose is much smaller than the maximum dose recommended by the manufacturer.

Sotalol
(Sotacor)

Supplied: tablets; 40, 80, 160, 200 mg

Dosage: 80 mg once or twice daily for 2 to 4 weeks; maximum 240 mg daily. Do not use in combination with diuretics, which may cause hypokalemia.

If bothersome adverse effects occur with a beta blocker, a switch to another may obviate symptoms sufficiently to allow continuation of this important class of cardioactive drug (see Chapter 1 for subtle differences and choice of beta blocker).

NITRATES

Mechanism of Antianginal Effect

The action of nitrates is given in Figure 2–8.

Nitrates act on so-called "nitrate receptors" believed to be structured on the myocyte. The mononitrates are unaffected by the liver, whereas iso-

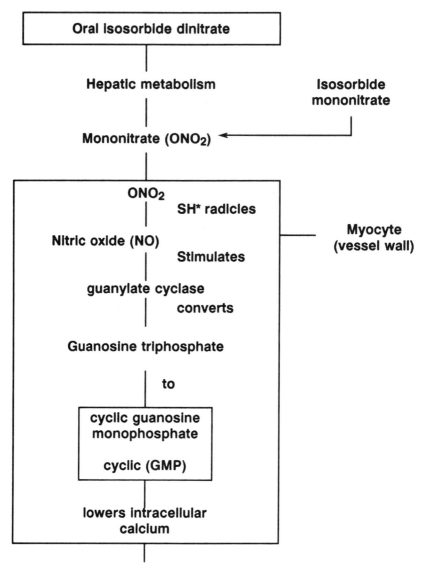

*SH = Sulfhydryl radicles required for formation of NO,
oxidized by excess exposure to nitrates become
depleted, leading to nitrate tolerance

FIG. 2–8. Nitrates' mechanism of action.

sorbide dinitrate undergoes extensive hepatic metabolism. Mononitrates, on entering the walls of veins and arteries, combine with sulfhydryl groups with the formation of nitric oxide, which activates guanylate cyclase to produce cyclic guanosine monophosphate, which in turn brings about relaxation of vascular smooth muscle at the doses commonly used, with maximal dilatation of veins and minimal dilatation of arteries. The profound venous dilatation causes reduction in preload and, at high nitrate dosage, a modest decrease in afterload occurs. Sulfhydryl groups become depleted by continued exposure to nitrates and tolerance develops with little or no resulting venous dilatation. Thus, 24-hour therapy with nitrates is of no value to the patient.

Nitrate tolerance occurs after 24 hours of IV nitroglycerin. Oral and transdermal preparations administered at regular intervals produce tolerance after a few days. A minimum daily 10-hour nitrate-free interval is necessary for the intracellular regeneration of sulfhydryl groups and to maintain the effectiveness of the nitrate preparation.

The "nitrate receptor" is not located in the endothelium and has no relation to the production of endothelium-derived relaxing factor (EDRF), now recognized as nitric oxide. The exact role of EDRF needs clarification. Endothelium-dependent coronary relaxation is impaired by atheroma, and reduced EDRF activity may allow increased smooth muscle response to constrictor agents. It appears that transmitters may stimulate EDRF, producing vasodilatation of large coronary vessels.

Nitrates are powerful venous dilators. As indicated, they reduce preload, thus decreasing ventricular volume and myocardial wall stress, and some diminution of myocardial oxygen demand occurs. At high doses, a small reduction in afterload occurs, but an increase in heart rate may then take place and increase oxygen demand. Effort tolerance is somewhat improved by the use of nitrates, especially if the patient with angina has concomitant left ventricular dysfunction.

The evidence of nitrates redistributing blood flow from epicardial to ischemic subendocardial regions is weak. Studies done in 1971 and 1975 supported this evidence, but another study completed in 1982 suggested otherwise.

Indications

- Second-choice management of Class 2 and 3 stable angina
- Angina with concomitant left ventricular dysfunction. Shortness of breath and effort tolerance may be improved by nitrate therapy
- Angina with concomitant mild or moderate hypertension
- Combination therapy with beta blockers or if beta blockers are contraindicated combined with verapamil or diltiazem
- Pre- and postoperative management of the cardiac patient undergoing surgery
- Intraoperative hypertension

Contraindications

- Hypertrophic cardiomyopathy, constrictive pericarditis, or cardiac tamponade
- Hypovolemia
- Right ventricular infarction
- Severe uncontrolled glaucoma with very high nitrate dosing, especially IV nitrates

Adverse Effects

Adverse effects include syncope, especially in the elderly, and an increased incidence with added ACE inhibitors, diuretics, alcohol, or alpha blockers. Tachycardia, mild palpitations, dizziness, and flushing commonly occur. Headaches are often bothersome; more than 25% of patients are intolerant and discontinue the drug. Indigestion and halitosis may occur. High-dose nitrates may cause a decrease in arterial oxygen tension and are relatively contraindicated in severe COPD and hypoxemic situations. Methemoglobinemia has been noted with prolonged high dosage and withdrawal symptoms have been observed with high-dose, longterm use.

Interactions

Heparin resistance with high nitrate dosage. ACE inhibitors, alpha blockers, and diuretics also decrease preload tachycardia may be increased when nitrates are used with dihydropyridine calcium antagonists.

Advantages

- Moderately effective agents for the management of stable angina
- Inexpensive, except for mononitrates and transdermal
- Very few contraindications or serious adverse effects, whereas patients must be carefully selected prior to the use of beta blockers, verapamil, and diltiazem

Disadvantages

The development of tolerance is a major disadvantage. Withholding nitrates at night is appropriate and trouble-free in the patient with mild exertional-only angina. However, all patients may not be protected during the early morning catecholamine surge. The use of beta blocking drug or, if these agents are contraindicated, a calcium antagonist is advisable to cover the nitrate-free interval in patients with rest angina who require 24-hour antianginal therapy. In patients with unstable angina already on triple therapy, IV nitroglycerin must be continued with titration of the dosage upward as needed for pain control, regardless of concerns of nitrate tolerance.

Nitroglycerin

Supplied: sublingual tablets; 0.15, 0.3, and 0.6 mg (in the UK, glyceryl trinitrate: 300, 500, 600 μg). spray; nitrolingual spray, 0.4 mg/metered dose, 200 doses/vial

Dosage: 0.3 mg is given if the systolic blood pressure is less than 130 mm Hg, 0.6 mg if greater than 130 mm Hg systolic.
The patient should be instructed on how and when to use nitroglycerin

- Sit and put one tablet under the tongue or use the sublingual spray. Avoid taking the drug while standing except when accustomed to such usage. Nitroglycerin is less effective when used with the patient lying, since less pooling occurs in the limbs and the drug is thus less effective in relieving pain
- Take a nitroglycerin tablet before activities that are known to precipitate angina
- Take a second tablet if pain is not relieved in 2 minutes. After taking the second nitroglycerin tablet, chew and swallow a junior aspirin (80 mg) or a regular 325 mg aspirin tablet. Aspirin is used here for its effect in preventing coronary thrombosis
- Go to the nearest emergency room if pain persists beyond 10 minutes, using a third nitroglycerin during transport if marked weakness or faint-like feeling is not present
- Take nitroglycerin for acute shortness of breath but not if the symptoms are dizziness or palpitations in the absence of pain
- Keep nitroglycerin tablets in dark, light-protected bottles. If exposed to light, they may only last a few months
- Use two bottles, one for stock supply with the cotton wool within a well-stoppered bottle, kept in the refrigerator. This will last 1 to 2 years. The second bottle containing no cotton wool should contain a month's supply and be refilled when needed

Isosorbide Dinitrate
(Isordil, Coronex, Cedocard, Iso-Bid, Sorbitrate)

Supplied: tablets; 10, 20, 30 mg. capsules; 40 mg

Dosage: 10 to 30 mg three times daily, preferable 1 hour before meals on an empty stomach. Maintenance 30 mg at approximately 7 a.m., 11 a.m., 3 p.m.: Allow a 10- to 12-hour nitrate-free interval to prevent tolerance.

Isosorbide Mononitrate
(Elantan 20, 40; Monit 20 mg; Mono-Cedocard 20, 40 mg; sustained release: Elantan LA, 50 mg; Imdur, 60 mg; Ismo, 20 mg)

Dosage: 1 tablet at approximately 7 a.m. and 2 p.m. daily; maximum 120 mg daily, or sustained release 1/2 to 2 tablets once daily.

Nitroglycerin

Supplied: oral tablets; 2.6 mg (Nitrong SR)

Dosage: 1 tablet at 7 a.m. and 2 p.m. daily.
Other nitrates and dosages are given in Table 2–5.

CALCIUM ANTAGONISTS

Verapamil is the most potent antianginal calcium antagonist but is not the safest agent for general use. The pharmacologic and clinical effects of calcium antagonists are given in Table 1–7. Verapamil is more effective than diltiazem because of a more prominent negative inotropic effect; in addition, verapamil causes a greater decrease in systemic vascular resistance. If beta blockers are contraindicated, verapamil is a reasonable choice, provided that there are no contraindications to the use of this agent.

Dihydropyridines have no electrophysiologic and minimal negative inotropic effects. The rapid-acting nifedipine capsule may cause an increase in heart rate and has been reported to increase anginal episodes. Undoubtedly, early studies were done using nifedipine capsules, which have a rapid onset of action and cause mild provocation of angina in some patients with stable angina. However, the administration of extended release formulations, e.g., Procardia XL (Adalat XL in Canada) virtually abolishes this adverse effect and allows the drug to be used freely in all patients with stable angina who are unable to take a beta blocking drug. Dihydropyridines are a rational choice for use in conjunction with beta blockers (see Table 1–7).

Diltiazem and dihydropyridines have about equal antianginal effects.

Calcium Antagonist Beta Blocker Combination

Verapamil should not be combined with a beta blocker since there is a high incidence of bradyarrhythmias, including life-threatening sinus arrest and asystole; heart failure may be precipitated.

Diltiazem combined with a beta blocker may cause sinus arrest or asystole. Although the occurrence is rare, caution is necessary and patients should be properly selected prior to prescribing this combination. Sinus bradycardia is not uncommon.

Dihydropyridines can be safely combined with beta blockers since they have no effect on the sinus or AV nodes. Care is needed when dihydropyridines or diltiazem is added to beta blockers in patients with left ventricular dysfunction, since heart failure can be precipitated.

Indications

- Consider calcium antagonists as second line in the management of stable angina, Class 2 and 3, advisable only when beta blockers are contraindicated or produce bothersome effects

Advantages

- More effective than nitrates in the management of angina and do not carry the risk posed by a 10-hour drug-free interval
- One-a-day preparation exists
- These agents do not decrease preload and are useful in angina patients with hypertrophic cardiomyopathy, in which nitrates are relatively contraindicated
- Angiographic studies, including the International Nifedipine Trial on Antiatherosclerotic Therapy (INTACT), have demonstrated that calcium antagonists appear to prevent progression of early atheromatous lesions and may cause some regression. Although the observed effect is quite modest, it could occasionally signify longterm gains for a wide range of patients with CHD. Ongoing studies will clarify this issue

Disadvantages

- Sinus node dysfunction, AV block with verapamil or diltiazem
- High incidence of constipation with verapamil
- Calcium antagonists do not significantly decrease the incidence of fatal myocardial infarction. Verapamil and diltiazem increase the risk of heart failure in patients with left ventricular dysfunction and should be avoided in this subset when the EF is less than 40%. Nifedipine may be given a trial in patients without overt heart failure and EF above 35% if a beta blocker is contraindicated. Calcium antagonists are commonly and appropriately used in this large group of cardiac patients in whom beta blockers, when used with due caution, are often effective, well tolerated, and likely to have salutary effects on prognosis. The calcium antagonists may, however, have to be used judiciously when beta blocking agents are ineffective or contraindicated

Dosages of calcium antagonists and the adverse effects of extended release calcium antagonists are shown in Tables 2–6 and 2–7.

Interactions

- Digoxin level is increased with verapamil, diltiazem, and nicardipine
- Verapamil and diltiazem interact with beta blockers, quinidine, disopyramide, amiodarone (Table 1–8)

Contraindications

- Aortic stenosis
- Sick sinus syndrome and AV block with verapamil and diltiazem
- Congestive heart failure or suspected left ventricular dysfunction
- Myocardial infarction with heart failure. EF less than 40% for verapamil and diltiazem; EF less than 35% for nifedipine
- Presence of marked beta blockade: avoid the use of verapamil or diltiazem

TABLE 2–6. DOSAGES OF CALCIUM ANTAGONISTS FOR ANGINA

PREPARATION	INITIAL	DOSAGE MAINTENANCE (daily mg)	MAXIMUM (daily mg)
Nifedipine Extended Release Procardia XL; Adalat XL (C) 30, 60, 90 mg tabs	30 mg *once daily*	60–90	90
Adalat PA 20 (C)	20 mg BID	40–80	80
Adalat Retard 20 mg (UK)	20 mg BID	40–80	80
Diltiazem 60, 120 mg tabs (30, 60, C)	60 mg TID	180–240	360
Cardizem 60, 90, 120 mg	60 mg TID	180–240	360
Cardizem SR (C) 60, 90, 120 mg capsules Tildiem (UK) 60 mg Adizem SR (UK), 120 mg	60–90 mg BID	180–240	360
Verapamil 80, 120 mg tablets	80 mg TID	240–360	360

BID = twice daily
TID = three times daily
C = Canada

TABLE 2–7. ADVERSE EFFECTS OF EXTENDED RELEASE CALCIUM ANTAGONISTS

ADVERSE EFFECTS	CARDIZEM SR* (%)	PROCARDIA XL (%)	VERAPAMIL SR (%)
% patients reporting	34.2	32.3**	
discontinuation rate	7.2	3.8**	
Edema	8.3	10***	2
Headache	4.9	15.8	3.8†
Dizziness	4.7	4.1	3.3
Flushing	2.3	≤1	<1
Constipation	0.7	3.3	7.3
Bradycardia	2.1	Nil	1.4
AV block first degree	1.6	Nil	≤1
third degree	Nil	Nil	0.8
Palpitations	1.3	≤1	Nil
Heart Failure	0.5	Nil	1.8

* From product monograph (Canada); Incidence 13% higher in patients 65 years or over
** Adalat PA 20
*** Dose dependent
† Average of three products

- Unstable angina: do not use nifedipine if a beta blocker cannot be used
- Wolff-Parkinson-White (WPW) syndrome with anterograde conduction through a bypass tract and/or WPW syndrome with atrial fibrillation (Chapter 6)
- Pregnancy and during lactation. Short-term nifedipine therapy has a

role in the management of severe hypertension during the third trimester (see Chapter 1)
• Porphyria

Nifedipine; Nifedipine Extended Release
(Procardia XL; Adalat XL 30, 60, 90 mg or Adalat PA 10, 20 in Canada; Adalat Retard 10, 20 in the UK)

Supplied: see Table 2–6

Dosage: Nifedipine extended release, 30 to 60 mg daily, usual maintenance 60 mg daily, increase to 90 mg if required. As outlined in Chapter 1, an extended release preparation is preferred because the capsule formulation causes a quick release and a higher incidence of adverse effects. The adverse effects of extended release calcium antagonists are listed in Table 2–7.

Pharmacokinetics
• Oral dose fully absorbed
• High first-pass metabolism, broken down by hepatic metabolism to inactive metabolites. Half-life about 5 hours
• The capsule and extended release formulation have an onset of action less than 20 minutes and 6 hours, with a peak effect of 1 and 6 hours respectively

Nicardipine
(Cardene)

Supplied: capsules; 20, 30 mg

Dosage: 20 mg three times daily, increase slowly, if needed, to 30 mg three times daily. The dose of 40 mg three times daily increases the risk of mild tachycardia and worsening of angina. The drug is partially eliminated by the kidney and the dose interval should be increased in renal failure.

Diltiazem

Supplied: tablets: Cardizem 60, 90, 120 mg (30 mg in Canada); Cardizem SR capsules 60, 90, 120 mg, Canada; Adizem SR 120 mg, Tildiem, UK; Anginyl, Dilzem, Herbesser, Tilazem, in other countries)

Dosage: 60 mg three or four times daily, increase slowly to 90 mg three times daily. The effective dose range is 240 to 360 mg daily. In the elderly or patients with renal dysfunction, give 30 to 60 mg twice daily.

Caution. Caution is required to carefully select patients prior to giving a combination of diltiazem and a beta blocker. The SR preparation appears to cause a higher incidence of adverse effects than the tablet formulation.

Avoid in patients with heart failure or with left ventricular dysfunction, EF less than 40%. Reduce dose in hepatic or renal dysfunction.

Pharmacokinetics

- About 90% absorbed
- Bioavailability 45%
- Onset of action after taking orally, 30 minutes
- Peak 1 to 2 hours
- Elimination half-life approximately 5 hours
- Extensively metabolized in the liver
- 40% excreted unchanged in the urine

Contraindications have been listed previously under Calcium Antagonists.

Adverse effects. AV block, bradycardia, liver dysfunction, hypotension, toxic erythema, depression, psychosis, mild ataxia.

Verapamil

Supplied: tablets; 80, 120 mg (Cordilox 40, 80, 160 mg; Berkatens 40, 120, 160 mg available in the UK)

Dosage: Initial, 80 mg twice daily; maintenance 80 to 120 mg three times daily. A higher dose is not advisable in angina. Reduce dose with hepatic dysfunction and renal failure.

Pharmacokinetics

- After oral dosing, 90% absorption from the gut
- Extensive first-pass hepatic metabolism
- 10 to 20% bioavailability
- Two hours to act, three hours to peak
- Elimination half-life 3 to 7 hours, with cirrhosis or renal failure activity prolonged beyond 10 to 16 hours
- 70% excreted in the urine as active metabolites, 5% unchanged
- Increased blood levels with hepatic dysfunction or with reduced hepatic flow, cimetidine use, and renal failure

Cautions. Avoid in acute myocardial infarction if bradycardia, AV block, hypotension, left ventricular failure, or left ventricular dysfunction with an EF less than 40% is present. Not advisable in patients taking beta blockers, except under close supervision in properly selected patients (see Contraindications of Calcium Antagonists).

Adverse effects. Severe constipation, hepatic dysfunction, edema, flushing, gynecomastia.

UNSTABLE ANGINA

PATHOPHYSIOLOGY

In the majority of cases of unstable angina, atheromatous plaques are eccentric with irregular borders and a narrow neck on angiography. A ruptured or fissured plaque with overlying platelet thrombus is a common finding confirmed on angioscopy and is often suspected from a hazy appearance on the angiogram. In addition, silent ischemia is frequently observed in patients with unstable angina, and prognosis is worse in this subset.

THERAPY

Figure 2–9 gives suggested steps in treating unstable angina.

- Aspirin, 325 mg, chewed or swallowed for a rapid effect, then 160 to 325 mg coated aspirin is given daily
- Heparin is commenced, 5,000 units and then continuous infusion (see later discussion and Chapter 11)
- Admission to a coronary care unit: monitor cardiac rhythm for 24 to 48 hours, total CK and CK-MB every 4 to 6 hours for 24 hours, ECG every 6 hours for 24 to 48 hours
- Bedrest with bedside commode, fasting 8 hours, allowed fluids only
- Blood pressure taken every 15 to 30 minutes for a few hours, then every 1 to 2 hours or as needed for 24 to 48 hours and more often if IV nitroglycerin is used
- The patient is encouraged to report any recurrence of pain, however mild
- 5% dextrose in water to maintain IV line

BETA BLOCKERS

If beta blockers are not contraindicated, give propranolol, 20 mg, every 4 hours or metoprolol, 50 mg, every 8 hours, then titrate quickly to right dose, usually metoprolol, 100 mg, every 12 hours or equivalent dose of another beta blocker. Hold dose if systolic blood pressure is less than 100 mm Hg or if pulse is less than 50 per minute. If pain is present and unrelieved by nitroglycerin, the first dose of a beta blocking drug can be given intravenously. The IV dosage of beta blockers is given in Table 2–8.

NITROGLYCERIN

- IV nitroglycerin dosage is given in Table 2–9. Commence with 5 to 10 μg/min, increase 5 to 10 μg/minute, every 5 or 10 minutes, if needed to 100 to 200 μg/minute. Titrate to eliminate all episodes of chest pain and do not lower the systolic blood pressure below 100 mm Hg. The dose is usually sufficient to reduce arterial pressure 10 to 15 mm Hg and up to 20 mm Hg in a hypertensive patient. These medications are prescribed

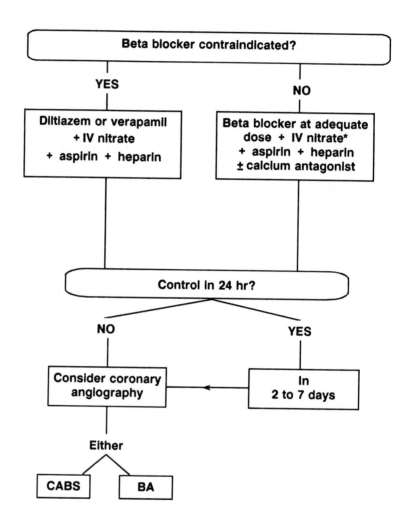

```
* =         Oral if IV not available
CABS =      Coronary artery bypass surgery
BA =        Balloon angioplasty
```

FIG. 2–9. Suggested steps in therapy for unstable angina.

TABLE 2–8. IV BETA BLOCKER DOSAGE	
DRUG	**DOSAGE**
Atenolol	2.5 mg rate of 1 mg/min repeated if necessary at 5-minute intervals to a maximum of 10 mg
Atenolol (IV infusion)	150 μg/kg over 20 minutes repeated every 12 hours if required
Esmolol (Infusion)	3–6 mg over 1 minute then 1 to 5 mg/minute, see text
Metoprolol	5 mg rate 1 mg/min repeated if necessary at 5-minute intervals to a maximum of 10–15 mg. Re-evaluate patient and ECG prior to each dose
Propranolol	1 mg rate of 0.5 mg/min repeated, if necessary, at 5-minute intervals to a maximum of 5–10 mg or 0.025–0.05 mg/kg over 15–30 minutes

Caution: The systolic blood pressure should not be allowed to fall less than 100 mm Hg or a 10–15 mm fall from baseline, or up to 25 mm Hg in hypertensives

with careful monitoring of blood pressure and pulse and a dose is withheld if the systolic blood pressure is 100 or less. Occasionally, a systolic pressure of 95 mm Hg is acceptable in a patient who was not previously hypertensive. The systolic pressure should not be allowed to drop more than 20 mm Hg from baseline levels. Although tolerance to IV nitroglycerin has been shown to occur after 24 to 48 hours of infusion, concern should not be given to the development of tolerance in patients with unstable angina; the IV nitroglycerin dose is titrated upward. This administration is often successful in controlling pain, especially when time is allowed: 24 to 48 hours to attain adequate therapeutic dosage of beta blockers and/or calcium antagonists

- Assess for anemia, hypoxemia, arrhythmia, or sinus tachycardia that can aggravate unstable angina
- Administer oxygen by nasal prongs (2 to 4 liters per minute) if the patient has concomitant shortness of breath or if hypoxemia is proven
- Thrombolytic therapy does not appear to improve morbidity and mortality and is not used routinely except if an obstructing thrombus is observed on angiography

CALCIUM ANTAGONISTS

These agents are added if the blood pressure reading allows this addition to be safely made. If a beta blocker is used, nifedipine extended release is the calcium antagonist of choice since the combination does not usually cause marked sinus bradycardia or AV block, which may be precipitated by verapamil and occasionally by diltiazem. If a beta blocking drug is contraindicated, give diltiazem 30 mg every 6 hours for 24 hours, then 60 mg every 6 hours, increasing if needed to 90 mg every 6 hours. Caution is needed when the triple combination is used, since all three drugs (beta blockers, nitrates, and calcium antagonists) can cause excessive reduction in blood pressure, which has the potential to worsen ischemia. Calcium

TABLE 2–9. NITROGLYCERIN INFUSION PUMP CHART*

DOSE (μg/min)	INFUSION RATE (ml/h)
5	0.75
10	1.5
15	2.3
20	3
25	3.8
30	4.5
40	6
50	7.5
60	9
80	12
100	15
120	18
140	21
160	24
180	27
200	30
220	33
240	36
260	39
280	42
300	45
320	48
340	51
360	54
380	57
400	60

Commence dosing 5 to 10 μg/minute, increase by 5 μg/minute every 5 minutes until relief of chest pain. Decrease the rate if systolic blood pressure is <100 mm Hg or falls >20 mm Hg below the baseline systolic or diastolic blood pressure <65 mm Hg.

* 100 mg nitroglycerin in 250 ml 5% dextrose/water
= 400 μg/ml

antagonists do not decrease mortality in patients with unstable angina. Nifedipine or other dihydropyridines should not be used alone or in combination with nitrates in patients with unstable angina since mortality might be increased. Verapamil or diltiazem should not be given if sinus node disease, bradycardia, AV block, heart failure, or left ventricular dysfunction is present.

ASPIRIN

Acetyl salicylic acid is known to be effective in decreasing mortality in patients with unstable angina. No trial is available to show its effectiveness with stable angina, although the Physicians' Study indicates a favorable trend, and many patients must be treated to observe a beneficial effect. However, patients with angina are at risk, and an 80-mg tablet or 160- to 325-mg enteric coated tablet daily or every second day is advisable if there are no contraindications.

HEPARIN

IV heparin is as effective as aspirin. Both agents cause approximately 50% decrease in the occurrence of infarction in patients with unstable angina. The combination of heparin and aspirin increases the risk of bleeding and, since the benefit of administration of both agents is unproven, combination therapy is of questionable wisdom.

A significant reduction in mortality greater than 50% has been documented in randomized studies utilizing aspirin. Paul Wood advocated the use of IV heparin for acute coronary syndromes during the late 1950s. A Northern Ireland study provided support for this notion. A Montreal study documented heparin's effectiveness as equal to aspirin and heparin is preferred for patients who are likely candidates for angioplasty and/or bypass surgery. Since aspirin, as opposed to heparin, carries a slightly greater risk of bleeding during bypass surgery, which may require transfusion, some units routinely use heparin in place of aspirin. If contraindications to the use of heparin exist, the patient is given 325 mg regular aspirin for immediate effect, followed by a 160- to 325-mg enteric coated aspirin daily, given with a gastric cytoprotective agent.

In the majority of cases, the emergency use of aspirin (325 mg) followed by short-term heparin, limited to 24 to 48 hours, followed by enteric coated aspirin, 160 to 325 mg daily is a reasonable compromise. Heparin is virtually always required in certain interventional situations; for example, when intra-arterial sheaths are left in place following certain angiographic procedures where angioplasty or repeat angioplasty is considered likely and during intra-aortic balloon counterpulsation in patients who are hemodynamically unstable en route to angioplasty or surgery.

PRINZMETAL'S (VARIANT) ANGINA

Coronary artery spasm (CAS) is a rare cause of angina in which spasm of the coronary artery occurs often without identifiable stimuli. However, in some patients, exposure to cold, smoking, emotional stress, aspirin ingestion, or cocaine usage may trigger coronary spasm. Discontinuation of nitrates or calcium antagonists may cause a worsening of spasm. Use of a beta blocker in the absence of vasodilator drugs may allow alpha activity with resulting vasoconstriction to predominate. However, although beta blockers may increase spasm, the risk of serious complications is likely to be small and is certainly not high enough to justify withholding this form of therapy from the great majority of patients with angina or even from those whose symptom pattern includes one or two atypical features, in case spasm is present.

All patients with variant angina should have coronary angiography since a significant number of them have underlying obstructive atheromatous coronary disease with spasm at the site of the lesion.

The clinical hallmarks of Prinzmetal's angina are

- Pain, usually at rest, often during sleep, (between 3 a.m. and 7 a.m.) and described as chronic angina at rest as distinct from unstable angina occurring at rest

- ECG shows ST segment elevation during pain
- Worsening of angina during beta blocker use
- Variable threshold angina

THERAPY

- Nitroglycerin tablets sublingually
- Cessation of smoking
- Aspirin may precipitate spasm and should be avoided if spasm is proven to be the cause of symptoms
- For chronic management, nitrates at high dosage allowing a 10-hour nitrate-free interval to prevent tolerance; the full 24-hour period at risk may not be covered. Calcium antagonists are preferred. Nifedipine, verapamil, or diltiazem are equally effective. For dosage, see Table 2–6. Occasionally, it is necessary to combine both a calcium antagonist and a nitrate
- If the patient is admitted to the hospital, commence IV nitroglycerin 5-20 µg/minute, see Table 2–9 (Nitroglycerin Infusion Pump Chart)
- IV heparin to prevent coronary thrombosis

A review of all trials using beta blocker monotherapy for coronary artery spasm shows neither exacerbation nor benefit. Beta blockers should not be withheld in patients with unstable angina at rest, except in patients who are known to have proven coronary artery spasm.

Calcium antagonists and nitrates do not appear to prevent death in patients with coronary artery spasm. Verapamil carries the risk of causing severe bradyarrhythmias. Some patients require coronary bypass surgery of their organic stenoses for control of symptoms. Mortality is increased in patients who have double or triple vessel disease with associated spasm compared to those with normal coronary arteries.

Patients with coronary artery spasm have episodes similar to cluster headaches and these may occur during a couple weeks per year. During this period, transdermal nitrate can be added to maintenance calcium antagonist for 14 hours daily, especially from bedtime to 11 a.m. if pain has been documented to occur most frequently at these times.

SILENT ISCHEMIA

Symptomless or painless myocardial ischemia is common in patients with ischemic heart disease. More patients die without warning or with only minutes of warning pain than from stable or unstable angina.

The incidence of silent ischemia is high in patients with unstable angina. Holter monitoring following noncardiac surgery in patients with stable angina and in post myocardial infarction patients has documented a high incidence of silent ischemia within the second to fourth day following surgery.

Patients with evidence of silent ischemia should be maintained on a beta blocker and aspirin and evaluated with exercise stress testing or noninvasive imaging technique such as thallium scintigraphy. Those with strongly positive exercise tests should be submitted to coronary angiography for consideration of an appropriate revascularization procedure. Drug treatment of patients with a diagnosis of silent ischemia should commence with enteric-coated aspirin, 160 to 325 mg daily; beta blockers are advisable to protect from death and infarction, although this therapy has not been proven in clinical trials in patients with silent ischemia. Nitrates and calcium antagonists do not offer this protection and beta blockers must remain the mainstay of therapy.

SPECIAL CASES OF ANGINA

Patients with angina may have concomitant underlying diseases, particularly hypertension, diabetes, chronic lung disease, peripheral vascular disease, and left ventricular dysfunction, which may alter the choice of antianginal medication. Guidelines that can assist with decision-making in the choice of drug therapy for special problem cases of angina are given in Table 2–10.

TABLE 2–10. CHOICE OF DRUG THERAPY FOR SPECIAL CASES OF ANGINA

CONCOMITANT DISEASE OR CLINICAL STATUS	DRUG OF CHOICE
Hypertension	Beta Blocker Calcium Antagonist* or combination
Asthma or COPD	Calcium Antagonist
Class III or IV Angina awaiting angioplasty or CABS	Triple therapy**
Heart Failure or ejection fraction <25%	Nitrates
Left Ventricular Dysfunction***	
moderate: EF 35 to 40%****	Nitrates + β-blockers (with care)
severe: EF 25 to 35%	Nitrates + small-dose Beta blocker (care)
Tendency to Bradycardia	Nifedipine ER + Nitrates or Acebutolol + Nitrates
Diabetic	
mild	Beta blocker + Nitrates
brittle, on insulin	Calcium antagonist
Hypertrophic Cardiomyopathy	Beta blocker or Verapamil
Mitral Valve Prolapse	Beta blocker
Peripheral Vascular Disease	
mild	Beta blocker
severe	Calcium Antagonist
Abdominal Aortic Aneurysm	Beta blocker
Heavy Smoker (won't quit)	Timolol, acebutolol, atenolol, metoprolol

* 2nd choice, nifedipine extended release
** Beta blocker, nifedipine extended release + nitrate
*** No overt heart failure
+ = plus
**** Diltiazem or verapamil contraindicated

INTERVENTIONAL THERAPY FOR ANGINA

Interventional therapy in the form of coronary angioplasty or CABS should be strongly considered in virtually all patients with unstable angina and in those with bothersome angina and/or functional Class 2 and 3 stable angina as illustrated in the decision-making algorithms (Figs. 2–4, 2–5, and 2–6). In several categories of patients, interventional therapy has advantages over medical therapy in amelioration of angina, a return to a normal lifestyle, and prolongation of life.

BALLOON CORONARY ANGIOPLASTY

Coronary angioplasty and CABS each have a definite role. It is advisable, however, to delay surgery for as long as possible in patients under age 65, where balloon angioplasty plays a major role. This is especially important since more than 10% of patients post bypass surgery require reoperation in 5 years and more than 50% of bypass grafts occlude after the tenth year. Moreover, longterm survival and symptomatic benefit following reoperation are far less favorable with a mortality rate exceeding 2%, as opposed to less than 1% with primary surgery.

Angioplasty can be successfully carried out only when acceptable angiographic lesions are documented (Table 2–11). More difficult lesions may be considered for dilation, but only if deemed necessary and carried out by a highly experienced team. Since many patients have lesions that are not suitable for angioplasty, bypass surgery is required for relief of symptoms and prolongation of life in some subsets.

Coronary angioplasty, when successful, and bypass surgery in similar symptomatic patients with severe proximal single vessel disease appear to give equally excellent 10-year results: mortality, 0.6% per year; myocardial infarction rate less than 1%. However, patients with single vessel disease with 50 to 60% vessel diameter narrowing have a good outcome with medical therapy, mortality less than 1% per year. In this subset, angioplasty with its predisposition for restenosis is not advisable unless angina is not

---

TABLE 2–11. ANGIOGRAPHICALLY ACCEPTABLE CORONARY BALLOON ANGIOPLASTY LESIONS

Proximal 70–95% stenosis*
Not totally occluded
Concentric
Discrete <10 mm length
Readily accessible
Nonostial
Location in nonangulated segment <45 degrees
Nontortuous
No major branch involvement
Absence of thrombus
Little or no calcification

* >60%

controlled with intensive medical therapy: intolerance to drugs, a strongly positive exercise test, or if thallium scintigraphy reveals a large area of ischemic myocardium.

The goal of angioplasty is pain relief. In complicated cases with multi-vessel disease or difficult lesions, the decision is made on an individual basis. As a general rule, patients do not undergo coronary angioplasty unless they are potential candidates for surgery, since bypass surgery will be required in about 3 to 5%. The indications and contraindications listed are in keeping with the AHA guidelines; complications are given in Table 2–12.

INDICATIONS

Patients with stable angina Class 2 and 3, Canadian Cardiovascular Society classification with good left ventricular function, EF greater than 40%, and acceptable angiographic lesions with symptoms

- Inadequately controlled by intensive medical therapy or in patients who have bothersome adverse effects of medications
- Proximal single vessel disease with a 70 to 95% stenosis
- Proximal single vessel disease with greater than 70% vessel diameter narrowing with a documented large area of viable myocardium involved, dominant artery, moderate or strongly positive exercise test, and symptoms uncontrolled with medical therapy

Patients with Class 1 angina with documented myocardial ischemia, a strongly positive exercise test, a large area of myocardium at risk, and documented 75 to 95% proximal single vessel disease should be considered for angioplasty.

Controversial indications include

- Double vessel disease with angina Class 1, 2, 3 in control with medical therapy, acceptable angiographic lesions, not high-grade proximal left anterior descending (LAD) obstruction with stenosis of another artery especially in patients under age 60 with EF greater than 40
- Young patients with unstable angina with suitable angiographic lesions and EF greater than 40%

CONTRAINDICATIONS

- Bypass surgical team not available
- Left main greater than 50% stenosis not protected by a patent bypass graft to the left anterior descending or left circumflex
- Triple vessel disease in symptomatic patients with strongly positive stress test, large area of variable myocardium at risk, or EF less than 40%
- Double vessel disease with high grade lesion proximal LAD with obstruction of another artery in association with a strongly positive stress test with EF less than 40%
- Calcified lesion

- Presence of thrombus
- Lesion with 50 to 60% vessel narrowing, thallium scintigraphy indicates small area of myocardium involved
- Low expected success rate in view of angiographic features of the lesion: eccentric, greater than 2 cm long, excessive tortuosity of proximal segment, extremely angulated or sharp bend, total occlusion
- Angiographic features suggest less than 80% chance of successful angioplasty, with a probable high restenosis rate and a moderate risk of occlusion: length 10 to 20 mm, eccentric, angulated segment greater than 45 degrees, moderate calcification or ostial location, total occluded artery marked tortuosity
- Angiographic features suggest less than 60% chance of successful dilatation and a very high risk of acute closure: a diffuse lesion greater than 20 mm in length, excessive tortuosity of the proximal segment, angulation greater than 90 degrees, complete occlusion

ELECTIVE ANGIOPLASTY PROTOCOL

- Patients are admitted overnight or fasting the day of the procedure
- Aspirin, 325 mg, plus diltiazem, 60 mg, prior to angioplasty
- After vascular access, give IV heparin, 7,500 to 10,000 units
- Dilatation to accomplish less than 50% residual stenosis
- Intravascular sheaths are removed approximately 3 hours post successful angioplasty
- Post angioplasty aspirin, 160 to 325 mg, plus diltiazem, 60 mg, four times daily, plus or minus nitrates. These medications do not significantly decrease the rate of restenosis, and a recent study indicates that the combination of aspirin and dipyridamole is not effective
- Discharge 12 to 24 hours later on enteric coated aspirin, 325 mg daily
- Advice on discontinuation of smoking, low saturated fat diet to maintain serum cholesterol less than 200 mg/dl (5.2 mmol/l) or, if needed, cholesterol-reducing agent (see Chapter 8).

LASER CORONARY ANGIOPLASTY

Within a few years, experience with percutaneous coronary excimer laser angioplasty (308 nm xenon chloride) and modification in laser catheter technology will allow application of this interventional therapy to coronary stenoses where balloon angioplasty is not feasible or with lesions where success is expected to be low with the balloon

- Aorto-ostial stenosis (good success rate)
- Calcified lesions
- Complete occlusions
- Greater than 10 mm, tubular or diffuse morphology
- Blocked saphenous vein graft

Information from studies in more than 1,400 patients indicates successful dilatation, i.e., less than 50% residual stenosis, in approximately 80% with about 50% of these requiring added balloon angioplasty at the same time.

In reported studies, the approximate complication rate includes:

- Dissection (12%), abrupt occlusion (4 to 6%), perforation (less than 2%)
- Myocardial infarction (3 to 5%)
- Death (less than 4%)

RESTENOSIS

Success in angiographically acceptable lesions indicates a greater than 20% increase in luminal diameter or a less than 50% residual stenosis. Approximately 90% of patients with proximal single vessel stenosis that is angiographically acceptable for dilation achieve successful angioplastic dilatation, although nearly 25% require a second dilatation, which is often successful.

Restenosis 3 to 6 months post coronary angioplasty occurs in approximately 30% of patients (Table 2–12). Fortunately, the second dilatation is often successful. Prevention of restenosis presents a major challenge. The process is not significantly prevented by aspirin, dipyridamole, ticlopidine, or omega 3 fatty acids and several test medications.

OTHER INTERVENTIONAL PROCEDURES

Various approaches to dealing with difficult atheromatous stenoses and balloon modifications are under way. Atherectomy is an experimental procedure that is often successful in the removal of atheromatous obstruction but has a high incidence of restenosis. The role of laser angioplasty and atherectomy should increase when therapy for the prevention of restenosis is proven effective. Coronary artery stents have a role in properly selected patients.

CORONARY ARTERY BYPASS SURGERY

The results and complications of CABS are given in Table 2–2. Overall mortality of CABS is about 1 to 2%, with 96% survival at one month and 95, 87, 76, and 60% at 1, 5, 10, and 15 years, respectively.

TABLE 2–12. COMPLICATIONS AND OUTCOME OF CORONARY BALLOON ANGIOPLASTY	
Death	<1%
Acute myocardial infarction	<2%
Emergency bypass surgery	<2%
Restenosis at 6 months	30%
Annual mortality rate	1%
Rate of nonfatal myocardial infarction	2%
5-year follow-up	
Symptomatic improvement	60%
No fatal or nonfatal myocardial infarction or coronary artery bypass surgery	80%

Approximately 50% of saphenous vein grafts occlude by 10 years postoperative. This incidence is highest in patients with hypertension, hyperlipidemia, diabetes, and in persistent smokers. Some studies indicate 40% occlusion at 10 years and approximately 25 to 40% for LAD vein grafts. Use of the internal mammary artery as a graft results in less than 15% occlusion at 10 years.

The most important advance in reduction of graft occlusion has resulted from the use of the left internal mammary artery. The artery is left attached to its origin from the left subclavian artery, mobilized, and anastomosed to the LAD artery. The 10-year occlusion rate is only 5% (Table 2–2).

Coronary artery bypass surgery protects from sudden death, with only a 5 and 10% incidence at 10 and 15 years, an important indicator of the role of ischemia in promoting this tragic outcome.

INDICATIONS

- For relief of angina uncontrolled by intensive medical therapy, especially if symptoms intensely hinder the patient's lifestyle
- Intolerance to drugs in severely symptomatic patients
- Patients with significant obstructive lesions considered angiographically unacceptable for balloon angioplasty

To relieve symptoms and prolong life in

- Left main coronary stenosis with 50% or more reduction in luminal diameter
- Proximal LAD equal to or greater than 75% plus a second vessel with greater than 50% overall diameter reduction
- Strongly positive exercise test, large area of myocardium involved in the ischemic process
- EF less than 40% but greater than 20% with two or three vessel disease
- Three vessel disease with EF less than 40% but higher than 20%. The internal mammary artery anastomosis to the LAD gives results superior to vein grafts and should be done in patients under age 65. Patients aged 70 and older should benefit sufficiently from a vein graft to the left anterior descending artery if angioplasty is not feasible

PREOPERATIVE AND POSTOPERATIVE MANAGEMENT

If the patient is receiving a beta blocker, a calcium antagonist, and IV nitroglycerin, these should be continued until the patient arrives in the operating room.

Guidelines for the administration of aspirin and effects include

- Aspirin should be discontinued 7 days prior to elective surgery for stable angina and 36 hours or more in patients with unstable angina. Heparin IV is administered instead of aspirin in patients with unstable angina who are being considered as candidates for CABS to prevent postoperative bleeding and reoperation caused by preoperative aspirin therapy
- Aspirin has proven effective in preventing occlusion of bypass grafts

TABLE 2–13. ASPIRIN PREVENTION OF VEIN GRAFT* OCCLUSION

	1 WEEK		1 YEAR	
	PLACEBO 98 (%)	ASPIRIN 102 (%)	PLACEBO (%)	ASPIRIN (%)
Occlusion	6.2	1.6	11.6	5.8
		p = 0.004		p = 0.013
New occlusion			7.4	4.3
				p = 0.013
Reoperation	1	4.8		
		p = 0.1		

Immediate postoperative aspirin is the treatment of choice
* Improves early graft patency, protects against further occlusion up to 1 year
Modified from: Gavaghan TP, et al.: Immediate postoperative aspirin improves vein graft patency early and late after coronary bypass graft surgery. Circulation, *83*:1526, 1991.

TABLE 2–14. EFFECTS OF PREOPERATIVE AND POSTOPERATIVE ASPIRIN ON VEIN GRAFT

	ASPIRIN	
	Preop (%)	6 hr Postop (%)
1-week occlusion	7.4	7.8
LAD occlusion	5.9	5.4
IM graft occlusion	0	2.4
		p = 0.036
Reoperation (another study)	6.6	1.7

IM = Internal mammary artery
Modified from: Goldman S, et al.: Starting aspirin therapy after operation. Effects on early graft patency. Circulation, *84*:520, 1991.

- Immediate postoperative aspirin therapy has been documented as the treatment of choice to prevent graft occlusion (see Table 2–13). In a successful study by Gavaghan, et al., aspirin (324 mg) dissolved in 30 ml water, administered within 1 hour of leaving the operating room by nasogastric tube and 90-minute clamp time, then 325 mg orally daily, reduced graft occlusion from 6.2 to 1.6% at one week and from 11.6 to 5.8% at the end of 1-year follow-up; reoperation rate was 4.8% in the aspirin group versus 1% in the placebo arm. Other studies confirm the 1-year benefit of aspirin administered up to 6 hours after surgery
- Aspirin causes a significant increase in postoperative bleeding and requirement for blood transfusion. Reoperation directly related to aspirin therapy given 1 hour postoperative was 4.8% versus 1% in the placebo arm in one study. In two well-run studies, reoperation was necessary in 2.4 and 1.7% of patients administered aspirin 6 hours after completion of surgery (Table 2–14). Aspirin is considered effective and relatively

safe when administered between 1 and 6 hours of leaving the operating room
- Aspirin orally, 160 to 325 mg daily, is continued for the lifetime of the patient if no contraindications or adverse effects ensue
- Significant bleeding occurs with low-dose aspirin in use. In the Physicians' 5-year follow-up study, aspirin (325 mg alternate day) caused significant melena in 364 (3.3%) of patients versus 246 (2.2%) in the placebo arm (p = 0.00001)

Vein graft occlusion is common, occurring in up to 50% occlusion 10 years post surgery (Table 2–2).
Risk factors for vein graft occlusion include

- Smoking: This must be discontinued
- Hyperlipidemia: This must be controlled with strict diet. Drug therapy is advisable if the LDL cholesterol exceeds 160 mg/dl (4 mmol/l). If the HDL cholesterol is less than 39 mg/dl (0.9 mmol/l), drug therapy is advised if the LDL cholesterol exceeds 140 mg/dl (3.6 mmol/l) (see Chapter 8)

The incidence of perioperative myocardial infarction was reduced by pretreatment with allopurinol in one study, and further clinical trials are required to confirm this important observation.

CASE STUDY: DECISION-MAKING IN MANAGING ANGINA

Case 1: A 46-year-old male with mild angina (Class 1 to 2), positive exercise test, 80 to 90% proximal stenosis of the left anterior descending artery. Choice of therapy: angioplasty preferred to surgery because of young age, and acceptable angiographic single vessel lesion (Fig. 2–5). If restenosis in 6 months, repeat angioplasty; if recurrent angina, proceed to CABS with left internal mammary artery to the left anterior descending, advisable in younger patients.

Case 2: A 52-year-old female with angina Class 2, positive exercise test, 90% proximal left anterior descending, 80% proximal right coronary artery dominant, EF greater than 40%, anterior wall hypokinesia. Choice of therapy: no clear answers concerning angioplasty versus surgery. If staged angioplasty chosen because of young age, acceptable angiographic lesion, and EF greater than 40%, proceed with dilatation of left anterior descending first (Fig. 2–5). CABS with internal mammary artery to left anterior descending can be done later, if needed, or if angioplasty results in occlusion.

If EF is less than 35%, choose CABS with internal mammary artery to the left anterior descending. Treat male and female the same.

Case 3: A similar scenario to Case 2 but the patient is older than 65 or EF is less than 40%, a vein graft should be used (Fig. 2–5 and 2–6).

Case 4: A 72-year-old female with a 90% proximal left anterior descending, 80% proximal right, 70% circumflex, Class 2 or 3 angina, positive stress test, EF between 30 and 40%. Choice of therapy: CABS using vein graft (Fig. 2–6).

Case 5: An 80-year-old patient in good health, an active golfer, with Class 3 angina that has been poorly controlled with intensive medical therapy. The EF is greater than 40%; a proximal left anterior descending artery 90% occluded. Choice of therapy: if the lesion is angiographically acceptable, angioplasty is advisable.

BIBLIOGRAPHY

Abrams J: Management of myocardial ischemia: Role of intermittent nitrate therapy. Am Heart J, *120*:762, 1990.

Bashour TT: Vasotonic myocardial ischemia. Am Heart J, *122*:1701, 1991.

Bourassa MG, Lespérance J, Eastwood C, et al.: Clinical, physiologic anatomic and procedural factors predictive of restenosis after percutaneous transluminal coronary angioplasty. J Am Coll Cardiol, *18*:368, 1991.

Cairns J, Gent M, Singer J, et al.: Aspirin, sulfinpyrazone, or both in unstable angina: Results of a Canadian multicenter trial. N Engl J Med, *313*:1369, 1985.

Chaitman BR, Ryan TJ, Kronmal RA, et al.: Coronary Artery Surgery Study (CASS): Comparability of 10 year survival in randomized and randomizable patients. J Am Coll Cardiol, *16*:1071, 1990.

Collins P, Fox KM: Pathophysiology of angina. Lancet, *335*:94, 1990.

Cook SL, Eigler NL, Shefer A, et al.: Percutaneous excimer laser coronary angioplasty of lesions not favourable for balloon angioplasty. Circulation, *84*:632, 1991.

Coplan NL: Evaluation of patients for coronary artery bypass surgery: The role of exercise testing. Am Heart J, *122*:1800, 1991.

Crea F, Pupita G, Galassi A, et al.: Comparative effects of theophylline and isosorbide dinitrate on exercise capacity in stable angina pectoris, and their mechanisms of action. Am J Cardiol, *64*:1098, 1989.

Diethrich E: Has excimer coronary laser angioplasty finally found a niche? Circulation, *84*: 939, 1991.

Dimas PA, Arora RR, Whitlow PL, et al.: Percutaneous transluminal angioplasty involving internal mammary artery grafts. Am Heart J, *122*:423, 1991.

Elkayam U: Tolerance to organic nitrates: Evidence, mechanisms, clinical relevance and strategies for prevention. Ann Intern Med, *114*:667, 1991.

Fifer MA: What does positron emission tomography teach us about coronary angioplasty? J Am Coll Cardiol, *18*:979, 1991.

Fitzgibbon GM, Leach AJ, Kafka HP, et al.: Coronary bypass graft fate: long-term angiographic study. J Am Coll Cardiol, *17*:1075, 1991.

Freeman MR, Langer A, Wilson RF, et al.: Thrombolysis in unstable angina. Randomized double-blind trial of t-PA and placebo. Circulation, *85*:150, 1991.

Frierson JH, Dimas AP, Whitlow PL, et al.: Angioplasty of the proximal left anterior descending coronary artery: Initial success and long-term follow-up. J Am Coll Cardiol, *19*:745, 1992.

Gavaghan TP, Gebski V, Baron DW: Immediate postoperative aspirin improves vein graft patency early and late after coronary artery bypass graft surgery. Circulation, *83*:1526, 1991.

Goldman S, Copeland J, Moritz T, et al.: Spahenous vein graft patency 1 year after coronary artery bypass surgery and effects of antiplatelet therapy. Results of a Veterans Administration Cooperative Study. Circulation, *80*:1190, 1989.

Goldman S, Copeland J, Moritz T: Starting aspirin therapy after operation. Circulation, *84*: 520, 1991.

Goldstein RE, Boccuzzi SJ, Cruess D, et al.: Diltiazem increases late-onset congestive heart failure in postinfarction patients with early reduction in ejection fraction. Circulation, *83*: 52, 1991.

Grossman W, Baim DS, eds. Cardiac Catheterization Angiography, and Intervention. 4th Ed. Philadelphia, Lea & Febiger, 1991.

Hermans WRM, Rensing BJ, Strauss BH, et al.: Prevention of restenosis after percutaneous transluminal coronary angioplasty: The search for a "magic bullet." Am Heart J, *122*:171, 1991.

Ivanhoe RJ, Weintraub WS, Douglas JS Jr., et al.: Percutaneous transluminal coronary angioplasty of chronic total occlusions. Primary success, restenosis, and long-term clinical follow-up. Circulation, *85*:106, 1992.

Johnson WD, Kayser KL, Brenowitz JB, et al.: A randomized controlled trial of allopurinol in coronary bypass surgery. Am Heart J, *121*:20, 1991.

Johnson DW, Kayser KL, Hartz AJ, et al.: Aspirin use and survival after coronary bypass surgery. Am Heart J, *123*:603, 1992.

Kaski JC, Tousoulis D, McFadden E, et al.: Variant angina pectoris. Role of coronary spasm in the development of fixed coronary obstructions. Circulation, *85*:619, 1992.

Kawanishi DT, Reid CL, Morrison EC, et al.: Response of angina and ischemia to long-term treatment in patients with chronic stable angina: A double-blind randomized individualized dosing trial of nifedipine, propranolol and their combination. J Am Coll Cardiol, *19*:409, 1992.

Khan M Gabriel: Angina. *In* Cardiac Drug Therapy. 3rd Ed. London, W.B. Saunders, 1992.

Khusrow N, Cragg DR, Strzelecki M, Friedman HZ, et al.: Angiographic risk factors for coronary restenosis following mechanical rotational artherectomy. J Am Coll Cardiol, *17*:218A, 1991.

Kirklin JW, Akins CW, Blackstone EH, et al.: ACC/AHA Task Force Report. Guidelines and indications for coronary artery bypass graft surgery. J Am Coll Cardiol, *17*:543, 1991.

Kishida H, Tada Y, Tetsuoh Y, et al.: A new strategy for the reduction of acute myocardial infarction in variant angina. Am Heart J, *122*:1554, 1991.

Kragel AH, Gertz SD, Roberts WC: Morphologic comparison of frequency and types of acute lesions in the major epicardial coronary arteries in unstable angina pectoris, sudden coronary death and acute myocaridal infarction. J Am Coll Cardiol, *18*:801, 1991.

Lessof MH, Evans JG, Joy MD, et al.: Report of a working group of the Royal College of Physicians. Cardiological intervention in elderly patients. J Royal Coll Physicians, *25*:197, 1991.

Lichtlen PR, Hugenholtz P, Rafflenbeul W, et al.: Retardation of the angiographic progression of coronary artery disease in man by the calcium channel blocker nifedipine. Results of the international nifedipine trial on antiatherosclerotic therapy (INTACT). Lancet, *335(8698)*: 1109, 1990.

Loaldi A, Polese A, Montorsi P, et al.: Comparison of nifedipine, propranolol and isosorbide dinitrate on angiographic progression and regression of coronary arterial narrowings in angina pectoris. Am J Cardiol, *64*:433, 1989.

Miranda CP, Liu J, Kadar A, et al.: Usefulness of exercise-induced ST-segment depression in the inferior leads during exercise testing as a marker for coronary artery disease. Am J Cardiol, *69*:303, 1992.

Motomura S, Zerkowski HR, Daul A, et al.: On the physiologic role of beta-2 adrenoceptors in the human heart: In vitro and in vivo studies. Am Heart J, *119*:608, 1990.

Naftilan AJ: Chemical atherectomy. Circulation, *84*:946, 1991.

Nobuyoshi M, Kimura T, Ohishi H, et al.: Restenosis after percutaneous transluminal coronary angioplasty: Pathologic observations in 20 patients. J Am Coll Cardiol, *17*:433, 1991.

Parmley WW, Nesto RW, Singh BN, et al.: Attenuation of the circadian patterns of myocardial ischemia with nifedipine GITS in patients with chronic stable angina. J Am Coll Cardiol, *19*:1380, 1992.

Parker JO: Controlled release isosorbide-5-mononitrate in angina pectoris: A comparison with standard formulation isosorbide dinitrate. Can J Cardiol, *7*:125, 1991.

Pepine CJ, Allen HD, Bashore TM, et al.: ACC/AHA guidelines for cardiac catheterization and cardiac catheterization laboratories. J Am Coll Cardiol, *18*:1149, 1991.

Peters RW, Muller JE, Goldstein S, et al.: For the BHAT Study Group. Propranolol and the morning increase in the frequency of sudden cardiac deaths. (BHAT Study) Am J Cardiol, *63*:1518, 1989.

Popma JJ, Califf RM, Topol EJ: Clinical trials of restenosis after coronary angioplasty. Circulation, *84*:1433, 1991.

Prakash C, Deedwania PC, Carbajal EV, et al.: Anti-ischemic effects of atenolol versus nifedipine in patients with coronary artery disease and ambulatory silent ischemia. J Am Coll Cardiol, *17*:963, 1991.

Reeves F, Bonan R, Côté G, et al.: Long-term angiographic follow-up after angioplasty of venous coronary bypass grafts. Am Heart J, *122*:620, 1991.

Rensing BJ, Hermans WRM, Deckers JW, et al.: Lumen narrowing after percutaneous transluminal coronary balloon angioplasty follows a near gaussian distribution: A quantitative angiographic study in 1,445 successfully dilated lesions. J Am Coll Cardiol, *19*:939, 1992.

Ryan TJ: A 10 year follow-up of single vessel angioplasty: Some important lingering questions. J Am Coll Cardiol, *16*:66, 1990.

Sahni R, Maniet AR, Voci G, et al.: Prevention of restenosis by lovastatin after successful coronary angioplasty. Am Heart J, *121*:1600, 1991.

Sanborn TA, Torre SR, Sharma SK, et al.: Percutaneous coronary excimer laser-assisted balloon angioplasty: Initial clinical and quantitative angiographic results in 50 patients. J Am Coll Cardiol, *17*:94, 1991.

Sanborn TA, Bitt JA, Hershman RA, et al.: Percutaneous coronary excimer laser-assisted angioplasty: Initial multicenter experience in 141 patients. J Am Coll Cardiol, *17*:169B, 1991.

Sanborn TA: Early limitations of coronary excimer laser angioplasty. J Am Coll Cardiol, *17*:995, 1991.

Savage MP, Goldberg S, Hirshfield JW, et al.: Clinical and angiographic determinants of primary coronary angioplasty success. J Am Coll Cardiol, *17*:22, 1991.

Schatz RA, Goldberg S, Leon M, et al.: Clinical experience with the Palmaz-Schatz coronary stent. J Am Coll Cardiol, *17*:155B. 1991.

Shah PK, Amin J: Low high density lipoprotein level is associated with increased restenosis rate after coronary angioplasty. Circulation, *85*:1279, 1992.

Solomon SA, Ramsay LE, Yeo WW, et al.: β Blockade and intermittent claudication: Placebo controlled trial of atenolol and nifedipine and their combination. Br Med J, *303*:1100, 1991.

Thadani U, Zellner SR, Glasser S, et al.: Double-blind, dose-response, placebo-controlled multicenter study of nisoldipine. Circulation, *84*:2398, 1991.

The Multicenter Diltiazem Postinfarction Trial Research Group: The effect of diltiazem on mortality and reinfarction after myocardial infarction. N Engl J Med, *319*:385, 1989.

Théroux P, Ouimet H, McCans J: Aspirin, heparin, or both to treat unstable angina. N Engl J Med, *319*:1105, 1988.

Vlay SC, Olson LC: Nifedipine and isosorbide dinitrate alone and in combination for patients with chronic stable angina: A double-blind crossover study. Am Heart J, *120*:303, 1990.

Wackers FJ: Adenosine or dipyridamole: Which is preferred for myocardial perfusion imaging? J Am Coll Cardiol, *17*:1295, 1991.

Weintraub WS, Ghazzal ZMB, Cohen CL, et al.: Clinical implications of late proven patency after successful coronary angioplasty. Circulation, *84*:572, 1991.

Wilson RF, Marcus ML, Christensen BV, et al.: Accuracy of exercise electrocardiography in detecting physiologically significant coronary arterial lesions. Circulation, *83*:412, 1991.

Yeung AC, Barry J, Orav J, et al.: Effects of asymptomatic ischemia on long-term prognosis in chronic stable coronary disease. Circulation, *83*:1598, 1991.

Yusuf S, Collins R, MacMahon S, et al.: Effect of intravenous nitrates on mortality in acute myocardial infarction: An overview of the randomised trials. Lancet, *1*:1088, 1988.

3

ACUTE MYOCARDIAL INFARCTION
M. Gabriel Khan

PATHOPHYSIOLOGIC IMPLICATIONS

An acute myocardial infarction (MI) is nearly always caused by occlusion of a coronary artery by thrombus overlying a fissured or ruptured atheromatous plaque. Coronary angiography performed during the early hours of infarction has confirmed the presence of total occlusion of the infarct-related artery in over 90% of patients. In a few, occlusion is incomplete or intermittent.

Highly thrombogenic substances are discharged from a ruptured plaque. In addition, exposed collagen provokes platelet aggregation. These and other undetermined mechanisms activate a thrombotic occlusion of the coronary artery.

It is not surprising, therefore, that aspirin, through inhibition of platelet aggregation, reduces the incidence of coronary thrombosis and is especially useful in prevention of the progression of unstable angina to thrombosis and MI. Aspirin is particularly useful when given at the onset of chest pain produced by infarction. Aspirin, however, does not block all pathways that relate to platelet aggregation. In addition, aspirin does not decrease the incidence of sudden death in patients with acute MI.

The increased morning incidence of acute MI documented in several studies of the diurnal variation of infarction is related to the early morning catecholamine surges, that induce platelet aggregation, and an increase in blood pressure and hydraulic stress that may lead to plaque rupture. Beta-adrenergic blockers have been shown to decrease the early morning peak incidence of acute infarction and sudden death.

Unfortunately, when an atheromatous plaque ruptures, the thrombogenic effect of plaque contents cannot be completely nullified by the inhibition of all aspects of platelet aggregation, and chemical agents that can arrest the effects of these thrombogenic substances deserve intensive study.

Two such agents, hirudin and agatroban, competitive inhibitors of thrombin, have been shown to be superior to heparin in preventing coronary thrombosis in experimental models and in patients with unstable angina. Preliminary studies in patients suggest that agatroban and hirudin administered with aspirin is effective in the prevention of coronary thrombosis and requires testing in clinical trials. These studies may pave the way to further research that may uncover newer types of antithrombotic agents, more specific and superior to the coumarins, in preventing coronary thrombosis. Importantly, agatroban does not prolong the bleeding time in patients after the administration of aspirin. The combination of a thrombin inhibitor, therefore, with aspirin and a beta blocking agent may cause a significant increase in survival of patients with coronary heart disease (CHD), and clinical trials are in progress.

Coronary artery spasm appears to play a relatively small role in the pathogenesis of coronary occlusion leading to infarction. Evidence of coronary vasoconstriction was found when angioscopy was performed shortly after infarction, and intermittent occlusion, presumably on a vasomotor basis, has been apparent in some cases. Vasoconstriction appears to be a secondary factor, however, and since sudden plaque rupture is now proven to be the initiating event causing coronary thrombosis, the mechanisms underlying plaque rupture and its prevention deserve intensive study to no lesser degree than the important aspect of prevention of atheroma formation.

Currently, the only therapy that has the potential to avert plaque rupture appears to be the use of a beta blocking agent to decrease cardiac ejection velocity. This action reduces hydraulic stress on the arterial wall that might be critical at the arterial site where the atheromatous plaque is predisposed to rupture (Fig. 2–7).

Occlusion of a coronary artery leads, in about 20 minutes, to death of cells in areas of severely ischemic tissue, which will usually become necrotic over 4 to 6 hours. Since early and late mortality are directly related to the size of the infarct, limitation of infarct size (or even prevention of necrosis) by means of thrombolytic therapy initiated at the earliest possible moment, is of the utmost importance. Therapy will be of very limited value if the delay exceeds 6 hours.

The ischemic zone surrounding the necrotic tissue provides electrophysiologic inhomogeneity that predisposes the occurrence of lethal arrhythmias. These arrhythmias are most common during the early hours after onset and contribute to one of the major mechanisms of sudden death.

Extensive myocardial necrosis is the major determinant of heart failure, papillary, septal, and freewall rupture, as well as cardiogenic shock, in which more than 35% of the myocardium is usually infarcted. The most effective means of reducing the extent of myocardial necrosis is the administration of thrombolytic therapy, aspirin, and a beta blocking agent shortly after the onset of symptoms of coronary thrombosis.

DIAGNOSIS

CHEST PAIN

- Usually lasts longer than 20 minutes and often persists for several hours. However, the pain of infarction can last for only 15 minutes and, occasionally, fatal infarction is ushered in by only a few minutes of severe

pain or even unheralded cardiac arrest. Infarction may be silent, particularly in diabetic patients and in the elderly
- Typically retrosternal and across the chest
- Variations of crushing, vise-like, heavy weight on the chest, pressure, tightness, strangling, aching
- At times, only a discomfort with an oppression and burning or indigestion-like feeling
- May radiate to the throat, jaws, neck, shoulders, arms, scapulae, or the epigastrium. At times, pain is centered at any one of these areas, e.g., the left wrist or shoulder without radiation
- Usually builds up over minutes or hours, as opposed to aortic dissection, in which pain has an abrupt onset like a gunshot

Associated symptoms and factors include

- Diaphoresis, cold clammy skin, apprehension
- Shortness of breath, nausea, vomiting, dizziness
- Presyncope and rarely syncope may occur due to bradyarrhythmias, especially in inferior MI
- Occasionally, no pain. A marked fall in blood pressure with associated symptoms, along with ECG findings, should suffice in making the diagnosis
- Painless infarcts (in about 10% of patients), especially in diabetics or the elderly. In these patients, associated symptoms are often prominent and serve as clues to diagnosis
- Over 50% of patients have a history of angina or prior infarction
- Approximately 33% of patients with acute infarction have no major risk factors: death of a parent or sibling prior to age 55, hypercholesterolemia, cigarette smoking, hypertension, or diabetes. Absence of these factors should not influence the diagnosis

PHYSICAL SIGNS

- Patient appears apprehensive, anxious, cold, clammy
- Area of chest pain may be indicated with a clenched fist
- Tachycardia 100 to 120/minute; an increase in blood pressure due to increased sympathetic tone is observed in slightly more than half of patients with anterior infarction
- Bradycardia below 60 beats/minute and a fall in blood pressure in about two-thirds of inferior infarcts; many of these patients become hypotensive, sometimes profoundly
- S4 gallop is common; S3 and S4 if in heart failure or cardiogenic shock
- Murmur of mitral regurgitation due to papillary muscle dysfunction
- Crepitations, more prominent over the lower third of the lung fields, may be present
- Positive hepatojugular reflux due to left ventricular failure
- Elevated jugular venous pressure due to left and right heart failure or a very high venous pressure in the presence of right ventricular infarction or cardiac tamponade

- Frequently, there are no abnormal physical signs, and this finding in a patient with suggestive symptoms should not decrease the level of suspicion that the patient may have an MI

Although sophisticated tests evolved in the 1980s to improve diagnostic accuracy, they are of limited value in the area of thrombolysis. Thus, a relevant history and correct interpretation of the electrocardiogram are of paramount importance in the implementation of early thrombolytic therapy, which will be of greatest benefit if given prior to creatine kinase (CK) elevation.

ELECTROCARDIOGRAM

DIAGNOSTIC FEATURES OF ACUTE MYOCARDIAL INFARCTION

- ST segment elevation of at least 1 mm in two or more limb leads or
- At least 2 mm ST elevation in two or more precordial leads

The above criteria, which have been used in several clinical trials of thrombolytic therapy, have become internationally standard and are considered diagnostic in patients with symptoms suggestive of acute MI. Where symptoms are not typical, the response to nitroglycerin is ascertained. Also, minimal ST segment elevation in black patients must be reassessed to exclude the occasional normal variant. There is clear recognition that Q waves may evolve early or late and cannot be relied upon for early diagnosis. Thus, the terms "transmural" and "nontransmural" have been abandoned and Q wave or non Q wave infarction cannot be categorized in the early phase.

In addition, later ECG signs of infarction include

- Diminution of R waves (poor R wave progression)
- Evolving Q waves
- The simultaneous presence of reciprocal ST segment depression is not diagnostic but tends to confirm the diagnosis
- Patients who are developing non Q wave infarction often manifest ST depression, and this finding cannot be distinguished from ischemia on the ECG

If the first electrocardiogram is not diagnostic of acute injury/infarction, the ECG is repeated every 30 minutes until diagnostic changes are observed or until the CK and/or CK-MB results are reported. If the ECG is equivocal and there is a strong clinical impression that acute MI is present, valuable confirmatory information may be obtained from an echocardiogram.

Because the initial abnormality may not be fully diagnostic in more than 40% of cases, it is imperative to correlate the findings with accurate historical details. In patients with chest pain, new or presumably new Q waves in two leads with ST elevation are diagnostic in over 85% of cases

- Q waves are fully developed in 4 to 12 hours and may manifest as early as 2 hours from onset of chest discomfort or associated symptoms
- Evolutionary ST-T changes occur during 12 to 24 hours but may be delayed up to 30 hours

- Inferior myocardial infarction ST elevation in lead 2, 3 and AVF with evolving Q waves and reciprocal depression in V_1-V_3. The latter depression may be due to reciprocal changes, but there is evidence to suggest that in some patients it is due to left anterior descending artery disease. The evolutionary changes in repolarization that occur with inferior infarction evolve more rapidly than with anterior infarcts
- Tachycardia may increase ischemic injury, causing elevation of the ST segment that must be differentiated from extension of infarction of pericarditis. Importantly, reciprocal depression does not occur in pericarditis.

NONDIAGNOSTIC ECG

Acute MI may be present with ECG changes that are nonspecific in 10 to 20% of cases and may result from

- Slow evolution of electrocardiographic changes, the tracing may remain normal for several hours
- Old infarction masking the electrocardiographic effect of a new infarct
- Inferior myocardial infarction associated with left anterior hemiblock in which R waves are expected to be small in leads 2, 3, AVF
- Left bundle branch block
- Apical infarction
- Posterolateral infarction is not usually associated with ST elevation or Q waves

ST elevation of infarction must be distinguished from the following

- Acute pericarditis where the ST segment elevation is not confined to leads referrable to an anatomic segmental blood supply. Thus, elevation in lead 1 is accompanied by elevation in leads 2, 3, AVF; the ST elevation is concave, as opposed to convex, upward with an injury current of infarction, and reciprocal depression is absent (see Chapter 13)
- Early repolarization changes may mimic infarction but are often observed mainly in leads V5 and V6 with a subtle "fish hook" configuration. This feature is common in blacks
- Left ventricular aneurysm, in which there may be permanent ST elevation
- Prinzmetal's (variant) angina: In this very uncommon condition, ST elevation resolves with relief of pain and/or responds to nitroglycerin

ECG AND LOCATION OF INFARCTION SITES

- Anteroseptal: ST elevation V_1, V_2, V_3
- Anterior: ST segment elevation V_2-V_4
- Extensive anterior: V_1-V_6, 1 AVL
- Anterolateral: V_4-V_6, 1 AVL
- Inferior: 2, 3, AVF
- Posterior infarction : Tall R waves V_1, V_2, upright T waves occasionally ST depression V_1-V_2 and often inferior or inferolateral infarct signs

- Right ventricular infarction: ST segment elevation V_2, V_4R, often associated with inferior infarction

ECG AND SIZE OF INFARCTION

The extent of ST segment elevation gives clues to infarct size, but the correlation is not close. The site of infarction influences mortality but is not as paramount as the size of infarction, which can be reasonably ascertained from the number of leads showing ST elevation, as follows

- Small MI: 2 or 3 leads
- Moderate: 4 or 5 leads
- Large: 6 or 7 leads
- Extensive: 8 or 9 leads

ECHOCARDIOGRAPHY IN ACUTE MYOCARDIAL INFARCTION

The echocardiogram is not required routinely in a first uncomplicated MI, especially where the history and ECG are typical or with non Q wave infarction.

INDICATIONS

- Patients with cardiogenic shock often require assessment to determine the presence of mechanical complications: septal rupture, severe mitral regurgitation, myocardial rupture, and tamponade. Color Doppler gives quick results and, with the unconscious patient, a transesophageal echocardiogram (TEE) is helpful and accurate
- To distinguish acute severe mitral regurgitation from papillary muscle rupture
- In patients with new left bundle branch block with typical chest pain and history suggestive of acute infarction, echocardiography assists with the diagnosis
- Patients with an atypical ECG pattern and clinical features of MI
- Suspected right ventricular infarction with high jugular venous pressure to assess right ventricular involvement and differentiate pericardial tamponade causing a high venous pressure
- Patients with extensive infarction, to assess the need for heparin or oral anticoagulant therapy for left ventricular thrombi
- In patients with moderate heart failure not clearing after two or more doses of furosemide, echocardiographic assessment of left ventricular systolic function is useful prior to beta blocker therapy. Although radionuclide ventriculography gives a more accurate assessment of the EF, the estimate obtained from echocardiography is usually adequate to assist with the evaluation of outcomes and therapy

PUBLIC EDUCATION AND PHYSICIAN INTERACTION

It is estimated that in areas where thrombolytic therapy is available, 20 to 30% of patients with acute MI in North America and about 40% in the UK receive such treatment.

Thrombolytic therapy has proven value and reduces mortality and morbidity. Timing of treatment, however, is of great importance, and a major benefit was observed in The Gruppo Italiano per lo Studio della Strepto chinasi Nell Infarto Miocardico (GISSI)-1 and The Second International Study of Infarct Survival (ISIS)-2, mainly in patients treated within 3 hours of onset. Some benefit is observed up to 4 hours, and small but significant benefit is seen up to 6 hours of onset, but only minimal decrease in mortality is observed between 6 to 12 hours. Therapy for patients seen in the 6- to 12-hour period depends on weighing the risks of therapy and potential benefits in terms of significant decrease in mortality versus serious adverse effects and justifiable cost. Although ISIS-2 shows a benefit from treating patients in the 6- to 12-hour period, only one patient of every 100 treated could be saved. Thus, so-called significant benefits are observed only when high numbers of patients are treated to attain a statistical p value. Patients seen between 6 and 12 hours of onset are treated mainly if there are symptoms and signs of ongoing ischemia. Patients and the public must be informed that thrombolytic therapy is usually meaningless if given after 6 hours of onset of symptoms. This statement may motivate some individuals. Tables 3–1 and 3–2 indicate the lifesaving potential of thrombolytic therapy and relation to treatment times. The physician must be aware that thrombolytic therapy begun after a 4-hour delay is usually too late to limit myocardial ischemia or necrosis and ventricular performance does not improve. Indeed, patency rates observed after 4 hours appear to be meaningless as far as EF or wall motion abnormalities are concerned.

A major undertaking is the education of patients and the community at large about the importance of minimizing delays between the onset of symptoms of suspected heart attack and attention in the emergency room

TABLE 3–1. TIMING OF THROMBOLYTIC THERAPY AND LIVES SAVED IN GISSI-1 AND ISIS-2

	GISSI-1*		ISIS 2**	
	Control	SK Treated	Control	SK & Aspirin Treated
Mortality: Mortality reduction:	5,860 13% 17.7% Lives saved 130/5852 2/100 treated Hours ≤3 3–6 6–9 6–24	5,852 10.7% Lives saved 3/100 2/100 1/123 —	8,595 11.8% 22.9% Lives saved 233/8595 3/100 treated Lives saved 4/100 2.6/100 1/100	8,592 9.1%

SK = Streptokinase
* = Modified from: Lancet, *1*:397, 1986
** = Modified from: Lancet, *2*:350, 1988

TABLE 3–2. ISIS-2: EFFECTS OF ASPIRIN AND STREPTOKINASE GIVEN WITHIN 4 HOURS AND WITHIN 24 HOURS OF ONSET OF MYOCARDIAL INFARCTION					
	PLACEBO (I)	SK	ASPIRIN	SK + ASPIRIN	PLACEBO (I) + TABLETS	NEITHER
35-day vascular mortality; therapy within 4 hours	12.3%	8.2%	8.9%	6.4%	13.1%	
Within 24 hours	12% 1029/8595	9.2% 791/8592	9.4% 804/8587	8% 343/4292	11.8% 1016/8600	13.3% 568/4300

I = infusion
SK = streptokinase
Modified from: Lancet, 2:350, 1988.
* Odds of death, 53% SD 8 Reduction; 2 p < 0.00001

of the nearest hospital. Preferably, initial treatment may be given by a paramedic unit prior to transport.

It is not easy to motivate healthy individuals, and efforts to educate the public in this area of their care have not been sufficiently fruitful. Leaflets and health booklets appear to have little impact. A concerted effort must be made by physicians' groups in individual communities in conjunction with audiovisual programs for the public. In addition, hospitals must adopt policies to enforce rapid triage in the emergency room; physicians must be encouraged to institute thrombolytic therapy within a few minutes of the patient's arrival. Programs to enable treatment to be initiated outside the hospital under the direction of a physician are being evaluated at certain centers, e.g., in Seattle and Sydney.

DELAYS TO BE AVOIDED

- Reaching the emergency room more than 6 hours after onset of symptoms: Patient and public education should address this issue
- Slow emergency room triage: Patients with chest pain should be allowed quick passage, not exceeding 1 minute delay at the so-called "triage area," to an area of the emergency room delineated for the rapid assessment of MI
- Waiting for attending physician
- Emergency room physician delay: The emergency room physician must be well trained to deal with patients who have chest pain. This physician must be allowed to give IV streptokinase or tissue plasminogen activator (tPA) to all those who qualify according to an approved, well-outlined hospital emergency room protocol for IV use of thrombolytic agents. The protocol must clearly show the indications and contraindications to IV streptokinase or tPA and the areas where a cardiologist's opinion should be sought. Tissue plasminogen activator should be available for

patients who are allergic to streptokinase or who have received streptokinase in the prior 9 months

- Waiting for coronary care unit (CCU) beds: Transfer is advisable after commencement of thrombolysis and initial hemodynamic stability is achieved. Thus, emergency rooms must be equipped to administer all functions that are available in the CCU
- Waiting 1 to 2 hours for CK, CK-MB enzyme results: The CK is not usually sufficiently elevated within the first 4 hours to establish the diagnosis of infarction and can be used only after the fact. The object is to reduce or, in some cases, prevent enzyme release by rapid reperfusion of ischemic myocardium

RISK STRATIFICATION

On admission, risk stratification (Table 3–3) assists in decision-making, especially when relative contraindications to thrombolytic therapy are present. Characteristics of patients with acute MI who, on admission, have a high risk of death or complications include

- Large infarcts usually associated with moderate to severe heart failure, pulmonary edema, with crackles observed over greater than one-third of the lower lung field
- An EF less than 35%
- Cardiogenic shock indicating a large infarct or mechanical complication and high mortality

TABLE 3–3. ACUTE MYOCARDIAL INFARCTION IN-HOSPITAL MORTALITY RISK STRATIFICATION

PARAMETERS	*APPROXIMATE MORTALITY %
Average	13
Age	
75–85	24
65–74	15
50–65	9
<50	<7
Cardiogenic shock	80
Large anterior** infarcts associated with	
a) Severe heart failure pulmonary edema	>30
b) Previous infarct and heart failure ejection fraction <30%	>25
c) Q wave anterior infarct heart rate >100/min blood pressure	>20
<110 mm Hg	
New left bundle branch block proven infarction	>20
Q wave anterior infarct uncomplicated	12
Q wave inferior	3
Non Q wave infarction	3
Q wave and age <55 uncomplicated	7
Non Q wave age <55	1

* Recent pooled trial results
** Anterior, anterolateral

- Over age 75: the 1-year mortality exceeds 30% versus less than 10% in patients under age 70
- New left bundle branch block
- New right bundle branch block with left ventricular failure
- Previous MI and recent infarction with heart failure

THERAPY

Immediate relief of pain is of paramount importance since pain enhances autonomic disturbances that may precipitate sudden death. All patients should take or be given noncoated aspirin, 162 to 325 mg, immediately and then enteric coated, 160 to 325 daily. This dosage proved very effective in ISIS-2 (Table 3–2) and ISIS-3; a 325-mg dose was used successfully in GISSI-2 (Table 3–1). An initial large dose of 325 mg is strongly recommended because a lower dose may still leave substantial thromboxane activity at this crucial period and may take a few days before achieving more than 95% of inhibition of platelet activity. Beta blockers are administered without delay if there are no contraindications, and thrombolytic therapy is commenced in properly selected patients. These treatment modalities will be discussed in this chapter. The reader is advised to consult Chapter 4 for a discussion of angioplasty and the management of complications of acute MI.

In all patients with uncomplicated infarction, treated with thrombolytic agents, a delayed strategy of coronary angiography is pursued in selected patients at about the sixth week post infarction with consideration for angioplasty or CABS, this subject is discussed in Chapter 4. A conservative strategy has evolved based on the result of the Thrombolysis in Myocardial Infarction (TIMI)-2 trial.

EMERGENCY MANAGEMENT

PAIN RELIEF

- Morphine: 4 mg IV over 1 minute, repeated if necessary at a dose of 2 to 5 mg every 5 to 30 minutes as needed at the rate of 1 mg/minute
- A beta blocker, preferably given IV for two doses then orally (see Table 3–4), if there is no contraindication. Beta blockade has been shown to abolish and may prevent recurrence of chest pain and decreases the need for morphine or nitroglycerin
- Nitroglycerin is usually given sublingually for two doses. Recurrence of chest discomfort after adequate administration of morphine and a beta blocker should prompt the use of IV nitroglycerin (see Pump Infusion, Table 2–9)

CONTROL OF EARLY LIFE THREATENING ARRHYTHMIAS

Lives can be saved by

- Prompt defibrillation or conversion of ventricular tachycardia (VT) by medical teams or paramedics

TABLE 3–4. DOSAGE OF BETA BLOCKERS IN ACUTE MYOCARDIAL INFARCTION*

IV**	ORAL DOSAGE 1ST 7 DAYS	1 WEEK TO 2 YEARS
Atenolol (IV 5 mg over 5 min, 10 min later 5 mg over 5 min)	10 min after last IV dose give 50 mg oral/daily	50 mg daily
Metoprolol (IV 5 mg at a rate of 1 mg/min 5 min later 2nd 5 mg bolus 5 min later 3rd 5 mg bolus)	8 hours after IV 25 to 50 mg twice daily	50 to 100 mg twice daily
Propranolol (IV not approved for MI in USA)	20 mg three times daily	80 mg long-acting, increasing to 160 mg once daily; maximum 240 mg daily
Timolol	5 mg twice daily	10 mg twice daily

* Contraindications: bronchial asthma, severe heart failure, systolic BP <100 mm Hg, 2nd- or 3rd-degree AV block
** Halt IV if the following events develop: heart rate <50/minute, 2nd- or 3rd-degree AV block, PR >0.24, systolic BP <95 mm Hg, marked shortness of breath, wheezes, or crackles >⅓ of the lung fields, or pulmonary capillary wedge pressure >22 mm Hg, if this parameter is being monitored.

- Lidocaine IV: Effective for the control of VT, but its prophylactic use is controversial, which is discussed later in this chapter
- Beta blockers: May be required as therapy independent of pain control to abolish ventricular arrhythmias or to prevent their occurrence, especially if these arrhythmias are catecholamine-induced. Also, these agents decrease the incidence of VF

Treatment of autonomic disturbances

- Monitoring of the cardiac rhythm is routine practice
- Autonomic disturbances are triggered by ischemic tissue as well as pain and may result in sinus tachycardia and tachyarrhythmias that are associated with inappropriate catecholamine release, thereby intensifying ischemia, which further increases release of catecholamines. Alternatively, bradycardia may occur and the associated hypotension may enlarge the infarct. This vicious cycle results in an increase in infarct size, which can culminate in progressive heart failure and shock
- Autonomic disturbances may be abolished by morphine and beta blockade
- Symptomatic bradycardias with pulse rates less than 40/minute are controlled with the judicious use of atropine (0.4 to 0.6 mg) IV given slowly every 5 to 10 minutes if needed, to a maximum of 2 mg

Caution: Do not increase the heart rate beyond 60/minute. Too rapid administration of atropine may result in sinus tachycardia in some patients and, rarely, VF may be precipitated.

NON-SPECIFIC THERAPY

- Oxygen 2 to 3 L/minute via nasal prongs is given during the first few hours until assessment is completed, then oxygen is continued if the patient is short of breath, tachypneic, or if there is proven hypoxemia. Pulmonary edema causes hypoxemia, but ventilation perfusion mismatch plays a role. Cessation of oxygen administration indicates to the patient that some improvement is occurring and helps to allay anxiety
- Diet: Fluids only for 8 to 12 hours until it is established that the infarction is uncomplicated, then light diet as tolerated with no added salt until the patient is discharged from the CCU
- A stool softener is routinely prescribed, e.g., docusate (100 to 200 mg) twice daily
- Bedrest and bedside commode for 24 hours, then washroom privileges and ambulation
- Anticoagulants: Subcutaneous heparin (5,000 to 10,000 U) every 12 hours if thrombolytic therapy is not being administered, see later discussion for the management of mural thrombi and embolism. IV heparin is advisable in patients who are expected to have slow ambulation, cardiogenic shock, and/or severe heart failure and in patients with embolization
- Mild sedation: Oxazepam (15 mg) or a similar agent at bedtime; some patients may require twice daily dosing
- Psychologic management is discussed in Chapter 4

RECOMMENDATIONS FOR BALLOON FLOTATION RIGHT HEART CATHETER

Hemodynamic monitoring is required only when information is not available clinically and is needed to assess the degree of cardiac decompensation or to guide the administration of pharmacologic agents.
Indications include

- Cardiogenic shock
- Severe heart failure
- Suspected mechanical complications: Ventricular septal or papillary muscle rupture, suspected severe mitral regurgitation, pericardial tamponade
- Diagnosis of right ventricular infarction when there is also a degree of left heart failure
- Progressive hypotension failing to respond to fluid administration in patients without pulmonary congestion

Avoid the use of the subclavian or internal jugular vein if thrombolytic therapy is required. Instead, use a brachial approach, basilic vein via a cutdown as an easily compressable vein. A strip chart recorder helps in identifying artifactual pressures and it is necessary to be able to display pressure wave forms since digital display may be misleading.

REDUCTION OF INFARCT SIZE AND MORTALITY

- Infarct-related vessel patency is best achieved with early thrombolysis using IV streptokinase, tPA, or front loading and/or combination therapy where indicated. See discussion under Thrombolytic Therapy
- Aspirin, 162 to 325 mg, enteric coated is administered daily. Aspirin administered at the onset of symptoms added to IV streptokinase was shown in ISIS-2 to cause a significant improvement in survival (see Table

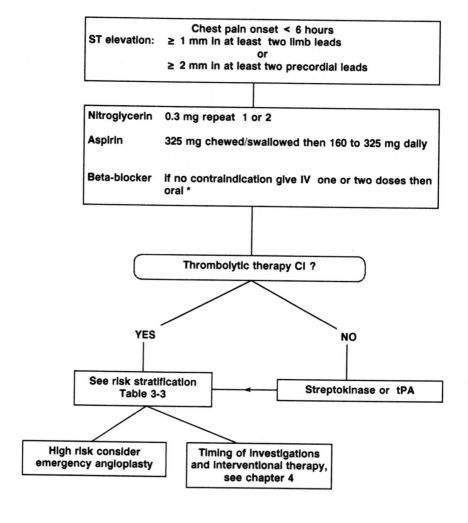

*   Table 3-4
CI =   Contraindicated
tPA = Tissue plasminogen activator

FIG. 3–1. Management of acute myocardial infarction: ECG ST elevation (probable evolution of Q wave infarct).

3–2). Aspirin reduces death by about 25% and the incidence of rein-farction by 50%. Also, aspirin is necessary following thrombolytic ther-apy to prevent reocclusion of the infarct-related vessel

• Beta blockade given at the earliest opportunity reduces infarct size and mortality. A beta blocking agent is advocated by the ACC/AHA Task Force and the early use of these agents for the management of acute MI has now been appropriately adopted worldwide. The above guidelines applied to patients with ST elevation (probable evolution to Q wave infarct) and ST depression (probable evolution to non Q wave infarct) are given in Figures 3–1 and 3–2

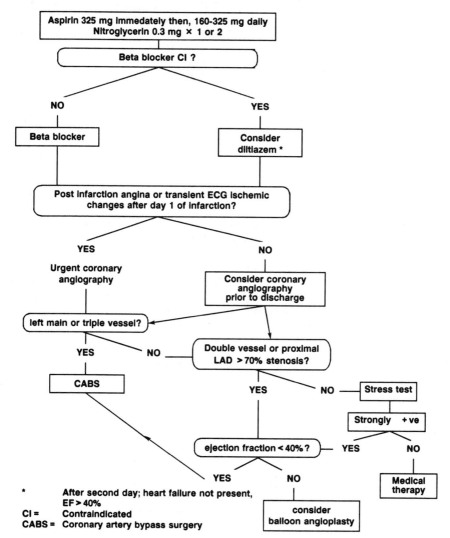

FIG. 3–2. Management of acute myocardial infarction: ECG ST depression (probable ev-olution to non Q wave infarct).

- Patients with large anterior infarcts considered high risk (Table 3–3), and in whom thrombolytic therapy is contraindicated or ischemia persists, should be considered for urgent coronary angiography and angioplasty if a highly skilled team is available (Fig. 3–1)

THROMBOLYTIC THERAPY

Optimal reduction in major events and mortality is achieved by thrombolytic therapy instituted within 3 hours of onset of symptoms (Table 3–1), and ISIS-2 confirms a salutary effect up to 4 hours (Table 3–2).

Pooled mortality results of recent trials in over 42,000 patients randomized 21,034 to thrombolytic therapy, 20,979 to placebo, was 10% in the treated group and 11.7% in the control group. These percentages account for 350 lives saved. The treatment of 21,000 patients saved 2 lives in 100 patients under age 60 treated within 6 hours from onset of symptoms, 7 lives in patients 60 to 69 years old, and 8 lives in those over age 70. Thus, the 70- to 75-year-old patients derived the greatest benefits from thrombolytic therapy.

There is currently no ideal thrombolytic agent. The three approved agents, streptokinase, tPA, and anistreplase (APSAC) are equally effective. The TIMI-1 study showed tPA and streptokinase to be equal in maximizing EF, limiting infarct size, and decreasing the incidence of events at 1-year follow-up.

Tables 3–1, 3–2, 3–5, and 3–6 give relevant results of GISSI-1, ISIS-2, GISSI-2, and ISIS-3.

No evidence of any real difference in 5-week mortality between streptokinase and tPA has been observed despite randomization of over 60,000 patients in ISIS-3 and GISSI-2. Assessment of global and regional left ventricular function 3 weeks after a first infarction indicates similar effects for streptokinase and tPA. However, tPA causes a minimal but significantly higher incidence of intracranial bleed compared to streptokinase (Fig. 3–3); tPA must be used in conjunction with IV heparin to achieve excellent

TABLE 3–5. TIMING OF THROMBOLYTIC THERAPY ON EVENTS, MORTALITY AND EFFECT OF HEPARIN* IN GISSI-2

HOURS	tPA	SK	HEPARIN	NO HEPARIN	TOTAL EVENTS**
≤3 Events	973/4449 21.9%	962/4481 21.5%			1935/8930 = 21.7
3–6 Events	454/1729 26.3%	430/1711 25.1%			884/3440 = 25.7
Deaths	556/6182 9%	536/6199 8.6%	518/6175 8.3%	574/6206 9.3%	

Modified from: Lancet, *336*:65, 1990
* Subcutaneous
** Death plus heart failure beyond 4 days, plus extensive left ventricular damage in the absence of heart failure; treatment <3 hours, maximum benefit

TABLE 3-6. EFFECTS OF ALLOCATED TREATMENT ON DEATHS IN DAYS 0–35 AMONG (i) ALL PATIENTS AND (ii) PATIENTS PRESENTING WITHIN 0–6 H WITH ST ELEVATION

	FIBRINOLYTIC COMPARISONS			Difference %SK–%tPA		Difference %SK–%APSAC	
	SK	tPA	APSAC	%	SD	%	SD
(i) All patients	13 780	13 746	13 773				
Any	1455 (10.6%)	1418 (10.3%)	1448 (10.5%)	0.24	0.37	0.05	0.37
(a) Timing							
Day 0–1	699 (5.1%)	649 (4.7%)	700 (5.1%)	0.35	0.26	−0.01	0.26
Day 2–7	357 (2.6%)	415 (3.0%)	378 (2.7%)	−0.43	0.20*	−0.15	0.19
Day 8–35	399 (2.9%)	354 (2.6%)	370 (2.7%)	0.32	0.20	0.21	0.20
(b) Antithrombotic allocation							
Aspirin plus sc heparin	726 (10.5%)	684 (10.0%)	722 (10.5%)	0.58	0.52	0.06	0.52
Aspirin alone	729 (10.6%)	734 (10.7%)	726 (10.6%)	−0.09	0.53	0.03	0.52
(ii) 0–6 h, ST elevation	8643	8571	8622				
Any	861 (10.0%)	822 (9.6%)	855 (9.9%)	0.37	0.45	0.05	0.46
(a) Timing							
Day 0–1	421 (4.9%)	389 (4.5%)	408 (4.7%)	0.33	0.32	0.14	0.33
Day 2–7	201 (2.3%)	236 (2.8%)	218 (2.5%)	−0.43	0.24	−0.20	0.23
Day 8–35	239 (2.8%)	197 (2.3%)	229 (2.7%)	0.47	0.24	0.11	0.25
(b) Antithrombotic allocation							
Aspirin plus sc heparin	425 (9.8%)	389 (9.1%)	427 (9.9%)	0.69	0.63	−0.13	0.64
Aspirin alone	436 (10.2%)	433 (10.1%)	428 (9.9%)	0.05	0.65	0.22	0.65

* 2p < 0.05.

From: ISIS-3: A randomised comparison of streptokinase vs. tissue plasminogen activator vs. anistreplase and of aspirin plus heparin vs. aspirin alone among 41,299 cases of suspected acute myocardial infarction. Lancet, 339:759, 1992.

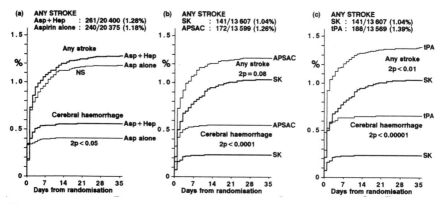

FIG. 3–3. Cumulative percentage with any stroke (upper lines) and with (definite or probable) cerebral hemorrhage in hospital up to day 35 or prior discharge. (a) All patients allocated aspirin plus heparin (thicker line) vs. all allocated aspirin alone; (b) all patients allocated streptokinase (SK) (thicker line) vs. all allocated APSAC; (c) all patients allocated SK vs. all allocated tPA. From: ISIS-3: A randomised comparison of streptokinase vs. tissue plasminogen activator vs. anistreplase and of aspirin plus heparin vs. aspirin alone among 41,299 cases of suspected acute myocardial infarction. Lancet, *339*:757, 1992.

late patency rates. This combination, however, increases the risk of intra-cerebral bleed. The slightly better survival rates observed with the combination of streptokinase, aspirin, and IV heparin versus streptokinase, aspirin, and subcutaneous heparin are offset by a slight increase in intra-cranial bleed. Indeed, most of this excess risk could be caused by IV heparin therapy. The ISIS-3 data suggest that patients receiving IV heparin gained no survival benefit but faced a doubling of the stroke risk regardless of which thrombolytic agent they were taking.

Because ISIS-2, GISSI-2, and ISIS-3 results indicate that the combination of streptokinase and aspirin is easy to administer and provides good results at low risk and low cost, this combination enjoys the status of standard therapy worldwide, except in the United States, where the combination of tPA and IV heparin is often administered. The results of the Global Utilization of Streptokinase and tPA for Occluded Coronary Arteries (GUSTO) study should provide some solution to the controversies and should define the role of IV heparin.

It must be reemphasized that although ISIS-3 showed that net clinical outcomes were the same with the streptokinase subcutaneous heparin combination and tPA plus subcutaneous heparin, controversy persists because it is claimed that ISIS-3 and GISSI-2 did not evaluate the "best" tPA regimen. In these studies, tPA was given for the standard period over 3 hours, in accordance with the manufacturers product monograph and prior successful clinical trials, but subcutaneous heparin was used in the majority of patients; IV heparin was started too late in the few patients given this combination. It is accepted that infarct vessel patency attained by tPA is maximized by IV heparin and reocclusion is decreased by IV heparin used for up to 6 days following tPA infusion. Front-loading and combination therapy holds promise, but more information is needed about the effects of variation and methods of administration of thrombolytic agents to obtain maximum salutary effects.

INDICATIONS FOR THROMBOLYTIC THERAPY

Guidelines for the administration of thrombolytic therapy are shown in Figure 3–4.

• Patients, 75 years old or under, seen within 6 hours of onset of symptoms with clinical and ECG diagnoses consistent with acute MI (with at least 2 mm ST elevation in one or more precordial leads or at least 1 mm ST elevation in two or more limb leads) are candidates for thrombolytic therapy

PROBABLE INDICATIONS

• Patients over age 75 in good general health should not be excluded if seen within 6 hours of pain onset where the impending infarction is large or extensive and there is no contraindication to thrombolytic therapy (Fig. 3–4). ISIS-3 indicated that patients over age 75 showed the greatest benefits. In patients under age 65, aged 65 to 76, and aged 75 to 85, in-hospital mortality was approximately 8, 18, and 30%, and with thrombolytic therapy, 6, 16, and 26%, respectively. However, thrombolytic therapy should be used with great caution in patients over age 80 because most studies indicate increased risk of major bleeding in this subset of patients. In one study, streptokinase caused a twofold increased risk of major hemorrhage that resulted in a mortality of 17% in patients over age 75 and 1% in those under age 75. It must be reemphasized that IV heparin and a thrombolytic agent in patients over age 80 should be used with caution until further large, randomized studies show proven benefit at low risk in these patients. When thrombolytic therapy is considered necessary in healthy patients over age 80 with large infarcts seen within 6 hours, the combination of aspirin and the cautious use of streptokinase is advisable, preferably without heparin use

• Patients with new left bundle branch block seen within 6 hours of onset of chest pain. This subset represents a high risk group and has been shown to gain beneficial results in the ISIS-3 study

• Patients with new right bundle branch block, proven acute infarction, associated with heart failure

• Patients seen within 6 to 12 hours from onset of symptoms with evidence of ongoing ischemia: Pain still present or stuttering episodes in the presence of continuing elevation of ST segments and CK and CK-MB elevation. Caution is required in patients seen between 6 and 12 hours because late reperfusion appears to increase the risk of myocardial rupture and it is necessary to weigh the risks involved

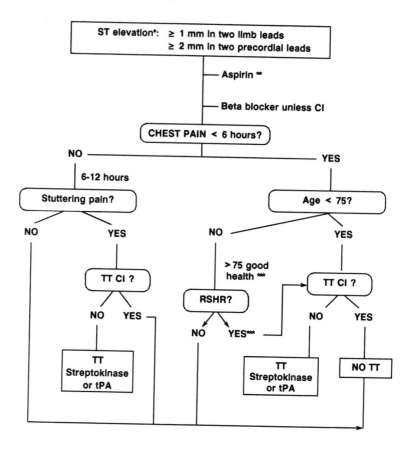

*	Probable Q wave infarct
**	Aspirin 160-325 mg, chewed/swallowed plus beta blocker IV or oral (see text)
CI =	Contraindicated
*** =	ACC/AHA task force report: J Am Coll Cardiol 16:269, 1990
RSHR =	Risk stratification, high risk (Table 3-3)
tPA =	Tissue plasminogen activator

FIG. 3–4. Guidelines for thrombolytic therapy.

CONTRAINDICATIONS TO THROMBOLYTIC THERAPY

Absolute contraindications include

- Active internal bleeding within the prior weeks
- Suspected aortic dissection
- Recent head injury or cerebral neoplasm
- Recent trauma, major surgery within 6 weeks
- Recent prolonged or clearly traumatic CPR
- History of cerebrovascular accident known to be hemorrhagic

- Non-hemorrhagic cerebrovascular accident within 2 months is a contraindication to streptokinase. The Activase product monograph lists a history of cerebrovascular accident as a contraindication
- Diabetic retinopathy or other ophthalmic hemorrhagic lesion
- Allergy to streptokinase or anistreplase or therapy with either drug from 5 days to 1 year previously (but not a contraindication to tPA)
- Acute pancreatitis
- Pregnancy
- Severe hypertension, blood pressure greater than 200/110 mm Hg

Relative contraindications

- Minor trauma or surgery beyond 2 weeks with low risk of bleeding
- Known bleeding diathesis or current use of anticoagulants
- Aneurysms
- Active peptic ulcer without bleeding, patient on medications
- History of severe hypertension under drug treatment; systolic greater than 180 mm Hg, diastolic greater than 110 mm Hg
- Significant liver dysfunction or esophageal varices
- Underlying malignancy
- Severe anemia
- Local tendency to bleeding (e.g., recent translumbar arteriography)
- Patients over age 75. (Caution is necessary because bleeding complications are common). However, patients over age 80 in robust health should receive thrombolytic therapy if they present with an anterior infarct, large infarction, or left bundle branch block
- Elderly patients who are confused, lethargic, or agitated

Complications of thrombolytic therapy include the following

- Bleeding, especially in patients requiring invasive procedures; intracranial bleeding reportedly occurs in 0.1 to 1.4% and is more common in patients over age 70
- Rarely myocardial and splenic rupture, aortic dissection, cholesterol embolization
- Rare hypotension and allergic reaction with streptokinase or anistreplase

Streptokinase
(Streptase, Kabikinase)

Action. Streptokinase combines with plasminogen to form plasminogen activator complex. The complex converts free plasminogen to plasmin, which causes fibrinogenolysis and independent lysis of fibrin (Fig. 3–5). Streptokinase also causes activation of fibrin-bound plasminogen; thus, two independent actions occur. The activator complex has a half-life of about 85 minutes, the extensive coagulation defect begins rapidly after administration, remains intense for about 4 to 8 hours, and dwindles over the following 36 to 48 hours.

About 65% coronary reperfusion rate is observed when 1.5 million units of the drug are given within 3 hours of onset of symptoms of infarction but a patency rate of 82% has been reported with a 3 million unit dose.

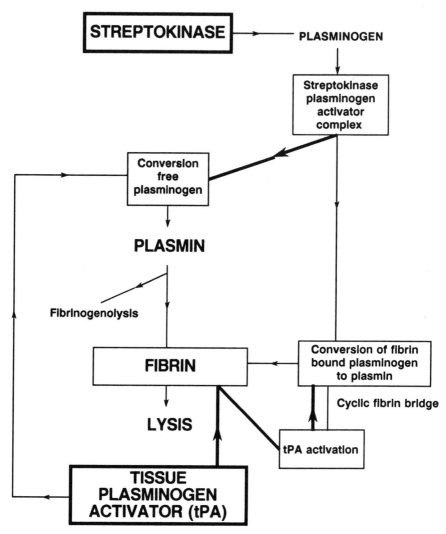

FIG. 3–5. Thrombolytic agents' mechanism of action.

The Intravenous Streptokinase in Acute Myocardial Infarction (ISAM) Trial has indicated that streptokinase administered within 6 hours of symptoms improved left ventricular function for up to 3 years in patients with anterior but not inferior infarction.

Dosage: See Table 3–7.

Adverse effects. Allergic reactions are seen in about 2% of patients. Edema, bronchospasm, angioneurotic edema, anaphylaxis reported in 0.1 to 0.5% with apparently no fatalities. Hypotension in less than 4%, for-

TABLE 3–7. DOSAGE OF THROMBOLYTIC AGENTS	
DRUG	**DOSAGE**
Streptokinase	1.5 million U in 100 ml 0.9% saline IV infusion over 30 to 60 minutes
Anistreplase (APSAC)	30 U in 5 ml sterile water or saline by slow IV bolus over 2 to 5 minutes
tPA (alteplase) (Manufacturer's dosage; product monograph 1990 to 1992)	6–10 mg IV bolus over 1–2 minutes then 50 mg IV infusion over 1 hour, 20 mg IV infusion over 2nd hour, 20 mg IV infusion over 3rd hour; 100 mg total dose
tPA (Clinical trial dosage 1991–92)	15 mg bolus 0.75 mg/kg over 30 minutes (not >50 mg) 0.50 mg/kg over 60 minutes (not >35 mg) Total dose ≤100 mg

tunately, does not appear to worsen if hypotension already exists. Splenic rupture and cardiac tamponade with shock have been reported. Also, there is occasionally a late transient renal effect with proteinuria. Management of internal bleeding complication requires the use of blood products, clotting factors, and antaguosin, a proteinase inhibitor (dosage: 200,000 to 1 million KIU IV, followed by 50,000 KIU per hour until bleeding is arrested).

Anistreplase
(Eminase)

Anisoylated Plasminogen-Streptokinase Activator Complex (APSAC) is a 1:1 molecular combination of plasminogen and streptokinase with a catalytic center protected by a chemical group.

Anistreplase is activated in the bloodstream; de-acylation to the active complex begins immediately and continues at a constant rate with a half-life of about 90 minutes. An advantage over streptokinase is the ease of administration by slow IV bolus. The drug produces about a 60% patency rate in about 40 minute with persistence of activity for 4 to 6 hours. This agent is as effective as streptokinase or tPA in achieving vessel patency and this effect is enhanced by routine aspirin use. Concomitant heparin therapy is not advisable.

ISIS-3 reportedly indicates that concomitant heparin therapy is not advisable because no significant improvement in survival occurs and the risk of cerebral hemorrhage is increased.

Dosage: See Table 3–7.

Tissue Plasminogen Activator
(tPA; Activase)

Tissue type plasminogen activator is the physiologic activator of plasminogen but has a higher affinity for fibrin-bound plasminogen. However, tPA's specificity for fibrin-bound plasminogen is relative and dose dependent. Activation of free plasminogen occurs with increasing dosage and blood levels of tPA (Fig. 3–5). Thus, bleeding complications are similar to streptokinase.

Because tPA therapy results in a significantly higher vessel patency rate than streptokinase and tPA was used in ISIS-3 without the necessary combination with IV heparin for 6 days, further randomized studies using different heparin regimens are in progress. The net clinical outcome (total death plus stroke) in ISIS-3 was similar (11.1%) in the streptokinase versus the tPA treated group. As outlined earlier, the GUSTO trial may help resolve some controversies. Also, the role of tPA front-loading of streptokinase and tPA with IV heparin combination with urokinase must be defined by large randomized trials; small studies indicate excellent patency rates and decreased reocclusion rates with the aforementioned front-loaded regimens. tPA has a rapid disappearance rate with a half-life of approximately 8 minutes; thus, it was initially believed that a prolonged IV infusion over 3 hours was necessary to achieve patency and this timing is still outlined in the product monograph. A dose of up to 100 mg over 90 minutes is being used in ongoing clinical trials. Plasma clearance is decreased with hepatic dysfunction and the drug is not advisable in patients who have hepatic disease.

Dosage: See Table 3–7.

Adverse effects. These are essentially the same as listed under streptokinase, except that allergic reactions do not occur.

BETA BLOCKER THERAPY

Acute coronary occlusion producing anteroseptal or anterior MI is often associated with sinus tachycardia. Necrotic tissue is surrounded for a time by a zone of severe myocardial ischemia and injury that causes pain. Both ischemia and pain initiate catecholamine release, and the vicious circle is perpetuated. During the early phase of infarction, the amount of myocardial damage is not fixed and a dynamic process is usually in evolution.

Beta blockers have a proven beneficial effect when relieving pain, ischemia, and injury current during the early phase of acute MI. Decreased mortality, modest reduction in infarct size, and decrease in the reinfarction rates have been documented in patients given IV beta blockers, followed by oral therapy from day 1 and for 30 to 90 days, as well as up to 2 years post infarction. The early reduction in mortality and infarction rates have been modest, but sufficiently significant to warrant early beta blocker therapy to all patients with anterior or anteroseptal infarcts, especially in those with sinus tachycardia, provided that the systolic blood pressure is greater than 100 mm Hg and there is no contraindication to beta blockade. If adverse effects are feared, esmolol IV is advisable since its action dissipates in about 10 minutes. However, in the United States, presently only metoprolol is approved for IV use during acute MI.

Dosage: See Table 3–4.

SALUTARY EFFECTS IN ACUTE MYOCARDIAL INFARCTION

The merits of beta-adrenergic blockade in ischemic syndromes are given in Figure 2–7.

- Decrease in heart rate prolongs the diastolic interval during which coronary perfusion normally occurs. Thus, an increase in blood flow may ensue to ischemic areas of myocardium. Necrotic tissue is not capable of salvage, but the area subject to infarction may remain ischemic for several hours, and increased perfusion to ischemic areas may limit the ultimate size of infarction
- Sinus tachycardia causes increased oxygen demand and can shift the balance in ischemic tissue toward necrosis; sinus tachycardia decreases VF threshold. Beta blockers relieve sinus tachycardia and associated hypertension and increase VF threshold; some trials showed reduction in the incidence of VF
- Beta blockers decrease phase 4 depolarization and thus suppress arrhythmias that may arise in ischemic tissue, especially when initiated by catecholamines
- Decrease in myocardial contractility decreases oxygen requirement
- Decrease in stress on infarcting tissue by the remaining myocardium appears to be responsible for the modest but important decrease in the incidence of early myocardial rupture due to acute infarction
- In patients given thrombolytics, there is currently no confirmation of experimental findings that viability of ischemic myocardium is prolonged. However, beta blockers greatly reduce the incidence of post-thrombolytic ischemic events in patients
- Where there is some residual patency of the infarcted-related artery, beta blockers do exert a strong anti-ischemic effect and will reduce infarct size; in this group of patients, perhaps equivalent to non Q wave infarction, beta blockers have been demonstrated to have a major impact on pain and serious events

Clinical trials have not adequately tested the use of beta blockers during the first 3 hours of onset of symptoms. The Metroprolol in Acute MI (MIAMI) trial is often quoted as showing a lack of effectiveness of early beta blocker use in reducing mortality. However, the mean treatment time was 11 hours. In ISIS-1, 80% of patients were treated up to 8 hours and less than 30% within 4 hours of onset, resulting in a 15% decrease in cardiovascular mortality with significant prevention of early myocardial rupture. Beta blockers were given to 720 patients at about 3 to 4 hours after onset of symptoms in TIMI II-B and resulted in a 47% decrease in the incidence of reinfarction in 6 days; also, the incidence of recurrent chest pain was significantly decreased. However, a decrease in mortality and myocardial rupture was not observed in TIMI II, probably due to the small number of patients studied, resulting in a type II error. Pooled trial results with the use of beta blockade covering mainly 4 to 6 hours from onset of symptoms indicate a 23% decrease in mortality occurring on day 1, then no significant decrease during the next few weeks.

Approximately 100 patients under age 70 must be treated with beta blockers within 6 hours of onset to save two lives. It must be emphasized that thrombolytic therapy produces similar results; 100 patients under age 70 must be treated with streptokinase in less than 6 hours to save two lives (see Table 3–1). Early beta blocker and thrombolytic therapy is complementary.

The ACC/AHA Task Force recommends beta blocker IV therapy to be given at the same time as aspirin, as soon as the diagnosis of acute MI is entertained. This is especially important in patients with anteroseptal and anterior myocardial infarction with a heart rate greater than 100 and/or systolic blood pressure greater than 110 mm Hg, where no contraindication to beta blockade exists. In this subset, beta blockers should be given in the emergency room at the same time as aspirin and sublingual nitroglycerin. No harm can ensue if the patient is not later selected for thrombolytic therapy. The concomitant use with a thrombolytic agent has been documented in TIMI II-B and other trials as safe and worthwhile. Beta blocker therapy from day 7 for 2 years is expected to save three lives annually per 100 treated (see Chapter 4).

INDICATIONS FOR BETA BLOCKERS

Early IV followed by oral beta blocker therapy should be strongly considered for all patients presenting with definite or probable acute infarction, in whom contraindications do not exist.

These agents are particularly strongly indicated in the following situations

- Sinus tachycardia unassociated with hypotension or clinically apparent heart failure
- Rapid ventricular response to atrial fibrillation or flutter
- Administration of thrombolytic agents: To prevent arrhythmias and/or ischemia and improve survival
- Recurrent ischemic pain
- Moderate impairment of left ventricular function with frequent or complex ventricular ectopy after the first week post infarction

NITROGLYCERIN

In patients with anterior infarction, there is evidence to suggest that IV nitroglycerin causes a slight decrease in mortality. The ACC/AHA Task Force considers the data inadequate to recommend the routine use of IV nitroglycerin in patients with uncomplicated acute myocardial infarction.

IV nitroglycerin is not recommended in patients with uncomplicated myocardial infarction. Cutaneous preparations have a role in some patients without hypotension for the relief of chest discomfort.

Indications

- Relief of chest pain unresponsive to morphine and beta blockers
- Stuttering pattern of pain indicating continued ischemia

- Moderate to severe heart failure or pulmonary edema complicating acute MI and pulmonary capillary wedge pressure greater than 20 mm Hg

Contraindications

- Hypovolemia
- Inferior infarction. Used cautiously only when needed to manage post infarction angina and/or pulmonary edema, since hypotension may be precipitated
- Right ventricular infarction
- Cardiac tamponade
- Significant hypoxemia. IV nitroglycerin may accentuate hypoxemia by increasing ventilation perfusion mismatch

Adverse effects. These include worsening of hypoxemia and severe hypotension that may increase ischemia. Preload reduction may cause hypotension. Rarely, nitrates precipitate bradycardia and hypotension responsive to atropine. Oral, cutaneous, and other nitrates are discussed further in Chapter 2.

Dosage: See Infusion Pump Chart, Figure 2–9. Commence with a 5 μg bolus injection then increase the dose by 5 to 10 μg/minute every 5 or 10 minutes to abolish chest pain and/or to achieve a mean arterial pressure decrease of 10% and a maximal decrease of 20% in hypertensive patients. The systolic blood pressure must not be allowed to fall under 95 mm Hg or diastolic less than 60 mm Hg. Heart rate should be maintained less than 110/minute. Nitrate tolerance develops after about 48 hours use of IV nitroglycerin, but in unstable patients, the dose is titrated up as required rather than leaving a nitrate-free interval.

Sublingual, oral, or transdermal nitrates are not advisable in the unstable patient since it is not possible to titrate their effects.

LIDOCAINE

In the first 24 to 48 hours, ventricular premature contractions (VPCs) and short runs of VT bear little relation to the occurrence of VF. R on T are an exception but usually appear less than 2 minutes before VF. Lidocaine is far from completely effective in preventing VF, and inexperienced staff are often tempted quite unnecessarily to push the dose to toxic levels to "control" VPCs, which are, in the main, quite harmless.

Probable indications

- Frequent VPCs, causing hemodynamic disturbance in the absence of bradycardia where atropine is advisable
- Sustained VT (see Fig. 6–4)
- Following VT occurring in the first 24 hours of infarction, lidocaine is given for 48 hours
- Post VF or for repetitive VF

Old indications, no longer accepted worldwide but still adopted in some CCUs in the United States, and included by the ACC/AHA Task Force 1990 as accepted indications, include

- Frequent VPCs greater than 6/minute in the presence of sinus tachycardia associated with anterior infarction, if needed after the judicious use of a short-acting beta blocker (esmolol or metoprolol)
- Multiform VPCs
- R on T or closely coupled VPCs
- Runs of three or more VPCs, nonsustained VT

Recent trials and meta-analysis suggest that lidocaine may actually increase mortality, and the use of lidocaine in these categories of patients is expected to dwindle throughout the United States. Contraindications include

- Sinoatrial dysfunction, which may precipitate sinus arrest
- Atrioventricular block, all grades, which can cause asystole
- Patients recovering from asystole
- Idioventricular rhythm
- Severe heart failure
- Porphyria
- Relative contraindications include sinus bradycardia

The prophylactic use of lidocaine in acute MI remains controversial in the United States and its widespread use has dwindled. The ACC/AHA Task Force 1990 states that the drug is recommended but remains controversial. The Task Force points out that the adverse effects of prophylactic lidocaine offset any benefit. The drug is associated with an increase in the occurrence of asystole. In the early hours of infarction, VF occurs in approximately 5% of patients and many patients must be treated to prevent some episodes of VF. A meta analysis of 14 randomized trials indicate that lidocaine reduced the incidence of ventricular fibrillation 33% without a decrease in mortality.

Indications for prophylactic lidocaine

- Some departments in the United States continue to advocate prophylactic lidocaine in patients under age 65 without previous heart failure seen within the first 6 hours of infarction
- In areas where facilities for monitoring cardiac rhythm and/or for defibrillation are lacking or inadequate, the drug has a role. In heavily monitored units, lidocaine is unnecessary, and the cost is not justified

Dosage: Bolus IV 1.0 to 1.5 mg/kg, 75 to 100 mg over 5 minutes, during which time a continuous infusion of 2 mg/min. for a 70- to 80-kg patient under age 70 is commenced (see Table 3–8). An additional bolus of 50% of the original amount given at 10 minutes after the first bolus prevents a dip in plasma level below the therapeutic range, which commonly occurs between 20 and 60 minutes after starting the infusion. In the elderly, bolus 0.75 mg/kg, then if needed, 25 to 30 mg IV bolus. Do not allow a time lapse of minutes between the bolus and commencement of the infusion, as in-

TABLE 3-8. LIDOCAINE (LIGNOCAINE) DOSAGE		
	NORMAL DOSAGE E.G.: 60–90 KG PATIENT	**HALVE DOSE: ELDERLY, CHF, SHOCK, HEPATIC DYSFUNCTION, CIMETIDINE, SOME BETA BLOCKERS, HALOTHANE**
1st IV Bolus	1.5 mg/kg	0.75 mg/kg
usually	100 mg	50 mg
2nd Bolus	0.75 mg/kg	0.5 mg/kg
usually	50 mg	25 to 30 mg
Concomitant infusion	2 to 4 mg/min	1 to 2 mg/minute
	(50 μg/kg/min)	(20 μg/kg/min)

Therapeutic level 1.5 to 5 μg/ml, 1.5 to 5 mg/L, 6 to 26 μmol/L
Seizures: levels >6 mg/L
* Hepatic metabolized beta blockers: propranolol, metoprolol

TABLE 3-9. WARNINGS TO AVOID LIDOCAINE (LIGNOCAINE) TOXICITY
1. Reduce bolus dose and infusion rate in the elderly (over age 70)
2. Determine the dose utilizing lean body weight
3. Decrease the dose in heart failure, hypotension, cardiogenic shock
4. Decrease dosage with hepatic dysfunction or concomitant use of cimetidine, propranolol, or drugs that decrease hepatic blood flow or metabolism
5. Previous seizure activity or central nervous system disease
6. Determine blood levels if infusion rates are high (≥4 mg/ml/min) or neurologic adverse effects

adequate blood levels may ensue. Halve the dose in patients with heart failure, shock, hepatic dysfunction, or concomitant use of a hepatic metabolized beta blocker or cimetidine (see Table 3–9).

If frequent multiform ventricular ectopy persists, resulting in hemodynamic disturbance, an additional bolus, 0.5 to 1 mg/kg, is given every 10 minutes for two or three doses if deemed necessary, and the infusion rate is increased to 3 mg/minute. Reevaluate the clinical situation including serum potassium, magnesium, presence of bradycardia or sinus tachycardia, and contraindications, and factors that increase lidocaine toxicity prior to increasing the rate to a maximum 4 mg/min for a patient less than 200 lbs (90 kg).

Adverse effects. The incidence of asystole appears to be increased by lidocaine use. Confusion, seizures, drowsiness, dizziness, lips or tongue numbness, slurred speech, muscle twitching, double vision, tremor, altered consciousness, respiratory depression or arrest, complete heart block in patients with impaired atrioventricular conduction, hypotension due to peripheral vasodilatation.

NON Q WAVE INFARCTION

The term "non Q wave infarction" is often used to embrace non-transmural infarction and the term "Q wave infarction" to denote transmural infarction. Because of anatomical inconsistencies, however, the use of the terms "transmural" and "non-transmural" are no longer recommended. The mortality and reinfarction rates of non Q wave and Q wave infarctions are given in Table 3–3 and 4–2. It is established that patients with non Q wave infarction represent a group at high risk for the occurrence of reinfarction within 3 months of hospital discharge.

Timolol has been shown to decrease mortality in patients with non Q wave infarction. All patients with non Q wave infarction should be treated with aspirin and a beta blocker if no contraindication exists to beta blockade. Patients who have good left ventricular function with an ejection fraction greater than 40% and in whom beta blockers are contraindicated, should receive diltiazem in addition to aspirin (Fig. 3–2). Patients with non Q wave infarction and post infarction angina or those who continue to have transient ischemic ECG changes from day 2 onward require urgent coronary angiography with a view to coronary angioplasty or bypass surgery.

Patients with uncomplicated non Q wave infarction are discharged on aspirin, a beta blocker, and/or diltiazem and with coronary angiography done within 4 weeks or earlier, depending on departmental preferences.

Exercise stress testing is not essential since virtually all patients with non Q wave infarction should be managed as for unstable angina with fairly urgent coronary angiography and assignment to coronary angioplasty or bypass surgery.

It is commonly stated that propranolol in the BHAT did not reduce the incidence of reinfarction or mortality in patients with non Q wave infarction. However, in that study, the number of patients with non Q wave infarction was small. Also, the salutary effects of propranolol are blunted by smoking, and this parameter was not taken into consideration in the study design or the interpretation of the results.

Beta blockers remain first-line drug therapy along with aspirin in the management of non Q wave infarction up to the moment of interventional therapy.

CALCIUM ANTAGONISTS

CALCIUM ANTAGONISTS FOR NON Q WAVE INFARCTION

In a very small study of 288 post-infarction patients treated with diltiazem, 11 patients died, as opposed to nine patients in the placebo group; diltiazem decreased infarction rates at 2 weeks. This small, short-term study has been used to advance the claim that diltiazem is the drug of choice in the management of non Q wave infarction. Physicians have extended the drug's use to other ischemic syndromes with the hope that the drug will prevent reinfarction, but without bearing in mind that the drug does not significantly decrease the cardiac death rate.

A second large, well-run study of 2,466 post-infarction patients treated with diltiazem showed an increase in total mortality due to diltiazem in patients with left ventricular dysfunction. Thus, diltiazem is not recommended in acute myocardial infarction, Q wave or non Q wave, if signs of left ventricular dysfunction are present or if the ejection fraction is less than 40% (Fig. 3–2). There was a trend in favor of a decrease in total events (death and/or reinfarction) in the small number of patients with non Q wave infarction treated for 1 year with diltiazem, but the evidence from this overall negative study is not sound enough to recommend diltiazem to all patients with non Q wave infarction. In the absence of ongoing chest pain, diltiazem has an uncertain role in the management of non Q wave infarction in patients with good left ventricular function, who are unable to take a beta blocking drug and in whom further interventional therapy in the form of angioplasty or bypass surgery is contraindicated because of underlying ill health or age (see Chapter 4).

OTHER INDICATIONS FOR CALCIUM ANTAGONISTS

It is clear that calcium antagonists have no role in the routine management of acute MI. Meta analysis indicates that this group of drugs does not significantly reduce infarct size, infarction rates, or mortality in patients with acute MI.

Nifedipine used without a beta blocking drug in patients with unstable angina may increase chest pain and shows no beneficial trend in mortality. Dihydropyridines should be avoided in patients with acute MI since they may increase heart rate and vasodilatation may cause a fall in blood pressure. Also, calcium antagonists may decrease blood pressure during the early hours of infarction. A decrease in blood pressure may contraindicate the use of lifesaving medications: beta blockers, thrombolytic agents, IV nitroglycerin, and/or ACE inhibitors.

Verapamil should not be used in patients with acute MI because of its negative inotropic effect and strong propensity to precipitate heart failure, sinus arrest, or asystole. The drug is advisable in selected patients with supraventricular tachycardia or atrial fibrillation with an uncontrolled ventricular response after a trial of beta blockers or digoxin in the absence of heart failure.

Diltiazem is not indicated in acute MI since it increases mortality in patients who manifest left ventricular dysfunction or in those with an ejection fraction less than 40%. Calcium antagonists are not advisable in patients with acute MI and concomitant, severe chronic obstructive pulmonary disease since these agents may increase hypoxemia.

BIBLIOGRAPHY

AIMS Trial Study Group: Long-term effects of intravenous anistreplase in acute myocardial infarction: Final report of the AIMS study. Lancet, *335*:427, 1990.

Anderson JL, Sherman G, Sorensen SG, et al.: Multicenter patency trial of intravenous anistreplase compared with streptokinase in acute myocardial infarction. Circulation, *83*:126, 1991.

Baim DS, Diver DJ, Feit F, et al.: Coronary angioplasty performed within the thrombolysis in myocardial infarction II study. Circulation, *85*:93, 1992.

Bassand J-P, Cassagnes J, Machecourt J, et al.: Comparative effects of APSAC and rt-PA on infarct size and left ventricular function in acute myocardial infarction. Circulation, *84*:1107, 1991.

Bates ER, Topol EJ: Limitations of thrombolytic therapy for acute myocardial infarction complicated by congestive heart failure and cardiogenic shock. J Am Coll Cardiol, *18*:1077, 1991.

Becker RC, Carrao JM, Harrington R, et al.: Recombinant tissue-type plasminogen activator: Current concepts and guidelines for clinical use in acute myocardial infarction. Part 1. Am Heart J, *121*:220, 1991.

Berger PB, Ryan TJ: Inferior myocardial infarction. Circulation, *81*:401, 1990.

Califf RM, Topol EJ, Stack RS, et al.: Evaluation of combination thrombolytic therapy and timing of cardiac catheterization in acute myocardial infarction - Phase 5 randomized trial. Circulation, *83*:1543, 1991.

Chesebro JH, Fuster V: Dynamic thrombosis and thrombolysis. Circulation, *83*:1815, 1991.

Clark RJ, Mayo G, Fitzgerald GA, et al.: Combined administration of aspirin and a specific thrombin inhibitor in man. Circulation, *83*:1510, 1991.

Cross DB, Ashton NG, Norris RM: Comparison of the effects of streptokinase and tissue plasminogen activator on regional wall motion after first myocardial infarction: Analysis by the centerline method with correction for area at risk. J Am Coll Cardiol, *17*:1039, 1991.

De Jaegere PP, Arnold AA, Balk AH, et al.: Intracranial hemorrhage in association with thrombolytic therapy. Incidence and clinical predictive factors. J Am Coll Cardiol, *19*:289, 1992.

Dreifus LS, Fisch C, Griffin JC, et al.: Guidelines for implantation of cardiac pacemakers and antiarrhythmia devices. Circulation, *84*:455, 1991.

Ellis SG, Van de Werf F, Ribeiro-daSilva E, et al.: Present status of rescue coronary angioplasty: Current polarization of opinion and randomized trials. J Am Coll Cardiol, *19*:681, 1992.

Ferlinz J: Acute myocardial infarction: Does the lack of Q waves help or hinder? J Am Coll Cardiol, *15*:1208, 1990.

Fuster V, Badimon L, Badimon JJ, et al.: The pathogenesis of coronary artery disease and the acute coronary syndromes. In Mechanisms of Disease. Edited by F.H. Epstein. N Engl J Med, *326*:310, 1992.

Ganz W: The quest for the ideal reperfusion strategy continues. Circulation, *83*:1818, 1991.

Grines CL, Nissen SE, Booth DC, et al.: A prospective, randomized trial comparing combination half-dose tissue-type plasminogen activator and streptokinase with full-dose tissue-type plasminogen activator. Circulation, *84*:540, 1991.

Gruppo Italiano per lo Studio della Streptochinasi Nell 'Infarto Miocardico (GISSI): Effectiveness of intravenous thrombolytic treatment in acute myocardial infarction. Lancet, *1*:397, 1986.

Gruppo Italiano per lo Studio della Sopravvivenza Nell 'Infarto Miocardico (GISSI-2): A factorial randomised trial of alteplase versus streptokinase and heparin versus no heparin among 12,490 patients with acute myocardial infarction. Lancet, *336*:65, 1990.

Gunnar RM: Response to ACC/AHA subcommittee to develop guidelines for the early management of patients with acute myocardial infarction. J Am Coll Cardiol, *17*:1237, 1991.

Gurwitz JH, Goldberg RJ, Gore JM: Coronary thrombolysis for the elderly? JAMA, *265*:1720, 1991.

Held PH, Teo KK, Yusuf S: Effects of tissue-type plasminogen activator and anisoylated plasminogen streptokinase activator complex on mortality in acute myocardial infarction. Circulation, *82*:1668, 1990.

Hogg KJ, Gemmill JD, Burns JMA, et al.: Angiographic patency study of anistreplase versus streptokinase in acute myocardial infarction. Lancet, *335*:254, 1990.

Honan MB, Harrell FE, Reimer KA, et al.: Cardiac rupture, mortality and the timing of thrombolytic therapy: A meta-analysis. J Am Coll Cardiol, *16*:359, 1990.

ISIS-2 (Second international study of infarct survival) Collaborative Group: Randomised trial of intravenous streptokinase, oral aspirin, both, or neither among 17,187 cases of suspected acute myocardial infarction: ISIS-2. Lancet, *2*:350, 1988.

ISIS-3 (Third International Study of Infarct Survival) Collaborative Group: A randomised comparison of streptokinase vs. tissue plasminogen activator vs. anistreplase and of aspirin plus heparin vs. aspirin alone among 41,299 cases of suspected acute myocardial infarction. Lancet, *339*:953, 1992.

Jansson J, Nilsson TK, Johnson O: von Willebrand factor in plasma: a novel risk factor for recurrent myocardial infarction and death. Br Heart J, *66*:351, 1991.

Karliner JS: Right bundle branch block after anterior myocardial infarction. J Am Coll Cardiol, *17*:864, 1991.

Kennedy G: Expanding the use of thrombolytic therapy for acute myocardial infarction. Ann Intern Med, *113*:907, 1990.

Lee RT, Grodzinsky AJ, Frank EJ, et al.: Structure-dependent dynamic mechanical behavior of fibrous caps from human atherosclerotic plaques. Circulation, *3*:1764, 1991.

MacMahon S, Collins R, Peto R, et al.: Effects of prophylactic lidocaine in suspected acute myocardial infarction. JAMA, *260*:1910, 1988.

McCall NT, Tofler GH, Schafer AI: The effect of enteric-coated aspirin on the morning increase in platelet activity. Am Heart J, *121*:1382, 1991.

Midgette AS, O'Connor GT, Baron JA, et al.: Effect of intravenous streptokinase on early mortality in patients with suspected acute myocardial infarction. Ann Intern Med, *113*:961, 1990.

Monrad ES: Thrombolysis: The need for a critical review. J Am Coll Cardiol, *18*:1573, 1991.

Morgan CD, Roberts RS, Haq A, et al.: Coronary patency, infarct size and left ventricular function after thrombolytic therapy for acute myocardial infarction: Results from the tissue plasminogen activator: Toronto (TPAT) placebo-controlled trial. J Am Coll Cardiol, *17*:1451, 1991.

Meuller HA, Cohen LS, Braunwald E, et al.: Predictors of early morbidity and mortality after thrombolytic therapy of acute myocardial infarction. Analyses of patient subgroups in the thrombolysis in myocardial infarction (TIMI) Trial, Phase II. Circulation, *85*:1254, 1992.

Muller DWM, Topol EJ: Selection of patients with acute myocardial infarction for thrombolytic therapy. Ann Intern Med, *113*:949, 1990.

Munkvad S, Jespersen J, Gram J, et al.: Depression of factor XII-dependent fibrinolytic activity characterizes patients with early myocardial reinfarction after recombinant tissue-type plasminogen activator therapy. J Am Coll Cardiol, *18*:454, 1991.

Neuhaus K-L, Von Essen R, Tebbe U, et al.: Improved thrombolysis in acute myocardial infarction with front-loaded administration of alteplase: Results of the rt-PA-APSAC Patency Study (TAPS). J Am Coll Cardiol, *19*:885, 1992.

Qiao J-H, Fishbein MC: The severity of coronary atherosclerosis at sites of plaque rupture with occlusive thrombosis. J Am Coll Cardiol, *17*:1138, 1991.

Renkin J, De Bruyne B, Benit E, et al.: Cardiac tamponade early after thrombolysis for acute myocardial infarction: A rare but not reported hemorrhagic complication. J Am Coll Cardiol, *17*:280, 1991.

Rapaport E: Should β-blockers be given immediately and concomitantly with thrombolytic therapy in acute myocardial infarction? Circulation, *83*:695, 1991.

Roberts R, Rogers WJ, Mueller HS, et al.: Immediate versus deferred β-blockade following thrombolytic therapy in patients with acute myocardial infarction. Circulation, *83*:422, 1991.

Roux S, Christeller S, Lüdin E: Effects of aspirin on coronary reocclusion and recurrent ischemia after thrombolysis: A meta-analysis. J Am Coll Cardiol, *19*:671, 1992.

Sane DC, Stump DC, Topol EJ, et al.: Racial differences in responses to thrombolytic therapy with recombinant tissue-type plasminogen activator. Circulation, *83*:170, 1991.

Sherry S: Fibrinolysis, Thrombosis and Hemostasis: Concepts and Perspectives. Philadelphia, Lea & Febiger, 1992.

Sherry S, Marder VJ: Streptokinase and recombinant tissue plasminogen activator (rt-PA) are equally effective in treating acute myocardial infarction. Ann Intern Med, *114*:417, 1991.

Sherry S, Marder VJ: Mistaken guidelines for thrombolytic therapy of acute myocardial infarction in the elderly. J Am Coll Cardiol, *17*:1237, 1991.

Sherry S: Creation of the recombinant tissue plasminogen activator (rt-PA) image and its influence on practice habits. J Am Coll Cardiol, *18*:1579, 1991.

Schweitzer P: The electrocardiographic diagnosis of acute myocardial infarction in the thrombolytic era. Am Heart J, *119*:642, 1990.

Tanswell P, Tebbe U, Neuhaus K-L, et al.: Pharmacokinetics and fibrin specificity of alteplase during accelerated infusions in acute myocardial infarction. J Am Coll Cardiol, *19*:1071, 1992.

The International Study Group: In-hospital mortality and clinical course of 20,891 patients with suspected acute myocardial infarction randomised between alteplase and streptokinase with or without heparin. Lancet, *336*:71, 1990.

The TIMI Study Group: Comparison of invasive and conservative strategies after treatment with intravenous tissue plasminogen activator in acute myocardial infarction: Results of the Thrombolysis in Myocardial Infarction (TIMI) Phase II Trial. N Engl J Med, *320*:618, 1989.

Topol EJ, Holmes DR, Rogers WJ: Coronary angiography after thrombolytic therapy for acute myocardial infarction. Ann Intern Med, *114*:877, 1991.

Topol EJ: Ultrathrombolysis. J Am Coll Cardiol, *15*:922, 1990.

Voth E, Tebbe U, Schicha H, et al.: Intravenous streptokinase in acute myocardial infarction (ISAM) trial: Serial evaluation of left ventricular function up to 3 years after infarction estimated by radionuclide ventriculography. J Am Coll Cardiol, *18*:1610, 1991.

Williams DO, Braunwald E, Knatterud G, et al.: One-year results of the thrombolysis in myocardial infarction investigation (TIMI) Phase II trial. Circulation, *85*:533, 1992.

Yarnell JWG, Baker IA, Sweetnam PM: Fibrinogen, viscosity, and white blood cell count are major risk factors for ischemic heart disease. Circulation, *83*:836, 1991.

Yusuf S, Wittes J, Probstfield J: Evaluating effects of treatment in subgroups of patients within a clinical trial: The case of non Q-wave myocardial infarction and beta blockers. Am J Cardiol, *66*:220, 1990.

4

COMPLICATIONS OF MYOCARDIAL INFARCTION AND POST-INFARCTION CARE

M. Gabriel Khan

Knowledge of the probable outcome after myocardial infarction (MI) is important in formulating an appropriate plan of management, as with Q wave versus non Q wave infarction. Therefore, the following presents information on risk stratification.

Acute MI in-hospital mortality is about 12 to 14% (Table 4–1). However, several characteristics alter the in-hospital and post-discharge mortality

- Age over 70
- Prior MI, angina, or heart failure is associated with a twofold or more increase in mortality
- Uncomplicated Q wave infarct with the absence of even mild heart failure has a 7 to 8% mortality
- Non Q infarcts, in contrast to Q wave infarction, have a lower in-hospital mortality (about 2%) but a threefold higher incidence of reinfarction within the following 3 months, and angina occurs in 33 to 66% of patients during the first year post discharge
- On admission to the hospital, 40 to 50% of patients with Q wave infarction have mild to moderate heart failure and the presence of this complication carries a twofold early mortality. Table 4–2 gives comparison outcomes in acute Q wave and non Q wave infarction. Overall, increasing age beyond 70 and the degree of heart failure or reduction in ejection fraction (EF) that relates to the size of infarction are the most telling predictors. Thus, frank pulmonary edema during day 1 and 2 prior to discharge or an EF less than 30% is most unfavorable
- Recurrence of ischemic symptoms after day 1 represents an unstable state and carries a high mortality if not appropriately managed

The complications of MI determine prognosis. The outcome can be improved, however, by appropriate pharmacologic therapy and by angioplasty or coronary artery bypass surgery (CABS) in properly selected patients. The complications of acute MI are listed in Table 4–3.

TABLE 4–1. ACUTE MYOCARDIAL INFARCTION: MORTALITY RISK STRATIFICATION

PARAMETERS	IN HOSPITAL	APPROXIMATE % 1 Year	3 Year	5 Year
Overall mortality	12–14	10–15		33*
Uncomplicated				
Anterior infarction	12	15	33	
Inferior infarction	3	5	12	
Complicated				
Anterior infarction				
Moderate heart failure	30	50	60	
Cardiogenic shock	80			
Ejection fraction				
<30%	30	50	60	
30–40%	15	25		
40–50%	5	15		
>50%	3			
Previous infarct	25	30	50	
Post-infarction Angina (Day 2 to 10)	20	20		
Anterior infarct				
Age >70	25			
Age <50	7			

* Unchanged 1960 to 1969, 1970 to 1979; (1980–1990 not available)

TABLE 4–2. COMPARISON OF OUTCOMES IN ACUTE Q WAVE AND NON Q WAVE INFARCTION

PARAMETERS	APPROXIMATE % Q Wave	Non Q Wave
Incidence prehospital	>90	<10
Mortality prehospital	Very high	Low
Incidence in hospital	80	20†
In hospital mortality		
All patients	12 (18)	6 (9)
First infarction	10 (15)	3 (5)
Incidence of moderate/severe heart failure	>20	<1*
Incidence of arrhythmias	High	Low
Incidence of post-infarction angina (12 months)	<40	>60
Reinfarction <3 months	6	10; 16**

* Except if previous Q wave infarction
** Pooled data prior to the use of aspirin, beta blockers, and diltiazem
† 10% in GISSI-2
( ) Pooled data, 1962 to 1988, prior to thrombolytic therapy and general use of aspirin and beta blockers.

TABLE 4–3. COMPLICATIONS OF MYOCARDIAL
INFARCTION

1. Heart Failure
2. Cardiogenic Shock
3. Recurrent Ischemia
   (a) Angina
   (b) Reinfarction
4. Early Mechanical Complications
   (a) Freewall rupture
   (b) Interventricular septal rupture
   (c) Mitral regurgitation
5. Late Mechanical Complications
   (a) Aneurysm
6. Electrical
   (a) Ventricular fibrillation
   (b) Ventricular tachycardia other tachyarrhythmias
   (c) Bradyarrhythmias, complete heart block
7. Left Ventricular Thrombus/Embolism
8. Psychologic

HEART FAILURE POST INFARCTION

The degree of heart failure is related to the size of the infarction. More than 50% of patients with anterior or anterolateral Q wave infarction show evidence of mild or moderate heart failure. Less than 10% of inferior infarcts manifest heart failure that usually dissipates quickly over 1 to 2 days. Approximately 25% of patients with extensive inferior infarction are complicated by right ventricular involvement and these patients often show signs of right-sided pump failure.

Mild to moderate left ventricular (LV) failure is observed in approximately 40% of patients admitted with acute infarction and is associated with a twofold increase in mortality. Frank pulmonary edema carries a fivefold mortality increase (see Table 4–1). Patients over age 70 with large anterior or anterolateral infarcts complicated by moderate to severe heart failure have a particularly poor prognosis.

Patients with severe heart failure due to acute MI have three possible outcomes

- Relief of pulmonary edema achieved over 1 to 3 days with the use of morphine, diuretics, and ACE inhibitors, plus or minus digoxin when mechanical complications are not present
- Heart failure refractory to drug therapy as outlined above persists, especially in patients with severe global hypokinesia, LV aneurysm, or mechanical complications
- Death due to malignant arrhythmias or mechanical complications

PATHOPHYSIOLOGY

Hemodynamic derangements occur due to five major determinants

- Severe LV systolic dysfunction is usually associated with very large areas of myocardial necrosis, especially when superimposed on an old infarction

- Significant ventricular diastolic dysfunction plays an important role, especially in patients with large infarcts, right ventricular infarction, old infarcts, or aneurysm
- Mechanical complications: Mitral regurgitation, septal, papillary, or rarely freewall rupture. In these situations, global LV function is generally well preserved; otherwise, the patient would have succumbed at the onset of the complication
- A variable area of mild myocardial ischemia and "stunned" myocardium usually surround the necrotic myocardium and can influence ventricular contractility and relaxation
- The exact incidence of painless ischemia among patients with heart failure in the presence of large infarction is unknown but appears to play a role within the first 48 hours of infarction. Painless ischemia is amenable to pharmacologic intervention with IV nitroglycerin and beta blockade
- Arrhythmias: Atrial fibrillation, atrial flutter, or other supraventricular tachycardias commonly precipitate or aggravate heart failure. The fast ventricular response reduces the time for ventricular filling as well as for coronary perfusion. In addition, the loss of atrial transport function reduces preload, especially important in patients with diastolic dysfunction

Mild interstitial edema is common during the first 12 hours of infarction and responds to bedrest, oxygen administration, morphine, and the judicious use of furosemide. In contrast to the more severe forms of failure discussed above, this situation is not associated with a poor outcome.

In the presence of a normal serum albumin, a pulmonary capillary wedge pressure exceeding 25 mm Hg results in pulmonary edema. Reduction of venous tone by nitrates, morphine, or the rapid loss of several hundred milliliters of urine with the aid of diuretics can reduce left atrial pressure by 10 to 15 mm Hg and thus prevent the formation of further pulmonary edema, provided that ventricular function is not too severely impaired by poor contractility or mechanical pump failure and cardiogenic shock does not supervene.

Factors that may precipitate heart failure in the patient admitted with acute myocardial infarction include

- Concomitant therapy with a calcium antagonist
- Antiarrhythmics, including disopyramide and procainamide
- Nonsteroidal anti-inflammatory drugs (NSAIDS)

THERAPY

MILD HEART FAILURE

Mild interstitial edema occurs in over 40% of patients with acute MI and responds to bedrest, oxygen, morphine and judicious use of furosemide.

Furosemide

Dosage: 20 to 40 mg IV; repeated with care to avoid potassium depletion suffices in the majority.

Diuretic therapy improves symptoms, but excessive volume depletion stimulates the renin angiotensin system and may paradoxically increase myocardial wall stress. It is advisable, therefore, to use a small dose of diuretic along with an ACE inhibitor if larger doses of a diuretic are considered necessary in the management of heart failure caused by LV dysfunction.

Morphine

Dosage: 4 to 8 mg IV at a rate of 1 mg/minute; repeat, if necessary, at a dose of 2 to 4 mg/min. It is important to allay anxiety. Patients at this stage may not complain bitterly of chest pain, but mild discomfort increases apprehension, which must be avoided. Morphine produces venous dilatation and thus reduces preload; in addition, the drug has a modest but important effect on elevating ventricular fibrillation (VF) threshold. Morphine should be avoided in patients with right ventricular infarction since all drugs that reduce preload are contraindicated in this setting.

Patients with mild heart failure, as discussed, represent about 25% of patients admitted and have about a 10% mortality. They do not require hemodynamic monitoring if they respond over a few hours to appropriate doses of furosemide and morphine. Some of these patients may require low-dose IV dobutamine via a peripheral vein, according to clinical status, before resorting to Swan-Ganz catheterization. In this subset of patients, if there is evidence of hypoperfusion with oliguria and/or a fall in systolic blood pressure less than 100 mm Hg or a fall greater than 30 mm from baseline, hemodynamic monitoring is necessary to guide pharmacologic intervention.

SEVERE HEART FAILURE

Patients with severe heart failure/early shock require the prompt insertion of a balloon flotation catheter.

The choice of a pharmacologic agent based on hemodynamic parameters is indicated in Table 4–4, and Figure 4–1 gives an algorithmic approach to management.

Severe heart failure and pulmonary edema, with pulmonary capillary wedge pressure exceeding 22 mm Hg and a low cardiac index less than 2.2 L/min/m^2, carry an in-hospital mortality of about 30% (see Table 4–1).

Intensive hemodynamic monitoring is essential in patients with severe heart failure. Large doses of pharmacologic agents and combination therapy are usually required

- Furosemide, 80 mg or more, in repeated doses if pulmonary edema is present with the wedge pressure greater than 24 mm Hg. The subsequent development of hypotension following an IV bolus of furosemide

TABLE 4–4. CHOICE OF PHARMACOLOGIC AGENTS IN PATIENTS WITH ACUTE MYOCARDIAL INFARCTION BASED ON HEMODYNAMIC PARAMETERS

DRUG EFFECT	FUROSEMIDE	IV NITRATES	DOBUTAMINE	DOPAMINE	NITROPRUSSIDE	ACE INHIBITORS
Preload	↓	↓	—	↑	↓	↓
Afterload	—	minimal ↓	minimal ↓	↑	↓	↓
Sinus tachycardia *Parameters*	No	Yes	minimal	Yes	Yes	no, minimal
Moderate heart failure PCWP ≥20 >24	Yes	Yes	Yes, if BP >70†	Yes, if BP <70 and oliguria (on dobutamine)	BP >110 and >6h* post infarction	Oral maintenance weaning nitroprusside
Severe heart failure PCWP >24 Cardiac index >2.5 L/min/m²	Yes	Yes if BP > 95	Yes if BP > 70	Yes if BP < 70‡	CI < 6h	Yes
Cardiogenic shock if BP <95	CI	CI	Yes IABP	Yes	CI	RCI**
Right ventricular infarction JVP ↑ PCWP >18 Cardiac index <2.5 L/min/m²	CI	CI	Useful with titrated volume infusion	Relative CI ↑PA pressure	CI	CI

Yes = useful
↓ = decrease
— = no change
↑ = increase
BP = systolic blood pressure mm Hg
* = Coronary steal during ischemic phase of infarction
** = See text
PCWP = Pulmonary capillary wedge pressure
IABP = Intra-aortic balloon pump
RCI = Relative contraindication
CI = Contraindication
† = See Fig. 16–2
‡ = Dopamine, dobutamine combination (see Ch. 16)

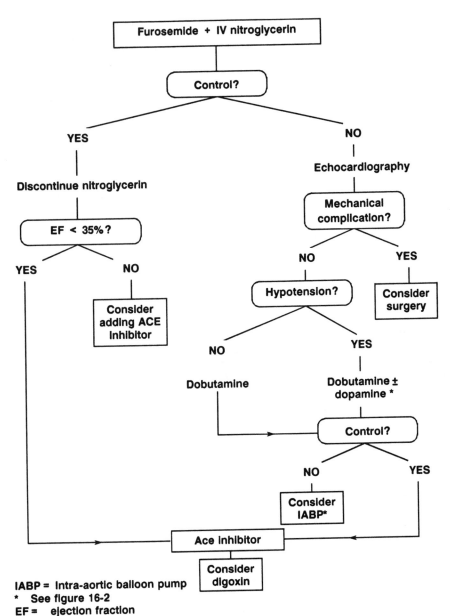

FIG. 4–1. Management of moderate to severe heart failure; acute myocardial infarction in sinus rhythm.

should alert the physician to the possibility of hypovolemia secondary to the diuretic or the presence of right ventricular infarction. Care is required in some patients with severe heart failure and concomitant cardiogenic shock to maintain a wedge pressure as high as 24 mm Hg provided that fulminant pulmonary edema is absent (Chapter 16)

- IV nitroglycerin is commenced if the systolic blood pressure is greater than 100 mm Hg, pulmonary capillary wedge pressure is greater than 20, and right atrial pressure is increased in the absence of right ventricular infarction. Titrate the dose to attain an optimal wedge pressure of 14 to 18 mm Hg without causing a fall in systolic blood pressure below 95 mm Hg or 10% from baseline (Table 2–9)
- A fall in blood pressure is best managed with the use of dobutamine in combination with nitroglycerin. Other inotropes carry no advantages over dobutamine; if severe hypotension is present, dopamine is added, but amrinone IV may be given a trial if severe hypotension is not present
- ACE inhibitors are given to all patients with EF less than 40% in the absence of hypotension (Figure 4–1) and considered for patients no longer in overt heart failure who are maintained on furosemide and with EF greater than 40%.

Dosage: Captopril 3 to 6.25 mg test dose; observe for 2 hours. If tolerated without a fall in blood pressure, give 12.5 mg twice daily. The dose is titrated slowly up to 25 mg, maximum 50 mg daily, over the following few days

Digoxin

Digoxin may increase oxygen demand, but in this situation with known high mortality, there is little reason to withhold digoxin. The area of infarction is a necrotic zone and there is no evidence to support the notion that digoxin increases infarct size. Improvement in cardiac function and hemodynamics may have a salutary effect on the peripheral ischemic zone. The concern of increasing infarct size is irrelevant if severe heart failure persists on the second day post infarction in the absence of recurrent chest pain or electrocardiographic signs of worsening ischemia. Digoxin is usually not advisable within the first 12 hours of infarction, when the risk of ischemia and arrhythmia is at its highest.

If the echocardiogram shows no mechanical defect or tamponade, digoxin is advisable for the management of severe heart failure or pulmonary edema. Also, when the patient is weaned off dobutamine, the action of digoxin is manifest. Patients with severe heart failure often require digoxin along with ACE inhibitors on discharge. Although the effect of digoxin on longterm survival post MI remains controversial, the risk of precipitating an arrhythmia with digoxin is low, as long as the serum potassium is maintained in the normal range. In patients who have been previously treated with diuretics, magnesium depletion may be a problem and should be addressed.

Dosage: Digoxin IV is not normally required, except where atrial fibrillation with a fast ventricular response requires control. With sinus rhythm and severe heart failure, give orally 0.5 mg immediately, then 0.25 mg at bedtime in patients under age 70 with normal renal function and in the absence of conditions in which there is an increased sensitivity to digoxin (see Table 5–3); follow with 0.25 mg daily. In patients over age 70 and those with slight elevation of serum creatinine, 1.3 to 2.3 mg/dl (115 to 203 μmol/l), the maintenance dose should be reduced to 0.125 mg daily after the second day (see Chapter 5). Digoxin is particularly useful in post-infarction patients who have systolic blood pressures less than 110 mm Hg. In these patients, nitrates or ACE inhibitors may further reduce systolic blood pressure and preload, causing decreased coronary and cerebral perfusion that may induce ischemia or presyncope.

ACE Inhibitors

ACE inhibitors have appropriately assumed a major role in the acute and chronic management of patients with post-infarction heart failure. These agents produce symptomatic improvement and also help prevent the recurrence of heart failure in patients with poor systolic function and an EF below 35%. They cause a modest decrease in mortality in patients with heart failure with chronic ischemic heart disease when used in conjunction with digoxin and diuretics (see Chapter 5).

The renin angiotensin system is activated during the early hours of MI and appears to be an important compensatory mechanism that serves to maintain blood pressure. The arterial vasoconstrictor effects of angiotensin II cause an unnecessarily great increase in afterload and ventricular wall stress, which initiate and perpetuate ventricular enlargement and an associated change in geometry with consequent further LV dysfunction. ACE inhibitors have been shown to attenuate these processes. Their effect on post-infarction ventricular remodeling may provide further salutary effects, even in the absence of heart failure, that may result in the reduction of cardiac mortality among patients with LV dysfunction. Clinical trials are in progress to establish whether the beneficial effects of these agents on ventricular size and shape are associated with an increase in longterm survival in the period of 1 to 2 years following acute MI. The Survival and Ventricular Enlargement (SAVE) trial indicates a beneficial trend in long-term survival in this category of patients treated with an ACE inhibitor.

At the present time, ACE inhibitors are indicated during recovery from acute MI if mild heart failure persists beyond day 3 and if not completely controlled with furosemide, morphine, and nitrates. ACE inhibitors should be given to the majority of patients who have severe heart failure or pulmonary edema. ACE inhibitors must be used with caution, however, in patients who develop post-infarction angina or other manifestations of worsening ischemia, because coronary artery perfusion beyond a critical stenosis may be reduced by these and other vasodilators.

Captopril

Dosage: 6.25 mg test dose or 3 mg if the blood pressure is marginal. If there is no decrease in blood pressure and the systolic blood pressure remains greater than 110 mm Hg, give 6.25 mg twice daily. The dose may be slowly increased over the next week to 12.5 mg twice or three times daily. A dose greater than 75 mg daily in the immediate post-infarction period is not advisable and appears to provide no added benefit. The majority of post-infarct patients require between 25 and 37.5 mg or the equivalent dose of enalapril to achieve beneficial effects without adverse side effects of hypotension and presyncope, which are easily precipitated by the addition of nitroglycerin or oral nitrates. The benefits of afterload reduction must be weighed against the risk of too dramatic a decrease in blood pressure and preload with consequent deleterious effects on coronary perfusion. Importantly, diastolic dysfunction is a feature of large infarcts and right ventricular infarction. In these settings, ACE inhibitors, nitrates, or other preload-reducing agents do not improve ventricular function and may be hazardous, especially in patents with right ventricular infarction. The dosage for enalapril is given in Chapter 5.

Contraindications (See Chapter 5)

- Severe anemia
- Unilateral renal artery stenosis in a solitary kidney or severe bilateral renal artery stenosis
- Hypotension
- Aortic stenosis

Interactions

- Except when the patient requires additional significant doses of loop diuretics, potassium supplements and potassium-sparing diuretics should not be given concomitantly with ACE inhibitors since severe hyperkalemia may ensue. Potassium supplementation may be hazardous, and close monitoring of serum potassium and serum creatinine is required because a sharp decline in renal function is sometimes seen
- Both nitrates and ACE inhibitors decrease preload and may precipitate presyncope or syncope

Intubation

Patients who manifest florid pulmonary edema and respond poorly to furosemide and IV nitroglycerin, with an arterial PaO_2 less than 50 or $PaCO_2$ greater than 50 mm Hg, require mechanical ventilation and positive-end expiratory pressure (PEEP) in addition to the other measures described. Caution: PEEP may decrease cardiac output and precipitate hypotension.

PUMP FAILURE AND SHOCK

There are two hemodynamic subsets of pump failure and patients may move from one subset to another. This chapter deals briefly with Subset I. Chapter 16 presents a more detailed discussion of cardiogenic shock.

The clinical spectrum of pump failure and shock embraces

- Poor peripheral perfusion with cold cyanotic extremities
- Obtundation

- Oliguria
- Weak pulse
- Cuff systolic blood pressure range
  Subset I—greater than 100 mm Hg
  Subset II—less than 90 mm Hg
- Patients with systolic pressures between 90 and 100 mm Hg may move toward Subset I or Subset II; close hemodynamic monitoring is necessary
- Symptoms and signs of LV failure

Salient therapeutic measures include

- Define the filling pressure of the left ventricle to exclude volume depletion. Various causes of preload reduction must be defined
- If the LV filling pressure is less than 15 mm Hg, give a rapid IV fluid challenge over a very short period to increase the filling pressure to the range 18 to 23 mm Hg. A prolonged infusion must be avoided, as it can worsen pulmonary congestion without increasing LV filling pressure appreciably

If volume depletion and preload-reducing factors are absent, management must rapidly progress to

- Relieving the load on the left ventricle with afterload-reducing agents but without decreasing blood pressure and perfusion to vital areas
- Improving myocardial oxygen supply-demand ratio with oxygen-sparing agents, reperfusion by thrombolysis, angioplasty, or finally resorting to CABS if these alternatives are technically feasible, if a substantial amount of viable myocardium is believed to persist in the ischemic region, and if the patient's condition permits. Two hemodynamic subsets in the spectrum of pump failure and shock can be defined by hemodynamic monitoring

SUBSET I

- LV filling pressure greater than 15 mm Hg
- Systolic blood pressure greater than 100 mm Hg
- Cardiac index less than 2.5 L/min/m²
- Evidence of peripheral hypoperfusion and some evidence of pulmonary congestion
  This category of patients have LV failure, and the systolic blood pressure range of 95 to 115 mm Hg allows the use of afterload- and preload-reducing agents, thus relieving the load on the left ventricle and favorably altering myocardial oxygen supply-demand ratio. Salutary effects are obtained with the administration of nitroglycerin, dobutamine, dopamine, or nitroprusside, depending on hemodynamic parameters (Table 4–4).

NITROGLYCERIN

Nitroglycerin has advantages over nitroprusside during the early hours of infarction since, at this stage, ischemia is often present. The drug is reserved for selected cases where continued ischemia is suspected of causing progression of infarction or LV dysfunction.

The drug reduces preload, which may be beneficial in some patients with severe pulmonary congestion but in whom blood pressure is reasonably well maintained. However, patients with pump failure and severe shock may have deleterious effects from too great a reduction in preload. Higher doses also reduce afterload. Thus, careful hemodynamic monitoring is essential when using pharmacologic agents that alter both preload and afterload.

Dosage: Commence with 5 μg/min via pump controlled infusion (see Nitroglycerin Infusion Pump Chart, Table 2–9). Increase by 5 μg/min every 10 minutes. Do not allow a fall in systolic blood pressure in excess of 10 mm Hg. The systolic blood pressure should not fall to less than 90 mm Hg.

If nitroglycerin alone causes improvement in the pump failure/shock syndrome, achieving an acceptable increase in cardiac output, continue the infusion for 24 to 48 hours. During this period, therapy with an ACE inhibitor is introduced.

If hypotension persists or worsens and preload is high, decrease the nitroglycerin infusion and add dobutamine 2 to 5 μg/kg/minute (Table 16–4). If the preload is low or blood pressure decreases more precipitously, dopamine should replace dobutamine (see Chapter 16).

DOBUTAMINE

Dosage: Commence with 2 μg/kg/min, increase slowly if needed to 5 μg; maximum of 10 μg/kg/min. If a 10 μg/kg/min dose of dobutamine fails to maintain blood pressure, a dopamine infusion should replace the dobutamine or a low-dose dobutamine/dopamine combination should be considered (see Chapter 16).

The intra-aortic balloon pump (IABP) is required in some cases when nitroglycerin, dobutamine, or dopamine does not halt hemodynamic deterioration and an aggressive approach is considered appropriate. See Table 4–5 for indications and contraindications for IABP.

TABLE 4–5. INDICATIONS AND CONTRAINDICATIONS FOR INTRA AORTIC BALLOON PUMP IN ACUTE MYOCARDIAL INFARCTION

INDICATIONS
1. Cardiogenic shock (selected cases)
2. Post-infarction angina (selected cases, stabilization for angiography)
3. Right ventricular infarction with refractory hypotension (consider IABP)
4. Early mechanical complications (Table 4–3) (if stabilization is necessary for interventional therapy)

CONTRAINDICATIONS
1. Severe peripheral vascular disease
2. Aortic aneurysm and aortic disease
3. If contraindications to anticoagulants exist

NITROPRUSSIDE

The drug is a powerful afterload-reducing agent and has a role, especially when the systolic blood pressure is in the range of 100 to 120 mm Hg, in the presence of pump failure/shock syndrome. The drug can replace nitroglycerin in patients presenting with pump failure/shock syndrome after 6 hours of infarction if ischemia is not present and afterload reduction is considered necessary.

Dosage: Commence with 0.4 μg/kg/min with close monitoring of arterial pressure, increase the infusion given by infusion pump, and titrate the dosage in increments of 0.2 μg/kg/min every 2 to 5 minutes (Table 1–10). A dose of up to 3 μg/kg/min should suffice to achieve salutary hemodynamic effects.

Caution. Severe hypotension is a major risk. Also, the drug may produce a coronary steal, reflex tachycardia, and hypoxemia. These serious adverse effects may worsen ischemia and infarction and increase mortality. Thus, in each patient, the benefits and risks must be weighed prior to introduction of nitroprusside.

Contraindications

- Hepatic dysfunction
- Severe anemia
- Severe renal failure
- Inadequate cerebral circulation

Adverse effects. Patients with liver disease may develop cyanide toxicity and if kidney disease exists, thiocyanate levels must be monitored when treatment is given for more than 2 days. Severe hypotension causing increased shock, retrosternal chest pain, or palpitations may occur. Great care is necessary to avoid accidental acceleration of the infusion. If acute cyanide poisoning occurs, amyl nitrite inhalations and IV sodium thiosulfate should be given. For further information on nitroprusside, see Chapters 1 and 16.

SUBSET II

- Systolic blood pressure less than 90 mm Hg
- LV filling pressure greater than 15 mm Hg
- Cardiac index less than 2.5 l/min/m^2

These parameters define patients with severe cardiogenic shock. Failure to stabilize the patient should prompt consideration of IABP and urgent coronary angiograms with a view to angioplasty or bypass surgery to enhance coronary perfusion or to correct underlying mechanical problems.

TABLE 4–6. RIGHT VENTRICULAR INFARCTION

1. High jugular venous pressure with clear lung fields (exclude tamponade)
2. Kussmaul's sign present >90%
3. a) ECG evidence of inferoposteror infarct,
   b) ST segment depression V_1, V_2, or elevation in V_4 R
4. PCWP normal
5. Right atrial and right ventricular pressure >10 mm Hg
6. *Ratio right atrial to PCWP >0.8

---

* Present in <33% of patients
PCWP = Pulmonary capillary wedge pressure

RIGHT VENTRICULAR INFARCTION

Right ventricular infarction is usually associated with inferoposterior infarction and, where present, frequently causes right-sided pump failure/shock. Approximately 25% of patients with inferior infarction show varying degrees of right ventricular infarction, but only those with a large affected area develop the characteristic signs. The diagnostic hallmarks of right ventricular infarction are given in Table 4–6. The right atrial and right ventricular diastolic pressures are greater than 10 mm Hg, the cardiac index is less than 2.5 l/min/m^2, and the LV filling pressure is normal or elevated.

The mechanism of shock in right ventricular infarction combines the following

• Acute right pump failure reduces the venous return to the left ventricle. Thus, decrease in LV preload is the principal mechanism for the decreased LV output
• Interventricular septal shift toward the left ventricle reduces left ventricular diastolic volume. Also, an increase in intrapericardial pressure occurs, which restricts LV filling and passively increases pulmonary artery pressure, thus increasing right ventricular afterload

In the presence of severe right-sided heart failure, it is necessary to exclude cardiac tamponade, which may occasionally give hemodynamic findings resembling those seen with right ventricular infarction, with equalization of diastolic pressures resulting from intrapericardial pressure due to a distended pericardium.

THERAPY OF RIGHT VENTRICULAR INFARCTION

Patients with extensive right ventricular infarction are very sensitive to volume depletion, and titrated volume infusion should be tried. The right ventricle is unable to deliver adequately the venous return to the left ventricle, however, and the reduced left ventricular preload results in decreased systemic output. Thus, volume infusion is often partially or even completely ineffective but must be tried judiciously.

• Dobutamine infusion should be commenced at 2 μg/kg/min and increased to a maximum of 10 μg/kg/min if needed (Table 16–5)

- Failure to respond to volume replacement and dobutamine is a strong indication for the use of IABP
- Sublingual or IV nitroglycerin is contraindicated in patients with right ventricular infarction since reduction in preload must be avoided
- Nitroprusside, as well as diuretics and ACE inhibitors, reduce preload and are not recommended
- Dopamine increases pulmonary vascular resistance and may increase right ventricular pump failure. Dobutamine is thus superior to dopamine in patients with right ventricular infarction although the hypotensive effect may limit the dose that can be tolerated

POST-INFARCTION ANGINA

Definite post-infarction angina occurring after day 1 to discharge, associated with new electrocardiographic changes and correctly interpreted as due to worsening ischemia, is an indication for coronary angiography with a view to possible intervention in the form of CABS or angioplasty according to the angiographic findings.

Careful selection of patients for this investigation, based on a diagnosis formulated by an experienced cardiologist or team, is essential to avoid a reflex angiographic rush to see the lesion.

Consider and exclude

- Pericarditis
- Esophagogastric origin of pain due to stress ulceration, esophagitis, and the effects of aspirin in individuals with so-called sensitive stomachs
- Some patients with a stuttering pattern of pain due to ischemia or reinfarction respond readily to beta-adrenergic blockers and/or IV nitroglycerin. In patients categorized at high risk for surgery, administration of tissue plasminogen activator (tPA) should be considered (see Chapter 3, discussion on thrombolytic therapy)

In the Thrombolysis in Myocardial Infarction (TIMI) Phase II Trial, the incidence of coronary angiography for presumed post-infarction ischema in tertiary and community hospitals was 48%, versus 32% that resulted in a greater frequency of angioplasty and bypass surgery, with no difference observed in end points of reinfarction or death at 40 days and 1 year. In TIMI II, within 42 days post infarction, investigations and major interventions were performed in tertiary care hospitals for presumed early recurrent ischemia as follows

- Coronary angiography: 48%
- Angioplasty: 18%
- CABS: 12%

The results of TIMI II indicate that the conservative strategy adopted in the community hospitals using thrombolysis during the early hours of acute MI resulted in a significantly lower number of invasive procedures being done than in the tertiary care setting, with no apparent deleterious consequences. This conservative strategy appears to be effective in the selection of patients with presumed post-infarction ischemia for consideration of angiography and major interventional therapy.

The surgical mortality and survival of patients with post-infarction angina with an EF greater than 50% are as good as those observed with elective surgery. When the EF is below 35% and perhaps as low as 25%, bypass surgery is preferred over angioplasty if the ischemic syndrome persists and lesions of the left main, triple vessel, or double vessel with left anterior descending proximal occlusion are observed on angiography.

In many of the above scenarios, decision-making is difficult; the goals and risks of the possible therapeutic approaches must be considered jointly by medical and surgical teams, with full understanding by the patient or family.

EARLY VENTRICULAR ARRHYTHMIAS

The mechanism of early infarction arrhythmias includes

- Disturbances of impulse generation/enhanced automaticity
- Disturbances of impulse conduction/reentry, focal conduction slowing
- Increased sympathetic and parasympathetic tone is a commonly prominent feature that influences the above underlying mechanisms

Precipitating factors are

- Ischemia with associated tissue acidosis and local increase in extracellular potassium concentration
- Catecholamine release: May induce arrhythmia as well as increase ischemia. Arrhythmias worsen ischemia and vice versa. Thus, a dynamic interplay perpetuates ventricular arrhythmias that may terminate in VF
- Hypokalemia from prior use of diuretics or induced by verapamil
- Hypomagnesemia due to diuretic use
- Hypoxemia
- Respiratory or metabolic acidosis or alkalosis
- Severe heart failure probably related to extensive infarction

VENTRICULAR PREMATURE CONTRACTION

Ventricular premature contractions (VPCs) occurring during the first 6 hours of infarction and requiring therapy are managed with lidocaine (see Chapter 6).

During the later hospital phase, frequent VPCs (more than 10/hour multifocal beats or couplets) may increase risk, but there is only limited evidence that antiarrhythmic therapy, other than beta blocking agents, prolongs life in these patients. The Cardiac Arrhythmia Suppression Trial (CAST) indicated an increase in mortality among these patients with the use of flecanide and encainide. Patients with this category of arrhythmia should be given a beta-adrenergic blocking agent such as metoprolol or timolol if there is no contraindication to the use of this class of drug. A study has shown improved survival among high-risk patients treated with amiodarone, but this finding requires confirmation (see Chapter 6).

SUSTAINED VENTRICULAR TACHYCARDIA

- Ventricular tachycardia (VT) asymptomatic or mild symptoms with the pulse present occurring during the first 24 hours of MI (rare at this time): Give lidocaine (lignocaine) IV 100 mg bolus. IV lidocaine infusion 2 to 3 mg/min is given for a time after conversion without waiting for recurrence (Fig. 6–4). If the drug is ineffective and the patient is hemodynamically stable, give procainamide IV 100 mg bolus at the rate of 20 mg/min and then 10 mg/min; maximum 24 mg/min not to exceed 1 g during the first hour. Procainamide has a negative inotropic effect and is not recommended for patients who manifest heart failure or with EF less than 40%. The drug is, therefore, reserved for patients who fail to respond to lidocaine or who have recurrent VT but who remain hemodynamically stable
- The cardioverter should be prepared and connected to the patient while drug therapy is in progress
- Failure to control with lidocaine or procainamide requires synchronized cardioversion (see Fig. 6–4)
- Any breakthrough should be treated by adding a beta blocker (if not already being administered) and, if needed, IV amiodarone 300 mg in 20 minutes, preferably via a central vein followed by 50 mg/hour for 6 to 12 hours, then 30 mg/hour if stable (see Chapter 6). IV amiodarone may cause hypotension and caution is required. With the availability of IV amiodarone, which is effective and has good tolerability, the use of bretylium has appropriately dwindled. If amiodarone IV is not available and VT or VF recurs, give bretylium, 5 mg/kg undiluted, rapidly as an IV bolus. Electrical defibrillation is then carried out. If VF persists, bretylium dosage is increased to 10 mg/kg and repeated, if needed. Caution: IV bretylium has not been shown to be superior to lidocaine. Bretylium causes severe hypotension, and epinephrine or norepinephrine must not be used concomitantly. Importantly, most early ventricular arrhythmias settle down, and lidocaine is stopped after about 24 hours
- VT no pulse present or hemodynamically unstable: Chest pain, shortness of breath, clouding of consciousness or obtundation, treat as VF (Fig. 6–4)

SUPRAVENTRICULAR ARRHYTHMIAS

The incidence of supraventricular arrhythmias in acute MI is shown in Table 4–7.

ATRIAL FIBRILLATION

Atrial fibrillation in acute MI is often precipitated by

- Large infarction of the atrium
- Chronic atrial enlargement
- Heart failure with atrial dilatation
- Acute mitral regurgitation

TABLE 4–7. INCIDENCE OF SUPRAVENTRICULAR TACHYCARDIA IN ACUTE MYOCARDIAL INFARCTION

	APPROXIMATE %
1. Atrial fibrillation	
(a) within 3 hours of infarction	3
(b) new onset first week	5
(c) known prior (chronic)	10
2. Atrial flutter	1–3
3. Ectopic atrial tachycardia (benign)	1–10 (transient)
4. Nonparoxysmal AV junctional tachycardia (benign arrhythmia relates to size of infarction)	5–15
5. Atrioventricular nodal reentrant tachycardia	Rare

- Increase catecholamines
- Acute pericarditis
- Hypoxemia
- Inferior infarction more commonly than anterior infarction, with occlusion of the right coronary or circumflex artery

Acute atrial fibrillation occurs within the first few hours of infarction in approximately 3% of patients and is often of short duration, lasting less than 2, 4, and 24 hours in 50, 75, and 95% of patients, respectively.

Atrial fibrillation is observed during the first few days of infarction in up to 15% of patients, and in 10%, the onset is prior to infarction.

Management of atrial fibrillation depends on the hemodynamic and proischemic effect of a rapid or uncontrolled ventricular response

- Hemodynamic compromise requires immediate electrocardioversion
- Asymptomatic patients or patients with heart failure with a moderate ventricular response and normal blood pressure should be slowly digitalized
- Digoxin may not reach peak effect for 8 to 24 hours depending on the dosing schedule, but a rapid-acting drug is not essential. Importantly, the other available agents are hazardous in this setting
- Patients not in prominent heart failure with systolic blood pressure greater than 110 mm Hg and rates of 120 to 150/minute can be managed with a beta blocking drug. A fast rate of 140 to 160/minute not causing hemodynamic compromise should respond to metoprolol or ultra-short-acting esmolol (see Table 3–4 for dosage)

The calcium antagonist verapamil slows the ventricular response, but the negative inotropic effect is more prominent than that of titrated small doses of esmolol or metoprolol and is not advisable in acute infarction unless the use of a beta blocker is absolutely contraindicated by severe asthma.

BRADYARRHYTHMIAS

Early occurring sinus bradycardia, symptomatic or associated with hypotension usually with rates less than 45/minute, should be managed with atropine. Similarly, second- or third-degree AV block occurring during the first few hours after onset of MI often responds to this agent. Also, patients with asystole should be given atropine.

Atropine

Dosage: 0.4 to 0.6 mg IV repeated if needed every 5 or 10 minutes to a maximum of 2 mg.

Caution. Rapid injection or too large a dose may cause unwanted sinus tachycardia and rarely VF. Dosage for asystole: 1 mg IV repeated in 2 to 5 minutes during which CPR should continue. Total dose: 2.5 mg over 30 minutes. In the latter situation, a large dose given promptly is essential, without concern for tachycardia causing increased myocardial oxygen demand.

Indications
- Sinus bradycardia associated with peripheral hypoperfusion, hemodynamic deterioration
- Frequent VPCs associated with sinus bradycardia
- All forms of AV blocks, 2nd or 3rd degree in patients with inferior MI, since they often respond if less than 8 hours post onset
- Asystole, along with CPR and preparation for pacing

Adverse effects. Hallucination, sinus tachycardia, rarely VT, and VF. Severe bradycardia due to Mobitz Type 2 or third-degree AV block not responding to atropine requires temporary pacing (see Chapter 18).

RECOMMENDATIONS FOR TEMPORARY PACEMAKER POST INFARCTION

Indications include

- Asystolic episodes
- Complete heart block, unless escape rhythm is present greater than 60/min and hemodynamics are good
- Right bundle branch block with left anterior or left posterior hemiblock or left bundle branch block developing during acute infarction can be managed with external pacer with chest pads on standby
- Mobitz Type 2 second degree AV block
- Mobitz Type 1 second degree AV block with hypotension or heart failure (see Chapter 18 for further details)

Pacemaker electrode insertion is not indicated in

- First-degree AV block
- Mobitz Type 1 second-degree AV block with normal hemodynamics
- Accelerated idioventricular rhythm with AV dissociation
- Bundle branch block known prior to the acute infarction

LATE VENTRICULAR ARRHYTHMIAS

It is advisable to obtain Holter recordings for all patients at 1 to 3 weeks post MI to assist in assessing the risk profile, especially if the EF is less than 40%. A 24- or 48-hour Holter study is indicated if the patient complains of palpitations, presyncope, syncope, or other symptoms. Holter monitoring is advisable in patients to document the presence of significant arrhythmia requiring consideration of drug therapy.

Late-occurring sustained VT is very ominous. Sustained VT or complex ventricular ectopy occurring during the weeks following infarction greatly increases the risk of sudden death. These potentially lethal arrhythmias require antifibrillary therapy.

Currently, it is not known what pharmacologic agent is best for post-MI patients at highest risk. Beta-adrenergic blockers are the only antiarrhythmic agents that have been proven to prevent cardiac death or sudden death. However, there is evidence from one study that amiodarone may improve survival rates.

The Basel Antiarrhythmic Study of Infarct Survival (BASIS) investigated the effects of prophylactic antiarrhythmic therapy in patients with asymptomatic complex ventricular arrhythmias post infarction. Low-dose amiodarone, 200 mg daily, was given over 1 year. Cumulative mortality rates were 13% in the control group, 5% in the amiodarone-treated group (p < 0.05), and 10% in the individually treated patients who were administered mexiletine, quinidine, propafenone, sotalol, disopyramide, or flecanide. (Treatment failures were given amiodarone.) Arrhythmic events were also reduced in the amiodarone group.

In contrast with the beneficial effects of beta blocking agents and possibly for amiodarone, other antiarrhythmic agents have been shown to increase mortality. Flecanide and encainide caused an increase in cardiac mortality observed in the CAST.

The management of patients with late nonsustained VT, at least in short runs, or complex ventricular arrhythmias is presently unsatisfactory. Suggestive steps include

- If a beta blocking drug is being administered as routine beta blocker post-MI prophylaxis, the dose should be increased: e.g., 100 mg metoprolol, 160 mg propranolol, 20 mg timolol, and 50 mg atenolol daily should be increased to 300, 240, 30, or 150 mg daily, respectively. A change from one of the aforementioned beta blocking agents to sotalol, 240 to 480 mg daily, may be effective and should be given a trial
- If beta blockers are ineffective, poorly tolerated, or are contraindicated because of asthma or very poor LV function, many cardiologists will go to amiodarone, oral or IV as appropriate, as the next choice because of the high frequency of failure with other drugs
- The third choice is mexiletine, which has a low proarrhythmic effect and a minimal negative inotropic action. The drug is, however, poorly effective

Amiodarone and other antiarrhythmic agents are used only under close supervision by using repeated Holter monitoring, and the usual precautions are observed when prescribing amiodarone (see Chapter 6). The combination of amiodarone and a beta blocking agent (except sotalol) has a role in patients with lethal arrhythmias, as discussed in Chapter 6. Failure of this trial therapy should prompt consideration of selecting alternative treatment

- A combination of antiarrhythmic agents guided by electrophysiologic (EP) testing, although the recommendation of antiarrhythmic therapy has several limitations
- Rare surgical excision of focus
- Catheter ablative techniques
- An implantable cardioverter-defibrillator, which has antibradycardia pacing and algorithms for pace termination of VT (see Fig. 18–15 and Chapter 18)

MECHANICAL COMPLICATIONS

Mechanical complications should be strongly suspected in patients who develop sudden hemodynamic deterioration especially from the second post-infarct day onward with no new ECG changes occurring. The incidence and associated mortality of these complications are given in Table 4–8.

SEVERE ACUTE MITRAL REGURGITATION

A transient mitral regurgitant murmur is often present with acute MI. Severe acute mitral regurgitation is uncommon, however, occurring in less than 3% of patients with acute MI, and is usually due to

- Papillary muscle rupture: Partial rupture of the tip or rarely the trunk
- Rupture of the chordae tendineae

Strongly suspected severe mitral regurgitation in the presence of acute inferior infarction on the second to fifth days in patients with pulmonary edema and/or hemodynamic deterioration developing out of proportion to the ECG changes. An EF in the normal range is typical of regurgitant flow. The posterior papillary muscle is most commonly affected with inferoposterior infarction
Physical signs include

- A new murmur of mitral regurgitation may be loud and rarely accompanied by a thrill. The murmur is usually loud, in the presence of papillary muscle rupture, but may be soft in patients with low cardiac output or shock syndrome
- Papillary muscle dysfunction: Mitral regurgitation is not usually severe. The systolic murmur may fluctuate in intensity from hour to hour and may be soft, loud, high-, or low-pitched; the murmur may stop abruptly well before the second heart sound
- The murmur caused by ischemia of the posterior papillary muscle radiates anteriorly, while that of the anterior papillary muscle radiates posteriorly to the axilla

TABLE 4–8. ACUTE MYOCARDIAL INFARCTION-MECHANICAL COMPLICATIONS INCIDENCE, TIMING AND MORTALITY

	% OF TOTAL ACUTE INFARCTS	INCIDENCE & TIMING	% OF TOTAL RUPTURE	% OF TOTAL IN-HOSPITAL MORTALITY	TYPE OF INFARCT
Cardiac rupture	3–10	Up to 50%; 2–3 days Up to 40%; day 1		20	
Free wall	2–8	10%; days 4–7 25%; day 1	85	15	
Papillary muscle rupture	1	75%; 3–5 days 25%; day 1–2 or 6–10	5	5	Commonly infero-posterior
Ventricular septal rupture	1–3	75%; 3–5 days 25%; 1–2 or 6–14	10	1–4	60% anterior 40% inferior
Severe mitral regurgitation	2%	1–5 days			
LV aneurysm	10–15	3 months			90% anterior 10% inferior

- The murmur of a flail leaflet may be well heard over the spine from the skull to the sacrum

Diagnosis and management include

- Echocardiography with continuous wave Doppler flow study has an important role
- If the Doppler flow study is in keeping with severe mitral regurgitation, proceed with catheterization. Large V waves on pulmonary capillary wedge and severe mitral regurgitation are observed on left ventriculography
- Patients with severe acute mitral regurgitation due to papillary muscle or chordal rupture require surgery. IABP provides support if needed during catheterization and to the operating room
- Patients with papillary muscle dysfunction and severe mitral regurgitation who are not hypotensive are managed with afterload-reducing agents. IV nitroglycerin has a role in relieving ischemia, as well as reducing preload, and causes minimal afterload reduction (see Chapter 16). Dobutamine and the use of IABP may be necessary to support blood pressure where needed while considering interventional therapy

PAPILLARY MUSCLE RUPTURE

Papillary muscle rupture occurs infrequently, in approximately 1% of patients with infarction, and accounts for 5% of myocardial rupture and 5% of all mortality from acute MI (Table 4–8).
Rupture of one of the smaller heads of the papillary muscle occurs much more commonly than rupture of a main trunk.
Diagnosis and therapy include

- Sudden deterioration of the patient's hemodynamic status, with pulmonary edema out of proportion to the extent of ECG changes, is common in patients with inferoposterior infarction
- A new mitral regurgitant murmur is usually loud
- The catastrophic event is usually fatal, but if severe mitral regurgitation and partial rupture of a papillary muscle are quickly detected by bedside Doppler echocardiography or transesophageal echocardiography (TEE) and catheterization confirms the diagnosis, then surgery carries the only hope of survival. Surgical mortality is 10 to 25%. Hemodynamic support using IABP may be required during catheterization and transport to the operating room
- Surgery involves replacement of the mitral valve, since the mitral apparatus is usually severely deranged and beyond repair
- Rupture of a papillary muscle main trunk is a catastrophic event and death ensues within the hour, a situation that is fortunately rare

FREEWALL RUPTURE

The two leading causes of in-hospital post-infarction mortality are

- Cardiogenic shock
- Myocardial rupture: This catastrophic event accounts for 10 to 20% of total in-hospital post-infarction mortality.

Importantly, myocardial rupture has been found in 38% of patients at autopsy in clinical trials of thrombolytic agents. Several clinical trials indicate that late administration, at 8 to 21 hours from onset of symptoms, increases the risk of cardiac rupture, especially in patients over age 70. The Gruppo Italiano per lo Studio della Streptochinasi nell' Infarto Miocardico (GISSI) trial has independently confirmed the relation between the risk of cardiac rupture and time to streptokinase therapy.
Free external cardiac rupture occurs in 3 to 10% of acute infarcts; peak incidence is within the first 72 hours, and up to 40% of cases occur within the first 24 hours of symptoms (Table 4–8)
Freewall rupture presents in four scenarios

- Acute free rupture
- Acute limited rupture
- Subacute rupture
- Chronic rupture

Associated factors include

- Vigorous contraction of surviving myocardium appears to be an important contributing factor
- Most commonly occurs after first infarction
- Mainly Q wave transmural infarcts and mainly anterior infarction
- Patients are usually over age 70
- Pre-existing hypertension
- More common in women
- Thrombolytic therapy given more than 7 hours after onset of symptoms, when necrosis is complete. Cardiac rupture is caused by extensive infarction and dissection of blood through the regions of transmural necrosis. Thrombolytic therapy may cause hemorrhage into areas of fresh necrosis and may promote dissection that could result in freewall rupture
- Use of anticoagulants or NSAIDS. NSAIDS cause vasoconstriction and may alter myocardial healing. Also, sodium and water retention adds to ventricular strain
- Early ambulation is an unproven association

Prevention plays a major role

- Early use of thrombolytic agents to ensure reperfusion in less than 6 hours of onset of symptoms
- Avoid late use of thrombolytic agents in patients over age 75 seen after the sixth hour with completed Q wave infarction, except where a stuttering pain pattern persists (see Indications for Thrombolytic Therapy in Patients over Age 75, Chapter 3)
- Reduce the force and velocity of ventricular contractility with the use of beta blocking agents. Importantly, beta blockers are the only available cardiac medications that have shown modest protection from myocardial freewall rupture. There are good theoretical reasons to justify their salutary effects in preventing this catastrophic occurrence in patients with first infarction (see Fig. 2–7). In the International Study of Infarct Survival (ISIS-I) Trial, causes of myocardial rupture were over 2.5-fold more frequent in the placebo group than in those administered IV atenolol. The Göteborg Metoprolol and MIAMI trials showed a similar trend. The Beta Blocker Heart Attack Trial (BHAT) showed a 43% decrease in early morning sudden deaths not believed to be caused by arrhythmias. Because it is rare to prevent death after freewall rupture has occurred, prevention of rupture is of utmost importance. An IV beta blocker such as esmolol, metoprolol, or atenolol should be given at the earliest opportunity, preferably within the first 2 hours of onset of symptoms.
- ACE inhibitors decrease afterload and may reduce ventricular work. However, although these agents are reported to favorably alter postinfarction remodeling, the effect in preventing myocardial rupture needs to be confirmed by multicenter randomized clinical trials.
- Nitrates cause moderate yet important sinus tachycardia and an increase in ejection velocity. Thus, these agents are not indicated in prevention and should be avoided after the first 6 hours of infarction, except where recurrence of ischemia is documented.

Acute freewall rupture is a catastrophic event; death occurs within minutes. Less than 50 successful surgical repairs of myocardial rupture have been reported.

Acute limited rupture of the thick spiral muscular layer may occur, but an intact outer longitudinal layer of muscle causes a precarious containment of the rupture. Transient cracks may occur in the thin longitudinal layer, causing pericardial effusion and tamponade but also closure of the small leak.

Immediate pericardiocentesis with derived benefit excludes the confounding diagnosis of pulmonary embolism, which may occur between days 2 to 8 and may occasionally present catastrophically and with electromechanical dissociation. Hemodynamic support using IABP may be necessary; the patient may be rushed to the operating room for correction of a defect, making survival possible.

Subacute rupture may cause hemorrhagic pericarditis due to a slow leak of blood and can present during the 2- to 8-day period. In this condition, a few hours are available to rapidly define the underlying lesion. As in other forms of pericarditis, the patient usually complains of severe chest pain increased on inspiration and recumbent posture with some relief by leaning forward. However, increasing signs of cardiac tamponade may be manifest (see Chapter 13). Initially, this condition may be difficult to differentiate from benign post-infarction pericarditis, but the latter does not cause hemodynamic compromise. Urgent pericardiocentesis is necessary. If some relief ensues, rapid surgical intervention can produce salutary results in these patients. Coronary bypass surgery or angioplasty in selected patients improve survival.

Chronic rupture with or without pseudoaneurysm is a rare occurrence. Circumferential adhesions and a layer of thrombus formation between the visceral and parietal pericardium may cause containment of the hemopericardium for days to weeks.

The abnormal bulge on the cardiac border, chest discomfort, or increasing heart failure may alert suspicion. Echocardiographic visualization and, occasionally, CT scanning and left ventriculography are indicated on an emergency basis to exclude this potentially correctable lesion.

VENTRICULAR SEPTAL RUPTURE

Ventricular septal rupture occurs in 1 to 3% of patients with acute infarction.

Associated features and hallmarks include

- Occurs in both anterior and inferior infarctions with concomitant infarction of the interventricular septum
- More common with first Q wave anterior or anteroseptal infarction
- Peak occurrence in 3 to 5 days, but up to 30% occur within 24 hours or up to 2 weeks post infarction (Table 4–8)
- Abrupt onset of hemodynamic deterioration often with cardiogenic shock from 12 hours to 14 days post infarction, in the absence of signs of tamponade or new ECG changes of reinfarction

- A new loud, harsh holosystolic murmur maximal at the left and right lower sternal border, often with spoke-wheel radiation
- A thrill occurs in up to 50% of cases
- The murmur may be maximal at the apex without a thrill and may be difficult to differentiate from acute mitral regurgitation
- Rupture usually occurs at the junction of the septum with anterior or posterior left ventricular freewall
- Right heart failure is more prominent than pulmonary edema
- Severe heart failure, yet a normal, supernormal, or only mild decrease in EF should be a clue to the diagnosis of the cause of cardiogenic shock occurring between days 2 and 14
- Echocardiography should confirm the diagnosis, and right-sided catheterization with oximetry should show an oxygen step-up in the right ventricle

The degree of hemodynamic compromise and the general health and age of the patient dictate the urgency and selection of pharmacologic and interventional therapy. Patients often come through angioplasty without problems on the IABP. Mortality exceeds 80% with medical therapy. Surgery should not be delayed for some weeks as was formerly recommended, even if the IABP produces some stability. This improvement is usually temporary, and although surgical mortality is high, repair of the lesion that is causing hemodynamic compromise gives the only hope of survival. Some centers use intraoperative angiography or angioscopy to define coronary occlusions for added management with CABS.

LEFT VENTRICULAR ANEURYSM

An angiographic left ventricular demarcated diastolic deformity with systolic dyskinesia defines a ventricular aneurysm.
Associated features and implications include

- Left ventricular aneurysm is observed in 10 to 15% of patients within 3 months post infarction
- ECG at this stage shows ST segment elevation greater than 1.5 mm in two or more of the following leads: V1 to V5 in approximately 33% of cases
- Usually seen with large Q wave anterior infarction and absence of LVH
- More than 75% involve the apical anteroseptal region
- Severe heart failure is often refractory to intensive cardiac drug therapy. Thus, these patients have a poor quality of life
- Three-month and 1-year mortalities are greater than 50 and 75%, respectively
- Most deaths are due to heart failure and lethal arrhythmias
- Low cardiac output state due to steal of stroke volume
- Elevated LV end diastolic pressure and pulmonary congestion due to LV diastolic volume overload
- Increased LV wall stress imposed by global remodeling secondary to aneurysmal dilatation; thus, angina may worsen

- The thinned myocardial wall is densely fibrotic, and variable calcification occurs
- Although significant benefit from surgery is far from invariable, aneurysmectomy carries advantages over medical therapy in patients under age 75 who are healthy enough to undergo aneurysmectomy and any necessary CABS if clear indications are present
- The thin yet tough fibrocalcific aneurysmal walls are not prone to rupture

ANEURYSMECTOMY

Indications include

- Surgery may not attain symptomatic benefit or prolong life and is carefully considered in younger patients with severe angina or intractable heart failure, refractory to optimal doses of digoxin, furosemide, and ACE inhibitor
- Patients with lethal or potentially lethal arrhythmias: Recurrent sustained ventricular tachycardia, VF, patients resuscitated from cardiac arrest. This group will include patients whose arrhythmias have not responded to amiodarone or in whom adverse effects and intolerance to amiodarone exist. Some patients in this category may benefit from multiple programmable pacemaker-cardioverter-defibrillator. Aneurysmectomy and map-guided focus resection are offered at some centers, while a few use aneurysmectomy and extensive cryoablation applied to surrounding areas (see Chapter 18)

Contraindications to surgery include

- Elderly patients, infirmity, or underlying disease
- Large aneurysm with no effective left ventricular cavity to generate adequate stroke volume following aneurysmectomy
- Poor contractility of the nonaneurysmal left ventricle

MEDICAL THERAPY FOR VENTRICULAR ANEURYSM

A large percentage of patients with left ventricular aneurysm must be managed with drug therapy because of contraindications to surgery.

- Management entails the judicious use of digoxin, furosemide, and ACE inhibitor and is discussed in Chapter 5
- Recurrent sustained VT or resuscitation from VF is best managed with low-dose amiodarone (see Chapter 6). Importantly, all antiarrhythmic agents, with the exception of amiodarone, mexiletine, and quinidine, have marked negative inotropic effects and may precipitate heart failure, especially in patients with poor contractility, poor LV systolic function, and an EF less than 25%. Quinidine is relatively safe in patients with low EF, but has poor efficacy. The unsatisfactory nature of the results obtained with Class I agents is undoubtedly amplified by a high incidence of proarrhythmic effects with the majority of these agents, especially in the presence of poor LV function. Quinidine decreases VF threshold and there is a definite indication that the drug increases mor-

tality. Mexiletine's weak action limits its usefulness. Amiodarone has low proarrhythmic effects and has a role in patients with life-threatening arrhythmias. The dose of amiodarone and adverse effects are given in Chapter 6

- Left ventricular thrombus occurs in over 80% of patients. However, the thrombus is usually laminated and well attached to the endocardium, and embolization occurs in less than 3%. If there is no contraindication, warfarin is given to increase the prothrombin time ratio 1.25 to 1.5 times the control or to achieve an international normalized ratio (INR) of 2–3, for a period of 6 months in patients with nonlaminated thrombus protruding into the LV cavity and for 3 months with nonlaminated, nonprotruding thrombi. Thereafter, enteric-coated aspirin is given. There is some evidence that aspirin can prevent occurrence of atrial and LV mural thrombi and it is advisable to give aspirin to patients with left ventricular aneurysm

DEEP VEIN THROMBOSIS/PULMONARY EMBOLISM/ SYSTEMIC EMBOLISM

Antithrombotic therapy is required during the first 10 days of acute MI. Thereafter, aspirin is continued indefinitely.

Antithrombotic therapy is required to prevent

- Deep vein thrombosis (DVT) and pulmonary embolism
- LV mural thrombus formation and systemic embolization
- Reinfarction, especially among patients with non Q wave infarction, since these patients are at high risk for reinfarction within 3 months
- Reocclusion after successful coronary reperfusion with thrombolytic therapy

Within 4 days of acute MI, DVT occurs in the lower limbs in some 15 to 25% of patients (see Table 4–9). An additional 10 to 15% of patients develop DVT in the ensuing 10 days. This early occurrence of DVT suggests the presence of a hypercoagulable state similar to that observed post surgery.

The post-infarction incidence of DVT increases with the presence of cardiogenic shock, heart failure, and prolonged immobilization beyond the fifth day. Age over 70 years carries a sixfold increase with an incidence of about 70%; this may be compared with an incidence of only 12% among patients under age 50.

Three randomized clinical trials with a total of 130 patients using subcutaneous heparin, started within 18 hours of the onset of acute MI and given for 10 days, showed a reduction of DVT from 24 to 4% in the treated patients.

RECOMMENDATIONS FOR PREVENTION OF DVT

On admission, subcutaneous heparin, 10,000 to 12,500 units every 12 hours, is advisable in all patients considered at high risk and who are not given aspirin along with a thrombolytic agent. Patients at high risk include

TABLE 4–9. DEEP VENOUS THROMBOSIS, VENTRICULAR THROMBOEMBOLISM FOLLOWING ACUTE MYOCARDIAL INFARCTION

PARAMETERS	APPROXIMATE INCIDENCE (%)
DVT patients	
age >70	72
<50	12
Timing of occurrence	
<4 days	15–25
5–15 days	5–15
1–15 days	20–40
Effect of early heparin therapy	<4
Pulmonary embolism	4
Early heparin	<1
Mural thrombus	
anterior infarcts	30
large anterior infarcts	50
Systemic embolism	<4
Effect of heparin (10,000 to 12,500 units SC 12 hourly)	<1
Effects of early aspirin	To be defined.

- Age greater than 70 years
- Q wave MI or suspected large anterior infarction
- Heart failure
- Cardiogenic shock
- Expected prolonged immobilization beyond 3 days
- Previous DVT or pulmonary embolism

The present use of aspirin and thrombolytic agents appears to have decreased the incidence of DVT and pulmonary embolism post MI.

Patients considered at high risk for developing DVT should be given subcutaneous heparin every 12 hours, along with aspirin, 162.5 mg daily. Heparin is given until the patient is discharged. Patients not considered at high risk for the development of DVT can be managed with aspirin.

Early ambulation from day 2 is crucial in the prevention of DVT and pulmonary embolism and must be enforced, except when cardiogenic shock and other mechanical complications preclude sitting out of bed from day 2. Table 4–10 gives an ambulation schedule suited for patients with uncomplicated MI. All patients, including those with heart failure, are best managed from the second post-infarct day from bed to chair and with leg and calf muscle exercises.

Studies done prior to the current era of early mobilization and use of aspirin plus or minus thrombolytic therapy have indicated a 4 to 5% incidence of post-MI pulmonary embolism. Thus, patients considered at low risk for developing DVT or pulmonary embolism, i.e., patients under age 65 with non Q wave infarcts, small infarcts, absence of heart failure, and ability to mobilize on day 2, can be given aspirin only to prevent DVT or pulmonary embolism. Patients given IV streptokinase should continue on

TABLE 4–10. UNCOMPLICATED POST MYOCARDIAL INFARCTION AMBULATION
DAY

DAY	
2	Lower limb exercises, sit in chair, use bedside commode
3	Bed to chair, walk to shower
4	Transfer from CCU, bathroom privileges, walk in room
5	Walk in corridor 100–200 feet
6	Blood pressure pre & post 200-foot walk
7	If no contraindications, predischarge (Naughton or similar protocol exercise test)
8	Discharge
9	Walk outside 50–100 yards, increase by 50–100 daily to
14	0.25-mile walks once or twice daily
21	1-mile walks
	Post-discharge exercise test

aspirin; low-dose subcutaneous heparin is continued from day 2 to discharge if the patient is considered at high risk for thromboembolism.

PREVENTION OF SYSTEMIC EMBOLISM

Mural thrombus occurs in approximately 20% of patients, but large anterior infarcts have an incidence as high as 60%. Systemic embolism occurs in less than 4%, and the incidence can be reduced to about 1% with subcutaneous heparin, 10,000 to 12,500 units, given subcutaneously for 10 days. The incidence of mural thrombus and systemic embolism is reduced by the early use of aspirin and streptokinase. Continued aspirin therapy appears to decrease the incidence of mural thrombus and systemic embolism.

If heparin is not contraindicated and thrombolytic therapy has not been given, it is advisable to give subcutaneous heparin to patients with large anterior infarcts or infarction, which include the apex of the heart.

Heparin

Dosage: 10,000 to 12,500 units subcutaneously every 12 hours given from admission for 10 days. Alternatively, IV heparin is used as part of the thrombolytic therapy regimen if tPA was the agent administered. Heparin is then continued for up to 6 days and followed by subcutaneous heparin. If aspirin only is being used, without thrombolytic therapy, reduce the dose of heparin to 7,500, to a maximum 10,000 units every 12 hours. The activated partial thromboplastin time should just exceed 1.5 but should not exceed twice the control. If echocardiography done prior to discharge shows the thrombus to be nonlaminated and protruding, oral anticoagulation with warfarin should be commenced and continued for 3 months. Most systemic emboli occur within the first 10 days of infarction and, after discharge, the majority occur in under 3 months. For thrombi associated with aneurysm, see the earlier section of this chapter.

PERICARDITIS

Approximately 40% of fatal MI show acute fibrinous pericarditis. The incidence of clinical pericarditis ranges from 5 to 25%. Pericarditis usually manifests during the second and fifth day post infarction, localized in the area overlying the infarct, but may diffusely involve the pericardial sac. Approximately 50% are symptomatic.

CLINICAL HALLMARKS

Diagnostic features include

- Mild to moderate pleuritic-type pain. Maximal over the precordium or substernal area with occasional or typical involvement of the trapezius ridges (one or both)
- Pain is made worse with recumbency, deep breathing, and body movement, and is improved by leaning forward
- Pain can be confused superficially with post-infarction angina. It is of paramount importance to distinguish the two conditions, since the latter usually requires interventional therapy beginning with coronary angiography, whereas pericarditis requires conservatism. Importantly, the pain of angina does not radiate to the trapezius ridges
- A pericardial friction rub is heard in 10 to 30% of cases. The rub is typically evanescent and may come and go over 1 to 2 days, may increase with inspiration or expiration, coughing, or swallowing, and is best heard with the diaphragm of the stethoscope with the patient leaning forward. The rub usually has two diastolic components: early, during the early diastolic phase, and late, due to atrial systole. A third component occurs during ventricular systole. However, occasionally only one component may be heard, and the rub must be distinguished from acute mitral regurgitation, in which a soft murmur is produced due to papillary muscle dysfunction. Pericardial friction rub has a superficial scratchy characteristic. The ECG is rarely of value in the diagnosis of post-MI pericarditis. During acute infarction, typical ECG findings are rare and cannot be relied upon for diagnosis
- Echocardiography is helpful in over 33% of patients who show pericardial effusion
- Pericarditis appears to be more common in patients with Q wave infarction

THERAPY

- Discontinue heparin if pericarditis is proven
- Treatment is indicated for pain even when no friction rub is present
- Aspirin in full doses, 650 mg three times daily, is useful, and NSAIDS should be avoided because indomethacin and similar agents may cause vasoconstriction and alter myocardial healing and appear to increase the incidence of myocardial rupture. Also, these agents cause retention of sodium and water

- Pericarditis presenting between 2 and 6 months of infarction occurs in less than 0.1% of patients. Fever, increased sedimentation rate, and increased titer of heart reactive antibodies may be present; NSAIDS are best avoided because they cause vasoconstriction and increase stress on the myocardium
- Late pericarditis is treated with aspirin. Failure to respond or relapses should be managed with a short course of prednisone with aspirin overlapping at least 2 weeks before prednisone is withdrawn

PREDISCHARGE EXERCISE TEST

The ACC/AHA Task Force Report 1990 states that the best time to obtain the exercise test depends on patient characteristics, physician preference, departmental policies, and local laboratory expertise. The report adds that maximal exercise testing at 3 weeks post-infarction is a cost-effective alternative to submaximal predischarge testing on day 7 to 14 and can be used for evaluation of functional capacity as well as prognostication. Timing and relevance of post-infarction exercise stress testing is given in Table 4–11.

The Task Force emphasizes that a 10- to 14-day predischarge test does not allow for the early sixth to seventh-day discharge of patients with uncomplicated infarction. The report appropriately states that the safety of predischarge submaximal testing is less well established and only evalu-

TABLE 4–11. TIMING AND RELEVANCE OF POST-INFARCTION EXERCISE STRESS TESTING

PARAMETERS	6–7 DAYS	10–14 DAYS	3 WEEKS
Functional test	Yes	Yes	Yes
Prolongs hospital stay >7 days	No	Yes	Not applicable
Requires very careful selection of patients	Yes	Yes	Not as stringent
Safety established	No	Somewhat	Yes
Standard for comparison	Not well established	Not well established	Yes
Confusion in interpretation	Yes	Yes	Little
Cost	High, 2 tests required*	2 tests required	Acceptable
Mainly low-risk group tested	Yes	Yes	Can test all grades if needed
Prognostic value	No (Probable in some)	No (Probable in some)	Yes: Attain ≥6 METS <3% 1-year mortality Attain ≤4 METS >12% 1 year mortality

* Predischarge and at 6 weeks

ates functional capacity in properly selected patients. Testing at 3 weeks has proven to be safe, and the 10- to 14-day delay caused in patients with uncomplicated infarction appears to be associated with rare instances of intercurrent death or reinfarction. In one study of 1,000 patients, using 3-week testing, 0.5% sustained a cardiac event: reinfarction occurred in five patients and cardiac death in two between the tenth day and 3 weeks. However, treadmill-induced deaths, although rare, tend to occur prior to 14 days post infarction. The results of a 3-week test can be correlated with that of several well documented studies

- Patients who complete 6 or more metabolic exercise equivalents (METs: one MET equals the amount of oxygen used at rest) and experience no electrocardiographic ischemic changes have a less than 3% 1-year mortality
- Inability to complete a treadmill workload of 4 METs is associated with a 6-fold increase in the risk of death or nonfatal reinfarction in the subsequent year
- Patients who fail to achieve peak systolic blood pressure greater than 110 mm Hg, increased systolic pressure greater than 10 mm Hg from baseline, have a poor prognosis
- Patients who develop greater than or equal to 2 mm ST segment depression persisting for more than 2 minutes at a heart rate of less than 120/min, have poor coronary reserve and should be considered for urgent interventional therapy

These conclusions are applicable to tests performed at 3 or 6 weeks but are of limited relevance to submaximal tests performed at 6 to 14 days post infarction. Fortunately, tertiary or community hospitals rarely keep uncomplicated infarct patients longer than 7 days. Thus, a 7- to 14-day predischarge test is not applicable to those patients with uncomplicated MI, who will have been discharged long before the test.

A study of patients admitted to early thrombolytic therapy indicates that predischarge exercise test results were not predictive of 5-year reinfarction or survival. In one study, exercise testing in the elderly incorrectly identified 57% of patients with multivessel disease. In addition, exercise testing in the post-infarct patient had a less than 80% sensitivity and, thus, may have missed 20% of patients at high risk for fatal or nonfatal reinfarction. Patients not suitable for predischarge exercise testing are indicated in Table 4–12.

Patients at high risk for fatal or nonfatal reinfarction post discharge include those with large anterior myocardial infarction, EF less than 35%, mild heart failure, post-infarction angina, non Q wave infarction right ventricular infarction, and patients aged 70 to 80, many of whom cannot complete a meaningful exercise test but may require bypass surgery.

In view of the limitations of stress testing, many cardiologists consider that patients with non Q wave infarctions require urgent coronary angiograms to define critical stenoses. It may be preferable to manage this large group of patients in this way rather than to perform discharge exercise testing (see Table 4–12 and Fig. 3–2).

TABLE 4–12. POST-INFARCTION PATIENT NOT SUITABLE FOR PREDISCHARGE EXERCISE TEST

	APPROXIMATE %
1. Postinfarction ischemia	>5
2. Age over 75, test probably not justifiable	>15
3. Moderate or severe heart failure or ejection fraction <35%	>15
4. Non Q wave infarction, manage as unstable angina, (see Fig. 3–2)	15
5. Presence of debility, serious underlying disease	5

Patients suitable for predischarge exercise testing include those with uncomplicated infarction, a low-risk group that could derive greater benefit from a 3- or 6-week post-discharge test.

Despite the limitations of exercise testing as a method of screening patients during the early post-MI period, therapeutic decisions may sometimes rest on the result; for example, recurring atypical pain and a lesion of uncertain significance in a noninfarct-related artery. In contrast to the predischarge testing, several categories of post-infarction patients are able to perform a 3- or 6-week test that is meaningful regarding advice on exercise, return to work, and consideration of interventional therapy. As outlined earlier, however, the timing of exercise stress testing depends on departmental preferences.

THALLIUM-201 SCINTIGRAPHY

Several studies have failed to show significant benefit from thallium 201 scintigraphy when added to predischarge or 6-week exercise testing. Dipyridamole-thallium scintigraphy has a small role in a select subset of patients who are unable to perform an exercise stress test 6 weeks post infarction. The test should not be used in patients with unstable angina, post-infarction angina, left bundle branch block, or heart failure and has no role in patients with uncomplicated myocardial infarction (see Chapters 2 and 17).

The sensitivity and specificity of thallium-201 photon emission computed tomography (SPECT) for detecting noninfarct-related coronary stenosis is approximately 60 and 45%, respectively. Thus, SPECT appears to give a limited diagnostic definition of post-infarction coronary disease, and further studies are needed to clarify its role.

ANGIOPLASTY

The TIMI-II trial indicates no difference in mortality or reinfarction in patients treated with thrombolytic therapy and urgent coronary angiography followed, where feasible, by angioplasty as compared with patients submitted to a strategy of delayed coronary angioplasty only when indicated. The sum of total mortality and nonfatal reinfarction within 42 days in patients treated with thrombolytic therapy and urgent coronary angioplasty was 11% and 10% in the conservative delayed coronary angioplasty group. In post-MI patients treated or nontreated with thrombolytic therapy, selection for angiography with a view to optimal intervention with angioplasty or CABS requires sound judgment on the part of the cardiologist; a team discussion is often involved in the decision.

Coronary angiography with a view to angioplasty or CABS is considered in the following categories of patients

* Post-infarction angina: Recurrent chest pain clearly related to ischemia
* Anterior infarcts and those considered at high risk for cardiac events (see Table 4–1)
* Cardiogenic shock
* With ischemic changes on predischarge or post-discharge exercise stress testing
* Non Q wave infarction
* With VF or sustained VT considered to be related to ischemia

The above categories of patients are selected for coronary angioplasty and dilatation of the infarct-related artery, provided that the coronary obstructed lesion is angiographically acceptable for balloon angioplasty and there is good ventricular function with an EF equal to or greater than 40%. In addition, patients seen within 6 hours of onset of infarction with cardiogenic shock with a proximal high-grade left anterior descending obstructive lesion benefit from urgent coronary angioplasty.

Patients over age 75 have a good success rate with coronary angioplasty, but hospital mortality is high, at about 6%, versus less than 2% in patients under age 65. However, there is a high recurrence rate of angina post dilatation, and longterm relief is therefore less common than in younger patients. In one study, 86% of elderly hospital survivors were still alive 4 years after angioplasty.

In patients who have severe limiting angina, coronary angioplasty affords significant relief of symptoms, sometimes in an otherwise intractable situation, although after 5 years, less than 30% are expected to be alive and free of Class III and IV angina.

Since less than 25% of patients with acute infarction presently qualify in North America (up to 40% in the UK) for thrombolytic therapy, there remains a significant number of patients who may benefit from primary angioplasty, especially those at moderate to high risk. Ongoing clinical trials should clarify management strategies. It is anticipated that more than 30% of patients can be selected for thrombolytic therapy, approximately 15% for early coronary angioplasty, and the remaining medium- to low-risk patients for medical therapy or revascularization on the basis of 3 or 6 weeks post-exercise testing.

Apart from reocclusion by thrombus and rare dissection, the major problem encountered with coronary angioplasty done within the first week of infarction is a high reocclusion rate, which was observed in several multicenter randomized studies. If reocclusion rates can be reduced, urgent coronary angioplasty in the early infarction setting could have a major role in the tertiary care setting, especially in patients in whom thrombolytic therapy is contraindicated. The high reocclusion rate may be related to a hypercoagulable state present in the first 4 days post infarction. In support of this proposition are the results of studies indicating an increased risk of thrombosis: left ventricular mural thrombus, deep vein thrombosis, and pulmonary embolism similar to the post-surgical state. The incidence of post-infarction DVT is 20 to 40%, an incidence that is higher than should be expected from a 2- to 4-day period of bed rest. Strategies to prevent rethrombosis following thrombolytic therapy and coronary angioplasty, therefore, merit intensive studies. The problem of late restenosis after successful coronary balloon or laser angioplasty is discussed in Chapter 2.

Post-angioplasty early reocclusion is not surprising, however. Trauma to the atheromatous plaque releases thrombogenic plaque contents and, with local endothelial damage, predisposes thrombosis. Heparin and/or aspirin are not sufficiently effective. New thrombin-specific inhibitors and other agents are being tested.

CORONARY ARTERY BYPASS SURGERY

In experienced hands, CABS is now considered a relatively safe, justifiable, and useful procedure in properly selected post-infarction patients at high risk for death or reinfarction. Patient selection has been discussed earlier under angioplasty. Patients who have an EF greater than 50% have a less than 1% mortality. Among patients who have an EF less than 40%, the mortality is higher, is in the range of 5 to 10% according to the degree of irreversible LV dysfunction, and is higher still in the elderly and other patients at special risk. Some of these patients require hemodynamic support with IABP to allow hemodynamic stability for angiography and CABS.

DISCHARGE MEDICATIONS

BETA BLOCKERS

If beta blockers were commenced during the early hours of MI and no adverse effects were apparent, the beta blockers should be continued. If not given at that time, beta blockers should be administered prior to discharge and maintained for at least 2 years. Studies indicate that this approach is highly beneficial and cost effective.

BETA BLOCKER CLINICAL TRIAL RESULTS

More than 15 beta blocker trials have been conducted on post-MI patients. However, several of these trials lack the methodology that is consistent with current practice in clinical trial design. Unacceptable meta analyses have been carried out using beta blocker trials that included few patients, some nonrandomized trials and trials in which beta blocker therapy was commenced later than 1 month post infarction.

Four clinical trials that meet most current acceptable standards are listed in Table 4–13. These trials indicate an impressive 33% reduction in mortality due to beta blocker therapy. Importantly, mortality reduction with

TABLE 4–13. MORTALITY REDUCTION IN BETA BLOCKER LONG TERM TRIALS				
TRIAL	PLACEBO MORTALITY	DRUG MORTALITY	RELATIVE REDUCTION (%)	p VALUE
Norwegian (1981)				
Timolol	152/939	98/945	35.5	<0.001
20 mg daily	16.2%	10.4%		
BHAT				
Propranolol	188/1921	138/1916	26.5	<0.01
180/240 mg daily	9.8%	7.2%		
Salathia (1985)				
Metoprolol	43/364	27/391	41.5	<0.05
200 mg daily	11.8%	6.9%		
APSI Trial (1988)				
Acebutolol	34/309	17/298		
400 mg daily	11.0%	5.7%	48	0.019
Total	417/3533	2801/3252		
	11.8%	7.9%	33	

propranolol is significantly less than that observed with timolol in smokers as emphasized in Chapter 2, the efficacy of hepatic-metabolized beta blockers is blunted by cigarette smoking. It is necessary to prescribe metoprolol or timolol to refractory smokers.

If there is no contraindication to beta blockade, virtually all post-MI patients should receive timolol, 10 mg twice daily, or acebutolol, 400 mg daily, or metoprolol, 100 to 200 mg daily. Propranolol, 180 to 240 mg daily, is advisable only in nonsmokers. The ACC/AHA Task Force recommends treatment to commence within the first few days of infarction and to continue for at least 2 years in virtually all patients if there are no contraindications to beta blockers.

It is estimated that 70% of post-infarction patients are suitable for beta blocker therapy. Up to 20% of post-infarction patients are unable to receive beta blockers because of contraindications, and a further 10% have relative contraindications.

Contraindications to longterm beta-adrenergic blockade include

• Severe LV failure
• Systolic blood pressure less than 100 mm Hg
• Heart rate less than 60/min
• Type I, II, or III AV block
• Asthma or severe chronic obstructive pulmonary disease

Some cardiologists do not prescribe beta blockers to so-called "low-risk" patients. However, risks are not accurately assured by stress testing. Because beta blockers are capable of producing about a 28% reduction in reinfarction rates, up to 67% reduction in sudden death, and a 33% decrease in mortality, it is advisable to prescribe these medications to virtually all patients who can tolerate the effects at the relatively low dosage indicated above. Acebutolol, metoprolol, and timolol, are better tolerated than propranolol and are preferred. If mild adverse effects occur, the drug dos-

TABLE 4–14. BETA BLOCKER REDUCTION OF EARLY MORNING SUDDEN CARDIAC DEATH

SUDDEN DEATHS	CONTROL	PROPRANOLOL	DECREASE
Total	78	60	23%*
5 to 8 a.m.	6	0	
5 to 11 a.m.	25	11	56%
11 to 4 a.m.	33	31	Similar

* Timolol: 67% reduction in sudden death
Modified from: Beta-Blocker Heart Attack Study Data. Am J Cardiol, *63*:1518, 1989.

age should be decreased slightly or a switch should be made to another beta blocking agent. Subtle but important differences of various beta blockers are discussed in Chapters 1 and 2. Patients should be encouraged to persist with therapy except when adverse effects are bothersome.

Protective effects of beta-adrenergic blockade appear to relate to their ability to actuate

• A decrease in early morning sudden cardiac death (see Fig. 2–7 and Table 4–14)
• A decrease in the incidence of early myocardial freewall rupture
• A decrease in lethal arrhythmias, yet causing only a modest suppression of VPCs
• An increase in VF threshold and a decrease in the incidence of VF
• Proven decrease in the incidence of fatal and nonfatal MI rates, possibly by decreasing hydraulic stress at the site of atheroma, thus preventing plaque fissuring and subsequent thrombosis. The action of beta blockers to attenuate the hemodynamic effects of catecholamine surges may protect a vulnerable atheromatous plaque from rupture and consequent coronary thrombosis that leads to fatal MI, sudden death, or nonfatal MI
• Prevention of early morning platelet aggregation induced by catecholamines and decreased early morning peak incidence of acute MI and sudden death (Table 4–14)
• Decreased renin activity. This may have salutary effects on ventricular remodeling. Decreased aneurysmal expansion may occur

In the United States, beta blocker usage in the post-infarction patient can prevent more than 15,000 deaths in the first year and up to 60,000 deaths over 5 years in patients at medium or high risk. The effectiveness of beta blockers in the low-risk post-infarction population is modest but worthwhile because it is occasionally difficult to correctly assign risks based on prognostic parameters including post-discharge exercise stress testing. In addition, beta blocking agents prevent sudden cardiac death, and it must be emphasized that aspirin does not prevent sudden cardiac death.

Adverse effects and dosage of beta blockers are given in Chapter 2.

ACETYL SALICYLIC ACID (ASPIRIN)

Dosage: Initial dose, regular aspirin, 325 mg, and then enteric-coated aspirin, 160 to 325 mg, once daily.

Indications
- Unstable angina
- Stable angina
- Onset of acute MI, 160 to 325 mg aspirin
- Post-MI prophylaxis
- Prevention of systemic embolization from atrial or ventricular thrombi
- Prevention of pulmonary embolism
- Prevention of fatal or nonfatal strokes in patients with cerebral transient ischemic attacks or post stroke
- Post CABS to prevent graft occlusion
- Lone atrial fibrillation in patients under age 70

Action. Aspirin irreversibly acetylates the platelet enzyme cyclooxygenase, thus preventing platelets from forming the powerful aggregating agent thromboxane A2, resulting in a decrease in platelet aggregation. One dose of 80 mg of aspirin inhibits cyclooxygenase for the 1-week lifespan of the circulating platelets. This action abolishes platelet aggregation that would occur in response to stimuli such as

- Collagen
- Arachidonate
- Second-phase aggregation by adenosine diphosphate (ADP) and epinephrine
- Aspirin, unfortunately, reduces the formation of the potent vasodilator prostacyclin, and the smallest possible dose is advisable, 80 to 160 mg daily, so as not to inhibit prostacyclin. Further studies will clarify the dose range. Currently, a dose of 160 to 325 mg daily is widely used in post-MI patients

Aspirin causes a reduction of the early morning incidence of acute MI but does not prevent sudden death (Table 4–15). The incidence of gastrointestinal bleeding is shown in Table 4–16.

NITRATES

Nitroglycerin is given to all patients upon hospital discharge, including patients with uncomplicated infarction.

Dosage: 0.3 mg. If pain occurs, the patient is advised to take the drug sublingually while sitting or propped up in bed to allow sufficient pooling of blood in the periphery. The drug must not be taken while standing because presyncope or syncope may occur, especially in patients on concomitant therapy with ACE inhibitors, diuretics, or calcium antagonists.

Oral nitrates are not prescribed routinely to post-MI patients, except for patients with post-infarction angina, who are unable to undergo coronary

TABLE 4–15. ASPIRIN REDUCTION OF EARLY MORNING MYOCARDIAL INFARCTION BUT NOT SUDDEN DEATH*

	ASPIRIN	PLACEBO	p VALUE
Fatal MI	10	26	0.007
Nonfatal MI	129	213	0.0001
Sudden death	22	12	0.08
Other coronary heart disease	24	25	
Stroke death	9	6	
Total cardiovascular death	81	83	
Total death	271	227	0.64

* 22,071 physicians aged 50–80: 325 mg aspirin alternate day over 5 years
Modified from: The Physicians' Health Study. N Engl J Med, *321*:129, 1989.

TABLE 4–16. GASTROINTESTINAL BLEED IN THE PHYSICIANS STUDY (22,071 PHYSICIANS)

	ASPIRIN	PLACEBO	p VALUE
Upper gastrointestinal	38	28	
Melena	364	246	0.00001
Transfusion	48	28	

Modified from: The Physicians' Health Study. N Engl J Med, *321*:129, 1989.

angioplasty or bypass surgery because of contraindications such as advanced age or serious underlying disease. Where required, oral nitrates are best used in combination with a beta blocker because they do not prevent reinfarction and have not been shown to decrease mortality. Dosage and other effects of nitrates are given in Chapter 2.

CALCIUM ANTAGONISTS

Calcium antagonists do not have a role during the early phase (first day) of acute MI (see Chapter 3). Prior to discharge, a few properly selected patients may require calcium antagonists. Importantly, calcium antagonists have not been shown to significantly decrease mortality in the post-infarction patient and are advisable only when beta blockers are contraindicated for the management of post-infarction angina. A meta analysis indicates that calcium antagonists do not reduce infarct size or mortality, and in some categories of patients, these agents increase the risk of death.

Indications for calcium antagonists in post infarction

- As an adjunct to beta blockers, because ischemia in some patients cannot be controlled with the judicious use of one of these drugs
- Patients with post-infarction angina in whom coronary angioplasty, bypass surgery, or beta blockers are contraindicated
- Hypertensive patients in whom beta blockers are contraindicated and blood pressure reduction is required. However, these patients are best

controlled with an ACE inhibitor so that decrease in blood pressure and ventricular remodeling are both addressed

There is no role for routine prophylactic verapamil during the first 2 years post MI. The Danish Study Group on Verapamil in Myocardial Infarction (DAVIT II) showed an 18-month mortality rate of 11.1% and 13.8% in the verapamil and placebo treated groups, respectively (p = 0.11).

Numerous post-infarction patients have been given diltiazem. This practice has been based on a small non Q wave infarction study. In the 1986 Non Q Wave Infarction Study, performed on 288 control patients and 288 patients given high-dose diltiazem, 360 showed a 51% reduction in reinfarction rates in patients with non Q wave infarction treated from day 1 for 14 days. This small study group did not show a decrease in mortality. A large multicenter study, however, involving 2,466 patients was completed in 1988 (see Table 4–17). This study showed no decrease in total cardiac mortality, and there was no significant decrease in reinfarction rates in patients with Q wave versus non Q wave infarction. A significant increase in mortality attributable to diltiazem was observed in patients with pulmonary congestion and left ventricular EF below 40%. The increase in mortality persisted during long-term therapy beyond 1 year.

In patients with an EF below 40%, heart failure occurred in 12% (39/326) of patients on placebo and in 21% (61/297) of patients receiving diltiazem (p = 0.004).

Only 514 patients with non Q wave were enrolled in this study. The cumulative 1-year cardiac event rate (death and/or nonfatal reinfarction was 9% in diltiazem-treated and 15% in placebo-treated patients). There was a small decrease in reinfarction rates only in patients treated up to 6 months. Reinfarction after 6 months occurred in 13 patients in the placebo group and in 14 in the treated group. Firm conclusions cannot be made from subgroup analysis of an overall negative study. Also, these studies were done prior to the era of widespread aspirin use in patients with MI.

Short-term, 1- to 3-month randomized trials need to be carried out in patients with non Q wave infarction treated with standard therapy, aspirin,

---

TABLE 4–17. DILTIAZEM IN ACUTE MYOCARDIAL INFARCTION, LONGTERM STUDY*

	PLACEBO PATIENTS	DILTIAZEM PATIENTS	COMMENTS
Cardiac deaths	124	127	
Noncardiac deaths	43	38	
Total mortality	167	166	
Reinfarction	116	99	
Total cardiac events	226	202	11% decrease p = 0.26
Ejection fraction <40%			
Heart failure occurrence	39	61	p < 0.004
	12%	21%	↑ HF due to diltiazem

Modified from: N Engl J Med, *319*:385, 1988 and Circulation, *83*:52, 1991.

and a beta blocker, compared with a group treated with diltiazem, to verify the benefits of diltiazem on early reinfarction rates. Until trial results are available, diltiazem in combination with aspirin has a small role in patients with non Q wave infarction who are unable to take a beta-blocking drug. In these patients, after the second post-infarction day, if heart failure is not present and the EF is greater than 40%, diltiazem may be administered for up to 6 months until interventional therapy, CABS or angioplasty, has been carried out (see Chapter 3 and Fig. 3–2).

Contraindications. Contraindications to calcium antagonists post infarction include

• Pulmonary congestion of all grades
• EF less than 40%
• Bradyarrhythmias, suspected sinus or AV node disease
• Hypotension

Caution. Do not combine beta blockers with calcium antagonists, except in carefully selected patients, in order to avoid heart failure and bradyarrhythmias (see Chapter 2). Care is needed when giving diltiazem to post-MI patients who show pulmonary congestion or LV dysfunction. The evidence indicating that diltiazem decreases reinfarction rates and non Q wave infarction is weak. Meta analysis of therapy with calcium antagonists in post-infarction patients has revealed an excess mortality (averaging 6%). This mortality is markedly increased if pulmonary congestion, LV dysfunction, or bradyarrhythmia is present.

ACE INHIBITORS

The beneficial effects of ACE inhibitors in the acute phase of infarction have been discussed earlier. A detailed discussion of these agents is given in Chapters 1 and 5. Only their prophylactic role will be considered in this section.

The renin angiotension aldosterone system is stimulated during acute infarction, and the degree of stimulation relates to the size of the infarct. Increase in renin activity appears to relate to an increase in mortality. This finding is, of course, to be expected because patients with large infarcts and EF less than 35% have high in-hospital and 1-year mortalities. LV dysfunction or concomitant decrease in blood pressure stimulates the renin angiotensin system.

Some degree of ventricular enlargement is detectable in over 40% of patients with Q wave transmural anterolateral infarction and is observed as early as 1 or 2 weeks after the event. Physical slippage and reorientation of myocyte bundles in the infarcted area occur, causing thinning and expansion. The left ventricle appears to undergo a variable amount of dilatation with some hypertrophy of the noninfarcted area.

Stimulation of the renin angiotensin system plays an important role in augmenting diastolic and systolic wall stresses, producing further left ventricular enlargement. The structural changes in the left ventricle, termed remodeling, appear to have some detrimental effects that may later increase the incidence of heart failure.

Fortunately, ACE inhibitors favorably influence remodeling and improve EF, and their use may be considered in post-infarct patients without overt heart failure but with EF less than 35%. This indication is being tested in ongoing clinical trials.

The Survival and Ventricular Enlargement Trial (SAVE) studied patients at an average of 11 days post infarction, with an average EF of 31%; 60% of patients were in Killip I and 40% Killip Class II. Patients randomized to treatment with captopril showed a significant 17% reduction in risk of death (p = 0.020) compared with the control group at 2-year follow-up.

Thus, captopril therapy (37.5 to 150 mg daily) is advisable, commencing between day 3 and discharge and continued for 1 to 2 years in patients with anterior infarction, large infarction, or EF less than 30%. Therapy in these patients reduces the incidence of hospitalization for heart failure and improves survival.

CHOLESTEROL-LOWERING AGENTS

Serum cholesterol and HDL cholesterol should be evaluated within a few days of admission to the hospital. These measurements can be done in a nonfasting state. If the serum cholesterol in patients under age 70 is greater than 240 mg/dl (6.2 mmol/l), the test should be repeated and decisions should be made based on the degree of elevations (see Chapter 8). In the Framingham post-MI study, patients with cholesterol levels greater than 7.11 mmol/l (274 mg/dl) proved to be at increased risk for reinfarction and cardiac mortality compared with patients who had cholesterol levels less than 5.2 mmol/l (200 mg/dl). An increased risk was not observed in patients with cholesterol levels of 5 to 7 mmol/l (193 to 270 mg/dl).

In-hospital diet should reflect the dietary advice given to the patient. Instructions on the value and use of a low saturated fat diet with an increase in polyunsaturated fatty acids, as outlined in the AHA guidelines or similar instructions, are appropriate for all patients.

In patients under age 65, an LDL cholesterol greater than 160 mg/dl (4 mmol/l) after 3 months of dietary counseling calls for therapy with a 3-hydroxy-3-methylglutaryl coenzyme A (HMG-CoA) reductase inhibitors: lovastatin, mevastatin, or pravastatin. A combination HMG-CoA reductase inhibitor and cholestyramine or colestipol may be necessary if cholesterol levels do not attain treatment goals.

Hyperlipidemia caused by beta blockers is often offered as a reason for not prescribing these medications. In the BHAT, propranolol, over a 1-year period, increased serum triglycerides by about 17% and lowered HDL cholesterol by about 6% (3 mg/dl; 0.06 mmol). There was no effect on total cholesterol or LDL cholesterol. The reduction in HDL is considered non-significant and does not significantly reduce the beneficial reductions in mortality and morbidity due to propranolol in the post-MI patient. The longterm reduction in the level of HDL by metoprolol is 0 to 7%. The reader is advised to see the discussion in Chapter 8 and to consider the salutary effects of beta-adrenergic blockers given in Figure 2–7. In the post-MI patient with moderate or severe hyperlipidemia, it is preferable to prescribe a beta blocker such as acebutolol that does not significantly alter HDL levels; advice on diet and, if needed, drug therapy to control the hyperlipidemic state should be given.

PSYCHOSOCIAL IMPACT OF THE HEART ATTACK

The emotional distress to the individual in the months following an acute MI is often as severe as the heart attack itself. The intense apprehension concerning an impaired quality of life, returning to work, and the ability to meet financial obligations poses a threat to the patient's well-being and must be considered of paramount importance by the treating physician and the medical, nursing, and social teams. Thus, psychologic intervention should be commenced during the first 24 hours after admission.

The patient and the family must be given information concerning diagnosis and proposed therapy. The patient should be given reassurance, especially if heart failure is not present with uncomplicated MI. The removal of an oxygen mask or nasal prongs if hypoxemia is absent serves to reassure the patient and family that improvement is underway.

Anxiety and depression may center around concerns about longterm disability or death and may persist for weeks to months in more than 50% of patients with infarction. It is imperative that the patient be allowed to discuss fears and inner feelings at this early stage and again prior to discharge. The reassuring tone of the patient's cardiologist or treating physician helps allay anxiety. Decisions concerning the length of hospital stay and, with uncomplicated infarction, an approximate date of return to work should be given as early as day 3, with the understanding that these are rough estimates of the timing that will materialize as long as the expected progress is continued. Early ambulation from day 2 also helps to allay anxiety.

A trainee, nurse, or social worker may attend to other aspects of discussion regarding family matters. Stress associated with the patient's employment should be thoroughly explored and advice and assistance should be given. Advice must be consistent to avoid discrepancies between the physician's recommendations and those of trainees or the nursing staff.

Although small doses of anxiolytic agents may be required during the first 2 days post MI, patients should be quickly weaned. Patients can usually overcome their emotional hurdles by clear advice from the nursing staff, and few patients require antidepressant drugs, which should be avoided where possible, because of their mild negative inotropic effect. Also, they may trigger arrhythmias, notably, torsades de pointes.

Uncomplicated infarct patients are usually discharged on the sixth or seventh day. Patients with mild heart failure usually require more time, and those with complications not requiring surgical intervention are often ready for discharge between the tenth and fourteenth days. Patients with uncomplicated infarction are advised to return to nonstressful work in 6 to 8 weeks; depending on complications, 10 weeks to 3 months may be required.

Sexual activities should be permitted within days or weeks of returning home. A low-level predischarge exercise test is reassuring if the patient is able to achieve a heart rate of about 120/min and to complete 4 METs of work without chest pain, marked shortness of breath, or ischemic changes. This functional test and knowledge of risk stratification should suffice to assure the patient that sexual activity can be resumed within days of discharge, but similar advice can be given to those patients who are expected to complete a low-level exercise test, based on risk stratification and common sense.

For the majority of sexually active individuals, intercourse is one of the most enjoyable, satisfying, and stress-relieving activities that life provides. The treating physician should encourage sexual activity, except in the obviously complicated cases, since this advice may convince the patient that all is proceeding well. This reassurance serves to control the fear of impending doom. Males must be reassured that heart attacks do not cause impotence and that the lack of intercourse for 3 to 6 weeks will not alter later sexual performance. It is important to explain to the patient that there is no reason to change to a different position; the most familiar position is usually best. This advice increases confidence in the male and allays anxiety in the female. Importantly, studies indicate that heart rate and blood pressure are not significantly affected by sexual position. The patient may also be reassured to learn that by 3 months after infarction, more than 80% of patients are able to engage in sexual performance with normal intensity and frequency.

REHABILITATION

Some patients require vocational and stress management counseling. Resumption of prior physical and sexual activity and engagement in some form of exercise program improves the patient's

- Morale
- Emotional, psychologic, and vocational status

Walking is the most commonly prescribed exercise activity for patients. Uncomplicated-infarct patients are expected to increase from 0.25 mile at week 2 to 1 mile at 3 weeks and, after a 3-month period, to have regular 1- to 2-mile brisk walks at least 6 days a week, in addition to normal activities. A brisk 1-mile walk twice daily, climbing three flights of stairs, and stretching exercises are advisable. Also advised is a 1-mile walk in 20 to 30 minutes over the first few weeks, followed, in energetic individuals, by the same distance covered in about 15 minutes. Healthy patients up to age 75 have been shown to improve their peak oxygen consumptional status by walking outdoors and/or in shopping or rehabilitation centers. From 3 weeks to 3 months, the patient is allowed activities beyond brisk walking.

Riding a stationary bike, simulated cross-country skiing, stretching exercises, or similar activities are common inexpensive modes of exercise. Many patients take pride in their ability to exercise, and this must be encouraged. The three- or six-week exercise test helps reassure the patient and indicates the level of activity desired and its safety.

Jogging and swimming, for interested patients, should commence after a 6-week exercise test. Jogging is built up slowly, one mile daily, increasing over months to three miles daily. Regular exercise is encouraged for at least 4 days of the week. Patients should refrain from weightlifting, rowing, and other static exercises.

SUPERVISED REHABILITATION PROGRAMS

These important programs require the services of

- Physician
- Nurse coordinator
- Physical therapist
- Social worker/psychiatrist

There is no proof from randomized trials that exercise training programs improve survival. However, improvement of muscle tone and the ability to perform employment activities and engage in a sporting hobby enhance quality of life.

Patients with Q wave infarction who are able to do greater than 4 METs predischarge exercise test or 6 METs at 3 or 6 weeks exercise testing (1 MET unit is equal to 3.5 ml oxygen consumed per kg body weight per minute) may participate in rehabilitation exercise programs. The patient should achieve 20 beats per minute above standing heart rate or increase 4 METs equivalent. Peak blood pressure should not exceed 140 mm Hg and heart rate should not exceed 140/min.

Only patients with moderate to severe heart failure, severe angina, inability to manage about 6 METs, and uncontrolled sustained VT or complex ventricular arrhythmias are denied access to exercise programs (Table 4–18). Participation is not allowed until residual ischemia has been managed by angioplasty or CABS, if feasible, and hypertension or arrhythmia has been controlled.

TABLE 4–18. CONTRAINDICATIONS TO EXERCISE TRAINING PROGRAMS FOR POST MYOCARDIAL INFARCTION PATIENTS*

1. Patients with suspected ischemia are deferred pending interventional therapy
2. Inability to manage about 6 METs at 3 or 6 weeks exercise stress testing
3. Overt or treated heart failure*
4. Suspect left ventricular systolic dysfunction, ejection fraction <35%
5. Systolic blood pressure <100 mm Hg
6. Bradyarrhythmia pulse <60 mm Hg not due to beta blockade, sinus or atrioventricular node dysfunction
7. New left bundle branch block during recent infarction; difficult to assess ischemic changes*
8. Ventricular arrhythmias (uncontrolled)
9. Uncontrolled systolic hypertension: systolic >200, diastolic hypertension >105 mm Hg
10. Significant valvular heart disease*

* Individual exercise prescriptions.

Patients should learn to take their pulse rate. An increase in pulse rate to 120 to 130 beats/minute should suffice. Patients on beta blockers should be advised not to exercise beyond the point of shortness of breath. The physician should also recognize the minority of patients in whom a very gradual program with only mild exercise is appropriate (see Table 4–18 for these categories and contraindications to exercise training programs).

BIBLIOGRAPHY

Abraham RD, Freddman SB, Dunn RF, et al.: Prediction of multivessel coronary artery disease and prognosis early after acute myocardial infarction by exercise, electrocardiography and thallium-201 myocardial perfusion scintigraphy. Am J Cardiol, *58:*423, 1986.

Barbash GI, Roth A, Hod H, et al.: Randomized controlled trial of late in-hospital angiography and angioplasty versus conservative management after treatment with recombinant tissue-type plasminogen activator in acute myocardial infarction. Am J Cardiol, *66:*538, 1990.

Boissel J-P, Leizorovicz A, Picolet H, et al.: Efficacy of acebutolol after acute myocardial infarction (The APSI Trial). Am J Coll Cardiol, *66:*24C, 1990.

Bonaduce D, Petretta M, Arrichiello P, et al.: Effects of Captopril treatment on left ventricular remodeling and function after anterior myocardial infarction: Comparison with digitalis. J Am Coll Cardiol, *19:*858, 1992.

Breithardt G, Cain ME, El-Sherif N, et al.: Standards for analysis of ventricular late potentials using high-resolution or signal-averaged electrocardiography. AHA Medical/Scientific Statement. Circulation, *83:*1481, 1991

Brugada P, Brongada J, Mont L, et al.: A new approach to the differential diagnosis of a regular tachycardia with a wide QRS complex. Circulation, *53:*1647, 1991.

Burkart F, Pfisterer, Kiowski W, et al.: Effects of antiarrhythmic therapy on mortality in survivors of myocardial infarction with asymptomatic complex ventricular arrhythmias: Basel antiarrhythmic study of infarct survival (BASIS). J Am Coll Cardiol, *16:*1711, 1990.

Butman SM: What would I want to know if my dad had a heart attack?: Good sense versus dollars and cents. J Am Coll Cardiol, *18:*1220, 1991.

Curtis JL, Houghton JL, Patterson JH, et al.: Propranolol therapy alters estimation of potential cardiovascular risk derived from submaximal postinfarction exercise testing. Am Heart J, *121:*1655, 1991.

DeBusk RF: Specialized testing after recent acute myocardial infarction. Ann Intern Med, *110:* 470, 1989.

DeBusk RF, Dennis CA: "Submaximal" predischarge exercise testing after acute myocardial infarction: Who needs it? Am J Cardiol, *55:*299, 1985.

Deckers JW, Fioretti P, Brower RW, et al.: Prediction of one-year outcome after complicated myocardial infarction: Bayersian analysis of predischarge exercise test results in 300 patients. Am Heart J, *113:*90, 1987.

De Vreede JJM, Gorgels APM, Verstraaten GMP, et al.: Did prognosis after acute myocardial infarction change during the past 30 years? A meta-analysis. J Am Coll Cardiol, *18:*698, 1991.

Chandrashekhar Y, Anand IS: Exercise as a coronary protective factor. Am Heart J, *122:*1723, 1991.

Dhingra RC: Electrophysiologic studies during acute myocardial infarction: Do they prognosticate? J Am Coll Cardiol, *18:*789, 1991.

Dickstein K, Barvik S, Aarsland T: Effects of long-term enalapril therapy on cardiopulmonary exercise performance after myocardial infarction. Circulation, *83:*1895, 1991.

Dusman RE, Stanton MS, Miles WM, et al.: Clinical features of amiodarone-induced pulmonary toxicity. Circulation, *82:*51, 1990.

Ellis SG, Muller DW, Topol EJ: Possible survival benefit from concomitant beta- but not calcium-antagonist therapy during reperfusion for acute myocardial infarction. Am J Cardiol, 66:125, 1990.

Feit F, Mueller HS, Braunwald E, et al.: Thrombolysis in Myocardial Infarction (TIMI) Phase II Trial: Outcome comparison of a "conservative strategy" in community versus tertiary hospitals. J Am Coll Cardiol, 16:1529, 1990.

Ferlinz J: Vagaries of predischarge exercise stress testing in acute myocardial ischemic syndromes. J Am Coll Cardiol, 18:684, 1991.

Figueras J, Cinca J, Valle V, et al.: Prognostic implications of early spontaneous angina after acute transminal myocardial infarction. Int J Cardiol, 4:261, 1983.

Fragasso G, Benti R, Sciammarella M, et al.: Symptom-limited exercise testing causes sustained diastolic dysfunction in patients with coronary disease and low effort tolerance. J Am Coll Cardiol, 17:1251, 1991.

Gavaghan TP, Gebski VG, Baron DW: Immediate postoperative aspirin improves vein graft patency early and late after coronary artery bypass graft surgery. Circulation, 83:1536, 1991.

Gheorghiade M, Schultz L, Tilley B, et al.: Natural history of the first non-Q wave myocardial infarction in the placebo arm of the Beta-Blocker Heart Attack Trial. Am Heart J, 122:1548, 1991.

Goldberg RJ, Gore JM, Alpert JS, et al.: Non-Q wave myocardial infarction: Recent changes in occurrence and prognosis—a community-wide perspective. Am Heart J, 113:273, 1987.

Goldman L: Electrophysiological testing after myocardial infarction. Circulation, 83:1090, 1991.

Goldstein RE, Boccuzzi SJ, Cruess D, et al.: Diltiazem increases late-onset congestive heart failure in postinfarction patients with early reduction in ejection fraction. Circulation, 83: 52, 1991.

Hilton TC, Miller DD, Kern MJ, et al.: Rational therapy to reduce mortality and reinfarction following myocardial infarction. Am Heart J, 122:1740, 1991.

Hod H, Lew AS, Keltai M, et al.: Early atrial fibrillation during evolving myocardial infarction: A consequence of impaired left atrial perfusion. Circulation, 75:146, 1987.

Hohnloser SH, Meinertz T, Dammbacher T, et al.: Electrocardiography and antiarrhythmic effects of intravenous amiodarone: Results of a prospective, placebo-controlled study. Am Heart J, 91:89, 1991.

Honan MB, Harrell FE, Reimer KA, et al.: Cardiac rupture, mortality and the timing of thrombolytic therapy: A meta-analysis. J Am Coll Cardiol, 16:359, 1990.

Jensen GVH, Torp-Pedersen C, Kober L, et al.: Prognosis of late versus early ventricular fibrillation in acute myocardial infarction. Am J Cardiol, 66:10, 1990.

Junt D, Sloman G, Pennington C: Effects of atrial fibrillation on prognosis of acute myocardial infarction. Br Heart J, 40:303, 1978.

Kennedy JW: Is there a role for multivessel coronary angioplasty early after acute myocardial infarction? J Am Coll Cardiol, 16:551, 1990.

Kulick DL, Rahimtoola SH: Risk stratification in survivors of acute myocardial infarction: Routine cardiac catheterization and angiography is a reasonable approach in most patients. Am Heart J, 121:641, 1991.

Lamas GA, Pfeffer MA: Left ventricular remodeling after acute myocardial infarction: Clinical course and beneficial effects of angiotensin-converting enzyme inhibition. Am Heart J, 121: 1194, 1991.

Lerman BB, Belardinelli L: Cardiac electrophysiology of adenosine: Basic and clinical concepts. Circulation, 83:1499, 1991.

Leclercq J-F, Coumel P, Denjoy I, et al.: Long-term follow-up after sustained monomorphic ventricular tachycardia: Causes, pump failure, and empiric antiarrhythmic therapy that modify survival. Am Heart J, 121:1658, 1991.

MacMahon S, Collins R, Peto R, et al.: Effects of prophylactic lidocaine in suspected acute myocardial infarction. JAMA, 260:1910, 1988.

Madsen EB, Gilpin E, Henning H, et al.: Prediction of late mortality after myocardial infarction from variables measured at different times during hospitalization. Am J Cardiol, 53:47, 1984.

Marzoll U, Kleiman NS, Dunn JK, et al.: Factors determining improvement in left ventricular function after reperfusion therapy for acute myocardial infarction: Primacy of baseline ejection fraction. J Am Coll Cardiol, *17*:613, 1991.

Matzer L, Kiat H, Friedmand JD, et al.: A new approach to the assessment of tomographic thallium-201 scintigraphy in patients with left bundle branch block. J Am Coll Cardiol, *17:* 1309, 1991.

Miranda CP, Herbert WG, Dubach P, et al.: Post-Myocardial Infarction Exercise Testing. Non-Q wave versus Q wave correlation with coronary angiography and long-term prognosis. Circulation, *84:*2357, 1991.

Morris DD, Rozanski A, Berman DS, et al.: Non-invasive prediction of the angiographic extent of coronary artery disease after myocardial infarction: Comparison of clinical, bicycle exercise electrocardiographic, and ventriculographic parameters. Circulation, *70:*192, 1984.

Moss AJ, Benhorn J: Prognosis and management after a first myocardial infarction. N Engl J Med, *322:*743, 1990.

Myers J: Predicting outcome in cardiac rehabilitation. J Am Coll Cardiol, *15:*983, 1990.

Ochi RP, Goldenberg IF, Airnquist A, et al.: Intravenous amiodarone for the rapid treatment of life-threatening ventricular arrhythmias in critically ill patients with coronary artery disease. Am J Cardiol, *64:*599, 1989.

Peters RW, Muller JE, Goldstein S, et al.: For the BHAT Study Group. Propranolol and the morning increase in the frequency of sudden cardiac deaths (BHAT Study). Am J Cardiol, *63:*1518, 1989.

Pfeffer MA, Braunwald E: Ventricular remodeling after myocardial infarction. Circulation, *81:* 1161, 1990.

Rankin AC, McGovern BA: Adenosine or verapamil for the acute treatment of supraventricular tachycardia? Ann Int Med, *114:*513, 1991.

Rapaport E: Should β-blockers be given immediately and concomitantly with thrombolytic therapy in acute myocardial infarction? Circulation, *83:*695, 1991.

Ridker PM, Manson JE, Buring JE, et al.: The effect of chronic platelet inhibition with low-dose aspirin on atherosclerotic progression and acute thrombosis: Clinical evidence from the Physicians' Health Study. Am Heart J, *122:*1588, 1991.

Simoons ML, Vos J, Tijssen JGP, et al.: Long-term benefit of early thrombolytic therapy in patients with acute myocardial infarction. 5-year follow-up of a trial conducted by the Inter-University Cardiology Institute of the Netherlands. J Am Coll Cardiol, *14:*1609, 1989.

Sloan MA, Plotnick GD: Stroke complicating thrombolytic therapy of acute myocardial infarction. J Am Coll Cardiol, *16:*541, 1990.

Stewart RE, Kander N, Juni JE, et al.: Submaximal exercise thallium-201 SPECT for assessment of interventional therapy in patients with acute myocardial infarction. Am Heart J, *121:* 1033, 1991.

Sutton JM, Topol EJ: Significance of a negative exercise thallium test in the presence of a critical residual stenosis after thrombolysis for acute myocardial infarction. Circulation, *83:* 1278, 1991.

The Danish Study Group on Verapamil in Myocardial Infarction: Secondary prevention with verapamil after myocardial infarction. Am J Cardiol, *66:*331, 1990.

The TIMI Study Group: Comparison of invasive and conservative strategies after treatment with intravenous tissue plasminogen activator in acute myocardial infarction: Results of the thrombolysis in myocardial infarction (TIMI) phase II trial. N Engl J Med, *320:*618, 1989.

Thompson RC, Holmes DR, Gersh BJ, et al.: Percutaneous transluminal coronary angioplasty in the elderly: Early and long-term results. J Am Coll Cardiol, *17:*1245, 1991.

Vane JR, Botting RM: Heart disease, aspirin, and fish oil. Circulation, *84:*2588, 1991.

Van Der Wall EE, Eenige Van MJ, Visser FC, et al.: Thallium-201 exercise testing in patients 6–8 weeks after myocardial infarction: Limited value for the detection of multivessel disease. Eur Heart J, *6:*29, 1985.

Wilson RF, Marcus ML, Christensen BV, et al.: Accuracy of exercise electrocardiography in detecting physiologically significant coronary arterial lesions. Circulation, *83:*412, 1991.

Wong ND, Wilson PWF, Kannel WB: Serum cholesterol as a prognostic factor after myocardial infarction: The Framingham Study. Ann Intern Med, *115:*687, 1991.

Wong S-C, Greenberg H, Hager WD, et al.: Effects of diltiazem on recurrent myocardial infarction in patients with non-Q wave myocardial infarction. J Am Coll Cardiol, *19:*1421, 1992.

5

HEART FAILURE
M. Gabriel Khan

Nearly 450,000 individuals die of heart failure in North America each year, and up to 40% of those die suddenly. At any given time, heart failure affects approximately 1% of the population. The incidence is rising because of the increase in the aging population, which is predisposed to heart failure. Also, better management and improved survival following acute myocardial infarction have created a large population of patients who may succumb to heart failure.

The term "heart failure" is preferred to "congestive heart failure," because manifestations of congestion may be absent at rest in some patients with moderate or severe left ventricular dysfunction. Indeed, there may be no clinical manifestations of forward or backward failure at rest.

The management of heart failure requires the application of five basic principles to actuate a salutary effect

- Ensure a correct diagnosis, excluding mimics of heart failure
- Determine the underlying heart disease, if possible, and treat
- Define precipitating factors, because heart failure can be a result of underlying disease and is often precipitated by conditions that can be prevented or easily corrected
- Understand the pathophysiology of heart failure
- Know the actions of the pharmacologic agents and their appropriate indications

DIAGNOSTIC HALLMARKS

SYMPTOMS

Dyspnea, orthopnea, paroxysmal nocturnal dyspnea, weakness, fatigue, edema, and an increase in abdominal girth are common complaints. Nocturnal angina may occur if severe ischemic heart disease is the underlying cause of heart failure.

PHYSICAL SIGNS

Signs of left ventricular failure include the following

- Crepitations (crackles) over the lower lung fields. Many patients are treated for heart failure based on the presence of crepitations. Heart

187

failure may be present without pulmonary crepitations, and importantly, crepitations may be present in the absence of heart failure. Crepitations that fail to clear on coughing may be due to atelectasis, fibrosis and restrictive lung disease, pneumonia, pneumocystis infection, lymphangitic carcinomatosis, and other causes of noncardiogenic pulmonary edema
- S3 gallop or summation gallop (S3 and S4). An S3 gallop may elude auscultation in patients with ischemic heart disease, although a corresponding movement associated with rapid diastolic filling may be visible on careful inspection of the precordium. An S3 or summation gallop is virtually always present in patients with dilated cardiomyopathy, even in the absence of heart failure.

Signs of right ventricular failure include the following

- An increase in jugular venous pressure greater than 2 cm above the sternal angle. Importantly, the most common cause of right ventricular failure is left heart failure, and signs of this should be sought
- A prominent V wave of tricuspid regurgitation or an A wave of atrial hypertrophy
- A positive hepatojugular reflux usually indicates a right atrial pressure greater than 9 mm Hg and a pulmonary capillary wedge pressure greater than 15 mm Hg where right heart failure is secondary to left heart failure
- Bilateral leg or sacral edema. Edema may be absent with severe heart failure, and when present, edema is often assumed to be due to heart failure. If a diagnosis of heart failure is not confirmed by other findings and a basic cause for heart failure is not present, consider the edema to be due to stasis, venous insufficiency, or deep venous thrombosis, of lymphangitic origin, or induced by drugs such as NSAIDS or calcium antagonists

CHEST X-RAY VERIFICATION

Look for

- Constriction of lower lobe vessels with dilatation of those in the upper lobes. This sign is observed with pulmonary venous hypertension in left ventricular failure, mitral stenosis, severe obstructive lung disease, or x-ray taken in the recumbent position
- Interstitial pulmonary edema: Pulmonary clouding, perihilar haze, Kerley B or A lines caused by edema and thickening of interlobular septa. Kerley B lines usually are localized to the periphery of the lower zones and appear as horizontal lines 1 to 3 cm in length and no wider than 0.1 to 0.2 cm. They occur transiently when pulmonary venous pressure exceeds about 22 mm Hg. A lines are less common, reflect thickened intercommunicating lymphatics, and appear as thin nonbranching lines, several inches in length, extending from the hilar region. The transient appearance of A and B lines is caused by left ventricular failure and may persist if the lymphatic channels are obstructed by tumor, choked by dust particles in pneumoconiosis, or thickened by fibrosing alveolitis or

hemochromatosis. They may be caused by viral infections or drug hypersensitivity
- Pleural effusions: Subpleural or free pleural, blunting of the costophenic angle, the right usually greater than the left
- Alveolar pulmonary edema, a butterfly pattern, may be unilateral
- Interlobar fissure thickening due to accumulation of fluid, seen best on the lateral film
- Dilatation of the central right and left pulmonary arteries
- Cardiomegaly

The heart size may be normal on chest x-ray, in many instances, with heart failure present due to

- Acute myocardial infarction in patients with ischemic heart disease. Cardiac dilatation may not take place in a transverse direction and patients with one or more old infarcts may present with heart failure and a normal heart size on chest radiograph. Hypokinetic, dyskinetic areas may be observed on inspection or palpitation of the chest wall and are readily observed on echocardiography
- Mitral stenosis
- Aortic stenosis in some patients
- Heart failure due to predominant diastolic dysfunction
- Cor pulmonale

The following radiologic mimics of heart failure should be excluded

- Lung infection, including all causes of adult respiratory distress syndrome
- Allergic pulmonary edema (heroin, nitrofurantoin)
- Lymphangitic carcinomatosis
- Uremia
- Increased cerebrospinal fluid pressure
- High altitude pulmonary edema
- Alveolar proteinosis

ELECTROCARDIOGRAPHIC ASSESSMENT

Scrutinize the electrocardiogram for

- Acute or old infarctions
- Recent ischemia (assess by serial ECGs)
- LV aneurysm: ST segment elevation in two contiguous leads present more than 3 months post infarction
- Bradyarrhythmias or tachyarrhythmias, particularly atrial fibrillation with a fast ventricular response
- Left or right ventricular hypertrophy
- Left atrial enlargement, which is an early sign of altered left ventricular compliance from left ventricular hypertrophy and a common feature of mitral regurgitation and/or mitral stenosis

ECHOCARDIOGRAPHIC EVALUATION

Echocardiography provides many diagnostic aids

- Decreased systolic function: An ejection fraction (EF) less than 35% is often seen in patients with moderate heart failure. The EF may not be decreased in patients with heart failure caused by mitral regurgitation or ventricular septal defect and in patients with ventricular diastolic dysfunction. The radionuclide evaluation of EF is more accurate than that of echocardiography, but the latter is superior in detecting the presence and significance of valvular lesions and specific chamber enlargement
- Ventricular wall motion abnormalities, global hypokinesia, and chamber enlargement
- An approximate assessment of pulmonary artery pressure is extremely useful
- Valvular abnormalities: Reasonably accurate assessment of the severity of mitral regurgitation and obstructive lesions can be ascertained by continuous wave Doppler (see Chapter 12)
- Exclude cardiac tamponade
- Assess pericardial effusion and pericardial calcification
- Diastolic dysfunction abnormalities
- Assess left ventricular hypertrophy, left atrial enlargement, and right ventricular hypertrophy
- The diagnosis of hypertrophic, dilated, or restrictive cardiomyopathy

ASSESS FOR UNDERLYING CAUSE OF HEART FAILURE

A complete cure may be a rare reward if a surgically correctable lesion is uncovered
- Left atrial myxoma
- Significant mitral regurgitation: May be missed because of the presence of a poorly audible murmur due to low cardiac output, thick chest wall, or chronic obstructive pulmonary disease
- Atrial septal defect
- AV fistula
- Constrictive pericarditis
- Cardiac tamponade: May simulate heart failure and must be excluded because usual heart failure medications, diuretics, ACE inhibitors, or nitrates can cause marked hemodynamic deterioration in patients with tamponade
- Pulmonary edema or heart failure is not a complete diagnosis. The basic cause must be stated as part of the diagnosis and an associated precipitant must be defined, if present

  It is necessary to make a systematic search for the following basic causes of heart disease.

Myocardial Damage

- Ischemic heart disease and its complications
- Myocarditis
- Cardiomyopathy

Ventricular Overload

Pressure overload

- Systemic hypertension
- Coarctation of the aorta
- Aortic stenosis
- Pulmonary hypertension

  Volume overload

- Mitral regurgitation
- Aortic regurgitation
- Ventricular septal defect
- Atrial septal defect
- Patent ductus arteriosus

Restriction and Obstruction to Ventricular Filling

- Right ventricular infarction
- Constrictive pericarditis
- Cardiac tamponade (although not truly heart failure)
- Restrictive cardiomyopathies (see Chapter 14)
- Specific heart muscle diseases (see Chapter 14)
- Hypertensive, hypertrophic "cardiomyopathy" of the elderly
- Mitral stenosis and atrial myxoma

Others

- Cor pulmonale, thyrotoxicosis, high output failure: AV fistula, peripartum cardiomyopathy, and beri-beri

SEARCH FOR PRECIPITATING FACTORS

- Reduction or discontinuation of medications, salt binge, increased physical and mental stress
- Increased cardiac work: Increasing hypertension (systemic or pulmonary), arrhythmias, pulmonary embolism, infections, increased activities, physical and emotional stress
- Progression or complications of the underlying disease: Acute myocardial infarction, left ventricular aneurysm, valvular heart disease with progression of stenosis or regurgitation
- Several drugs may precipitate heart failure: Alcohol, NSAIDS, beta blockers, corticosteroids, disopyramide, procainamide, propafenone

and other antiarrhythmics, verapamil, diltiazem, nifedipine or other dihydropyridine calcium antagonists, adriamycin, daunorubicin, mithramycin. Excessive alcohol intake can significantly decrease left ventricular contractility

PATHOPHYSIOLOGIC IMPLICATIONS

In the majority of patients with heart failure, cardiac output is reduced due to poor left ventricular systolic function. However, left ventricular systolic function may be relatively normal in some patients with valvular regurgitant lesions, hypertensive heart disease, and restrictive cardiomyopathy, in which diastolic dysfunction plays a major role in causing heart failure (Fig. 5–1).

Heart failure is a syndrome identified by well-defined symptoms, signs, and/or hemodynamic findings caused by an abnormality of cardiac function

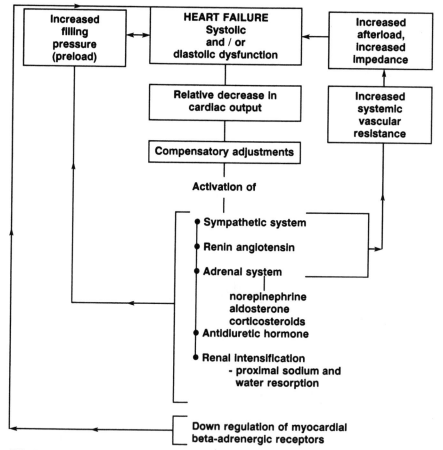

FIG. 5–1. Pathophysiology of heart failure.

that results in a relative decrease in cardiac output and compensatory renal and neurohormonal adjustments (Fig. 5–1).

Cardiac output is the product of stroke volume and heart rate. Stroke volume is modulated by

- Preload
- Myocardial contractility
- Afterload

PRELOAD

Preload is the extent of fiber stretch during diastole and is clinically represented by the end diastolic volume. The left ventricular end diastolic or filling pressure is closely related, although in a nonlinear fashion to end diastolic volume, and is an indication of left ventricular preload. In the absence of obstruction to blood flow through the pulmonary veins and into the ventricle, the left ventricular end diastolic pressure is in turn reflected by the pulmonary capillary wedge pressure or pulmonary artery end diastolic pressure.

DECREASE PRELOAD AND DIASTOLIC DYSFUNCTION

The affected ventricle may contract well if adequately filled but may relax poorly, resulting in a diastolic dysfunction that is more prominent than the commonly occurring systolic dysfunction.

An increase in ventricular diastolic stiffness impedes diastolic stretch and causes failure to adequately fill the ventricle. Conditions that alter ventricular compliance, causing diastolic dysfunction, a decrease in preload, and thus, a decrease in cardiac output, include

- Myocardial infarction (although systolic dysfunction is the main abnormality)
- Cardiac tamponade
- Constrictive pericarditis
- Hypertensive heart disease
- Restrictive cardiomyopathy
- Dilated cardiomyopathy
- Specific heart muscle disease, e.g. amyloid
- The aging heart
- Hypertensive, hypertrophic "cardiomyopathy" of the elderly

Age and some cardiac diseases appear to cause changes in the cross-linking of intercellular connective tissue. Alteration in myocardial collagen occurs with hypertensive and coronary heart disease (CHD). Approximately 15% of patients with heart failure have mainly diastolic dysfunction with relatively preserved EF. Over 70% of patients with heart failure have systolic dysfunction and about 15% have both systolic and diastolic dysfunction.

In patients with predominant diastolic dysfunction, the heart size and EF are often normal. The heart fills less and empties less, and the percent ejected may be relatively normal, but the stroke and cardiac index are decreased.

Since a decrease in preload exists in the above conditions, the use of preload-reducing agents is relatively contraindicated. Hemodynamic and clinical deterioration may ensue with the use of diuretics, nitrates, ACE inhibitors, nitroprusside, or prazosin.

AFTERLOAD

Afterload is represented by left ventricular wall end systolic stress, which must be overcome to allow ejection of blood from the ventricle. An increase in afterload signifies an increase in myocardial oxygen demand.

Afterload is determined by

- The radius of the ventricle (A)
- Left ventricular end systolic pressure (B)
- Arteriolar resistance or impedance (C)

Afterload is highly dependent on A and B. In turn, B is dependent on cardiac index and C. A decrease in systolic vascular resistance or a fall in blood pressure is not identical with a decrease in afterload. Also, a decrease in systemic vascular resistance is not synonymous with a decrease in arterial blood pressure, as a compensatory increase in cardiac output occurs to maintain blood pressure. The peripheral systolic pressure may be maintained because of colliding reflected pressure waves, despite a fall in central systolic blood pressure.

Conditions causing an increase in afterload include

- Aortic stenosis
- Pulmonary stenosis
- Coarctation
- Hypertension
- All causes of heart failure, because of activation of the renin angiotensin and sympathoadrenal system

Left ventricular dysfunction and heart failure due to systolic dysfunction improve with therapy directed at

- A decrease in afterload, which improves ventricular emptying at a lowered demand for oxygen
- A judicious decrease in preload, in order to decrease symptoms caused by pulmonary congestion but without bringing about an unwanted fall in cardiac output or a marked stimulation of the renin angiotensin system

MYOCARDIAL CONTRACTILITY

A decrease in myocardial contractility or systolic dysfunction is commonly caused by CHD, especially in patients with large areas of infarction. Rarely, dilated cardiomyopathy and myocarditis are implicated, and with late stage volume overload due to valvular regurgitant lesions, myocardial damage occurs, culminating in pump failure.

COMPENSATORY ADJUSTMENTS IN HEART FAILURE

The body responds to the abnormality of cardiac function and a relative decrease in cardiac output by bringing several homeostatic mechanisms into action (Fig. 5–1). This situation is similar to the body's reaction to severe bleeding over several hours, but the results are, of course, less than completely appropriate in heart failure.

COMPENSATORY ADJUSTMENTS

- The activation of the sympathetic system causes an increase in heart rate, force, and velocity of myocardial contraction in order to increase stroke volume and cardiac output. An increase in systemic vascular resistance occurs in order to maintain blood pressure. The body's homeostatic response (indicated in Fig. 5–1) is appropriate but often not sufficient to compensate for the decrease in cardiac index and increased filling pressures. It is, in fact, counterproductive in some ways. Also, sympathetic stimulation causes sodium and water retention and an increase in venous tone in order to increase filling pressure that enhances preload, provided that there is no restriction to ventricular filling
- The renin angiotensin system is stimulated. Patients with mild heart failure show little or no evidence of stimulation of the renin angiotensin system. Stimulation of the system is observed in response to treatment with diuretics and is seen in untreated patients with more severe degrees of heart failure. The secretion of renin causes angiotensin I to be converted by angiotensin converting enzyme to the vasoconstrictor angiotensin II. This action occurs in the circulation and in the tissues

Angiotensin II supports systemic blood pressure and cerebral, renal, and coronary perfusion through

- Arteriolar vasoconstriction and an increase in systemic vascular resistance
- Stimulation of central and peripheral effects of the sympathetic system
- Marked resorption of sodium and water in the proximal nephron
- Enhanced aldosterone secretion, which brings about sodium and water retention in the renal tubules, distal to the macula densa. Since the distal tubules only handle about 2% of the nephron's sodium load, this latter contribution is small, compared to proximal sodium resorption, but is a final tuning of sodium balance
- Stimulating thirst and vasopressin release, thereby increasing total body water

Renal blood flow is preserved by selective vasoconstriction of postglomerular efferent arterioles. The adjustments, however, made to maintain blood pressure and cerebral, coronary, and renal perfusion, cause a marked increase in afterload, which unnecessarily increases cardiac work and myocardial oxygen demand. Thus, heart failure may worsen.

THE RENAL RESPONSE

It must be reemphasized that the renal homeostatic mechanisms are similar to those for heart failure, with a decrease in cardiac output, and for severe bleeding, which lowers blood pressure. The design of nature appears to protect systemic blood pressure in order to maintain adequate cerebral and renal perfusion in situations such as hemorrhage, where this reaction is productive.

Sodium and water retention occurs in the proximal tubule. The sensors that activate this response in heart failure are undetermined. Sensors are possibly linked to baroreceptors in the heart and to aortic arch and low-pressure sensors in the ventricle and atria, as well as at the level of the nephron and macula densa. Failure of the neurohumoral response and renal adjustment would result in a fall in blood pressure and deprivation of cerebral, coronary, and renal perfusion.

The compensatory neurohumoral response thus increases afterload to some extent, in order to maintain adequate systemic blood pressure. The intense sodium and water retention and the increase in venous tone bring about an increase in filling pressure (Fig. 5–1) in an attempt to increase myocardial fiber stretch during diastole, that is, an increase in preload.

NONSPECIFIC THERAPY

- Bedrest is necessary for patients with New York Heart Association (NYHA) Class IV or acute heart failure requiring admission to the hospital. Most patients are able to walk to the bathroom, with assistance, but some may require a bedside commode for the first 24 hours. It is important to quickly ambulate in order to avoid deep vein thrombosis and pulmonary embolism
- Heparin, 5,000 units subcutaneous every 12 hours, is advisable until the patient is mobilized. This is an effective strategy to prevent thromboembolism and is especially indicated in patients at high risk
- In patients ill enough to be admitted to the hospital and suspected of having hypoxemia because of a history of orthopnea, paroxysmal nocturnal dyspnea, and symptoms of pulmonary congestion or when hypoxemia is proven by arterial blood gas analysis, oxygen is given for 12 to 24 hours. Arterial blood gas analysis is not necessary in the majority of patients with heart failure. Oxygen, 2 to 3 l/min, by nasal prongs is usually adequate. When deterioration occurs despite appropriate therapy and in patients with chronic lung disease and heart failure, arterial blood gas analysis is necessary. In the latter situation, oxygen is given utilizing a controlled low-flow oxygen system, such as a Venturi mask, commencing with 28% oxygen for a few hours with repeat blood gas analysis. If there is no increase in $PaCO_2$ and the PaO_2 content is satisfactory, a switch can be made to nasal prongs for patient comfort.
- Overweight patients with heart failure benefit from weight reduction. The physician or nurse should advise the patient regarding a weight reduction diet. Occasionally, the assurances of a weight loss clinic are rewarding. The physician must have a basic understanding of salt intake

to confidently advise the patient. All patients with heart failure must be given relevant information on the importance of sodium restriction; a formal diet sheet or dietary consultation is not usually required. Diet sheets are not practical. Booklets prepared by the AHA and other organizations should be made available to the patient. Patients must recognize that salt added to meals at the table is only a minor part of the daily salt consumption and that increased salt in the diet can precipitate heart failure and an expensive admission to hospital. The body requires about 500 mg sodium daily. The average daily intake of salt (sodium chloride) ranges from 8,000 to 12,000 mg daily; the sodium content of which is approximately 40%, i.e., 3,000 to 5,000 mg. One teaspoon of table salt contains 5,000 mg sodium chloride and 2,000 mg sodium. Most patients with heart failure can be managed satisfactorily on a diet containing less than 5,000 mg sodium chloride and 2,000 mg sodium. A 1-gram-sodium diet requires the use of a diet sheet and a strict salt intake; this is extremely difficult to follow and is not advisable, except in patients with refractory heart failure. Instructions to the patient should include the following. No salt should be added in cooking or at the table. The patient should be aware of the sodium content of various foods. Table 1–1 lists a few commonly used foods and their sodium content in order to indicate the marked differences, e.g., 1 teaspoonful of garlic salt contains 2,000 mg sodium, garlic powder contains 2 mg sodium, and a large dill pickle contains about 1,900 mg sodium. Importantly, foods that are not salty to taste may have a high salt content. Fast foods such as one hamburger or one portion of fried chicken contain 1,000 mg sodium. Canned soups must be avoided, because they usually contain 500 to 1,000 mg sodium per 250 ml. A simple aid in controlling sodium intake is checking product labels. If the salt content is greater than 500 mg or if the word "sodium" is listed among the first four ingredients, then it is a high-sodium product and should be avoided. If the patient cannot avoid the use of canned foods, tuna, salmon, vegetables, and similar products should be rinsed under running water and the liquid should be drained. Some high-sodium foods not listed in Table 1 include onion salt, celery salt, seasoned salts, soy sauce, salted crackers, rye rolls, salted popcorn, pretzels, waffles, hot dogs, salted pork, TV dinners, sardines, smoked fish, and all smoked meats. Patients are usually motivated by the advice that watching the diet carefully will assist in using fewer pills and may prevent admission to hospital

WHICH DRUG OR DRUG COMBINATION TO CHOOSE

In clinical practice, an appropriate drug or combination for patients with heart failure due to ventricular systolic dysfunction requires consideration of the patient's functional class. It is appropriate to utilize the NYHA functional class since several major clinical trials have incorporated this parameter in study design. Also, most physicians are conversant with the use of this clinical classification. Objective measurements or metabolic classifications relate well to this functional classification, albeit, not exactly. Indeed, the clinical classification provides a guide to prognosis that is reflected by clinical trials and can be used to compare trial results. Consequently, the following discussion is centered on studies utilizing patients assigned according to NYHA classification. Studies that have a mixture of Class II to IV patients clearly distort scientific evaluation.

NYHA FUNCTIONAL CLASS

- Class I: Asymptomatic on ordinary physical activity associated with maximal oxygen (VO_2) consumption greater than 20 ml/kg/min
- Class II: Symptomatic on ordinary physical activity with maximum VO_2 of 16 to 20 ml/kg/min
- Class III: Symptomatic on less than ordinary physical activity with maximum VO_2 of 10 to 15 ml/kg/min
- Class IV: Symptomatic at rest or on any activity with maximum VO_2 of less than 10 ml/kg/min

DRUG THERAPY, NYHA CLASS IV HEART FAILURE

The Cooperative North Scandinavian Enalapril Survival Study (CONSENSUS) studied only NYHA Class IV heart failure patients. In 253 randomized patients, the 6-month mortality was 44% in patients treated with diuretics and a digoxin combination and 26% in patients given enalapril in addition, ($p < 0.002$). Forty-two percent of the group treated with added ACE inhibitors showed an improvement in functional class, compared with 22% in the control group ($p = 0.001$). A significant reduction in mortality attributable to ACE inhibitor therapy was observed mainly during the first 6 months.

The CONSENSUS trial had too few patients in the placebo group between 6 months and 2 years to allow firm conclusions to be made regarding the beneficial effects of ACE inhibitors beyond 6 months in patients with Class IV heart failure.

In a study by Fonarow, et al. in 117 Class IV patients enrolled for transplantation, sudden cardiac death occurred in only three captopril-treated patients, compared with 17 of 60 hydralazine-treated patients ($p = 0.01$). At 8 ± 7 months follow-up, the actuarial 1-year survival rate was 81 and 51% in the captopril-treated and hydralazine-treated patients, respectively ($p = 0.05$). Patients in both groups received diuretics, digoxin, and isosorbide dinitrate. It must be emphasized however, that eight patients in the captopril and 16 in the hydralazine group received a Type 1 antiarrhythmic agent, which could have increased the sudden death rate in the hydralazine group. There were other defects in methodology in this study.

The current recommendation to treat NYHA Class IV heart failure patients with diuretics, digoxin, and an ACE inhibitor for life is appropriate, given the short life expectancy of Class IV patients, and is, of course, supported by the obvious symptomatic benefit, improved survival, and decrease in sudden death that results from therapy in most patients.

DRUG THERAPY, NYHA CLASS II AND III HEART FAILURE

- Clinical trials have confirmed that monotherapy with diuretics, digoxin, or ACE inhibitors is not satisfactory for NYHA Class II patients in sinus rhythm who have an EF less than 35% and who have had overt heart failure
- There are sufficient data that strongly indicate that these patients should be managed with triple therapy: diuretic, digoxin, and ACE inhibitor. It is this combination that has been shown in both the studies of left ventricular dysfunction (SOLVD) and the Veterans Administration Cooperative Vasodilator Heart Failure Trial (VHeFT) II to improve survival, and in the SOLVD, significant reduction in hospitalization for recurrent heart failure was achieved
- In the few patients in whom ACE inhibitors are contraindicated or cause adverse effects, the diuretic digoxin combination should suffice
- If angina or active ischemia is documented, the combination of diuretic, digoxin, and nitrate is preferable because ACE inhibitor therapy has been shown to cause an increase in angina in these patients
- When exercise performance is not improved by diuretic, digoxin, and ACE inhibitor therapy, the dose of ACE inhibitor should be halved and intermittent oral nitrate should be administered. Caution is necessary with this combination because a sharp decrease in preload may result in syncope or presyncope

Because clinical trials that have proven triple therapy effective have incorporated NYHA class and EF into their methodology, and because decisions in the management of heart failure require a sound knowledge of the extent of left ventricular systolic function, a brief discussion of the relevance of EF is appropriate. Except in patients with atrial fibrillation, radionuclide estimation of EF is more accurate than echocardiographic evaluation of left ventricular systolic function. Echocardiography is preferred, however, because it provides other important information on cardiac structure and function. It must be emphasized that the EF may be normal in patients with mitral regurgitation and/or diastolic dysfunction and is not an accurate measurement of left ventricular systolic function in these patients. In areas where facilities for these investigations are not available, the physician should use the following parameters to assist with estimation of left ventricular systolic function

- Post heart failure patients in sinus rhythm stabilized on diuretic and digoxin therapy, who can be graded as NYHA Class III or IV, usually have severe impairment of left ventricular systolic function and an EF less than 35%
- Heart failure patients in sinus rhythm stabilized on diuretics and digoxin, who can be graded as Class II and who have a recurrence of heart failure in the absence of hypertension, valvular obstruction, or arrhythmia with a fast ventricular response, are expected to have significant impairment of left ventricular systolic function and an EF near 35%

In practice, an exact EF measurement is seldom required for the day-to-day management of patients with NYHA Class III and IV heart failure and in many patients graded as Class II. All patients in sinus rhythm Class II and III, who have had heart failure and who have an EF less than 35%, are expected to derive major benefits from triple therapy diuretic, digoxin, and ACE inhibitor.

The clinician should no longer think in terms of diuretic/digoxin versus diuretic/ACE inhibitor in Class III patients. This statement also applies to Class II patients who have had a recurrence of heart failure or are known to have a moderate degree of left ventricular systolic dysfunction or an actual EF measurement equal to or less than 35%. As stated earlier, these patients have been shown to have an improvement in survival and a decrease in hospitalizations when administered triple therapy (diuretics, digoxin, and ACE inhibitor). Studies that support or are relevant to the above recommendations will be discussed briefly. These studies include the following

- CONSENSUS
- SOLVD
- VHeFT-I and VHeFT-II
- Captopril-Digoxin Multicenter Research Group (MRG) Study
- The Canadian Enalapril Versus Digoxin Study Group
- The Hy-C Trial: Effect of direct vasodilation with hydralazine versus angiotensin-converting enzyme inhibition with captopril on mortality in advanced heart failure was discussed under NYHA Class IV heart failure

The CONSENSUS study has shown that triple therapy is lifesaving in Class IV patients, as discussed earlier.

SOLVD studied heart failure patients who had EFs equal to or less than 35%; 1,284 patients who had overt heart failure with EF less than 35% were randomly selected to receive enalapril 2.5 to 20 mg plus conventional therapy, and 1,285 patients were randomly assigned to a control group to receive conventional therapy. Approximately 30% of the study group were in NYHA Class III. At an average follow-up of 41 months, in Class III patients, there were 182 (47%) deaths in the enalapril group and 201 (51%) deaths in the placebo group. Total mortality in the enalapril group was 452 (35%) versus 510 (39.7%) in the placebo arm, a 16% risk reduction (p = 0.0036). Enalapril therapy resulted in a significant decrease in hospitalizations; overall, 971 patients in the placebo group required hospitalization versus 683 patients in the enalapril group. Mortality reduction was highest at 24 months of therapy, when the risk reduction was 23% (Table 5–1). Although Class III patients did not achieve major mortality reduction, hospitalizations were decreased. In SOLVD, enalapril therapy resulted in a significant reduction in mortality in NYHA Class II patients, who comprised 56.7% of the study group. There were 219 (30%) deaths in the enalapril group and 254 (35%) in the placebo group.

The small VHeFT-I studied 459 Class III and some Class II heart failure patients for 48 months. The control group of 273 patients received diuretics and digoxin, 183 patients were treated with added prazosin, and 186 patients received isosorbide dinitrate (ISDN)-hydralazine added to diuretics and digoxin. No decrease in mortality was observed with the use of prazosin. This clinical trial and others confirmed that prazosin is not useful

TABLE 5–1. EFFECT OF TREATMENT ON MORTALITY AND HOSPITALIZATION FOR CONGESTIVE HEART FAILURE, AND PROPORTION OF PATIENTS TAKING ANGIOTENSIN-CONVERTING–ENZYME INHIBITORS AFTER VARIOUS PERIODS*

MONTHS OF FOLLOW-UP	MORTALITY			DEATH OR HOSPITALIZATION FOR HEART FAILURE			PROPORTION TAKING INHIBITORS†	
	Placebo	Enalapril	Risk Reduction (95% CI)	Placebo	Enalapril	Risk Reduction (95% CI)	Placebo	Enalapril
	number		*percent*	*number*		*percent*	*percent*	
3	69	47	33 (2–53)	164	92	46 (30–57)	6	91
6	126	91	29 (8–46)	259	150	45 (33–55)	10	88
12	201	159	23 (5–37)	401	262	40 (30–48)	12	86
24	344	277	23 (10–34)	559	434	30 (21–38)	20	83
36	450	396	16 (4–27)	680	555	28 (19–35)	23	82
48	504	443	17 (5–27)	731	607	27 (18–34)	30	83
Overall‡	510	452	16 (5–26)	736	613	26 (18–34)	—	—
			$Z = 2.69; p = 0.0036$			$Z = 5.65; p < 0.0001$		

*The 95% confidence intervals (CI) correspond to a two-sided p value of <0.05 or a one-sided p value of <0.025. Risk reductions were calculated by the log-rank test from the data available at each specific time.

†Values shown for 3 and 6 months were based on data obtained after the visits at 4 and 8 months, respectively. The inhibitors were angiotensin-converting–enzyme inhibitors.

‡The total numbers of deaths were 518 and 458 when deaths after January 31, 1991, but before the patients' last visits, were included. See notes to Table 2.

From: Yusuf S, et al.: The SOLVD Investigators: Effect of enalapril on survival in patients with reduced left ventricular ejection fractions and congestive heart failure. N Eng J Med, 325:297, 1991.

and not advisable for the management of heart failure. The ISDN-hydralazine group showed a significant decrease in mortality, 26% at 2 years, compared to a 34% mortality in the control arm. The 4-year mortality reached a questionable level of significance. However, the message was clear that vasodilator therapy improves survival. Also, exercise tolerance was improved by the ISDN-hydralazine combination.

VHeFT-II randomized 804 Class II and III heart failure patients who had EF less than 0.45 (mean at baseline = 0.29). Enalapril (10 to 20 mg) added to standard therapy diuretic-digoxin was compared to ISDN-hydralazine added to standard therapy. Enalapril therapy resulted, at the end of 2-year follow-up, in a significant reduction in mortality (18% versus 25% [p = 0.016] in the ISDN-hydralazine arm). The incidence of sudden death was reduced mainly in Class II patients. Only ISDN-hydralazine therapy, however, resulted in an increased body oxygen consumption at peak exercise. The venodilator effect of ISDN is more potent than enalapril at the dose administered. This may have contributed to the ISDN-hydralazine improvement in exercise performance since hydralazine therapy alone does not improve this parameter.

The Captopril-Digoxin MRG study compared the effects of placebo, digoxin, or captopril added to maintenance diuretic therapy at 6 months in 300 Class II and III heart failure patients, left ventricular EF mean of 25%. Results are listed in Table 5–2. Digoxin significantly increased EF, compared to diuretics alone or a diuretic-captopril combination. Exercise time was increased and recurrence of heart failure was reduced by digoxin. The study had several drawbacks, however. In particular, the two groups were not identical, the number of Class III patients was twice as high in the digoxin-diuretic group as in the captopril-diuretic group. Also, 30 patients who deteriorated when digoxin was withdrawn were not randomized, thereby biasing the study against digoxin (see further discussion under digoxin).

The Canadian enalapril versus digoxin study randomized NYHA Class II or III heart failure patients who were stabilized on furosemide to receive

TABLE 5–2. CAPTOPRIL-DIGOXIN MULTICENTER RESEARCH GROUP STUDY*

PARAMETERS	DIURETIC	DIURETIC + DIGOXIN	DIURETIC + ACE INHIBITOR
Increase in EF	0.9%	4.4%	1.8%
Exercise time (seconds)	40	55	77
Recurrence of heart failure (not due to myocardial infarction)	20%	10%	10%

* 300 patients; New York Heart Association Class II and III heart failure
% = Approximate percentage
(Data obtained from JAMA *259*:1988)

enalapril (72) and digoxin (73). The radionuclide mean EF at baseline was 30% ($\pm$12%). After 14 weeks in the enalapril group, 13 patients showed improvement, 50 had no change, and 9 deteriorated, versus 14, 37, and 22 patients, respectively, in the digoxin group (p < 0.025). Heart failure recurred in 2 enalapril- and 7 digoxin-treated patients, a nonsignificant difference. Left ventricular systolic function and exercise time improved significantly in both treatment groups, with no significant difference between the enalapril and digoxin groups.

Current recommendations for the management of NYHA Class II and III heart failure patients include the following

- Diuretics at small to medium doses (furosemide, 40 to 80 mg)
- Digoxin for patients in sinus rhythm as well as for those in atrial fibrillation
- ACE inhibitor (captopril, 25 to 75 mg, or enalapril, 5 to maximum 20 mg daily, or the equivalent dose of another ACE inhibitor)
- ISDN in patients with impaired exercise capacity or ischemia persisting after judicious titrated dosage of diuretics, digoxin, and ACE inhibitor. ISDN should be added at a small dose (15 mg), increasing slowly over weeks to 30 mg if needed at 7 AM, 12 noon, and 5 PM daily. A small dose is advisable to avoid presyncope. An intermittent dose schedule is used to avoid nitrate tolerance

The addition of ISDN is encouraged if ischemia is present or in patients with impairment of exercise capacity. It must be emphasized that ISDN is added only when the furosemide dosage has been increased for several weeks without benefit, in patients who are observed to have electrolyte abnormalities or gout with increased diuretic dosage, or for documented ischemia. Many patients on furosemide, 40 to 80 mg, tolerate an increase to 120 mg daily, given for several days to weeks. When clinical benefit is achieved, a small decrease in furosemide dosage usually maintains relief of symptoms and signs of heart failure. ISDN should be avoided if ischemia is not present, because headaches and dizziness are bothersome and a fourth drug constitutes polypharmacy.

DRUG THERAPY, NYHA CLASS I HEART FAILURE

Patients with mild left ventricular systolic dysfunction who are asymptomatic generally do not require treatment with a diuretic, digoxin, or ACE inhibitor. The role of ACE inhibitors in Class I patients, especially following acute MI, is presently being evaluated in the Survival and Ventricular Enlargement (SAVE) Following Myocardial Infarction Study. This is a double-blind, placebo-controlled parallel study designed to evaluate the efficacy of captopril in reducing mortality and the deterioration of left ventricular EF in patients following MI. More than 20,000 patients within 3 to 16 days of MI, with an average EF of 31% by radionuclide ventriculography or without overt heart failure or post-infarction angina, were randomized and followed for 2 years. The SAVE data showed a 17% reduction in risk of death compared with the control group (p = 0.020). Fewer patients in the captopril-treated group required hospitalization for the occurrence of heart failure (see Chapter 4). The SOLVD prevention arm showed that enalapril administered to patients without overt heart failure and an EF less than 35% caused a 37% reduced risk of developing heart failure and hospitalizations, but no significant changes in mortality or infarction rates were observed.

FUNCTIONAL CLASS AND ANGINA

A placebo-controlled study of the effects of captopril in heart failure patients with concomitant angina showed reduced exercise tolerance and an increase in angina and consumption of nitroglycerin in the captopril-treated group. These adverse effects were related to the hypotensive effects of the ACE inhibitor. This finding is not surprising since ACE inhibitors are contraindicated in patients with critical stenosis of the carotid and renal arteries. In angina-free patients with heart failure, critical coronary stenoses are mainly restricted to arteries that supply infarcted, hypocontractile segments. Angina occurs if coronary stenoses exist in arteries that supply actively contracting myocardial segments. Poor diastolic perfusion pressure to these segments precipitates angina. Because vasodilators act mainly on arterioles in the viscera, skin, and muscle, a major drawback of these agents is that although they may increase cardiac output and favorably decrease afterload and myocardial oxygen requirement, delivery of blood to critical vascular beds (e.g. the brain, heart, kidneys, and exercising muscle) may not occur.

Coronary perfusion occurs during diastole. The fall in diastolic blood pressure produced by ACE inhibitor therapy in patients with left main stenosis or in those with greater than 80% stenosis may worsen ischemia and mortality.

DIURETICS

The main action of diuretics is to decrease preload. Although this effect does not improve cardiac output or survival, diuretics are still first-line agents in the management of heart failure because they ameliorate bothersome, congestive symptoms and prevent costly hospitalization. As discussed earlier, they can be used alone as first-line therapy in patients with NYHA Class II heart failure with mild systolic dysfunction, especially when heart failure is precipitated by a reversible cause such as pneumonia, infection, arrhythmia, or NSAIDS. These patients are often controlled with a diuretic only and maintained without ACE inhibitor or digoxin therapy. Further reasons for the choice of diuretics in various grades of heart failure are given under the previous section regarding which drugs to choose.

FUROSEMIDE

This well-known loop diuretic is the most commonly used agent in the management of heart failure. The drug has been given to millions of patients worldwide since 1964. It is easy to use orally and intravenously and, other than electrolyte imbalance, has negligible side effects.

Indications
- IV furosemide is indicated for pulmonary edema and severe heart failure with poor oral absorption or due to hypertensive emergency
- Oral therapy is indicated as monotherapy for NYHA Class II heart failure patients as monotherapy or in combination with digoxin and/or ACE inhibitors in selected patients
- NYHA Class III and IV heart failure patients, in combination with digoxin and ACE inhibitors
- Heart failure due to acute myocardial infarction (IV or oral)

Contraindications
- Cardiac tamponade
- Right ventricular infarction
- Hepatic failure
- Uncorrected hypokalemia [less than 3.5 mEq (mmol)/l]
- Hypersensitivity to furosemide, sulfonamides, or sulfur-containing compounds
- Women of child-bearing potential, except in life-threatening situations in which IV furosemide is necessary. Furosemide has caused fetal abnormalities in animal studies and is not recommended for maintenance therapy.

Action. Furosemide inhibits sodium and chloride reabsorption from the ascending limb of the loop of Henle, with weak effects in the proximal tubule, which excretes the drug. IV furosemide has a venodilator effect; thus, preload reduction occurs within minutes and relief of symptoms may occur before the appearance of increased urinary flow. The potency of action allows furosemide and other loop diuretics to retain beneficial effects in renal failure patients with glomerular filtration rates as low as 10 ml/min. Thus, in patients with elevated serum creatinine, greater than 2.3 mg/dl (203 μmol/l), furosemide retains activity, whereas thiazides, except metolazone, are not effective.

Supplied: tablets; 20, 40, 80, 500 mg. ampules available in 10 mg/ml, 20 mg/2 ml, 40 mg/4 ml, and 250 mg/25 ml

Dosage: IV 20 to 80 mg given as a slow IV bolus, 20 mg/min.

Caution. If renal failure is present, do not exceed 4 mg/min to prevent ototoxicity.

For acute heart failure of mild to moderate severity in patients with acute MI, small doses are advisable (20 to 40 mg IV repeated 1 to 2 hours after careful assessment), in order not to decrease cardiac output or produce further stimulation of the renin angiotensin system (see Chapters 3 and 4).

For acute heart failure in patients with known NYHA Class III or IV, large doses may be required, depending on the extent of pulmonary congestion and the degree of respiratory distress (80 mg IV followed by 80 to 120 mg in 2 to 4 hours and repeated every 8 or 12 hours as needed;

maintenance 40 to 120 mg once daily). Larger dosages may be required if urinary output is poor or if chronic renal failure is present (with serum creatinine greater than 2.3 mg/dl, 203 μmol/l) or if severe pulmonary congestion with respiratory distress persists (with a jugular venous pressure greater than 5 cm), having excluded cardiac tamponade or mimics of heart failure. See earlier discussion on this topic.

Maintenance dose should be given before 9 A.M. daily. Split doses are rarely needed at 7 A.M. and 3 P.M. The afternoon dose should not be given later than 3 P.M. in order not to disturb the patient's sleep. It is preferable to give 160 mg once daily rather than 80 mg twice daily since the tubules may be resistant to the 80 mg dose in patients with severe heart failure. Doses beyond 160 mg are preferably divided into 120 mg in the morning and 80 mg in the afternoon. Patients with Class IV ventricles and graded as NYHA Class IV require at least 120 mg in one day, alternating with 80 mg the next day to achieve adequate control.

Patients who require a dose of furosemide greater than 40 mg daily to prevent pulmonary congestion and shortness of breath should be digitalized or an ACE inhibitor should be prescribed. Patients with Class III and Class IV NYHA heart failure require management with furosemide (average 80 to 120 mg daily), along with digoxin and ACE inhibitor therapy.

Always maintain the serum potassium above 4 mEq (mmol)/l. Patients who require large doses of furosemide beyond 80 mg daily benefit from ACE inhibitor therapy, which normalizes serum potassium. When the combination is used, potassium supplements or potassium-sparing diuretics should not be given, except with carefully monitored serum potassium levels. Also, salt substitutes contain potassium and can cause hyperkalemia. Periodic measurements of serum potassium are advisable for all patients taking daily diuretics.

Adverse effects. Hypokalemia, hypersensitivity in patients allergic to sulfur compounds, very rarely leukopenia, thrombocytopenia, precipitation of gout, hypocalcemia, hypomagnesemia.

Drug interactions. Cephalosporin or aminoglycoside antibiotics may show increased nephrotoxicity in patients with renal dysfunction when given large doses of loop diuretics. An increased reabsorption of lithium may occur, resulting in lithium toxicity; with chloral hydrate, hot flushes, sweating, and tachycardia may occur; NSAIDS antagonize the action of loop diuretics as well as thiazides; the effect of tubocurarine is increased.

ETHACRYNIC ACID

Supplied: tablets; 50 mg. vials; 50 mg

Dosage: oral 50 to 150 mg daily, IV 50 mg diluted with 50 ml of 5% dextrose in water given slowly.

Ethacrynic acid is recommended when there is failure of a response to large doses of furosemide or when sulfonamide sensitivity exists. The drug causes slightly more chloride loss than furosemide and has slightly more adverse effects. However, uric acid elevation appears to occur less frequently than with thiazides or furosemide. Warfarin's anticoagulant effect is increased by ethacrynic acid.

BUMETANIDE

Supplied: tablets; 0.5, 1, and 5 mg. ampules; 2, 4, 10 ml (500 μg/ml)

Dosage: oral 0.5 to 1 mg daily, increase if needed to 2 to 5 mg daily. In patients with renal failure, 5 mg or more may be required. IV 1 to 2 mg repeated in 30 minutes to 1 hour if needed.

The drug has similar actions to furosemide but is reported to cause less magnesium loss (1 mg bumetanide is equivalent to 40 mg furosemide). The drug is more nephrotoxic than furosemide, and its use should be avoided with cephalosporins and aminoglycosides.

THIAZIDE DIURETICS

See Chapter 1 for products and dosage. Thiazide diuretics are advisable mainly in patients with NYHA Class II heart failure. However, hypokalemia occurs in up to 30% of patients and as many as 50% with chlorthalidone. Also, hypomagnesemia often occurs and goes undetected. Potassium-sparing diuretics retain potassium and magnesium, and are useful in patients with mild heart failure (NYHA Class II). The patient may benefit from a potassium-sparing diuretic given 3 to 4 days per week only.

MODURETIC

The formulation contains hydrochlorothiazide (50 mg) and amiloride (5 mg) available in the United States, United Kingdom, and elsewhere. Moduret, which also contains 50 mg hydrochlorothiazide and 5 mg amiloride, is available in Canada. Moduret 25, hydrochlorothiazide (25 mg) and amiloride (2.5 mg) is available in UK and Europe. This is an excellent combination, and the use of 1 to 2 tablets daily sufficiently conserves potassium and magnesium and allows for the use of a small dose of hydrochlorothiazide. Amiloride is the only diuretic that possesses salutary antiarrhythmic properties in certain situations.

DYAZIDE

Supplied: tablets; 25 mg hydrochlorothiazide, 50 mg triamterene

Dosage: 1 tablet daily. A larger dose is not advisable, since 50 mg hydrochlorothiazide may cause hypokalemia, even in the presence of a small dose of triamterene. The drug is contraindicated in patients with renal calculi.

Caution. Potassium-sparing diuretics may cause serious hyperkalemia when used in conjunction with ACE inhibitors, potassium supplements, or salt substitutes. Patients with maturity-onset diabetes may develop hyporeninemic hypoaldosteronism, which causes hyperkalemia in patients with a normal serum creatinine. Potassium-sparing diuretics may increase this effect. Spironolactone may cause gynecomastia, and tumorigenicity in rats has been noted; although this finding may not apply to humans, care is needed with the use of this drug. Spironolactone's onset of action occurs in a few days, and split doses are necessary. Thus, spironolactone is not advisable for maintenance therapy in patients with heart failure.

METOLAZONE

Supplied: tablets; 2.5, 5, 10 mg

Dosage: 2.5 to 5 mg once daily; maximum 10 mg (rarely indicated). This thiazide diuretic has a unique property of retaining effectiveness when other thiazides become ineffective with glomerular filtration rate less than 30 ml/min. The combination of metolazone and furosemide is very useful in patients with refractory heart failure who fail to respond to large doses of furosemide or ethracrynic acid. In one reported study, in 15 of 17 patients with severe failure refractory to loop diuretics, digoxin, and ACE inhibitors, substantial improvement occurred, allowing discharge from the hospital. This potent combination is useful, but hypokalemia is often pronounced. Intermittent therapy (metolazone twice weekly) may help avoid this effect. In this situation, however, combination with an ACE inhibitor or potassium supplement often becomes necessary.

ACETAZOLAMIDE
(Diamox)

Supplied: tablets; 250 mg

Dosage: 250 mg three times daily for 4 days once or twice monthly. This carbonic anhydrase inhibitor has a weak diuretic action, which dissipates in 3 or 4 days. The drug is useful in the management of hypochloremic metabolic alkalosis in the presence of a normal serum potassium. The patient with refractory heart failure on furosemide and potassium-sparing diuretics or ACE inhibitors may show a typical electrolyte abnormality: potassium 4 to 5 mEq (mmol)/l, chlorides less than 92 mEq (mmol)/l, CO_2 greater than 30 mEq (mmol)/l. The addition of acetazolamide to furosemide and ACE inhibitors 3 days weekly maintains diuresis with correction of normokalemic, hypochloremic, metabolic alkalosis.

The drug is contraindicated in patients with severe cirrhosis, metabolic acidosis, renal failure, and renal calculi.

DIGITALIS

DIGOXIN
(Lanoxin)

After more than 200 years of use and controversies in the 1970s regarding its efficacy and role, digoxin has been fully restored as the only oral positive inotropic agent available that significantly improves symptoms, signs, EF, and other hemodynamic parameters in patients with all grades of acute, recurrent, or chronic heart failure with salutary effects occurring when combined with a diuretic and/or ACE inhibitor.

Clinicians who have used this drug for over 30 years in patients with ventricular systolic dysfunction (NYHA Class III and IV heart failure) recognize the effectiveness of the drug when combined with diuretics and have documented the recurrence of heart failure when digoxin is discontinued. An S3 or summation gallop present during several days of treatment with diuretics and ACE inhibitors disappears within days of digitalization. Also, objective hemodynamic data are now available that clearly indicate the drug's salutary effects.

Digoxin has been shown to further improve cardiac function in patients with abnormal hemodynamic variables when stabilized on diuretics and ACE inhibitors. In 11 patients in sinus rhythm with severe heart failure stabilized on digoxin and vasodilators, IV digoxin increased EF by 38% from 0.21 to 0.29, the mean cardiac index rose 30%, and pulmonary wedge pressure decreased by 29%. Six patients who had persistent hemodynamic evidence of left ventricular dysfunction when given appropriate doses of diuretic and vasodilators responded dramatically to digoxin. Patients with the most severe left ventricular dysfunction showed the most hemodynamic improvement.

Although potentially serious, genuine digoxin toxicity is very rare. Conclusions drawn from poorly designed studies in the 1970s and early 1980s incorrectly overestimated the incidence of digoxin toxicity. The drug has few adverse effects and rare toxicity when used under the supervision of a physician. As discussed earlier, this economical one-a-day inotropic agent, when combined with diuretics, has an important role in the management of all grades of heart failure, usually in combination with an ACE inhibitor.

In the Milrinone Multicenter Trial Group, mainly NYHA Class III heart failure patients using the mean dose of furosemide 90 mg, only 46% of patients switched from digoxin to placebo completed the full 3-month study, versus 77% of those treated with digoxin. Exercise tolerance and EF were improved by digoxin.

In a randomized, double-blind crossover study of digoxin and placebo in 28 heart failure patients, NYHA Class II and III, digoxin increased fractional shortening and walking distance and reduced cardiothoracic ratio. Importantly, during the placebo period, all seven treatment failures occurred.

In a double-blind, placebo-controlled study, 16 of 46 patients with proven heart failure deteriorated 4 days to 3 weeks upon stopping digoxin.

In the CONSENSUS and other trials of NYHA Class III and IV heart failure patients, digoxin was used with a diuretic, plus or minus vasodilator. In Class III and IV patients, the combination of diuretics and vasodilators has not been shown to be superior to diuretics plus digoxin, and triple therapy constitutes rational therapy.

The use of vasodilators is limited in patients with severe heart failure complicated by relative hypotension. Patients with severe heart failure commonly have lowered blood pressure or hypotension and often require doses of furosemide equal to or greater than 80 mg. ACE inhibitors carry the risk of producing or increasing hypotension in a significant number of these patients. They may cause coronary insufficiency, may increase angina, syncope, and renal failure, and may increase mortality in patients with critical stenosis of the carotid, renal, or coronary arteries. Digoxin, undoubtedly, has a role in patients with severe heart failure.

Contraindications
- Patients with sick sinus syndrome or AV block of all grades

Cautions. Many physicians avoid the use of digoxin in the first 24 hours of MI, except in the management of patients with atrial fibrillation with hemodynamic compromise, in whom electrical cardioversion is preferred. The drug can be used judiciously in smaller initial doses within the first 24 hours of infarction if moderate to severe heart failure is unimproved with the use of furosemide and nitrates and/or if dobutamine is not available.

Indications
- Heart failure associated with atrial fibrillation
- Patients in sinus rhythm: Severe heart failure due to systolic dysfunction, particularly patients with NYHA Class III or IV, regardless of the presence of an S3 gallop. In these patients, the drug is combined with diuretics and ACE inhibitors
- As part of triple therapy in patients with NYHA Class II heart failure and EF less than 35%
- As the second-line agent for management of NYHA Class II heart failure patients with EF greater than 35% in combination with diuretics. Salutary effects are equal to those of ACE inhibitors combined with diuretics
- Where ACE inhibitors are contraindicated because of hypotension, renal failure, or bothersome adverse effects
- Patients with angina or NYHA Class II, III, or IV heart failure requiring furosemide dosage greater than 40 mg daily. Studies indicate that ACE inhibitors may worsen angina and are relatively contraindicated in these patients.
- The drug can be used, if indicated, in pregnancy and during breastfeeding

Action
- Inotropic effect: Digoxin increases the force and velocity of myocardial contraction and improves the EF. It combines with and partially inhibits the sodium pump, the enzyme sodium, and potassium-activated adenosine triphosphatase (Na K ATPase) located in the sarcolemmal membrane of the myocardial cell and increases the availability of intracellular calcium to contractile elements resulting in enhanced myocardial contractility. This effect causes the Frank-Starling function curve to move upward and to the left
- Increase of vagal activity and a modest decrease in sympathetic activity slow conduction velocity in the AV node. This action is important in

slowing the ventricular response in atrial fibrillation and the termination of paroxysmal supraventricular tachycardia (PSVT). Mild slowing of the sinus rate occurs due to the mild decrease in sympathetic activity
• Increase in Phase 4 diastolic depolarization increases the activity of ectopic pacemakers

Pharmacokinetics. About 66% of the oral tablet dose is absorbed mainly in the stomach and the upper small bowel. Following absorption, the drug is widely distributed, but binding to skeletal muscle is particularly important because a low muscle mass in the elderly calls for a smaller loading dose. The mean serum half-life is approximately 36 hours. It is advisable to wait until equilibration is reached to obtain a digoxin level that represents myocardial concentration. After IV and oral dosing, wait at least 3 hours and 6 hours, respectively, before obtaining a serum digoxin assay. Dosing at bedtime is advisable so that an assay during a morning assignment would be appropriate.

Bioavailability is reduced as a result of decreased absorption due to

• Malabsorption syndrome
• Colestipol, cholestyramine, Metamucil (or similar agents)
• Antacids, metoclopramide, phenytoin, phenobarbital

Absorption is enhanced by Lomotil and decreased intestional motility.

An increased serum digoxin level may result from antibiotics, especially Neomycin, and some broad-spectrum antibiotics that may eliminate Eubacterium lentum, which partially metabolizes digoxin to inactive dihydrodigoxine and may thus cause increased digoxin absorption. However, this effect occurs in less than 10% of patients. Digoxin levels are also increased by quinidine, some calcium antagonists, and amiodarone.

Excretion is by the kidneys. Thus, undetected or unnoticed renal insufficiency is the commonest cause of digoxin toxicity.

After 1 mg oral dosing, peak onset of action occurs in 1 to 6 hours, with serum levels usually exceeding 1 μg/ml; maximum inotropic action is observed in 4 to 6 hours.

Dosage: 0.5 to 1 mg over 24 hours prescribed as follows

• Orally: 0.5 mg immediately, 0.25 mg every 12 hours for two doses, followed by an appropriate maintenance dose depending on age, renal function, and presence or absence of conditions that increase sensitivity to the drug (Table 5–2). If such conditions are present, halve the initial dose (or 0.25 mg twice daily) for 2 days, followed by maintenance dosage depending on age or renal function. In the UK, the British National Formulary recommendation is 0.125 to 0.25 mg twice daily for about 1 week and then once daily, having regard to renal function. However, 0.5 mg daily for 1 week may cause toxicity if an unsuspected decrease in creatinine clearance is present, especially in the elderly, or if sensitivity exists. Also, in patients less than age 70 with normal renal function, the initial 0.25 mg daily dose may not achieve adequate levels or salutary effects for several weeks

- Rapid oral method for atrial fibrillation with a ventricular response: 110 to 140/minute in patients with heart failure not receiving digoxin. Caution: The patient is reassessed prior to each dose and the order for the drug is then written: 0.5 mg immediately, 0.25 mg every 4 or 6 hours for three doses, followed by maintenance
- IV therapy for atrial fibrillation with a fast ventricular response greater than 150/min where urgent digitalization is required in the absence of definite daily digoxin use in the previous week and the exclusion of sick sinus syndrome: 0.5 mg IV slowly over 10 minutes with ECG monitoring, reassess before each dose, 0.25 mg over 10 minutes every 2 to 4 hours for two or three doses, followed by maintenance. It is often necessary to give 1.25 to 1.5 mg over 12 hours to obtain satisfactory control of the ventricular response. Occasionally, higher doses are necessary to achieve a ventricular response less than 110/min, followed by maintenance dose. Alternatively, verapamil or a beta blocker administered orally may be added to control a fast ventricular rate

Alternatively, it is recommended (in the UK) that digoxin is given by IV infusion (0.75 to 1 mg in 50 ml) over 2 or more hours when rapid control of atrial fibrillation is required.

Suggested maintenance dosage with normal serum creatinine

- Age less than 70 (0.25 mg daily preferably at bedtime)
- Age greater than 70 (0.125 mg at bedtime)

In patients with atrial fibrillation requiring further control of ventricular response, a 0.125-mg daily dose in addition to the maintenance dose indicated is often necessary. A 0.1875-mg tablet is available in some countries and is a convenient once daily dose.

If renal failure is present, obtain a direct measurement of the creatinine clearance or determine the clearance by utilizing the lean body weight, age, sex, and serum creatinine.

Caution. Digoxin toxicity may occur in patients with known or unsuspected renal dysfunction, and especially in the elderly, in whom creatinine clearance is frequently reduced in the presence of a normal serum creatinine. In patients under age 70 with serum creatinine of 1.3 to 2.3 mg/dl (115 to 203 μmol/l), give 0.125 mg on alternate days and assess digoxin levels in about 10 days. In patients over age 70 with abnormal serum creatinine above 2.3 mg/dl (203 μmol/l), it is advisable to avoid digoxin use because toxicity is a major concern. In this situation, treatment with diuretics and vasodilators is indicated and digoxin is relatively contraindicated. If needed, digitoxin can be used.

DIGITOXIN

Supplied: tablets; 0.1, 0.15 mg

Dosage: 0.05 to 0.15 mg daily with no loading dose. The drug is metabolized by the liver and is excreted in the gut. The half-life is 4 to 6 days; if digitoxin toxicity occurs, it is prolonged. Levels are not usually increased in a patient with hepatic or renal dysfunction. Therapeutic levels are 10 to 25 ng/ml, and toxic levels are greater than 35 ng/ml.

DIGITALIS TOXICITY

Studies done in the 1970s and early 1980s that evaluated the incidence of digitalis toxicity and mortality had serious flaws in their design. In a 1980–1988 Henry Ford Hospital study, digoxin intoxication was a discharge diagnosis in 106 patients in the hospital, with 35,000 admissions and 1.7 million annual clinic visits per year. A thorough analysis revealed only 43 cases of the 106 as definite intoxication; 20 had life-threatening arrhythmias, and 5% required temporary pacing. The mortality rate in the definitely intoxicated patients was 2 of the 43 patients (4.6%), compared to 14 of 31 patients (41%) reported in a 1971 study. A 1987 review of 563 patients receiving digoxin and admitted for heart failure showed that only 4 of the 27 diagnosed as digoxin toxicity were definitely intoxicated (an incidence of 0.8%).

A decrease in the incidence of definite or serious digitalis intoxication has materialized because of physician awareness of the pharmacokinetics: absorption, binding, distribution, and excretion of the drug. In particular, the hazard in patients with renal dysfunction, including elderly patients with unsuspected impaired renal function with a normal serum creatinine, has sharply curtailed digitalis toxicity.

A lean skeletal mass, especially in the elderly, carries two important connotations

- Digoxin binds to skeletal muscle; thus, in individuals with lean, skeletal mass, more digoxin is available in the serum for myocardial binding. Therefore, there is a higher probability of toxicity in patients with lean skeletal mass, especially if renal dysfunction inhibits elimination of the drug
- Low skeletal muscle mass in the elderly reflects a lowered serum creatinine that leads the physician to believe that renal function is normal, when creatinine clearance may be reduced by 50% or more

Reduction of the maintenance dose in patients with conditions that increase sensitivity to digoxin (Table 5–3) and the appropriate use of digoxin serum assay are important precautionary measures. Conditions that increase or decrease the bioavailability of digoxin, particularly drugs that cause interactions, are listed in Table 5–4.

Symptoms and signs of digitalis intoxication include

- GI: Nausea, anorexia, vomiting, diarrhea, abdominal pain, weight loss
- CNS: Visual hallucinations; blue, green, or yellow vision; blurring of vision and scotomas; dizziness, headaches, restlessness, insomnia, and rarely mental confusion and psychosis
- Cardiac: There is a spectrum from occurrence of arrhythmia in digoxin free state, through latent arrhythmia precipitated by digoxin, to arrhythmia directly secondary to digoxin. First-, second- or third-degree AV block; sinus pause greater than 2 seconds; paroxysmal atrial tachy-

TABLE 5-3. CONDITIONS IN WHICH THERE IS AN
INCREASED SENSITIVITY TO DIGOXIN AND
CONSERVATIVE DOSING IS RECOMMENDED

1. Elderly patients (age >70)	8. Hypercalcemia
2. Hypokalemia	9. Hypocalcemia
3. Hyperkalemia	10. Myocarditis
4. Hypoxemia	11. Low skeletal mass
5. Acidosis	12. Hypothyroidism
6. Acute myocardial infarction	13. Amyloidosis
7. Hypomagnesemia	

From: Khan, M Gabriel: Cardiac Drug Therapy. 3rd Ed. London, W.B. Saunders, 1992.

TABLE 5-4. DIGOXIN INTERACTIONS

Increase serum levels
  Quinidine displaces digoxin at binding sites, decreases renal elimination
  Verapamil, diltiazem, nicardipine, felodipine, amiodarone, propafenone
    ACE inhibitors may decrease renal elimination
  NSAIDS decrease renal elimination
    Lomotil, probanthine decrease intestinal motility
  Erythromycin, tetracycline eliminate eubacterium lentum
  Spironolactone, digoxin assay falsely elevated
  Electrophysiologic interactions may occur with amiodarone, diltiazem, verapamil
Decrease serum levels or bioavailability
  Antacids, metoclopramide, cholestyramine, colestipol
  Metamucil, neomycin, phenytoin, phenobarbital, salicylazosulfapyridine

---

cardia with block (ventricular rate is often 90 to 120/min; the P waves may be buried in the T waves); accelerated junctional rhythm; ventricular premature beats, bigeminal or multifocal; ventricular tachycardia; and rarely VF. Table 5–5 shows the incidence of arrhythmias caused by digoxin toxicity. In addition, deterioration in heart failure may be due to digoxin toxicity

Serum Digoxin Assay

No single serum digoxin concentration drawn at the appropriate time interval, more than 6 hours after oral dosing, can indicate toxicity reliably, but the likelihood increases progressively through the range 1.5 to 3 ng/ml or μg/l (1.2 to 3.5 nmol/l). Concentrations above 3 ng/ml must be avoided. Levels less than 1.5 ng/ml drawn at the appropriate time are rarely associated with toxicity, except in patients with myocardial sensitivity as listed in Table 5–3. Digoxin toxicity in the patient with the absence of the conditions listed and a level less than 1 ng/ml is so rare as to exclude the diagnosis. Reviews indicate that digoxin-intoxicated patients had a mean serum digoxin level of 3.3 ng/ml.

TABLE 5–5. MAJOR MANIFESTATIONS OF DIGOXIN TOXICITY	
	%
A. Non-life-threatening arrhythmias	
Multifocal VPCs	30
1° AV Block	15
Supraventricular tachycardia	25
B. Life-threatening arrhythmias	
3° AV Block	25
2° AV Block	15
Ventricular tachycardia	20
Ventricular fibrillation	10
Asystole	8
C. Noncardiac	
Nausea & vomiting	50
Hyperkalemia*	25

* Due to renal failure and/or inhibition of the sodium pump

Serum digoxin levels are often not necessary and are overused or drawn at an inappropriate time interval.
Suggested indications for assay include

- Known or suspected renal impairment or elderly patients with renal dysfunction. An assay is advisable every 3 months
- Symptoms or signs suggesting toxicity, especially in the presence of hypokalemia or conditions in which there is increased sensitivity to digoxin (Table 5–3)
- In patients over age 70 with a normal serum creatinine and no signs of renal disease, assay at least twice yearly if the maintenance dose exceeds 0.125 mg daily. If the dose is 0.125 mg daily, a level once yearly should suffice
- Concomitant use of digoxin with drugs that increase serum levels (Table 5–4)

Management of Digitalis Toxicity

- Discontinue digoxin
- Replace potassium if hypokalemia is present. Hold diuretics until serum potassium is in the normal range
- Clarify conditions that increase sensitivity to digoxin (Table 5–3). Toxicity is likely to be present if suggestive symptoms are manifest and if there is a precipitating cause for renal impairment or if the serum creatinine is elevated
- Assess digoxin level
- Assess ECG signs: Digitalis effect does not mean toxicity. (See bradyarrhythmias and tachyarrhythmias as listed under Adverse Effects)

Drug therapy is indicated for

- Arrhythmias causing a threat to life, hemodynamic deterioration, or worsening of heart failure. The incidence of digoxin-induced arrhythmias is given in Table 5–5

Bradyarrhythmias

Sinus bradycardia, second-degree AV block, and sinoatrial dysfunction are managed with atropine 0.4, 0.5, or 0.6 mg IV every 5 minutes to maximum of 2 mg. Failure to respond to atropine or the presence of third-degree AV block is an indication for digoxin-specific Fab antibody fragments or temporary pacing (see Chapter 18).

Caution. Potassium chloride is relatively contraindicated with bradyarrhythmias as potassium and digoxin synergistically depress conduction and may precipitate a higher degree of AV block. If the serum potassium is in the range of 3.0 to 3.8 mEq(mmol)/l, potassium should be given intravenously at a rate less than 10 mEq(mmol)/hour; a serum potassium less than 3 mEq/l may require an infusion rate greater than 10 mEq(mmol)/hour and continuous monitoring of the cardiac rhythm is necessary.

Tachyarrhythmias

VT, multifocal VPCs, or atrial tachycardia with block in the presence of hypokalemia.

Potassium chloride. IV 40 to 60 mEq(mmol) in 1 liter of 0.9% or half normal saline over 4 hours, except in patients with renal insufficiency or in patients with AV block, because an increase in potassium may increase the degree of AV block. Potassium chloride is diluted in 5% dextrose in water if heart failure is present. Magnesium sulfate may be of value in suppressing some cases of VT by blocking calcium currents that are involved in after depolarization.

Lidocaine. Considered the drug of choice for control of ventricular arrhythmias secondary to digoxin intoxication after the correction of hypokalemia. The short duration of action and relatively low toxicity and availability are major advantages. Lidocaine is not indicated for junctional tachycardias because it is not effective.

Dosage: 1.5 mg/kg, 50 to 100 mg with a simultaneous infusion of 1 to 3 mg/minute and repeat bolus in 10 minutes.

If lidocaine fails to control the tachyarrhythmia and if there are no contraindications, a beta blocking drug may be tried cautiously (see Tables 3–8 and 3–9 for IV dosage).

Phenytoin is no longer recommended in the treatment of digitalis toxicity, and the use of beta blockers has dwindled with the availability of digoxin-specific Fab antibody fragments.

Digoxin-Specific Fab Antibody Fragments

The treatment of digitalis toxicity has been revolutionized since the value of digoxin-specific Fab fragments was proven. The preparation is obtained from sheep immunized with a digoxin-serum albumin conjugate. The intact antibody is then cleaved with papain to yield digoxin-specific Fab fragments that are isolated and purified. The purified immunoglobulin G, antibody, has a high specificity and affinity for digoxin. The digoxin-specific antibodies bind to digoxin and accelerate digoxin removal from cellular membranes. Because the digoxin is bound, it is rendered inactive. The entire body load of digoxin is bound and pulled back into the blood stream; thus, the serum digoxin level may be high, but the bound level is inactive. Fab fragments are excreted by the kidneys with a half-life of 16 to 20 hours.

In a multicenter study of 150 patients with potentially life-threatening digitalis toxicity, administration of digoxin-specific Fab antibody fragments caused amelioration of symptoms and signs of digitalis toxicity in 80%; 10% of patients were unimproved and 10% showed no response. A treatment response was observed within 20 minutes, and by 60 minutes, more than 75% of patients showed a salutary response. Most patients showed complete recovery within 4 hours. Approximately 3% of patients had a recurrence of toxicity within 7 days, especially patients receiving less than the estimated adequate dose of Fab. Patients with severe digoxin toxicity may have hyperkalemia due to renal failure and/or inhibition of the sodium pump.

Hyperkalemia or an increasing serum potassium level is an important predictor; clinical trials suggest that as potassium levels rise, mortality rates increase. Digitalis-induced hyperkalemia suggests imminent cardiac arrest; in these patients, mortality is high and Fab fragments are urgently advised. If serum potassium exceeds 5 mEq/l (mmol/l) in the presence of signs and symptoms of digitalis intoxication, digoxin-immune Fab is immediately indicated. Fab fragments are indicated for digoxin toxicity and have been successful with digitoxin overdose.

In patients with life-threatening tachyarrhythmias or bradyarrhythmias, the early use of digoxin-specific antibody is strongly recommended; pacing can be avoided.

Supplied: (Digibind) powder for preparation of infusion; vial, 40 mg

Dosage: 2 to 3 vials, 80 to 120 mg: an estimated adequate dose is calculated using the patient's body weight and serum digoxin level if toxicity is due to therapy or based on the amount ingested for patients with overdose. (See product monograph.)

Adverse effects. These are uncommon. Hypokalemia is observed in less than 5% of patients and allergic reaction occurs in less than 1%.

Caution. Rapid onset of hypokalemia should be anticipated following reversal of toxicity by Fab fragments. IV potassium chloride should be given as needed to avoid hypokalemia.

ACE INHIBITORS

When heart failure occurs, sensors in the heart, the aortic arch, and arterioles of the juxtaglomerular apparatus actuate a host of neurohormonal responses that are necessary for the perfusion of vital tissues, especially of the brain, heart, and kidneys. These responses, initiated by sympathoadrenal activation and enhanced by stimulation of the renin angiotensin system, result in marked vasoconstriction, which increases systemic vascular resistance in order to maintain central blood pressure. Unfortunately, an increase in systemic vascular resistance increases afterload and contractile myocyte energy costs.

Components of the renin angiotensin system are not only confined to the kidney, adrenals, liver, and blood but are also present in several tissues, including the heart, brain, pituitary gland, uterus, gut, salivary glands, ovaries, testes, and placenta. Angiotensin is synthesized in many tissues as well as in the circulation. Thus, some ACE inhibitors have tissue site of action, the importance of which requires further evaluation.

ACE inhibitors prevent formation of the vasoconstrictor angiotensin II and, at the appropriate dose, provide sufficient vasodilatation to bring about reduction in afterload and decrease in systolic ventricular workload. Thus, ACE inhibitors play a major role as second-line drug therapy for heart failure (NYHA Class II, III, and IV). Although these agents have greatly improved the management and survival of heart failure patients, they do not replace loop diuretics as first-line agents and are used in combination with a diuretic, with or without added digoxin therapy; see earlier discussion of drug therapy, NYHA class II, III, and IV heart failure.

Available ACE inhibitors include captopril and enalapril, which are approved for the management of heart failure in the United States; in the UK and Europe, lisinopril, perindopril, quinapril, and ramipril are available.

The dosages and the pharmacologic profile of ACE inhibitors are given in Tables 1–2 and 1–3.

ACTION OF ACE INHIBITORS

Renin release causes the conversion of angiotensinogen to angiotensin I. ACE inhibitors are competitive inhibitors of angiotensin converting enzyme and thus prevent the conversion of angiotensin I to angiotensin II, which brings about

- Marked arteriolar vasodilatation; thus, a fall in systemic vascular resistance, afterload, and blood pressure
- Decreased sympathetic activity and reduced release of norepinephrine. This action causes further vasodilatation. It also prevents the usual increase in heart rate observed with vasodilators of the non-ACE-inhibitor category
- Decreased aldosterone secretion; thus, enhancement of sodium excretion with potassium retention
- Suppression of vasopressin release with free water loss, resulting in some protection from severe dilutional hyponatremia

- Accumulation of bradykinin, causing a release of vasodilator prostaglandins and further vasodilatation
- Reduced hyperuricemia resulting from uricosuric effect

Captopril
(Capoten)

Supplied: tablets; 12.5, 25, 50, and 100 mg

Dosage: 6.25 mg test dose (a 3 mg test dose is administered to the elderly or patients considered at risk for hypotension). Observation is necessary for the next 2 to 4 hours; blood pressure should be taken every 15 to 30 minutes for 1, 2, or 3 hours post dosing. If there is no occurrence of hypotension or presyncope, give 6.25 mg twice daily for the first day, increase to 12.5 mg twice daily for 1 to 2 days, and then over days to weeks, increase to the usual maintenance dose of 37.5 to 50 mg daily (maximum of 75 mg daily). A dose in excess of 75 mg provides little added benefit. Marked lowering of the diastolic blood pressure may occur with doses exceeding 50 mg daily, causing a decrease in coronary perfusion that may worsen angina or silent ischemia, an effect that could increase mortality in patients with angina. If symptoms and signs of heart failure persist, it is wise to increase the dose of loop diuretic and add digoxin, followed by the addition of a nitrate preparation. Caution is necessary to avoid hypotension and syncope. In addition, metolazone added to loop diuretic therapy improves diuresis in patients who appear to be partially resistant to moderate doses of loop diuretics; a trial of metolazone may provide salutary effects in patients with Class IV heart failure refractory to loop diuretic, digoxin, and ACE inhibitors.

The renin angiotensin system is blocked by a captopril dosage of about 25 mg and, allowing for renal clearance, a daily dose of 25 to 50 mg is usually sufficient to achieve salutary effects. It is often necessary to discontinue diuretics or halve the dose to allow the introduction of an ACE inhibitor at an appropriate dose. When the patient is stabilized on captopril (25 to 37.5 mg daily), the dose of loop diuretics can be increased as required to relieve congestion and shortness of breath. In renal failure, the dose interval is increased according to the creatinine clearance, so that a once daily dose should suffice for a patient who has a 50% decrease in creatinine clearance or a serum creatinine at the upper limit of normal or at maximum 2.3 mg/dl (203 µmol/l). The serum creatinine is an approximation of renal function, and caution is necessary in patients with renal failure.

Enalapril
(Vasotec; Vasotec or Innovace, UK)

Supplied: tablets; 5, 10, 20 mg

Dosage: 2.5 mg orally and observe for 2 to 6 hours. If there is no hypotension, give 2.5 mg twice daily for a few days, and increase slowly over days or weeks to 5 mg to a maximum of 10 mg twice daily. If heart failure is refractory, systolic pressure exceeds 120 mm Hg and active ischemia is not present; a maximum dose of 20 mg in the morning and 10 mg at night may be tried cautiously. In patients with severe heart failure, the dose can be increased more rapidly when under supervision with careful monitoring of blood pressure to avoid hypotension. As with captopril, the dose is often given one daily in patients with very mild renal dysfunction or in patients over age 70. It is advisable to reduce the dose of loop diuretics prior to giving the first dose of enalapril, as with other ACE inhibitors.

An initial effect of hypotension is usually observed within 1 to 2 hours after administration of captopril and within 2½ to 5 hours with enalapril. Withdrawal of diuretics does not always prevent marked hypotension or syncope, and caution is required at all times with the initiation of ACE inhibitor therapy.

Lisinopril
(Prinivil, Zestril; Zestril, Carace, UK).

Supplied: 2.5, 5, 20 mg

Dosage: In the UK, for heart failure, 2.5 mg daily under close hospital supervision; usual maintenance is 5 to 15 mg daily for heart failure.

Quinapril
(Accupro, available in UK and Europe)

Dosage: Initial dose of 2.5 mg under close hospital supervision, maintenance dose of 5 to 10 mg daily in two divided doses for heart failure, 5 mg to a maximum of 20 mg oral daily.

Ramipril
(Altace; Tritace: not yet approved for heart failure in the US)

Dosage: Initial dose of 1.25 mg daily, increase over 1 to 2 weeks; maintenance dose is 2.5 to 5 mg daily.

Caution. With the use of ACE inhibitors, caution is necessary in patients with stenosis in a solitary kidney or in patients with suspected tight renal artery stenosis because acute renal failure may be precipitated. Renal circulation in patients with severe bilateral renal artery stenosis or stenosis in a solitary kidney is critically dependent on high levels of angiotensin II. In these situations, ACE inhibitors markedly decrease renal blood flow and may worsen renal failure, causing a sharp elevation in serum creatinine. Thus, patients showing a sharp rise in serum creatinine during the first few days following commencement of ACE inhibitors are at high risk for occlusion of the renal circulation, and the drug should be discontinued immediately.

Maturity-onset diabetic patients with hyporeninemic, hypoaldosteronism may develop severe hyperkalemia. ACE inhibitors should not be given concurrently with potassium supplements, salt substitutes, or potassium-sparing diuretics unless measurements of serum potassium levels indicate that this is necessary; then supervision is required.

CONTRAINDICATIONS

- Aortic stenosis
- Renal artery stenosis of a solitary kidney or severe bilateral renal artery stenosis
- Severe carotid artery stenosis
- Heart failure associated with unstable angina restrictive cardiomyopathy or hypertrophic cardiomyopathy with obstruction
- Severe anemia
- Pregnancy and during breastfeeding

Relative contraindications include patients with collagen vascular diseases or concomitant use of immunosuppressives, because neutropenia and agranulocytosis observed with ACE inhibitors appear to occur more often in these patients.

Interactions may occur with acebutolol, allopurinol, hydralazine, NSAIDS, pindolol, procainamide, tocainide, and immunosuppressives.

ADVERSE EFFECTS

These include the following

- Hypotension
- Hyperkalemia in patients with renal failure and/or diabetes
- Cough in about 10% of patients; may be prostaglandin mediated, as it may be abolished by use of NSAIDS
- Angioedema of the face, mouth, tongue, or larynx may occur in approximately 0.2% of patients and can be fatal
- Pruritus and rash in about 10% of patients
- Loss of taste (apparently specific for sulfhydryl compounds) in approximately 7% of patients
- Mouth ulcers, neurologic dysfunction, and proteinuria in about 1% of patients with pre-existing renal disease
- Neutropenia and agranulocytosis (rare, occur mainly in patients with serious intercurrent illness, particularly immunologic disturbances, altered immune response, or collagen vascular disease)
- Occasionally wheeze, myalgia, muscle cramps, hair loss, impotence, decreased libido, hepatitis, pemphigus, or the occurrence of antinuclear antibodies

NITRATES

Nitrates are used extensively, and perhaps inappropriately, in the management of NYHA Class III and IV heart failure. Small trials have been carried out using continuous nitrate, and it is now known that nitrate tolerance develops after 48 hours of use. Probable clinical benefits are observed only when a nitrate-free interval is provided. Unfortunately, intermittent therapy produces a high incidence of intolerable headaches. Clinical trials are not available to document significant effects of oral nitrates on morbidity and mortality when the drug is added to standard therapy, digoxin, and diuretics. Hemodynamic parameters are not improved, except with the use of IV nitroglycerin.

Five clinical trials have used oral nitrates in the management of NYHA Class II and III heart failure. Studies conducted in 1978 and 1980, 8 and 12 weeks, respectively, showed no clinical differences between oral nitrates and placebo. A study using a parallel group design in 30 patients with congestive cardiomyopathy followed for 1 year showed no difference in ventricular function and exercise tolerance after 6, 9, and 12 months of therapy. In another study, deaths due to heart failure occurred more frequently in patients treated with oral nitrates. VHeFT-1 showed a modest improvement in survival at 2 years of isosorbide dinitrate (ISDN) and hydralazine added to digoxin-diuretic versus digoxin-diuretic therapy. VHeFT-II patients received hydralazine (37.5 mg) four times daily and ISDN (40 mg) four times daily. The 2-year result indicated that enalapril was superior to the combination of hydralazine and ISDN in reducing mortality, but peak VO_2 on exercise capacity was somewhat better during the first 2 years with the use of ISDN-hydralazine. However, the importance of the effect of ISDN in comparison with that of hydralazine in producing this result is unknown. Surprisingly, this study utilized continuous nitrate therapy. Thus, there are no definite scientific data to support the widespread belief that nitrates are effective in the management of NYHA Class III and IV heart failure. The drug is not indicated for Class II heart failure, except in the management of angina patients with heart failure.

Oral nitrates are therefore reserved for patients who are unable to take ACE inhibitors or in properly selected patients with Class III and IV heart failure who continue to have recurrence of pulmonary congestion, shortness of breath, poor effort tolerance, or manifestations of cardiac ischemia when on maintenance digoxin, loop diuretics, and ACE inhibitors. When added to ACE inhibitors, serious hypotension may occur, which may produce syncope or cerebral circulatory insufficiency. Caution is therefore necessary with the combination of nitrates and ACE inhibitors.

A study indicates that ACE inhibitors may prevent nitrate tolerance during longterm therapy. The sulfhydryl group was apparently not essential, because enalapril gave similar results to captopril. However, another study failed to support this observation and further studies are required.

CALCIUM ANTAGONISTS

Calcium antagonists should not be given to patients with moderate to severe left ventricular systolic dysfunction. Verapamil has a marked negative inotropic effect and may precipitate heart failure. The negative inotropic effect of diltiazem is not as intense, but the drug increases the incidence of heart failure in patients with left ventricular dysfunction. Dihydropyridines can cause depression in left ventricular systolic function, although this effect is partially ameliorated by the increase of sympathetic activity.

However, dihydropyridines have often precipitated heart failure and caution is necessary with these drugs. Worsening of heart failure of a serious nature requiring hospitalization has been reported for all calcium antagonists. Thus, nifedipine is no longer recommended in patients with mild or moderate heart failure, as deterioration occurs in a significant number of patients. The combination of a pure vasodilator, nifedipine or other dihydropyridine, with isosorbide dinitrate as a venodilator appears to be a rational approach, but it is nonetheless unsafe. Complementary hemodynamic and clinical benefits are not observed with the combination of nifedipine and isosorbide dinitrate. Caution: calcium antagonists are hazardous in patients with heart failure and are contraindicated for heart failure of all grades.

The propensity of dihydropyridine calcium antagonists to cause heart failure appears to be determined by their significant hypotensive and sympathohormonal effects. Activation of the renin angiotensin system and stimulation of sympathetic activity are undesired effects.

In a study of 23 patients with NYHA Class II and III heart failure (mean EF of 20%; stabilized on diuretics and digoxin and then given nefidipine 20 mg four times daily, plus ISDN up to 40 mg four times daily, with follow-up for 8 weeks), nifedipine caused clinical deterioration necessitating hospitalization in 24% of patients. Hospitalization was necessary in 26% of patients during combined therapy with nitrates. No patient deteriorated, however, during treatment with ISDN alone. Also, the Multicenter Diltiazem Post Infarction Trial showed worsening of heart failure and increased mortality in patients treated with diltiazem after Q wave myocardial infarction complicated by left ventricular dysfunction (EF less than 40%).

OTHER AGENTS FOR HEART FAILURE

MILRINONE

Milrinone is a non-glycoside, non-beta-agonist inotropic agent with about 20 times the inotropic potency of amrinone. However, several clinical studies have indicated an increase in mortality from the use of this drug. The Promise Trial, a large multicenter randomized study was halted 5 months prior to completion because of an excess of 43 deaths in patients treated with milrinone. Patients with NYHA Class IV heart failure showed an up to 54% increase in mortality and about a 30% increase in risk occurred in milrinone-treated patients.

It is quite clear that milrinone and similar inotropic agents are hazardous; no further trials are expected with this group of inotropic agents. Amrinone IV is, however, occasionally used in intensive care units for patients resistant to other inotropes; its administration is monitored closely. Trials indicate that this agent has no advantages over dobutamine.

BETA BLOCKERS

Beta-adrenergic blocking drugs have a role to play in properly selected patients with heart failure. Some patients with dilated cardiomyopathy show benefit with the use of very small doses of metoprolol. Labetalol and bucindolol have additional vasodilator effects and have shown salutary effects in some patients. Carvedilol is a new non-selective beta blocker that, like labetalol, has additional alpha$_1$ blocking, thus vasodilating, properties. A preliminary study with this drug in patients with NYHA Class II and III heart failure indicates improvement in exercise time, pulmonary artery wedge pressure, and symptomatic improvement. The results of randomized trials should clarify the role of beta blockers in carefully selected patients with heart failure (see Chapter 14 for suggested dosage of beta blockers in heart failure). It must be emphasized that it is pure beta-adrenergic blockade that actuates the major salutary effects in heart failure and the benefits are enhanced by added alpha$_1$ blocking effects.

ATRIAL NATRIURETIC PEPTIDE

The effects of IV infusion of this peptide in patients with dilated cardiomyopathy and severe heart failure causes the expected modest increase in urine and sodium output. However, in one acute study, after two hours of infusion, one of four patients treated had a severe sinus tachycardia, another had sinus bradycardia. Arrhythmias disappeared soon after cessation of the infusion. There is little hope that atrial natriuretic factor will be of value in the management of heart failure or hypertension. The drug has a mild diuretic effect with a negligible influence on hemodynamics and sympathoadrenal function. Unfortunately, the peptide can only be given parenterally and appears to have adverse effects on the sinus node.

IBOPAMINE

This drug stimulates dopaminergic and beta receptors in the heart and blood vessels, which results in vasodilatation and a mild positive inotropic effect. Stimulation of presynaptic dopaminergic receptors reduces sympathetic outflow. Also, the drug inhibits the renin angiotensin system and appears to have a natriuretic effect. These effects produce a reduction in systemic vascular resistance and inhibition of the sympathoadrenal system and may prove useful in the management of heart failure patients. Ibopamine via its metabolite epinine has been shown to significantly reduce the sympathoendocrine activation seen in heart failure. Exercise tolerance has shown improvement during short-term (2- to 6-month) studies. The results of longterm trials are awaited.

TRIMETAZIDINE

This piperazine derivative has been shown to have antianginal properties. The drug is believed to raise the ischemic threshold without vasodilation or chronotopic effects. Also, a direct effect on energy metabolism and antioxidant properties appears to confer salutary effects in patients with heart failure.

A 6-month, double-blind, placebo-controlled study in 20 patients with severe myocardial dysfunction secondary to ischemic heart disease (NYHA Class III and IV heart failure) indicates improvement in dyspnea, increase in EF, and significant amelioration of angina. All patients treated with trimetazidine gained one stage on the NYHA classification, as opposed to only one patient improved with placebo. At 6 months, the difference was statistically significant, (p < 0.001). The drug may have a role in patients with heart failure, angina, or silent ischemia and should be assessed in large randomized trials.

PULMONARY EDEMA

Cardiogenic causes include

- Pulmonary edema, commonly accompanied by left-sided heart failure, which may result from or be precipitated by complications of ischemic heart disease, atrial fibrillation with uncontrolled ventricular response, other tachyarrhythmias, hypertension, mitral regurgitation or aortic valve disease, and dilated cardiomyopathy
- Mitral stenosis and, rarely, left atrial myxoma

Noncardiogenic causes include

- Adult respiratory distress syndrome due to pneumonias, severe trauma, toxins, allergens, smoke inhalation, gastric aspiration, hemorrhagic pancreatitis (see Chapter 28)
- Drugs, narcotic overdose, severe hypoalbuminemia, uremia, and neurogenic causes. Lymphagitic carcinomatosis may mimic left ventricular failure

THERAPY FOR CARDIOGENIC PULMONARY EDEMA

- Oxygen must be given at high concentrations to maintain an adequate PaO$_2$
- Furosemide (80 to 120 mg IV) usually produces an effect in 10 minutes due to the drug's venodilator action, which produces a reduction in preload followed in 30 minutes to 1 hour by diuresis that lasts for about 2 hours. If the response is not adequate, a further dose of 40 to 120 mg IV is given, provided that hypotension is not present. A higher dose is usually required if severe renal failure is present
- Morphine remains an extremely useful drug to allay anxiety and relieve discomfort. Also, the drug causes pooling of blood in the periphery. Morphine is advisable, provided that severe respiratory insufficiency or untreated severe hypothyroidism is absent. Dosage: 3 to 5 mg IV at a rate of 1 mg/min. Repeat as needed at 15- to 30-minute intervals to a total dose of 10 to 15 mg/hour
- Treat underlying problems such as severe hypertension: give captopril or nitroprusside (see Nitroprusside Infusion Pump Chart, Table 1–10)
- Manage cardiac arrhythmias and administer digoxin to reduce the ventricular response in atrial fibrillation
- Nitroglycerin: If the systolic blood pressure is greater than 100 but less than 120 mm Hg, give 0.3 mg sublingually; give 0.6 mg for systolic pressure greater than 120 mm Hg. The application of a transdermal

preparation, e.g., 1- to 1.5-inch nitropaste, or patch formulation is useful following the sublingual dose. However, transdermal application produces variable absorption and must not be relied upon within the first hour. Both sublingual and transdermal preparations should be avoided if the systolic pressure is less than 100 mm Hg. In severe cases, IV nitroglycerin is recommended (see Infusion Pump Chart, Table 2–9, Chapter 2)

- Nitroprusside is indicated if pulmonary edema is due to severe hypertension or mechanical complications of acute MI (see Infusion Pump Chart, Table 1–10, and Chapter 16)
- Aminophylline should not be used routinely. It has a role if bronchospasm and/or diaphragmatic fatigue are present. The drug increases the diuretic effect of furosemide and has mild anti-ischemic effects. The incidence of life-threatening arrhythmias caused by the judicious use of aminophylline has been exaggerated and has resulted in a decrease in the use of this agent, which has a role when the cardiac adverse effects of albuterol (salbutamol) or other beta agonists must be avoided. Dosage: 2 to 4 mg/kg IV over 20 minutes, then infusion 0.3 to 0.5 mg/kg/hour. The smaller dose is used in the elderly or in patients with hepatic dysfunction (see Tables 20–5 and 20–6)
- Rotating venous tourniquets can be temporarily beneficial in patients with severe pulmonary edema unresponsive to standard therapy listed above. Tourniquets should be placed several inches distal to the groin and shoulders, and only three of the four tourniquets should be inflated at one time, to approximately 10 mm Hg below the diastolic pressure; one should be released every 15 to 20 minutes
- Dobutamine is indicated if the above measures fail to control pulmonary edema in the presence of mild hypotension and severe left ventricular systolic dysfunction; dobutamine is superior to amrinone IV (see Chapter 16). If respiratory failure complicates pulmonary edema, dopamine should be avoided because this agent may cause constriction of pulmonary veins, which results in an increase in pulmonary capillary hydrostatic pressure and lung fluid accumulation. Dosage: 2.5 to 7.5 μg/kg/min (see Infusion Pump Chart, Table 16–5)
- Digoxin: see earlier sections of this chapter. Digoxin is required if atrial fibrillation or flutter with a rapid ventricular rate is present; slower rates (100 to 120/min) may require slowing in patients with severe mitral stenosis
- Endotracheal intubation and mechanical ventilation may be required for patients with respiratory failure: if PaO_2 cannot be maintained at or near 60 mm Hg despite 100% O_2 at 20 liters/minute or if there is progressive hypercapnia (see Chapter 29). Identify and treat precipitating factors, especially acute MI, arrhythmias, and infection

Non-cardiogenic pulmonary edema is discussed in Chapter 28.

BIBLIOGRAPHY

Anderson B, Blomström-Lundqvist C, Hedner T: Exercise hemodynamics and myocardial metabolism during long-term beta-adrenergic blockade in severe heart failure. J Am Coll Cardiol, *18*:1059, 1991.

Albers GW, Atwood JE, Hirsh J: Stroke prevention in nonvalvular atrial fibrillation. Ann Intern Med, *115*:727, 1991.

Anand IS, Kalra GS, Ferrari R, et al.: Hemodynamic, hormonal, and renal effects of atrial natriuretic peptide in untreated congestive cardiac failure. Am Heart J, *118*:500, 1989.

Antman EM, Wenger TL, Butler VP, Jr., et al.: Treatment of 150 cases of life-threatening digitalis intoxication with digoxin-specific fab antibody fragments. Circulation, *81*:1744, 1990.

Brennan FJ, Brien JF, Armstrong PW: Plasma concentration time course and pharmacological effects of a standardized oral amiodarone dosing regimen in humans. Can J Cardiol, *7*:117, 1991.

Braunwald E: ACE inhibitors–A cornerstone of the treatment of heart failure. New Engl J Med, *325*:351, 1991.

Brottier L, Barat JL, Combe C, et al.: Therapeutic value of a cardioprotective agent in patients with severe ischemic cardiomyopathy. Eur Heart J, *11*:207, 1990.

Cheng TO: Cardiac failure in coronary heat disease. Am Heart J, *120*:396, 1990.

Cleland JGF, Henderson E, McLenachen J, et al.: Effect of captopril, an angiotensin-converting enzyme inhibitor in patients with angina pectoris and heart failure. J Am Coll Cardiol, *17*: 733, 1991.

Cohn JN, Johnson G, Ziesche S, et al.: A comparison of enalapril with hydralazine-isosorbide dinitrate in the treatment of chronic congestive heart failure. N Engl J Med, *325*:303, 1991.

Das Gupta P, Broadhurst P, Raftery EB, et al.: Value of carvedilol in congestive heart failure secondary to coronary artery disease. Am J Cardiol, *66*:1118, 1990.

Davies RF, Beanlands DS, Nadeau C, et al.: Enalapril versus digoxin in patients with congestive heart failure: A multicenter study. J Am Coll Cardiol, *18*:1602, 1991.

Devereux RB: Toward a more complete understanding of left ventricular afterload. J Am Coll Cardiol, *17*:122, 1991.

Editorial: Digoxin: New answers: New questions. Lancet, *2*:79, 1989.

Editorial: Calcium antagonist caution. Lancet *337*:885, 1991.

Elkayam U, Roth A, Mehra A, et al.: Randomized study to evaluate the relation between oral isosorbide dinitrate dosing interval and the development of early tolerance to its effect on left ventricular filling pressure in patients with chronic heart failure. Circulation, *84*:2040, 1991.

Elkayam U: Tolerance to organic nitrates: Evidence, mechanisms, clinical relevance, and strategies for prevention. Ann Intern Med, *114*:667, 1991.

Ellison DH: The physiologic basis of diuretic synergism: Its role in treating diuretic resistance. Ann Intern Med, *114*:886, 1991.

Fonarow GC, Chelimsky-Fallick C, Warner Stevenson L, et al.: Effect of direct vasodilation with hydralazine versus angiotensin-converting enzyme inhibition with captopril on mortality in advanced heart failure: The Hy-C trial. J Am Coll Cardiol, *19*:842 1992.

Gheorghiade M, Hall V, Lakier JB, et al.: Comparative hemodynamic and neurohormonal effects of intravenous captopril and digoxin and their combinations in patients with severe heart failure. J Am Coll Cardiol, *13*:134, 1989.

Gheorghiade M, Fergurson D: Digoxin. A neurohormonal modulator in heart failure. Circulation, *84*:2181, 1991.

Grossman W: Diastolic dysfunction in congestive heart failure. N Engl J Med, *325*:1557, 1992.

Hagemeijer F: Intractable heart failure despite angiotensin-converting enzyme inhibitors, digoxin and diuretics: Long-term effectiveness of add-on therapy with pimobendan. Am Heart J, *122*:517, 1991.

Hickey AR, Wenger TL, Carpenter VP, et al.: Digoxin immune fab therapy in the management of digitalis intoxication: Safety and efficacy results of an observational surveillance study. J Am Coll Cardiol, *17*:590, 1991.

Jessup M: Beta-adrenergic blockade in congestive heart failure: Answering the old questions. J Am Coll Cardiol, *18*:1067, 1991.

Kameyama T, Asanoi H, Ishizaka S, et al.: Ventricular load optimization by unloading therapy in patients with heart failure. J Am Coll Cardiol, *17*:199, 1991.

Kiyingi A, Field MJ, Pawsey CC, et al.: Metolazone in treatment of severe refractory congestive cardiac failure. Lancet, *335*:29, 1990.

Lamas GA, Pfeffer MA: Left ventricular remodeling after acute myocardial infarction: Clinical course and beneficial effects of angiotensin-converting enzyme inhibition. Am Heart J, *121*: 1194, 1991.

Lichstein E, Hager WD, Gregory JJ, et al.: Relation between beta-adrenergic blocker use, various correlates of left ventricular function and the chance of developing congestive heart failure. J Am Coll Cardiol, *16*:1327, 1990.

Mahdyoon H, Battilana G, Rosman H, et al.: The evolving pattern of digoxin intoxication: Observations at a large urban hospital from 1980 to 1988. Am Heart J, *120*:1189, 1990.

Packer M: Are nitrates effective in the treatment of chronic heart failure? Antagonists's viewpoint. Am J Cardiol, *66*:458, 1990.

Packer M: Calcium channel blockers in chronic heart failure. Circulation, *82*:2254, 1990.

Packer M: Lack of relation between ventricular arrhythmias and sudden death in patients with chronic heart failure. *85*:I–50, 1992.

Packer M, Carver JR, Rodeheffer RJ, et al.: Effect of oral milrinone on mortality in severe chronic heart failure. N Engl J Med, *325*:1468, 1991.

Packer M, Kukin ML: Management of patients with heart failure and angina: Do coexistent diseases alter the response to cardiovascular drugs? J Am Coll Cardiol, *17*:740, 1991.

Rahimtoola SH: The pharmacologic treatment of chronic congestive heart failure. Circulation *80*:693, 1989.

Sharpe N, Smith H, Murphy J, et al.: Early prevention of left ventricular dysfunction after myocardial infarction with angiotensin-converting-enzyme inhibition. Lancet, *337*:872, 1991.

Sochowski RA, Dubbin JD, Naqvi SZ: Clinical and hemodynamic assessment of the hepatojugular reflux. Am J Cardiol, *66*:1002, 1990.

SOLVD Investigators: Effect of enalapril on survival in patients with reduced ventricular ejection fractions and congestive heart failure. N Engl J Med, *325*:293, 1991.

Taylor SH, Cicchetti V: Efficacy of ibopamine in the treatment of heart failure. Am Heart J, *120*:1583, 1990.

6

ARRHYTHMIAS

M. Gabriel Khan

MANAGEMENT GUIDELINES

Accurate differentiation of ventricular and supraventricular tachycardia is essential for appropriate management. The electrocardiographic diagnostic points for tachyarrhythmias are shown in Tables 6–1 and 6–2. It is important to designate the tachycardia as narrow QRS or wide QRS and then determine whether the rhythm is regular or irregular. Figure 6–1 indicates an algorithmic approach for the diagnosis of wide QRS complex tachycardia.

The common underlying diseases causing arrhythmia are listed in Table 6–3. The treatment of these conditions may cause amelioration and/or prevention of arrhythmia recurrence. The severity of the underlying diseases, particularly the degree of left ventricular (LV) dysfunction, may dictate the choice of antiarrhythmic agent and the outcome. The prognosis of ventricular arrhythmias is closely linked to the degree of LV dysfunction: an ejection fraction (EF) greater than 50% carries an excellent prognosis; 40 to 50%, a fair prognosis, is commonly associated with benign arrhythmias; 30 to 39% is often associated with potentially lethal arrhythmias; and less than 30% indicates a poor prognosis.

Adverse effects of drug therapy are clearly related to the degree of LV dysfunction. Drugs that may be used in patients with an EF less than 30%, and other ranges of EFs, are given in Table 6–4. Determining the EF is essential to the management of ventricular arrhythmias. Echocardiographic assessment is useful, because it assists with detection of valvular lesions, segmental areas of hypocontractility, the extent of ischemic heart disease (IHD), cardiomyopathy, and other diseases. Although echocardiographic EF is subject to some error and radionuclide EF is preferred by some, the former has practical advantages in assessing structural defects and is cost effective. In addition, the radionuclide EF is inaccurate in patients with atrial fibrillation and both methods yield falsely high EFs in patients with mitral regurgitation.

The emergency management of arrhythmias calls for a quick assessment of

- The hemodynamic status: Is the blood pressure less than 90 mm Hg and are there signs of peripheral hypoperfusion?

229

TABLE 6-1. DIFFERENTIAL DIAGNOSIS OF NARROW QRS TACHYCARDIA	
REGULAR	**IRREGULAR**
1. AVNRT Rate = 140–220 P waves usually buried and not apparent in the QRS or less commonly retrograde P barely visible in terminal QRS or very early ST segment, inverted in II III AVF 2. WPW with AV reentry, negative P wave Lead I suggest left-sided bypass tract Marked alternation in QRS amplitude highly suspect WPW 3. PAT with block, AR 150–200 VR usually <140 P wave often buried in T Isoelectric intervals between P waves 4. Sinoatrial tachycardia Average rate = 140/minute Sinus P waves present: Upright P waves in the ST segment 5. Atrial flutter AR = 250–350 often 300/minute VR often 150–160/minute Conduction ratio often 2:1 Sawtooth pattern leads II, AVF Sharp-pointed "P" waves in V_1 6. Ectopic atrial tachycardia	1. Atrial fibrillation R–R intervals completely irregular Absent P waves 2. Atrial flutter: AR >250 Variable AV conduction 3. Multifocal atrial tachycardia (MAT) Three different P wave morphologies in any lead, variable P–P, PR, RR intervals Atrial rate = 100–200/minute R–R intervals completely irregular; may progress to AF

AVNRT = AV nodal reentrant tachycardia
AR = atrial rate
VR = ventricular rate
AF = atrial fibrillation
VR = 240–300 suggests WPW

- The symptomatic status: Chest pain, shortness of breath, presyncope, syncope or clouding of consciousness
- Cardiac decompensation: Signs of heart failure

PRECIPITATING FACTORS AND CLINICAL SETTINGS

An essential step in the management of arrhythmia is to rapidly define the clinical setting and correct a precipitating cause, in order to obviate the need for antiarrhythmic therapy or to appraise and prevent deleterious proarrhythmic effects of these agents.

Precipitating factors and/or clinical settings include

- Ischemia: As with acute myocardial infarction (MI) or acute myocardial ischemia

TABLE 6–2. WIDE QRS TACHYCARDIA

REGULAR	IRREGULAR
1. Ventricular tachycardia Hallmarks a. Absence of an RS complex in all precordial leads b. QRS duration: R to S interval >100 msec* in one precordial lead RBBB QRS >140 msec* LBBB QRS >160 msec* c.† AV dissociation (cannon waves in neck) excludes atrial but not nodal tachycardia Suggestive Features: d. Positive concordance (except WPW type A) e. Left axis − 90 to + 180 (−60 to −90 suggest VT) f. QS or rS in V₆ (R to S, ratio <1) or net negative QRS in V₆ g. V₁ "Left rabbit ear" taller than the right: slurred downslope of S wave in V₁ strongly suggests VT 2. SVT with known Right or LBBB 3. SVT with aberrant conduction: visible on aberrant atrial ectopic: small normal q: qRs in V₆ 4. Atrial flutter: with wide QRS‡ with WPW§ (rare) 5. WPW anterograde through bypass tract§ (resembles VT)	1. Atrial fibrillation and WPW rate (200–300/min with aberrancy§) 2. AF and prior intraventricular conduction defect on recent ECG

* milliseconds
† AV block or dissociation excludes bypass tract
‡ AF treated with Class IC or IA agents may induce this arrhythmia
§ RR <205 milliseconds suggests WPW, treat as VT

TABLE 6–3. COMMON UNDERLYING DISEASES CAUSING ARRHYTHMIAS

1. Ischemic heart disease
   Acute myocardial infarction
   Myocardial ischemia
   Left ventricular aneurysm
2. Cardiomyopathies
3. Rheumatic and other valvular
4. Myocarditis
5. Sinus and atrioventricular node diseases
6. Bypass tract
7. Congenital heart disease
8. Pulmonary diseases: All causes of hypoxemia
9. Endocrine: Thyrotoxicosis
10. Hypokalemia in patients with heart disease and/or concomitant use of antiarrhythmic agents

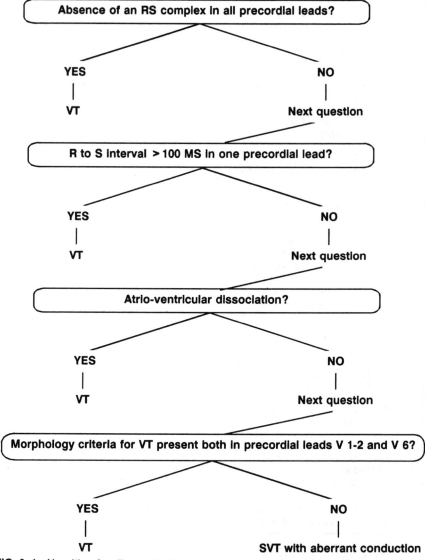

FIG. 6–1. Algorithm for diagnosis of a tachycardia with a widened QRS complex. From: Brugada P, et al.: A new approach to the differential diagnosis of a regular tachycardia with a wide QRS complex. Circulation, *83*:1651, 1991.

- Those characterized by myocardial reperfusion: Post-thrombolytic therapy in acute MI, balloon deflation during coronary angioplasty, release of coronary artery spasm
- Hypotension
- Sick sinus syndrome or AV block
- Heart failure

TABLE 6–4. EJECTION FRACTION MAY DICTATE CHOICE OF ANTIARRHYTHMIC AGENT		
GROUP I	**GROUP II**	**GROUP III**
Ejection fraction (EF) <30% only safe agents* Amiodarone Mexiletine Quinidine Beta blockers†	EF >30% Beta blockers and agents used for Group 1*	EF >40% Agents given under Group I, II plus Class IA, IB Propafenone‡ Flecanide‡ Verapamil Diltiazem

* All other agents: hazard of precipitating heart failure
† Used judiciously in properly selected patients, absence of overt heart failure, EF down to 25%
‡ Limited indications (see text)

- Hypokalemia, hypomagnesemia, hyperkalemia
- Alkalemia, e.g., may develop rapidly in ventilated patients
- Acidemia
- Hypoxemia
- Pulmonary disease, cor pulmonale, atelectasis, pneumothorax, and carcinoma of lungs: May precipitate atrial flutter or atrial fibrillation
- Infection
- Fluctuations in autonomic tone
- Acute blood loss
- Thyrotoxicosis
- Digoxin toxicity
- Proarrhythmic effects of antiarrhythmic drugs: Quinidine and other Class IA drugs may cause torsades de pointes, also rarely caused by Class III agents and sotalol and extremely rarely caused by amiodarone. More typical monomorphic ventricular tachycardia (VT) and other lethal arrhythmias may be initiated by antiarrhythmic drugs
- Beta agonist
- Theophylline
- Ruptured esophagus: May initiate atrial flutter or atrial fibrillation

MECHANISM OF THE ARRHYTHMIA

The mechanism of the arrhythmia is usually

- A disturbance of impulse generation (enhanced automaticity or ectopic tachyarrhythmia)
- A disturbance of impulse conduction (reentrant arrhythmia). Most of the evidence suggests that reentry is the mechanism for sustained VT

The mechanism often is not known when deciding on treatment. Other prerequisites that may influence the choice of appropriate therapy include knowledge of the mode of action of the selected antiarrhythmic drug, adverse effects to be anticipated, and possible outcomes of such therapy (salutary, life threatening, or proarrhythmic).

PROARRHYTHMIC EFFECTS OF ANTIARRHYTHMIC AGENTS

Proarrhythmia connotes that antiarrhythmic agents can worsen existing arrhythmias or induce new ones. The early and late proarrhythmic effects of the antiarrhythmic drug to be chosen must be carefully considered. Because proarrhythmia may be life threatening, the physician must consider the degree of risk and justify the need for antiarrhythmic drug therapy.

Early proarrhythmia is observed in up to 5, 10, and 25% of patients with benign, potentially lethal, and lethal arrhythmia, respectively. Importantly, late proarrhythmia is even more worrisome. The incidence of late proarrhythmia for encainide and flecainide is known to be substantial. The incidence for amiodarone is very low, but for other agents (except beta blockers), the incidence is unknown and may be substantial. Most available antiarrhythmic agents have not been studied for the incidence of late proarrhythmia in well-controlled, randomized, multicenter longterm trials.

Factors that increase the incidence of proarrhythmic effects include

- Prior cardiac arrest, ventricular fibrillation (VF), or sustained VT
- Prolonged QTc
- Severity of LV dysfunction. Patients with EF less than 30% have a high incidence of early and late proarrhythmia, perhaps because of the propensity for the occurrence of heart failure. More than 85% of lethal arrhythmias occur in patients with severe underlying heart disease and EF less than 30% and with a 20 to 40% incidence of recurrence over 2 years. Table 6–5 indicates the arrhythmic agent and type of proarrhythmic effect

Basic mechanisms and precipitating factors for proarrhythmia include

- Prolongation of the action potential duration and QTc, particularly in the setting of hypokalemia or bradycardia: commonly seen with Class IA agents and with Class III agents occurring mainly with sotalol, which prolongs the action potential duration maximally in the presence of bradycardia. Although the QT interval is prolonged by amiodarone, proarrhythmic effect is very low
- Incessant VT, ventricular flutter, often terminating in VF, usually with Class IC antiarrhythmics. However, if conduction is severely depressed, Class IA agents may induce incessant VT
- Rapid increase in already high dose of Class IC agents
- Severe LV dysfunction, EF less than 30%
- Concomitant administration of potassium-losing diuretic
- Atrial fibrillation treated with Class IA or IC agent

The results of outcomes of proarrhythmia during antiarrhythmic therapy include

- Nonserious increase in frequency of nonsustained VT or ventricular premature beats (VPCs) without hemodynamic deterioration

TABLE 6–5. TYPES OF PROARRHYTHMIC EFFECTS INITIATED BY ANTIARRHYTHMIC AGENTS	
ANTIARRHYTHMIC AGENTS	**ARRHYTHMIA**
	Torsades de Pointes
Class IA	+ + +
Class III	
Amiodarone	± mainly with associated hypokalemia or bradycardia
Sotalol	+
	+ + + with hypokalemia or with bradycardia
	Incessant Monomorphic VT
Class IC	+ + + +*
Class IA	+ +
Class IB	Rare
	Ventricular Flutter VF
	Polymorphic VT
Class IC	+ +*

4 (+) Strongly proarrhythmic
* May be extremely resistant to cardioversion

- Hemodynamic deterioration with nonsustained VT
- New onset sustained VT or VF
- Antiarrhythmic death

It must be reemphasized that the late proarrhythmic characteristics of antiarrhythmic agents are currently unknown and present bothersome problems with decision-making concerning the selection of an appropriate agent. The absence of early proarrhythmia bears no relationship to the drug's propensity to produce late deleterious proarrhythmia.

The Multicenter Cardiac Arrhythmia Pilot Study (CAPS) was instituted to ensure the safety and feasibility of chronic suppressive therapy for asymptomatic VPCs after MI in prevention of cardiac arrhythmic death; encainide and flecainide were studied and were determined to be safe and effective in completely suppressing VPCs. Yet, the subsequent Cardiac Arrhythmic Suppression Trial (CAST) showed that in the long term, encainide and flecainide produced considerably more deaths than placebo because of serious proarrhythmia that occurred late and progressively throughout the 15 months or more of study. Careful analysis suggests that fresh ischemia in the presence of these agents may have been the major triggering factor for arrhythmia.

Electrophysiologic (EP) studies, as well as frequent Holter monitoring, appear to be of little value in predicting late proarrhythmia. Thus, there are few guidelines to direct physicians to avoid late proarrhythmia caused by antiarrhythmic drugs, with the exception of information gleaned from therapy with four agents used extensively for the past 15 or more years: beta blockers (safe), amiodarone and mexiletine (relatively safe), and quinidine (hazardous). In the face of such a dilemma, the physician's assessment of the risk benefit ratio of initiating antiarrhythmic drug therapy is a worthwhile strategy.

SUPRAVENTRICULAR ARRHYTHMIAS

AV NODAL REENTRANT TACHYCARDIA (AVNRT)

Paroxysmal supraventricular tachycardia (PSVT) is most often due to AVNRT and is one of the most frequently encountered arrhythmias in clinical practice. In patients under age 35, PSVT usually occurs in an otherwise normal heart and has a good prognosis. However, AVNRT is not uncommon with organic heart disease, due to ischemic, rheumatic, or other valvular heart disease, and rarely can be life threatening. The onset and termination are abrupt; heart rate varies from 140 to 220/minute, with regular rhythm (Table 6–1).

TERMINATION OF THE ACUTE ATTACK

Carotid Sinus Massage, Patient Rhythm Monitored

- Response is either reversion to sinus rhythm or no effect at all, in contrast to atrial flutter, where slowing of heart rate virtually always occurs
- Not recommended in the elderly or in patients with known or highly suspected carotid disease or digitalis toxicity
- With the patient supine (head slightly hyperextended, turned a little toward the opposite side), locate the right carotid sinus at the angle of the jaw. Apply firm pressure in a circular or massage fashion for 2 to 6 seconds, using the first and second fingers. It is necessary to monitor the cardiac rhythm and gauge exactly when to stop massage because asystole, although rare, can occur. If unsuccessful, massage the left carotid sinus after an interval of 2 minutes to allow acetylcholine to be manufactured in the AV node. (If asystole occurs during the procedure, ask the patient to cough and/or give the patient one or more light chest thumps, which usually reverses transient asystole.)

Caution: never massage for more than 10 seconds.

Other vagal maneuvers include Valsalva maneuver or squatting and Valsalva, putting a finger into the throat to initiate a gag reflex, immersion of the face in cold water, taking a drink of cold water, or elevating the legs against a wall.

Caution: never apply eyeball pressure because retinal detachment may occur.

DRUG THERAPY

Suggested steps in treating AVNRT are given in Figure 6–2 and are based on the clinical setting: the presence of cardiac pathology, particularly LV dysfunction, acute MI, or hypotension, which contraindicate the use of verapamil. In patients with acute MI, an IV beta blocking agent, especially short-acting esmolol, is advisable if there is no contraindication to the use of a beta blocking drug.

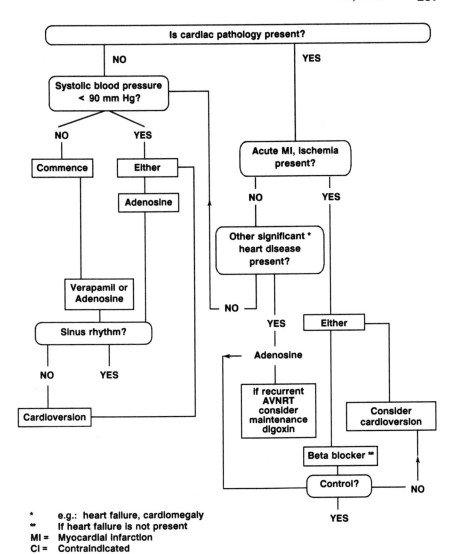

FIG. 6–2. Suggested steps in how to treat AV nodal reentrant tachycardia (AVNRT). From: Khan M Gabriel: Management of cardiac arrhythmias. *In* Cardiac Drug Therapy. 3rd Ed. London, W.B. Saunders, 1992.

Electrical cardioversion is indicated for PSVT causing hemodynamic compromise. Digoxin is indicated if heart failure is present. In the absence of acute MI, adenosine can be used for reversion and, if needed, digoxin can be considered for maintenance therapy; digoxin is an obvious choice in patients with heart failure. Verapamil is contraindicated with hypotension and if significant cardiac pathology is present, especially in patients with cardiomegaly or known or suspected LV dysfunction.

In patients with AVNRT and a virtually normal heart, the arrhythmia is usually well tolerated for 12 to 24 hours. If no response is obtained from vagal maneuvers, IV verapamil or adenosine is indicated; the choice depends on the presence or absence of hypotension. Verapamil can cause hypotension and is contraindicated if systolic blood pressure is less than 90 mm Hg. Adenosine has the advantage of not causing hypotension.

When adenosine is contraindicated because of the presence of asthma or known sensitivity, then phenylephrine has a role in young patients with PSVT complicated by hypotension but not severely compromised.

Recommendations for the Management of AVNRT: Which Drug to Choose

Verapamil is inexpensive and remains first choice for uncomplicated cases (see contraindications for verapamil). Adenosine has a major role in patients where contraindications or even relative contraindications exist in the use of verapamil, mainly because of adenosine's short half-life (less than 2 seconds) as opposed to that of verapamil (6 hours). Although adenosine has a high incidence of minor adverse effects, serious side effects are rare. Table 6–6 indicates the agent of choice (adenosine versus verapamil) for the management of PSVT. Median time to termination, 20 seconds for adenosine versus 80 seconds for verapamil, is only important in patients with hemodynamic compromise because PSVT is usually well tolerated. Both drugs are effective, causing reversion to sinus rhythm in up to 90% of patients. Recurrence of tachycardia is slightly more common after the use of adenosine, but a second dose of adenosine often proves effective.

TABLE 6–6. ADENOSINE VERSUS VERAPAMIL FOR THE MANAGEMENT OF PAROXYSMAL SUPRAVENTRICULAR TACHYCARDIAS

PARAMETERS	FIRST CHOICE	SECOND CHOICE
Uncomplicated cases ventricular rate <220/min	Verapamil	Adenosine
Hypotension		
mild	Adenosine	Verapamil after pretreatment with calcium chloride or gluconate
moderate/severe	Adenosine	Verapamil CI
Left ventricular dysfunction heart failure cardiomegaly	Adenosine	Verapamil CI
Suspect pre-excitation (AVRT)	Adenosine	Verapamil CI
Wide QRS		
? aberrancy	Adenosine	Verapamil CI
Ectopic or multifocal atrial tachycardia	Verapamil	Adenosine ineffective

CI = contraindicated
R = relative
HF = heart failure

Adenosine assists in the diagnosis of atrial flutter and recording of lead V_1 and lead 2 is advisable for diagnosis and during attempted conversion, as with all antiarrhythmic agents. Morphology in V_1 (Table 6–1 and 6–2) is vital to arrhythmia diagnosis and has been advocated since the early 1970s. However, the majority of hospitals, including teaching centers, continue to record mainly lead 2. In the setting of PSVT, V_1 may reveal type A Wolff-Parkinson-White (WPW) syndrome. Also, adenosine IV injection during sinus rhythm may reveal latent pre-excitation, usually type A, dominant R wave in V_1 that highlights the presence of a left-sided bypass tract in this condition.

Patients who have latent pre-excitation due to left-sided pathway are particularly likely to develop rapid ventricular rates, if atrial fibrillation supervenes, with degeneration to ventricular fibrillation, a situation that can be precipitated by verapamil. In patients with anterograde conduction over an anomalous pathway, verapamil is known to cause an increase in ventricular response because of reflex sympathetic stimulation and may dangerously accelerate the ventricular response in patients with atrial fibrillation or atrial flutter. Although adenosine can increase the ventricular response to pre-excited arrhythmias, the effect lasts less than 3 seconds due to the short half-life of the drug.

Verapamil produces some slowing of the ventricular response in atrial fibrillation but does not usually change the rate in patients with atrial flutter. Adenosine usually produces a higher grade of AV block; thus, atrial activity may be exposed, revealing the diagnosis of atrial flutter.

Verapamil

Verapamil mainly delays conduction in the slow, anterograde AV nodal pathway in patients with AVNRT or in the AV node in patients with AV reentrant, reciprocating tachycardia (AVRT). Verapamil is effective in converting these arrhythmias in over 87% of patients.

Dosage: Verapamil (5 mg IV) is given slowly over 2 minutes or over 3 minutes in the elderly and with the continuous monitoring of cardiac rhythm and blood pressure. Use 2.5 mg initially if LV function is believed to be slightly impaired. A bolus injection that achieves therapeutic plasma concentration causes reversion to sinus rhythm in 5 to 10 minutes. Resistance to termination or recurrence of arrhythmia without a marked fall in blood pressure should be managed with an additional 2.5- to 5-mg dose, 10 minutes after the first dose. Occasionally, an IV infusion is used, 1 mg/min to a total of 10 mg over 20 minutes with blood pressure monitoring. Mild hypotension is not a contraindication to the use of verapamil, but adenosine, if available, is preferred. If adenosine is not available, further hypotension due to verapamil can be avoided by the administration of calcium chloride or calcium gluconate (10 ml of a 10% solution over 5 to 10 minutes) prior to verapamil bolus (over 3 minutes or preferably by infusion, 1 mg/min for 10 minutes). If the patient is taking a beta blocking drug, adenosine is preferred or verapamil should be reduced to 5 mg IV given over 5 minutes in an attempt to avoid severe bradycardia and hypotension. If sinus arrest or AV block occurs, give calcium chloride or gluconate and atropine (0.5 to 1 mg IV repeated, if required, to a total dose of 2 mg).

Contraindications
- Patients with hypotension, systolic blood pressure less than 95 mm Hg
- Heart failure of all grades
- Patients with suspected LV dysfunction, particularly patients with cardiomegaly or an EF less than 40%
- Sick sinus syndrome
- Suspected digitalis toxicity
- Beta blockade
- Concomitant use of disopyramide or amiodarone
- Wide QRS tachycardia, unless identical complexes of intraventricular conduction delay seen on previous ECG while in sinus rhythm
- Atrial flutter or fibrillation complicating WPW syndrome; patients with atrial fibrillation and an anterograde conducting accessory pathway. In this situation, verapamil, causing vasodilatation and reflex sympathetic stimulation, may accelerate the ventricular response through the accessory pathway leading to VF and hemodynamic collapse. The rapidity of the ventricular response 250 to 300 beats per minute should alert the physician to the underlying bypass tract with anterograde conduction
- Patients with latent preexcitation, usually type A with dominant R wave in V_1. These patients may develop rapid ventricular rates if atrial fibrillation supervenes and verapamil is given intravenously

Adverse Effects. Hypotension, heart failure, sinus arrest, AV block, asystole, and acceleration of the ventricular response in patients with atrial fibrillation or atrial flutter complicating WPW syndrome.

Adenosine
(Adenocard)

This ultra short-acting agent has decreased the need for IV verapamil, digoxin, or beta blockers in the acute management of PSVT.

Dosage: Using a peripheral vein: 6 mg by rapid IV bolus injection over 2 seconds rapidly flushed into a peripheral vein; if given via an IV line, the drug should be given as proximal as possible and followed by a rapid saline flush. Termination of the arrhythmia is expected in less than 1 minute, and the action of the drug lasts for less than 30 seconds after injection. A second bolus injection of 12 mg is repeated 2 minutes after the first if the arrhythmia persists or recurs. The 12-mg dose may be repeated in 2 to 5 minutes, if required, and may be given via a larger vein than used in prior IV injection. Further recurrence of the arrhythmia calls for alternative therapy. In 10 to 30% of cases, arrhythmia recurs within minutes of the first injection of adenosine. A smaller dose is required if the drug is given through a central vein. A dose of 6 mg administered through a central vein in the same patient may have a potent effect, whereas a 12-

mg dose may be ineffective when administered through a small peripheral vein. The drug should be used cautiously in patients with right to left shunting and must not be administered into the distal port of a balloon flotation catheter.

Action. The drug has a depressant effect on the SA node and slows impulse conduction through the AV node. These effects appear to be mediated at the cellular level by an increase in potassium and a decrease in calcium conductance. These electrophysiologic effects are not antagonized by atropine.

After IV quick bolus injection, adenosine has a rapid onset of action within 5 to 30 seconds and converts up to 90% of PSVTs to sinus rhythm. The drug has a very short half-life (less than 2 seconds) because it is avidly taken up and metabolized by adenosine deaminase in endothelial and red blood cells. Intracoronary adenosine and papaverine induce a similar degree of coronary vasodilatation. When given a continuous low-dose infusion, adenosine causes coronary vasodilatation without significant effects on the sinoatrial or AV nodes and has a role similar to dipyridamole in conjunction with thallium-201 scintigraphy. The coronary vasodilator effect, which is similar to dipyridamole, is the likely explanation for the occurrence of chest pain provoked in patients with angina. Chest pain in patients without significant obstructive coronary disease appears to be due to abnormalities of adenosine feedback or metabolism. Also, during severe ischemia or MI, the marked release of endogenous adenosine may explain some incidences of bradycardia and AV block resistant to atropine, which, however, respond to theophilline, an adenosine antagonist.

With AVNRT, the reentry circuit is located within or just above the AV node and is formed by a slow pathway with a short refractory period often conducting anterogradely and a fast pathway with a long refractory period conducting retrogradely. The drug is also effective for AV reciprocating tachycardia in which an extra-nodal pathway forms the retrograde portion of the circus movement and the AV node, constitutes the anterograde limb. Adenosine, as other drugs that are effective for termination of reentrant supraventricular arrhythmias, delays conduction or increases refractoriness in either the anterograde or retrograde limb of the reentry circuit (usually the former).

Indications. Adenosine is indicated for the termination of AVNRT and AV reentrant reciprocating tachycardia. The drug causes termination of these arrhythmias in over 90% of cases. It is the agent of first choice for these arrhythmias in patients with hypotension or other situations where rapid conversion to sinus rhythm is needed or as an alternative to electrical cardioversion. Adenosine is also indicated in patients with PSVT that fail to terminate with a 10-mg dose of verapamil or when contraindications or relative contraindications to verapamil exist.

The drug has advantages over verapamil in patients with AV reentrant tachycardia utilizing an accessory pathway in the reentry circuit; adenosine may unmask latent pre-excitation when sinus rhythm is restored and can only produce very transient episodes of rapid pre-excited arrhythmia, as opposed to verapamil, which is contraindicated in these situations. Thus, adenosine is much safer than verapamil for use in patients with WPW or suspected WPW arrhythmias.

Adenosine, in decreasing AV conduction, unmasks atrial flutter and assists with diagnosis. Adenosine also has a role in patients with suspected supraventricular tachycardia with aberration. In patients with misdiagnosed ventricular tachycardia, verapamil may precipitate heart failure and other life-threatening complications. Adenosine, in this situation, causes reversion if the rhythm is due to AV nodal reentry and its effect on ventricular tachycardia is transient and not detrimental because of its ultra-short half-life. This agent is not effective in ectopic atrial tachycardia and multifocal atrial tachycardia.

Adenosine appears to have an important role and is relatively safe in infants with rapid PSVT with hemodynamic compromise, because repeat electrical cardioversion with 20 joules can cause deleterious effects on the myocardium at this age. Adenosine pediatric dosage: 50 μg/kg increase at 50 μg/kg increments, if needed to 150 μg/kg (not included in the drug's product monograph but appears to be relatively safe at this dose range). Studies have indicated the drug to be effective for the acute termination of PSVT in children, especially when repeated electrical cardioversion is hazardous.

Adenosine indications may be limited by cost; adenosine is 60 times more expensive than verapamil. A multicenter study indicated that a 12-mg dose is usually required to achieve about a 90% success in conversion of the arrhythmia to sinus rhythm at a cost of $30 compared with $.50 for 10 mg verapamil. Also, there is a high incidence of recurrence of the arrhythmia within minutes of the first successful conversion. The incidence varies from 10 to 33%; a second injection is usually successful.

Contraindications
- Second- or third-degree AV block, except in patients with a functioning pacemaker
- Sinus node disease
- Known hypersensitivity to adenosine
- Asthma
- Chronic pulmonary disease with theophylline usage
- Unstable angina
- Acute MI: Not given in the product monograph; the drug may cause a steal similar to dipyridamole and is best avoided until further trials document safety

Adverse effects. Minor adverse effects occur in 30 to 60% of patients. It is wise to advise the patient that minor transient adverse effects may occur, lasting from 30 seconds to 1 minute. These effects include facial flushing, dyspnea, chest pain or pressure, mild bronchospasm in patients with chronic lung disease, and less commonly, nausea, vomiting, headache, transient hypotension, and sinus pauses with ventricular standstill of several seconds.

Caution. Safety in patients with LV dysfunction due to CHD is not established and caution is needed. A dose of 12 mg may be ineffective if given through a small peripheral vein, but 6 mg given through a central vein may have a potent effect. Do not administer the 12-mg dose through a central vein or porthole of a balloon flotation catheter. Avoid the use of adenosine in the presence of a prolonged QT interval because induced bradycardia may promote the precipitation of torsades de pointes.

Interactions
- Dipyridamole markedly enhances the sinoatrial and AV nodal effects of adenosine. Dipyridamole decreases cellular uptake of adenosine, thereby inhibiting its metabolism. This interaction may be important in patients being given oral dipyridamole
- Aminophylline, caffeine, and other methyl xanthines completely antagonize adenosine.

Esmolol

Esmolol has an ultra-short action that confers major advantages over propranolol, atenolol, and metoprolol. The onset of action is rapid. The drug is quickly metabolized by esterases of red blood cells and has a half-life of 9 minutes that is unaffected by renal failure, heart failure, or hepatic dysfunction. The drug is cardioselective and has the same contraindications as other beta blocking agents.

Indications. Management of uncomplicated cases of PSVT not terminated by adenosine and when adenosine or verapamil are contraindicated, especially during acute MI or other ischemic syndromes.

Dosage: Initial loading infusion of 3 to 40 mg (usually 6 mg), IV infusion over 1 minute (30 to maximum 500 μg/kg given over 1 minute), and then maintenance infusion 1 to 5 mg/min (maximum 50 μg/kg/min). If mild hypotension is present, the maintenance dose should be reduced to 1 to 3 mg/min.

Adverse effects. Mild transient hypotension occurs in less than 25% of patients, more commonly in those with systolic blood pressure less than 100 mm Hg, and improvement occurs within minutes of discontinuing the IV infusion.

Propranolol

Dosage: 1 mg IV given over 2 minutes, repeated every 5 minutes to a maximum of 5 mg

Metoprolol IV

Dosage: 5 mg bolus over 3 minutes, then if required after 5 minutes, an additional bolus is given, and repeated if needed 5 to 10 minutes later

Phenylephrine

This alpha-agonist increases blood pressure, and the ensuing vagal activity results in sinus rhythm and has a role only in young patients with a normal heart when the systolic blood pressure is less than 90 mm Hg, when adenosine is not available, when contraindications exist to the use of verapamil, or when cardioversion is felt to be undesirable.

Dosage: 0.1 mg in 5 ml of 5% dextrose water given IV over 2 minutes. Repeat in 2 or 3 minutes. Allow 1 to 3 minutes after each bolus for the blood pressure to return to the baseline value before giving an additional bolus. Maximum dose = 0.5 mg. If this fails to produce sinus rhythm but stabilization of blood pressure is achieved, verapamil or esmolol can then be administered.

Digoxin

If rapid restoration of sinus rhythm is not considered essential, digoxin is advisable if there is associated hypotension, cardiomegaly, or signs of heart failure caused by LV dysfunction. Digoxin takes more than 2 hours, however, to have an effect and is not recommended where rapid restoration of sinus rhythm is required. Adenosine for termination and digoxin for maintenance therapy are advisable in some patients (Fig. 6–2).

Dosage: In the absence of digoxin use during the previous week, 0.5 mg IV by infusion over 10 minutes followed, if required, in 30 minutes by 0.25 mg, 0.25 mg 2 to 4 hours later, and then oral 0.25 mg once daily.

Chronic Management of PSVT

This is needed only in patients with bothersome episodes, e.g., occurring several times annually. If WPW syndrome and structural heart diseases are excluded, one tablet of verapamil (80 mg) may be taken during acute attacks if vagal maneuvers fail. The earlier the drug is taken, the greater the efficacy. An additional 80-mg tablet may be taken 1 hour later if the arrhythmia persists and is well tolerated. If this is not effective, the patient is advised to go to the emergency room, where IV verapamil or adenosine can be given safely.

Patients with frequent episodes, e.g., monthly and requiring frequent visits to the emergency room, deserve daily medications. Digoxin is economical and has a role as a one-a-day tablet. A beta blocker usually is effective in over 75% of patients. Verapamil, although widely used, has only a modest prophylactic effect. One-half of a 240-mg sustained release verapamil tablet may be tried and appears to be effective in about 33% of patients. Sotalol may be more effective than the other agents but must not be used concomitantly with diuretics that decrease serum potassium. If episodes remain bothersome, catheter modification of the atrioventricular junction with radiofrequency energy is indicated (see Chapter 18).

PAROXYSMAL ATRIAL TACHYCARDIA (PAT) WITH BLOCK

An atrial rate less than 200 excludes atrial flutter (see Table 6–1). If the heart rate is 90 to 120/minute with a normal serum potassium and symptoms of angina and dyspnea are absent, no immediate treatment is required. If the serum potassium is less than 3.5 mEq(mmol)/l and a high degree of AV block is absent, give potassium chloride IV (60 mEq) in 1 liter normal saline over 5 hours. In recent years with more intelligent use of digoxin this arrhythmia has become uncommon with digoxin use.

MULTIFOCAL ATRIAL TACHYCARDIA

Multifocal atrial tachycardia (MAT) and other ectopic atrial tachycardias are usually seen in patients with

- Chronic lung disease
- Hypoxemia
- Theophylline toxicity
- IHD
- Myocarditis

Therapy should be directed at the underlying cause. If tachycardia is symptomatic or causes cardiac embarrassment, give verapamil (2.5 to 5 mg IV, repeated in 30 minutes). IV verapamil is usually successful and 80 mg orally three of four times daily can be administered until the underlying problem resolves. Often, the arrhythmia causes no hemodynamic disturbances, especially at rates of 100 to 130/minutes and requires no drug therapy, or the initial dose of verapamil can be given orally. Magnesium sulfate is effective in some patients. Arrhythmias due to triggered activity or increased automaticity appear to be partly due to potassium flux from cells; magnesium has a direct effect on potassium channels and increases intracellular potassium.

A beta blocker, especially metoprolol (IV, then orally) is more effective than verapamil, but caution is necessary to avoid the use of beta blockers in patients with COPD. In patients in whom arrhythmia is not terminated by a beta blocker, verapamil, or treatment of the underlying cause and remains bothersome, amiodarone orally may prove effective after a few weeks of administration. Caution: Amiodarone is not generally recommended for non-life-threatening arrhythmias.

ATRIAL FLUTTER

Atrial flutter is usually due to underlying cardiac pathology, particularly ischemic heart disease, MI, and valvular heart disease. Noncardiac disturbances may initiate atrial flutter: hypoxemia caused by pulmonary embolism, pneumothorax, chronic lung disease, and thyrotoxicosis. Removal of the underlying cause may be followed by spontaneous reversion to sinus rhythm.

The mechanism of this arrhythmia is still not clarified. A reentrant mechanism in the right atrium is the currently accepted mechanism for the common (Type 1) atrial flutter.

Atrial flutter is easily converted to sinus rhythm by synchronized DC shock, 20 joules increased to 50 joules, if required. This should be carried out early if the patient is hemodynamically compromised, has symptoms or signs of ischemia or a ventricular response greater than 200/minute, or is known or suspected of having WPW syndrome. For patients with a ventricular rate less than 200/minute, esmolol, propranolol, or metoprolol may be used to slow the ventricular response. Digoxin often converts atrial flutter to atrial fibrillation and slows the ventricular response. Verapamil may reduce the ventricular response, but conversion to sinus rhythm rarely occurs. Verapamil, digoxin, and beta blockers are contraindicated in patients with WPW presenting with atrial flutter or atrial fibrillation. In this setting, verapamil or digoxin may precipitate VF. Rapid atrial pacing is effective in terminating atrial flutter, but in drug-refractory cases, cardioversion is usually employed.

Flecainide

This drug is expected to convert atrial flutter to sinus rhythm in less than 20% of patients and, therefore, is not sufficiently effective to recommend its use. Caution is needed because doses of 25 to 50 mg twice daily have precipitated incessant sustained VT, incessant atrial flutter with rapid ventricular rates, VT, heart failure, and a high incidence of noncardiac adverse effects.

Propafenone

Conversion to sinus rhythm is expected in less than 33% of patients given propafenone. The effect is slightly better than flecanide, with fewer adverse effects, but this agent may cause ventricular acceleration and hemodynamic depression. Propafenone may have a role in a small number of properly selected patients but should be administered under the guidance of a cardiologist and with continuous ECG monitoring in a CCU setting.

Dosage: 2 mg/kg IV infusion over 10 minutes.

Contraindications
- Heart failure or LV dysfunction
- Asthma or COPD
- Conduction defects, bundle branch block, second- or third-degree AV block
- Sinus node dysfunction, severe bradycardia
- Electrolyte disturbances
- Hypotension
- Myasthenia gravis
- Pregnancy

CHRONIC ATRIAL FLUTTER

If the arrhythmia is resistant to pharmacologic therapy or synchronized DC shock, digoxin is indicated to control the ventricular response, especially if structural heart disease or chronic lung disease is present. Anticoagulants are not indicated for patients with atrial flutter undergoing cardioversion or in those with chronic atrial flutter because cardiac systemic thromboembolism usually does not occur.

ATRIAL FIBRILLATION

In patients with cardiac pathology, the overall prevalence rate of atrial fibrillation is 4%. Atrial fibrillation is present in more than 50% of patients with mitral stenosis or heart failure. Diagnosis is readily made from the electrocardiogram. Causes of atrial fibrillation include CHD, rheumatic and other valvular heart disease, hypertension, cardiomyopathies, cor pulmonale, pulmonary embolism, thyrotoxicosis, sick sinus syndrome producing tachyarrhythmias and bradyarrhythmias, WPW syndrome, alcohol abuse, post-thoracotomy, esophago-jejunostomy, ruptured esophagus, carbon monoxide poisoning, and idiopathic.

Investigations should include echocardiogram to confirm underlying causes and evaluate left atrial size. Two-dimensional echocardiography may miss atrial thrombus detected by transesophageal echocardiography (TEE).

Caution: atrial fibrillation with a fast ventricular rate greater than 220/minute, often with wide QRS complex, occurs in up to 10% of patients with WPW syndrome. In this subset of patients, digoxin, beta blockers, and calcium antagonists plus lidocaine are contraindicated since VF may be precipitated (see later discussion of WPW Syndrome).

Digoxin

Digoxin is used in the majority of patients to control the ventricular response, except when ventricular rate is greater than 220/minute, probably due to WPW syndrome. In symptomatic patients with ventricular rate of 150 to 220/minute: give digoxin IV 0.5 mg slowly under ECG monitoring, followed by 0.25 mg IV every 2 hours to control the ventricular response. A total dose of 1 to 1.25 mg is usually necessary if the patient has not taken digoxin in the past 2 weeks. For patients who have taken digoxin within 1 week, a dose of 0.125 mg IV should be tried, followed by an additional 0.125 mg after 2 hours if needed, followed by maintenance doses (0.25 to 0.375 mg daily). In the elderly or in patients with mild renal dysfunction, give 0.125 mg daily. This dose is stabilized using the apical rate as a guide and not resorting to the inappropriate use of digoxin serum levels (see Chapter 5). In some patients, digoxin fails to prevent activity-induced tachycardia and verapamil or a beta blocker causes a satisfactory reduction of fast heart rates.

In the absence of significant LV dysfunction, sotalol is worth a trial because often this agent adequately controls the ventricular response. The serum potassium must be maintained above 4 mEq(mmol)/l, especially if digoxin or sotalol is being administered. If sotalol or another beta blocker causes bradycardia, a trial of pindolol (2.5 mg twice daily, increased if needed to 7.5 mg twice daily) added to digoxin often causes reduction of a fast ventricular response with minimum likelihood of precipitating symptomatic bradycardia. Patients with recent onset of atrial fibrillation should be anticoagulated if no contraindication exists.

Conversion to sinus rhythm may be achieved in some patients if it is believed to be desirable: conversion may be achieved after full digitalization and control of ventricular response by adding quinidine (200 to 300 mg) every 6 hours, or if ventricular function is unimpaired, disopyramide may be used instead of quinidine. In view of the hazards associated with these agents, sotalol (although not FDA approved) is now frequently used and seems at least as effective. Conversion to sinus rhythm is achieved in about 50% of patients. DC cardioversion should be utilized in individuals with suspected WPW syndrome or heart rate greater than 220 with unstable patients and acute MI with hemodynamic compromise; DC conversion is also deemed necessary in patients with severe aortic stenosis or cardiomyopathy in whom atrial transport function is of great importance. Amiodarone has a role in the latter subset of patients (see Chapter 14) and in others with failed drug therapy or poor LV function.

The main indication for pharmacologic or DC cardioversion in patients with chronic atrial fibrillation and advanced heart disease and left atrial enlargement is the possibility of obtaining a hemodynamic benefit.

Flecainide

Flecainide IV is more effective than a combination of digoxin and quinidine in converting paroxysmal atrial fibrillation to sinus rhythm. The drug is effective mainly in patients with atrial fibrillation of recent onset (less than 6 weeks) or in patients with small atria (less than 4 cm).

Dosage: IV bolus 2 mg/kg over 10 minutes, followed by oral treatment 200 to 300 mg daily, maximum 400 mg daily. Flecainide given orally is useful in preventing recurrence of paroxysmal AF, but the drug's use may be hazardous and caution is required. The manufacturers no longer recommend the drug for benign or potentially lethal arrhythmias, and its use is restricted to the management of patients with post-cardiac surgical atrial fibrillation in an intensive care setting. The CAST initiated this recommendation. The drug must not be used in patients with heart failure, poor ventricular function, and/or conduction defects.

It is advisable to combine a Class IC or IA agent with digoxin when attempting to convert paroxysmal atrial fibrillation because failure to slow conduction in the AV node may precipitate rapid life-threatening tachycardia. Fatalities have been reported with the use of IA or IC drugs when used without prior administration of digoxin. It is well established that quinidine must not be used alone to convert atrial fibrillation since atrial flutter with 1:1 AV conduction may supervene, resulting in hazardous ventricular rates exceeding 240/minute.

Zehender, et al. studied 40 patients with atrial fibrillation persisting for 4 weeks up to 2 years. Sinus rhythm was achieved by treatment with quinidine, quinidine plus verapamil, or amiodarone in 5 (25%), 11 (55%), and 12 (60%) of patients, respectively.

The combination of small dose quinidine (480 mg/day) and verapamil (240 mg/day) provided safe and effective maintenance of sinus rhythm in 60% of patients over a 2-year follow-up. Initial conversion to sinus rhythm was successful mainly in patients with atrial fibrillation of less than 12 months duration, left atrial size less than 55 mm.

SYNCHRONIZED DC CARDIOVERSION

- DC cardioversion is usually contraindicated in atrial fibrillation duration greater than 1 year because sinus rhythm is usually not maintained
- Patients with atrial fibrillation less than 1 week usually regain atrial function after conversion
- Cardioversion is often not considered worthwhile with chronic atrial fibrillation duration exceeding 1 year because less than 60% and 33% of patients remain in sinus rhythm 1 week or 1 year post conversion. But conversion is often attempted where heart failure or other symptoms of low cardiac output warrant an aggressive approach
- Embolization occurs in about 2% of patients
- DC conversion is not advisable in patients with suspected digitalis toxicity because of the risk of precipitating VF, but titrated energy doses are permissible in addition to other measures such as potassium administration
- Patients with sick sinus syndrome may develop prolonged post-conversion pauses, which often can be terminated by a series of chest thumps
- In patients with left atrial size greater than 5 cm, sinus rhythm is usually not maintained. A report, however, indicates that left atrial size greater than 5 cm does not appear to be a major determinant of failure to maintain sinus rhythm post conversion. Again, the decision depends on the importance of restoring sinus rhythm
- Amiodarone has been shown to cause reversion and maintenance of sinus rhythm for up to 3 months in approximately 60% of patients with atrial size less than 6 cm
- For DC conversion, anticoagulants are not generally used if atrial fibrillation has less than 24-hour duration
- If atrial fibrillation is greater than 24 hours duration and conversion is necessary, oral anticoagulants are given. In patients with duration slightly over 24 hours, IV heparin for 72 hours may be an acceptable compromise. In a study by Arnold, et al., in 454 patients undergoing direct current cardioversion, the incidence rate of embolism in nonanticoagulated patients with atrial fibrillation average duration 6 ± 4 days was 1.32% (six patients), compared with no embolic complications in patients who received oral anticoagulants to maintain a prothrombin time equal to or greater than 15 seconds. Nonanticoagulated patients with atrial flutter undergoing cardioversion did not have embolic complications, which supports the standard recommendation that patients with atrial flutter do not require anticoagulants during conversion or for longterm therapy. When anticoagulants are commenced in patients with atrial fibrillation undergoing cardioversion, these agents should be con-

tinued for at least 3 weeks post conversion because mechanical atrial systole with peak A wave velocity returns only after about 3 weeks post conversion to sinus rhythm

- Digoxin is maintained for the period before conversion and is interrupted 24 to 48 hours prior to conversion
- Light anesthesia, IV diazepam, midazolam, or thiopental with a standby anesthesiologist is necessary

Quinidine or disopyramide given immediately after conversion and continued to increase the chance of perpetuating sinus rhythm is not of proven value.

However, as discussed earlier, the combination of low-dose quinidine (480 mg/day) and verapamil (240 mg/day) has been shown to maintain sinus rhythm in up to 60% of patients followed for 2 years, and this combination is advisable in properly selected patients. Verapamil must not be used in patients with heart failure or EF less than 40%.

Sotalol has not been adequately compared with other agents but may be tried in patients with EF greater than 30%. Amiodarone is reserved for patients with EF less than 30% in whom the maintenance of sinus rhythm is considered essential.

CHRONIC ATRIAL FIBRILLATION

Slowing of the ventricular response with digitalis suffices in the majority. Younger patients, who have a fast ventricular response during daily activities or on exercise, gain further benefit with the addition of small doses of oral verapamil, half of a 240-mg SR, or a one-a-day beta blocker, preferably atenolol or sotalol if available, for use as an antiarrhythmic agent.

ROLE OF ANTICOAGULANTS

Patients with recent onset and paroxysmal atrial fibrillation should be anticoagulated if there is no contraindication in order to prevent embolization. In patients with chronic atrial fibrillation and structural heart disease systemic embolization is expected in more than 33% of patients over a period of 5 years. Risk of embolization is about 20% higher in patients with rheumatic heart disease and congestive cardiomyopathy; thus, anticoagulation is strongly recommended in patients with structural heart disease.

In patients under age 60 who have lone atrial fibrillation (absence of cardio-pulmonary disease or hypertension), the risk of stroke is less than 0.5% per year; if hypertension is included, as in the Framingham Study, the risk of stroke increases to 2.6% per year in older patients (mean age: 70 years).

In the Copenhagen Atrial Fibrillation, Aspirin, Anticoagulant (AFASAK) study of 1,000 patients with nonrheumatic atrial fibrillation, the stroke reduction risk was 58% for oral anticoagulants and only 16% for aspirin. In the Stroke Prevention in Atrial Fibrillation (SPAF) study, stroke risk reduction was 67% for anticoagulants and 42% for aspirin, but this was an interrupted study and a direct comparison of warfarin and aspirin was not done; aspirin reduced the stroke rate mainly in younger patients (under age 60). Aspirin (162 to 325 mg daily) has a role in patients less than age 70 with lone atrial fibrillation if relative contraindications to anticoagulants exist; 165 mg enteric-coated tablet is available in the United States. Ongoing studies will clarify guidelines for therapy of lone atrial fibrillation.

WOLFF-PARKINSON-WHITE SYNDROME

The electrocardiographic changes in WPW Syndrome are not always typical and depend on the distance between the sinoatrial node and the accessory pathway; the resulting conduction times are also important: intra-atrial, AV node-His, bundle branch, and accessory pathway. Thus, when AV nodal conduction is slowed, electrocardiographic features are more prominent and less apparent during exercise or when the accessory pathway is distant from the sinoatrial node.

Electrocardiographic hallmarks include

- A PR interval less than 0.12 second is observed in up to 80% of cases. In approximately 20% of patients, the PR interval is 0.12 second or slightly longer, especially with advancing age
- A QRS equal to or greater than 0.12 second is not necessary for the diagnosis; in about 20% of cases, the QRS duration is less than 0.11 second
- A delta wave is not always present
- Occasionally, a pseudo infarction pattern "Q in leads 2, 3 or AVF" is present
- R wave as the sole or main deflection in V1, V2 referred to as Type A WPW suggests left ventricular localization of the bypass tract
- Type A pattern and a negative delta wave in leads 2, 3 and AVF; consider posteroseptal bypass tract
- Type A and isoelectric or negative delta in one of the following leads: 1, AVL, V_5, V_6, consider a left lateral bypass tract
- A negative P wave in lead 1 during tachycardia suggests a left-sided bypass tract
- In so-called "Type B WPW," an S or QS is the dominant deflection in V_1, V_2 and may be mistaken for incomplete LBBB or voltage criteria for left ventricular hypertrophy. Type B pattern is more commonly seen with right-sided bypass tracts. The terms "Type A and Type B" are no longer considered important hallmarks, but they are ingrained in history and may serve to remind the physician of certain scenarios, e.g., tall R in V1 is not always due to right ventricular hypertrophy or true posterior MI but may be due to pre-excitation, also Type B is present in up to 25% of cases of Ebstein's anomaly
- Atrial fibrillation occurs in 15 to 39% of cases and rarely exhibits a fast ventricular response (240 to 300) that may precipitate VF. Fortunately, the bypass tract pathway usually has a longer refractory period than the AV node. If the refractory period is very short, rapid rates (cycle length as short as 0.2 second, ventricular rate of 300/minute) may occur. During spontaneous or induced atrial fibrillation, patients with an increased risk for VF have a mean shortest RR interval less than 205 milliseconds

- Rarely, atrial flutter is manifest
- Very rarely a wide QRS regular tachycardia may be caused by multiple mechanisms, including the antidromic form of tachycardia
- A clearly observed retrograde P wave in the ST segment is suggestive of WPW tachyarrhythmia, whereas in AVNRT, the P wave is usually lost in the QRS complex and is rarely seen in the ST segment
- The presence of alternation in QRS amplitude during tachycardia suggests the participation of a bypass tract
- Rate-related LBBB, consider WPW

Also, patients can have two or more pathways with reciprocation using them and not the AV node, or may have AVNRT with conduction to the ventricles by the bypass tract.

ORTHODROMIC CIRCUS MOVEMENT TACHYCARDIA

The most common orthodromic arrhythmia in WPW syndrome is a circus movement in which the reentrant circuit uses the AV node in the anterograde direction and the accessory pathway in the retrograde direction and is a reciprocating tachycardia. This situation is present in over 85% of WPW arrhythmia. Rarely, a spontaneous change occurs in some patients from orthodromic to the rare antidromic tachycardia.

ANTIDROMIC CIRCUS MOVEMENT TACHYCARDIA

This uncommon but clinically important form of tachyarrhythmia occurs in 7 to 15% of patients with WPW, and over 66% have multiple bypass tracts. In antidromic WPW, the tachycardia uses the accessory pathway in the anterograde direction and the AV node in the retrograde direction resulting in rapid wide QRS tachycardia.

Atié et al. reported dizziness and syncope in 61 and 50% of patients with antidromic tachycardia and in less than 10% of patients with orthodromic tachycardia; atrial fibrillation and VF occurred in 16 and 11% of patients. The anterograde refractory period of the bypass tract in patients with VF was less than 200 milliseconds. Atrial fibrillation may present with rapid ventricular rates, R-R less than 205 milliseconds with a wide QRS complex. Table 6–7 gives types of tachyarrhythmias observed with WPW and their approximate incidence.

TABLE 6–7. TYPES AND APPROXIMATE INCIDENCE OF TACHYARRHYTHMIAS IN WPW SYNDROME	
TACHYCARDIA	**APPROXIMATE %**
1. AVRT	60
2. Atrial fibrillation	15–39
3. Atrial flutter	1
4. Regular wide complex QRS indistinguishable from VT (Atrial flutter or BBB during AVRT)	1
5. Ventricular flutter VF	3

ASSOCIATED DISEASES AND MIMICRY

- There is an increased incidence of WPW in patients with hypertrophic cardiomyopathy and echocardiographic assessment is advisable in all patients with WPW
- Approximately 25% of Ebstein abnormality has a Type B ECG pattern
- Q waves in 2 of the 3 inferior leads 2, 3 and AVF may be incorrectly diagnosed as inferior infarction
- Absence of R in V_1 and initial Q in V2, simulate anteroseptal infarction
- Tall R waves in V_1 may incorrectly suggest right ventricular hypertrophy or true posterior infarction
- High QRS voltage may incorrectly suggest left ventricular hypertrophy (LVH)
- Type B or Type A ECG pattern can be mistaken for incomplete left bundle branch or right bundle branch block, respectively

RISK STRATIFICATION

WPW patients at high risk for potentially lethal arrhythmias include

- All patients with PSVT with ventricular rates greater than 240/minute, regular or irregular, narrow or wide QRS. The average heart rate in patients with PSVT due to AVNRT is about 170/minute and 200/minute with WPW
- Atrial fibrillation with ventricular response greater than 240/minute
- Atrial flutter with a ventricular response greater than 240/minute
- Alternation between AVRT and atrial fibrillation
- WPW with hypertrophic cardiomyopathy
- Family history of WPW and/or sudden death
- A short anterograde refractory period (less than 240 to 270 milliseconds) is a setting for ventricular rates greater than 280 and precipitation of VF if atrial fibrillation supervenes. A refractory period greater than 270 milliseconds is indicated by blockade of conduction through the bypass tract utilizing IV procainamide 10 mg/kg given over 5 minutes with the patient in sinus rhythm

Patients who may have hazardous patterns require electrophysiologic testing with consideration for ablative therapy and are discussed in Chapter 18.

DRUGS AND INCREASED RISK

- Digoxin decreases the refractory period of the bypass tract, may increase the ventricular rate in patients with atrial fibrillation or flutter leading to ventricular fibrillation, and is best avoided unless the patient has been screened by electrophysiologic testing
- Verapamil may also decrease the refractory period and cause a similar life-threatening situation. Also, verapamil causes vasodilatation and increasing sympathetic stimulation may enhance rapidity of the ventricular response

- Lidocaine may also increase sympathetic stimulation and increase the ventricular response
- Beta blockers, digoxin, verapamil, and diltiazem slow conduction in the AV node and should be avoided in patients unless there is proof that the arrhythmia is truly WPW presenting with AVRT, orthodromic tachycardia. These agents should not be given to patients to prevent PSVT unless the diagnosis is clarified, the patient is regarded at low risk of developing anterograde conduction over the bypass tract, and the refractory period of the accessory pathway is greater than 270 milliseconds.

These agents are all contraindicated in patients with WPW presenting with atrial fibrillation or atrial flutter or with a wide QRS complex tachycardia. Patients considered at low risk for developing potentially lethal arrhythmias include

- Intermittent pre-excitation
- Disappearance of pre-excitation during exercise. A decrease in pre-excitation, however, occurs normally with exercise and must not be taken as an index of low risk
- The documentation that the refractory period of the bypass tract is greater than 270 milliseconds as indicated by response to IV procainamide or amaline. Procainamide and amaline must not be given to patients with hypertrophic cardiomyopathy and WPW tachyarrhythmia

THERAPY

- The emergency room management of AVRT in patients with WPW: Adenosine rapid bolus injection as indicated in the previous section regarding management of AVNRT
- Patients with rapid ventricular response greater than 240/minute should be managed with IV procainamide. Caution: Avoid in patients with hypertrophic cardiomyopathy. In tachycardia, which could be pre-excited, e.g., atrial fibrillation or flutter, procainamide up to 10 mg/kg IV over 30 minutes, maximum 1 g in 1 hour is advisable, provided that the patient is not hypotensive and does not develop hypotension. Failure to convert the arrhythmia or hemodynamic deterioration is an indication for prompt electrical conversion

Amiodarone has a role in the prevention of paroxysmal atrial fibrillation with rapid rates. Failure to respond is an indication for electrophysiologic studies with a view to ablative therapy (see Chapter 18).

BRADYARRHYTHMIAS

Severe bradycardia producing symptoms is usually treated with atropine 0.5 to 0.6 mg, repeated every 2 minutes to a maximum of 2 to 2.4 mg. However, when atropine is used to treat asystole prior to pacing, a dose of 1 mg is given immediately followed by an additional 1 mg after 2 minutes. Mobitz Type 2 block or third-degree AV block, as well as sick sinus syndrome, must be managed with pacing. This topic is dealt with in Chapter 18. Where pacing is delayed, give isoproterenol IV cautiously with the cardioverter available.

VENTRICULAR ARRHYTHMIAS

GRADES OF VENTRICULAR ARRHYTHMIA

The following grades of ventricular arrhythmia determine outcomes from low risk to high risk: benign arrhythmias to potentially lethal and lethal arrhythmias. This grading is important for decision-making concerning appropriate therapy

- VPCs: Unifocal
- VPCs: Multifocal
- VPCs: Couplets, runs, or salvos, 3 to 5 consecutive beats
- Nonsustained VT: A run of three or more consecutive beats lasting less than 30 seconds and not associated with hemodynamic deterioration
- Sustained VT: Runs equal to or greater than 30 seconds or associated with unstable cardiovascular symptoms or signs (chest pain, shortness of breath, syncope, or clouding of consciousness); sustained VT is considered potentially lethal
- VF or resuscitation from cardiac arrest: Lethal arrhythmias

The outcome and prognosis of ventricular arrhythmias are clearly related to EF. An arrhythmia associated with an EF less than 30% has a poor prognosis compared with the same arrhythmia and EF greater than 50%.

VENTRICULAR PREMATURE CONTRACTIONS AND POTENTIALLY LETHAL ARRHYTHMIAS

A spontaneous significant decrease in benign and potentially lethal VPCs occurs in more than 33% of patients; this favorable outcome should not be ascribed to administered agents.

The use of antiarrhythmic agents must be justified in the given individual by the presence of symptoms or proven benefit on prognosis because the occurrence and consequence of late proarrhythmias with antiarrhythmic agents other than ecainide and flecainide are currently unknown. It is the late proarrhythmic effects of antiarrhythmics that are bothersome since the short-term pre-CAST study showed encainide and flecainide to be nearly devoid of early proarrhythmic effects. However, the subsequent CAST showed longterm therapy to be disastrous in patients eligible for the trial. As well, the study indicates that virtual suppression of VPCs does not prevent sudden cardiac death.

Table 6–8 gives guidelines for the management of ventricular arrhythmias. Arrhythmia in a normal heart rarely requires therapy. VPCs (bigeminy couplets, triplets and nonsustained VT) do not require drug therapy. If symptoms are bothersome, it is advisable to give a trial of a beta blocking drug and to reassure the patient.

Patients with potentially lethal arrhythmias (arrhythmia in an abnormal heart, e.g., underlying IHD) should be managed with a beta blocking drug.

TABLE 6–8. GUIDELINES FOR THE MANAGEMENT OF VENTRICULAR
ARRHYTHMIAS

BENIGN ARRHYTHMIA	POTENTIALLY* LETHAL	LETHAL (MALIGNANT ARRHYTHMIA)
Normal heart: VPCs, couplets, Bigeminy	Abnormal heart e.g., post myocardial infarction: Frequent VPCs multifocal, Nonsustained VT	a. Cardiovascular collapse b. Post cardiac arrest (VF)
↓	↓	EP Studies: In approximately 25% of cases, can initiate
No treatment reassurance	EF >30%; No overt CHF	and suppress with drug or combination and improve
If symptoms very bothersome or VT normal heart	↓ Beta blocker† ↓ Not controlled and symptomatic	outcome ↓
↓		In majority EF <30% trial sotalol† or
Beta blocker and reassurance; consider Mexiletine 2nd choice	Mexiletine (unproven to improve survival) ↓ Not controlled ↓ Consider ↓ Amiodarone‡	Amiodarone or Amiodarone + beta blocker§ or Multiprogrammable implantable pacemaker-cardioverter-defibrillator, especially if EF ≤25% (see Chapter 18) or ablative treatment
		c. Torsades de pointes (see text)

* Only beta blockers significantly prolong life; amiodarone appears to do so only in the absence of heart failure
† Used judiciously, EF down to 25% (see text)
‡ Flecainide, encainide, moricizine, and propafenone not recommended for benign or potentially lethal arrhythmias.
§ Not sotalol

If symptoms are bothersome and are not controlled by adequate doses of a beta blocker, then substitution or addition of mexiletine, which has a low proarrhythmic effect, is advisable. Sotalol may be helpful when other beta blockers fail. Encainide and flecainide were used to treat this type of patient in the CAST study and are no longer recommended based on the result of that study. Propafenone has mild beta blocking properties and slightly fewer proarrhythmic effects than encainide and flecainide; the longterm proarrhythmic dangers of propafenone are not yet known, however, and the use of the drug in this situation is not advisable.

VENTRICULAR TACHYCARDIA AND LETHAL ARRHYTHMIAS

As emphasized earlier in this chapter, the distinction of VT from supraventricular tachycardia with aberrant conduction is crucial to appropriate management. Diagnostic steps are given in Figure 6–1 and Tables 6–1 and 6–2. When doubt exists, a wide QRS tachycardia should be treated as VT.

A separation of VT into monomorphic and polymorphic appearance aids in clinical recognition of the various types of VT

A

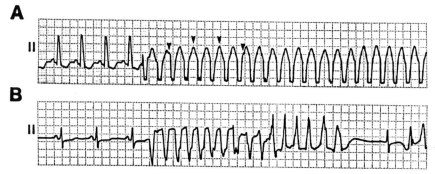

B

FIG. 6–3. Monomorphic versus polymorphic ventricular tachycardia. Recordings from electrocardiographic bipolar lead II showing monomorphic versus polymorphic QRS morphology. *Panel A*: Spontaneous onset of a monomorphic ventricular tachycardia. Note identical beat-to-beat QRS configuration. The arrows depict the dissociated P waves, which at times modify QRS morphology. *Panel B*: Polymorphic ventricular tachycardia characterized by beat-to-beat changes in QRS appearance. From: Akhtar M: Clinical spectrum of ventricular tachycardia. Circulation, *82*:1562, 1990.

- Monomorphic implies an identical beat-to-beat QRS configuration with the QRS morphology at times being modified by dissociated P waves (Fig. 6–3). The substrate for monomorphic VT is usually within the vicinity of a healed MI and sometimes associated with LV aneurysm, dilated cardiomyopathy, and rarely, in association with no overt structural heart disease
- Polymorphic VT is characterized by beat-to-beat changes in QRS morphology; at times, the beat-to-beat changes in QRS appearance may be subtle, and a true polymorphic pattern may be revealed only after careful study of rhythm strips from multiple leads. Polymorphic VT is represented by two clinical scenarios that will be discussed later
- Torsades de pointes
- Polymorphic VT in the absence of QT prolongation

The settings of lethal arrhythmias include sustained VT or VF in patients with severe underlying heart disease. More than 90% of patients in this category have poor LV function with EF less than 35%. Over 80% of these arrhythmias are found in patients with EF less than 30%; there is a high incidence of recurrent lethal arrhythmias. At the other extreme, a few have these arrhythmias in the presence of a structurally normal heart "primary electrical disease."

The management of sustained VT is given in Figure 6–4.

- If the pulse is present and the patient is hemodynamically stable, give lidocaine (lignocaine) 100 mg bolus IV and an immediate infusion up to 3 mg/minute (see Tables 3–8 and 3–9). If the arrhythmia is not controlled, repeat a 75-mg bolus of lidocaine; if sinus rhythm is not restored, but the patient remains hemodynamically stable, a trial of procainamide is advisable

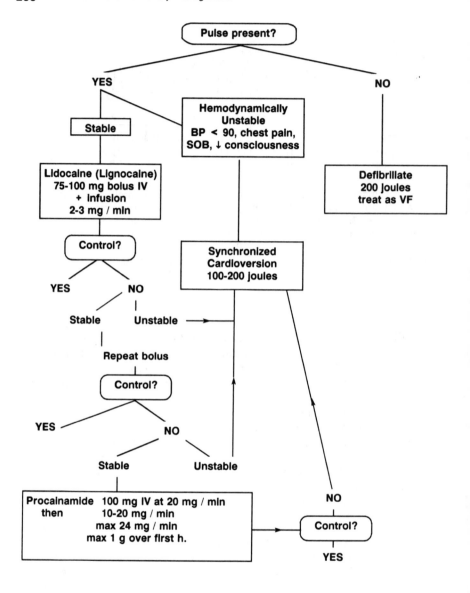

*Sustained = VT > 30 sec or unstable signs.

FIG. 6–4. Management of sustained* ventricular tachycardia.

- In patients with a palpable carotid or femoral pulse but who are hemodynamically unstable (blood pressure less than 90 mm Hg, chest pain, shortness of breath, or clouding of consciousness), immediate synchronized cardioversion using 100 to 200 joules should be carried out
- In patients with an absent carotid or femoral pulse, prompt defibrillation

utilizing 200 joules should be carried out, as in treatment of VF (Fig. 6–4)

Table 6–9 lists the serious adverse effects of antiarrhythmic agents with an emphasis on their role as dictated by negative inotropic effects, their ability to precipitate heart failure, the propensity for serious adverse effects, and their efficacy with lethal arrhythmias. It must be reemphasized that patients with an EF less than 30% are not able to tolerate most antiarrhythmic agents. Only amiodarone, mexiletine, and quinidine are considered safe. Quinidine has very limited efficacy against lethal arrhythmias, however. The drug decreases the VF threshold, has a strong proarrhythmic potential, and appears to increase mortality. The judicious use of beta blockers has a role in these patients.

Table 6–10 gives drug dosages of antiarrhythmic agents. The maximum doses given are less than that indicated by the manufacturer but are consistent with current clinical practice. A review of the literature indicates that dosages beyond those given in Table 6–10 should be used only under strict supervision with caution in patients with renal dysfunction or in the elderly.

TORSADES DE POINTES

Torsades de pointes implies twisting of the QRS points around the baseline. As with other polymorphic forms of VT, typically there is a beat-to-beat change in QRS morphology (Fig. 6–3). This life-threatening arrhythmia is also termed "atypical ventricular tachycardia." The short bouts of VT persist for 5 to 30 seconds with R wave direction changing every few beats. The arrhythmia is usually initiated by VPCs, with a long coupling time and following a long R-R interval, but falls on the T wave because of the prolonged QT interval. Rates of 150 to 300/minute are not unusual, and the arrhythmia frequently terminates spontaneously. However, the arrhythmia is likely to deteriorate into VF or VT and syncope or clouding of consciousness.

The absolute value of the QTc is inaccurate in predicting the recurrence of torsades de pointes. With reported amiodarone cases, the QTc values range from 0.43 to 0.87 seconds. However, with agents other than amiodarone, at a QT interval of 0.60 seconds or more, torsades de pointes is often precipitated by Class IA agents or by sotalol.

Precipitating factors include

- Most commonly caused by Class IA agents: quinidine, disopyramide, procainamide, and rarely sotalol (particularly if hypokalemia or hypomagnesemia are present)
- Amiodarone may cause the arrhythmia, but the occurrence is extremely rare, and only about 60 cases have been reported in the literature
- Phenothiazines, tricyclic antidepressants, and importantly, the commonly used antibiotic, erythromycin
- Prenylamine, lidoflazine
- Hypokalemia, hypomagnesemia, hypocalcemia
- Myocardial ischemia/infarction

TABLE 6–9. DRUGS FOR VENTRICULAR ARRHYTHMIAS, ADVERSE EFFECTS, AND EFFICACY WITH LETHAL ARRHYTHMIAS

DRUG	NEGATIVE INOTROPIC EFFECT	PRECIPITATES HEART FAILURE?	SERIOUS SIDE EFFECTS	EFFICACY WITH LETHAL ARRHYTHMIAS
Quinidine	+	No EF <25 yes+	Yes proar- rhyth- mic+ + + precipitates tor- sades, VF, platelets ↓	Minimal
Procainamide IV oral	 + + + + +	Yes if EF <40	Yes agranulocyto- sis+ lupus, tor- sades	Poor
Disopyramide	+ + + +	Yes if EF <40	No precipitates torsades +	Poor
Mexiletine	+	No EF <25, yes	No High minor ef- fects Low proar- rhythmic +	Minimal
Tocainide	+	EF <25 yes+	Yes agranulocyto- sis+ + + pulmonary alveolitis	Poor pulmonary
Encainide*	+ +	Yes if EF <30+	No, but proar- rhyth- mic+ + +	Poor if EF <30
Flecainide*	+ + +	Yes if EF <35	No, but proar- rhyth- mic+ + + +	Not recom- mended if EF <35
Propafenone	+ + +	Yes if EF <35	Yes rare agranulo- cytosis+ proarrhythmic + +	Not if EF <35
Amiodarone	+	No EF <25 yes+	Yes low proar- rhythmic +	Yes+ + +
Beta blocker	+ +	Yes if EF <35	No not proar- rhythmic**	Yes + + +

EF = ejection fraction (%)
+ + + + = maximum effect
+ = minimal effect
* Not recommended for benign or potentially lethal arrhythmias
** Except sotalol mildly proarrhythmic

TABLE 6–10. ANTIARRHYTHMIC DRUG DOSAGE	

Quinidine: 200-mg test dose: If no hypersensitivity, syncope, or ↓ BP, 200–400 mg q 4h × 4 doses then q 6h then long-acting forms
Procainamide: 375–500 mg q 3h × 1 wk then, q 4h × 2–4 months. RF*
Disopyramide: 300 mg, then 150 mg q 6h. RF*
SR 300 mg bid
Mexiletine: 200–400 mg then 2h later 200–250 mg q 8h
RF* or MI q 12h or q 24h
or elderly: 100–150 mg BID
Encainide: 25 mg q 8h × 7 days, then
35mg q 8h × 7 days, then
50 mg q 8h max 200 mg daily. RF* caution
Flecainide: 50–200 mg bid max 400 mg daily
RF* caution
Sotalol:† 160–240 mg daily × 1–7 days, then 160–240 mg once or twice daily. (investigational 320 to 720 mg daily for lethal arrhythmias, see table 6–8 and text) RF*
Amiodarone: 200 mg tid or QID × 1–2 wk then 200 bid × 4–6 wk reduce weekly dose‡ by about 400 mg every 4 weeks until patient is taking 200 mg on 5–7 days per week (final maintenance according to Holters)

* Renal Failure: increase dosage interval
† Other beta blocker dosages (see Table 1–3)
‡ Higher doses previously used in USA cause increased pulmonary toxicity
BID = twice daily
TID = three times daily
QID = four times daily
h = hours
q = every

- Congenital long QT syndromes
- Myocarditis
- Bradycardia in association with prolonged QT interval
- Bepridil
- Chloroquine
- Organophosphate insecticides
- Astemizole
- Adenosine (see cautions for the use of adenosine)
- Liquid protein diets
- Subarachnoid hemorrhage

In most cases of acquired long QT syndrome, at least two of these factors are required simultaneously.

THERAPY OF TORSADES

- Immediately identify and withdraw the offending agent: antiarrhythmics and other drugs known to increase the QT interval
- Rapidly correct potassium and magnesium deficiency
- Magnesium sulfate (1 to 2 g) is usually highly successful, even in the absence of magnesium deficiency, 2 g (10 ml of a 20% solution) is given IV over 10 minutes and is followed by 4 g over 4 to 8 hours as an infusion of 30 mg/minute. Also, a low serum potassium is corrected by potassium

chloride infusion. Magnesium is a cofactor of membrane sodium, potassium, adenosine, triphosphatase, or sodium pump known to keep the intracellular potassium level constant. Magnesium sulfate given IV at higher doses occasionally causes marked hypotension. The substance also has a mild negative inotropic action. Patients with moderate to severe renal failure generally have high magnesium levels, and great caution is required in this situation

- Accelerating the heart rate is the simplest and quickest method to shorten the QT interval
- Temporary transvenous pacing is the safest and most effective method of management since the heart rate can be quickly and easily controlled for long periods. If available, atrial or atrial ventricular sequential pacing is preferable, but ventricular pacing is a simple procedure and the catheter obtains a more stable position with reliable capture. As an immediate measure, transthoracic pacing may be used while preparations are being made for electrode placement. If there is chronic bradycardia, the patient progresses to permanent atrial sequential pacing
- An infusion of isoproterenol (2 to 8 μg/min) is sometimes used if pacing is not readily available. This agent is carefully infused to increase the heart rate to about 120/minute. Isoproterenol is contraindicated in acute MI, angina, or severe hypertension. However, isoproterenol infusion needs to be carefully monitored to maintain a heart rate of 100 to 120. Myocardial ischemia may be precipitated, and the drug may precipitate VT or VF
- Amiodarone has been successfully used to manage torsades de pointes precipitated by sotalol or Class IA agents. This approach requires further confirmation, however
- Patients with congenital QT prolongation syndrome are best managed with beta-adrenergic blockers because these agents reduce mortality. Phenytoin has a role if beta blockers are contraindicated. Resistant cases are managed with permanent pacing plus beta blockers or left stellate ganglionectomy. Isoproterenolol is contraindicated in the congenital QT prolongation syndrome
- Hemodialysis to remove sotalol has been used successfully in a patient with torsades de pointes precipitated by sotalol at therapeutic level and normal serum potassium and with failure to respond to magnesium sulfate, isoproterenolol, and overdrive pacing

Importantly, prevention of torsades depends on the removal of the cause and maintenance of normal serum potassium. Amiloride has Class III antiarrhythmic activity; the drug retains potassium and is the diuretic of choice in patients treated with agents that have the propensity to prolong QT interval.

It is important to recognize that polymorphic VT associated with a prolonged QT interval is termed "torsades de pointes." When polymorphic VT occurs, however, in the absence of prolonged QT, the condition must not be managed as torsades de pointes. It is important to differentiate the two conditions. The majority of patients with polymorphic VT and normal QT intervals have underlying CHD and are managed in the manner described earlier in this chapter.

Accelerating the heart rate shortens the QT interval. Thus, sympathetic stimulation with physical exertion or excitement often controls the acquired form of torsades de pointes. Sudden acceleration of heart rate, however, tends to provoke the occurrence of torsades de pointes in patients with congenital long QT syndrome. Although beta blockers do not usually shorten the QT interval, they are the agents of choice in this syndrome and have been shown, in symptomatic patients, to reduce mortality. In patients with congenital long QT syndrome, with or without deafness, torsades de pointes represents the predominant form of VT. Agents that shorten the QT, e.g., calcium, potassium, lidocaine, and digitalis, are not effective. Because syncope or sudden death occurs in these patients, consideration must be given for intervention with left cervicothoracic sympathetic ganglionectomy or an automatic implantable cardioverter defibrillator if events are not prevented by beta blockade.

ANTIARRHYTHMIC AGENTS

CLASSIFICATION

A knowledge of the electrophysiologic classification of antiarrhythmics is useful in understanding arrhythmia suppression, drug combinations, proarrhythmia, and some adverse effects.

A modification of Vaughan Williams electrophysiologic classification of antiarrhythmic drugs is given in Table 6–11. Several electrophysiologic effects of these agents are not accounted for by their class action and considerable overlap exists.

- Amiodarone has powerful Class III and IA actions, as well as significant Class II and IV effects. Although the drug prolongs the QT interval, the clinical effect is different from QT prolongation caused by sotalol and Class IA agents. Amiodarone brings about a more uniform action potential throughout the myocardium, enhancing electrophysiologic homogeneity, which appears to protect from lethal arrhythmias. Sotalol placed as a Class III or Class II agent leads to a false notion; it is perhaps preferable to place sotalol in a class of its own (Class IIIA) as opposed to an assignment of Class II with other beta blockers. The antiarrhythmic effect of bretylium is mainly due to chemical sympathectomy; the drug does not alter the action potential directly as other Class III agents do
- Class I drugs inhibit influx of sodium into the cardiac myocyte (Fig. 6–5). Class IA: Quinidine, disopyramide, and procainamide slow phase 0 and prolong the duration of the action potential
- Class IB: Lidocaine, mexiletine, and tocainide have relatively little effect on phase 0, cause minimal narrowing of the action potential, and decrease repolarization time. They do slow conduction and delay repolarization in certain situations
- Class IC: Flecainide, encainide, and propafenone slow phase 0 but have little or no effect on action potential duration. However, these agents have a marked inhibitive effect on His-Purkinje conduction, increasing

TABLE 6–11. ELECTROPHYSIOLOGIC CLASSIFICATION OR ANTIARRHYTHMIC DRUGS*

CLASS	EFFECT ON THE ACTION POTENTIAL (AP)†

I. Sodium channel blockers
  A. Sodium channel (+ +); blocks
    potassium efflux (+)
      Disopyramide
      Quinidine
      Procainamide
	Slows phase zero (+ +)
	Moderately prolongs the AP:
	↑ repolarization time, ↑ QT

B. Sodium channel (+)
    Other effects
    Lidocaine (lignocaine)
    Mexiletine
    Moricizine (also IA IC actions)
    Tocainide
	Minimal slowing phase zero (+)
	Minimal narrowing of the AP
	↓ repolarization time

C. Sodium channel (+ + + +)
    Encainide
    Flecainide
    Lorcainide
    Propafenone
	Marked slowing phase zero:
	Marked depression of upstroke
	Marked inhibitory effect on HIS-Purkinje
	  conduction:
	↑ QRS duration
	Shortens AP but only of Purkinje fibers:
	  marked depression on conduction.‡
	Repolarization time unchanged.‡

II. Inhibition of the effects of
  sympathetic stimulation
  Beta-adrenergic blockers
	No effect on AP or repolarization.§
	↓ phase 4 spontaneous depolarization:
	Decrease automaticity

III. Potassium channel efflux blockade
  Amiodarone + + + +, Also
  sodium block. Sotalol (+ +) (No
  sodium block and usual Class II
  effects)
  Bretylium partly Class III
	Slows phase zero (Class I effect)
	Markedly prolongs the AP:
	Markedly prolongs repolarization time.
	↑ QT; Amiodarone brings about a more
	  uniform AP throughout the
	  myocardium:
	Enhances EP homogeneity

IV. Calcium channel blockers	No effect
V. Alinidine	Investigational

* Modified from Vaughan Williams
† See Fig. 6–5
‡ May explain proarrhythmic effect
§ Except sotalol, Class III effect
  + = Minimal effect
+ + + + = Maximal effect
  K = Potassium

QRS duration. These agents shorten the action potential, but only in Purkinje's fibers, and thus cause marked depression of conduction. Also, repolarization time is unchanged. These latter effects may explain the proarrhythmic effects of these agents

- Class II agents, the beta-adrenergic blocking drugs, inhibit sympathetic stimulation. They cause, therefore, a decrease in phase 4 diastolic depolarization in spontaneously discharging cells, which results in a decrease in automaticity. Beta blockers cause an important increase in VF

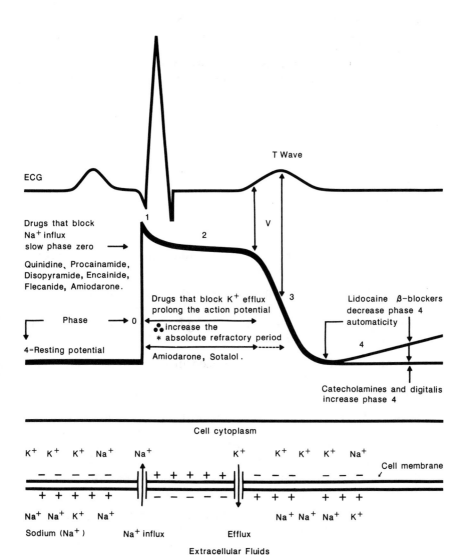

T Wave

ECG

Drugs that block
Na$^+$ influx
slow phase zero →

Quinidine, Procainamide,
Disopyramide, Encainide,
Flecanide, Amiodarone.

1

2

V

Drugs that block K$^+$ efflux
prolong the action potential

Phase → 0

4=Resting potential

⁘ increase the
∗ absoloute refractory period

Amiodarone, Sotalol.

3

Lidocaine β-blockers
decrease phase 4
automaticity

4

Catecholamines and digitalis
increase phase 4

Cell cytoplasm

K$^+$ K$^+$ K$^+$ Na$^+$ Na$^+$ K$^+$ K$^+$ K$^+$ K$^+$ Na$^+$

Cell membrane

– – – – –   + + + + +   – – –   – – –

+ + + + +   – – – – –   + + +   + + +

Na$^+$ Na$^+$ K$^+$ Na$^+$ Na$^+$ Na$^+$ Na$^+$ K$^+$

Sodium (Na$^+$)   Na$^+$ influx   Efflux

Extracellular Fluids

Caption:

∗   Absolute refractory period = During phases 1 and 2 a stimulus
    evokes no response : an arrhythmia cannot be triggered

V = Vulnerable period

FIG. 6–5. Antiarrhythmic drug action. From: Khan, M Gabriel: Cardiovascular system,
pharmacology. *In* Encyclopedia of Human Biology. Vol. 2. Edited by R Dulbecco. San
Diego, Academic Press, Inc., 1991, pp. 167–177.

threshold. Sympathetically mediated acceleration of impulses through the AV node are blocked. These agents have no effect on the action potential or repolarization time. Sotalol is the only beta blocking agent with Class III effects
- Adenosine causes an increase in potassium and a decrease in calcium conductance and should not be associated with Class IV calcium antagonists

CLASS IA

Class IA agents include
- Disopyramide
- Quinidine
- Procainamide

Disopyramide

Supplied: capsules; 100 and 150 mg and controlled release. Rythmodan Retard, 250 mg; Norpace CR, 150 mg

Dosage: Loading dose 300 mg, then 100 to 150 mg every 6 hours or sustained action 250 to 300 mg twice daily. IV (not approved in the USA): 2 mg/kg over 15 minutes, then 1 to 2 mg/kg by infusion over 45 minutes; maintenance = 0.4 mg/kg/hour.

Caution. The dose should be reduced in severe renal failure, heart failure, and in the elderly.

The action of the drug is given in Table 6–11 and Figure 6–5.

Adverse effects. The drug has a powerful negative inotropic effect and may precipitate heart failure in patients with LV dysfunction. Disopyramide has strong anticholinergic activity, precipitates urinary retention, and is contraindicated in patients with glaucoma, prostate hypertrophy, myasthenia gravis, heart failure, and renal failure. The drug may cause sinus node depression and torsades de pointes.

Indications. Disopyramide may have a role in the management of potentially lethal arrhythmias that are bothersome and not responsive to beta blockers but must only be used in patients with near normal EF and those with no suspicion of LV dysfunction. The drug has a role in the management of antidromic and orthodromic tachycardia or atrial fibrillation and flutter in patients with WPW syndrome because it inhibits anterograde and retrograde conduction in the accessory pathway.

Procainamide

Supplied: capsule; 250, 375, 500 mg. sustained release tablets; 250, 500, 750, 1,000 mg

Dosage: 500 mg oral loading dose, 375 to 500 mg every 3 hours for 24 hours, and then sustained release 500 mg every 6 hours for a 60-kg patient

(750 mg every 6 hours for patients over 60 kg) for a maximum of 6 months. IV dosage: 100 mg bolus at a rate of 20 mg/minute, followed by 10 to 20 mg/minute to a maximum of 1 g over the first hour; maintenance = 1 to 4 mg/minute.

Indications

• Management of ventricular tachycardia that fails to terminate with a second bolus of lidocaine (lignocaine). Chronic oral therapy is not advisable because the drug does not improve survival in this category of patients with ventricular arrhythmias. If the drug is prescribed, it should generally not be given for longer than 6 months because of the incidence of drug-induced lupus and the occurrence of agranulocytosis, albeit rare.

Adverse effects. The IV preparation has moderate negative inotropic effects, and the oral preparation has a mild risk of precipitating heart failure. Torsades de pointes is not uncommon. Lupus occurs in over 33% of patients treated beyond 6 months; agranulocytosis appears to occur more commonly with the sustained release preparation.

Interactions. ACE inhibitors may enhance immune effects; cimetidine increases procainamide levels.

Quinidine

Supplied: tablets; 200, 300 mg (Quinidine bisulphate: 250 mg)

Dosage: Quinidine sulphate 200-mg test dose; observe for 4 hours, if there is no hypersensitivity reaction, give 200 to 400 mg every 3 hours for three or four doses and then every 6 hours. When the arrhythmia is stabilized, a control release preparation can be used: quinidine bisulphate 250 mg, usual maintenance 500 mg twice daily, sustained release tablets 325 mg (1 to 2 tablets twice daily).

Action. The drug is a sodium channel blocker that slows phase 0 of the action potential, blocks potassium efflux, and moderately prolongs the action potential, resulting in an increase in repolarization time and prolongation of the QT interval. The drug has an anticholinergic effect, facilitates AV conduction, and may cause an increase in the ventricular response in patients with atrial flutter or atrial fibrillation if the AV node has not been previously blocked by digitalis.

Pharmacokinetics

• After oral dosing, peak plasma levels: 1 to 3 hours
• Half-life: 7 to 9 hours
• Hepatic metabolism with minimal renal elimination
• Therapeutic blood levels: 2 to 5 µg/ml (3 to 5.5 µmol/l)

Indications

- Occasional use for conversion of atrial fibrillation to sinus rhythm following digitalization in properly selected patients
- Post-electrical cardioversion, quinidine may be used for maintaining sinus rhythm but is of limited value
- Recurrent sustained VT, often in combination with another agent as part of electrophysiologically guided regime. The drug has not been shown to prolong survival in patients with potentially lethal arrhythmias and is rarely indicated in the management of ventricular arrhythmias. A meta-analysis suggests that quinidine has an adverse effect on mortality

Adverse effects. First-dose idiosyncrasy, diarrhea, nausea, angioedema, thrombocytopenia, hepatitis, agranulocytosis, torsades de pointes, especially in patients with hypokalemia. The drug decreases VF threshold and may increase the risk of VF. Precipitation of sustained VT and cardiac arrest may occur. Rare hypersensitivity angiitis with coronary artery dissection has been reported.

Contraindications

- Heart block, torsades de pointes caused by QT prolongation
- Sick sinus syndrome
- Bundle branch block
- Myasthenia gravis
- Hepatic failure
- WPW with atrial fibrillation or flutter

Interactions

- Serum digoxin levels increase
- Amiodarone and quinidine should not be given concomitantly, since torsades de pointes may be precipitated. Verapamil and diltiazem increase quinidine plasma levels
- Warfarin action may be enhanced
- Phenytoin decreases quinidine blood levels

Caution. For all Class IA agents, hypokalemia must be corrected for maximum efficacy and to prevent torsades de pointes.

CLASS IB

Class IB agents include

- Lidocaine (lignocaine)
- Mexiletine
- Moricizine
- Tocainide

Lidocaine
(Lignocaine, UK)

IV lidocaine has remained the mainstay of therapy for the acute management of VT.

Dosage: IV bolus 1.0 to 1.5 mg/kg (75 to 100 mg) given over a few minutes with the immediate institution of lidocaine infusion at 2 to 3 mg/minute. A second bolus of 50 to 75 mg is given 5 minutes later, and a third bolus is given if arrhythmia recurs with simultaneous increase in the infusion rate. The maximum rate of 4 mg/minute should only be used after careful reevaluation of the clinical situation and rationale for the use of lidocaine. Infusion rates greater than 2 mg/minute should not be used in the presence of heart failure and in the elderly (see Tables 3–8 and 3–9).

Action. The drug causes minimal slowing of phase 0, causes a minimal narrowing of the action potential, resulting in a decrease in repolarization time, and as with other Class IB agents, does not prolong the QT interval. The drug depresses spontaneous phase 4 depolarization and has no significant negative inotropic effect, a factor that makes this agent extremely useful. The drug acts by slowing conduction selectively on diseased or ischemic tissue and thus has a major role in the management of ventricular arrhythmias during acute MI and ischemia, where enhancement of conduction block appears to interrupt reentry circuit. Prolongation of refractoriness following premature beats has been demonstrated with other drugs in this class (mexiletine), and this may be a useful property. The effectiveness of lidocaine is decreased in the presence of hypokalemia and bradycardia, which must be corrected.

Pharmacokinetics

- After bolus IV injection, the drug acts within minutes and the action lasts only for 5 to 10 minutes because of rapid de-ethylation by liver microsomes. Thus, plasma levels are increased with liver dysfunction and a decrease in hepatic blood flow, as may occur with heart failure, the elderly, cimetidine, propranolol, and other hepatic-metabolized beta blockers (Table 3–9)
- Therapeutic blood levels: 1.4 to 5 mg/l (1.4 to 5 μg/ml or 6 to 26 μmol/l) levels greater than 6 mg/l are associated with seizures and central nervous adverse effects

Indications

- Sustained VT
- Digitalis-induced ventricular arrhythmias
- Ventricular arrhythmias caused by tricyclic antidepressants and phenothiazine
- The drug may be used during pregnancy for the management of VT, although it does cross the placenta
- Indications for use in acute MI are discussed in Chapters 3 and 4

Contraindications

* Second- or third-degree AV block
* Idioventricular rhythm, sinus node dysfunction
* Bradycardia of less than 50/minute

Adverse effects. Sinus arrest may appear in patients with sick sinus syndrome; third-degree AV block may be precipitated in patients with impaired atrioventricular conduction; vomiting, twitching, seizures.

Interactions

* Cimetidine
* Hepatic-metabolized beta-adrenergic blocking agents
* Phenytoin decreases lidocaine blood levels

Mexiletine
(Mexitil)

Supplied: capsules; 150, 200, 250 mg

Dosage: orally, initial dose 200 to 400 mg, followed by 200 to 250 mg every 8 hours (over 12 hours with severe renal failure, hepatic dysfunction, acute MI, or in the elderly).

Mexiletine is a weak antiarrhythmic agent and rarely shows salutary effects in the treatment of lethal arrhythmias. However, because of its weak negative inotropic effect, a low proarrhythmic potential, and the absence of serious adverse effects (Table 6–10), the drug may be combined, in properly selected cases, with amiodarone, sotalol, or quinidine if sinus node disease, hypotension, bradycardia, AV block, hypokalemia, or other contraindications are absent. The drug can precipitate heart failure in patients with severe LV dysfunction with EF below 25%.

Action. The drug causes minimal slowing of phase 0, minimal narrowing of the action potential, decreases repolarization time, and does not lengthen the QT interval.

Pharmacokinetics

* The drug is well absorbed orally
* Peak plasma levels in 2 to 4 hours
* The drug is lipophilic and high brain concentration accounts for prevalent CNS adverse effects
* Half-life of 9 to 16 hours may be prolonged to 19 to 26 hours in patients with heart failure, acute MI, and liver dysfunction
* About 15% of the drug is excreted unchanged in the urine. Some unchanged drug is reabsorbed, therefore, in patients with severe renal impairment creatinine clearance less than 10 ml/min), the dose interval should be increased
* Effective plasma concentration: 0.75 to 2.0 mg/l (0.75 to 2 µg/ml or 3.5 to 9.3 µmol/l)

Contraindications

- Severe LV failure
- Hypotension
- Bradycardia or sick sinus syndrome
- AV block
- Hepatic or severe renal failure and epilepsy

Adverse effects. Bradycardia and transient AV block, hypotension, confusional state, seizures, tremor, diplopia, ataxia, nystagmus, dysarthria, parasthesia, psychiatric disorders, nausea, gastric irritation may occur in up to 70% of patients and jaundice, hepatitis, and blood disorders have been reported.

Interactions. Phenytoin is an inducer of hepatic enzymes and decreases mexiletine blood levels; theophylline levels may increase.

Tocainide

Supplied: 400, 600 mg

Dosage: Oral 400 to 600 mg two or three times daily. IV 0.5 to 0.75 mg/kg/min for 15 to 30 minutes, i.e., 500 to 750 mg by IV infusion over 15 to 30 minutes with ECG monitoring, followed immediately by 400 to 600 mg orally, and then maintenance. (IV tocainide is not approved in the USA.) Reduce the dose and increase the dosing interval in renal failure patients.

Action. The drug has a similar action to lidocaine with very mild negative inotropic effect. Over 40% of the drug is excreted unchanged by the kidney and the half-life is 25 to 30 hours; therefore, the dose must be reduced and the time interval must be increased in patients with renal failure.

Adverse effects. Agranulocytosis, interstitial pulmonary alveolitis, lupus syndrome, and a high incidence of GI and CNS effects.

Indications. Life-threatening ventricular arrhythmias, refractory to other agents and indicated only after electrophysiologic testing.

Contraindications

- AV block and severe heart failure. The drug is best avoided in patients with renal failure and hepatic dysfunction, and weekly blood counts are essential for the first 3 months of therapy
- Hypersensitivity may cause second- or third-degree AV block in the absence of an artificial pacemaker
- Atrial fibrillation or flutter in nondigitalized patients because of the danger of producing rapid ventricular rates
- Moderate to severe renal failure or severe hepatic dysfunction

Moricizine
(Ethmozine)

Moricizine is a phenothiazine derivative that appears to control some life-threatening ventricular arrhythmias.

Action. Moricizine is considered a Class IB agent but has IA and IC effects. Unlike lidocaine, moricizine has no effect on the slope of phase 4 depolarization, except in ischemic Purkinje fibers; the sodium channel blocking effect is similar to IA agents. The drug prolongs the PR interval and QRS duration but usually does not change the QT interval (IC effects). Phenothiazines usually increase the QT interval and predispose torsades de pointes, which may occur, albeit rarely, with moricizine.

The drug has mild negative inotropic effects and can precipitate heart failure in patients with moderately severe LV dysfunction (EF less than 30%).

<u>Dosage:</u> Oral 200 to 300 mg every 8 hours.

Pharmacokinetics

- Good bioavailability if taken on an empty stomach
- Extensive hepatic metabolism; half-life of 2 to 5 hours prolonged in renal dysfunction
- Renal elimination and, thus, dose reduction or increased intervals are advisable with moderate or severe renal failure

Interactions

- Cimetidine
- Hepatic-metabolized beta blockers

Adverse effects. Dizziness, headaches, GI upset, and proarrhythmia in patients with severe LV dysfunction, although the incidence is much less than that observed with flecainide and encainide; rarely AV block, intraventricular conduction defects.

The conclusion of CAST indicates no salutary benefits from the use of moricizine in post-infarction patients with complex VPCs.

CLASS IC

Class IC agents include

- Encainide
- Flecainide
- Lorcainide
- Propafenone

Indications for Class IC agents include

- Paroxysmal atrial fibrillation in properly selected cases in combination with digoxin

The use of Class IC agents is limited by their proarrhythmic effects highlighted by the CAST study, which indicated a significant increase in mortality in patients with post-infarction ventricular arrhythmias treated with encainide or flecainide.

Several reports indicate the effectiveness of Class IC agents in conversion to sinus rhythm of paroxysmal atrial fibrillation, a bothersome and sometimes incapacitating arrhythmia. Physicians are tempted to use flecainide or propafenone because of their low frequency of noncardiac adverse effects. However, their use is fraught with danger, since over 15% of patients treated with supraventricular arrhythmias have been reported to develop very serious cardiac adverse effects. These deleterious effects may occur early or several months later, and patients at risk cannot be predicted.

Type IC agents slow atrial conduction with little effect on anterograde AV nodal refractoriness. The atrial rate is slowed and the rhythm may regularize to atrial flutter, resulting in fewer impulses penetrating the AV node, which may permit one-to-one AV conduction with a rapid ventricular response. This may precipitate hypotension, the resulting sympathetic release further facilitates AV nodal conduction. Hypotension may induce MI, or heart failure may be precipitated because of a fast ventricular response and negative inotropic effects of the drug.

Class IC agents are not warranted for ventricular arrhythmias because the salutary effects of these agents are poor and adverse effects are hazardous. There is little indication for their use with atrial fibrillation, except in properly selected cases of paroxysmal atrial fibrillation less than 48-hour duration (for example, post cardiac surgery). Conversion is expected in more than 80% with normal LV function and with prior digitalization to avoid a 1:1 response that is well recognized with quinidine and Class IA agents. Class IC drugs are not sufficiently effective with atrial flutter to justify their use (see earlier discussion).

Propafenone is slightly less effective than flecainide, causing reversion to sinus rhythm in patients with paroxysmal atrial fibrillation and in about 70% of patients where atrial fibrillation is present for less than 48 hours. Flecainide causes about an 80% reversion to sinus rhythm. Propafenone appears to be safer than flecainide for IV conversion. However, the drug must be avoided in patients with bronchospasm.

Propafenone is useful in patients with WPW and anterograde conduction over the bypass tract. Patients with this rare presentation with rapid ventricular rates are best treated with electrical cardioversion followed by electrophysiologic studies and selection of an appropriate antiarrhythmic agent, usually amiodarone followed, if needed, by ablative therapy (Chapter 18).

Flecainide

Supplied: tablets; 400 to 600 mg (UK, 100 to 200 mg)

Dosage: Oral 25 mg twice daily, increasing to 50 to 100 mg twice daily. After several weeks or months, give a maximum of 200 mg twice daily. In the elderly, half of the above dose is advisable; the dose must be reduced with renal or hepatic impairment. IV 2 mg/kg over 30 minutes (maximum 150 mg with continuous cardiac monitoring) followed, if needed, by infusion of 1.5 mg/kg/h for 1 hour, then reduce to 100 to 250 μg/kg/hour for up to 24 hours. Do not exceed 600 mg in 24 hours, then, if justifiable, transfer to oral therapy.

Contraindications

• Sinus node dysfunction
• AV block
• Heart failure, LV dysfunction, EF less than 35%
• History of MI
• Nonsustained VT

Adverse effects. Noncardiac adverse effects are rare (dizziness, visual disturbances, GI upset). Serious life-threatening cardiac arrhythmias may be precipitated because of a high proarrhythmic effect and atrial flutter with one-to-one conduction as discussed previously.

Interactions

• Beta blocker combinations may increase LV dysfunction
• Verapamil or diltiazem may increase the incidence of heart failure as well as AV disturbances
• Disopyramide may increase the risk of heart failure
• Flecainide plasma levels increase with amiodarone

Propafenone

Supplied: tablets; 150 to 300 mg

Dosage: 150 mg three times daily after food, increase after a few weeks, if needed, to 300 mg two or there times daily for individuals over 70 kg. For elderly patients or those under 70 kg, half of the above dose is advisable. Patients should be under direct hospital supervision with ECG monitoring and blood pressure control during institution of therapy.

Indications

• Paroxysmal atrial fibrillation (see earlier discussion)
• The drug is rarely effective with ventricular arrhythmias and safety of longterm use is not established

Contraindications

• Heart failure, patients with moderate or severe LV dysfunction, EF less than 35%
• Bradycardias, sinus or AV node disease, bundle branch block
• Asthma or chronic obstructive pulmonary disease

- Myasthenia gravis
- Pregnancy

Caution. In patients with heart failure, hepatic and renal impairment, pacemakers, or in elderly patients, propafenone increases thresholds and dramatically widens paced-QRS complex. The drug is not advisable in pregnancy.

Adverse effects. These include proarrhythmias, fatal VT, taste disturbances, and, rarely, agranulocytosis, hepatitis, and lupus syndrome.

Interactions

- Beta blockers, since propafenone has beta blocking properties
- Digoxin levels are increased
- Increased effects of oral anticoagulants

CLASS II DRUGS

The beta-adrenergic blocking agents are effective antiarrhythmic agents that have no proarrhythmic effects, with the exception of sotalol, which has Class III effects.
Beta blockers

- Are effective in all grades of ventricular arrhythmias
- May not completely suppress VPCs, nevertheless, in the same individual, the occurrence of sustained VT or VF may be prevented
- Are particularly useful for ventricular arrhythmias initiated by ischemia or catecholamine release
- Are effective for supraventricular arrhythmias (this has been discussed earlier in this chapter)

Atenolol, acebutolol, and nadolol at doses of 100, 600, and 120 mg, respectively, have proven to be effective in suppression of ventricular arrhythmias. Both acebutolol (600 mg) and atenolol (100 mg) have been shown to be as effective as quinidine in controlling ventricular arrhythmias and more effective than quinidine in suppressing exercise-induced ventricular arrhythmias. In one study, sotalol and propranolol caused up to 65 and 44% reduction in VPCs, respectively, but sotalol caused up to 99% reduction of ventricular couplets versus less than 50% reduction with propranolol administration.

Several clinical trials have shown sotalol to be a well-tolerated, effective antiarrhythmic agent in patients at high risk for sudden death. The drug is often effective in patients who did not benefit from multiple-drug treatment. A dose of sotalol ranging from 160 to 720 mg with a mean dose of 240 mg is usually required for suppression that is more frequent in patients with VF, 58 versus 24% in patients with VT. When sotalol is used, it is necessary to maintain a normal serum potassium. Thiazide diuretics should not be used in combination. If a diuretic is necessary, it is advisable to give amiloride (see later discussion in this chapter).

Often, a combination of acebutolol (200 to 400 mg) or nadolol (40 to 80 mg) with amiodarone proves effective and safer than amiodarone combined with a Class I agent.

In general, beta blockers are avoided in patients with EF less than 30% because heart failure may be precipitated. However, recent trials indicate the benefit and relative safety of beta blockers in the management of patients with EF as low as 25%, who are at high risk for sudden death following episodes of monomorphic VT, and a judicious trial of a beta blocking drug is advisable in these patients. The use of beta-adrenergic blocking agents to prevent sudden cardiac deaths in patients at risk will increase because of the failure of all antiarrhythmic agents to prevent sudden cardiac death. Also, the use of amiodarone has not resulted in a reduction in sudden cardiac death in patients with a low EF and/or heart failure. It is appropriate, therefore, that several clinical trials are in progress to document the salutary effects of beta blockers on sudden cardiac death.

Evidence supports the extensive use of beta blockers for the prevention of sudden cardiac death in patients with life-threatening arrhythmias and in patients with left ventricular dysfunction and in others at high risk

- In the Norwegian MI study, timolol showed an impressive 67% reduction in sudden cardiac death in patients treated from approximately day 7 and followed up for 2 years
- In the BHAT, beta blockers caused a greater reduction of sudden cardiac death than placebo in post-MI patients with either a history of prior heart failure or the emergence of heart failure. These agents also caused a reduction in early morning sudden cardiac death and infarction, possibly because of their ability to suppress the effects of early morning catecholamine surge and resulting increased platelet aggregation, heart rate, blood pressure, arterial hydraulic stress, and plaque rupture (see Fig. 2–7)
- The incidence of VF in patients with acute MI was significantly reduced in patients treated with metoprolol compared to controls. Beta blockers cause a salutary increase in VF threshold and have been used since the 1960s in the management of recurrent VF (see Chapter 7)
- In animals with induced myocardial ischemia, beta blockers have been shown by Lynch, et al. to protect against digoxin sensitization of the myocardium to catecholamine-induced ventricular arrhythmias. Animals treated with beta blockers and digoxin revealed a reduction in the incidence of sudden cardiac death, compared to animals treated with digoxin
- In animal studies of MI, Inoue and Zipes have demonstrated that in the areas distal to the zone of infarction, there is a supersensitivity to catecholamines
- Dellsperger, et al. have shown that in dogs with induced left ventricular hypertrophy, although ACE inhibitors and beta blockers have similar hemodynamic effects, the incidence of sudden cardiac death caused by ischemia was only decreased by the beta blocking drug
- Lipophilic beta blockers achieve brain concentration and are superior to hydrophilic agents in the prevention of cardiac death in animals (see

Chapter 1). Randomized clinical trials support this experimental work. Metoprolol, propranolol, timolol, and acebutolol are the only beta blockers proven effective in reducing the incidence of total deaths and/or sudden cardiac deaths in patients, and these are lipophilic beta blocker agents. Thus, a lipophilic beta blocker with Class III effect may find a role in the prevention of death, and further research and clinical trials are required to resolve these important issues

CLASS III

Class III agents include amiodarone, sotalol, bretylium, bethanidine, and possibly amiloride. Both amiodarone and sotalol have become widely accepted for use in patients with lethal arrhythmias: their role has increased because of the findings of the CAST. As outlined earlier, sotalol is particularly effective in patients whose presenting arrhythmia was VF and may be given a trial in patients with EF above 30%; some patients without overt heart failure and EF as low as 25% have been successfully treated.

Beta blockers, particularly sotalol with type III activity, are the only antiarrhythmics that have been shown to cause prolongation of life in patients with potentially lethal or lethal arrhythmias. Amiodarone appears to improve survival in post-infarction patients with lethal arrhythmias but not in patients with heart failure. It is not surprising therefore, that over 30 Class III agents are currently under development. It is appropriate that the role of Class III agents, including those with associated beta-adrenergic blocking effects, is increasing and that of Class I agents should dwindle because of proarrhythmia and lack of their ability to prolong life.

Amiodarone
(Cordarone)

Action. Amiodarone blocks the efflux of potassium from myocytes and markedly prolongs the action potential, thus increasing repolarization time and the effective refractory period.

Although the QT interval is prolonged, torsades de pointes is, in fact, a rare complication of amiodarone, mainly because the drug enhances homogeneity of the action potential throughout the myocardium. Amiodarone does not encourage calcium-mediated oscillations of membrane potential at the end of the action potential (afterdepolarizations). Undoubtedly, the absolute value of the QTc interval does not predict the occurrence of torsades de pointes, although the amplitude and stability of the T-U segments probably do. Amiodarone also blocks sodium channels and slows phase 0 of the action potential. The drug noncompetitively blocks alpha and beta receptors, resulting in vasodilatation and mild beta blockade. Fortunately, the drug has a very mild negative inotropic action that allows its use in patients with lethal arrhythmias who often have underlying severe LV dysfunction with EF less than 30% although the drug does not appear to prolong life in these patients.

The benzofuran derivative has two atoms of iodine and a structure similar to thyroxine. A 200-mg tablet contains more than 50 times the daily requirement of 150 μg of iodine.

Supplied: tablets; 200 mg. ampules; 150 mg

Dosage: IV for life-threatening arrhythmias: infusion up to 5 mg/kg, usually 300 mg over 2 hours with ECG monitoring often given over 30 minutes if life is threatened (maximum dose = 1.2 g in 24 hours). Central venous cannulation is required for prolonged infusion. Additional 150-mg boluses can be given if required during the infusion. Caution: hypotension may occur.

Oral: 200 mg three or four times daily for 2 weeks, 200 mg twice daily for 4 to 6 weeks, and then, if arrhythmia is controlled, reduce the dose by about 400 mg every 4 weeks, i.e., decrease from 14 to 10 tablets weekly, reducing from 9 to 5 tablets at intervals of about 4 weeks. Reduction of dosage is guided by 24- or 48-hour Holter monitoring with a goal of 5 to 7 tablets weekly to avoid longterm toxicity.

Pharmacokinetics

- About 50% of the oral dose is absorbed; bioavailability ranges from 20 to 80%
- Plasma levels occur in 6 to 12 hours
- The lipophilic compound is extensively metabolized to desethyl amiodarone, which has pharmacologic activity. The drug is highly bound (95%) to protein, and widespread distribution occurs in most tissues, especially the liver, lungs, and adipose tissue. The concentration in the myocardium is about 20 to 40 times that in plasma
- The volume of distribution is high; an adequate loading dose is necessary
- The half-life is about 30 to 110 days
- With dosages of 200 mg, three or four times daily, a therapeutic effect is observed in 1 to 4 days but increases up to 6 months; the action of the drug may persist for more than 50 days after cessation of therapy, although most side effects show a decrease after 4 to 7 days, depending on the oral loading dose
- When given intravenously, a therapeutic effect is observed within a few minutes
- A therapeutic effect shows poor correlation with the therapeutic plasma levels (0.75 to 2.0 μg/ml, up to about 95% of which is bound to plasma proteins). These levels, as well as metabolite levels, (desethylamiodarone 1.1 ± 0.5 μg/ml) however, assist with monitoring of toxicity
- A loading dose of 10 to 12 g in the first 2 weeks and maintenance of 400 mg daily 5 days weekly reportedly showed steady-state plasma amiodarone and desethylamiodarone concentrations of 1.7 ± 1.3 and 1.1 ± 0.5 μg/ml, respectively, only after about 1 month of therapy. Patients usually experience therapeutic benefits to amiodarone at plasma concentrations less than 1.0 μg/ml, and toxicity is not often manifest with concentrations less than 2.0 μg/ml

- The action of the drug appears to relate to tissue stores, and myocardial concentration is important

Indications

- Lethal ventricular arrhythmias (Tables 6–8 and 6–9): Sustained VT, recovery from VF or cardiac arrest
  Patients with a first occurrence of lethal arrhythmias in the absence of precipitating factors have about a 50% mortality. Survivors have a high mortality; some subsets of patients have a mortality of over 90% in 1 year. The overall mortality in survivors of cardiac arrest is about 66% over 5 years. In these high-risk patients, amiodarone has a role. Alternatively, an antiarrhythmic device may be implanted (Chapter 18).
  The Basel Antiarrhythmic Study of Infarct Survival (BASIS) indicated that in patients at high risk for sudden death (i.e., potentially lethal arrhythmias), amiodarone at a low dose (200 mg daily) caused a decrease in mortality in the first year in post-MI patients (see Chapter 4).

- For conversion of acute atrial fibrillation to sinus rhythm, especially in patients with hypertrophic cardiomyopathy
- Paroxysmal atrial fibrillation that is highly symptomatic with rapid ventricular rates refractory to other therapy and deemed bothersome and incapacitating
- WPW: Management of atrial fibrillation or atrial flutter with rapid ventricular rates due to anterograde conduction over the accessory pathway. In this subset, the drug is worth a trial prior to consideration of ablative therapy (see Chapter 18)

Contraindications

- Sinus bradycardia, sinus node disease, or AV block (requires pacing to allow amiodarone therapy)
- Hypokalemia
- Severe hepatic dysfunction
- Iodine sensitivity
- Pregnancy and breastfeeding
- Porphyria

Interactions

- Class IA antiarrhythmic agents prolong the QT interval and may include torsades de pointes; also, erythromycin increases the QT interval and must not be given concomitantly
- Oral anticoagulant activity is increased
- Verapamil and diltiazem may produce sinus arrest or AV block
- Digoxin levels increase
- Quinidine levels increase
- Sotalol should not be used in combination, but any of the available beta blocking drugs can be combined with amiodarone, provided that contraindications to both drugs are not present

- Tricyclics and phenothiazines, including moricizine, may induce torsades de pointes
- Thiazide diuretics should be avoided since they may produce hypokalemia and increase the risk of torsades, unless covered by potassium supplements or ACE inhibitors
- Beta blocking agents interact with amiodarone, which has weak beta blocking properties, and mild bradycardia may occur. These two agents, out of necessity, are commonly used in combination, especially if the patient has a pacemaker

Adverse effects

- Cardiac side effects: Severe bradyarrhythmias, asystole, and rarely torsades de pointes, especially in patients with a low serum potassium. Approximately 60 cases of torsades de pointes associated with the use of amiodarone have been reported in the literature. Most of these cases were induced by multifactorial causes, the majority having hypokalemia, hypomagnesemia, or the concomitant use of antiarrhythmics, phenothiazines, or tricyclics. The drug has been used in a patient to successfully treat torsades de pointes caused by sotalol-thiazide combination; despite further prolongation of the QT interval from 0.56 to 0.72 seconds, amiodarone was successful in causing reversal to sinus rhythm. The incidence of serious proarrhythmic effects in patients administered amiodarone is less than 1%
- Hypothyroidism or, less often, hyperthyroidism occurs in about 5% of patients. Asymptomatic corneal microdeposits developed in most patients after about 3 months of therapy. A few patients complain of halo or blurred vision, which disappears on lowering the dose of amiodarone
- Hepatitis with grossly elevated transaminase levels occurs very rarely but may progress to cirrhosis, which may be fatal, and immediate discontinuation of amiodarone is necessary if hepatic transaminases rise to greater than three times normal. Mild elevations of liver function tests rarely occur when plasma amiodarone levels are less than 2 μg/ml
- Photosensitivity, metallic taste, nausea, and vomiting
- Slate gray skin, rarely seen, is related to high loading and maintenance doses
- Nervous system effects are common, especially sleep disturbances, twitching, paresthesia that usually responds to decreased dosage
- Pulmonary infiltrates and alveolitis should occur in less than 1% of patients with modern conservative dosing schedules, but the patient should be warned of the risks and the need to obtain chest x-rays in the event that dyspnea develops
- High loading dose of 800 mg for 6 weeks followed by maintenance of 600 mg daily for several months has been shown to have toxicity in over 50% of patients: pulmonary infiltrates (5%), neurologic involvement (35%), abnormal liver function tests (20%) with high-dose therapy, and pulmonary toxicity may be seen as early as 1 to 3 months but may be delayed from 1 to 5 years. With low-dose therapy as outlined, adverse effects requiring withdrawal appear to occur in less than 25% of patients.

These effects are usually reversible within days to weeks of cessation of amiodarone therapy
- Severe hypotension during IV bolus injection is avoided by giving the drug as infusion over 1 to 2 hours, although IV infusion given over 30 minutes is often required for life-threatening arrhythmias

Monitoring necessary. Because of the high potential for adverse effects, the drug should be administered in the hospital or outpatient setting under close supervision. Monitor at 2 to 4 weeks for 2 to 4 months, assessing the following

- Serum potassium and magnesium levels: If a diuretic is necessary, ensure that a potassium-sparing diuretic is being used. In patients with heart failure on furosemide, supplemental potassium is necessary, or the use of amiloride adequately conserves potassium; also, amiloride has antiarrhythmic properties that appear useful in the suppression of VT
- ECG for bradyarrhythmias and QT prolongation
- Liver function tests
- Free T4, TSH, and T3
- Digoxin serum assay and the dose of digoxin should be halved. If oral anticoagulants are used concomitantly, the dosage should be halved and a close scrutiny of the international normalized ratio (INR) or prothrombin time is necessary
- Amiodarone and desethylamiodarone plasma levels
- Request chest x-rays at 3 and 6 months, then every 6 months or annually thereafter, or earlier if dyspnea occurs in order to detect pulmonary toxicity, peripheral and apical or bilateral diffuse interstitial or alveolar infiltrates. Baseline pulmonary function tests are advisable and should be repeated if pulmonary symptoms occur. Although the role of pulmonary function tests still appears doubtful, the cost of a baseline test is justifiable in patients who are given a potentially toxic agent that has proven benefits. A greater than 15% decrease in diffusion capacity assists in identifying patients who have amiodarone pulmonary toxicity if they are symptomatic. Since pulmonary function test results vary considerably, their routine use is not recommended in asymptomatic patients. Higher mean desethylamiodarone levels, but not amiodarone levels, are observed in patients who develop pulmonary toxicity. However, hepatic and neuromuscular adverse effects are related to high desethylamiodarone and amiodarone plasma levels
- Holter monitoring early in the course of therapy confirms arrhythmia suppression and is useful to screen for intermittent bradycardia

Bretylium

Dosage: For the management of recurrent VF, 5 mg/kg undiluted is given rapidly; increase, if needed, to 10 mg/kg. This bolus is followed by electrical defibrillation. Maintenance = 5 to 10 mg/kg every 8 hours. If the arrhythmia recurs and there is no hypotension, increase the dose to 10 mg/

kg. In hemodynamically stable patients, bretylium may be given diluted in 50 mg over 10 minutes or as a continuous infusion of 1 to 2 mg/minute (maximum dose = 30 mg/kg).

Action. This sympathetic ganglion-blocking agent concentrates in the terminal sympathetic neurons, producing a chemical sympathetectomy such that norepinephrine release is completely inhibited. Also, the drug has Class III activity in Purkinje's fibers, has no effect on phase 0, and does not prolong the action potential. Thus, repolarization time and increased QT interval do not occur. The drug increases VF threshold and has an antifibrillatory action. Bretylium may cause severe hypotension. The drug has a half-life of about 7 hours.

Indications

• For the management of recurrent VF refractory to electrical cardioversion and IV lidocaine. However, its use has now been largely superseded by amiodarone

Caution. The drug must not be given concomitantly with norepinephrine, epinephrine, or other sympathomimetics.

Adverse effects. Hypotension, nausea, and vomiting commonly occur.

OTHER ANTIARRHYTHMIC AGENTS
Amiloride

This agent is a diuretic that is commonly used in combination with a thiazide (Moduret, Moduretic). This guanidium compound has antifibrillatory and antiarrhythmic properties similar to bethanidine. Amiloride prolongs the action potential without altering phase 0. Amiloride appears to have beneficial effects in the management of some patients with sustained VT and is the diuretic of choice in patients who require a diuretic and when the combination with Class IA and Class III agents is necessary.

Dosage: 10 mg tablets once daily, increase if needed to 20 mg daily. Amiloride appears to have a low incidence of adverse effects and may have a role in patients with LV dysfunction treated with furosemide and amiodarone to control lethal arrhythmias. The addition of amiloride to furosemide enhances diuretic action but conserves potassium and magnesium.

BIBLIOGRAPHY

Akhtar M, Avitall B, Jazayeri M, et al.: Role of implantable cardioverter defibrillator therapy in the management of high-risk patients. Circulation, 85:(suppl I):I-131, 1992.
Akhtar M: Clinical spectrum of ventricular tachycardia. Circulation, 82:1561, 1990.
Albers WG, Atwood JE, Hirsh J, et al.: Stroke prevention in nonvalvular atrial fibrillation. Ann Intern Med, 115:727, 1991.

Alboni P, Ratto B, Cappato R, et al.: Clinical effects of oral theophylline in sick sinus syndrome. Am Heart J, *122*:1361, 1991.

Allen BJ, Brodsky MA, Capparelli EV: Magnesium sulfate therapy for sustained monomorphic ventricular tachycardia. Am J Cardiol 64:1202, 1989.

Antman EM, Beamer AD, Cantillon C, et al.: Therapy of refractory symptomatic atrial fibrillation and atrial flutter: A staged care approach with new antiarrhythmic drugs. J Am Coll Cardiol, *15*:698, 1990.

Arnold AZ, Mick MJ, Mazurek RP, et al.: Role of prophylactic anticoagulation for direct current cardioversion in patients with atrial fibrillation or atrial flutter. J Am Coll Cardiol, *19*:851, 1992.

Atié J, Brugada P, Brugada J, et al.: Clinical and electrophysiologic characteristics of patients with antidromic circus movement tachycardia in the Wolff-Parkinson-White syndrome. Am J Cardiol, *66*:1082, 1990.

Beckman KJ, Parker RB, Hariman RJ, et al.: Hemodynamic and electrophysiological actions of cocaine. Effects of sodium bicarbonate as an antidote in dogs. Circulation, *83*:1799, 1991.

Brennan FJ, Brien JF, Armstrong PW: Plasma concentration time course and pharmacological effects of a standardized oral amiodarone dosing regimen in humans. Can J Cardiol, *7*:117, 1991.

Brodsky M, Doria R, Allen B, et al.: New-onset ventricular tachycardia during pregnancy. Am Heart J, *123*:933, 1992.

Brugada P, Brugada J, Mont L, et al.: A new approach to the differential diagnosis of a regular tachycardia with a wide QRS complex. Circulation, *83*:1649, 1991.

Burkart F, Pfisterer M, Kiowski W, et al.: Effect of antiarrhythmic therapy on mortality in survivors of myocardial infarction with asymptomatic complex ventricular arrhythmias: Basel antiarrhythmic study of infarct survival (BASIS). J Am Coll Cardiol, *16*:1711, 1990.

Cairns, JA, Connolly SJ, Gent M, et al.: Post-myocardial infarction mortality in patients with ventricular premature depolarizations. Canadian Amiodarone Myocardial Infarction Arrhythmic Trial Pilot Study. Circulation, *84*:550, 1991.

Cairns JA, Connolly SJ: Nonrheumatic Atrial Fibrillation. Risk of stroke and role of antithrombotic therapy. Circulation, *84*:469, 1991.

Calkins H, Niklason L, Sousa J, et al.: Radiation exposure during radiofrequency catheter ablation of accessory atrioventricular connections. Circulation, *84*:2376, 1991.

Camm AJ, Sneddon JF: High-energy His bundle ablation, a treatment of last resort. Circulation, *84*:2187, 1991.

CAST Investigators (Cardiac Arrhythmia Suppression Trial): Preliminary report. Effect of encainide and flecainide on mortality in a randomized trial of arrhythmia suppression after myocardial infarction. N Engl J Med, *321*:406, 1989.

Chen P-S, Pressley JC, Tang ASL, et al.: New observations on atrial fibrillation before and after surgical treatment in patients with the Wolff-Parkinson-White syndrome. J Am Coll Cardiol, *19*:974, 1992.

Chesebro JH, Fuster V, Halperin JL: Atrial fibrillation - Risk marker for stroke. New Engl J Med, *323*:1556, 1990.

DiMarco JP, Miles W, Akhtar M, et al.: Adenosine for paroxysmal supraventricular tachycardia: Dose ranging and comparison with verapamil. Assessment in Placebo-Controlled, Multicenter Trials. Ann Intern Med, *113*:104, 1990.

Duff HF, Lestor WM, Rahmberg M: Amiloride. Antiarrhythmic and electrophysiological activity in the dog. Circulation, *78*:1469, 1988.

Duff HF, Mitchell LB, Kavanagh KM, et al.: Amiloride. Antiarrhythmic and electrophysiologic actions in patients with inducible sustained ventricular tachycardia. Circulation, *79*:1257, 1989.

Dusman RE, Stanton MS, Miles WM, et al.: Clinical features of amiodarone-induced pulmonary toxicity. Circulation, *82*:51, 1990.

Ellenbogen KA, O'Callaghan WG, Colavita PG, et al.: Wolff-Parkinson-White syndrome. Applied Cardiol, May/June: 21, 1986.

Fan W, Peter CT, Gang ES, et al.: Age-related changes in the clinical and electrophysiologic characteristics of patients with Wolff-Parkinson-White syndrome: Comparative study between young and elderly patients. Am Heart J, 122:741, 1991.

Friday KJ, Jackman WM, Lee IK, et al.: Sotalol-induced torsades de pointes successfully treated with hemodialysis after failure of conventional therapy. Am Heart J, 121:601, 1991.

Furberg CD, Yusuf S: Antiarrhythmics and VPD suppression. Circulation, 84:928, 1991.

Garratt C, Linker N, Griffith M, et al.: Comparison of adenosine and verapamil for termination of paroxysmal junctional tachycardia. Am J Cardiol, 64:1310, 1989.

Gettes LS: Electrolyte abnormalities underlying lethal and ventricular arrhythmias. Circulation, 85(suppl I):I-70, 1992.

Gonzales A, Sager PT, Akil B, et al.: Pentamidine-induced torsades de pointes. Am Heart J, 122:1489, 1991.

Greene HL, Roden DM, Katz RJ, et al.: The cardiac arrhythmia suppression trial: First CAST . . . then CAST-II. J Am Coll Cardiol, 19:894, 1992.

Guccione P, Paul T, Garson A: Long-term follow-up of amiodarone therapy in the young: Continued efficacy, unimpaired growth, moderate side effects. J Am Coll Cardiol, 15:1118, 1990.

Herre JM, Sauve MJ, Malone P, et al.: Long-term results of amiodarone therapy in patients with recurrent sustained ventricular tachycardia or ventricular fibrillation. J Am Coll Cardiol, 13:442, 1989.

Hohnloser SH, Meinertz T, Dammbacher T, et al.: Electrocardiographic and antiarrhythmic effects of intravenous amiodarone: Results of a prospective, placebo-controlled study. Am Heart J, 121:89, 1991.

Hood MA, Smith WM: Adenosine versus verapamil in the treatment of supraventricular tachycardia: A randomized double-crossover trial. Am Heart J, 123:1543, 1992.

Huang WKS, Tan de Guzman WL, Chenarides JG, et al.: Effects of long-term amiodarone therapy on the defibrillation threshold and the rate of shocks of the implantable cardioverter-defibrillator. Am Heart J, 122:720, 1991.

Kennedy HL: Late proarrhythmia and understanding the time of occurrence of proarrhythmia. Am J Cardiol, 66:1139, 1990.

Kerber RE, Kienzle MG, Olshansky B, et al.: Ventricular tachycardia rate and morphology determine energy and current requirements for transthoracic cardioversion. Circulation, 85:158, 1992.

Klein LS: Radiofrequency catheter ablation, safety and practicality. Circulation, 84:2594, 1991.

Knilans TK, Prystowsky EN: Antiarrhythmic drug therapy in the management of cardiac arrest survivors. Circulation, 85(suppl I):I-118, 1992.

Kuck K-H, Schlüter M: Single-catheter approach to radiofrequency current ablation of left-sided accessory pathways in patients with Wolff-Parkinson-White syndrome. Circulation, 84:2366, 1991.

Kubac G, Klinke WP, Grace M: Randomized double blind trial comparing sotalol and propranolol in chronic ventricular arrhythmia. Can J Cardiol, 4:355, 1988.

Lazzara R: Amiodarone and torsade de pointes. Ann Intern Med, 111:549, 1989.

Leclercq J-F, Coumel P, Denjoy I, et al.: Long-term follow-up after sustained monomorphic ventricular tachycardia: Causes, pump failure, and empiric antiarrhythmic therapy that modify survival. Am Heart J, 121:1685, 1991.

Lee MA, Morady F, Kadish A, et al.: Catheter modification of the atrioventricular junction with radiofrequency energy for control of atrioventricular nodal reentry tachycardia. Circulation, 83:827, 1991.

Lerman BB, Belardinelli L: Cardiac electrophysiology of adenosine. Circulation, 83:1499, 1991.

Levine JH, Mellitis ED, Baumgardner RA: Predictors of first discharge and subsequent survival in patients with automatic implantable cardioverter-defibrillator. Circulation, 84:558, 1991.

MacMahon S, Collins R, Peto R, et al.: Effects of prophylactic lidocaine in suspected acute myocardial infarction. An overview of results from the randomized, controlled trials. JAMA, 260:1910, 1988.

Marcus FI: The hazards of using type IC antiarrhythmic drugs for the treatment of paroxysmal atrial fibrillation. Am J Cardiol, *66*:366, 1990.

Mattioni TA, Zheutlin TA, Sarmiento JJ, et al.: Amiodarone in patients with previous drug-mediated torsades de pointes. Ann Intern Med, *111*:574, 1989.

McComb JM: Review. Clinical cardiac electrophysiology: The last 10 years. Int J Cardiol, *33*: 351, 1991.

Mehta AV, Chidambaram B: Efficacy and safety of intravenous and oral nadolol for supraventricular tachycardia in children. J Am Coll Cardiol, *19*:630, 1992.

Meissner MD, Akhtar M, Lehmann MH, et al.: Nonischemic sudden tachyarrhythmic death in atherosclerotic heart disease. Circulation, *84*:905, 1991.

Morganroth J, Bigger JT: Pharmacologic management of ventricular arrhythmias after the cardiac arrhythmia suppression trial. Am J Cardiol, *65*:1497, 1990.

Morganroth J, Goin JE: Quinidine-related mortality in the short-to-medium-term treatment of ventricular arrhythmias. A Meta-Analysis. Circulation, *84*:1977, 1991.

Moss AJ, Robinson J: Clinical features of the idiopathic long QT syndrome. Circulation, *85*(suppl I):I-140, 1992.

Myers M, Peter T, Weiss D, et al.: Benefit and risks of long-term amiodarone therapy for sustained ventricular tachycardia/fibrillation: Minimum of three-year follow-up in 145 patients. Am Heart J, *119*:8, 1990.

Nalos PC, Ismail Y, Pappas JM: Intravenous amiodarone for short-term treatment of refractory ventricular tachycardia or fibrillation. Am Heart J, *122*:1629, 1991.

Ochi RP, Goldenberg IF, Almquist A, et al.: Intravenous amiodarone for the rapid treatment of life-threatening ventricular arrhythmias in critically ill patients with coronary artery disease. Am J Cardiol, *64*:599, 1989.

O'Reilly M: Chronic use of acebutolol in the treatment of cardiac arrhythmias. Am Heart J, 4:1185, 1991.

Pitt B: The role of β-adrenergic blocking agents in preventing sudden cardiac death. Circulation, *85*(suppl I):1-107, 1992.

Pritchett EL, DaTorre SD, Platt ML: Flecainide acetate treatment of paroxysmal supraventricular tachycardia and paroxysmal atrial fibrillation: Dose-response studies. J Am Coll Cardiol, *17*:297, 1991.

Rankin AC, McGovern BA: Adenosine or verapamil for the acute treatment of supraventricular tachycardia? Ann Intern Med, *114*:513, 1991.

Rankin AC, Oldroyd KG, Chong E, et al.: Adenosine or adenosine triphosphate for supraventricular tachycardias? Comparative double-blind randomized study in patients with spontaneous or inducible arrhythmias. Am Heart J, *119*:316, 1990.

Rankin AC, Pringle SD, Cobbe SM, et al.: Amiodarone and torsades de pointes. Am Heart J, *120*:1482, 1990.

Rankin AC, Pringle SD, Cobbe SM: Acute treatment of torsades de pointes with amiodarone proarrhythmic and antiarrhythmic association of QT prolongation. Am Heart J, *119*:185, 1990.

Rossi AF, Burton DA: Adenosine in altering short- and long-term treatment of supraventricular tachycardia in infants. Am J Cardiol, *65*:685, 1989.

Rosenheck S, Sousa J, Calkins H, et al.: Comparison of the results of electrophysiologic testing after short-term and long-term treatment with amiodarone in patients with ventricular tachycardia. Am Heart J, *121*:1693, 1991.

Saksena S, Poczobutt-Johanos M, Castle LW, et al.: Long-term multicenter experience with a second-generation implantable pacemaker-defibrillator in patients with malignant ventricular tachyarrhythmias. J Am Coll Cardiol, *19*:490, 1992.

Salerno DM: Quinidine. Worse than adverse? Circulation, *84*:2196, 1991.

Schwartz PJ, Locati EH, Moss AJ, et al.: Left cardiac sympathetic denervation in the therapy of congenital long QT syndrome. Circulation, *84*:503, 1991.

Schlüter M, Kuck K-H: Catheter ablation from right atrium of anteroseptal accessory pathways using radiofrequency current. J Am Coll Cardiol, *19*:663, 1992.

Singh SN, Cohen A, Chen Y, et al.: Sotalol for refractory sustained ventricular tachycardia and nonfatal cardiac arrest. Am J Cardiol, 62:399, 1988.

Singh BN: When is QT prolongation antiarrhythmic and when is it proarrhythmic? Am J Cardiol, 63:867, 1989.

Stratmann HG, Kennedy HL: Torsades de pointes associated with drugs and toxins: Recognition and management. Am Heart J, 113:1470, 1987.

Suttorp MJ, Kingma JH, Jessurun ER: The value of Class IC antiarrhythmic drugs for acute conversion of paroxysmal atrial fibrillation or flutter to sinus rhythm. J Am Coll Cardiol, 16:1722, 1990.

The Boston Area Anticoagulation Trial for Atrial Fibrillation Investigators: The effect of low-dose warfarin on the risk of stroke in patients with nonrheumatic atrial fibrillation. New Engl J Med, 22:1505, 1990.

Tobé TJ, de Langen Lees DJ, Bink-Boelkens ME, et al.: Late potentials in a bradycardia-dependent long QT syndrome associated with sudden death during sleep. J Am Coll Cardiol, 19:541, 1992.

Tzivoni D, Banai S, Schuger C, et al.: Magnesium sulfate therapy for sustained monomorphic ventricular tachycardia. Circulation, 77:392, 1988.

Viskin S, Belbassen B: Acute management of paroxysmal atrioventricular junctional reentrant supraventricular tachycardia: Pharmacologic strategies. Am Heart J, 120:180, 1990.

Wang Y, Scheinman MM, Chien WW, et al.: Patients with supraventricular tachycardia presenting with aborted sudden death: Incidence, mechanism and long-term follow-up. J Am Coll Cardiol, 18:1711, 1991.

Weiss JN, Nademanee K, Stevenson WG, et al.: Ventricular arrhythmias in ischemic heart disease. Ann Intern Med, 114:784, 1991.

Wellens HJJ: Atrial flutter: Progress, but no final answer. J Am Coll Cardiol, 17:1235, 1991.

Wilson JS, Podrid PJ: Side effects from amiodarone. Am Heart J, 121:158, 1991.

Yee R, Klein GJ, Leitch JW, et al.: A permanent transvenous lead system for an implantable pacemaker cardioverter-defibrillator. Nonthoracotomy approach to implantation. Circulation, 85:196, 1992.

Zehender M, Hohnloser S, Müller B, et al.: Effects of amiodarone versus quinidine and verapamil in patients with chronic atrial fibrillation: Results of a comparative study and a 2-year follow-up. J Am Coll Cardiol, 19:1054, 1992.

Zipes DP: The long QT interval syndrome. A rosetta stone for sympathetic related ventricular tachyarrhythmias. Circulation, 84:1414, 1991.

7

CARDIAC ARREST
M. Gabriel Khan

Sudden cardiac death is defined as a sudden natural death caused by cardiac disease that is associated with the following

- An abrupt loss of consciousness within 1 hour of onset of acute symptoms
- Known or unknown preexisting heart disease
- Unexpected time and mode of death

Hinkle and Thaler classified cardiac death as

- Class I: An arrhythmic death if circulatory failure follows the disappearance of the pulse. In these situations, the nature of the terminal illness is an acute cardiac event in more than 98% of victims, and ventricular fibrillation (VF) or asystole has been observed to be the terminal event in approximately 83% and 17% of patients, respectively
- Class II: Circulatory failure death if the disappearance of the pulse is preceded by circulatory failure. This scenario is common in patients with terminal illnesses and usually is associated with a terminal bradyarrhythmia; asystole and VF have been observed in 67% and 33% of these patients, respectively

Cardiac arrest is defined as the abrupt cessation of cardiac pump function that will result in death, which may be averted if prompt intervention is instituted. A number of cardiac disorders cause lethal tachyarrhythmias or failure of formation or transmission of the cardiac impulse that results in cardiac arrest, but the mechanisms that initiate these fatal arrhythmias are mostly unknown and are diverse.

The basic cardiac causes of cardiac arrest include

- VF or pulseless ventricular tachycardia (VT): in at least 80%
- Asystole: 10%
- Electromechanical dissociation (EMD): 5%
- Myocardial rupture, cardiac tamponade, acute disruption of a major blood vessel, and acute mechanical obstruction to blood flow

The following underlying diseases or disturbances may result in cardiac arrest

287

- Approximately 75% of all cases of cardiac arrest involve the rupture of an atheromatous plaque with overlying thrombus, causing occlusion or distal embolization of a major coronary artery. Cardiac arrest in coronary disease may occur with little or no warning (plaque emboli), during the acute phase of myocardial infarction (MI) (occlusion), or later, caused by an arrhythmia circuit that may respond to trigger factors (catecholamines, ischemia, hypokalemia, critically timed VPCs) to precipitate VF. A history of ischemic heart disease is present in up to 50% of patients; in a significant number of these patients, atheromatous coronary disease is silent until the time of the event
- Aortic stenosis
- Hypertrophic cardiomyopathy
- Dilated cardiomyopathy
- Complete heart block or sinoatrial disease
- WPW syndrome in patients with very short refractory period of the bypass tract
- Torsades de pointes in patients taking antiarrhythmic drugs or in those with prolonged QT syndromes (congenital or acquired)
- Structural abnormalities such as pulmonary embolism, aortic dissection

Rarely, a sudden cardiac death due to electrical dysfunction occurs without discernible cardiac pathology (Primary Electrical Disease). Current information strongly indicates that coronary artery spasm, latent pre-excitation, and prolonged QT syndromes do not play a role in patients with idiopathic VF. Physical and mental stress appears to be implicated in less than 33% of cases of idiopathic VF.

Pathogenesis of the syndrome of sudden death during sleep in young, apparently healthy Southeast Asian males is undetermined and appears to be unrelated to idiopathic VF in "normal" hearts. Wellens, et al. suggest that because of the rarity of sudden arrhythmic death and the unexplained mechanisms in the absence of heart disease, a worldwide registry of these patients must be maintained.

"CHAIN OF SURVIVAL" CONCEPT

Although an emergency coronary care system designed to get the defibrillator promptly to the patient via emergency vehicles was devised and put into practice by Pantridge and Geddes in Belfast as long ago as 1966 (and was quickly accepted in the United States), the concept has only gradually gained acceptance in a number of countries. The AHA state-of-the-art review, "Improving Survival from Cardiac Arrest: The Chain of Survival Concept," is a timely one

- Early access
- Early cardiopulmonary resuscitation (CPR)
- Early defibrillation
- Early advanced care

Since prompt defibrillation is the single most effective lifesaving intervention for the majority of victims of cardiac arrest, the Advanced Cardiac

Life Support Subcommittee and the Emergency Cardiac Care Committee of the AHA have approved the widespread distribution of semiautomated external defibrillators, which are now required items in all ambulances or emergency vehicles engaged in the transit of cardiac patients. It is a logical approach to have these lifesaving devices in housing complexes, stadiums, and at all large public gatherings, shopping centers, etc. The AHA has endorsed the position that all first-responding hospital and nonhospital personnel (doctors, nurses, medical technicians, paramedics, firefighters, volunteer emergency personnel and several other categories in the population) be trained in the use of and be permitted to operate a defibrillator. Zipes indicates that the time to defibrillation and/or pacing may be shortened by developing external devices that incorporate the automatic approaches to arrhythmia recognition and therapy available in the multiprogrammable implantable pacemaker-cardioverter-defibrillator. These devices should become as accessible as fire extinguishers. A similar call for the widespread distribution of defibrillators was made by Pantridge and the late Dr. Grace in the early 1970s.

CARDIOPULMONARY RESUSCITATION

Unless immediate defibrillation is possible (for example, in the CCU), early CPR is essential. Importantly, late CPR and/or late advance support must be avoided. Although in Seattle up to 20% of prehospital VF patients survive, in other areas of the United States, less than 10% of all cardiac arrest patients in or out of the hospital survive and, unfortunately, up to 50% of these patients have been observed to have a neurologic deficit. Thus, unless the arrest is witnessed and CPR can be instituted within 4 minutes with a defibrillator available within 8 minutes, caution is necessary. If CPR cannot be instituted within 4 minutes, it is advisable to allow the patient to die in peace. In the elderly or in patients with noncardiac underlying disease such as stroke, terminal renal failure, cancer, or other chronic disease, the final arrhythmia is not unexpected and does not constitute true cardiac arrest. When appropriate in these situations, families and patients should be aware of the possibilities in advance.

CPR TECHNIQUE

- Rapidly establish that the patient is unconscious, unresponsive
- Promptly verify that the patient is not breathing
- Determine that the pulses are absent in the large arteries
- Immediately commence CPR (Fig. 7–1)

MANAGEMENT OF VENTRICULAR FIBRILLATION

Immediate defibrillation within 2 to 4 minutes of witnessed cardiac arrest and following either minimal or no CPR is the most important single therapy that may rescue patients in cardiac arrest, without producing tragic iatrogenic brain damage from attempting full CPR and the unavoidable hesitations that occur in many settings of cardiac arrest

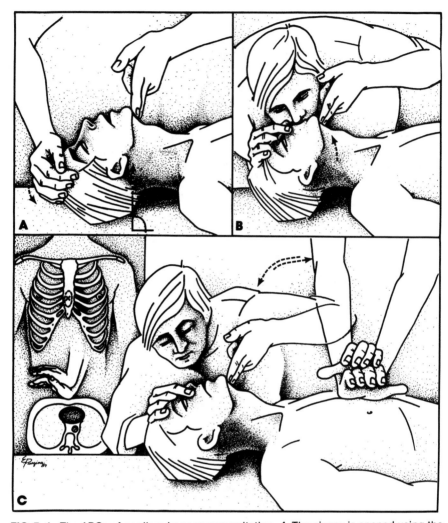

FIG. 7–1. The ABCs of cardiopulmonary resuscitation. *A.* The airway is opened using the heat tilt/chin lift technique. *B.* Breathing: the victim's nostrils are pinched closed and the rescuer breathes twice into the victim's mouth. *C.* Circulation: if no pulse is present, external chest compression is instituted at 80 to 100/minute. Two rescuers: 5 compressions to 1 ventilation. One rescuer: 15 compressions to 2 ventilations. Modified from: Khan M Gabriel: Cardiac Drug Therapy. 3rd Ed. London, W.B. Saunders, 1992.

- Turn the monitor power on
- Apply conductive medium to defibrillator paddles and evaluate rhythm with the "quick look" paddles
- If VF is present, turn defibrillator power on: be certain that the defibrillator is not in synchronous mode
- Select energy and charge the defibrillator

Apply quick look paddles or press analyze:* VF confirmed switch to defibrillator (DF)
Non-synchronized

Immediate		
1st shock	200 joules (J)	Check pulse, rhythm
		VF: CPR; recharge DF
2nd shock	300 J	VF persists: recharge DF
3rd shock	360 J	CPR
	Epinephrine 1 mg IV bolus	IV line, intubate
4th shock	360 J	VF: CPR, for 1 min (allow
	Lidocaine 100 mg IV	drug action)
5th shock	360 J	VF
	Epinephrine** 1 mg IV	VF persists, assess pH
6th shock	360 J	VF: CPR
	Lidocaine 50 mg IV	allow 2 min
7th shock	360 J	VF: arrest > 10 min ph < 7.1
	NaHCO₃ 50 mEq IV bolus	
8th shock	360 J	VF: CPR or Bretylium 5 mg/
	Lidocaine 50–75 mg IV bolus	kg allow 2–4 min
9th shock	360 J	Conversion successful
	Lidocaine 50 mg IV + simultaneous	
	infusion 2 mg/min.	

* Semi-automated external defibrillator.
** Repeat every 5 minutes.

FIG. 7–2. Management of VF or pulseless VT.

- Defibrillate using 200 joules (see Figure 7–2). During recharging the defibrillator or administration of IV bolus drugs, CPR must be continued. Immediate defibrillation for the patient with VF is the key to success; intubation, establishment of IV lines, and administration of medications should commence only if the first series of DC shocks fails to restore a spontaneous circulation

If a defibrillator is immediately available and defibrillation is achieved within 4 minutes of a cardiac arrest, longterm survival rates of 20 to 30% are possible. However, without prompt defibrillation, the survival rate ranges from 1 to 5% and is not acceptable.

Paramedic systems have been shown to achieve defibrillation in an average of 12 minutes, which is considered to be late defibrillation, resulting in about a 10% survival rate. Several countries and many communities in the United States have approved the use of semiautomated defibrillators by emergency medical technicians trained as first responders, after completion of a 40-hour training program. It is feasible to train ambulance personnel, firefighters, police officers, emergency volunteers, security guards, airline crews, designated attendants at stadiums, etc.

The operation of semiautomatic devices does not demand complex learning skills in rhythm analysis, and operation of the device can be mastered within hours. A single control activates the defibrillator to quickly analyze the cardiac rhythm, indicates that a shock is required, and on command, charges and delivers the shock.

In four communities in the United States, survival rates for patients in VF increased from an average of 4 to 18% with the use of emergency defibrillators by medical technicians.

DRUG THERAPY FOR CARDIAC ARREST

EPINEPHRINE

Epinephrine and other cardiac arrest drugs and their dosages are listed in Table 7–1. Salutary effects of epinephrine are

- Increased myocardial contractility
- Elevated perfusion pressure
- Possible conversion of EMD to electromechanical coupling
- Improved chances for defibrillation
- Improved blood flow to the heart and brain when sinus rhythm is restored

Epinephrine is the drug of first choice, administered as an initial 1-mg IV bolus after the third shock fails to defibrillate. Intracardiac epinephrine is not recommended, except when IV or intratracheal routes are not possible.

Failure to defibrillate should prompt the use of high-dose epinephrine (0.1 to 0.2 mg/kg). This dosage has been shown to be useful in establishing successful resuscitation, and many clinicians have switched to this regimen: 2, 4, 6, and 8 mg given at 1-minute intervals; the action of the drug is apparent within 1 minute.

A high dose of epinephrine is necessary to maintain adequate diastolic blood pressure in order to produce adequate coronary and cerebral perfusion. The drug produces peripheral arteriolar constriction and an increase in systemic vascular resistance, thus increasing aortic and coronary diastolic perfusion pressure. Also, coronary artery dilatation occurs. Some studies indicate that phenylephrine or methoxamine may be superior to epinephrine for the management of cardiac arrest.

Indications

- Fine VF is made coarse and more susceptible to removal by electrical countershock
- VF that fails to respond to countershock may respond following epinephrine
- Asystole and pulseless idioventricular rhythms
- Electromechanical dissociation

LIDOCAINE
(Lignocaine)

Lidocaine is given, after a fourth shock fails to defibrillate, as a 100-mg IV bolus followed, after about 1 minute of CPR, by a 360-joule shock. If defibrillation is successful, give a 50-mg bolus of lidocaine and an infusion

TABLE 7–1. CARDIAC ARREST DRUGS

DRUG	DOSAGE	SUPPLIED	COMMENT
Epinephrine	IV bolus 1 mg repeated q 5 min. Tracheobronchial 10 ml (1:10,000)	10 ml (1 mg in 1:10,000 dilution)	Do not give with $NaHCO_3$ in same IV
Sodium Bicarbonate	IV bolus 1 mEq (mmol)/kg, usually 50 mEq (mmol) initially; then ½ initial dose q 10 to 15 min	50 ml of 8.4% = 50.0 mEq (mmol) 1 Amp = 44 mEq	Not used routinely. Recommended for trial after 7th shock, pH <7.1, or 10 min. in asystole
Atropine	In asystole 1 mg q 2–5 min (max of 2.5 mg) Bradycardia 0.5 mg q 5 min to 2 mg	10 ml = 1 mg 5 ml = 0.5 mg (UK, 1 ml amp = 0.6 mg or 1 mg)	
Lidocaine	75–100 mg IV bolus simultaneous infusion 2–3 mg/ min	50 mg in 5 ml (1%) 100 mg in 10 ml (1%) 100 mg in 5 ml (2%)	
Bretylium Tosylate for VF	5 mg/kg IV bolus (undiluted). If countershock fails, repeat 10 mg/kg (max 30 mg/kg)	500 mg in 10 ml amp (UK 50 mg/ml; 2 ml amp)	Hypotension Do not give epinephrine or norepinephrine simultaneously
Propranolol for VF	USA: 1 mg over 2–5 min (q 2–5 min to max 5mg) UK: 1 mg over 2 min (q 2 min to max 5 mg)		Useful in recurrent VF if lidocaine fails
Calcium Chloride	2.5 to 5 ml 10% (5–7 mg/kg 250– 500 mg) IV bolus	10 ml 10% $CaCl_2$	Not recommended in cardiac arrest, except with hyperkalemia or post verapamil Do not give with $NaHCO_3$

q = every
Modified from: Khan, M Gabriel: Cardiac Drug Therapy. 3rd Ed. London, W.B. Saunders, 1992.

at 2 mg/min immediately (1 to 3 mg/min is the lower dose for the elderly or those with heart failure, see Tables 7–1, 3–8, and 3–9). An additional bolus is given 10 minutes later to maintain therapeutic lidocaine levels. Lidocaine is preferred to bretylium because trials have not shown bretylium to be superior and lidocaine does not produce severe hypotension, which is often seen with bretylium.

SODIUM BICARBONATE

This agent is no longer recommended for routine use during cardiac arrest of brief duration. However, after about 10 minutes of CPR and if a seventh shock fails to result in defibrillation, an IV bolus of sodium bicarbonate (50 mEq) is advisable. The drug should not be used simultaneously with calcium chloride or epinephrine. In the UK, sodium bicarbonate is usually given after failure of the fifth shock.

CALCIUM CHLORIDE

Calcium chloride is no longer recommended. The drug may be useful

- If asystole is caused by verapamil. Give 2.5 to 5 ml 10% calcium chloride or gluconate IV bolus
- In the management of hyperkalemia causing arrest
- The substance is, however, of no value in EMD

BRETYLIUM

Bretylium may be given if a third bolus of lidocaine fails. Give 5 mg/kg IV rapid bolus, then wait 2 to 4 minutes before attempting defibrillation. If conversion fails, give 10 mg/kg bolus, wait 5 to 10 minutes, and continue CPR before attempting further defibrillation because occasionally, bretylium may take 5 to 10 minutes to be effective. Unfortunately, by that time, the heart is likely to be atonic. As discussed in Chapter 6, the role of bretylium has appropriately dwindled with the availability of amiodarone.

AMIODARONE

Amiodarone is useful in the management of cardiac arrest. A 150- to 500-mg bolus over 5 to 10 minutes, followed by 10 mg/kg/24 hours (0.5 mg/ml) continuous infusion. Amiodarone is superior to bretylium and is advisable if it is necessary to continue resuscitative measures (see Chapter 6 for discussion on amiodarone).

BRADYARRHYTHMIAS - ASYSTOLE OR EMD

Severe symptomatic bradycardia is usually treated with atropine, 0.5 to 0.6 mg repeated every 2 minutes to a maximum of 2.4 mg. When atropine is used to treat asystole prior to pacing, a dose of 1 mg is given immediately, followed by an additional 1 mg after 2 minutes. In severe bradycardia or

AV block without a QRS complex, atropine is worth a trial. No harm can ensue, as if VF is precipitated by atropine; defibrillation may produce a stable rhythm to allow coronary perfusion prior to pacing. Be aware that VF may masquerade as asystole. Thus, rotate the monitoring electrodes and check the monitor to ensure that VF is not present. Give epinephrine with the hope that fibrillation may ensue, and then countershock.

Asystole in a heart that was beating forcefully minutes prior to the occurrence of asystole may complicate anterior infarction, and pacing may be lifesaving. However, asystole in the atonic heart (agonal) and EMD are usually due to irreversible myocardial damage and prognosis is very poor.

Management of EMD

- Commence CPR
- IV line
- Epinephrine (1 mg IV bolus)
- Intubate
- Assess for cardiac rupture and tamponade

Search for extracardiac causes of EMD

- Inadequate ventilation, including intubation of right main stem bronchus and tension pneumothorax
- Poor perfusion: Hypovolemia (jugular venous pressure decreased), give fluid challenge. If the JVP is markedly elevated, suspect cardiac tamponade or massive pulmonary embolism
- Severe acidosis or hyperkalemia

CPR should be continued with the hope that one of these factors may be correctible. Mobitz Type 2 block and complete heart block must be managed with ventricular pacing (see Chapter 18). If there is asystole or severe bradycardia unresponsive to atropine continue CPR, give epinephrine 1 mg IV or endotracheal and then 2, 4, 6, 8 mg at 1 minute intervals. If there is no response, consider pacing. For severe hypotension with mild bradycardia, dopamine is advisable (see Infusion Pump Chart, Table 16–6).

BIBLIOGRAPHY

Cobb LA, Eliastam M, Kerber, RE, et al.: Report of the American Heart Association Task Force on the future of cardiopulmonary resuscitation. Circulation, *85*:2346, 1992.

Cummins RO, Ornato JP, Thies WH, et al.: Improving survival from sudden cardiac arrest: The "Chain of Survival" concept. Circulation, *83*:1832, 1991.

Dimarco JP: Management of sudden cardiac death survivors: Role of surgical and catheter ablation. Circulation, *85*(suppl I):I-125, 1992.

Echt DS, Cato EL, Coxe DR: pH-Dependent effects of lidocaine on defibrillation energy requirements in dogs. Circulation, *80*:1003, 1989.

Forgoros RN, Elson JJ, Bonnet CA: Long-term outcome of survivors of cardiac arrest whose therapy is guided by electrophysiologic testing. J Am Coll Cardiol, *19*:780, 1992.

Gray WA, Capone RJ, Most AS: Unsuccessful emergency medical resuscitation—Are continued efforts in the emergency department justified? N Eng J Med, *325*:1393, 1991.

Hinkle LE, Thaler JH: Clinical classification of cardiac deaths. Circulation, *65*:457, 1982.

Hurwitz JL, Josephson ME: Sudden cardiac death in patients with chronic coronary heart disease. Circulation, *85*(suppl I):I-143, 1992.

Kerber RE: Statement on early defibrillation. From The Emergency Cardiac Care Committee, American Heart Association. Circulation, *83*:2233, 1991.

Lazzam C, McCans JL: Predictors of survival of in-hospital cardiac arrest. Can J Cardiol, *7*: 113, 1991.

Pantridge JF, Geddes JS: Cardiac arrest after myocardial infarction. Lancet, *i*:807, 1966.

Pantridge JF, Geddes JS: A mobile intensive-care unit in the management of myocardial infarction. Lancet, *ii*:271, 1967.

Ruskin JN: Role of invasive electrophysiological testing in the evaluation and treatment of patients at high risk for sudden cardiac death. Circulation, *85*(suppl I):I-152, 1992.

Schwartz PJ, La Rovere MT, Vanoli E: Autonomic nervous system and sudden cardiac death. Experimental basis and clinical observations for post-myocardial infarction risk stratification. Circulation, *85*(suppl I):I-77, 1992.

Viskin S, Belhassen B: Idiopathic ventricular fibrillation. Am Heart J, *120*:661, 1990.

Weaver WD: Resuscitation outside the hospital—What's lacking? N Eng J Med, *325*:1437, 1991.

Wellens HJJ, Lemery R, Smeets JL, et al.: Sudden arrhythmic death without overt heart disease. Circulation, *85*(suppl I):I-92, 1992.

Zipes DP: Sudden cardiac death. Furture Approaches. Circulation, *85*(suppl I):I-160, 1992.

8

HYPERLIPIDEMIA
M. Gabriel Khan

ELEVATED BLOOD CHOLESTEROL

A total blood cholesterol level less than 200 mg/dl (5.2 mmol/l) is considered desirable. Individuals with cholesterol levels greater than 350 mg/dl (9 mmol/l) are at high risk for the development of premature atheromatous occlusion of the coronary arteries and early manifestations of ischemic heart disease; fortunately, this scenario is uncommon and the attention given to familial hypocholesterolemia in the 1960s to early 1980s is being focused on mild and moderate elevations of blood cholesterol. However, recommendations concerning the management of borderline high blood cholesterol varies in different countries. The Canadian guidelines are not as aggressive as those of the United States, and the guidelines of the United Kingdom are even more conservative.

The recommendations of the Adult Treatment Panel of the National Cholesterol Education Program (NCEP) for Classification of Patients are listed in Table 8–1. Borderline high blood cholesterol levels are 200 to 239 mg/dl (5.17 to 6.18 mmol/l). Most heart attacks occur in individuals with levels between 210 and 240 mg/dl (5.5 to 6.2 mmol/l), and approximately 50% of adult Americans have cholesterol levels in this range. The average cholesterol level for North Americans is about 212 mg/dl (5.5 mmol/l). In these individuals with borderline high blood cholesterol, a low level of high density lipoprotein (HDL) cholesterol further increases the risk for coronary heart disease (CHD) (Fig. 8–1).

The emphasis, therefore, must be placed on the general population, in which mild to moderate elevation of total cholesterol associated with a low HDL cholesterol is a common health problem. Indeed, mild hypertension is a parallel marker and the conditions often coexist, thus increasing CHD risk, which is compounded by cigarette smoking in individuals who may have a "genetic," albeit unproven, predisposition to develop more intense atheromatous coronary occlusions than others with similar levels of cholesterol and blood pressure (Table 8–2).

A level of total cholesterol greater than 240 mg/dl (6.2 mmol/l) is considered high blood cholesterol. Approximately one-third of adult North Americans have high blood cholesterol and are at especially high risk for CHD.

297

TABLE 8-1. RECOMMENDATIONS OF THE ADULT TREATMENT PANEL OF THE NATIONAL CHOLESTEROL EDUCATION PROGRAM FOR CLASSIFICATION OF PATIENTS

CLASSIFICATION BASED ON TOTAL CHOLESTEROL	CLASSIFICATION BASED ON LDL CHOLESTEROL
<200 mg/dl (<5.17 mmol/l) Desirable blood cholesterol	<130 mg/dl (<3.36 mmol/l) Desirable LDL cholesterol
200–239 mg/dl (5.17–6.18 mmol/l) Borderline-high blood cholesterol	130–159 mg/dl (3.36–4.11 mmol/l) Borderline–high-risk LDL cholesterol
≥240 mg/dl (≥6.21 mmol/l) High blood cholesterol	≥160 mg/dl (≥4.13 mmol/l) High-risk LDL cholesterol

LDL: low density lipoprotein
From the National Cholesterol Education Program, Adult Treatment Panel, January 1988.
From: Carleton RA, et al.: Report of the expert panel on population strategies for blood cholesterol reduction. Circulation, *83*:2161, 1991.

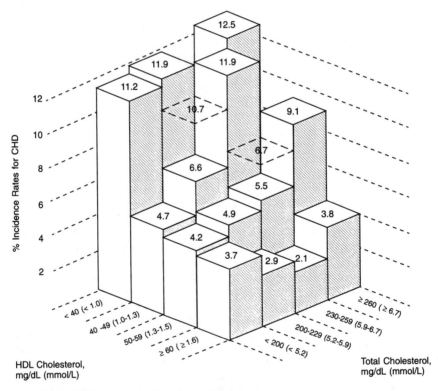

FIG. 8-1. Incidence of coronary heart disease (CHD) in 4 years by high-density lipoprotein cholesterol (HDL-C) and total plasma cholesterol level for men and women free of cardiovascular disease. Modified from: Castelli WP, et al.: Incidence of coronary heart disease and lipoprotein cholesterol levels. The Framingham Study. JAMA, *256*:2837, 1986.

TABLE 8–2. CHD RISK FACTORS OTHER THAN LDL CHOLESTEROL
• Male sex • Family history of premature CHD (definite myocardial infarction or sudden death before age 55 in a parent or sibling) • Cigarette smoking • Hypertension • Low HDL cholesterol concentration (below 35 mg/dl, 0.9 mmol/l confirmed by repeat measurement) • Diabetes mellitus • History of definite cerebrovascular or occlusive peripheral vascular disease • Severe obesity (≥30% overweight)

CHD: coronary heart disease; LDL: low density lipoprotein; HDL: high density lipoprotein.
From: The National Cholesterol Education Program Report of the Expert Panel on Detection, Evaluation, and Treatment of High Blood Cholesterol in Adults. United States Department of Health and Human Services, Public Health Service, National Heart, Lung and Blood Institute. Publication No. (NIH) 88-2925 Bethesda, MD, 1988 (with permission).

The Framingham Study indicated that post-infarction patients with cholesterol levels greater than 7.11 mmol/l (274 mg/dl) were at increased risk for reinfarction, death from CHD, and mortality when compared to patients with cholesterol levels below 5.17 mmol/l (200 mg/dl). Intermediate cholesterol levels of 5 to 7 mmol/l generally were not associated with increased risk.

LOW DENSITY LIPOPROTEIN CHOLESTEROL

The low density lipoprotein (LDL) cholesterol is the main culprit in CHD, but its measurement is more costly than that of total cholesterol. While total cholesterol can be measured in the nonfasting state, the measurement of LDL cholesterol requires a 12- to 14-hour fasting specimen for accurate determination of the triglyceride level, which is required for the estimation of the LDL cholesterol. An LDL cholesterol less than 130 mg/dl (3.36 mmol/l) is desirable, 130 to 159 mg/dl (3.36 to 4.11 mmol/l) is considered borderline high risk, and a level greater than 160 mg/dl (4.13 mmol/l) is considered high risk (see Table 8–1). It must be reemphasized that a greater than 12-hour fasting specimen is necessary because triglyceride estimation must be performed in the fasting state.

The LDL cholesterol is derived as follows:

LDL (mg/dl) = total cholesterol − HDL − (triglyceride ÷ 5)
LDL (mmol/l) = total cholesterol − HDL − (triglyceride ÷ 2.2)

If the triglyceride value is above 400 mg/dl (4 mmol/l), LDL cholesterol estimation using the above formula is not accurate.

HIGH DENSITY LIPOPROTEIN CHOLESTEROL

Table 8–2 lists CHD risk factors, other than LDL cholesterol. An HDL cholesterol level is vital in decision-making concerning the management of hyperlipidemia. Data from the Framingham Study indicate that the mortality risk from CHD increases as HDL cholesterol levels decrease. The average risk of mortality from CHD is at a level of 40 mg/dl (1 mmol/l). Every 1% increase in HDL cholesterol decreases CHD risk by about 2%, and each 1% reduction in total cholesterol should produce a 2% reduction in CHD risk. The Framingham 4-year surveillance study data illustrated in Figure 8–1 show the joint predictive impact of HDL cholesterol and total plasma cholesterol in the incidence of CHD in patients over age 49. The HDL cholesterol shows a strong inverse association with incidence of CHD at all levels of total cholesterol including levels under 200 mg/dl (5.2 mmol/l). The 12-year follow-up indicates that the relationship does not diminish appreciably with time. The study confirms that nonfasting HDL cholesterol and total cholesterol are related to development of CHD in both men and women over age 49.

The HDL cholesterol, as well as total cholesterol, is not affected by food eaten within prior hours; thus, a nonfasting specimen is not required. Importantly, a nonfasting specimen allows the sample to be taken immediately after the physician consultation and saves the time and cost of a return visit to a laboratory. The HDL estimation is recommended if the initial total cholesterol level is greater than 200 mg/dl (5.2 mmol/l). A CHD relative risk is less than 0.5 if the total cholesterol is 220 mg/dl and the HDL cholesterol is greater than 85 mg/dl (2.2 mmol/l), but the risk increases to 2.5 with an HDL cholesterol less than 35 mg/dl (0.9 mmol/l). Thus, an HDL level between 55 and 85 mg/dl (1.4 to 2.2 mmol/l) is desirable, a level less than 35 mg/dl (0.9 mmol/l) is undesirable.

TOTAL CHOLESTEROL/HDL RATIO

A total cholesterol/HDL ratio greater than 4.5 is associated with increased risk of CHD. Most agree that a ratio greater than 6 requires action. The total cholesterol to HDL ratio is important but is not always as reliable as the individual values of total cholesterol, LDL, and HDL.

ELEVATED BLOOD TRIGLYCERIDES

Triglyceride-rich, very low density lipoproteins (VLDL) are secreted by the liver. The VLDL surface coat contains apolipoprotein (apo) B and other lipoproteins. VLDL triglycerides undergo hydrolysis by lipoprotein lipase. VLDL remnants have one or two fates

- Direct removal by the liver
- Degradation into LDL by lipolytic removal of remaining triglycerides

Triglyceride levels greater than 300 to 500 mg/dl (3 to 5 mmol/l) are considered borderline and levels greater than 500 mg/dl (5 mmol/l) are considered high. A positive role for high triglyceride levels in CHD still remains to be proven. The association is weak; thus, triglycerides are not routinely measured as a screening test. Since increased triglyceride and low levels of HDL cholesterol are closely associated, the independent contribution of triglyceride disappears once the risk of HDL has been taken into account.

INVESTIGATIONS AND DECISION-MAKING

Request a nonfasting total cholesterol level, since it is the most cost-effective method of screening and is sufficient for initial estimation of cardiovascular risk. Total cholesterol is the only test recommended by the expert panel of NCEP for screening programs. It must be reemphasized that food has no immediate effect on total cholesterol for HDL measurements, so fasting is not necessary for their determination. Also, the nonfasting request saves time and cost.

For population screening, guidelines are as follows

- Total cholesterol less than 200 mg/dl (5.2 mmol/l), a repeat test is recommended in about 5 years
- Total cholesterol 200 to 240 mg/dl (5.2 to 6.2 mmol/l). These individuals may be regular patients or referred from community screening programs; the physician must be aware of the guidelines and procedure for further assessment

The estimation for total cholesterol is repeated, along with HDL, in a nonfasting state at some time in the following months. If this confirms borderline high cholesterol, the patient is called in for an assessment. If the HDL cholesterol is less than 35 mg/dl (0.9 mmol/l) or two or more risk factors (as outlined in Table 8–2) are present, the steps outlined below should be followed before proceeding with treatment.

Total serum cholesterol greater than 240 mg/dl (6.2 mmol/l): request a full lipid analysis (total, LDL, and HDL cholesterol and triglyceride) with the patient fasting 14 hours.

Although dietary advice is always given, it is necessary to exclude underlying causes for hyperlipidemia before proceeding to therapy.

DETERMINE THE CAUSE OF HYPERLIPIDEMIA

DIETARY FACTORS

Total cholesterol levels from 200 to 320 mg% (5.2 to 8.3 mmol/l) result from a complex interaction of polygenic and environmental factors. Although it is often assumed that excess dietary saturated fat intake is a major cause of elevated cholesterol levels, there is evidence that genetics is an important factor in most cases.

A dietary history of increased saturated fat and/or total cholesterol intake must be ascertained.

UNDERLYING DISEASES

Relevant underlying disease must be defined and controlled. Diabetes mellitus, hypothyroidism, pancreatitis, nephrotic syndrome, obstructive jaundice, biliary cirrhosis, and dysproteinemia may be implicated in a minority of patients. In these patients, a thorough physical examination should record the presence or absence of xanthelasma of the eyelids, xanthoma tendinosum, tuberosum, and planum. These lesions are mainly observed in patients with familial genetic severe hyperlipidemia, which is rare. Approximately 0.1% of the general population has a genetic abnormality characterized by cellular LDL receptor deficiency. These patients are at very high risk for development of premature IHD. Total cholesterol is often in the range of 350 to 1,000 mg/dl (9 to 25 mmol/l). If the situation is suspected, screen first-degree relatives, parents, siblings, and children.

MEDICATIONS

Hormones, estrogens, progestins, contraceptive pills, and anabolic steroids commonly alter lipid levels. In a menopausal woman, hormone deficiency will increase total cholesterol. Replacement therapy with premarin (0.625 mg), along with dietary measures, may suffice. Importantly, replacement hormone increases HDL cholesterol levels.

Diuretics (thiazides) may cause a mild elevation in total cholesterol (1 to 4%) and a slight lowering of HDL (approximately 1 to 10%). This effect is minimal, however, and occurs in less than 10% of individuals. Chronic treatment for more than 2 years usually produces no significant elevation in total cholesterol or decrease in HDL, and modest changes have been exaggerated.

Except for the documented significant increase in triglycerides, the longterm effects of beta-adrenergic blockers on HDL cholesterol have been poorly studied. Beta blockers, with the exception of those with intrinsic sympathomimetic activity (ISA), increase triglyceride levels from 10 to 30%. However, the evidence linking triglycerides to an increased risk of CHD is extremely weak and is considered unproven. It is clear that LDL cholesterol is not increased by beta blockers.

Longterm effects of beta blockers on HDL cholesterol are conflicting. Results of several studies evaluating the effect of beta blockers on HDL cholesterol have not been consistent. The pooled results of clinical trials published in 1989 include studies using few patients followed for 1 to 9 months. Table 8–3 shows beta blocker effects on lipid profile in patients followed up to 1 year. In one study of eight patients administered 400 mg acebutolol daily, a 13% decrease in HDL cholesterol was observed at 6 months, but at 1 year, the decrease was only 2%. Pooled results of 15 trials published prior to 1988 reveal that acebutolol increased HDL levels versus placebo by approximately 1.5%. Evidence to support the relatively neutral lipid effect of ISA beta blockers was provided by the Treatment of Mild Hypertension Study (TOMHS); acebutolol (400 mg) administered daily to 77 patients caused no significant change in HDL after 1 year of therapy.

Metoprolol has shown no effect on HDL in one well-run study and a decrease of 6% in another.

There is little doubt that beta blockers with mild ISA administered longterm cause no significant changes in HDL, LDL, or total cholesterol. Undoubtedly, mild ISA is not harmful to the cardiovascular system. Acebutolol, which has mild ISA, caused a 48% decrease in post-infarction mortality in patients followed for 10 months. In patients with hyperlipidemia, therefore, acebutolol is the beta blocker of choice.

TABLE 8–3. BETA-ADRENERGIC BLOCKER EFFECTS ON LIPID PROFILE				
	PERCENTAGE CHANGE			
BETA BLOCKER	HDL	LDL	Total Cholesterol	Triglyceride
Acebutolol				
15 studies to 1988	↑ 1.5			
TOMHS trial	NS		↓ 7	
8 patients*	↓ 2	↓ 8	7	↑ 7
Atenolol				
87 patients*	↓ 14	NS	NS	↑ 38
Metoprolol				
pooled trials	↓ 0–6	NS	NS	↑ 0–10
Propranolol				
46 patients*	↓ 13	NS	NS	
BHAT	↓ 6			
pooled trials	↓ 6	NS	NS	↑ 20
Pindolol				
pooled	↑ 1–5	NS	↓ 2	↓ 7

     * = 1-year study
   NS = No significant change
TOMHS = Treatment of mild hypertension study
 BHAT = Beta Blockers Heart Attack Trial
    ↑ = Increase
    ↓ = Decrease

DIETARY MANAGEMENT

Dietary modification is expected to decrease an elevated blood cholesterol by 7 to 15%, depending on the degree of adherence to a low saturated fat, low cholesterol diet and the previous intake of these substances. Some individuals have a marked increase in total cholesterol in response to dietary cholesterol, whereas in others, an increase in saturated fat or cholesterol intake has little or no effect. Of interest is the report of an 88-year-old man who consumed 25 eggs daily for over 50 years with maintenance of a normal serum cholesterol level. This is a common story relayed by many elderly individuals who may have sustained a very high intake of cholesterol and saturated fats over prolonged periods. In some individuals, a decrease in cholesterol absorption, an increased transformation, and excretion of bile acid serve to maintain total cholesterol in the desired range. Also, conversion of cholesterol to bile acid activates an upregulation of LDL receptor activity, permitting further clearance of blood cholesterol. Thus, genetic differences in response to the amount of dietary saturated fat appear to be important, and hypercholesterolemic individuals appear to be more sensitive to its presence.

Dietary change brings about a salutary effect in only some individuals, but a consistent effort must be made to enforce the change, especially because drug therapy entails costs and risks of adverse effects and because compliance is poor with the use of bile acid sequestrants, fibrates, or nicotinic acid. Fortunately, elevations of triglycerides are virtually always controlled by restriction of carbohydrates and alcohol, weight reduction, and exercise.

Several clinical trials have documented the effect of the dietary approach in significantly reducing total cholesterol. Approximately 28% of Americans with elevated total cholesterol appear to respond to dietary cholesterol and saturated fat restriction with a 10 to 15% decrease in cholesterol. In London, the incidence of hypercholesterolemia and response to diet appear to be similar to that observed in Americans. The number of civil servants in London with cholesterol levels less than 200 mg/dl (5.2 mmol/l) rose from 5 to 29% with a simple cholesterol-lowering diet. The average level of cholesterol while following the diet was approximately 220 mg%, with an approximately 10% salutary response to diet.

The following dietary plan is adapted from the 1991 Report of the Expert Panel on Population Strategies for Blood Cholesterol Reduction.

STEP 1 THERAPEUTIC DIET

The Expert Panel recommends the following

- An average of 30% or less of total calories from total fat
- Saturated fatty acids should not exceed 10% of total calories
- 20% of total calories should be derived from the combination of polyunsaturated fatty acids and monounsaturated fatty acids. Polyunsaturated fatty acids should not exceed 10% of total calories. Since the average diet of an adult male living in North America contains approximately 36% calories from fat, a reduction of 6 to 7% is feasible and allows dietary calorie levels adequate to maintain a desirable body weight
- Less than 300 mg cholesterol daily
- Carbohydrates 50 to 60% of total calories
- Protein 10 to maximum 15% of calories
- Avoid: organ meats such as liver, kidney, sweetbreads, heart, or brain; heavily marbled steaks, salt pork, or duck; whole milk or whole milk products, cream, lard, and nonvegetable margarine; coconut oil or products containing coconut oil (such as nondairy creamers), palm oil, peanut oil, rapeseed oil, or peanut butter (see Table 8–4)
- Use sparingly: luncheon meat, sausage, bacon, hamburger, spare ribs, butter, cheese made from whole milk or cream, pie, chocolate pudding, ice cream, or whole milk pudding. One egg yolk contains about 225 to 250 mg cholesterol, depending on the size of the egg. Thus, four to five eggs per week should suffice for adequate nutrition as well as enjoyment. Lobster should be used without abundant butter. Nuts to avoid include cashews, peanuts and Brazil nuts
- Recommended foods: fruits, whole grain products, beans, peas, vegetables, cereals; low-fat dairy products, including skim or low-fat milk, skim or low-fat butter (skim milk is a good source of calcium); fish such as salmon, mackerel, tuna, or cod, which contain an abundance of omega-3 fatty acids; moderate amounts of chicken without skin and lean red meat (up to 6 oz.) two or three times weekly. Shrimp contain a fair

TABLE 8–4. SATURATED FAT AND CHOLESTEROL CONTENT OF FOODS

ITEM	CHOLES-TEROL (mg)	TOTAL FAT (g)	SATU-RATED FAT (g)	NOT RECOM-MENDED	**RECOM-MENDED	USE SPAR-INGLY
MEATS						
beef liver	395	10	3		X	
kidney	725	11	4		X	
sweetbread	420	21	–		X	
lean beef	82	5	2			**
roast beef						
e.g., rib	85	33	14	X		¢
rump	85	21	9		X	
stewing	82	27	11	X		¢
" lean	82	9	4			**
ground	85	18	8	X		¢
steak						
sirloin	85	25	10	X		¢
" lean	85	5	2			**
veal	90	12	5			**
lamb, lean	90	7	4			¢
chop & fat	110	33	18		X	
ham						
fat roasted	80	28	7		X	
boiled						
sliced	80	18	5			¢
pork chop	80	30	12		X	
chicken						
breast & skin	72	6	1			**
drumstick	80	9	2			**
(fried)						
turkey	80	5	2			**
FISH						
sole	45	1	trace			**
trout	50	13	3			**
tuna	60	7	2			**
salmon						
fresh	42	7	1			**
canned	32	11	2			**
mackerel	85	10	2			**
halibut	54	6	trace			**
crabmeat	91	1	trace			¢
shrimp	130	1	trace			¢
lobster (450 g)	80	1	trace			¢
DAIRY PRODUCTS						
30 ml butter	460	25	16		X	
egg (50 g)	275	6	2			¢
substitute	0	0	0		**	
buttermilk†	10	2	1			
yogurt (250 ml)	16	3	2			**
whole milk						
250 ml	35	9	5			¢
2%	20	5	3			**
skim milk	trace	trace	trace			**
ice cream						
vanilla reg. (125ml)	32	8	5			¢
rich (125 ml)	46	12	8		X	

TABLE 8–4. (*cont.*)

ITEM	CHO- LES- TEROL (mg)	TOTAL FAT (g)	SATU- RATED FAT (g)	POLY- UNSAT- URATED	NOT RECOM- MENDED	**REC- OM- MENDED	USE SPAR- INGLY
butter	30	11	7	trace			¢
lard	12	13	5	1	X		
cheese (1 oz)							
brick	27	8	6	trace			¢
blue	24			"		¢	
cheddar	30	10	6	"			¢
cottage†	2	.6	.5	"		**	
skim milk,	0	trace	trace	trace		**	
processed,							
1 oz (30 g)							
OILS							
corn oil	0	14	1	7		**	
rapeseed	0	14	1	3	X		
safflower	0	13	1	10		**	
sunflower	0	14	1	9		**	
soyabean	0	14	2	7		**	
coconut	0	14	12	.2	X		
palm	0		7	.2	X		
olive	0	14	2	1		**	
peanut		14	2	4	X		
NUTS							
almonds	0	16	1	3		**	
brazil nuts	0	22	5	8	X		
cashews	0	13	3	2	X		
coconut	0	13	11	trace	X		
peanuts	0	17	3	4	X		
peanut butter	0	7.5	1.5	2	X		
pecans	0	21	2	5			¢
walnuts	0	19	2	11		**	

* Quantity is 3 oz (90 g) unless specified; 15 ml = one tablespoonful.
** Foods recommended contain less than 5 g saturated fat per 3 oz
† Low-fat milk, 2%.
From: Khan, M Gabriel: Is cholesterol important again? *In* Heart Attacks, Hypertension and Heart Drugs. Toronto, McClelland-Bantam Inc., 1990. By permission of McClelland-Bantam Inc.

amount of cholesterol but no saturated fatty acids, provided that they are not fried in a batter. Vegetable oils such as safflower, sunflower, soybean, corn, and olive oil are recommended, but coconut, palm, rapeseed, and peanut oils are not. Walnuts contain a high amount of polyunsaturated fatty acid but are low in saturated fat. Oat bran has little specific cholesterol-lowering effect and is not superior to low fiber dietary grain supplements

STEP 2 THERAPEUTIC DIET

• An average of 25% of total calories (or less) from total fat
• Less than 7% of total calories from saturated fat
• Cholesterol 200 to 250 mg daily

The Step 2 diet is recommended for patients with cholesterol elevated to 275 to 310 mg/dl (7.1 to 8 mmol/l) after a 6-month to 1-year trial of the Step 1 diet. The Step 2 diet is, therefore, mainly required for patients with severe familial hyperlipidemia in conjunction with drug therapy.

DRUG THERAPY

Drugs are utilized only after an adequate trial of dietary therapy, a concerted effort by the patient and physician, and/or the assistance of a dietician or lipid clinic fail to adequately lower total cholesterol or LDL cholesterol to the desired level. Figure 8–2 shows appropriate guidelines for the management of elevated blood cholesterol.

Because of the uncertain potential for longterm effects of medications, pharmacologic treatment is usually reserved for patients with severe familial hyperlipidemia and for other cases of hypercholesterolemia when 6-month dietary management and weight reduction produce an inadequate response. When drugs are prescribed, dietary restrictions must be continued. Dietary therapy can achieve only about a 10% lowering of total cho-

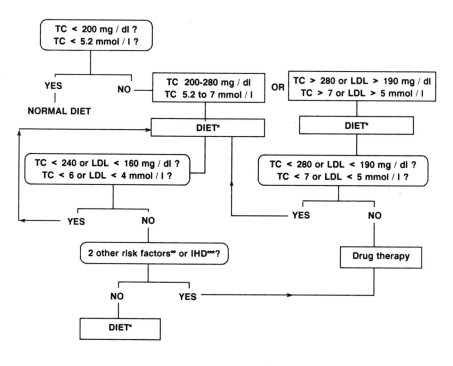

TC	= Total Cholesterol
*	= Step one therapeutic diet, see text
**	= Table 8-2
***	= Presence of coronary angioplasty or bypass surgery
IHD	= Ischemic heart disease

FIG. 8–2. Guidelines for management of high total or LDL cholesterol.

lesterol but can reduce triglyceride levels in most individuals from 25 to 50%.

The United States Expert Panel on Detection, Evaluation and Treatment of High Blood Cholesterol in Adults recommends that drug therapy be considered in the following situations

- LDL cholesterol equal to or greater than 190 mg/dl (5 mmol/l) or a total cholesterol greater than 280 mg/dl (7 mmol/l)
- LDL cholesterol greater than 160 mg/dl (4 mmol/l) or total cholesterol greater than 240 mg/dl (6.2 mmol/l) and the presence of two or more risk factors (Table 8–2)
- LDL cholesterol greater than 160 mg/dl (greater than 4 mmol/l) and manifestations of CHD: angina, MI, the presence of previous coronary angioplasty or coronary artery bypass surgery

Since it is difficult for the human brain to recall decimals, the important numbers to remember for LDL cholesterol, 4.13 and 4.9 mmol/l, have been altered to 4 and 5 mmol/l (Fig. 8–2).

Some lipidologists advise drug therapy for LDL cholesterol greater than 3.4 mmol/l (130 mg/dl) in patients who have angina or who have had a heart attack, coronary angioplasty, or bypass surgery.

HMG-CoA REDUCTASE INHIBITORS

Available agents include lovastatin, simvastatin, and pravastatin. These agents are competitive inhibitors of 3-hydroxy-3-methylglutaryl coenzyme A (HMG-CoA) reductase, the enzyme catalyzing the early rate limiting step in the biosynthesis of cholesterol, conversion of HMG-CoA to mevalonate. A modest reduction in intracellular cholesterol occurs, resulting in an increase in the number of hepatic LDL receptors that bring about clearance of circulating LDL cholesterol. In a well-designed, randomized study of 2,845 individuals, lovastatin caused a 24 to 40% decrease in LDL cholesterol, a 17 to 29% decrease in serum cholesterol, a 10 to 19% decrease in triglyceride level, and an increase of 6.6 to 9.5% in HDL level at dosages of 20 mg and 80 mg daily over a 48-week period. The LDL cholesterol goal of 160 mg/dl (4 mmol/l) was achieved in 80 and 96% of those treated with 20 mg and 80 mg, respectively. These agents cause no significant changes in triglyceride levels; a modest decrease (if any) may be observed. In the 48-week Expanded Clinical Evaluation of Lovastatin (EXCEL) Study of 8,245 patients with total cholesterol levels of 240 to 300 mg/dl (6.2 to 7.8 mmol/l) and LDL cholesterol greater than 160 mg/dl (4.1 mmol/l), the average changes from baseline for lovastatin (20, 40, and 80 mg daily) were −24%, −32%, and −40% for LDL cholesterol and 6.6, 7.9, and 9.5% for HDL cholesterol. The 20-mg twice-daily dose produced a more favorable trend compared to 40 mg each evening for both LDL and HDL cholesterol. An increase in the frequency of muscle symptoms with creatine kinase elevations was seen only in the 80-mg-daily group.

Some regression and prevention of progression of atheroma have been observed with the use of HMG-CoA reductase inhibitors.

Lovastatin
(Mecavor)

Supplied: tablets; 10, 20, 40 mg

Dosage: 10 to 20 mg given as a single dose with the evening meal. Increase, if needed, to 20 mg twice daily after checking for efficacy and for increased hepatic transaminases and creatine kinase elevation. The physician should endeavor not to exceed a dose of 60 mg daily, given as 20 mg with breakfast and 40 mg with the evening meal. The manufacturer's maximum of 80 mg daily is advisable if a trial of a combination of lovastatin (60 mg) and a bile acid resin fails to attain therapeutic goals. The 40-mg dose is expected to decrease LDL cholesterol by about 30%; a 60 or 80 mg dose is expected to cause a 35 and 40% reduction in LDL cholesterol.

Contraindications
- Women of childbearing age
- Pregnancy
- Breastfeeding
- Hepatic disease
- Concomitant use of cyclosporin, erythromycin, or other cytotoxic drugs
- Concomitant use of nicotinic acid or fibrates
- Porphyria
- Patients with myopathy or individuals engaging in strenuous physical exertion
- Patients under age 18

Adverse effects. Headaches in about 10%, stomach pain, flatulence, diarrhea, constipation, nausea, hepatic dysfunction with increased hepatic transaminases (2%), chest pain due to stomach disturbance or muscular aches. A flu-like illness with myalgia, elevation of creatine kinase, myopathy (0.5%), and rhabdomyolysis has been observed in patients receiving concomitant niacin, gemfibrozil, other fibrates, cyclosporin, and other immunosuppressive drugs. Lens opacity observed in animals given high doses has not been a clinical problem, although minor lens opacification occurs. Rash is uncommon. Baseline transaminase, creatine kinase, and opthalmology assessment are advisable. If more than a twofold increase in transaminases occurs, the drug should be discontinued.

Caution. Avoid in renal transplant patients on cyclosporin or immunosuppressives. In patients receiving oral anticoagulants, reduction in the dose of warfarin is usually required. Severe myositis may cause hyperkalemia in patients with renal insufficiency, particularly including long-standing diabetics who are also on ACE inhibitors.

Simvastatin
(Zocor)

Supplied: 5, 10, 20, 40 mg

Dosage: 5 to 10 mg with the evening meal, increase if needed in 8 to 12 weeks to 20 mg daily to a maximum of 40 mg once daily. Twice-daily dosing provides no added benefit. This is the most potent HMG-CoA reductase inhibitor because of its binding affinity for the reductase enzyme. Adverse effects and contraindications are the same as those for lovastatin. No effect on lens transluency has been observed.

Pravastatin
(Pravachol; Lipostat, UK)

Supplied: tablets; 10, 20 mg

Dosage: 10 mg with the evening meal, increase over 2 to 4 months to a maximum of 40 mg once daily or 20 mg twice daily. Contraindications are the same as those outlined for lovastatin. Adverse effects are similar, but hyperuricemia, urinary frequency, thrombocytopenia, leukopenia, and leukocytosis have been observed, albeit rarely. No lens disturbances have been recorded.

Pravastatin is a hydrophilic compound and has primarily a hepatic site of action with little influence on cholesterol synthesis in other tissues. The fact that it does not cause cataracts in dogs at 100 mg/kg is probably related to its hydrophilic property. Contraindications and adverse effects are similar to those listed for lovastatin.

CONCOMITANT THERAPY: HMG-CoA REDUCTASE INHIBITORS AND BILE ACID BINDING RESINS

Several trials utilizing the combination of lovastatin, simvastatin, and pravastatin with cholestyramine or colestipol in patients uncontrolled by one agent alone have indicated a marked additive effect. The HMG-CoA reductase inhibitor must be given 1 hour before or 4 hours following the resin because bile acid resins interfere with absorption of these agents. The combination of simvastatin (40 mg) and cholestyramine (16 g daily) lowered total cholesterol 37%, versus 29% with simvastatin alone.

Although these agents decrease triglycerides slightly, they are not indicated when triglycerides are elevated beyond 500 mg/dl (5 mmol/l).

BILE ACID BINDING RESINS

Bile acid binding resins have been available for the past 35 years. Their disagreeable taste, however, causes poor patient compliance. The use of bile acid binding resins declined with the advent of HMG-CoA reductase inhibitors, but they have a role as combination therapy in patients with severe hyperlipidemia, as outlined earlier.

The Lipid Research Clinic trial showed no decrease in cardiac or total mortality with the use of cholestyramine. Thirty cardiac deaths occurred in the cholestyramine-treated patients, versus 38 deaths in the control group. This nonsignificant difference has been labeled a 24% reduction in risk. The 7-year follow-up revealed 155 total events, nonfatal infarction and cardiac deaths, in patients treated with cholestyramine, versus 187 events in 1,900 patients given placebo (p < 0.05). Of interest, there were seven violent or accidental deaths in treated patients, versus four in controls. Total mortality was not significantly reduced by 7 years of cholestyramine therapy. Thus, drug therapy must be carefully weighed in terms of cost, adverse effects, and ability to prolong life. It is estimated that a lifetime reduction of total cholesterol with the use of dietary cholesterol and saturated fat restriction would prolong life an average of a few days to 1 year. Cholestyramine causes only a 7 to 19% reduction in total cholesterol, a reduction similar to that achieved with diet, and at an estimated cost ranging from $50,000 to $1 million per year of lives saved, depending on the duration of therapy. A similar lack of prolongation of life has been observed in the 5-year Helsinki study using gemfibrozil.

Action. Bile acid binding resins are not absorbed from the GI tract and act by binding bile salts in the gut; they are, therefore, bile acid sequestrants. This action causes cholesterol catabolism to bile acids and a decrease in serum LDL cholesterol. A decreased concentration of intrahepatic cholesterol stimulates the activity of LDL receptors that increase hepatic uptake of circulating LDL cholesterol.

Cholestyramine

Dosage: 4 g (1 packet) twice daily with meals for 1 to 2 weeks, then 8 g two or three times daily. It is advisable to prepare the daily dose at night; the bile acid binding resin is mixed with a noncarbonated beverage or orange drink and stored in the refrigerator for use the next day at meal times. Questran Light has an orange flavor and requires only about 75 ml liquid per packet; this preparation has improved the palatability of the product. A candy bar preparation is also available.

Medications, especially digoxin, oral anticoagulants, diuretics, beta blockers, thyroid hormone, and HMG-CoA reductase inhibitors, must be administered 1 hour before or 4 hours following the resin to prevent interference with absorption.

Adverse effects. Constipation, abdominal cramps, and rarely mild malabsorption of fat soluble vitamins; hypoprothrombinemia is rare, and a mild increase in triglycerides may occur. Thus, the drug should not be used in patients with triglyceride levels greater than 500 mg/dl (5 mmol/l).

Contraindications. Complete biliary obstruction.

Colestipol
(Colestid)

Dosage: 5 g one to two times daily in liquid; increase, if necessary, at intervals of about 2 months to 25 g daily. The adverse effects and contraindications are similar to that of cholestyramine.

FIBRATES

These agents are activators of the enzyme plasma-lipoprotein-lipase. Fibrates cause, at most, a modest decrease in total cholesterol or LDL cholesterol. A 1 to 15% reduction in serum cholesterol, a 30 to 50% reduction in triglycerides, and a 10 to 15% increase in HDL cholesterol have been observed in most studies. However, fenofibrate appears to reduce total cholesterol significantly more than that observed with bezafibrate and gemfibrozil.

Fibric acid derivatives, particularly clofibrate, have been widely used for the management of hyperlipidemia since 1964. Clofibrate has had extensive trials that failed to show significant reduction in cardiac or total mortality. Also, undesirable adverse effects and the advent of new agents have rendered this agent obsolete.

Gemfibrozil

The second fibric acid to gain widespread acceptance is gemfibrozil.

Supplied: capsules; 300 mg

Dosage: 300 to 600 mg 30 minutes before morning and evening meals.

Action. Gemfibrozil is a chemical homologue of clofibrate. The drug decreases hepatic production of VLDL triglyceride. Gemfibrozil causes a 30 to 40% reduction in triglycerides but only 2 to 10% reduction in serum cholesterol and a 5 to 12% increase in HDL cholesterol. Gemfibrozil has a small role in the management of severe hypercholesterolemia.

Indications
- Severe hypertriglyceridemia, greater than 1,000 mg/dl (10 mmol/l), that is unresponsive to dietary measures, exercise, and cessation of alcohol. In these patients, treatment is necessary to prevent pancreatitis
- Type III hyperlipoproteinemia that is associated with marked elevation of triglycerides
- Individuals with high total cholesterol, in the range of 250 to 300 mg/dl (6.5 to 7.9 mmol/l), and who have two risk factors other than LDL, one of which is a low HDL less than 35 mg/dl (0.9 mmol/l)

The use of gemfibrozil in patients with moderate hypercholesterolemia has gained support because of the results of the Helsinki Heart Study, which enrolled 4,081 men (40 to 50 years of age) who were free of coronary symptoms. A 10% increase in HDL occurred from a baseline of 47 mg/dl, and an 11% decrease from baseline of total cholesterol (290 mg/dl). At the end of 5 years, there was no reduction in cardiac or total mortality; there were 61 nonfatal myocardial infarcts and seven fatal infarcts in the placebo group, with 40 nonfatal and three fatal infarcts in the gemfibrozil-treated group (a 1.4% absolute difference). Thus, gemfibrozil therapy over 5 years is expected to improve the individual's chance of not having a cardiac event from approximately 96% to a little more than 97%, which is a 34% decrease in cardiac event rates, but without causing significant improvement in survival. Thus, several hundred individuals must be treated with gemfibrozil to prevent one infarct. A much larger study, over a longer period, enrolling patients with moderate hypercholesterolemia and HDL cholesterol less than 35 mg/dl (0.9 mmol/l), appears to be appropriate to establish the beneficial effects of this form of therapy.

Adverse effects. These include bloating, cramps, diarrhea, muscle aching, eczema, increase in liver function tests, rarely a mild increase in blood sugar, and impotence. The lithogenic activity appears to be less than that of clofibrate, but gallstone formation is increased and costly monitoring is necessary. In the Helsinki Study, there were 10 violent or accidental deaths in patients treated with gemfibrozil versus four in controls. Also, 81 GI operations were required in the treated patients, versus 53 in the placebo group ($p < 0.02$). The association with intracerebral bleed as well as hepatobiliary cancers is not established but is a concern.

The physician must persist with dietary advice for a prolonged period and should justify the use of fibric acid derivatives, taking into account the adverse effects, the necessity for careful monitoring of hepatobiliary complications, and the cost-effectiveness in terms of prevention of some nonfatal infarcts without the prolongation of life.

Caution. Reduce oral anticoagulant dose. Do not combine with HMG-CoA reductase inhibitors because of the risk of severe myositis and rhabdomyolysis. The drug is renally excreted. Reduce dose to 300 mg daily with renal failure.

Contraindications. Hepatic impairment, alcoholism, gallstones, pregnancy.

Clofibrate

This drug has been used mainly for lowering triglycerides. With the advent of gemfibrozil and other fibrates, clofibrate has been rendered obsolete because of its adverse effects.

Bezafibrate

Supplied: tablets; 200 mg

Dosage: 200 mg twice daily, with or after food. The drug can be taken once daily.

Contraindications. Severe renal or hepatic impairment, hypoalbuminemia, primary biliary cirrhosis, gall bladder disease, nephrotic syndrome, pregnancy.

Adverse effects. Nausea, abdominal pain, myositis, urticaria, headache, impotence.

Bezafibrate causes a fall in glucose levels; also, an increase in serum creatinine occurs and monitoring is necessary. Longterm trials are necessary to document efficacy in reducing mortality and to assess adverse effects. The drug may cause alopecia.

Interactions
- Oral anticoagulants: The dosage of anticoagulants should be reduced with careful management of prothrombin time or INR
- HGM-CoA reductase inhibitors: Severe myositis and rhabdomyolysis have been observed with the combination of fibrates and lovastatin, with marked elevation of serum potassium, which may be life threatening

Fenofibrate

Supplied: capsule; 100 mg

Dosage: 100 mg once or twice daily, maximum 400 mg daily. This prodrug is converted to fenofibric acid. The drug appears to reduce total cholesterol significantly more than other fibrates.

The drug has been shown to cause a reduction in total cholesterol, reduced LDL cholesterol of up to 20%, and increased HDL cholesterol by an average of 20%. Triglycerides are reduced significantly by an average of 50%.

Adverse effects. GI disturbances and dermatologic adverse effects occur in 7 to 14% of patients. In a 5-year trial, 1% of patients were withdrawn from medication due to adverse effects. Fenofibrate may increase cholesterol excretion in the bile, causing cholelithiasis. If cholelithiasis is suspected during treatment therapy, ultrasound of the gallbladder is indicated. If gallstones are present, fenofibrate should be discontinued. Thus, it is wise to perform this procedure prior to commencing therapy. Several adverse effects are similar to those observed with clofibrate. A dose 12 times that used in humans has been shown to be tumorigenic in the liver of male rats. Abnormal liver function tests with an elevation of transaminases and an increase in alkaline phosphatase have been observed but normalized on discontinuation of the drug. Test liver function monthly and then annually or if there are symptoms that suggest hepatic dysfunction. Rash, pruritus, urticaria or erythema, weight loss, impotence, alopecia, pancreatitis, hepatitis, and creatine kinase elevations may occur but subside on discontinuation of the drug.

Contraindications
- Severe renal or hepatic impairment. Fibrates are excreted by the kidney and should be used with caution in patients with renal dysfunction
- Gallbladder disease
- Hypersensitivity to fenofibrate
- Pregnancy, women of childbearing potential, and during lactation
- Primary biliary cirrhosis

Fibrates may potentiate the effects of oral anticoagulants.

NICOTINIC ACID

Supplied: 50, 100, 500 mg. Assess transaminases and glucose levels.

Dosage: 50 mg with the evening meal for 1 week, with 325-mg coated aspirin taken 30 minutes prior to prevent flushing. Increase to 100 mg twice daily and, over months, slowly increase from 100 to 500 mg tid, always after meals. Assess biochemistry and if there are no complications, increase to a maximum of 500 mg three times daily.

Adverse effects. Although the drug causes significant reduction in serum cholesterol and triglycerides, with a mild increase in HDL cholesterol, it has a small place in clinical practice because of the extent of its adverse effects and the number of tablets that must be taken daily. Adverse effects include flushing, pruritus, nausea, abdominal pain, diarrhea, hepatic dysfunction, jaundice, exacerbation of diabetes, gout, palpitations, arrhythmias, hypotension, rarely pigmentation, and optic neuritis with blurred vision. Acute hepatitis is a dangerous complication of niacin therapy, presenting with a flu-like illness with fatigue, malaise, anorexia, pruritis, and jaundice. The sustained-release preparations cause more frequent hepatic dysfunction than the short-acting tablet. A case has been reported of a patient who developed fulminant liver failure after switching from 1-year therapy with nicotinic acid to a sustained-release preparation.

Caution. Do not use in combination with HMG-CoA reductase inhibitors, because severe myositis may occur. Avoid the drug in patients with acute MI, heart failure, gallbladder disease, jaundice, liver disease, peptic ulcer, and diabetes. Treatment with aspirin decreases flushing. Aspirin can be discontinued when tolerance occurs and flushing abates, but the aspirin dose should be increased along with increases in nicotinic acid.

The drug has a small role in the management of familial combined hyperlipoproteinemia, where cholesterol remains greater than 320 mg/dl and triglycerides greater than 1500 mg/dl.

Nicotinic acid is claimed to be one of the few lipid-lowering drugs that have been shown to prolong life. However, only an 11% reduction in all-cause mortality and a 12% decrease in CHD death were observed in the 15-year Coronary Drug Project. These results hardly justify the use of nicotinic acid, except in rare instances.

ELEVATED SERUM TRIGLYCERIDES

A triglyceride level up to 300 mg/dl (3.0 mmol/l) is considered to be within normal limits. Most laboratories report the upper limit of normal as 250 mg/dl (2.5 mmol/l). Treatment of hypertriglyceridemia becomes urgent if triglyceride levels are above 1,000 mg/dl (10 mmol/l) because of the risk of pancreatitis and avascular necrosis of the femoral head. Fortunately, control is nearly always achieved with a low carbohydrate diet. Weight loss almost always reduces triglyceride levels. Alcohol abuse is one of the most common causes of high triglyceride levels and cessation of alcohol is necessary for control. Failure to reduce levels to less than 1,000 mg/dl (10 mmol/l) is an indication for drug therapy usually with gemfibrozil along with weight reduction diet, increase in exercise, and cessation of alcohol. The evidence linking triglycerides directly with an increased risk of CHD is unproven, and therapy is not indicated with the aim of reducing the risk.

BIBLIOGRAPHY

Alderman JD, Pasternak RC, Sacks FM, et al.: Effect of a modified, well-tolerated niacin regimen on serum total cholesterol, high density lipoprotein cholesterol and the cholesterol to high density lipoprotein ratio. Am J Cardiol, *64*:725, 1989.

Bachorik PS, Cloey TA, Finney CA, et al.: Lipoprotein-cholesterol analysis during screening: Accuracy and reliability. Ann Intern Med, *114*:741, 1991.

Boissel J-P, Leizorovics A, Picolet H, et al.: Efficacy of acebutolol after acute myocardial infarction (The APSI Trial). Am J Cardiol, *66*:245C, 1990.

Bradford RH, Shear CL, Chremos AN, et al.: Expanded clinical evaluation of lovastatin (EXCEL) study results. I. Efficacy in modifying plasma lipoproteins and adverse event profile in 8,245 patients with moderate hypercholesterolemia. Arch Intern Med, *151*:43, 1991.

Brett AS: Treating hypercholesterolemia. How should practicing physicians interpret the published data for patients? N Eng J Med, *321*:676, 1989.

Byington RP, Worthy J, Craven T: Propranolol-induced lipid changes and their prognostic significance after a myocardial infarction: The beta-blocker heart attack trial experience. Am J Cardiol, *65*:1287, 1990.

Carleton RA, Dwyer J, Finberg L, et al.: Report of the expert panel on population strategies for blood cholesterol reduction. Circulation, *83*:2154, 1991.

Clucas A, Miller N: Effects of acebutolol on the serum lipid profile. Drugs, *36*(Suppl2):41, 1988.

Frick MH, Elo O, Haapa K, et al.: Helsinki Heart Study: Primary-Prevention trial with gemfibrozil in middle-aged men with dyslipidemia. N Engl J Med, *317*:1237, 1987.

Genest J, McNamara JR, Ordovas JM, et al.: Lipoprotein cholesterol, apolipoprotein A-I and B and lipoprotein (a) abnormalities in men with premature coronary artery disease. J Am Coll Cardiol, *19*:792, 1992.

Gotto AM: Cholesterol intake and serum cholesterol level. N Engl J Med, *324*:912, 1991.

Grundy SM, Vega GL: Causes of high blood cholesterol. Circulation, *81*:412, 1990.

Israel DH, Gorlin R: Fish oils in the prevention of atherosclerosis. J Am Coll Cardiol, *19*:174, 1992.

Keenan JM, Fontaine PL, Wenz JB, et al.: A randomized, controlled trial of wax-matrix sustained-release niacin in hypercholesterolemia. Arch Intern Med, *151*:1424, 1991.

Larosa JC, Cleeman JI: Cholesterol lowering as a treatment for established coronary heart disease. Circulation, *85*:1229, 1992.

Manninen V, Tenkanen L, Koskinen P, et al.: Joint effects of serum triglyceride and LDL cholesterol and HDL cholesterol concentrations on coronary heart disease risk in the Helsinki Heart Study. Implications for treatment. Circulation, *85*:37, 1992.

Mascioli SR, Grimm RH, Neaton JD, et al.: Characteristics of participants at baseline in the treatment of mild hypertension study (TOMHS). Am J Cardiol, *66*:32C, 1990.

Mullin GE, Greenson JK, Mitchell MC: Fulminant hepatic failure after ingestion of sustained-release nicotinic acid. Ann Int Med, *111*:253, 1989.

O'Connor P, Freely J, Shepherd J: Lipid lowering drug. Br Med J, *300*:667, 1990.

Roberts WC: Recent studies on the effects of beta blockers on blood lipid level. Am Heart J, *117*:709, 1989.

Schnaper HW: Acebutolol effects on lipid profile. Am J Cardiol, *66*:49C, 1990.

Shear CL, Franklin RA, Stinnett S, et al.: Expanded clinical evaluation of lovastatin (EXCEL) study results. Effect of patient characteristics on lovastatin-induced changes in plasma concentrations of lipids and lipoproteins. Circulation, *85*:1293, 1992.

Stampfer MJ, Sacks FM, Salvini S, et al.: A prospective study of cholesterol apolipoproteins, and the risk of myocardial infarction. New Eng J Med, *325*:373, 1991.

Suh I, Shaten J, Cutler JA, et al.: Alcohol use and mortality from coronary heart disease: The role of high-density lipoprotein cholesterol. Ann Intern Med, *116*:881, 1992.

Swain JF, Rouse IL, Curley CB, et al.: Comparison of the effects of oat bran and low-fiber wheat on serum lipoprotein levels and blood pressure. N Engl J Med, *322*:147, 1990.

Wong ND, Wilson PWF, Kannel WB: Serum cholesterol as a prognostic factor after myocardial infarction: The Framingham Study. Ann Intern Med, *115*:687, 1991.

9
INFECTIVE ENDOCARDITIS
M. Gabriel Khan

The diagnosis of infective endocarditis must be considered and excluded in all individuals with a heart murmur and fever of unknown origin. Infection of the heart valves may be caused by bacteria and, less commonly, fungi, Coxiella, or Chlamydia.

DIAGNOSIS

A few hours or days of fever, chills, and rigors are common with acute bacterial endocarditis (ABE). An insidious onset over weeks with fever, malaise, chills, and weight loss indicates subacute bacterial endocarditis (SBE).

PREDISPOSING FACTORS

In a patient with a murmur and a fever of undetermined origin, one of the following precipitating or predisposing factors, if present, should produce a high index of suspicion of infective endocarditis

- Known valvular heart disease, especially rheumatic, bicuspid aortic valve or mitral valve prolapse, with significant regurgitation
- Prosthetic valve
- Marfan's, floppy valve
- Recent dental or oropharyngeal surgical procedure
- Genitourinary instrumentation or surgery of the respiratory tract
- IV addict
- Congenital heart disease: Patent ductus, ventricular septal defect, Fallot's tetralogy, coarctation
- Prolonged use of IV catheters and hyperalimentation
- Patient with burns
- Inflammatory and other bowel disease, suspect Streptococcus bovis. If this organism is isolated, exclude polyposis and carcinoma of the colon
- Hemodialysis

Infective endocarditis may occur, however, in the absence of previously known valvular disease or other precipitating factors, especially in elderly patients.

PHYSICAL SIGNS

- A heart murmur is usually present with SBE, absent in 1 to 5%
- A murmur may be absent in up to 15% of patients with ABE and not heard in about 33% of individuals with right-sided endocarditis, especially if care is not taken to listen for the murmur of tricuspid regurgitation: Holosystolic at the lower left sternal border and increased with inspiration or elicitation of the hepatojugular reflux
- A change in the quality or grade of the murmur is an unreliable indicator
- Intermittent medium- to high-grade fever is usually prominent, but in elderly or immunocompromised patients, fever may be mild or absent. Normal body temperature is lower in the elderly, 97°F (36°C) as opposed to 98°F (37°C) in individuals under age 70. However, these patients may feel chills
- Finger clubbing takes about 6 weeks to appear, is seen only with SBE, and disappears a few weeks after successful treatment
- Osler's nodes, although uncommon, are pathognomonic, manifest as exquisitely painful, yellowish or erythematous subcutaneous papules, pea- to almond-sized on the palms and soles. Lesions disappear in 1 to 5 days and may be seen during adequate therapy
- Petechiae with pale centers may be observed on everting the upper eyelids. They may be seen in the oropharynx or on the trunk, hands, and feet as retinal cotton wool exudates, canoe-shaped hemorrhages with white spots in their center (Roth's spots)
- Splinter hemorrhages may be due to trauma and occur in other conditions, but an increase in their numbers is relevant
- Splenomegaly is observed in about 50% of patients with SBE and in about 15% of those with ABE. The enlarged spleen may be painful and tender and can rupture. An ultrasound is advisable in all cases of suspected infective endocarditis
- Pigmentation: Subtle changes in skin coloration; pasty, cafe au lait complexion is an important sign and reverts to normal after treatment
- Janeway lesions are rarely observed: 1 to 4 mm painless flat erythematous macules, nontender on the palms and soles, blanch on pressure

UNDERLYING DISEASE

The underlying disease in left-sided native valve endocarditis is rheumatic in over 50% of cases and mitral valve prolapse in up to 15%; endocarditis on a bicuspid aortic valve is not uncommon. The incidence of underlying rheumatic valvular disease is higher in Southeast Asia, Africa, the Middle East, and Latin America, where rheumatic disease is still common.

INVESTIGATIONS

- Four to six blood cultures are taken over a 1- to 2-hour period and carry a 90% chance of recovering organisms
- Urinalysis often shows mild hematuria or increased red blood cells and few red blood cell casts

- Increased creatinine, urea, or blood urea nitrogen is nonspecific
- The erythrocyte sedimentation rate (ESR) is virtually always elevated and can be 75 to 110 mm/hour (Westergren) with SBE
- The rheumatoid factor is positive in approximately 50% of patients
- Anemia is seen in more than 30% of patients with SBE
- The white blood count may be slightly increased or remain normal. There is almost always a shift to the left, however, with an increase in band forms
- It is advisable to check the Gram's stain of the blood, buffy coat for organisms
  A sterile blood culture is observed in up to 25% of cases due to
- Prior antibiotic therapy
- Fastidious organisms as with slow-growing streptococci
- Fungal infection; request fungal precipitins
- Q fever; serology should be requested
- Chlamydia infection

BACTERIA CAUSING ENDOCARDITIS

- Staphyloccus aureus is responsible for over 85% of cases of acute endocarditis. Of 113 patients with infective endocarditis observed at the University of Massachusetts Medical Center (1981 through 1988), 45 (40%) had S. aureus with a 28% mortality versus 9% in the non-S. aureus group. S. aureus causes up to 25% of cases of native valve endocarditis
- Streptococcus pneumoniae causing acute fulminant endocarditis is now rare. Gonococcus, pseudomonas, and Streptococcus marcescens may cause right-sided acute endocarditis
- Streptococci are implicated in 60 to 80% of cases. Alpha hemolytic streptococcus, excluding Streptococcus pneumoniae designated S. viridans, includes Streptococcus milleri, Streptococcus mutans, Streptococcus salivarius originating in the upper respiratory tract and some in the upper GI tract
- Fecal streptococci, commonly termed "enterococci," cause up to 10% of infective endocarditis, but with a higher incidence in the geriatric population. The organisms include varieties of Streptococcus fecalis and, rarely, Streptococcus fecium and Streptococcus durans, often penicillin resistant; Streptococcus bovis is an exception because it is often sensitive to penicillin
- Nutritionally variant streptococci: Streptococcus anginosis, Streptococcus mitis, and similar oganisms require special media for their growth
- Other organisms include Staphylococcus epidermidis, proteus species, Haemophilus influenzae, parainfluenzae, fusobacterium, and brucella
- Escherichia coli commonly cause bacteremia and septicemia, but rarely cause endocarditis

ECHOCARDIOGRAPHY

Transthoracic two-dimensional echocardiography detects approximately 63% of vegetations (see Table 9–1). Staphylococcus aureus and some streptococci may produce small lesions of less than 5 mm, which are poorly detectable by transthoracic echocardiography.

TABLE 9–1. DETECTION OF VEGETATIONS BY TRANSESOPHAGEAL VS. TRANSTHORACIC 2D ECHOCARDIOGRAPHY				
	OVERALL	>10 mm	6 to 10 mm	<5 mm
TEE	100%	100%	100%	100%
Transthoracic 2D Color Doppler	63%	70%	65%	25%

Transesophageal echocardiography (TEE) is superior to the transthoracic technique and can be crucial to the management of endocarditis. Transthoracic two-dimensional Doppler echocardiography gives poor detection of prosthetic heart valves, especially in the mitral position, and of calcific sclerotic native valves. Vegetations that are less than 5 mm, 6 to 10 mm, or greater than 10 mm are observed in 25%, 65%, and 70%, respectively, by transthoracic technique. This is 100% for all lesions utilizing TEE (Table 9–1).

TEE is a semi-invasive procedure, and a benefit risk calculation should precede its use. In patients with suspected endocarditis, TEE has a role in the following

- Failure of transthoracic echocardiography to show vegetations in patients strongly suspected of having endocarditis
- All prosthetic heart valves
- Calcific sclerotic native valves
- Valvular destruction secondary to infective endocarditis, especially perivalvular abscesses

Complication of TEE include bronchospasm, arrhythmias, and rarely pharyngeal bleeding. Contraindications to TEE are given in Chapter 12.

THERAPY

It is imperative that therapy be started immediately after four to six blood cultures are taken and relevant clinical information is forwarded to the microbiology laboratory. It is important to have a personal discussion with the microbiologist, because some organisms require special culture medium and techniques.

Vegetations that are less than 1 cm are usually cured by 4 to 6 weeks of antibiotic therapy. Vegetations greater than 1 cm that do not respond to 3 weeks of antibiotic therapy often necessitate valve surgery.

Therapy and prognosis are related to the underlying disease and sensitivity of the organism. See Chapter 24 for a detailed description of antimicrobial agents and the preferred or alternative therapy for various microorganisms.

Empiric therapy can be tailored based on the following

NATIVE VALVE ENDOCARDITIS

- In patients with native valve endocarditis, SBE presentation in patients under age 65 require obvious coverage of S. viridans, which is the causative organism in up to 70% of cases and fecal streptococci in up to 15%:

penicillin (2 million units every 4 hours IV) plus gentamicin (1.3 to 2 mg/kg every 8 hours IV), until the organism has been defined and sensitivities and the minimum inhibitory concentration (MIC) of the drug against the isolated organism are known.

GERIATRIC ENDOCARDITIS

- As above, but in elderly patients, fecal streptococci are more common and occur in up to 25% of patients; it is advisable to use: Ampicillin/ sulbactam (2 g every 4 hours) plus gentamicin (1.3 to 2 mg/kg every 8 hours). Penicillin is the second choice and an alternative to ampicillin/ sulbactam, provided the SBE is present for less than 3 months. See further discussion of fecal streptococcal endocarditis. The dose interval of aminoglycosides must be increased in patients over age 65 or in individuals with renal impairment and titrated to blood levels to avoid renal and ototoxicity. A predose level (trough) greater than 2 μg/ml (2 mg/l) reflects decreased excretion rate and accumulation of the drug: extend the dosing interval. Keep predose level 1 to 2 μg/ml. Peak level 30 minutes post infusion 6 to 10 μg/ml, depending on sensitivities and type of organism

ACUTE ENDOCARDITIS

- Acute presentation obviously requires coverage for Staphylococcus aureus which causes more than 90% of ABE and up to 50% occurring on valves not known to be abnormal, especially bicuspid aortic valves: cloxacillin (2 g IV every 4 hours for 4 to 6 weeks) or nafcillin (2 g IV every 4 hours for 4 to 6 weeks) or flucloxacillin (2 g IV every 4 hours)

ORGANISM ISOLATED AND SENSITIVITIES DETERMINED

When the microorganism has been isolated and antibiotic sensitivities are available, an appropriate antibiotic combination is selected and changes are made, if needed, to the initial choice of antibiotic. Organisms that commonly cause endocarditis and appropriate antibiotic combinations include the following

- S. viridans of Streptococcus bovis: If the MIC to penicillin is less than 0.1 mg/1, give: penicillin (IV 2 million U every 4 hours for 2 weeks), then amoxicillin (orally 500 mg every 6 hours for 2 weeks) or ampicillin/sulbactam (2 g every 6 hours for 2 weeks IV), then amoxicillin (orally 500 mg every 6 hours for 2 weeks)
- Partially sensitive S. viridans or S. bovis, MIC penicillin greater than 0.1 mg/l: penicillin (3 million U every 4 hours IV) plus gentamicin (1.3 to 2 mg/kg every 8 hours IV for 2 to 4 weeks) or, from the third week, amoxicillin (500 mg orally every 6 hours for 2 weeks)
- Streptococcus fecalis, Streptococcus fecium, Streptococcus durans, or similar fecal streptococci are difficult to eradicate: If the length of illness is less than 3 months, it is advisable to give ampicillin/sulbactam (IV 2

to 3 g every 6 hours for 4 weeks) plus gentamicin (1.3 to 2 mg/kg every 8 hours) and monitor levels and adjustment for renal function. Gentamicin is given for 4 weeks. Wells, et al. have shown that combinations of penicillin or ampicillin and the beta-lactamase inhibitor sulbactam were significantly more active than a group of antibiotics tested against beta-lactamase-producing gentamicin-resistant Enterococcus fecalis. In the management of fecal enterococcal endocarditis, a beta-lactam beta-lactamase inhibitor combination is strongly recommended. Ampicillin should not be used without sulbactam. Although vancomycin and imipenem-cilastatin may be beta-lactamase stable, these agents are only bacteriostatic against enterococci. Only one apparent cure has been reported using vancomycin in a patient with Enterococcus fecalis (beta-lactamase-producing aminoglycoside-resistant) endocarditis. If the duration of illness is greater than 3 months, give ampicillin and gentamicin intravenously for 4 weeks, then amoxicillin (500 mg) every 6 hours orally for at least 2 weeks, because relapse is common with less than 4 weeks of therapy. In patients with illness less than 3 months, success has been obtained with the combination of high-dose penicillin and gentamicin for 4 weeks, as observed in a study of 40 patients. If duration of symptoms is more than 3 months, however, penicillin is not advisable because in a series of 16 patients treated for 4 weeks with penicillin, and gentamicin, there were 7 relapses and 4 deaths. If penicillin is used, it should be combined with the beta-lactamase inhibitor sulbactam. In the elderly, the dose of gentamicin combined with ampicillin or penicillin should be 1 mg/kg every 8 hours and adjusted further if renal function is impaired. Aim for peak levels of 6 to 8 μg/ml; if the peak is greater than 10 μg/ml, decrease the dose. If the range is too high (greater than 2 μg/ml), extend the dosing interval. The combinations of ampicillin or penicillin and the beta-lactamase inhibitor sulbactam have been shown to be the most active antimicrobials tested against gentamicin resistant beta-lactamase-producing Streptococcus fecalis and have proven useful in the treatment of S fecalis endocarditis. Beta-lactamase stable vancomycin and imipenem-cilastatin are mainly bacteriostatic against fecal streptococci. Daptomycin is an investigational antimicrobial that has shown activity against some gentamicin resistant S. fecalis.

- Other less common organisms causing endocarditis are treated according to sensitivities; suggested combinations are given in Table 9–2

In the UK, S. viridans or Streptococcus bovis infection are managed with 2 weeks of penicillin and gentamicin IV, then oral amoxicillin (500 mg every 6 hours) for at least 2 weeks

- Staphylococcus aureus: Methicillin-sensitive strains constitute the majority of cases of S. aureus endocarditis and are treated with nafcillin or cloxacillin (at doses given above) or flucloxacillin (IV 2 g every 4 hours) plus gentamicin (1.3 to 2 mg/kg every 8 hours IV), the dose to be monitored by levels. The dose is reduced in elderly patients and those with renal dysfunction, while the dosing interval is increased. Gentamicin is discontinued after 1 week, and nafcillin or flucloxacillin IV is continued for 3 to 4 weeks. The length of treatment is usually from 4 to 6 weeks.

TABLE 9–2. ORGANISMS CAUSING ENDOCARDITIS AND SUGGESTED
ANTIBIOTIC THERAPY*

ORGANISMS	ANTIBIOTIC, FIRST CHOICE	ALTERNATIVES
S. viridans	Penicillin-G	Penicillin + gentamicin, Penicillin + streptomycin
Streptococcus faecalis	Ampicillin/sulbactam + gentamicin	Penicillin + gentamicin, Penicillin + streptomycin
Streptococcus bovis	Penicillin	
Staphylococcus aureus	Nafcillin or cloxacillin or flucloxacillin	Vancomycin or Teicoplanin
Staphylococcus epidermidis	Vancomycin	Teicoplanin, Nafcillin
Gram-negative: Pseudomonas aeruginosa	Tobramycin + imipenem**	Piperacillin or ceftazidime or aztreonam + tobramycin
Xanthomonas maltophilia	Ciprofloxacin	Trimethoprim + SMX
Serratia marcescens	Cefotaxime or Imipenem + gentamicin	Aztreonam
Escherichia coli	Ampicillin/sulbactam + gentamicin	Imipenem Aztreonam
Proteus	Ampicillin/sulbactam + gentamicin	
Klebsiella pneumoniae	Cefuroxime + gentamicin	Imipenem Aztreonam
Bacteroides and Fusobacterium	Imipenem or Cefotetan	High-dose penicillin + Clindamycin High dose penicillin +
Salmonella	Chloramphenicol	Ampicillin
Gonococcus	Penicillin	
Enterobacter	Cefotaxime or Imipenem or Aztreonam + gentamicin	Surgery often necessary
Coxiella burnetti	Cotrimoxazole + rifampin	Tetracycline
Chlamydia	Erythromycin (trimethoprim + sulfamethoxazole)	
Fungi	Amphotericin B alone or + 5-fluorocystosine (if organism sensitive)	Surgery usually necessary

* See Chap. 24
** With Cilastatin
+ = plus

In the UK, S. aureus endocarditis is usually treated with IV flucloxacillin from 4 to 6 weeks and gentamicin IV for 14 days.
• Streptococcus pneumoniae is highly sensitive to penicillin and is managed with penicillin G (2 million units every 4 hours) for 2 or more weeks

In all cases of endocarditis, predisposing factors such as genitourinary tract pathology and poor dental hygiene must receive adequate therapy. For patients allergic to penicillin or methicillin-resistant Staphylococcus aureus, give: vancomycin (15 mg/kg IV every 12 hours given slowly over

6 hours) for 4 to 6 weeks. Monitor serum levels, peak 20 to 40 μg/ml 2 hours post completion of infusion, trough levels 5 to 10 μg/ml. Reduce dose and increase the dosing interval in renal failure.

PROSTHETIC VALVE ENDOCARDITIS

Infective endocarditis occurs in approximately 3% of patients within the first year of surgery and thereafter in about 1% per year. Depending on the region, prosthetic valve endocarditis accounts for 10 to 30% of all cases of endocarditis. The incidence is highest in the first 2 months, and the most common organisms at that stage are Staphylococcus epidermidis (in 25% to 30%) and Staphylococcus aureus (in 20% to 25% of cases). Staphylococcus epidermidis continues to be an important organism during the ensuing years but with a decreased incidence. Within the first 2 months, gram-negative organisms, fungi, diptheroids, and enterococci are infecting organisms. Staphylococcus epidermidis is nearly always methicillin resistant, and the use of vancomycin is necessary.

Dosage: Vancomycin 15 mg/kg IV every 12 hours in combination with gentamicin 1 to 1.2 mg/kg IV every 8 hours; the addition of rifampin 300 mg orally every 8 hours may cause a modest improvement in the cure rate but increases the incidence of toxicity.

Late prosthetic valve endocarditis should be treated in a similar method, as outlined, pending results of culture and sensitivities since the offending organism is usually Streptococcus viridans, fecal streptococci, Staphylococcus aureus, Staphylococcus epidermidis. Fungal infections, however, are uncommon with late cases.

As outlined earlier, TEE is superior to transthoracic echocardiography and plays an important role in the diagnosis of prosthetic valve endocarditis.

INDICATIONS FOR SURGERY

- Hemodynamic deterioration
- Signs of prosthetic valve dysfunction assessed by TEE
- Occurrence of heart failure
- Uncontrolled infection
- Conduction disturbances or suggestive ring abscesses
- Large vegetation caused by fungal infection
- Recurrent emboli
- Relapse after adequate medical therapy

RIGHT-SIDED ENDOCARDITIS

Right-sided endocarditis is most common in IV drug addicts and may present with a pneumonic illness. Infecting organisms include

- Staphylococcus aureus in over 60%
- Staphylococcus epidermidis in 10%
- Pseudomonas and Serratia in up to 10%

Systemic emboli are not as threatening as with left-sided endocarditis, and the outcome of medical therapy for 4 to 6 weeks is generally good; therefore, there is less need for surgical intervention. Table 9–1 lists a selection of antibiotics for the management of pseudomonas and other organisms. Imipenem is partially inactivated in the kidney and is therefore administered with a specific enzyme inhibitor, cilastatin, which blocks its renal metabolism (See Chapter 24).

BACTERIAL ENDOCARDITIS PROPHYLAXIS

Recent recommendations from the AHA on the antibiotic prophylaxis of endocarditis are given in Tables 9–3 through 9–7. Recommendations from the Endocarditis Working Party of the British Society for Antimicrobial Chemotherapy are indicated in Table 9–8.

The recent changes include the following relevant points

- The AHA has adopted the British 1984 recommendation to replace penicillin with amoxicillin for dental procedures: amoxicillin 3 g orally is given 1 hour prior to dental procedures, including professional cleaning, then 1.5 g 6 hours later
- Patients allergic to penicillin who can take oral medications are given the choice of erythromycin or clindamycin, 300 mg 1 hour prior and 150

TABLE 9–3. PREVENTION OF BACTERIAL ENDOCARDITIS–CARDIAC CONDITIONS*

Endocarditis prophylaxis recommended
  Prosthetic cardiac valves, including bioprosthetic and homograft valves
  Previous bacterial endocarditis, even in the absence of heart disease
  Surgically constructed systemic-pulmonary shunts or conduits
  Most congenital cardiac malformations
  Rheumatic and other acquired valvular dysfunction, even after valvular surgery
  Hypertrophic cardiomyopathy
  Mitral valve prolapse with valvular regurgitation
Endocarditis prophylaxis not recommended
  Isolated secundum atrial septal defect
  Surgical repair without residua beyond 6 months of secundum atrial septal defect, ventricular septal defect, or patent ductus arteriosus
  Previous coronary artery bypass graft surgery
  Mitral valve prolapse without valvular regurgitation†
  Physiologic, functional, or innocent heart murmurs
  Previous Kawasaki disease without valvular dysfunction
  Previous rheumatic fever without valvular dysfunction
  Cardiac pacemakers and implanted defibrillators

* This table lists selected conditions but is not meant to be all-inclusive.
† Individuals who have a mitral valve prolapse associated with thickening and/or redundancy of the valve leaflets may be at increased risk for bacterial endocarditis, particularly men who are 45 years of age or older.
From: Dajani AS, et al.: Prevention of bacterial endocarditis. Recommendations by the American Heart Association. JAMA, *264(22)*:2920, 1990. Copyright 1990, American Medical Association.

Infective Endocarditis **327**

TABLE 9-4. PREVENTION OF BACTERIAL ENDOCARDITIS-DENTAL OR SURGICAL PROCEDURES*

Endocarditis prophylaxis recommended
  Dental procedures known to induce gingival or mucosal bleeding, including professional cleaning
  Tonsillectomy and/or adenoidectomy
  Surgical operations that involve intestinal or respiratory mucosa
  Bronchoscopy with a rigid bronchoscope
  Sclerotherapy for esophageal varices
  Esophageal dilatation
  Gallbladder surgery
  Cystoscopy
  Urethral dilatation
  Urethral catheterization if urinary tract infection is present†
  Urinary tract surgery if urinary tract infection is present†
  Prostatic surgery
  Incision and drainage of infected tissue†
  Vaginal hysterectomy
  Vaginal delivery in the presence of infection†
Endocarditis prophylaxis not recommended‡
  Dental procedures not likely to induce gingival bleeding, such as simple adjustment of orthodontic appliances or fillings above the gum line
  Injection of local intraoral anesthetic (except intraligamentary injections)
  Shedding of primary teeth
  Tympanostomy tube insertion
  Endotracheal intubation
  Bronchoscopy with a flexible bronchoscope, with or without biopsy
  Cardiac catheterization
  Endoscopy with or without gastrointestinal biopsy
  Cesarean section
  In the absence of infection for urethral catheterization, dilatation and curettage, uncomplicated vaginal delivery, therapeutic abortion, sterilization procedures, or insertion or removal of intrauterine devices

---

* This table lists selected procedures but is not meant to be all-inclusive.
† In addition to prophylactic regimen for genitourinary procedures, antibiotic therapy should be directed against the most likely bacterial pathogen.
‡ In patients who have prosthetic heart valves, a previous history of endocarditis, or surgically constructed systemic-pulmonary shunts or conduits, physicians may choose to administer prophylactic antibiotics even for low-risk procedures that involve the lower respiratory, genitourinary, or gastrointestinal tracts.
From: Dajani AS, et al.: Prevention of bacterial endocarditis. Recommendations by the American Heart Association. JAMA, *264(22)*:2920, 1990. Copyright 1990, American Medical Association.

mg 6 hours post procedure. This is a major improvement in prophylaxis, since erythromycin (at 800 mg as advised by the AHA or 1500 mg by the British group) causes severe nausea and/or abdominal discomfort. Also, the drug is not extremely effective for fecal streptococci

- Prophylaxis for mitral valve prolapse has caused confusion over the past 10 years. The AHA advises prophylaxis only for individuals with mitral regurgitation, i.e., presence of a mid to late or holosystolic murmur. Men over age 45 tend to develop progressive mitral regurgitation more frequently than women (see Chapter 12). Mild to moderate mitral re-

TABLE 9-5. RECOMMENDED STANDARD PROPHYLACTIC REGIMEN FOR DENTAL, ORAL, OR UPPER RESPIRATORY TRACT PROCEDURES IN PATIENTS WHO ARE AT RISK*

DRUG	DOSING REGIMEN†
Standard regimen	
Amoxicillin	3.0 g orally 1 hour before procedure; then 1.5 g 6 hours after initial dose
Amoxicillin/penicillin-allergic patients	
Erythromycin	Erythromycin ethylsuccinate, 800 mg, or erythromycin stearate, 1.0 g orally 2 hours before procedure; then half the dose 6 hours after initial dose
or	
Clindamycin	300 mg orally 1 hour before procedure and 150 mg 6 hours after initial dose

* Includes those with prosthetic heart valves and other high-risk patients.

† Initial pediatric doses are as follows: amoxicillin, 50 mg/kg; erythromycin ethylsuccinate or erythromycin stearate, 20 mg/kg; and clindamycin, 10 mg/kg. Follow-up dose should be one half the initial dose. **Total pediatric dose should not exceed total adult dose.** The following weight ranges may also be used for the initial pediatric dose of amoxicillin: <15 kg, 750 mg; 15–30 kg, 1,500 mg; and >30 kg, 3,000 mg (full adult dose).

From: Dajani AS, et al.: Prevention of bacterial endocarditis. Recommendations by the American Heart Association. JAMA, *264(22):*2920, 1990. Copyright 1990, American Medical Association.

TABLE 9-6. ALTERNATE PROPHYLACTIC REGIMENS FOR DENTAL, ORAL, OR UPPER RESPIRATORY TRACT PROCEDURES IN PATIENTS WHO ARE AT RISK

DRUG	DOSING REGIMEN†
Patients unable to take oral medications	
Ampicillin	Intravenous or intramuscular administration of ampicillin, 2.0 g, 30 minutes before procedure; then intravenous or intramuscular administration of ampicillin, 1.0 g, *or* oral administration of amoxicillin, 1.5 g, 6 hours after initial dose
Ampicillin/amoxicillin/penicillin-allergic patients unable to take oral medications	
Clindamycin	Intravenous administration of clindamycin, 300 mg, 30 minutes before procedure and intravenous or oral administration of 150 mg 6 hours after initial dose
Patients considered high risk and not candidates for standard regimen	
Ampicillin, gentamicin, and amoxicillin	Intravenous or intramuscular administration of ampicillin, 2.0 g, plus gentamicin, 1.5 mg/kg (not to exceed 80 mg), 30 minutes before procedure; followed by amoxicillin, 1.5 g orally 6 hours after initial dose; alternatively, the parenteral regimen may be repeated 8 hours after initial dose
Ampicillin/amoxicillin/penicillin-allergic patients considered high risk	
Vancomycin	Intravenous administration of 1.0 g over 1 hour, starting 1 hour before procedure; no repeated dose necessary

* Initial pediatric doses are as follows: ampicillin, 50 mg/kg; clindamycin, 10 mg/kg; gentamicin, 2.0 mg/kg; and vancomycin, 20 mg/kg. Follow-up dose should be one half the initial dose. **Total pediatric dose should not exceed total adult dose.** No initial dose is recommended in this table for amoxicillin (25 mg/kg is the follow-up dose).

From: Dajani AS, et al.: Prevention of bacterial endocarditis. Recommendations by the American Heart Association. JAMA, *264(22):*2921, 1990. Copyright 1990, American Medical Association.

TABLE 9–7. PREVENTION OF BACTERIAL ENDOCARDITIS–REGIMENS FOR GENITOURINARY/GASTROINTESTINAL PROCEDURES

DRUG	DOSING REGIMEN*
Standard regimen	
Ampicillin, gentamicin, and amoxicillin	Intravenous or intramuscular administration of ampicillin, 2.0 g, plus gentamicin, 1.5 mg/kg (not to exceed 80 mg), 30 minutes before procedure; followed by amoxicillin, 1.5 g orally 6 hours after initial dose; alternatively, the parenteral regimen may be repeated once 8 hours after initial dose
Ampicillin/amoxicillin/penicillin-allergic patient regimen	
Vancomycin and gentamicin	Intravenous administration of vancomycin, 1.0 g, over 1 hour plus intravenous or intramuscular administration of gentamicin, 1.5 mg/kg (not to exceed 80 mg), 1 hour before procedure; may be repeated once 8 hours after initial dose
Alternate low-risk patient regimen	
Amoxicillin	3.0 g orally 1 hour before procedure; then 1.5 g 6 hours after initial dose

* Initial pediatric doses are as follows: ampicillin, 50 mg/kg; amoxicillin, 50 mg/kg; gentamicin, 2.0 mg/kg; and vancomycin, 20 mg/kg. Follow-up dose should be one half the initial dose. **Total pediatric dose should not exceed total adult dose.**
From: Dajani AS, et al.: Prevention of bacterial endocarditis. Recommendations by the American Heart Association. JAMA, *264(22)*:2921, 1990. Copyright 1990, American Medical Association.

TABLE 9–8. RECOMMENDATIONS FOR ENDOCARDITIS PROPHYLAXIS IN THE UK

(1) *Dental Extractions, Scaling, or Periodontal Surgery Under Local or No Anesthesia*
  (a) For patients not allergic to penicillin and not prescribed penicillin more than once in the previous month:
  Amoxycillin
    Adults: 3 g single oral dose taken under supervision 1 hour before dental procedure
    Children under 10: half adult dose
    Children under 5: quarter adult dose
  (b) For patients allergic to penicillin:
  Erythromycin stearate
    Adults: 1.5 g orally taken under supervision 1–2 hours before dental procedure plus 0.5 g 6 hours later
    Children under 10: half adult dose
    Children under 5: quarter adult dose
  or
  Clindamycin
    Adults: 600 mg single oral dose taken under supervision 1 hour before dental procedure
    Children under 10: 6 mg/kg body weight single oral dose taken under supervision 1 hour before dental procedure

(*Continued*)

TABLE 9–8. (*cont.*)

Under general anesthesia
(c) For patients not allergic to penicillin and not given penicillin more than once in the previous month:
Amoxycillin intramuscularly
Adults: 1 g in 2.5 ml 1% lignocaine hydrochloride just before induction plus 0.5 by mouth 6 hours later
Children under 10: half adult dose
or
Amoxycillin orally
Adults 3 g oral dose 4 hours before anesthesia followed by a further 3 g by mouth as soon as possible after operation
Children under 10: half adult dose
Children under 5: quarter adult dose
or
Amoxycillin and probenecid orally
Adults: amoxycillin 3 g together with probenecid 1 g orally 4 hours before operation
Special risk patients who should be referred to hospital:
  (i) Patients with prosthetic valves who are to have a general anesthetic
  (ii) Patients who are to have a general anesthetic *and* who are allergic to penicillin or have had a penicillin more than once in the previous month
  (iii) Patients who have had a previous attack of endocarditis
  Recommendations for these patients are:
(d) For patients not allergic to penicillin and who have not had penicillin more than once in the previous month:
  Adults: 1 g amoxycillin intramuscularly in 2.5 ml 1% lignocaine hydrochloride *plus* 120 mg gentamicin intramuscularly just before induction: then 0.5 g amoxycillin orally 6 h later
  Children under 10: amoxycillin, half adult dose; gentamicin 2 mg/kg body weight
(e) For patients allergic to penicillin or who have had penicillin more than once in the previous month:
  Adults: vancomycin 1 g by slow intravenous infusion over 60 min followed by gentamicin 120 mg intravenously just before induction or 15 min before the surgical procedure
  Children under 10: vancomycin 20 mg/kg intravenously, gentamicin 2 mg/kg intravenously
(2) *Surgery or Instrumentation of Upper Respiratory Tract*
Recommended cover is as for 1*(a)* or 1*(e)*, but any postoperative antibiotic may have to be given intramuscularly or intravenously if swallowing is painful.
(3) *Genitourinary Surgery or Instrumentation*
For patients with sterile urine the suggested cover is directed against fecal streptococci and is as for 1*(d)* or 1*(e)* above. If the urine is infected prophylaxis should also cover the pathogens involved.
(4) *Obstetric and Gynecological Procedures*
Cover is suggested only for patients with prosthetic valves, and is as for 1*(d)* or 1*(e)* because of the risk from fecal streptococci
(5) *Gastrointestinal Procedures*
Cover is suggested only for patients with prosthetic valves and is as for 1*(d)* or 1*(e)*.

From: Simmons, NA et al.: Antibiotic prophylaxis of infective endocarditis. Recommendations from the Endocarditis Working Party of the British Society for Antimicrobial Chemotherapy. Lancet, *335*:89, 1990.

gurgitation is observed as frequently in women as in men, however, and requires antibiotic prophylaxis. Echocardiographic documentation is thus not necessary. If doubt exists in patients with a click, the echocardiographic findings of billowing leaflets are not an indication for antibiotics, except where there is actual mitral valve prolapse, thickening, or redundancy of valve leaflets (see Chapter 12). The British group recommends prophylaxis for mitral valve prolapse only when it is associated with a murmur

- Procedures not requiring prophylaxis include injection of local anesthetic into the gum, fiber optic bronchoscopy, endotracheal intubation, and GI endoscopy with biopsy. However, prophylaxis is advised in patients with prosthetic heart valve for all procedures, including endoscopies. Cases of endocarditis have been reported rarely in patients with prosthetic heart valve undergoing gastroscopy or other GI endoscopic procedures with or without biopsy. Endocarditis in patients with prosthetic heart valve carries a 50% mortality and must be prevented at all costs. Endocarditis prophylaxis has been shown to be effective. In a study of 533 consecutive patients with prosthetic heart valves, 229 patients given prophylaxis prior to 287 procedures resulted in no cases of endocarditis, versus six cases of endocarditis in 304 patients undergoing 390 procedures without prophylaxis
- Patients with prosthetic heart valves are at high risk and require IV antibiotics for most procedures, including low-risk procedures
- The prophylaxis advised by the AHA for genitourinary procedures has undergone a minimal but useful change: amoxicillin (3 g orally 1 hour prior and 1.5 g 6 hours post) instead of ampicillin and gentamicin IV in patients considered at low risk

BIBLIOGRAPHY

Arber N, Militianu A, Ben-Yehuda A, et al.: Native valve staphylococcus epidermidis endocarditis: Report of seven cases and review of the literature. Am J Med, *90*:758, 1991.

Aufiero TX, Waldhausen JA: Early surgery for native left-sided endocarditis. J Am Coll Cardiol, *18*:668, 1991.

Birmingham GD, Rahko PS, Ballantyne F: Improved detection of infective endocarditis with transesophageal echocardiography. Am Heart J, *123*:774, 1992.

Chan K-L: Usefulness of transesophageal echocardiography in the diagnosis of conditions mimicking aortic dissection. Am Heart J, *122*:495, 1991.

Child JS: Infective endocarditis: Risks and prophylaxis. J Am Coll Cardiol, *18*:337, 1991.

Dajani AS, Bisno AL, Chung KJ: Prevention of bacterial endocarditis. Circulation, *83*:1174, 1991.

Daniel WG, Erbel R, Kasper W, et al.: Safety of transesophageal echocardiography. A multicenter survey of 10,419 examinations. Circulation, *83*:817, 1991.

Glazier JJ, Verwilghen J, Donaldson RM, et al.: Treatment of complicated prosthetic aortic valve endocarditis with annular abscess formation by homograft aortic root replacement. J Am Coll Cardiol, *17*:1177, 1991.

Jaffe WM, Morgan DE, Pearlman AS, et al.: Infective endocarditis, 1983–1988: Echocardiographic findings and factors influencing morbidity and mortality. J Am Coll Cardiol, *15*:1227, 1990.

Kay D: Prevention of bacterial endocarditis: Ann Intern Med, *114*:803, 1991.

Martin RP: The diagnostic and prognostic role of cardiovascular ultrasound in endocarditis: Bigger is not better. J Am Coll Cardiol, *15*:1234, 1990.

Middlemost S, Wisenbaugh T, Meyerowitz CM, et al.: A case for early surgery in native left-sided endocarditis complicated by heart failure: Results in 203 patients. J Am Coll Cardiol, *18*:663, 1991.

Roberts WC, Kishel JC, McIntosh CL, et al.: Severe mitral or aortic valve regurgitation, or both, requiring valve replacement for infective endocarditis complicating hypertrophic cardiomyopathy. J Am Coll Cardiol, *19*:365, 1992.

Sanabria TJ, Alpert JS, Goldberg R, et al.: Increasing frequency of staphylococcal infective endocarditis. Arch Intern Med, *150*:1305, 1990.

Sanfilippo AJ, Picard MH, Newell JB, et al.: Echocardiographic assessment of patients with infectious endocarditis: Prediction of risk for complications. J Am Coll Cardiol, *18*:1191, 1991.

Shively BK, Gurule FT, Roldan CA, et al.: Diagnostic value of transesophageal compared with transthoracic echocardiography in infective endocarditis. J Am Coll Cardiol, *18*:391, 1991.

Steckelberg JM, Murphy JG, Ballard D, et al.: Emboli in infective endocarditis: The prognostic value of echocardiography. Ann Intern Med, *114*:635, 1991.

Takeda S, Pier GB, Kojima Y, et al.: Protection against endocarditis due to Staphylococcus epidermidis by immunization with capsular polysaccharide/adhesin. Circulation, *84*:2539, 1991.

Wells VD, Wond ES, Murray BE, et al.: Infections due to beta-lactamase-producing, high-level gentamicin-resistant faecalis. Ann Intern Med, *116*:285, 1992.

10

AORTIC DISSECTION

M. Gabriel Khan

DISSECTION OF THE ASCENDING AORTA

Dissection involving the ascending aorta has an extremely high mortality (up to 1% per minute, 60% in 60 minutes). Thus, time-consuming investigations that are not sufficiently sensitive or specific, such as CT scans, must be forsaken. Emergency surgery carries the only hope of survival for the unfortunate patient with dissection of the ascending aorta, and immediate accurate diagnosis is mandatory to guide interventional therapy. Presently, the quickest, most accurate diagnostic procedure is transesophageal echocardiography (TEE), which can be performed at the bedside, in the ICU, or in the operating room. A study by Nienaber, et al. indicates a role for magnetic resonance imaging (MRI) as the noninvasive standard for the diagnosis (see discussion of investigations).

Dissection involving the ascending aorta, Type I of DeBakey, accounts for up to 66% of all aortic dissection. Usually, the intimal tear is located just above the aortic valve. It is very rare for the dissection to start or end in the transverse arch, so there is usually no need for arch repair, which requires hypothermic arrest and carries a high mortality. Also, it is more important to know where the tear ends than where it starts.

Type II of DeBakey may be regarded as a subgroup of Type I in which dissection is confined to the ascending aorta. Type III of DeBakey accounts for up to 25% of all aortic dissections, in which the tear usually ends just distal to the left subclavian artery; the dissection is confined to the descending aorta, and rupture may occur into the left pleural space, causing a left hemothorax.

DIAGNOSTIC HALLMARKS

Diagnosis must be prompt. Clues include

* Sudden onset of severe chest and/or interscapular pain, like a "gunshot," whereas in acute myocardial infarction (MI), pain builds up gradually over several minutes
* Tearing, ripping pain
* Pain may spread to other areas as dissection advances

333

- A shock-like state: cool, clammy, and vasoconstricted; impaired sensorium, yet the blood pressure may be in the normal range. Occasionally, the blood pressure is high
- Hypotension, an ominous sign usually from external rupture
- Syncope, usually indicates rupture into the pericardial space with cardiac tamponade; pericardial effusion heralds an extremely poor prognosis
- A new, loud aortic diastolic murmur
- An aortic thrill is a strong diagnostic point if present
- Sternoclavicular joint pulsation
- Loss of one or more pulses or pulses that come and go
- Blood pressure difference in arms if the left subclavian is affected
- Ischemic neuropathy due to ischemia of the limbs
- Signs of stroke
- Paraparesis or paraplegia, may occur with marked decrease in blood supply to the cord
- The scenario may mimic arterial embolism
- May be associated with MI if the dissection extends to coronary vessels. In this clinical setting, thrombolytic agents are contraindicated

When features are less typical in the presence of central chest pain, a diagnosis of MI is considered. The lack of developing Q waves and the absence of ST segment elevation in the majority of cases, especially in association with an elevated blood pressure in the presence of a shock-like state, should prompt the diagnosis of dissection. The early absence of an increase in creatine kinase (CK) and CK-MB does not exclude acute MI and estimation is not relevant for the urgent diagnosis of dissection.

PREDISPOSING FACTORS AND ASSOCIATIONS

- The majority of patients with aortic dissection are hypertensive and over age 60. Hypertension coexists in up to 80% of patients and is more common in Type III distal dissections. Hypertension accelerates the mild degree of aortic medial degeneration that occurs with normal aging
- Normotensive younger patients usually have associated underlying disease of the aortic root. Marfan's syndrome is the leading cause of aortic dissection in patients under age 40. Other causes include giant cell arteritis, lupus erythematosus, relapsing polychondritis, and Ehlers-Danlos, Turner's, and Noonan's syndromes
- A congenital bicuspid valve appears to be present in up to 7% of patients with aortic dissection, versus 1.5% in the general adult population with a tricuspid aortic valve. The bicuspid valve is at least five times more common in patients with aortic dissection than in those individuals with a tricuspid aortic valve
- Approximately 15% of patients with coarctation of the aorta succumb to aortic dissection
- The male to female ratio is 3:1; up to 40% of dissections in women occur in the third trimester of pregnancy and in the subsequent few weeks, in conjunction with other factors that predispose dissection

INVESTIGATIONS

Investigations are limited to estimation of the hemoglobin, serum creatinine and potassium, chest x-ray, and ECG to exclude MI. There is no need to await CK-MB results

- Chest x-ray may show moderate widening of the aorta: an aortic bulge, double densities from superimposition of the false chamber and aorta
- TEE is done urgently, in the emergency room, ICU, or operating room suite prior to the surgical procedure. A precursory screening transthoracic echocardiogram may be carried out. This test has a sensitivity of about 82%. Erbel, et al. have shown TEE to have a sensitivity of 99% and a specificity of 98%. CT scans have a sensitivity of only 60%.
  In a series by Ballal, et al., TEE compared with the diagnostic gold standard, aortography, correctly diagnosed aortic dissection in 33 of 34 patients (sensitivity 97%, specificity 100%). There were no false diagnoses by TEE.
- MRI has a role when patient access can be rapidly achieved. In a series of 53 patients studied utilizing TEE, MRI, angiography, intraoperative and necropsy findings, Nienaber, et al. showed both TEE and MRI to have a sensitivity of 100% and specificity of 68 and 100%, respectively. False positive TEE occurred mainly in patients with ascending dissection and was caused by extensive plaque formation and reverberations in an ectatic vessel. Multiplanar echocardiographic imaging may overcome these deficiencies of TEE. Because retrograde angiography requires the injection of contrast that has a potential risk of aortic dissection, TEE and MRI have definite roles. MRI can be considered the noninvasive standard for the diagnosis of thoracic aortic dissection. However, experience of the image reader, techniques to deal with infusion pumps, customized tubings, extensions for mechanically ventilated patients, transportation, improved accessibility, and MRI time must be addressed. Surgeons usually will proceed to surgery based on MRI diagnosis. In the Nienaber, et al. study, the aforementioned drawbacks of MRI did not increase individual risk; this was a special study, however, and does not reflect the situation that exists in most hospitals

THERAPY

For Type I and II dissection, emergency surgery is a necessity if life is to be salvaged. Because it is extremely rare for the dissection to end or start in the transverse arch, there is usually no need for arch repair, which requires hypothermic arrest and results in an increase in surgical mortality.
Contraindications to surgery include

- Cancer or other underlying severe debilitating disease
- Age over 80 unless in robust health
- Neurologic complications of dissection

EMERGENCY DRUG THERAPY

Short-term stabilization is attempted in the emergency room and in the operating room utilizing beta blockade, nitroprusside, or trimethaphan.

Nitroprusside

Dosage: IV 0.2 to 2 μg/kg/min, i.e., 12 to 120 μg/min for a 60-kg patient, (see Table 1–10, Nitroprusside Pump Chart). The aim is to reduce the blood pressure to the lowest possible level yet preserve cardiac, cerebral, and renal perfusion. An intra-arterial cannula is advisable to accurately monitor blood pressure.

Trimethaphan
(Arfonad)

The drug is indicated if beta-adrenergic blockade is contraindicated.

Dosage: Via infusion pump 1 to 2 mg/minute and then increase, if required, to 2 to 4 mg/minute. Keep the head of the patient's bed elevated 45° to enhance the orthostatic effects of the drug. Trimethaphan does not significantly increase the velocity of ventricular contraction, and no appreciable rate of rise of aortic pressure occurs. However, rapid tachyphylaxis occurs and the drug may precipitate respiratory arrest, tachycardia, and ileus.

Alpha blockers, diazoxide, or hydralazine are contraindicated because they cause tachycardia and increase cardiac ejection velocity and rate of rise of aortic pressure that predispose rupture.

Beta-Adrenergic Blockers

Beta-adrenergic blockade is of benefit because it decreases the velocity and force of myocardial contraction and reduces the rate of rise of aortic pressure, which is a major factor in determining extension of the dissection. Nitroprusside increases the velocity of ventricular contraction, the rate of pressure rise, and hence, the need for combination with a beta-adrenergic blocker.

Esmolol

Dosage: IV infusion, 5 to 40 mg over 1 minute (30 to 500 μg/kg/minute), then maintenance 1 to 5 mg/minute (maximum 50 μg/kg/minute). If hypotension is present or develops, decrease the maintenance dose to 1 to 3 mg/minute.

Propranolol

Dosage: 0.5 mg/min IV at 2- to 5-minute intervals to a maximum of 5 mg then 0.05 to 0.15 mg/kg every 4 to 6 hours (see Table 3–4).

Metoprolol

Dosage: 1 mg/min at 5-minute intervals to a maximum of 15 mg repeated every 6 to 8 hours

Atenolol

Dosage: IV infusion 150 μg/kg over 20 minutes repeated every 12 hours if required.

DISSECTION OF THE DESCENDING AORTA

Some time is available here for diagnostic workup with aortic arteriograms and, in some patients, MRI or CT scan if immediately available. In patients with dissection of the descending aorta, as opposed to those with ascending dissection, ischemic heart disease is often present and coronary arteriography is required.

Blood pressure is aggressively controlled with nitroprusside and beta blockers, and surgery should proceed in 12 to 48 hours. If spinal involvement is present, the patient and next of kin must thoroughly understand that that spinal problems may not be helped.

There is no need to surgically correct all descending dissections, but close follow-up with CT scan is necessary. If widening occurs, surgery should be prompt.

MARFAN'S SYNDROME

Patients with Marfan's Syndrome may develop aortic root dilatation, aortic regurgitation, and aneurysm of the ascending aorta. Patients may survive for several years.

Management includes intensive control of blood pressure. Beta-adrenergic blockers must be given to all patients with aneurysms, even if the blood pressure is in the normal range. Alpha blockers and hydralazine are contraindicated. Surgery is indicated if the aneurysm exceeds 5 cm. The outlook is bleak, however, even with surgery.

The non-Marfan patient with an asymptomatic, ascending aortic aneurysm should be submitted to surgery if the aneurysm is greater than 6 cm.

POST-SURGERY FOLLOW-UP

Aggressive control of blood pressure is necessary. The blood pressure must be kept fairly low and the rate of rise of aortic pressure must be decreased with the use of beta-adrenergic blockers. With all types of dissection, intensive post-surgery follow-up is essential. Patients with ascending dissection repair should be followed monthly with TEE for 3 months; descending aortic dissection necessitates CT scanning or MRI to assess enlargement. A false lumen is invariably present with some flow and is not an indication for surgery, except when the false lumen widens considerably.

Postoperative late deaths are usually due to rupture; thus, close monitoring of both surgical and medical patients is necessary.

BIBLIOGRAPHY

Ballal RS, Nanda NC, Gatewood R, et al.: Usefulness of transesophageal echocardiography in assessment of aortic dissection. Circulation, *84*:1903, 1991.

Debakey ME, Hendy WS, Cooley DA, et al.: Surgical management of dissecting aneurysm of the aorta. J Thorac Cardiovasc Surg, *49*:130, 1965.

DeSanctis RW, Doroghazi RM, Austen WG, et al.: Aortic dissection. N Engl J Med, *317*:1060, 1987.

Editorial: Acute Aortic Dissection. Lancet, 2:827, 1988.

Fenoglio JJ, Jr., McAllister HA, Jr., DeCastro CM, et al.: Congenital bicuspid aortic valve after age 20. Am J Cardiol, *39*:164, 1977.

Hirata K, Triposkiadis F, Sparks E, et al.: The Marfan Syndrome: Abnormal aortic elastic properties. J Am Coll Cardiol, *18*:57, 1991.

Nienaber CA, Spielmann RP, von Kodolitsch Y, et al.: Diagnosis of thoracic aortic dissection. Magnetic resonance imaging versus transesophageal echocardiography. Circulation, *85*:434, 1992.

Reed D, Reed C, Stemmerman G, et al.: Are aortic aneurysms caused by atherosclerosis? Circulation, *85*:205, 1992.

Roberts CS, Roberts WC: Dissection of the aorta associated with congenital malformation of the aortic valve. J Am Coll Cardiol, *17*:712, 1991.

Roberts CS, Roberts WC: Aortic dissection with the entrance tear in abdominal aorta. Am Heart J, *121*:1834, 1991.

11

DEEP VENOUS THROMBOSIS
M. Gabriel Khan

Deep venous thrombosis (DVT) occurring in the lower limbs is often impossible to diagnose from the history and physical examination. Some patients present with pain and swelling of the calf or thigh, and others are asymptomatic. The venous occlusion causes chronic passive congestion, and the muscle tissue becomes swollen with edema; a variable inflammatory response and perivascular hemorrhage may occur.

Differential diagnosis includes muscle tear, muscle cramps, ruptured Baker's cyst, external compression cellulitis without lymphangitis, and post-phlebitic syndrome. The presence of risk factors lends strong support to the diagnosis: e.g., previous DVT, soft tissue injury, the postoperative state, pregnancy, post partum, sudden immobilization for over 3 days, fractured lower limb, obesity, oral contraceptives, estrogens, underlying malignancies, heart failure, dehydration.

Inciting factors are

- Venous stasis
- Endothelial injury
- Hypercoagulability

Because pulmonary embolism occurs commonly in patients with thrombosis of the femoral and iliac veins, this situation is considered serious and life threatening. Below-the-knee deep venous thrombosis that fails to extend above the knee rarely embolizes. It must be emphasized, however, that the incidence of postphlebitic syndrome is 30 to 40% with calf vein thrombosis.

INVESTIGATIONS

- Venography is the investigation of choice for DVT
- Impedance plethysmography (IPG) detects thrombosis above the knee. Because only approximately 30% of acute calf vein thrombi later extend above the knee, a first negative IPG would reveal the extension later if the test was repeated on day 2, days 5 to 7, and if needed, on days 10 to 14. If the IPG becomes positive, anticoagulation is commenced. Trials have shown this method to be effective, especially because extension

above the knee is uncommon after day 7. In clinical practice, however, it is often difficult to arrange such tests for patients, except in specialized centers. Extension of thrombosis may occur and go unnoticed prior to the second or third IPG testing. IPG cannot distinguish old from fresh thrombi. Also, false positive results occur with heart failure, compression by pelvic tumor, or a gravid uterus. Thus, loopholes exist that may allow medicolegal action. The IPG method of managing DVT is suited to some teaching hospitals

- Duplex scanning: Real-time B mode Doppler ultrasound imaging carried out by experienced staff is useful in detecting above-knee thrombosis, but an incomplete venous obstruction may not be detected

THERAPY

After verifying a normal prothrombin time (PT) or international normalized ratio (INR), activated partial thromboplastin time (PTT), and platelets, commence the following.

HEPARIN

Dosage: IV bolus 100 units/kg, usually 5,000 to 7,500 units, then a continuous infusion of 15 to 25 units/kg/hour (set up as suggested in Table 11–1). In practice, it is convenient to add 20,000 units of heparin to 1 liter of 0.9% saline or 5% dextrose water for cardiac patients. This diluted so-

TABLE 11–1. CONTINUOUS INFUSION HEPARIN		
RATE (ml/hr)	**UNITS (/hr)**	**UNITS (/24 hrs)**
1. 21	840	20,160
2. 25	1000	24,000
3. 28	1120	26,880
4. 30	1200	28,800
5. 32	1280	30,720
6. 34	1360	32,640
7. 36	1440	34,560
8. 38	1520	36,480
9. 40	1600	38,400
10. 42	1680	40,320
11. 44	1760	42,240
12. 46	1840	44,160
13. 48	1920	46,080
14. 50	2000	48,000

20,000 units of heparin in 500 ml of 5% dextrose in water. If noncardiac, dilute in 0.9% saline. 1 ml equals 40 units.
* For each heparin order, specify both the rate of flow and the dose in units per hour.
Commence with No. 4, 1200 units/hr and adjust to maintain activated PTT at 1.5 to 2.5 times control value (usual therapeutic range 60 to 85 seconds; see text for the use of a nomogram).

lution of heparin (20 units/ml) is safer for general use than a 40- to 50-units/ml solution, which can cause life-threatening hemorrhage if the infusion pump becomes defective and heparin is infused inadvertently. However, a 40 units/ml solution is commonly used. The physician should specify the rate of flow (e.g., 30 ml/hour) and the dose (1,200 units/hour) (Table 11-1). Commence the infusion at 1,200 units/hour. Check the PTT 6 hours after the bolus injection, and then increase or decrease the infusion to maintain the activated PTT 1.5 to 2.5 times the mean control range that corresponds to a plasma heparin level of 0.2 to 0.4 units/ml (maximum 0.5 units/ml by protamine titration). The United States pharmaceutical units may be approximately 12% more potent than the international units used elsewhere. If either massive DVT or thromboembolism is suspected, the PTT should be determined 1 hour after the bolus dose. If the PTT is near the control value, another bolus of heparin should be administered, because these patients may have a more rapid heparin clearance.

Cruickshank, et al. have devised a standard heparin nomogram for the adjustment of IV heparin dosage. After a 5,000 unit bolus, their advice is as follows

- Commence with IV heparin infusion 32 ml/hour, 1280 units/hour (No. 5, Table 11-1)
- If the 6-hour PTT is 50 to 59, increase the rate 3 ml/hour and repeat the PTT in 6 hours
- If the PTT is 60 to 85, no change in rate, repeat the PTT next morning
- If the PTT is 86 to 95 decrease the rate 2 ml/hour, repeat PTT the next morning
- If the PTT is 96 to 120, hold the infusion for 30 minutes, decrease the rate 2 ml/hour, repeat the PTT in 6 hours
- If the PTT is greater than 120, hold the IV for 60 minutes, decrease the rate 4 ml/hour, and repeat the PTT in 6 hours
- If during the first 48 hours of therapy the PTT is subtherapeutic, less than 50 despite a heparin dose of 1,440 units/hour or greater, administer a heparin bolus of 5,000 units and increase the rate 5 ml/hour

At 24 to 48 hours after the start of heparin therapy, a therapeutic PTT was achieved in 66 and 81%, versus 37 and 58% in a heparin control group. The nomogram has proven useful. A specific thromboplastin (Actin FS) was used to devise the nomogram, which could be adapted to other reagents; it is necessary to compare either the test reagents and the Actin FS reagent or the test reagent and the heparin assay.

When the PTT is in the desired range, monitor PTT once daily. The platelet count should be evaluated after the third day of heparin therapy.

Action. The anticoagulant activity of heparin requires a cofactor, antithrombin III. Heparin binds to lysine sites on antithrombin III and converts the cofactor from a slow inhibitor to a very rapid inhibitor of thrombin. The heparin-antithrombin III complex inactivates thrombin and factor X, as well as a number of coagulation enzymes. The principal anticoagulant effect of heparin-antithrombin III appears to be caused by inhibition of thrombin-induced activation of factor V and factor VIII. Almost 20 times more heparin is required to initiate fibrin-bound thrombin than to inactivate free thrombin. Thus, the prevention of the extension of venous thrombosis requires much higher concentrations of heparin than the prevention of thrombus formation.

Also, heparin inhibits some aspects of platelet function and increases the permeability of vessel walls. Heparin is poorly absorbed from the gut and must be given parenterally. Heparin bound to endothelial cells is internalized and depolymerized, and desulfation occurs in mononuclear phagocytes. The elimination route of heparin remains uncertain. The agent has an apparent half-life of approximately 30 and 60 minutes after a 25- and 75-units/kg IV bolus, respectively.

It is advisable to continue to treat patients with heparin IV if immobilization or precipitating factors persist. For below-the-knee DVT, 14 days of subcutaneous calcium heparin appears to cause greater resolution of thrombosis compared to continuous heparin and deserves consideration. Calcium heparin, 250 units/kg subcutaneous twice daily and adjusted to maintain PTT 1.5 to 2 times the control, has a role in below-the-knee DVT.

Adverse effects. Thrombocytopenia caused by heparin occurs in up to 4% of patients. It is believed to be the result of immune sensitization to a heparin-platelet complex. This complication is associated with life-threatening arterial or venous thrombosis. Platelet counts should be assessed in patients administered heparin IV for a period longer than 3 days. Osteoporosis may occur after 5 months of therapy. Alopecia is a rare adverse effect.

Interactions. High-dose IV nitroglycerin may increase the required dose of heparin possibly because of an alteration in the antithrombin III molecule.

Contraindications
- Hemophilia and other hemorrhagic disorders
- Peptic ulceration, severe uncontrolled hypertension, severe hepatic disease, cerebral aneurysm, recent ophthalmic surgery, and pregnancy.

ORAL ANTICOAGULANTS

Coumarins induce anticoagulation by inhibiting vitamin K epoxide reductase, which causes an accumulation of hepatic and circulating vitamin K epoxide and a depletion of vitamin KH_2, limiting the carboxylation and biologic function of vitamin-K-dependent coagulant proteins (prothrombin, factors VII, IX, and X) and anticoagulant proteins (protein C and protein S).

Warfarin, a 4-hydroxycoumarin compound, has some anticoagulant effect within 12 to 24 hours, but peak activity is approximately 72 hours, because it takes time to impair the biologic function of coagulant protein and to clear circulating clotting factors.

Because the half-life of factor VII is about $6\frac{1}{2}$ hours and that of II, IX, and X is several days, peak warfarin effect is delayed (72 to 96 hours).

Importantly, protein C has a half-life as short as factor VII, and with depletion during the first 24 to 48 hours of anticoagulant therapy, there is a theoretically heightened risk of thrombosis in the first 12 hours of therapy. Therefore, for optimal salutary effects, heparin must be administered for 12 hours before giving warfarin.

Because protein C has a short half-life, a 5-day overlap of IV heparin and warfarin is necessary to prevent a potentially thrombogenic effect, which can be caused by low levels of protein C during the period when the levels of factors II and X are normal (during the first 4 days of warfarin therapy).

Adverse effects. Bleeding is common with prothrombin ratio greater than 2 or INR greater than 3.5; if the INR is less than 3 with an International Sensitivity Index (ISI) of 2.3, search for an underlying cause of bleeding. The risk of bleeding is increased in patients over age 65 and those who have occult GI lesions, renal failure, anemia from other causes, a history of cerebral vascular disease, ingestion of aspirin or nonsteroidal anti-inflammatory agents. Rarely, skin necrosis occurs due to extensive thrombosis of capillaries and venules in subcutaneous tissue. The pathogenesis of this unusual complication, which occurs between the third and seventh day of therapy, is undetermined but appears to be linked to the decrease in biologic activity of protein C caused by coumarins.

Contraindications
- Peptic ulcer or recent GI bleeding, pregnancy, severe and controlled hypertension, bacterial endocarditis

MONITORING OF ORAL ANTICOAGULANT EFFECT

Measurement of the INR is recommended by the World Health Organization (WHO) and has become established in the UK and Europe, but has been adopted by only a minority of hospitals and laboratories in North America, where most physicians have used a prothrombin time ratio of 1.5 to 2.0 since the early 1970s and more recently 1.4 to 1.7, with further changes in the thromboplastins used. Physicians who have inadvertently continued to use the 1948 AHA guideline prothrombin ratio of 2.0 to 2.5 have noted an increased incidence of bleeding.

The laboratory-determined INR is the prothrombin time ratio that reflects the result that would have been obtained if the WHO reference thromboplastin had been used to perform the test in that laboratory.

$$INR = \left(\frac{\text{patient PT}}{\text{control PT}}\right)^{ISI}$$

The INR is based, therefore, on two contributing factors: prothrombin time ratio and the ISI. The ISI is a measure of the responsiveness of a given thromboplastin to reduction in the vitamin-K-dependent coagulation factors. All reagent manufacturers should provide the laboratory with the ISI value.

Rabbit-brain thromboplastins have an ISI of 2.0 to 2.6, and the INR should be determined with the consistent use of sensitive thromboplastins

TABLE 11–2. SUGGESTED THERAPEUTIC RANGE OF INR AND CORRESPONDING PROTHROMBIN TIME RATIO FOR ANTICOAGULATION

CLINICAL SITUATION	PROTHROMBIN TIME RATIO	INR	ISI
Deep venous thrombosis	1.4–1.7	2–3	2.0
	1.4–1.6	2–3	2.3
	1.3–1.5	2–3	2.6
Atrial fibrillation	1.4–1.6	2–3	As above
Prosthetic heart valves:			
mechanical	1.5–1.9	2.3–3.6	2.0*
tissue	1.4–1.5	2–2.3	

INR = International Normalized Ratio
ISI = International Sensitivity Index
* The laboratory should state the ISI of the thromboplastin used. (see Table 11–3, INR nomogram)

with similar ISI values. An INR of 2 to 3, the desired range of anticoagulation for the majority of clinical situations, utilizing a thromboplastin with an ISI of 2.3, gives a corresponding prothrombin ratio of 1.4 to 1.6. This is considered a moderate intensity regimen that is adequate for the treatment of DVT. The suggested range of INR and the prothrombin time ratio for the management of some clinical situations are shown in Table 11–2; see Table 11–3, prothrombin time ratio, INR conversion chart; INR nomogram.

WARFARIN FOR DEEP VENOUS THROMBOSIS

DVT that extends to the mid thigh but is noniliofemoral, occurring in patients where the precipitating factors are removed and early mobilization is attained, can be treated with early administration of oral anticoagulants. Warfarin is begun on the second night following the commencement of heparin, at which time the diagnosis is usually confirmed by venography and the therapeutic level of heparin has been well maintained for more than 24 hours. Because warfarin may take from 24 to 96 hours to achieve anticoagulation and the biologic activity of protein C is markedly limited within the first 24 hours of warfarin therapy, resulting in an enhanced early thrombogenic state, Hull and Raskob advise that it is necessary to overlap the heparin and warfarin for 5 days to prevent the potentially thrombogenic effect caused by the presence of nearly normal levels of factors II and X during the first 3 or 4 days of warfarin therapy. A similar duration of heparin therapy is obtained if an order is written to discontinue IV heparin when the prothrombin time or INR is in the therapeutic range for 2 full days.

Warfarin

Dosage: 10 mg daily for 2 days, the third and daily dose is titrated to maintain the INR (2 to 3) or prothrombin time ratio (1.4 to 1.6, prothrombin time 1.4 to 1.6 times the control). The prothrombin time is often 16 to 19 seconds when the control prothrombin time is 12 seconds.

TABLE 11–3. INR NOMOGRAM

Pt ratio	1.2	1.4	1.6	1.8	2.0	2.2	2.4	2.6	2.8	3.0
3.0	3.74	4.66								
2.9	3.59	4.44								
2.8	3.44	4.23	5.19							
2.7	3.29	4.02	4.90							
2.6	3.15	3.81	4.61							
2.5	*3.00**	3.61	4.33	5.20						
2.4	*2.86*	3.41	4.06	4.83						
2.3	*2.72*	3.21	3.79	4.48	5.29					
2.2	*2.58*	3.02	3.53	4.13	4.84					
2.1	*2.44*	*2.82*	3.28	3.80	4.41	5.16				
2.0	*2.30*	*2.64*	3.03	3.48	4.00	4.59	5.28			
1.9	*2.16*	*2.26*	*2.79*	3.18	3.61	4.10	4.67	5.31		
1.8	*2.02*	*2.28*	*2.56*	*2.88*	*3.24*	3.64	4.10	4.61	5.19	5.83
1.7	1.89	*2.10*	*2.34*	*2.60*	*2.89*	3.21	3.57	3.97	4.42	4.91
1.6	1.76	1.93	*2.12*	*2.33*	*2.56*	*2.81*	3.09	3.39	3.73	4.10
1.5	1.63	1.76	1.91	*2.07*	*2.25*	*2.44*	*2.65*	*2.87*	3.11	3.38
1.4	1.50	1.60	1.71	1.83	1.96	*2.10*	2.24	2.40	*2.57*	*2.74*
1.3†	→1.37	→1.44	→1.52	→1.60	→1.69	→**1.78**	1.88	1.98	*2.08*	*2.20*
1.2	1.24	1.29	1.34	1.39	1.44	↑1.49	1.55	1.61	1.67	1.73
1.1	1.12	1.14	1.16	1.19	1.21	↑1.23	1.26	1.28	1.31	1.33
	1.2	1.4	1.6	1.8	2.0	↑**2.2**	2.4	2.6	2.8	3.0

Range of ISI values for most commercial thromboplastins

* Italic numbers = Most Common INR Values
The nomogram is used to determine the INR from observed prothrombin ratio.
† Bold = Example (arrows): An observed ratio of 1.3 with thromboplastin of ISI 2.2 equals an INR of 1.78.
Adapted from: Leclerc J: Venous Thromboembolic Disorders. Philadelphia, Lea & Febiger, 1990.

When the prothrombin time ratio or INR is in the desired range, overlap heparin for an additional 2 full days. Thus, heparin is given for a total of 5 to 6 days. With this method of heparin/warfarin therapy, the patient is usually ready to discharge on the sixth day. A recent study has indicated that 9 to 10 days of heparin therapy is not superior to 5 days of heparin with overlapping warfarin in patients with submassive venous thrombosis. The short course of heparin reduces the length of hospital stay and is an important patient cost consideration but is not recommended for iliac vein thrombosis or major pulmonary embolism.

The warfarin dose should be given at bedtime; this allows the physician or nurse to alter the dose based on the result of the prothrombin time ratio or INR obtained during the day.

For iliofemoral thrombosis or major pulmonary embolus, warfarin is commenced on the fifth night of heparin therapy, which with 5 days overlap, results in 10 days of heparin therapy. Warfarin is usually continued for 3 months, and the prothrombin time ratio is maintained in the range of 1.5 to 1.75 (INR = 2 to 3.2). Patients with isolated calf DVT are treated for 3 months, and the prothrombin time ratio is maintained at 1.4 to 1.5 (INR = 2 to 3). Patients presenting with a second DVT are treated for 1

TABLE 11–4. ORAL ANTICOAGULANTS–DRUG INTERACTIONS

1. Drugs that may enhance anticoagulant response

Alcohol	Naproxen
Alopurinol	Neomycin
Aminoglycosides	Penicillin (large doses IV)
Amiodarone	Phenformin
Ampicillin	Phenylbutazone
Anabolic steroids	Phenytoin
Aspirin	Propylthiouracil
Cephalosporins	Propafenone
Chloral hydrate	Quinidine
Chloramphenicol	Sulfinpyrazone
Chlorpromazine	Sulfonamides
Chlorpropamide	Tetracyclines
Chlortetracycline	Tolbutamide
Cimetidine	Tricyclic antidepressants
Ciprofloxacin	Verapamil
Clofibrate (fibrates)	

2. Drugs that may decrease anticoagulant response

Co-trimoxazole	Antacids
Danazol	Antihistamines
Dextrothyroxine	Barbiturates
Diazoxide	Carbamazepine
Dipyridamole	Cholestyramine
Disulfiram	Colestipol
Erythromycin	Corticosteroids
Ethacrynic acid	Cyclophosphamide
Fenclofenac	Dichloralphenazone
Fenoprofen	Disopyramide
Flufenamic acid	Glutethimide
Fluvoxamine	Griseofulvin
Liquid paraffin	Mercaptopurine
Mefenamic acid	Oral contraceptives
Methotrexate	Pheneturide
Metronidazole	Phenobarbitone
Monoamine oxidase inhibitors	Primidone
Nalidixic acid	Rifampicin
	Vitamins K_1 and K_2

Modified from: Khan, M Gabriel: Cardiac Drug Therapy. 3rd Ed. London, W.B. Saunders, 1992.

year. Patients with recurrent DVT and underlying risk factors are administered warfarin indefinitely. Patients with a stable anticoagulant response should be maintained with an estimation of INR or prothrombin time every 4 weeks. Drugs that may increase or decrease anticoagulant activity are listed in Table 11–4.

THROMBOLYTIC THERAPY

Acute massive pulmonary embolism and iliac or iliofemoral vein thrombosis, the latter of less than 14 days duration, should be managed with thrombolytic therapy to prevent a 60 to 70% incidence of postphlebitic syndrome and/or pulmonary embolism.

Streptokinase

Dosage: Loading dose, 250,000 units IV over 30 minutes, maintenance infusion 100,000 units/hour for 48 to 72 hours in patients with iliofemoral vein thrombosis. In patients with pulmonary embolism, the infusion is continued from 12 to 24 hours. Following the infusion, the PTT should be maintained at 1.5 to 2 times the control with the use of heparin (Table 11–1). Contraindications for streptokinase or thrombolytic therapy are given in Chapter 3.

Urokinase

Although it is more expensive than streptokinase, urokinase is nonantigenic and IV therapy is given for a much shorter duration.

Dosage: IV bolus of 4,000 IU/kg over 10 minutes and continuous infusion of 4,000 IU/kg/hour. Noninvasive studies should show a response in 24 hours. Continue the infusion as long as there is continued improvement. Discontinue the infusion if no improvement is observed in 24 hours or if there is no clot resolution over a 24-hour period. tPA also works well in this condition (see Chapter 30 for dosage).

HYPERCOAGULABILITY AND THROMBOEMBOLISM

Congenital and, more commonly, acquired abnormalities are associated with a high incidence of thrombotic complications and must be sought by careful history, physical, and laboratory investigations in patients with recurrent thromboses or thrombosis occurring in the absence of the usual trigger factors.

Congenital hypercoagulable disorders are rare and include

* Antithrombin III deficiency: In the homozygous setting, death occurs in infancy due to overwhelming thrombosis. The heterozygote state may present in the third decade of life or later. An increase in the partial thromboplastin time to 1.5 to 2 times the control, observed after a bolus and infusion of heparin over 6 hours, excludes significant antithrombin III deficiency so that assay of antithrombin III is not required
* Protein C deficiency: Presents as purpura fulminans neonatalis; rarely, thrombotic tendency is manifest in the late teens and early adulthood. Protein C is a vitamin-K-dependent protein. Patients presenting as young adults with recurrent DVT or with spontaneous abortions or coumarin skin necrosis require protein C assay
* Protein S deficiency: a rare vitamin-K-dependent protein with manifestations similar to protein C deficiency

Acquired hypercoagulability is associated with the following conditions

* Street drugs, which increase platelet count and adhesiveness
* Blood group A_1: Individuals with blood group A appear to have an elevated prothrombin and factor VIII and a significant decrease in an-

tithrombin III activity. These abnormalities are mainly observed in the subtype A_1, which represents less than 5% of the total population
- Birth control pills or estrogen therapy
- Surgical treatment, which usually triggers an increase in factor VIII, a decrease in protein C, and increased adhesiveness
- Several cancers, particularly pancreatic, stomach, large gut, and prostate, induce clotting by increasing coagulability, which is believed to be related to a decrease in platelet antithrombin, an increase in fibrinogen, and a decrease in antithrombin III activity
- Lupus erythematosus: A lupus anticoagulant, the presence of which can be detected in the laboratory, is present in up to 10% of cases, but its role in thrombus formation is unclear

The majority of patients suspected of hypercoagulable state should be referred to a hematologist for further evaluation and advice.

BIBLIOGRAPHY

Altman P, Rouvier J, Gurfinkel E, et al.: Comparison of two levels of anticoagulant therapy in patients with substitute heart valves. J Thorac Cardiovasc Surg, *101*:427, 1991.

Choonora IA, Malia RG, Haynes BP, et al.: The relationship between inhibition of vitamin K 2,3-epoxide reductase and reduction of clotting factor activity with warfarin. Br J Clin Pharmacol, *25*:1, 1988.

Curickshank MK, Levine MN, Hirsh J, et al.: A standard heparin nomogram for the management of heparin therapy. Arch Intern Med, *51*:333, 1991.

Gallus A, Jackaman J, Tillett J, et al.: Safety and efficacy of warfarin started early after submassive venous thrombosis or pulmonary embolism. Lancet, *2*:1293, 1986.

Gent M, Blakely JA, Easton JD, et al.: The Canadian American Ticlopidine Study (CATS) in thromboembolic stroke. Lancet, *1*:8649, 1989.

Hirsh J: Review article: Oral anticoagulant drugs. N Engl J Med, *324*:1865, 1991.

Hull RD, Raskob GE, Rosenbloom D, et al.: Heparin for 5 days as compared with 10 days in the initial treatment of proximal venous thrombosis. N Engl J Med, *322*:1260, 1990.

Hirsh J: Drug therapy: Heparin. N Engl J Med, *324*:1565, 1991.

International Committee for Standardization in Haematology, International Committee on Thrombosis and Haemotosis. ICSH/ICTH recommendations for reporting prothrombin time in oral anticoagulant control. Thromb Haemost, *53*:155, 1985.

Leclerc J: Venous Thromboembolic Disorders. Philadelphia, Lea and Febiger, 1990.

Levine MN, Hirsh J, Gent M, et al.: Prevention of deep vein thrombosis after elective hip surgery. Ann Intern Med, *114*:545, 1991.

Love PE, Santoro SA: Antiphospholipid antibodies: Anticardiolipin and the lupus anticoagulant in systemic lupus erythematosus (SLE) and in non-SLE disorders. Ann Intern Med, *112*:682, 1990.

Lynch DM, Howe SE: Heparin-associated thrombocytopenia: Antibody binding specificity to platelet antigens. Blood, *66*:1176, 1985.

Mohiuddin SM, Hilleman DE, Destache CJ, et al.: Efficacy and safety of early versus late initiation of warfarin during heparin therapy in acute thromboembolism. Am Heart J, *123*: 729, 1992.

Poller L: Progress in standardization in anticoagulant control. Hematol Rev, *1*:225, 1987.

Poller L: Laboratory control of oral anticoagulants. Br Med J, *294*:1184, 1987.

Saour JN, Sieck JO, Mamo LAR, et al.: Trial of different intensities of anticoagulation in patients with prosthetic heart valves. N Engl J Med, *322*:428, 1990.

Zucker S, Cathey MH, Sox PJ, et al.: Standardization of laboratory tests for controlling anticoagulant therapy. Am J Clin Pathol, *53*:348, 1970.

12

VALVULAR HEART DISEASE AND RHEUMATIC FEVER

M. Gabriel Khan

AORTIC STENOSIS

The causes of aortic stenosis and the average survival of patients are given in Tables 12–1 and 12–2.

Rheumatic aortic stenosis is now uncommon, except in Asia, Africa, the Middle East, and Latin America. The patient's age at the time of diagnosis usually gives a reasonable assessment of the underlying disease. Diagnosis prior to age 30 is typical of congenital aortic stenosis. In patients over age 70, calcific aortic sclerosis due to degenerative calcification is common, and significant stenosis develops in up to 5% of these individuals. A bicuspid valve occurs in 2 to 3% of the population, with a male to female ratio of 4:1, and is predisposed to degenerative calcification. Between age 30 and 70, calcification of a bicuspid valve is the most common cause of aortic stenosis, and much less frequently, cases of rheumatic valvular disease are encountered.

PHYSICAL SIGNS OF SIGNIFICANT AORTIC STENOSIS

- A systolic crescendo–decrescendo murmur best heard at the lower left sternal border, the second right interspace, or occasionally at the apex, with radiation to the neck
- The longer the murmur and the later the peak of the crescendo–decrescendo, the greater the gradient
- The intensity of the murmur, in the absence of significant aortic regurgitation, is usually Grade 3 or greater, except if cardiac output is low, as with heart failure; then, even a Grade 2 murmur may be in keeping with severe stenosis. Aortic regurgitation increases flow across the aortic valve and may produce a loud systolic murmur without stenosis
- An absent or very soft aortic component of the second sound (A2)
- An S4 gallop is usually present and is highly significant in patients under age 50

349

TABLE 12–1. CAUSES OF AORTIC VALVULAR STENOSIS	
Biscuspid calcific	60%*
Degenerative calcific	15%
Rheumatic	20%*
Other	5%

* Reverse in Asia, Africa, Middle East, Latin America

TABLE 12–2. AVERAGE SURVIVAL IN PATIENTS WITH MODERATE OR SEVERE AORTIC STENOSIS	
CLINICAL PARAMETERS	**SURVIVAL YEARS**
Left ventricular failure	1.5 to 2
Severe shortness of breath	2
Mild shortness of breath	3 to 4
Syncope	3
Angina	4 to 5

- A thrill is commonly present over the base of the heart or the carotid arteries; this indicates a murmur of Grade 4 or louder and may relate to the severity of aortic stenosis if aortic regurgitation is absent
- A thrusting, forceful apex beat of left ventricular hypertrophy (LVH); the apex beat is usually not displaced, except in patients with concomitant aortic regurgitation or with terminal left ventricular (LV) dilatation
- The carotid or brachial pulse in patients under age 65 shows a typical delayed upstroke. In the elderly, loss of elasticity in arteries often masks this important sign

INVESTIGATIONS

ELECTROCARDIOGRAM

The ECG in patients with moderate to severe stenosis often shows features of LVH

- S wave in V1, plus R in V5 or V6 or greater than 35 mm
- SV3, plus R in AVL greater than 20 mm Hg
- Left atrial enlargement
- ST-T change typical of LV strain: The ascending limb of the T wave is steeper than the descending in leads V5 and V6, with a lesser change in V4
- Left bundle branch block

CHEST X-RAY

Concentric LVH occurs; thus, the chest x-ray usually shows a normal heart size, with some rounding of the left lower cardiac border and apex, and occasionally some posterior protrusion in the lateral view may suggest

LVH. The heart size may be increased if cardiac failure supervenes or with concomitant aortic regurgitation. A common hallmark of valvular aortic stenosis is poststenotic dilatation of the ascending aorta.

ECHOCARDIOGRAPHY

The severity of aortic stenosis can be determined by continuous wave Doppler echocardiography. This technique agrees with data obtained from catheterization in up to 85% of cases.

Moderate to severe aortic stenosis is indicated by the following

- Doppler peak systolic pressure gradient greater than 60 mm Hg in the presence of a normal cardiac output
- Maximal instantaneous Doppler gradient greater than 60 mm Hg (range = 64 to 165 mm Hg)
- Peak systolic flow velocity greater than 4 m/s (range often observed = 4 to 7 m/s)
- Valve mean gradient greater than 40 (range in several clinical studies = 40 to 120 mm Hg)
- Valve area less than about 0.75 cm^2 in an average-sized adult, 0.4 cm^2/m^2 of body surface area, severe or critical stenosis (Table 12–3)

Valve area greater than 1.5 cm^2 indicates mild aortic stenosis, 0.75 to 1.4 cm^2 indicates moderate stenosis.

THERAPY

Because medical therapy is said to play a small role in management and the consequences of valve surgery may be life threatening, the timing of valve replacement requires accurate knowledge of the natural history of significant aortic stenosis, as well as careful attention to details in the patient's history and the sound appraisal of information gathered from Doppler echocardiography correlated with catheterization data.

It is now clear that more sophisticated echo Doppler techniques are available and can, in over 80% of patients, dispense with catheterization data. However, since valve surgery is a lifesaving but hazardous procedure, it

TABLE 12–3. HEMODYNAMIC PARAMETERS FOR SEVERE AORTIC STENOSIS

	AORTIC VALVE AREA* (cm^2)	AORTIC VALVE AREA INDEX (cm^2/m^2)	PEAK SYSTOLIC GRADIENT (mm Hg)	MEAN GRADIENT (mm Hg)
Severe stenosis	<0.75	<0.4	≥80	≥70
Probable severe	0.75–0.9	0.4–0.6	50–79	40–69
Uncertain	>0.9 to 1.2	>0.6	<50	<40

* = In an average-sized adult

is vital to gather information from all sources, including catheterization, to allow for sound decision-making when surgery is being contemplated. In certain patients, ancillary information about the state of the coronary arteries is of cardinal value in reaching a therapeutic decision. Importantly, in a recent study comparing echo Doppler with catheterization data to determine the timing for valve surgery, agreement varied from a 92% level for aortic regurgitation to 90% for mitral stenosis, but only 83% and 69% for aortic stenosis and mitral regurgitation, respectively.

NATURAL HISTORY

Significant aortic stenosis has a variable natural history. An elderly patient with moderately severe degenerative calcific aortic stenosis may progress rapidly to a more severe status with life-threatening symptomatology. Some patients with rheumatic or bicuspid valve calcification with moderate to severe stenosis may remain asymptomatic for several years. Less than 5% of asymptomatic patients with moderate or severe acquired aortic stenosis die suddenly, but even in these patients, a careful history taken weeks prior to death often elicits some symptomatology, albeit minimal. Thus, minimally symptomatic patients with moderate or severe aortic stenosis must be followed closely with attention to careful history, physical examination, assessment of electrocardiography, Doppler echocardiographic data, and Holter monitoring. The aortic valve index and a decrease in ejection fraction (EF) are important parameters.

When symptoms are manifest, the natural history can be anticipated. Patients with LV failure or severe breathlessness have a less than 2-year survival (Table 12–2). Mild shortness of breath or syncope indicate a 3-year survival, and angina without other manifestations usually indicates a 4- to 5-year survival in the absence of significant IHD. Angina may, of course, be due to IHD in some patients with mild to moderate aortic stenosis.

Thus, decision-making in the management of symptomatic patients is straightforward.

PATIENTS WITH SYMPTOMATIC SEVERE AORTIC STENOSIS

The echocardiographic findings usually indicate a valve area less than 0.7 cm^2 in an average-sized adult and Doppler peak systolic pressure gradient greater than 60 mm Hg, with a maximal instantaneous gradient in the range of 64 to 145 mm Hg. If the cardiac output is low or the valve gradient appears inadequate to account for symptomatology, the valve area index should be calculated (Table 12–3).

Patients with LV failure or LV dysfunction require emergency surgery. Others require prompt surgery. During the waiting period, dental work under antibiotic coverage should be completed. The patient should be instructed concerning the risk and strictness of longterm anticoagulant regimen.

Diuretics are indicated if heart failure is present and digoxin is used if systolic dysfunction is documented. Heart failure is not a contraindication to surgery.

Coronary angiography is necessary in patients over age 35 or in those with chest pain.

PATIENTS WITH SYMPTOMATIC MODERATE AORTIC STENOSIS

Patients who have a valve area of 0.75 to 1.4 cm^2 are usually categorized as having moderate aortic stenosis. However, the situation in patients with valve area of 0.75 to 1 cm^2 is regarded by some as a "fool's paradise" (see Table 12–3). Some determine severe stenosis by valve area of 0.9 cm^2 or less and/or valve area index equal to or less than 0.6 cm^2/m^2. Patients who have moderate aortic stenosis, if minimally symptomatic, should be regarded as being at high risk for development of complications during the following one or two years, especially if the EF is less than 50% or if there is hemodynamic evidence of LV decompensation. In a study of 66 patients who had moderate aortic stenosis, 31% with minimal symptoms experienced serious complications within 4 years. Also, patients who have EF less than 50% at catheterization appear to have up to a 64% chance of complications due to aortic stenosis over a 4-year period. The absence of severe symptoms does not ensure a favorable outcome. The elderly, mildly symptomatic patients with degenerative calcific aortic stenosis of a moderate degree is at high risk. Thus, if underlying diseases such as respiratory failure, stroke, renal failure, anemia, or cancer are not present, surgery is recommended.

MEDICAL MANAGEMENT

Medical therapy is required for the following

• Careful supervision of asymptomatic patients with moderate or severe aortic stenosis
• Follow-up of patients with mild aortic stenosis
• Rheumatic fever and bacterial endocarditis prophylaxis

ASYMPTOMATIC SEVERE AORTIC STENOSIS

Patients with truly asymptomatic severe aortic stenosis evaluated at valve area less than 0.75 cm^2 and having the other echocardiographic parameters listed earlier require close and careful follow-up. A careful history should be taken at each visit, supplemented by inquiry of a spouse, close relative, or friend. The patient may deny mild to moderate shortness of breath. Activities may be decreased by the patient in order to prevent significant breathlessness. The patient must be warned to report any change in breathlessness, dizziness, chest pressure, or discomfort on mild or moderate exertional activities, including walking up stairs. Any change in symptomatology or increase in electrocardiographic or echocardiographic features of LVH and increase in pressure gradient or decrease in valve area, require consideration of urgent surgical intervention.

A cardiologist or internist should assess the patient every 2 or 3 months with a thorough cardiac examination, ECG, and Holter monitor. Echocardiography is advisable at least every 6 months. Many truly asymptomatic patients can be followed for 1 to 4 years, but with the assurance that rapid access to a known surgical team is available if the mildest symptom or distress is noted by the patient. The patient should be instructed to present immediately to the emergency room for admission if any of the following symptoms appear

- Change in breathing pattern on usual or moderate activities
- Chest discomfort or pain on moderate activities or at rest
- Dizziness or presyncope
- Sudden paroxysm of cough with frothy sputum
- Fever, chills, or symptoms of chest infection

Not all cardiologists agree with the concept of conservative therapy and watchful care in patients who have asymptomatic severe aortic stenosis. One option is to offer surgery, which can be performed at low risk to these patients in some centers. However, Braunwald has severely criticized this approach and has cautioned that operative treatment is the most common cause of sudden death in asymptomatic patients with aortic stenosis. In a study by Pellika, et al., sudden death did not occur among 113 asymptomatic patients who had isolated aortic stenosis followed for a total of 188 patient years, but two of the 30 asymptomatic patients subjected to valve surgery died suddenly within 2 weeks of intervention. Therefore, in these patients, timing for surgery should be individualized and surgery should be considered if any one of the following parameters is manifest

- LV dysfunction at rest with EF less than 50%
- The patient is very active and must continue strenuous physical work or must maintain professional athletic standards. It is likely, however, that this category of patients would be symptomatic
- If painless ischemia, potentially lethal arrhythmias, or pulmonary hypertension is documented in the absence of other valve lesions. Of course, valve replacement should not be delayed until overt heart failure has supervened

ASYMPTOMATIC PATIENTS WITH MODERATE AORTIC STENOSIS

Truly asymptomatic patients with moderate aortic stenosis are not offered surgery but should be followed closely for a change in effort tolerance and breathlessness or other cardiac complications.

The patient should be advised to carry on with activities that are normal and to report any changes immediately.

Patients with a moderate degree of aortic stenosis should be considered at high risk if they are mildly symptomatic, especially if the EF is decreased or if there is hemodynamic evidence of LV decompensation.

MILD AORTIC STENOSIS

The valve area in patients with mild aortic stenosis exceeds 1.5 cm². Individuals are usually asymptomatic. The patient is advised that aortic valve replacement may be required in 5 to 15 years. But, an operation may never be required. The patient should continue with normal activities, except for competitive sports.

In all categories of aortic stenosis, the prevention of rheumatic fever is necessary if the underlying disease is believed to be rheumatic in origin. Patients under age 40 suspected of having rheumatic heart disease are given prophylaxis 200,000 units of penicillin G orally twice daily or 1.2 million units of benzathine penicillin intramuscually monthly. Prophylactic therapy is continued at least to age 40 and/or after 20 years from the previous episode of rheumatic fever.

SURGICAL THERAPY

Mechanical obstruction to the LV outflow due to significant aortic stenosis is a pressure overload situation that leads to progressive LVH, LV strain, and finally heart failure or sudden death. Symptoms due to obstruction of outflow are usually the main indications for valve replacement in patients with moderate or severe aortic stenosis (see Table 12–4). In the majority of these patients, the valve area is less than 1.0 cm^2 and the peak systolic gradient is greater than 60 mm Hg. Fortunately, the hypertrophied myocardium often retains mechanical efficiency, and once the valve is replaced, significant improvement in ventricular systolic performance occurs in the majority of patients. Thus, heart failure is not a contraindication to valve replacement. Patients with LV failure due to severe aortic stenosis and

---

TABLE 12–4. INDICATIONS FOR AORTIC PROSTHETIC VALVE SURGERY

PARAMETERS	INTERVENTION
Severe Aortic Stenosis Aortic Valve area < 0.75 cm^2 Valve area Index < 0.4 cm^2/m^2 *Symptomatic patients*	
a. Heart failure or dyspnea	Emergency surgery
b. LV dysfunction or EF $< 50\%$	Urgent surgery
c. Angina	Urgent surgery
d. Syncope	Urgent surgery (Within a few weeks)
Asymptomatic patients Valve area as above Hemodynamic deterioration	No surgery
a. Left ventricular dysfunction	Fairly urgent (Within a few months)
b. Ejection fraction $< 50\%$	
c. Cardiomegaly or LVH on: ECG or echocardiography	
Moderate Aortic Stenosis Valve area 0.75 to 1.4 cm^2 *Symptomatic*	
Heart Failure	Urgent surgery
Other symptoms or LV dysfunction or EF $< 50\%$ (Follow up monthly)	Fairly urgent (Within a few months)
Truly asymptomatic (Follow up at least every 2 months)	Surgery (1–5 years) (if becomes symptomatic)

followed for over 1 year because of intercurrent illness contraindicating surgery usually regain adequate LV function with later valve replacement. Since mortality is over 50% in 1 year in patients with heart failure, surgery should be done promptly.

Indications for valve replacement

- LV failure
- Shortness of breath
- Angina
- Presyncope or syncope not due to preload-reducing agents or other causes of syncope (see Chapter 15)

Patients with chest pain or those over age 35 require coronary angiography to assess the degree of atheromatous coronary stenosis and suitability for coronary artery bypass surgery. Young patients with left anterior descending disease should be offered left internal mammary artery to left anterior descending anastomosis or graft; in patients over age 65, vein graft is appropriately recommended by the ACC and the AHA Task Force.

Contraindications to surgery include

- Serious underlying disease, especially respiratory failure, cancer, severe renal failure, cerebrovascular accident with residual stroke, contraindication to anticoagulant therapy
- Age over 80 is a relative contraindication, except in patients with robust health and excellent cerebral status. Severe intercurrent illness should weigh heavily against surgery, except in patients with heart failure due only to severe aortic stenosis with a valve area less than 0.75 cm². Because angina may require a combination of valve replacement and bypass surgery if there is coronary artery obstruction, care must be taken to individualize the selection. The patient and family must understand the risks.

PROSTHETIC VALVE CHOICE

Problems exist with all types of valve prostheses; none is ideal. Scientific studies have indicated a superiority of mechanical valves over bioprosthetic valves, especially in patients under age 30 or at all ages in the mitral position, and mechanical valves are the obvious choice in patients with atrial fibrillation in whom anticoagulation is already necessary (Table 12–5). Importantly, Collins points out that of 1,117 isolated mitral valve replacements done at Brigham and Women's Hospital since 1971, 620 (54%) had atrial fibrillation and a need for anticoagulation. Bloomfield reiterates that 60% of mitral valves currently implanted in patients in the United States are mechanical; in 1988, the UK Registry reported that 68% of mitral valves implanted were mechanical. The surgeon's background and personal preferences, however, often dictate the choice of valve, taking into consideration the patient's age and the possible presence of contraindications to anticoagulant therapy. In underdeveloped countries, a mechanical valve is still considered first choice, because it is preferable to monitor anticoagulation than to run the risk of two operations in 20 years, since reop-

CLINICAL PARAMETERS	MECHANICAL VALVE	BIOPROSTHESIS
Age <30	First choice	Not recommended
Anticoagulant necessary as in atrial fibrillation	Natural choice	Not recommended
Anticoagulant contraindicated	Not recommended	First choice
Aortic valve replacement		
age 30 to 70	First choice	Second choice
over age 70*, sinus rhythm	Second choice	First choice
Mitral (all ages)	First choice	May be considered in patients over age 70 in sinus rhythm

TABLE 12–5. CHOICE OF VALVE PROSTHESIS

* Higher risk of bleeding with anticoagulants, and average life span 10 years

eration carries a higher than 10% mortality and is costly. In the aortic position, it is expected that the durability of the mechanical valve is superior for use over a 10- to 20-year period because of a high reoperation rate with the use of bioprosthetic valves. The major disadvantage of mechanical valves is the small risk of bleeding due to anticoagulant therapy and this must be weighed against possible reoperation over 7 to 15 years with a bioprosthetic valve.

It is well established that reoperation is required much more frequently with bioprosthetic valves, but the complications of thromboembolism, endocarditis, and valve obstruction are similar. A bioprosthetic valve may be considered a reasonable choice in patients over age 70 whose life expectancy may be shorter than that of the bioprosthesis. In patients in whom anticoagulants are contraindicated or compliance is expected to be poor, a prosthetic valve is appropriate. In women who intend to become pregnant, a bioprosthetic valve is advisable but a mechanical valve with the use of heparin subcutaneously for the first 4 months and during the last few weeks of pregnancy is an alternative.

Accelerated calcification of glutaraldehyde-treated bioprosthetic valves in patients under age 30 is of concern. However, cryopreserved tissue valves are being tested and appear to maintain tissue flexibility with considerably less tendency to calcify.

Two studies compared the mechanical valve with the bioprosthesis. The Veterans Administration (VA) study reported 10-year follow-up in 575 patients randomized between mechanical valve and bioprosthesis: reoperation for primary valve failure was necessary in 35 patients fitted with bioprostheses, compared to 19 patients with mechanical valves; repeat surgery was performed for perivalvular regurgitation in only 6 bioprosthetic versus 13 mechanical valves. There was a significantly higher incidence of bleeding due to anticoagulant therapy in patients with mechanical valves.

A 12-year comparison in Scotland of the Bjork-Shiley spherical disc valve with bioprosthesis in 261 mitral, 211 aortic, and 61 in both positions indicated no difference in reoperation or survival at 5 years. However, at 12 years, reoperation was necessary in 68 (37%) patients with bioprosthetic valve and 17 (8.5%) with mechanical valve. Porcine valve failure was usually due to rupture of one or more cusps, causing severe regurgitation, with a much greater risk in the mitral position. Importantly, 16 patients died as a result of reoperation for porcine valve replacement. Also, valve failure may cause death before further surgical intervention. Using death and reoperation as endpoints for an actuarial assessment of survival with the original prosthesis intact, the survival rate in patients with Bjork-Shiley prostheses was 48%, versus a 30% survival rate in patients 12 years after porcine valve replacement. This effect was significant for mitral valves but inconclusive for the aortic position.

As a result of the study, the Scottish group advises that a bioprosthesis appears to be contraindicated in the mitral position; replacement in young patients should be with a mechanical valve, but an aortic bioprosthesis has a role in patients over age 70 who are in sinus rhythm.

COMPLICATIONS OF VALVE REPLACEMENT

The major differences in complication rates in mechanical and bioprosthetic valves relate to the incidence of primary valve failure and major bleeding; primary valve failure is very high with bioprosthesis after 5 years and major bleeding is a drawback of the mechanical valve (see Table 12–6).

Primary Valve Failure

Primary valve failure due to central valvular regurgitation or nonthrombotic obstruction occurs in up to 12% of bioprosthetic valves and 6.6% of mechanical valves, as observed in the 10-year VA Study. The reoperation rate in the Scottish study was 37% and 8.5% for bioprosthetic and mechanical valve, respectively, followed for a mean of 12 years (Table 12–6).

Major Bleeding

Major bleeding was significantly greater in patients fitted with mechanical versus bioprosthetic valves in the 10-year VA Study, and this was also true (19% versus 7%) in the 12-year Scottish study. These figures are in agree-

---

TABLE 12–6. PROSTHETIC VALVE COMPLICATIONS

CLINICAL PARAMETER	MECHANICAL VALVE (%)	BIOPROSTHETIC (%)
Reoperation		
Veterans Administration* (10 year)	6.6	12
Scottish Study** (12 year)	8.5	37
Major bleeding (12 year)	19	7
Perivalvular leak	4.5	2
Major embolism	8.8	9
Endocarditis	3.7	4.6
Survival rate (12 year)	51.5	44.4

Modified from: *J Am Coll Cardiol, *176(2)*:41A, 1991. **N Engl J Med, *324*:573, 1991.

ment with other studies that indicate an incidence of major bleeding of 1 to 2% per year with fatal intracranial bleed in 0.05 to 0.2% annually. Genitourinary, gastrointestinal, or retroperitoneal bleeding occurs at a rate of about 0.5% per patient year. Bleeding complications are related to inappropriate anticoagulant control. See later discussion of anticoagulants, Chapter 11, and Table 11–3.

Valve Obstruction due to Thrombosis and/or Pannus Formation

Thrombotic occlusion occurs more often with poor anticoagulation but may occur with apparently adequate control. The incidence of thrombosis with the Bjork-Shiley convexo-concave model was excessive, and in addition, this model, introduced in 1979, was withdrawn from the market due to a high rate of strut fracture.

Valve obstruction due to thrombosis or pannus is very rare but is the most serious complication, occurring in 0.5 to 4.5% per patient year. In a reported study, inadequate anticoagulation appeared to be an important factor, present in up to 70% of the 100 patients with obstructed valves. In that series of 2,100 St. Jude and 1,892 Medtronic-Hall valves followed over a 10-year period, 100 patients underwent prosthetic valve declotting and excision of pannus resulting in a successful outcome.

Features of valve obstruction may be

- Insidious with mild symptoms of breathlessness over 1 to 2 weeks
- A subacute presentation with shortness of breath at rest for hours to a few days
- Abrupt hemodynamic collapse often causing death

Valve obstruction must be rapidly excluded in all patients with prosthetic heart valves who show new or worsening symptoms, especially shortness of breath on mild exertion or at rest. Valve obstruction is usually due to thrombosis in up to 54%, chronic pannus associated with thrombosis in approximately 30%, and isolated pannus only in approximately 16% of patients.

The diagnosis should be straightforward in patients with shortness of breath at rest and a low output state. A change in prosthetic sounds, an absence of normal clicks on auscultation, or the development of a murmur should be followed by a prompt cinefluoroscopy or radiological screening if the occluder has a radio opaque marker. Echocardiography, particularly transesophageal echocardiography (TEE), is an alternative approach, and the delay associated with catheterization may prejudice prompt surgical intervention in this life-threatening situation. Thrombolytic agents have a role in some patients.

Streptokinase

Dosage: IV 250,000 to 500,000 units over 30 to 60 minutes followed by infusion 100,000/h for 24 to 72 hours has had salutary effects and may avoid surgery in some patients with a subacute presentation in the absence of hemodynamic collapse. See Chapter 3 for further advice on thrombolytic therapy.

Urokinase

Dosage: 150,000 units over 30 minutes, and then 75,000 to 150,000 units/h over 24 to 48 hours.

Caution. Embolization of thrombotic material may occur, and the usual precautions with the use of thrombolytic therapy should be enforced (see Chapter 3).

Systemic Embolization

The incidence of systemic thromboembolism is less than 2% and about 4% annually for aortic and mitral valve prostheses, respectively, utilizing mechanical or bioprosthetic valves.

Small strokes, transient ischemic attacks with dysphasia, paraesthesia or mild weakness of the face or limb, visual disturbances, syncope, and rarely hemiplegia may occur. Small emboli to the kidneys or limbs may sometimes go unrecognized. Emergency embolectomy of a limb vessel is rewarding; thus, diagnosis must be prompt. An embolus to the kidney causes a sharp, marked rise in lactic dehydrogenase (LDH).

If embolization occurs, anticoagulants are commenced in patients with bioprosthetic valves, and with mechanical valves, dipyridamole (75 to 100 mg three times daily) is added to existing anticoagulant therapy.

Bacterial Endocarditis

Prosthetic valve endocarditis causes a high mortality of up to 62% with medical therapy and a somewhat lower fatality rate of less than 40% with valve replacement. The incidence is approximately the same for mechanical and bioprosthetic valves (0.7% per patient year). In the Scottish study over 12 years, endocarditis occurred in 3.7 and 4.6% of patients with mechanical and bioprosthetic valves, respectively. The organism involved and the therapy of prosthetic valve endocarditis are discussed in Chapter 9.

Hemolysis

Hemolysis is extremely rare with current mechanical prostheses. A small increase in LDH occurs but can increase dramatically when significant hemolysis occurs, as with paravalvular leak or strut fracture resulting in anemia, increased indirect bilirubin, reticulocytosis count, and hemosiderinuria.

Hemodynamic malfunction in a bioprosthesis with strut dislodgement or paravalvular leak may cause a 20 to 50 g/l fall in hemoglobin over a 1-week period with hemoglobinuria and myoglobinuria that can be mistaken for hematuria and prompt urologic investigation.

A marked rise in the LDH is seen without hemolysis in patients with renal infarction due to embolism.

PROSTHETIC VALVE FOLLOW-UP

The follow-up of a patient with a prosthetic valve includes a careful history and physical examination. Auscultation for changes in heart sounds, alteration in valve clicks, and the appearance of regurgitant murmurs and gallops is important. Investigations include ECG, chest x-ray, complete blood count, and LDH. 2D Doppler echocardiography is done at least annually; a TEE is more reliable and is advisable if a valve complication is unresolved by the aforementioned investigations (see later discussion of TEE).

Anticoagulants

Anticoagulation control must be verified, and drugs that interact with oral anticoagulants should be discontinued or dosing should be modified (see Table 11–4). Anticoagulant therapy should achieve the following

- Prothrombin time (PT): Assess biweekly until stable, then monthly. Maintain at 1.5 to 1.9 times the control value for mechanical valves, and 1.4 to 1.5 for tissue valves. (Thromboplastin International Sensitivity Index (ISI) of 2.0). See Table 11–3
- International Normalized Ratio (INR): Maintain at 2.3 to 3.6 for mechanical valves and 2 to 2.3 for tissue valves.

It is important to note that the reagent used in the UK is a brain thromboplastin and the prothrombin-time ratio is therefore not comparable. Care is necessary, therefore, to avoid increased incidence of fatal hemorrhage with the use of different standards of anticoagulant control. The 1948 AHA recommendation that the targeted therapeutic range for anticoagulant therapy should be equivalent to a prothrombin-time ratio of 2.0 to 2.5 is no longer valid. The less sensitive thromboplastins introduced in the 1970s have resulted in an only recently recognized increase in the degree of oral anticoagulation in the United States, which has caused an increase in clinically significant bleeding. The higher incidence of bleeding in the VA valve replacement study, compared to the Scottish study, is believed to be due to the higher level of anticoagulation used in that study. The laboratory should report the prothrombin-time ratio and provide information on the ISI of the thromboplastin used. This system will lead to better anticoagulant control. Also, the physician can make clinically meaningful comparisons of efficacy and safety of oral anticoagulant therapy and compare results of various studies. Alternatively, the INR system using more sensitive thromboplastins should be adopted (see Table 11–2, 11–3 and Chapter 11 for further information and discussion of anticoagulant control).

Transesophageal Echocardiogram

TEE is an expensive procedure, twofold more than transthoracic 2D color Doppler echocardiography, but is superior in many areas of clinical decision-making and advisable for patients who have had valve replacements especially in the following situations

- Prosthetic valves, especially in the mitral position, are not well visualized with the transthoracic procedure, because metal or plastic create artifacts and shadows. Thus, where problems are suspected with mitral valve prosthesis, TEE is superior
- TEE is best to quantify the degree of mitral regurgitation, because the esophagus is immediately posterior to the left atrium
- Vegetations of bacterial endocarditis: Observed in 100% with TEE, compared to less than 60% with transthoracic 2D (Chapter 9)
- To detect abscess formation in aortic valve ring
- To detect the source of cardiac emboli from prosthetic valve

BALLOON AORTIC VALVULOPLASTY

The results of balloon aortic valvuloplasty have been disappointing. If the procedure is contemplated, the patient and family must clearly understand that the procedure is usually only palliative, in order to avoid false expectations. A 7.5% in-hospital mortality was observed post valvuloplasty in 492 patients, and the report of the Mansfield Scientific Balloon Aortic Valvuloplasty Registry indicates a 64% 1-year survival rate and a 43% event-free survival rate. The success rate of valvuloplasty was approximately 86%; the procedure resulted in a small but significant increase in aortic valve area, from 0.50 to 0.90 cm^2, and a decrease in aortic valve gradient, from 62 to 33 mm Hg. Modest clinical benefit is expected; lessening of symptoms occur in up to 66% of patients, and 28% are asymptomatic. Undoubtedly, symptomatic elderly patients who derive the most palliation from aortic balloon valvuloplasty include those who have

- The most severe aortic stenosis, especially at a valve area less than 0.6 cm^2
- A low output
- A low gradient state

These very ill patients have a high surgical mortality; when valve surgery is contraindicated, valvuloplasty can be carried out with the same mortality as in patients with a higher aortic valve gradient.

The procedure is performed by utilizing an exchange guidewire technique, usually from the femoral artery, to advance the balloon-tipped catheter across the aortic valve orifice. Valve dilatation results from cracking and splitting calcific plaques and separation of commissural fusion utilizing a single or double balloon technique.

Complications occurring in 492 patients include the following

- Restenosis occurred in approximately 50% at 6 to 12 months
- 31 patients (6.3%) had catastrophic complications; death occurred in 24 (77%) of the 31 patients

Complications observed were

- Ventricular perforation: 1.8% (67% were fatal)
- Acute aortic regurgitation: 0.8%
- Fatal cardiac arrest: 2.6%

- Cardiac tamponade (nonfatal)
- Fatal cerebral event: 0.4%
- Limb amputation: 0.6%

Despite these complications, the procedure will undoubtedly undergo refinements because palliation is sometimes needed to prevent patient suffering or to make the patient fit for some other lifesaving procedure. Aortic valve replacement has a 5% mortality in young healthy patients. However, in patients aged 60 to 70, the 30-day mortality exceeds 15%, and in those over age 80, the 30-day mortality exceeds 30%. Mortality is even higher in elderly patients who have heart failure or depressed ventricular function, concomitant CHD, renal dysfunction, or other debilitating disease. Thus, in these patients and symptomatic patients with low gradient, low output state, the procedure will likely remain of value for properly selected patients.

CONGENITAL AORTIC VALVULAR STENOSIS

INDICATIONS FOR AORTIC VALVE COMMISSURAL INCISION

Commissural incision is recommended in symptomatic and asymptomatic children and adolescents with severe congenital bicuspid aortic valve stenosis, valve area index less than 0.75 cm^2/m^2. This procedure has an acceptably low mortality rate of less than 1%. Progressive calcification of the incised valve may occur over the next 10 to 20 years. Nevertheless, it is best to defer valve replacement until severe aortic stenosis with symptoms occurs. Balloon aortic valvuloplasty at age 60 to 85 as discussed above has a very restricted application but appears to have a relatively good effect in childhood congenital noncalcified valvular aortic stenosis. A series involving 25 patients between 3 and 21 years of age showed a decrease in peak systolic gradient from 112 ± 35 mm Hg to 44 ± 21 mm Hg, and valve area index increased from 0.3 cm^2/m^2 ± 0.07 to 0.69 cm^2/m^2 ± 0.2. There were three restenoses over 18 months.

Balloon aortic valvuloplasty may be rewarding as a temporary, palliative, cost-justifiable procedure in some countries in children and adolescents with severe congenital aortic valvular stenosis.

AORTIC REGURGITATION

Over the past 25 years, there has been a major change in the pattern of underlying conditions associated with diseases causing aortic regurgitation. Whereas rheumatic fever and syphilis comprised 70% and 20% of cases, respectively, they now account for less than 30% and 1%. With the fall in prevalence of these diseases, bicuspid valve, endocarditis, and diseases causing aortic root dilation have emerged as the common causes (Table 12–7).

DIAGNOSTIC HALLMARKS

With chronic aortic regurgitation, the left ventricle tolerates regurgitant volume overload and compensates adequately; an asymptomatic period of from 10 to 30 years is not uncommon. Many patients with a moderate

TABLE 12–7. CAUSES OF AORTIC REGURGITATION

ACUTE	CHRONIC
Bacterial endocarditis	Rheumatic
Aortic dissection	Endocarditis
Prosthetic valve surgery	Congenital: bicuspid valve, ventricular septal defect,
Aortic balloon valvuloplasty	sinus of valsalva aneurysm
Trauma	Aortic root dilatation: connective tissue disorder: Mar-
Rheumatic fever	fan's, ankylosing spondylitis, Reiter's syndrome,
	rheumatoid arthritis, lupus erythematosus
	Takayasu aortitis, cystic medionecrosis myxomatous
	degeneration, psoriatic arthritis, Behcet's syndrome,
	relapsing polychondritis, giant cell arteritis, osteo-
	genesis imperfecta, ulcerative colitis
	Whipples disease
	Hypertension
	Arteriosclerosis
	Syphilis

degree of aortic regurgitation deny shortness of breath on walking 3 to 5 miles and/or three flights of stairs. Complaints of shortness of breath on exertion, fatigue, palpitations, or dizziness are generally associated with moderate or severe regurgitation over a prolonged period or severe regurgitation of recent onset. Rarely, angina with diaphoresis occurs as the diastolic blood pressure falls, frequently at night, causing a decrease in coronary perfusion. Symptoms and signs of heart failure at rest are late manifestations.

PHYSICAL SIGNS

Hallmarks on physical examination include

- Typical collapsing pulse: Water-hammer or Corrigan's pulse or a bounding pulse. The underlying mechanism is a rapid rise in upstroke followed by an abrupt collapse due to a quick diastolic runoff from the arterial tree. Indeed, all conditions that cause a brisk runoff produce a collapsing or bounding pulse (Table 12–8). The collapsing quality is detected by the examiner placing his or her fingers or palm closed firmly over the radial pulse with the entire limb extended to the ceiling. Pulsus bisferiens, a double peak to the pulse, may be observed with the combination of aortic regurgitation and significant aortic stenosis
- The patient's head often bobs with each cardiac pulsation
- The blood pressure reveals a wide pulse pressure due to an increase in systolic blood pressure and a diastolic that is often less than 50 mm Hg. Occasionally, Korotokoff sounds persist to zero with diastolic arterial pressure still greater than 60 mm Hg
- Arterial, neck pulsations are usually prominent
- Quincke's sign: Exerting mild pressure on the nail beds brings out intermittent flushing

TABLE 12–8. CAUSES OF A COLLAPSING BOUNDING PULSE	
CARDIAC CAUSES	NONCARDIAC CAUSES
Aortic regurgitation	Arterovenous fistula
Patent ductus arteriosus	Paget's disease
	Pregnancy
	Fevers
	Thyrotoxicosis
	Vasodilator drugs

- Finger pulsations: Collapsing pulsations in the finger pulps or tips
- Traube's sign: Pistol-shot sounds over the femorals
- Duroziez's sign: Compression of the femoral artery proximal to the stethoscope produces a systolic murmur and a diastolic murmur with distal compression.

The apex beat is virtually always displaced downward and outward to the left, indicating LV enlargement in patients with moderate or severe aortic regurgitation. A diastolic thrill may be palpated in the second right interspace or third interspace at the left sternal border, where the murmur of aortic regurgitation is most prominent.

Hallmarks on auscultation include

- Typical high-pitched blowing, early decrescendo murmur begins immediately after the aortic second sound (A2). The early decrescendo murmur beginning immediately after A2 is unmistakable to the trained ear and is best heard with the diaphragm pressed firmly against the chest, with the patient leaning forward and the breath held in deep expiration. The listener should then listen to the murmur with the patient breathing normally and in the recumbent position in order to train the ear for detection of the softest diastolic murmur
- The degree of aortic regurgitation correlates best with the duration of the murmur and may be pan-diastolic with severe regurgitation
- Perforation of an aortic cusp may change the quality of the murmur to one that resembles the cooing of a dove
- A mid or late diastolic rumble at the apex, the Austin Flint murmur, may be heard as the regurgitant jet hits the anterior mitral leaflet, as it opens and closes during diastole. The leaflet's shuddering can be heard with the stethoscope or observed with the help of Doppler echocardiography
- The A2 may be increased, decreased, or normal, and the accompanying aortic systolic murmur and thrill may represent flow rather than stenosis

ECG

The ECG commonly shows nonspecific ST-T wave changes, and with LVH, the pattern of LVH with volume overload is often present.

CHEST X-RAY

In patients with moderate or severe aortic regurgitation, dilatation of the left ventricle with elongation of the apex inferoposteriorly is almost invariably visible. Progressive further enlargement occurs over years in patients with severe aortic regurgitation. Dilatation of the ascending aorta is common in Marfan's syndrome and other causes of aortic root dilatation (Table 12–7). The typical appearance of linear eggshell calcification of the ascending aorta is a hallmark of syphilitic aortitis, which is now rare.

ECHOCARDIOGRAPHIC FINDINGS

- Detection of the type of aortic valve abnormality and underlying disease, e.g., aortic regurgitation due to bicuspid valve or vegetations caused by endocarditis
- Left ventricular chamber dimensions: estimates of LV volume and ventricular function measurements (LV end systolic dimensions, LV end diastolic dimensions, fractional shortening or EF)
- Dilatation of the aortic root
- Aortic dissection
- Other valve disease
- Other associated states, e.g., perivalvular abscesses in infective endocarditis

MANAGEMENT OF ACUTE AORTIC REGURGITATION

Acute aortic regurgitation causing hemodynamic instability requires immediate aortic valve replacement. TEE gives accurate, rapid diagnostic information if adequate data cannot be obtained from conventional echocardiogram. Some stability is attempted with the use of nitroprusside, and if aortic dissection is diagnosed, an IV beta blocking agent is given prior to TEE or on the way to the operating room (see Chapter 10). Patients with bacterial endocarditis who are hemodynamically stable should be managed with appropriate antibiotics and surgery should be deferred for 2 weeks, provided the patients respond. The development of first-degree AV block on the ECG is an ominous sign and suggests perivalvular abscess formation, which demands early operation if the diagnosis is confirmed.

MANAGEMENT OF CHRONIC AORTIC REGURGITATION

Medical therapy plays an important role, since the timing of valve surgery presents an ongoing challenge for both physician and patient. A review of the natural history of the condition indicates that

- More than 75% of patients with moderate aortic regurgitation survive for at least 5 years
- More than 50% are alive 10 years after diagnosis
- More than 90% of patients with relatively mild aortic regurgitation survive over 20 years

- As with aortic stenosis, the occurrence of heart failure carries about a 2-year survival, while for angina survival is about 5 years

A VA study, completed in 1991, comparing the survival of 102 medically treated and 147 surgically treated patients with severe aortic regurgitation, and followed for 7.5 years, indicated that valve replacement may not prolong survival in these patients.

Valve replacement should be considered prior to irreversible myocardial deterioration. However, because timing is often difficult, close follow-up of the patient with minimal or absent symptoms is essential.

PHARMACOLOGIC AGENTS OF VALUE

Nifedipine

The unloading effect of nifedipine has been recently shown to be capable of reversing LV dilatation and hypertrophy, and this agent may delay the need for valve surgery. In a study of 72 patients followed for 12 months, LV end diastolic volume index decreased from 136 ± 22 to 110 ± 19 ml/m², $p < 0.01$, and LV mass decreased from 142 to 115 g/m² (Fig. 12–1). A 25% reduction of the mean LV wall stress and an increase in EF from 60 to 72% were observed.

Nifedipine is superior to hydralazine, which does not decrease left ventricular mass or significantly decrease LV end diastolic or systolic dimensions. It appears that afterload reduction with nifedipine in patients with moderate to severe aortic regurgitation and normal LV function can achieve a 5-year survival rate approaching 87%. The 5-year survival rate for aortic valve replacement is approximately 72%, and the surgical mortality is 5%.

Nifedipine is given preferably as the extended release preparation: Procardia XL or Adalat XL, 30 mg once daily (see Chapter 1, Dosage). The extended release formulation is preferable since the nifedipine capsule causes an early and transient peak effect; also, adverse effects are more frequent than those observed with the sustained release preparation.

Nifedipine has a mild negative inotropic effect that is somewhat offset by sympathetic stimulation. Verapamil and diltiazem are contraindicated because of their negative inotropic effects and their propensity to cause bradycardia, which can worsen nocturnal angina or heart failure. Indeed, all vasodilators are not alike and hydralazine has not proven useful. Prazosin and other alpha₁ blockers are contraindicated because postural hypotension and increased heart rate may occur; these agents do not decrease LV mass or favorably alter LV systolic or diastolic dimensions.

ACE inhibitors have not been tested, but caution is necessary since these agents have a marked lowering effect on diastolic blood pressure, which may worsen diastolic coronary perfusion in patients with aortic regurgitation, a situation that is prone to occur during sleep and can be deleterious in patients with significant, concomitant atheromatous coronary stenoses. These agents have been shown to be harmful in patients with angina and in patients with heart failure in the presence of aortic regurgitation; ACE inhibitors should be avoided in patients who manifest angina or silent

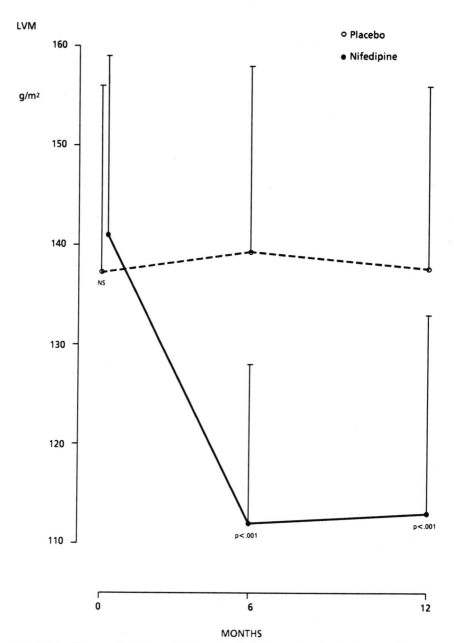

FIG. 12–1. Changes in left ventricular mass (LVM) over time for the two study groups. LVM did not change in patients treated with placebo but decreased significantly in the nifedipine-treated patients. From: Scognamiglio R, et al.: Longterm nifedipine unloading therapy in asymptomatic patients with chronic severe aortic regurgitation. J Am Coll Cardiol, *16*:424, 1990.

ischemia. Calcium antagonists, unlike ACE inhibitors, do not usually cause a reduction in blood pressure in normotensive individuals (see Chapter 1).

Digoxin

Digoxin should be given to all patients with moderate or severe aortic regurgitation, whether or not they are symptomatic.

Digoxin increases resting EF. Peak exercise EF increases with both digoxin and nifedipine but not with hydralazine. The combination of digoxin and nifedipine improves chronic hemodynamics in symptomatic and asymptomatic patients with severe regurgitation. The combination requires testing in randomized trials in patients with severe aortic regurgitation with normal LV systolic function.

TIMING OF VALVE REPLACEMENT

- There is a general agreement that symptomatic patients with severe chronic aortic regurgitation should have valve surgery in the absence of contraindications
- Valve surgery is not indicated in asymptomatic patients with severe chronic aortic regurgitation who have good effort tolerance and normal LV function

Between these two extremes are a large group of patients for whom firm data comparing the effect of prognosis of medical with surgical management are lacking, and widely accepted criteria or a task force consensus that may guide the physician are absent.

Patients with moderate or severe aortic regurgitation should be followed at least every 3 months. A careful history is necessary, including questioning of a spouse or relative who may be able to describe symptoms that are denied by the patient. A cardiovascular examination and ECG are done at each visit. Echocardiography is advisable every 6 months if LV end systolic dimension is greater than 50 mm or if fractional shortening is less than 30%. A biannual exercise test is useful to assess functional capacity.

If symptoms manifest (dyspnea on mild or moderate exertion, orthopnea, or chest discomfort), cardiac catheterization is necessary for verification of echocardiographic dimensions with a view to surgery.

Patients with prolonged severe LV dysfunction and marked LV dilatation are not expected to benefit from surgery. Although there are not fixed rules that would indicate clear contraindications, surgery generally is not advisable in patients who have

- EF less than 30%
- Prolonged severe LV dysfunction (18 months or more)

In these patients, symptoms, signs, and hemodynamic parameters of LV dysfunction may persist or worsen after successful valve replacement. Patients with EF less than 45% and less than 1 year of LV dysfunction usually have a successful postoperative outcome, but those with EF less than 45% and prolonged LV dysfunction (more than 18 months) have a poor postoperative survival. Repeated radionuclide or echocardiographic assessment of EF and end systolic volume, especially at rest, is necessary for decision-making. It must be emphasized that radionuclide EF is not accurate in patients with atrial fibrillation.

The role of the cardiologist is to consider interventional therapy prior to the occurrence of significant LV dysfunction. At this stage of careful follow-up, surgery is offered if LV function is impaired, if exercise capacity is reduced, or if LV dimensions are "highly abnormal" or show significant deterioration. Management of the asymptomatic patient with severe aortic regurgitation, depressed LV function, and abnormal dimensions, as indicated, should be individualized.

UNFAVORABLE LEFT VENTRICULAR DIMENSIONS

The following echocardiographic or catheter dimensions may be used to help serve in decision-making regarding timing for valve surgery. No single estimation should be accepted for making decisions. Marked changes or rate of change at 3- or 6-month visits should guide the physician

- LV end systolic dimension between 50 and 55 mm Hg. A dimension greater than 55 mm usually indicates LV dysfunction and, as outlined earlier, one does not wait for such ominous signals
- LV end diastolic dimension greater than 70 mm
- LV end systolic volume index greater than 60 ml/m²; greater than 90 ml/m² indicates severe LV dysfunction
- LV end diastolic volume index 140 to 150 ml/m²; greater than 180 ml/m² indicates severe LV dysfunction
- EF less than 50% or fractional shortening less than 30%: Fractional shortening less than 25% indicates severe LV dysfunction. LV EF less than 45% represents moderately severe LV dysfunction, and less than 35% indicates very severe dysfunction

The asymptomatic patient with severe aortic regurgitation should meet one or more of the above criteria and, in addition, should show a marked change 4 to 6 months prior in order to be regarded as a candidate for surgery.

It must be reemphasized that no single measurement is ideal and that most of them must be obtained to enable the cardiologist to apply the best clinical judgment, taking into account other variables such as age, occupation, and intercurrent illness.

Preparations for surgery include attention to dental work under antibiotic cover. Coronary angiography is necessary in patients over age 35 or in those with angina.

The choice of prosthetic heart valve is discussed in this chapter under aortic stenosis. Elective valve surgery has a 3 to 6% operative mortality and emergency surgery over 10%. The 5-year survival for valve implant ranges from 60 to 85%.

MITRAL STENOSIS

Mitral stenosis is almost always due to previous rheumatic fever. It takes 2 or more years following the rheumatic episode for sufficient fibrosis and thickening of the valve to produce the typical murmur. Most patients remain asymptomatic for 15 to 20 years following an episode of rheumatic fever, which is subclinical in over 50%.

Over the past 30 years, the problem of rheumatic valve disease has shown a marked decline in North America, the UK, and Europe. However, the disease is still endemic in much of Asia, Africa, the Middle East, Latin America, and the West Indies. Indeed, in these countries, significant mitral stenosis may emerge within a few years of the initial acute rheumatic fever and result in symptomatic disease in juveniles and young adults.

SYMPTOMS

The patient with mild mitral stenosis, valve area 1.6 to 2.0 cm^2, may develop mild dyspnea on moderate to severe exertion but is usually able to do all normal chores and lifestyle is not altered. Symptoms progress slowly, if at all, over the next 5 to 10 years. However, infection, pregnancy, or tachycardias, including atrial fibrillation, may precipitate severe dyspnea.

Patients with moderately severe mitral stenosis, valve area 1 to 1.5 cm^2, usually have symptoms that affect or interfere with daily living. Dyspnea due to progressive pulmonary venous hypertension becomes bothersome. Breathlessness is precipitated by moderate activity such as walking 100 yards briskly, walking up an incline, or even running slowly for 20 yards. Some patients with mild mitral stenosis may reduce activities and tolerate symptoms for several years. Pulmonary infection or atrial fibrillation often precipitates pulmonary congestion, emergency room visits, or hospitalization. Cough, shortness of breath, wheeze, and hemoptysis may mimic bronchitis for several months because the subtle signs of mitral stenosis can be missed by the untrained auscultator. Palpitations are usually due to atrial fibrillation, and some patients may present with a very rapid tachycardia or systemic embolization.

Severe mitral stenosis, valve area less than 1 cm^2 and valve area index less than 1 cm^2/m^2, usually causes symptoms on mild exertion. The patient presents with one or more of the following symptoms: progressive dyspnea, palpitations, marked fatigue, and occasionally cough, hemoptysis, hoarseness, or chest pain. Progression may be rapid with increasing edema, orthopnea, paroxysmal nocturnal dyspnea, and marked breathlessness. However, some patients tolerate dyspnea and are able to continue work that is not strenuous, at their own pace, for 3 to 12 months prior to interventional therapy. Fortunately, with mitral stenosis, patients with the most bothersome symptoms benefit the most from mitral valvotomy.

Some patients present with progressive symptoms and signs of low cardiac output and right heart failure with only mild pulmonary congestive features as a result of reactive hyperplasia of pulmonary arterioles and pulmonary arterial hypertension, a scenario appropriately termed "protected" mitral stenosis. At the other extreme, some patients present with florid pulmonary edema associated with only passive pulmonary arterial hypertension and mild or absent right heart failure, which is considered "unprotected" mitral stenosis. A mixture of protected and unprotected mitral stenosis is commonly observed.

PHYSICAL SIGNS

- On inspection, a malar flush is common in the presence of longstanding, moderately severe mitral stenosis
- A lower left parasternal lift of heave due to right ventricular hypertrophy may be present
- The apex beat is tapping in quality, usually not displaced
- A diastolic thrill localized to the apex beat may be palpated
- Auscultation reveals a loud slapping first heart sound and is so typical that it warns the examiner to search for other signs of mitral stenosis. Immobility of the cusps reduces this valuable sign
- The pulmonary second sound is intensified and this vibration associated with pulmonary valve closure is often palpable with significant pulmonary arterial hypertension
- An opening snap, a sharp high-pitched sound, is a hallmark of mitral stenosis. The opening snap is best heard with the diaphragm pressed firmly just internal to the apex beat and occurs from 0.04 to 0.14 seconds after the second heart sound. The opening snap may be heard over a wide area and, with severe mitral stenosis, usually occurs less than 0.08 seconds following the second heart sound, audible immediately rather than following a definite gap. The opening snap disappears if the valve becomes heavily calcified and nonpliable
- The loud slapping first heart sound and opening snap produce a particular cadence that alerts the examiner
- The opening snap is followed by a low-pitched, mid-diastolic rumbling murmur that is associated, if there is sinus rhythm, with presystolic accentuation, best heard with the bell lightly applied over the apex beat. The murmur often is localized to an area the size of a coin and can easily be missed; it is brought out by exercising the patient and listening with the patient lying on the left side. Occasionally, critical mitral stenosis may cause a marked reduction in transmitral flow, and the murmur may be hardly audible. There is evidence that in these cases, the disease and contracted chordae increase the impedance to ventricular filling so that the reduced mitral valve area is no longer the limiting factor
- The severity of mitral stenosis correlates best with the length of the murmur rather than the intensity

INVESTIGATIONS

CHEST X-RAY HALLMARKS

- Straightening of the left heart border due to left atrial enlargement
- Larger than normal double density, seen through the right half of the cardiac silhouette, indicating left atrial enlargement

- Elevation of the left main stem bronchus caused by distension of the left atrium with widening of the angle between the two main bronchi
- Redistribution: Restriction of lower lobe vessels and dilatation of the upper lobe vessels
- If heart failure is present, signs of interstitial edema are present: Kerley B lines due to lymphatic engorgement and fibrosis, perihilar haze, and eventually frank pulmonary edema is observed
- Fluroscopy is no longer commonly done, but shows posterior displacement of the barium-filled esophagus
- The heart size on posteroanterior x-ray is generally normal or near-normal, and the lateral film should be assessed for right ventricular enlargement: "creeping up the sternum"

ELECTROCARDIOGRAPHIC HALLMARKS

- Signs of left atrial enlargement are common with moderate and severe mitral stenosis: broad bifid P waves in lead 2 and, more specifically, an increase in the P terminal force ($PTFV_1$) equal to or greater than 40 millisec/mm, measured in V_1 (area subtended by the terminal negative portion of a biphasic P wave). Hazen, et al. have shown that when $PTFV_1$ is greater than 40 millisec/mm, 95% of individuals had left atrial size greater than 4 cm; when $PTFV_1$ is equal to or greater than 60 millisec/mm, 75% had left atrial size greater than 6 cm
- Right axis deviation 90 to 150 degrees reflects severe mitral stenosis
- Right ventricular hypertrophy may be present with severe stenosis but does not correlate well with the degree of pulmonary hypertension
- Atrial fibrillation is common with moderate longstanding rheumatic disease, with the left atrial size exceeding 4.5 cm, and is characteristically coarse in appearance

Electrocardiographic stress testing is of value in selected patients who are suspected of denying symptoms with the presence of a moderate degree of stenosis; functional capacity can be assessed.

ECHOCARDIOGRAPHIC ASSESSMENT

- The mitral diastolic gradient can be defined
- Excellent quantification of mitral valve orifice area
- Left atrial enlargement is uniformly present, and the size can be accurately determined
- The degree of calcification of the mitral valve leaflets can be verified
- Decreased posterior leaflet movement is often observed
- The degree of right ventricular enlargement can be documented
- Left ventricular size is expected to be small
- Right ventricular systolic pressures reflect the degree of pulmonary hypertension
- The degree of concomitant mitral regurgitation can be assessed

A flat E to F slope or EF slope less than 10 mm/sec may indicate severe mitral stenosis, but this measurement is no longer used for quantitating the degree of obstruction. Marked alteration of the E to F slope may be observed in patients with aortic stenosis and regurgitation with no evidence of mitral stenosis and in patients with impaired LV filling caused by reduced LV compliance.

MEDICAL THERAPY FOR MITRAL STENOSIS

All patients should receive prophylaxis for the prevention of rheumatic fever for at least 25 years from the acute episode and up to age 45, whichever is the longest. Although pure mitral stenosis is rarely the site of endocarditis, trivial mitral regurgitation is often present and endocarditis prophylaxis should be strongly enforced (see Chapter 9).

MILD MITRAL STENOSIS

Patients are usually asymptomatic and should be followed annually. A chest x-ray and echocardiogram are done initially, or if needed because of worsening symptomatology. Then, about every 5 years should suffice.

No treatment is indicated, except for advice on mild dietary salt restriction and avoidance of excessive weight gain and physically strenuous occupations.

MODERATE MITRAL STENOSIS

Moderate mitral stenosis, valve orifice area 1 to 1.5 cm^2, is usually mildly symptomatic. Salt restriction is advisable. Potassium-sparing diuretics such as Moduretic (Moduret) ameliorate shortness of breath and prevent potassium and magnesium loss (see Chapter 5). If palpitations are bothersome or short runs of supraventricular tachycardia are documented, a small dose of a beta blocking drug is useful: metoprolol 25 to 50 mg twice daily, atenolol 25 mg daily, or an equivalent dose of another beta blocker should suffice. Digoxin is not indicated for patients with sinus rhythm or heart failure with pulmonary congestion, except as prophylaxis against fast ventricular rates and pulmonary edema if atrial fibrillation develops.

Chest infections must be vigorously treated because hypoxemia increases pulmonary hypertension and may precipitate right heart failure. Also, tachycardia may precipitate pulmonary edema.

If the patient is managing daily chores and enjoying a near normal lifestyle, the interventional approach can await some progression of the disease or symptoms but is not delayed in very active patients who need to engage in strenuous work or sport. Marked limitation of lifestyle in such individuals may require early corrective measures. A patient with moderate mitral stenosis should be followed at least twice yearly, but annual echocardiography should suffice.

SEVERE MITRAL STENOSIS

Severe mitral stenosis, valve area corrected for body surface area (valve area index) less than 1 cm^2/m^2, usually requires interventional therapy within 3 to 6 months to abolish symptoms or decrease complications and/or progressive increase in pulmonary vascular resistance.

ATRIAL FIBRILLATION

Atrial fibrillation with a fast ventricular response decreases LV filling and may precipitate pulmonary congestion. Digoxin is indicated to control the ventricular response. Digoxin is discussed in detail in Chapter 5. If palpitations remain bothersome and the heart rate cannot be controlled with digoxin, as often occurs in very active individuals, the addition of a small dose of beta blocking drug is useful. The latter agents can also be used to decrease sinus tachycardia that is easily provoked in some patients without atrial fibrillation. Many physicians regard the development of atrial fibrillation as an indication for intervention when stenosis is of moderate severity, because the prospects for permanent restoration of sinus rhythm decrease rapidly with time from onset of arrhythmia.

ANTICOAGULANTS

The patient with atrial fibrillation must be anticoagulated, if no contraindication exists, because systemic embolization is common. Warfarin is given to maintain the prothrombin time, 1.25 to 1.5 times the control or INR 2 to 3, (see Chapter 11 for advice on anticoagulant control). These tests are done at least every two weeks until stabilized, then monthly should suffice. If contraindications to anticoagulant therapy exist, enteric-coated aspirin (325 mg daily) is advisable.

HEART FAILURE AND PULMONARY EDEMA

Pulmonary edema and right heart failure usually require admission for control (see Chapter 5).

INTERVENTIONAL MANAGEMENT

Balloon valvuloplasty or surgery to relieve valvular obstruction is indicated for most symptomatic patients who have moderate to severe mitral stenosis, valve orifice less than 1 cm^2, as determined by Doppler echocardiography. The results of this technique correlate sufficiently well with catheterization data. Cardiac catheterization is not required in patients under age 40, in whom ischemic heart disease is not present or suspected, and who have typical, clinical features of mitral stenosis that are confirmed by Doppler echocardiography.

Mild mitral stenosis, valve area 1.6 to 2.0 cm^2, often remains minimally symptomatic for 5 to 10 years or more. However, as explained earlier, in countries where rheumatic valve disease is endemic, tight mitral stenosis may emerge at a faster rate in the adolescent or young adult.

Moderately severe mitral stenosis, valve area 1 to 1.5 cm^2, usually does not require intervention, but decisions must be individualized. In these patients, intervention may be required

- For symptomatic young patients engaged in strenuous activity
- If atrial fibrillation supervenes

- To allow a further pregnancy in a patient who manifested pulmonary edema in a previous pregnancy

Elective procedures are sometimes performed in women who anticipate pregnancy, but relief of obstruction may be required during the second and third trimester of pregnancy, because the valve orifice is no longer large enough to permit the necessary increase in cardiac output to occur without an unacceptable rise in left atrial and pulmonary venous pressures. Interventional therapy may take the form of

- Surgical closed commissurotomy
- Surgical open commissurotomy
- Balloon valvuloplasty
- Valve replacement

SURGICAL OPEN VERSUS CLOSED COMMISSUROTOMY

Closed mitral commissurotomy was the technique of choice until the early 1970s for patients with severe mitral stenosis with noncalcified pliable valves. Open commissurotomy has largely replaced the closed technique, except in much of Asia, Africa, Latin America, and the West Indies, where closed valvotomy has remained the treatment of choice.

Undoubtedly, there will be a resurgence of closed commissurotomy in North America and Europe based on the recent survey entitled "Outcome Probabilities and Life History after Surgical Mitral Commissurotomy." In this study, Hickey, et al. compared the outcome in 236 open and 103 closed commissurotomies performed between 1967 and 1988. The survival rate at 1 month, 1 year, 5 years, and 10 years was 99.7%, 99%, 95%, and 87%, respectively, with outcomes being similar after closed and open commissurotomy. Thus, both techniques provide excellent relief, although eventual restenosis is usual over the ensuring 10 to 20 years or more post mitral valvotomy. Mitral valve replacement was required in 22% within 10 years of commissurotomy. In the entire study group, thromboembolism occurred in 33 (10% of 339 patients) and 9 (2.6%) patients had significant cerebral embolism.

Moderate to severe mitral stenosis accompanied by mild to moderate mitral regurgitation is not uncommon, and open repair with limited opening of the Tubbs dilator is a considered option for this category of patients.

TECHNIQUE FOR CLOSED SURGICAL COMMISSUROTOMY

The right index finger is inserted into the left atrium via an incision in the left atrial appendage. A Tubbs dilator, which has been introduced via a purse string stitch in the anterolateral LV freewall near the apex, but not directly into the apex, is guided by the finger into the mitral valve. Four dilatations, commencing at 2.5 cm and terminating with 4 cm, are performed, followed by amputation or ligation of the left atrial appendage.

The experienced surgeon is able to assess the degree of splitting and the degree of regurgitation (if any) after each dilatation.

TABLE 12–9. COMPLICATIONS OF MITRAL BALLOON VALVULOPLASTY	
CLINICAL PARAMETERS	**COMPLICATIONS, INCIDENCE (%)**
Mortality	2.7
Emergency surgery	6.7
Cardiac tamponade	6.7
Embolism	2.7
Significant mitral regurgitation	13
Emergency valve replacement	4
Restenosis	16
Iatrogenic atrial septal defect	20 to 87

MITRAL BALLOON VALVULOPLASTY

Percutaneous mitral balloon valvuloplasty appears to give hemodynamic results that are comparable with surgical closed commissurotomy, as shown by an 8-month follow-up study. The valve area is increased 100% from 1 cm^2 to 2 cm^2 in up to 77% of cases. A mortality of up to 2.7% has been reported by the Valvuloplasty Registry. The National Heart, Lung and Blood Institute (NHLBI) 30-day follow-up report on 738 patients indicates an 83% overall clinical improvement and mortality of 3%; 4% of patients require valve surgery. An iatrogenic atrial septal defect (ASD) has been reported to occur in 20 to 87% of patients depending on criteria used for defining the ASD, which takes up to 6 months to close. However, the defect is usually small, the magnitude of the shunt being less than 2:1, and only few of these ASDs are clinically significant. Currently, complication rates are still high (see Table 12–9). The procedure should be done only by highly trained and experienced operators. In such hands, the procedure is first choice in appropriately selected patients for relief of severe mitral stenosis.

Mitral balloon valvuloplasty must have a mortality less than 1% to be considered an acceptable alternative to surgical commissurotomy. The proper selection of patients and technical aspects are changing such that morbidity and mortality from the procedure are expected to fall.

PATIENT SELECTION

The patient selection for mitral balloon valvuloplasty is crucial to obtaining a salutary effect with a minimum number of complications. The patients are usually selected based on 2D echocardiographic results. Ideally, the patients should have

- Very symptomatic severe mitral stenosis, mitral valve area less than 1 cm^2
- Noncalcified, mobile valve with no subvalvular fibrosis (echo score less than 8): Valve rigidity, valve calcification, thickening, and subvalvular fibrosis are graded from 0 to 4, and the points are added together. The best candidates are patients who have an echo score less than 8

Contraindications

* Bleeding disorder: Abnormal prothrombin time, prolonged partial thromboplastin time, increased bleeding time (the patient must discontinue aspirin compounds for at least 1 week prior to the procedure)
* Left atrial or appendage thrombus
* Recent embolization
* Severe mitral valve calcification of subvalvular fibrosis
* Moderate or severe mitral regurgitation
* Cardiothoracic deformity

TEE has a role in obtaining information needed for the selection of patients for balloon valvuloplasty such as calcification, thickening, mobility, and subvalvular fibrosis. Atrial or appendage thrombus is best visualized with TEE. The technique is also of value in assessing the magnitude of the ASD following the procedure.

MITRAL VALVE REPLACEMENT

Mitral valve replacement utilizing prosthetic valve implant may be required because of the presence of moderate to severe mitral regurgitation coexisting with mitral stenosis. Replacement may also be selected for management of heavily calcified and immobile valves, which are often conical in shape, when they are considered to be beyond repair at the time of surgery. In general, a mechanical valve is preferred in the mitral area. See earlier discussion of prosthetic valve choice and Table 12–5. In up to 50% of patients, atrial fibrillation is present; a mechanical valve is a natural choice because anticoagulants are necessary. In the young female who may wish to become pregnant, a bioprosthesis is sometimes recommended. However, a mechanical valve can be used in this situation with discontinuation of oral anticoagulants; heparin can be used subcutaneously for the first 4 months of pregnancy and again for the last 3 weeks. Importantly, in the young patient, accelerated calcification of a bioprosthesis may occur. Calcification, as well as pannus formation, may require a second operation.

MITRAL REGURGITATION

While mitral stenosis is nearly always due to rheumatic disease, mitral regurgitation is a common valvular lesion that is caused by a number of conditions that alter the mitral valve apparatus: valve leaflets, annulus, chordae, and papillary muscles. Common causes of acute and chronic mitral regurgitation are given in Table 12–10.

ACUTE MITRAL REGURGITATION

Acute mitral regurgitation commonly occurs during acute MI, which causes papillary muscle dysfunction, and less commonly, chordal or papillary muscle rupture (see Chapter 4). Other causes of acute mitral regurgitation are listed in Table 12–10.

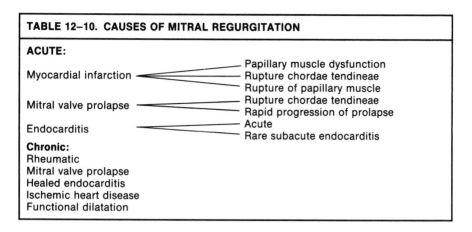

TABLE 12–10. CAUSES OF MITRAL REGURGITATION

ACUTE:

Myocardial infarction — Papillary muscle dysfunction / Rupture chordae tendineae / Rupture of papillary muscle

Mitral valve prolapse — Rupture chordae tendineae / Rapid progression of prolapse

Endocarditis — Acute / Rare subacute endocarditis

Chronic:
Rheumatic
Mitral valve prolapse
Healed endocarditis
Ischemic heart disease
Functional dilatation

CHRONIC MITRAL REGURGITATION

Patients may tolerate a mild to moderate degree of mitral regurgitation for 5 to 20 or more years without the appearance of heart failure. Chronic volume overload, however, causes slow progressive dilatation and mild hypertrophy of the left ventricle. Characteristically, a loud holosystolic murmur is heard maximal at the apex with radiation to the axilla, accompanied by a third heart sound gallop if regurgitation is moderate to severe. In patients with posterior papillary muscle dysfunction causing mitral regurgitation, however, the murmur radiates anteriorly and is best heard at the left sternal border without radiation to the axilla.

Mild to moderate shortness of breath indicates pulmonary congestion or LV dysfunction and should be managed with afterload-reducing agents, particularly ACE inhibitors to encourage forward flow at the expense of regurgitation; small doses are advisable: captopril, 6.25 mg twice daily for several days, increasing slowly to avoid hypotension to a maintenance of 37.5 mg twice daily (maximum 75 mg in 2 or 3 divided doses or equivalent doses of enalapril).

If concomitant ischemic heart disease with angina is present and LV dysfunction is not severe, nifedipine is preferred to ACE inhibitors; in these patients, ACE inhibitors may increase angina. Also, digoxin and the judicious use of diuretics in combination with nifedipine may cause some beneficial effects prior to consideration of early valve repair or valve replacement.

Atrial fibrillation with a rapid ventricular response is managed with digoxin and anticoagulants to prevent embolization.

Progressive dyspnea is a late stage and heart failure should be anticipated and prevented by timely surgical intervention.

SURGICAL TREATMENT

The timing of valve surgery, whether it is repair or valve replacement for chronic mitral regurgitation, remains a trial in decision-making as with that of aortic regurgitation. Patients with mitral valve prolapse and acute complications are often suitable for valve repair.

There is an increasing tendency to attempt valve reconstruction. It is advisable to repair as many and as often as feasible, but success depends on the skill of the surgeon. For mitral stenosis and regurgitation, many valves are beyond repair and require replacement.

Surgery should be considered in patients who have moderately severe mitral regurgitation prior to the development of severe pulmonary arterial hypertension and prior to a fall in EF to less than 50%. The interpretation of EF has to be adjusted downward to take into account the low impedance to retrograde flow resulting from mitral regurgitation. A patient with severe mitral regurgitation and an EF less than 40% will have a prohibitively high surgical mortality and will fare better with afterload reduction and digoxin. Because of the problems of assessing EF in the presence of mitral regurgitation, other parameters of LV function have been used, including end systolic volume index greater than 50 ml/m².

If surgery is done prior to the manifestations of the aforementioned parameters, survival, functional class, and LV systolic function should show significant improvement. If mitral regurgitation is moderately severe and LV dysfunction is present, it is hazardous to procrastinate. Early surgery is preferable.

In patients with predominant posterior leaflet prolapse, repair of the posterior leaflet followed by insertion of a nonflexible ring, as recommended by Carpentier, appears to be successful in preventing postoperative systolic anterior motion of the mitral valve.

In some patients with heavily calcified valves, the mitral valve annulous can be decalcified and valve repair, decalcification, and annuloplasty should be considered based on Doppler echocardiographic data. TEE gives a more accurate visualization of the mitral valve, however, and is advisable in potential candidates; the latter is justifiable and cost-effective, especially in view of the difficult decision as to timing of surgery.

The tricuspid valve is also often severely incompetent; tricuspid annuloplasty is advisable in such cases.

Intraoperative TEE is of considerable value in assessing valve repair. The surgeon ensures excellent coapting edges and lines of closure; if the geometry is ideal, saline is pumped into the ventricle.

MITRAL VALVE PROLAPSE

Mitral valve prolapse is said to be a common condition affecting an estimated 5% of the United States population. The incidence of mitral valve prolapse has been exaggerated because of the inclusion of a large number of patients with a normal variant of mitral valve closure but with correct coaptation; leaflets may only billow slightly into the left atrium with normal coaptation. Also, the appearance may result from the normal saddle shape of the normal mitral ring.

The minor variant with a click, without a murmur and nondiagnostic echocardiographic features commonly labeled mitral valve prolapse, is subject to interpretation and this "normal variant" disappears after age 40. Probably because of the inclusion of normal variants with billowing leaflets without true prolapse, the incidence of mitral valve prolapse is reported to be as high as 30% at age 10 to 20, 15% at age 30, 10% at age 50, 3% at age 70, and less than 1% at age 80. Under age 30, the female to male ratio is 3:1, but at age 70, both men and women are about equal. The incidence of significant mitral valve prolapse is about 6% in adult women and 3% in men.

Genuine mitral valve prolapse has a familial incidence of about 33% as noted in first-degree relatives.

Causes of mitral valve prolapse

- In developed countries, the common underlying process is a degenerative nonrheumatic condition of unknown etiology described as a dyscollagenosis or myxomatous degeneration of the mitral valve. An increase in the spongiosa, myxomatous tissue, in the middle layer of the mitral valve leaflet, encroaches upon the fibrosa. The anterior and posterior leaflets become elongated, thickened, voluminous, and grossly redundant. The chordae become thin and elongated and have a propensity to rupture. Herniation of the posterior leaflet above the anterior leaflet may occur. A mural endocardial fibrous plaque is often observed beneath the posterior leaflet in patients who die suddenly from mitral valve prolapse. The mitral valve annulus is often dilated in patients with significant regurgitation, and in those patients who die suddenly, calcification and fibrosis of the annulus appears to be a common finding
- Myxomatous changes and mitral valve prolapse are associated with Marfan's, Ehlos-Danlos syndrome, and osteogenesis imperfecta
- Rheumatic heart disease, where this disease is still endemic. A dilated annulus allows elongation of chordae with, sometimes, prolapse of the anterior leaflet, but marked billowing or redundancy of leaflets are unusual
- Papillary muscle dysfunction due to ischemic heart disease

SYMPTOMS

The majority of patients are asymptomatic. Dyspnea is rather vague, often occurs at rest, and is commonly out of proportion with the degree of mitral regurgitation that is usually asymptomatic in over 80% of patients. Extreme fatigue, dizziness, anxiety, panic disorders, palpitations, presyncope, syncope, and chest pain may occur without a satisfactory explanation. Psychogenic factors play a role in the varied symptomatology.

Some symptoms relate to the presence of autonomic dysfunction with increased levels of circulating catecholamine, a hyperadrenergic state, and in some patients, increased vagal activity is present. In this condition, there is a tendency for the sinus rate to increase steeply in the early part of exercise, and the high frequency of palpitations has been attributed to this pattern of response in these patients. It is not surprising, therefore, that Holter monitoring commonly shows sinus tachycardia, when palpitations are a complaint.

SIGNS

One or multiple mid or late systolic clicks of nonejection type may be constant or intermittent, changing with posture or maneuvers, but do not prove the existence of mitral valve prolapse. The timing of clicks may be misinterpreted as gallop sounds, but apart from their timing, clicks can be differentiated from a third heart sound by the high-pitched quality and by being most audible with a diaphragm. In some patients, the click is followed by a murmur; in others, only a murmur is present. The murmur has typical features

- A typical late systolic murmur is unmistakable and confirms the diagnosis
- The murmur is usually crescendo-decrescendo, and the auscultator gets the impression that the murmur is occurring synchronously with the second heart sound, and the murmur often extends through the aortic second sound
- A whoop, a short honking sound, or a sound of other musical quality may highlight the murmur, which changes in intensity depending on LV volume and blood pressure
- The late systolic murmur or click is heard earlier and made louder by the following maneuvers that reduce LV volume: standing, tilting upright, valsalva, and tachycardia. Amylnitrite decreases ventricular volume and blood pressure; therefore, the murmur is heard earlier but is made softer
- The murmur or clicks are heard later and are softer with maneuvers that increase LV volume or decrease blood pressure: squatting, bradycardia, beta blocking agents. Thus, the physician should listen to the patient lying, standing, and squatting because the murmur may be heard only on standing. With more severe mitral regurgitation, the duration of the murmur is longer and may become pansystolic
- When chordal rupture occurs, the murmur changes in quality and radiation
- The posterior mitral leaflet often has three scallops; rupture of the chorda to the middle scallop of the posterior leaflet is the most common chordal rupture. The resulting murmur radiates anteriorly and is maximal at the lower left sternal border and radiates toward the upper right sternal edge. The crescendo-decrescendo quality may simulate an aortic systolic murmur. However, the late timing of the murmur of mitral valve prolapse is a distinguishing feature that differentiates the murmur from the early timing of aortic valvular murmurs
- Chordal rupture of the anterior leaflet causes the murmur to radiate to the posterior axilla
- The flail mitral valve produces a loud murmur, the intensity of which is characteristically accentuated over the spine and may be heard from the occiput to the sacral spine
- The mitral regurgitant jet can be identified by TEE; it moves in a counterclockwise direction with flail anterior leaflet and clockwise with posterior leaflet involvement

Approximately 15% of patients with mitral valve prolapse have skeletal abnormalities: "straight back," pectus excavatum or carinatum, scoliosis, or some features of Marfan's syndrome.

COMPLICATIONS

SEVERE MITRAL REGURGITATION

Severe mitral regurgitation occurs in approximately 10% of patients with true mitral valve prolapse and is five times more common in men over age 45 than in women. Although mitral valve prolapse occurs most commonly in women, severe mitral regurgitation requiring surgery occurs in about 5% of men and less than 1.5% of women. Chordal rupture is a common occurrence in patients with severe mitral regurgitation.

ARRHYTHMIAS

Arrhythmias commonly occur and include VPCs, atrial ectopics, PSVT, and occasionally atrial fibrillation. Lethal arrhythmias have been reported (see Chapter 6).

SUDDEN DEATH

Sudden death, although rare, occurs in healthy young active individuals and is unexplained. Table 12–11 lists clinical and morphologic features in 15 patients who died suddenly secondary to mitral valve prolapse. These data and a review of previously reported studies on 63 patients indicate that patients with mitral valve prolapse who die suddenly have the following clinical and morphologic hallmarks

- Women aged 21 to 51, without significant mitral regurgitation (70%)
- Dilated mitral valve annulus (80%)
- Elongated anterior mitral valve leaflet (over 80%)
- Abnormal elongated posterior mitral leaflet, and often there is herniation of the posterior leaflet above the anterior leaflet (approximately 80%)
- Fibrous endocardial plaque under the posterior mitral valve leaflet (up to 75%)
- Significant, moderate to severe prolapse of the mitral valve (53%)
- Raptured chordae (33%)
- Significant, moderate or greater mitral regurgitation (10%)
- Mitral regurgitant murmur (50%)
- A click is present (only 25 to 37%)
- Arrhythmia (over 50%); VPCs (about 33%)

ENDOCARDITIS

The exact incidence of endocarditis in patients with true mitral valve prolapse is unknown but is estimated to be in the range of 1 in 6,000 in all patients with mitral valve prolapse and about 1 in 2000 of those patients with mitral regurgitation (see Chapter 9).

TABLE 12–11. CLINICAL AND MORPHOLOGIC FEATURES IN 15 PATIENTS DYING

Pt No.	Age (yr)	Race	Gender	MVP Diagnosed Clinically	The Marfan Syndrome	Location of Death	Last Activity	AUSCULTATORY FINDINGS SC	SM	SH
1	16	W	M	+	+	Basketball court	Sitting after playing	–	+	0
2	18	W	F	+	0	Home	Arguing	–	0	0
3	21	W	F	+	0	Work	Talking on phone	–	–	0
4	23	W	F	+	0	Work	Drinking water	+	+	0
5	26	W	F	+	0	Work	Talking	+	+	0
6	30	B	M	0	0	Work	Sitting alone	–	–	–
7	30	W	M	0	0	Golf course	Playing golf	–	–	0
8	40	W	F	0	+	Home	Playing with children	–	–	0
9	47	W	F	0	0	Home	Gardening	–	–	0
10	51	W	M	+	0	Restaurant	Sitting after fast dancing	+	+	0
11	53	W	F	+	0	Church	Sitting	–	–	0
12	53	W	F	0	0	Restaurant	Getting up to dance	–	–	–
13	55	W	F	+	0	Home	Standing	+	+	0
14	55	W	M	+	0	Home	Sleeping	–	+	0
15	69	W	F	0	0	Home	–	–	–	–

* This patient had survived a cardiac arrest 2 years earlier; † this patient had a history of paroxysmal atrial tachycardia. AML = anterior mitral leaflet; B = black; CHF = congestive heart failure; F = female; FO = fossa ovale; HW = heart weight; M = male; MVP = mitral valve prolapse; MAC = mitral annular calcification; PFO = patent foramen ovale; PML = posterior mitral leaflet; Pt = patient; SC = systolic click; SH = systemic hypertension; SM = systolic murmur;

SYSTEMIC EMBOLIZATION

Transient ischemic attacks (TIAs), stroke, retinal arteriolar occlusions, and amaurosis fugax are rare complications of mitral valve prolapse due to embolization of bland emboli: the exact incidence has not been accurately assessed.

THERAPY

GENERAL ADVICE AND MANAGEMENT OF ARRHYTHMIAS

The physician must be careful in reassuring patients with mitral valve prolapse syndrome. Patients with billowing leaflets without genuine prolapse rarely get severe mitral regurgitation and should be reassured. Palpitations due to VPCs or occasionally runs of SVT usually require no drug therapy. Following reassurance, if episodes of VPCs or SVT are bothersome and Holter monitoring demonstrates multiform VPCs, couplets or runs, non-sustained VT or short bouts of SVT, a very small dose of a beta blocking drug is appropriate and is the safest remedy. Metoprolol (25 to 50 mg twice daily) or atenolol (25 to 50 mg once daily) is advisable since they cause less fatigue than propranolol. Sotalol (80 to 160 mg once daily) is useful, but fatigue and the propensity to precipitate torsades de pointes, albeit rare, do not justify its use in this benign condition. Potentially lethal arrhythmias are rare with mitral valve prolapse and require higher doses of beta blockers

SUDDENLY SECONDARY TO MITRAL VALVE PROLAPSE

CHF	VPCS on ECG	HW (g)	MV Anulus (cm)	TV Anulus (cm)	AML Length (cm)	PML Length (cm)	Chords Missing	Grade of MVP (1–3+)	Plaque Under PML	MAC (0–4+)	VC	PFO	Redundant of Membrane
0	+	325	12.5	12	3	2.5	+	2	0	0	–		–
0	+*	220	9.6	11.5	2	1.5	0	1	+	0	0	0	
0	–	360	14	–	3	1.5	+	2	0	1	–		–
0	–	280	10	9	2.5	2	0	3	+	0	+		+
0	0†	265	12	11	3	3	0	3	+	0	+		+
0	–	570	15.5	13	3	2.5	0	3	+	0	0		0
0	–	475	10	11	3	2	0	1	+	0	0		0
0	–	355	13	12	–	–	+	2	0	2	–		+
0	+	445	12.5	12.5	2.5	2	0	3	+	0	0		0
0	0	500	10.5	12	2	1.5	0	1	0	0	0		0
0	+	325	12.6	10.5	2.5	3	0	2	+	3	0		0
0	–	390	13.6	11	3.5	3	0	3	+	1	+		+
0	+	390	13	13	3	2.5	+	3	+	0	0		0
+	+	670	>12	14	3.5	2	0	3	+	0	+		0
0	–	400	15.4	14.5	2.5	3	+	3	+	0	0		0

TV = tricuspid valve; VC = valvular competent; VPC = ventricular premature complex; W = white; + = present; 0 = absent; – = no information available.
From Dollar AL, et al.: Morphologic comparison of patients with mitral valve prolapse who died suddenly with patients who died from severe valvular dysfunction or other conditions. J Am Coll Cardiol, *17*:921, 1991.

(see Chapter 6). Chest pain requires reassurance or the use of enteric-coated aspirin (325 mg daily). If pain is bothersome or "angina like," a beta blocking drug should be administered with avoidance of nitrates, which reduce ventricular volume and thus increase the prolapse.

SYSTEMIC EMBOLIZATION

Small, bland emboli consisting of platelet and fibrin, which form in relation to the slightly abnormal valve apparatus, may cause TIAs or stroke. Management is with enteric-coated aspirin (160 to 325 mg daily) or one-quarter of a regular 325-mg aspirin daily. If TIAs continue, it is advisable to add dipyridamole (75 mg tid); this agent is more effective when given on an empty stomach or 30 minutes before meals. The drug is expensive and of unproven value but appears to have a salutary effect when combined with aspirin. The drug is ineffective when used without aspirin.

MITRAL REGURGITATION

Severe mitral regurgitation due to mitral valve prolapse is managed with surgical reconstruction where possible, but in some cases, valve replacement is necessary. The same considerations apply as in other varieties of mitral regurgitation as discussed earlier in this chapter.

RHEUMATIC FEVER

Rheumatic fever is now rare in North America and the Western world but is still prevalent in Asia, the Middle East, Africa, and Latin America and is the most commonly acquired heart disease in childhood.

CLINICAL FEATURES

The peak incidence is from age 5 to 15; rheumatic fever is uncommon under age 5 and virtually unknown under age 2. Symptoms are manifest 2 to 3 weeks after Group A streptococcal pharyngitis, which causes a hyperimmune reaction in susceptible individuals.

Symptoms and signs include

- Fever for 2 to 3 weeks
- Anorexia
- Weight loss
- Arthritis occurs in over 80% of patients and is more pronounced in older patients. It takes the form of flitting or migratory polyarthritis. Pain, redness, and swelling usually occur in large joints, knees, elbows, wrists, and shoulders; notably, the latter joint is rarely involved in other arthritides. A single joint is inflamed for about 1 day to 1 week only; the pain resolves completely and then moves on to the second joint. There is typically no deformity of joints
- Sinus tachycardia
- Subcutaneous nodules occur in up to 12% of cases
- Erythema marginatum in up to 10% of individuals. This is an effervescent, nonpruritic rash with pink circumscribed circles with a pale center mainly involving the trunk
- Sydenham's chorea (St. Vitus dance) may last for weeks to months and rarely for a few years
- Pancarditis is more common in the young, who have minimal or no arthritis. When rheumatic fever "licks" the joints, the disease often spares the heart
- New murmurs, friction rub, cardiomegaly, and heart failure indicate pancarditis
- An apical pansystolic murmur Grade I-II is common with valvular involvement and is usually accompanied by the Carey-Coombs murmur: A short, low-pitched rumbling, mid diastolic apical murmur, and its presence serves to distinguish the systolic murmur of carditis from common innocent systolic murmurs that are typically early or mid systolic vibratory murmurs or a scratchy short ejection systolic murmur located between the pulmonary area and the lower left sternal edge
- First-degree AV block or, rarely, bundle branch block occurs

THERAPY

ACUTE PHARYNGITIS

Prophylaxis of rheumatic fever requires aggressive treatment of the initial attack of pharyngitis with oral penicillin G, 500 mg immediately then 250 mg four times daily for 10 days, or intramuscular benzathine penicillin G,

1.2 million units in patients over 60 lbs. and 600,000 units for patients less than 60 lbs. Erythromycin (250 mg four times daily) or clindamycin (150 mg every 8 hours) is administered to patients allergic to penicillin.

ARTHRITIS

This is controlled with enteric-coated aspirin (100 mg/kg daily) in four divided doses to achieve a blood level of 20 to 25 mg/dl. Corticosteroids should be avoided because they produce no better results than aspirin.

PANCARDITIS

Modified bedrest is necessary for several weeks until signs of carditis are improved or unchanging. The sedimentation rate should revert to normal, and the C-reactive protein should become negative.

Enteric-coated aspirin should be given if fever and carditis is present, as well as for arthritis. Corticosteroids are not usually indicated and are used only if carditis is progressive with manifestation of cardiomegaly and heart failure. When required, prednisone (60 to 80 mg per day; 1.0 to 1.5 mg/kg/day) is administered in four doses for a period of 4 to 6 weeks. The dose is then reduced slowly with maintenance of aspirin. The possibility of steroid rebound may be reduced by employing aspirin as overlapping therapy with steroids for 2 to 3 weeks, during which time the steroids are weaned off. Pericarditis should be managed with aspirin.

SECONDARY RHEUMATIC FEVER PREVENTION

It is important to prevent recurrence since valvular damage is more intense with each recurrence of rheumatic fever. Management is with benzathine penicillin G (1.2 million units intramuscularly every 4 weeks), commonly used in North America and Europe, but in endemic areas, three weekly injections are advisable. Penicillin is continued for at least 20 years after the initial attack of rheumatic fever or to age 45, whichever occurs first. Patients allergic to penicillin are treated with sulfonamides: 1 g of oral sulfadiazine daily for patients over 60 lbs. and 0.5 g once daily for patients under 60 lbs., with liberal fluid intake.

BIBLIOGRAPHY

Alam M, Sun I: Superiority of transesophageal echocardiography in detecting ruptured mitral chordae tendineae. Am Heart J, *121*:1819, 1991.

Bassand J-P, Schiele F, Bernard Y, et al.: The double-balloon and Inoue techniques in percutaneous mitral valvuloplasty: Comparative results in a series of 232 cases. J Am Coll Cardiol, *18*:982, 1991.

Bisno AL: Group A streptococcal infections and acute rheumatic fever. N Engl J Med, *325*:783, 1991.

Bloomfield P, Wheatley DJ, Prescott RJ, et al.: Twelve-year comparison of a Bjork-Shiley mechanical heart valve with porcine bioprostheses. N Engl J Med, *324*:573, 1991.

Braunwald E: On the natural history of severe aortic stenosis. J Am Coll Cardiol, *15*:1018, 1990.

Calderwood SB, Swinski LA, Waternaux CM, et al.: Risk factors for the development of prosthetic valve endocarditis. Circulation, 72:31, 1985.

Campbell DB, Waldhausen JA: "Conservative" aortic valve intervention: Thwarted again! J Am Coll Cardiol, 16:631, 1990.

Casale P, Block PC, O'Shea JP, et al.: Atrial septal defect after percutaneous mitral balloon valvuloplasty: Immediate results and follow-up. J Am Coll Cardiol, 15:1300, 1990.

Chen CR, Hu SW, Chen JY, et al.: Percutaneous mitral valvuloplasty with a single rubber-nylon balloon (Inoue balloon): Long-term results in 71 patients. Am Heart J, 120:561, 1990.

Cohn LH: Statistical treatment of valve surgery outcomes: An influence on the evaluation of devices as well as practice. J Am Coll Cardiol, 15:574, 1990.

Cohn JN, Archibald DG, Ziesche S, et al.: Effect of vasodilator therapy on mortality in chronic congestive heart failure: Results of a Veterans Administration Cooperative Study. N Engl J Med, 314:1547, 1986.

Corin WJ, Murakami T, Monrad S, et al.: Left ventricular passive diastolic properties in chronic mitral regurgitation. Circulation, 83:797, 1991.

Crawford MH, Souchek J, Oprian CA, et al.: Determinants of survival and left ventricular performance after mitral valve replacement. Circulation, 81:1173, 1990.

Department of Health & Social Security. The United Kingdom Heart Valve Registry Report 1988. London, Crown Copyright, 1991.

Deviri E, Sareli P, Wisenbaugh T, et al.: Obstruction of mechanical heart valve prostheses: Clinical aspects and surgical management. J Am Coll Cardiol, 17:646, 1991.

Ferguson JJ, Garza RA, Mansfield Scientific Aortic Valvuloplasty Registry Investigators: Efficacy of multiple balloon aortic valvuloplasty procedures. J Am Coll Cardiol, 17:1430, 1991.

Fields CD, Slovenkai GA, Isner JM: Atrial septal defect resulting from mitral balloon valvuloplasty: Relation of defect morphology to transseptal balloon catheter delivery. Am Heart J, 119:568, 1990.

Frankl WS: Valvular heart disease: The technologic dilemma. J Am Coll Cardiol, 17:1037, 1991.

Fredman CS, Pearson AC, Labovitz AJ, et al.: Comparison of hemodynamic pressure half-time method and Gorlin formula with Doppler and echocardiographic determinations of mitral valve area in patients with combined mitral stenosis and regurgitation. Am Heart J, 119:121, 1990.

French JW: Aortic and pulmonary artery stenosis: Improvement without intervention? J Am Coll Cardiol, 15:1631, 1990.

Galloway AC, Gross EA, Baumann G, et al.: Multiple valve operation for advanced valvular heart disease: Results and risk factors in 513 patients. J Am Coll Cardiol, 19:725, 1992.

Goodman D, Kimbiris D, Linhart JW: Chordae tendineae rupture complicating the systolic click–late systolic murmur syndrome. Am J Cardiol, 33:681, 1974.

Hammermeister KE, Sethi GK, Oprian C, et al.: Comparison of occurrence of bleeding, systemic embolism, endocarditis, valve thrombosis and reoperation between patients randomized between a mechanical prosthesis and a bioprosthesis. Results from the VA randomized trial. J Am Coll Cardiol, 17:362A, 1991.

Hammermeister KE, Oprian C, Hur K: Valve replacement does not appear to prolong survival in aortic regurgitation patients. J Am Coll Cardiol, 17:41A, 1991.

Hammermeister KE, Sethi GK, Oprian C, et al.: Comparison of outcome an average of 10 years after valve replacement with a mechanical versus a bioprosthetic valve results of the VA randomized trial. J Am Coll Cardiol, 17:41A, 1991.

Hazen MS, Marwick TH, Underwood DA: Diagnostic accuracy of the resting electrocardiogram in detection and estimation of left atrial enlargement: An echocardiographic correlation in 551 patients. Am Heart J, 122:823, 1991.

Herrmann HC, Kleaveland JP, Hill JA, et al.: The M-Heart percutaneous balloon mitral valvuloplasty registry: Initial results and early follow-up. J Am Coll Cardiol, 15:1221, 1990.

Hickey MSJ, Blackstone EH, Kirklin JW, et al.: Outcome probabilities and life history after surgical mitral commissurotomy: Implications for balloon commissurotomy. J Am Coll Cardiol, 17:29, 1991.

Himelman RB, Kusumoto F, Oken K, et al.: The flail mitral valve: Echocardiographic findings by precordial and transesophageal imaging and Doppler color flow mapping. J Am Coll Cardiol, 17:272, 1991.

Hirata K, Triposkiadis F, Sparks, et al.: The Marfan syndrome. Cardiovascular physical findings and diagnostic correlates. Am Heart J, 123:743, 1992.

Isner JM: Acute catastrophic complications of balloon aortic valvuloplasty. J Am Coll Cardiol, 17:1436, 1991.

Kawanishi DT, Rahimtoola SH: Catheter balloon commissurotomy for mitral stenosis: Complications and results. J Am Coll Cardiol, 19:191, 1992.

Kennedy KD, Nishimura RAS, Holmes DR, et al.: Natural history of moderate aortic stensis. J Am Coll Cardiol, 17:313, 1991.

Khandheria BK, Seward JB, Oh JK, et al.: Value and limitations of transesophageal echocardiography in assessment of mitral valve prosthesis. Circulation, 83:1956, 1991.

Klues HG, Statler LS, Wallace RB, et al.: Massive calcification of a porcine bioprosthesis in the aortic valve position and the role of calcium supplements. Am Heart J, 121:1829, 1991.

Lefèvre T, Bonan R, Serr A, et al.: Pertucaneous mitral valvuloplasty in surgical high risk patients. J Am Coll Cardiol, 17:348, 1991.

Lund O: Preoperative risk evaluation and stratification of long-term survival after valve replacement for aortic stenosis. Reasons for earlier operative intervention. Circulation, 82: 124, 1990.

Nashef SAM, Sethia B, Turner MA, et al.: Bjork-Shiley and Carpentier Edwards valves: A comparative analysis. J Thorac Cardiovasc Surg, 93:394, 1987.

National Heart, Lung, and Blood Institute Balloon Valvuloplasty Registry: Complications and mortality of percutaneous balloon mitral commissurotomy. Circulation, 85:2014, 1992.

NHLBI Balloon Valvuloplasty Registry Participants: Percutaneous Balloon Aortic Valvuloplasty. Acute and 30-day follow-up results in 674 patients from the NHLBI balloon valvuloplasty registry. Circulation, 84:2383, 1991.

Nishimura RA, Holmes DR, Michelle MA, et al.: Seminar on balloon aortic valvuloplasty - III. Follow-up of patients with low output low gradient hemodynamics after percutaneous balloon aortic valvuloplasty: The Mansfield Scientific Aortic Valvuloplasty Registry. J Am Coll Cardiol, 17:828, 1991.

O'Connor BK, Beekman RH, Rocchini AP, et al.: Intermediate-term effectiveness of balloon valvuloplasty for congenital aortic stenosis. A prospective follow-up study. Circulation, 84: 732, 1991.

O'Neill WW: Seminar on balloon aortic valvuloplasty - 1. Introduction. J Am Coll Cardiol, 17:187, 1991.

Patel JJ, Shama D, Mitha AB, et al.: Balloon valvuloplasty versus closed commissurotomy for pliable mitral stenosis: A prospective hemodynamic study. J Am Coll Cardiol, 18:1318, 1991.

Pellikka PA, Nishimura RA, Bailey KR, et al.: The natural history of adults with asymptomatic, hemodynamically significant aortic stenosis. J Am Coll Cardiol, 15:1021, 1990.

Rahko PS: Doppler and echocardiographic characteristics of patients having an Austin Flint murmur. Circulation, 83:1940, 1991.

Rahimtoola SH: Vasodilator therapy in chronic severe aortic regurgitation. J Am Coll Cardiol, 16:430, 1990.

Roger VL, Tajik J, Bailey KR, et al.: Progression of aortic stenosis in adults: New appraisal using Doppler echocardiography. Am Heart J, 119:331, 1990.

Rao PS, Wilson AD, Sideris EB, et al.: Transcatheter closure of patent ductus arteriosus with buttoned device: First successful clinical application in a child. Am Heart J, 121:1799, 1991.

Rao V, Tong C, Ivanov J, et al.: Mitral valve replacement: Mechanical versus bioprosthetic valves - A clinical review. Can J Cardiol, 7:259, 1991.

Reeder GS, Nishimura RA, Holmes DR, et al.: Patient age and results of balloon aortic valvuloplasty: The Mansfield Scientific Registry Experience. J Am Coll Cardiol, 17:909, 1991.

Rodriguez AR, Kleiman NS, Minor ST, et al.: Factors influencing the outcome of balloon aortic valvuloplasty in the elderly. Am Heart J, 120:373, 1990.

Savage DD, Garrison RJ, Devereux RB, et al.: Mitral valve prolapse in the general population: Epideuriologic features. The Framingham Study: Am Heart J, *106*:571, 1983.

Sheikh KH, Bengtson JR, Scott J, et al.: Intraoperative transesophageal Doppler color flow imaging used to guide patient selection and operative treatment of ischemic mitral regurgitation. Circulation, *84*:594, 1991.

Shrivastava S, Das GS, Dev V, et al.: Follow-up after percutaneous balloon valvuloplasty for noncalcific aortic stenosis. Am J Cardiol, *65*:250, 1990.

Slater J, Gindea AJ, Freedberg RS, et al.: Comparison of cardiac catheterization and Doppler echocardiography in the decision to operate in aortic and mitral valve disease. J Am Coll Cardiol, *17*:1026, 1991.

Stein PD, Collins JJ Jr., Kantrowitz A: Antithrombotic therapy in mechanical and biological prosthetic heart valves and saphenous vein bypass grafts. Chest, *89*:465, 1986.

Stoddard MF, Arce J, Liddell NE, et al.: Two-dimensional transesophageal echocardiographic determination of aortic valve area in adults with aortic stenosis. Am Heart J, *122*:1415, 1991.

The Captopril-Digoxin Multicenter Research Group: Comparative effects of captopril and digoxin in patients with mild to moderate heart failure. JAMA, *159*:539, 1988.

The CONSENSUS Trial Study Group: Effects of enalapril on mortality in severe congestive heart failure: Results of the Cooperative North Scandinavian Enalapril Survival Study (CONSENSUS). N Eng J Med, *316*:1429, 1987.

The National Heart, Lung, and Blood Institute Balloon Valvuloplasty Registry Participants. Multicenter experience with balloon mitral commissurotomy. NHLBI balloon valvuloplasty registry report on immediate and 30-day follow-up results. Circulation, *85*:448, 1992.

Tornos MP, Permanyer-Miralda G, Evangelista A, et al.: Clinical evaluation of a prospective protocol for the timing of surgery in chronic aortic regurgitation. Am Heart J, *120*:649, 1990.

Turi ZG, Reyes VP, Raju BS, et al.: Percutaneous balloon versus surgical closed commissurotomy for mitral stenosis. Circulation, *83*:1179, 1991.

Tuzcu EM, Block PC, Griffin BP, et al.: Immediate and long-term outcome of percutaneous mitral valvotomy in patients 65 years and older. Circulation, *85*:963, 1992.

Tuzcu EM, Block PC, Palacios IF: Comparison of early versus late experience with percutaneous mitral balloon valvuloplasty. J Am Coll Cardiol, *17*:1121, 1991.

de Vries AG, Hess J, Witsenburg M, et al.: Management of fixed subaortic stenosis: A retrospective study of 57 cases. J Am Coll Cardiol, *19*:1013, 1992.

13

PERICARDITIS/MYOCARDITIS

M. Gabriel Khan

PERICARDITIS

The common causes of pericarditis are listed in Table 13–1. The division into obvious causes based on the presence of an easily recognizable underlying disease, and causes that are not obvious, but easily excluded by history and physical and nonspecific due to viral infections, provides for easy recall.

CLINICAL HALLMARKS

Chest pain is typically

- Retrosternal or left precordial
- Occasionally radiates to the trapezius ridge (a radiation that does not occur with angina)
- May radiate to the neck or left arm and may simulate angina or myocardial infarction (MI)
- At times localized to the epigastrium or left upper quadrant
- Sharp, pleuritic, but may be described as an oppressive, dull, vague ache
- Increased by deep inspiration, coughing, swallowing, recumbency
- Relieved by sitting and leaning forward

Genuine shortness of breath or forced, shallow breathing due to pain as well as palpitations are common features. Underlying infection may cause fever and myalgia.

A pericardial friction rub is characteristically

- Heard between the lower left sternal edge and apex
- Localized to any area or over most of the precordium
- Heard with the diaphragm pressed firmly against the chest wall, with the patient leaning forward with the breath held
- Absent if effusion develops

TABLE 13–1. CAUSES OF PERICARDITIS

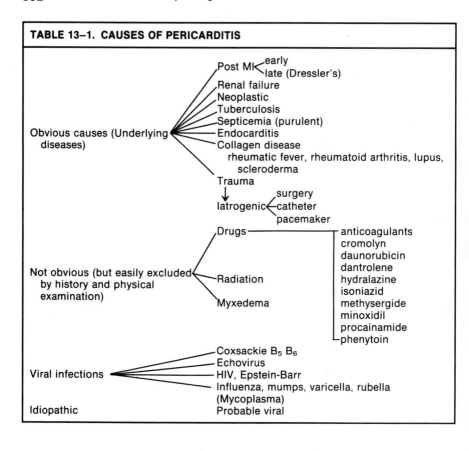

TABLE 13–2. ELECTROCARDIOGRAPHIC CLUES TO PERICARDITIS

STAGE I (hours to days)	Widespread ST segment elevation 2–5 mm concave upward LI, II, III, V_2–V_5; reciprocal depression AVR V_1
STAGE II (few days later)	ST and PR segments isoelectric, upright or flattened T
STAGE III	After normalization of ST segment, diffuse T wave inversion occurs
STAGE IV (days to weeks)	T waves normalize, rarely remain inverted

ELECTROCARDIOGRAPHIC FINDINGS

The four stages of the electrocardiographic abnormalities are given in Table 13–2

- Since tachycardia is common and may be the only electrocardiographic finding if ST elevation has resolved and the T waves remain normal
- ST segment elevation, when present, is concave upward with no T wave inversion, whereas with MI, the ST segment is convex, often with Q

waves present and the T waves begin to invert before the ST segment normalizes

Echocardiography is necessary to detect and quantitate associated pericardial effusion and in assessing tamponade.

IDIOPATHIC AND VIRAL PERICARDITIS

Most cases of idiopathic pericarditis are caused by viral infections (Table 13–1). The patient should be hospitalized and observed for tamponade. The occurrence of tamponade is manifested by

- Hemodynamic compromise
- Elevation of the jugular venous pressure
- Pulsus paradoxus and usually hypotension, which may mask pulsus paradoxus

Echocardiography is helpful in confirming the diagnosis or tamponade. Pericardiocentesis is not done routinely, even with moderate-sized effusions, if tamponade is not present. If pain is bothersome, the patient should rest in bed and chair for a few days, followed by slow ambulation over 1 to 2 weeks.

MANAGEMENT OF PAIN

- Usually relieved by aspirin or other nonsteroidal anti-inflammatory drugs (NSAIDS): Ibuprofen, 400 mg every six or eight hours, or Indomethacin, 25-50 mg every eight hours, or Naproxen, 250 mg three times daily for 4 to 10 days
- Modified bedrest and increasing dosage of NSAIDS with adequate gastric cytoprotection usually brings relief of pain without major adverse effects. It is not advisable to commence corticosteroids solely for the relief of pain, because these agents may increase viral replication.

CORTICOSTEROIDS

Corticosteroids are indicated when there is total failure of high-dose NSAIDS used over several weeks and with relapsing pericarditis not controlled by NSAIDS.

Dexamethasone

<u>Dosage:</u> IV 4 mg may relieve pain in a few hours.

Prednisone

<u>Dosage:</u> 60 mg daily for a few days, decrease by 10 mg every 3 to 5 days until a dose of 15 mg is reached. If symptoms are controlled, it is advisable to give 15 mg on alternate days for 5 days, and then 10 mg alternate days for 5 days, 5 mg alternate days for 5 days, and discontinue. The course of prednisone should be tapered as quickly as feasible. NSAIDS

are added at adequate dosage when the corticosteroid dose has reached 15 mg daily, and gastric cryoprotective agents are used if there is a history of previous peptic ulceration or if gastric symptoms are present.

RECURRENT PERICARDITIS

Approximately 25% of patients experience recurrence; if effusion develops, the risk of tamponade is high in this subset. In the absence of heart failure or tamponade, patients with severe recurrent chest pain unrelieved by adequate doses of NSAIDS may require corticosteroids for control of pain, fever, and shortness of breath. Alternate-day therapy carries less risk of adverse effects.

PERICARDITIS DUE TO SPECIFIC CAUSES

POST-INFARCTION PERICARDITIS

Acute pericarditis occurs in approximately 10% of patients within 12 hours to 10 days after infarction. The pain may be confused with post-infarction angina, extension of infarction, or pulmonary embolism. Most cases occur on the third or fourth day post infarction. Chest pain is best treated with aspirin. NSAIDS such as indomethacin, ibuprofen, and naproxen should be avoided because they appear to interfere with the healing of infarcted tissue and have been shown to cause infarct expansion and accelerate remodeling.

Dressler's Syndrome occurs in less than 0.1% of patients, usually weeks or months after MI, and may be an immune reaction. Pleuritic chest pain, fever, friction rub, leukocytosis, and increased sedimentation rate simulates nonspecific pericarditis. Enteric-coated aspirin, 650 mg two or three times daily for 1 to 2 weeks, should suffice. If pain remains bothersome or is recurrent, NSAIDS should be given a trial. Occasionally, corticosteroids are necessary and should be given as prescribed under Nonspecific Pericarditis.

PURULENT PERICARDITIS

Purulent pericarditis usually occurs during septicemia caused by pneumococcus, meningococcus, hemophilus, gonococcus, and other organisms. Pericardiocentesis is indicated in patients suspected of purulent pericarditis in order to isolate microorganisms and determine sensitivities and the appropriate choice of antibiotics. Cardiothoracic surgical assistance often is required for open pericardial drainage or creation of a pericardiopleural window.

TUBERCULOUS PERICARDITIS

In Asia, Africa, the Middle East, Latin America and some nonindustrialized countries, tuberculosis is the most common cause of pericarditis. In North America and Europe, tuberculosis is responsible for about 4%, 7%, and

6% of acute pericarditis, tamponade, and constrictive pericarditis, respectively.

Diagnosis requires isolation of myocobacterium tuberculosis in pericardial fluid or a histologic examination of pericardial tissue or proven active tuberculosis in other organs.

Tuberculous pericarditis is more common in blacks, is commonly seen in patients with AIDS, and has a peak incidence in patients between 30 and 60 years of age.

Symptoms and signs include

- Cough
- Weight loss
- Dyspnea, occasionally orthopnea
- Fever, chills, and night sweats may be present for several months before signs of pericarditis occur
- Cardiomegaly
- A pericardial friction rub plus signs of tamponade may develop
- Hepatomegaly occurs in over 90% of patients
- Ascites is fairly common
- Cardiac arrhythmias, especially atrial fibrillation or flutter

Echocardiographic and computed tomography examination may reveal pericardial effusion and pericardial thickening.

The patient should be hospitalized, observed for tamponade, and given therapy with isoniazid (300 mg), pyridoxine (50 mg), rifampin (600 mg), and ethambutol (15 mg/kg) daily for at least 9 months, allowing a minimum of 6 months of drug treatment following culture conversion. The combination of isoniazid (300 mg) and rifampin (600 mg) daily for 9 months has been shown to produce a satisfactory response in 95% of patients with extrapulmonary tuberculosis.

Corticosteroid Therapy

Corticosteroid therapy is indicated for recurrent or persistent pericardial effusion in patients receiving adequate courses of antituberculous therapy. This therapy may cause the avoidance of pericardial resection, which appears to be required in 7 to 40% of patients adequately treated with antituberculous drugs. Although some series show a high incidence of pericardial constriction, pericardiectomy is not routinely recommended. In a study by Strang, et al., only 17 of 240 patients treated with prednisolone in addition to antituberculous drugs for 11 weeks required pericardiectomy, and prednisolone therapy reduced overall mortality from 14 to 3%.

Dosage: Prednisone or prednisolone, 40 to 60 mg daily in two divided doses.

UREMIC PERICARDITIS

Pericardiocentesis is required only if there is suspicion of purulent infection or tamponade. The condition usually subsides with more frequent dialysis. Recurrent effusions uncontrolled by dialysis may respond to instillation of triamcinolone into the pericardial sac.

The instillation of sclerozing agents is of benefit in some patients with neoplastic pericarditis.

CARDIAC TAMPONADE

Tamponade may occur acutely secondary to

- Chest trauma: An individual who has sustained recent chest trauma and appears in shock with increased venous pressure should be suspected of having cardiac tamponade
- Acute MI with freewall rupture
- Dissecting aneurysm

Acute or subacute presentations occasionally occur with

- Neoplastic involvement
- Nonspecific pericarditis
- Uremia or purulent infections

Sudden progressive severe shortness of breath, chest tightness, or dysphagia may herald the shock-like state. The jugular venous pressure (JVP) is usually elevated; hypotension and tachycardia are usually present.

DIAGNOSTIC HALLMARKS

Significant pulsus paradoxus is usually detectable, except when severe hypotension or elevation of the diastolic pressure of either ventricle is present; for example, with uremic pericarditis and hypertension. Thus, the physician should not be lulled into a sense of false security by the absence of paradoxus. Pulsus paradoxus is an exaggeration of the normal inspiratory decline of systemic arterial pressure. To determine the presence of significant pulsus paradoxus, the patient's respirations are observed while slowly deflating the blood pressure cuff. Initially, the Korotkoff sound is heard only on expiration, but as the cuff pressure is lowered, Korotkoff sounds are heard during inspiration; the difference in systolic blood pressure recorded at the commencement of the Korotkoff sounds in inspiration and expiration is an estimate of pulsus parodoxus. Normally, this difference is less than 10 mm Hg. Pulsus paradoxus greater than 12 mm Hg is significant. Muffled heart sounds represent another hallmark.

Pulsus paradoxus may be observed in several conditions, including

- Severe COPD
- Status asthmaticus
- Pneumothorax
- Massive pulmonary embolism

However, in COPD and asthma, the JVP falls normally on inspiration. With right ventricular infarction, the venous pressure is high but increases on inspiration (Kussmaul's sign), and pulsus paradoxus is absent. Massive pulmonary embolism may produce a shock-like state with markedly elevated jugular venous pressure and represents a diagnostic challenge but the clinical setting usually assists in differentiating the two conditions.

Cardiac tamponade and cardiogenic shock secondary to acute MI may be difficult to differentiate, and both may occur during the course of massive infarction. Heart sounds may be faint in both conditions.

Severe heart failure causing marked elevation of jugular venous pressure can be confused with cardiac tamponade. It is important to differentiate the two conditions, since the use of diuretics is contraindicated in the presence of tamponade. Because the most common cause of right heart failure is left heart failure, pulmonary congestion is usually detectable with the presence of crackles, third heart sound, radiologic evidence of pulmonary congestion, and LV failure. Pulsus paradoxus is not a feature of severe heart failure, and the presence of a V wave in the venous pulse indicates tricuspid regurgitation.

Cardiac regional tamponade causing hemodynamic deterioration may occur within the first 2 weeks of cardiac surgery or in conditions causing adhesions and loculation. In these situations, pulsus paradoxus may be absent and the echocardiogram may fail to show effusion all around the heart. In patients with suspected cardiac tamponade, urgent echocardiography is mandatory.

Echocardiographic features include

* An early finding of right atrial collapse, which occurs in most cases except regional tamponade, in which right or left atrial collapse may be observed
* Right ventricular collapse

THERAPY

Management of tamponade involves the maintenance of an adequate preload so as to generate stroke volume. Thus, diuretics and preload-reducing agents such as nitrates and ACE inhibitors must be avoided. Volume expansion with saline and even transfusion with packed red cells may provide hemodynamic stability until pericardiocentesis is accomplished. It is important to maintain volume expansion so that right atrial pressure may be maintained above intrapericardial pressure in order to prevent right atrial or ventricular collapse.

Pericardiocentesis carried out by an experienced cardiologist under echocardiographic control or by a cardiac thoracic surgeon is necessary. An indwelling pericardial catheter with multiple side holes may be used for drainage and for installation of antibiotics, triamcinolone, or chemotherapeutic agents. Failure of pericardiocentesis is usually due to a posteriorly located effusion. Reaccumulation of fluid and recurrent tamponade are indications for subxiphoid pericardial window drainage carried out by a cardiothoracic surgeon.

CONSTRICTIVE PERICARDITIS

The proper management of constrictive pericarditis begins with correct diagnosis. Common causes include

* Neoplastic disease, especially carcinoma of lung or breast asbestosis and lymphoma

- Mediastinal irradiation
- Nonviral pericardial infections
- Viral pericarditis
- Tuberculosis
- Post-cardiac surgery
- Chest trauma
- Connective tissue diseases
- Chronic renal failure and dialysis

DIAGNOSTIC HALLMARKS

If the jugular venous pressure is both markedly and chronically elevated and the history and physical examination fail to suggest an apparent cardiac cause in the presence of a small quiet heart, then a restrictive syndrome must be considered, the most common cause being constrictive pericarditis. Neck vein examination should reveal Kussmaul's sign, which may be difficult to elicit when the venous pressure is severely elevated. The venous pulse usually has a prominent y-descent, coincident with the early rapid diastolic filling of the ventricle. A prominent x-descent, coincident with filling of the atrium, is often observed in patients with sinus rhythm. The exaggerated x- and y-descents give the venous pressure a characteristic M- or W-shaped pattern (Table 13–3).

Auscultation should reveal the presence of an early high-frequency third heart sound (S3) caused by abrupt cessation of early diastolic filling. This sound, referred to as a pericardial knock, occurs earlier than the conventional third heart sound of heart failure and has a sharp, high-pitched quality that is easily heard with the diaphragm and may mimic an opening snap or early filling sound heard in endomyocardial fibrosis.

Atrial fibrillation occurs in approximately 33% of cases of constrictive pericarditis.

The presence of marked ascites, occurring days to weeks before the presence of significant edema, points strongly to constrictive pericarditis and serves to distinguish the condition from heart failure, in which prominent edema occurs and is followed weeks later by mild ascites. In a few patients with longstanding constriction and congestion, protein-losing gastroenteropathy may ensue.

DIFFERENTIAL DIAGNOSIS

Patients who present with noncalcific constrictive pericarditis pose a diagnostic problem.

Heart Failure

Heart failure not caused by constrictive pericarditis can be difficult to differentiate. The presence of a pericardial knock and marked ascites developing prior to leg edema favor the diagnosis of constrictive pericarditis. Also, severe heart failure causing chronically elevated jugular venous pressure is invariably associated with tricuspid regurgitation and prominent v

TABLE 13–3. CONSTRICTIVE PERICARDITIS VS. RESTRICTIVE CARDIOMYOPATHY

	CONSTRICTIVE PERICARDITIS	RESTRICTIVE CARDIOMYOPATHY
Clinical Features		
Heart size	Usually normal	Usually large
Heart impulse	Quiet	LV and/or right ventricular dilatation
JVP	M pattern*	M pattern
Kussmaul's sign	Present	Present
Systolic (v) waves	Absent	Present (tricuspid regurgitation)
Systolic murmurs	Rare	Common
S3 gallop**	Present	Present (except in amyloid)
Chest X-Ray	Clear lung fields	Similar
	Normal heart size	Similar or moderately enlarged
	Pericardial calcification (50%)	Rare
		Myocardial calcification not uncommon
ECG	P mitrale	Uncommon
	Atrial fibrillation 33%	Common
	Conduction defects uncommon	Common
	Flat or inverted T waves common	Widespread T wave inversion common
	May show low voltage	Low voltage common
	Q waves very rare	QS precordial leads, pseudoinfarction pattern common
Echocardiogram	Thickened pericardium	
	Calcified pericardium	No pericardial calcification, myocardial calcification
	Normal septal motion	
Systemic Disease (associated)	Tuberculosis	Amyloid; sarcoid; tuberculosis (See text)
CT or MRI scan	Thickened pericardium	Normal pericardium

* Due to exaggerated x- and y-descents
** Pericardial knock

waves. The heart size is usually normal with constrictive pericarditis, and calcification may be apparent, depending on the causation.

Right Ventricular Infarction

Right ventricular infarction may produce a similar picture. However, right ventricular infarction usually presents in the setting of an acute MI and often with inferoposterior involvement. The condition is acute and presents with a high jugular venous pressure associated with hypotension. Constrictive pericarditis is a chronic condition with insidious appearance of symptoms and signs.

Right Atrial Myxoma

Myxoma should produce a prominent a wave in the venous pulse and requires echocardiographic exclusion.

Restrictive Cardiomyopathy

Restrictive physiology due to amyloid and endomyocardial fibrosis may mimic the hemodynamic findings of constrictive pericarditis. Table 13–3 gives diagnostic points for constrictive pericarditis versus restrictive cardiomyopathy. The presence of cardiac enlargement, prominent murmurs, and/or tricuspid regurgitation with prominent systolic v waves supports the diagnosis of restrictive cardiomyopathy. Electrocardiographic findings may be similar in both conditions, but pseudoinfarction pattern favors restrictive disease. Diagnosis can be difficult if pericardial calcification or pericardial thickening is not observed on echocardiography or CAT scan or in patients with left ventricular diastolic pressures equal to right ventricular diastolic pressures. Magnetic resonance imaging (MRI) may be helpful in identifying thickening of the pericardium. In patients with suspected myocardial disease, endomyocardial biopsy is desirable.

INVESTIGATIONS

A few or all of the following investigations may be required to be certain of the diagnosis

- Chest x-ray may show pericardial calcification, especially of the apex and posteriorly, which is best seen on lateral views; the heart size is usually normal
- ECG is virtually always abnormal but nonspecific and shows diffuse flat or inverted T wave in over 75%; the depth of inversion of the T waves is usually proportional to the degree of pericardial adherence to the myocardium, which may make stripping difficult; low voltage is present in approximately 50% of cases, along with abnormal P waves, P-mitrale if in sinus rhythm. Atrial fibrillation is present in approximately 33% of patients
- Echocardiography is of limited value in identifying thickened pericardium, unless calcification is present. Doppler echocardiography shows typical Doppler features in both mitral and hepatic vein flow in approximately 85% of patients with constriction amenable to surgery
- Ultrafast cine-computed tomography and/or MRI give fairly accurate assessment of pericardial thickness, pericardial impingement on the right ventricle, and the degree of dilation of the vena cavae and hepatic veins
- Cardiac catheterization findings are listed in Table 13–4. Elevation and equalization of all diastolic pressures and the dip and plateau or square root sign are typical findings, but these may be observed in some patients with restrictive cardiomyopathy; as outlined above, CT and MRI are useful in differentiating these two categories of patients (see Fig. 13–1 and Table 13–3)

TABLE 13–4. CATHETERIZATION DATA		
PARAMETERS	CONSTRICTIVE PERICARDITIS	RESTRICTIVE CARDIOMYOPATHY
Diastolic pressure	Equalization of early & late diastolic pressures	LV > right* Rarely LV-right and resembles constrictive pericarditis
LVEDP-RVEDP ≤6 mm Hg (predictive value 87%)**	Usual finding (few exceptions)	Usually >6, but significant overlap
LA pressure	Equal right	Higher than right; may equalize with severe tricuspid regurgitation
RV pressure square root sign	Always present: early dip and plateau during diastole	Present, but may disappear with therapy
Pulmonary hypertension	Mild	Moderate or severe
RV systolic pressure ≤52 mm Hg** (predictive value 71%)	Usual finding	Wide range (30 to 85 mm Hg)
RVEDP/RV systolic ≥0.38** (predictive value 83%)	Usual finding	Variable, significant overlap

LV = left ventricular
RV = right ventricular
EDP = end diastolic pressure
LA = left atrial
 * = both measured simultaneously
** = modified from Vaitkus PT, Kussmaul WG: Constrictive pericarditis versus restrictive cardiomyopathy: A reappraisal and update of diagnostic criteria. Am Heart J, *122*:1431, 1991.

- It is important to avoid diuretics prior to catheter studies, because sodium and water loss may cause equalization of left and right ventricular filling pressures in patients with restrictive cardiomyopathy

THERAPY

Surgical pericardiectomy is needed when medical therapy, with the judicious use of diuretics and digoxin for control of the ventricular response in patients with atrial fibrillation, fails to reduce markedly elevated jugular venous pressure and when symptoms are persistent and bothersome. Early surgical mortality is approximately 5%. In patients with severe calcific disease, recovery may be delayed for weeks or months. If constriction and restriction are both present, pericardiectomy may not cause symptomatic improvement.

MYOCARDITIS

Acute myocarditis is a disease that can cause a fulminant illness that may result in functional impairment or death. Myocarditis appears to be a precursor in some patients with dilated cardiomyopathy.

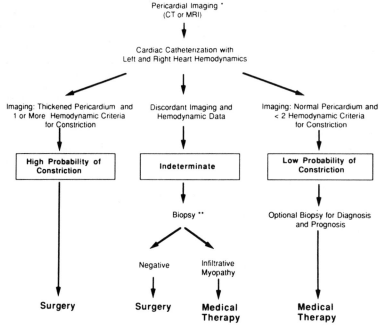

FIG. 13–1. Algorithm for evaluating patients with a clinical profile consistent with constriction or restriction. *If chest x-ray films reveal a calcified pericardium, more sophisticated imaging modalities (i.e., CT or MRI) are unnecessary. **If endomyocardial biopsy is unavailable, surgery should be pursued in this setting. From: Vaitkus PT, et al.: Constrictive pericarditis versus restrictive cardiomyopathy: A reappraisal and update of diagnostic criteria. Am Heart J, *122*:1431, 1991.

PATHOGENESIS

It appears that viruses may induce myocarditis in genetically susceptible individuals. In humans, viral involvement and a later immunologic modulation appear to be important. Viral myocarditis can be induced in genetically susceptible mice by viruses and can be prevented by vaccines or by interferon.

CLINICAL HALLMARKS

A viral illness in the preceding weeks is observed in over 85% of cases. Any one or more of the following may be manifest

- Chest pain in over 20% of patients, associated with pericarditis and its signs and symptoms
- Palpitations in approximately 33%
- Tachypnea
- Fatigue
- Symptoms and signs of heart failure

- Small pericardial effusion
- An easily heard S3 gallop is commonly present with acute myocarditis and is an expected finding in patients with significant myocardial involvement
- Subclinical illness is not uncommon
- ECG shows ST-T wave changes, often with low T wave and QRS voltage. Conduction detects and atrial or ventricular arrhythmias commonly occur
- Creatine kinase (CK) and CK-MB may simulate MI, but with a different time course
- Chest x-ray

Myocardial biopsy is rarely required, except for research purposes or prior to prescribing immunotherapy. A negative gallium scan is reassuring, because it excludes myocarditis in over 96% of all cases. Also, a negative gallium predicts a negative myocardial biopsy. In a multicenter study, only 9.4% of 2,000 patients with presumed myocarditis had a positive biopsy.

PREDICTION OF OUTCOME

More than 90% of patients recover completely over days, weeks, or months. Thus, in the majority, treatment is chiefly observation and support. In a few cases, heart failure is manifest and clears over weeks with conventional antifailure therapy. Rarely, heart failure becomes progressively worse and is unabated, except when corticosteroids or cyclosporin cause some amelioration.

Nonsustained ventricular arrhythmias should not be treated with antiarrhythmics, because these agents may cause deterioration due to their negative inotropic and, proarrhythmic effects. In the presence of lethal or potentially lethal arrhythmias, the use of amiodarone may be lifesaving, but its widespread prophylactic use cannot be recommended (Chapter 6).

Pacing may be required if Mobitz Type II or complete AV block develops (Chapter 18).

HEART FAILURE THERAPY

- Modified bedrest; i.e., bed to chair for one week, then slow ambulation over weeks
- Avoid digoxin because there is increased sensitivity; thus, the drug is used only for atrial fibrillation with a fast ventricular response or with severe heart failure along with furosemide and ACE inhibitors
- Diuretics must be used judiciously, taking care to prevent potassium and magnesium depletion
- ACE inhibitors are necessary to decrease afterload and appear to provide salutary effects
- Corticosteroids are advisable if symptoms persist or continue to progress in an unabated fashion. Corticosteroids may be given a trial, especially if the illness is beyond 3 weeks. During the first few weeks, there is a fear that corticosteroids may increase viral replication and worsen myocarditis

A nonrandomized study involving 13 children with biopsy-proven myocarditis showed benefit from corticosteroid therapy. However, a recently completed multicenter randomized study using corticosteroids and cyclosporin in patients with biopsy-proven myocarditis showed no improvement in survival or LV function. Thus, a conservative approach is suggested, except where life appears to be threatened.

BIBLIOGRAPHY

Dutt AK, Moers D, Stead WW: Short-course chemotherapy for extrapulmonary tuberculosis: Nine years experience. Ann Intern Med, *104*:7, 1986.

Chan KY, Iwahara M, Benson LN, et al.: Immunosuppressive therapy in the management of acute myocarditis in children: A clinical trial. J Am Coll Cardiol, *17*:458, 1991.

Fowler NO: Tuberculous pericarditis. JAMA, *266*:99, 1991.

Getz MA, Subramanian R, Logemann T, et al.: Acute necrotizing eosinophilic myocarditis as a manifestation of severe hypersensitivity myocarditis. Ann Intern Med, *115*:201, 1991.

Levine MJ, Lorell BH, Diver DJ, et al.: Implications of echocardiographically assisted diagnosis of pericardial tamponade in contemporary medical patients: Detection before hemodynamic embarrassment. J Am Coll Cardiol, *17*:59, 1991.

Mason JW: Distinct forms of myocarditis. Circulation, *83*:1110, 1991.

Oh JK, Hatle L, Seward JB, et al.: Sensitivity of Doppler echocardiography for constrictive pericarditis. J Am Coll Cardiol, *17*:49A, 1991.

Shabetai R: Changing concepts of cardiac tamponade. J Am Coll Cardiol, *12*:194, 1988.

Strang JIG, Kakaza HHS, Gibson DG, et al.: Controlled clinical trial of complete open surgical drainage and of prednisolone in treatment of tuberculosis pericardial effusion in Transkei. Lancet, *2*:759, 1988.

Talwar KK, Kumar K, Chopra P, et al.: Cardiac involvement in nonspecific aortoarteritis (Takayasu's arteritis). Am Heart J, *122*:1666, 1991.

Tunick PA, Nachamie M, Kronzon I: Reversal of echocardiographic signs of pericardial tamponade by transfusion. Am Heart J, *119*:199, 1990.

Vaitkus PT, Kussmaul WG: Constrictive pericarditis versus restrictive cardiomyopathy: A reappraisal and update of diagnostic criteria. Am Heart J, *122*:1431, 1991.

14

CARDIOMYOPATHY, SPECIFIC HEART MUSCLE DISEASE

M. Gabriel Khan
John F. Goodwin

Cardiomyopathy is defined as heart muscle disease of unknown cause. Cardiomyopathies are classified as follows

- Hypertrophic
- Dilated
- Restrictive

Heart muscle disease from known causes, particularly infiltrative or systemic disease, formerly termed secondary cardiomyopathy, is currently referred to as specific heart muscle disease and is discussed at the end of this chapter.

HYPERTROPHIC CARDIOMYOPATHY

Hypertrophic cardiomyopathy (HCM) refers to a condition in which massive ventricular hypertrophy occurs in the absence of any definite cause. The term hypertrophic cardiomyopathy is preferred, because not all affected patients have idiopathic hypertrophic subaortic stenosis or features of hypertrophic obstructive cardiomyopathy. Approximately 33% of patients have no significant left ventricular (LV) outflow tract gradient at rest or on provocation.

The myofibrillar disarray commonly seen in HCM is believed to be caused by an aberration of catecholamine function in the heart of the embryo. Familial cases show an autosomal dominant trait linked to chromosome 14q1.

PATHOPHYSIOLOGY

- Most patients show asymmetric hypertrophy of the septum and a hypertrophied nondilated left and/or right ventricle. But the septum may be diffusely hypertrophied or only in its upper, mid, or apical portion. Hypertrophy extends to the freewall of the left ventricle

- Decreased compliance and incomplete relaxation of the left ventricle cause impedance to diastolic filling
- Rapid, powerful contraction of the hypertrophied left ventricle expels most of its contents in the first half of systole. This hyperdynamic systolic function is apparent in most patients with HCM
- The anterior leaflet of the mitral valve is displaced toward the hypertrophied septum, causing obstruction in midsystole. Mitral regurgitation is virtually always present in the obstructive phase of the disease. Therefore, the sequence of events is: eject, obstruct, leak. A variable LV outflow pressure gradient at rest occurs in approximately 35% of patients. A further 25% develop a similar gradient precipitated by conditions that increase myocardial contractility or decrease ventricular volume. Thus, diuretics and other causes of hypovolemia and preload-reducing agents that reduce the volume of the small ventricular cavity may worsen outflow tract obstruction
- Fibrosis and occlusive disease in small coronary arteries and arterioles may occur. The major coronary arteries are wide and patent unless occlusive atherosclerotic coronary disease occurs as a chance association

CLINICAL HALLMARKS

SYMPTOMS

- Dyspnea caused by raised left ventricular end diastolic pressure
- Angina resulting from reduced diastolic coronary perfusion
- Presyncope or syncope during exercise, normal activities, or at rest, not simply related to failure to increase cardiac output on exercise
- May present with palpitations or symptoms and signs of heart failure

Table 14–1 gives the predominant symptoms and signs and their approximate incidence.

SIGNS

General physique is usually normal and well developed. The palpable left atrial beat preceding the left ventricular thrust is a most important sign, since it can occur in the absence of gradient or murmur.

The murmur has typical features

- Crescendo-decrescendo starts well after the first heart sound and ends well before the second. It is best heard between the apex and left sternal border
- Radiates poorly to the neck or axilla, if at all
- Intensity increases with maneuvers or drugs that decrease preload (valsalva, standing, amyl nitrate) and decreases in intensity with an increase in afterload (squatting, hand grip, phenylephrine)
- Easy to distinguish from aortic valvular stenosis, in which the murmur starts soon after the first heart sound and radiates well to the neck

A mitral regurgitant murmur is often heard in the last half of the systole with radiation to the axilla. It is usually associated with an outflow tract gradient. A mitral diastolic rumble may be detected.

TABLE 14-1. CLINICAL HALLMARKS OF HYPERTROPHIC CARDIOMYOPATHY

SYMPTOMS AND SIGNS	APPROXIMATE INCIDENCE (%)	FACTORS
Dyspnea	80	Diastolic dysfunction
Angina	60	Decreased coronary reserve, small vessel disease, or associated CHD
Presyncope	50	Even at rest
Syncope	20	Post-exertional and normal activities
Sudden death/annual		
Adult	2.5	Mainly arrhythmic
Children	6	
Annual mortality	4	
Brisk carotid upstroke	90	
Atrial fibrillation	15	
Left atrial beat	50	
Left ventricular thrust	60	
4th heart sound	50	
3rd heart sound	30	
Systolic murmur, late onset crescendo-decrescendo	90	Begins well after S1 Little or no radiation to neck or axilla, outflow gradient
Mitral systolic murmur	50	Mitral regurgitation, radiates to axilla

It must be emphasized that the physical examination may be relatively unremarkable in HCM; attention is necessary to elucidate three subtle signs

- Rapid carotid upstroke
- Abnormal cardiac impulse
- Gallop sounds

HCM causes a brisk carotid upstroke because of the dynamic LV emptying, giving an ill-sustained quality. Whereas aortic valvular stenosis produces a slow-rising pulse, pulsus tardus et parvus, with a delayed carotid upstroke.

Supraventricular arrhythmias occur in 20 to 50% of patients and ventricular arrhythmias occur in almost all patients.

SUDDEN DEATH

Unfortunately, the pathophysiologic mechanism of sudden death remains unresolved. Patients presumed to be at risk for sudden death include those who

- Are under 20 years of age at time of diagnosis
- Are under 20 years of age and have a family history of HCM and sudden death
- Have potentially lethal ventricular arrhythmias, sustained ventricular tachycardia (VT), nonsustained VT, and frequent multiform ventricular ectopics

- Have a history of syncope
- Have severe exertional dyspnea or orthopnea in association with ventricular arrhythmias

Studies indicate that death cannot be predicted adequately by these conventional criteria. They are an increased risk. The presence of sustained or nonsustained VT, multiform ventricular ectopy reflects a high risk, but in childhood, the absence of potentially lethal ventricular arrhythmias on 48-hour Holter monitoring must not be interpreted as a lowered risk. Mildly symptomatic or asymptomatic patients who die suddenly have marked left ventricular hypertrophy. Some evidence indicates that mildly symptomatic patients who have HCM with mild left ventricular hypertrophy have a low incidence of sudden cardiac death. The commencement of atrial fibrillation with loss of atrial function may precipitate pulmonary edema or hypotension.

ATRIAL FIBRILLATION IN HCM

Atrial fibrillation occurs in approximately 15% of patients with HCM. The loss of atrial systole with a fast ventricular response may precipitate pulmonary edema and, occasionally, severe hypotension. The outcome for patients with HCM and atrial fibrillation is not as bleak as envisaged in the 1970s and 1980s, however. The outlook is not significantly worse for patients with atrial fibrillation and failure to convert than it is for patients with sinus rhythm. Functional class does deteriorate with the onset of atrial fibrillation, but it improves with conversion and control of ventricular response or when chronic atrial fibrillation with controlled ventricular response is achieved.

INVESTIGATIONS

CHEST X-RAY

The chest x-ray may be normal but often shows some left atrial enlargement; the left ventricle ranges from normal to severe enlargement. Aortic valve calcification is absent in HCM, but annular calcification of the mitral valve occurs.

ELECTROCARDIOGRAM

ECG findings

- Virtually always abnormal (95%) in patients with significant symptomatic HCM and about 80% abnormal in asymptomatic patients
- Atrial fibrillation in 15%; an additional 33% have paroxysmal episodes
- Other supraventricular and ventricular arrhythmias, nonsustained VT is common, but sustained VT occurs in approximately 3%
- Deep, narrow Q waves in about 30% in leads II III AVF, V5-V6 or in I AVL V5-V6, rarely V1-V3 which may mimic infarction
- Intraventricular conduction delay in over 80%

- High QRS voltage left ventricular hypertrophy (LVH)
- Diffuse T wave changes in some patients or T waves of LVH
- Giant inverted T waves, very high precordial QRS voltage with apical HCM
- ST segment depression in some
- PR interval occasionally short; pre-excitation may be seen

ECHOCARDIOGRAM

Two-dimensional echocardiographic observation of a LV myocardial segment of 1.5 cm or more thickness in a normal-sized adult is considered diagnostic, if there is no other evident cause (Table 14–2 gives echocardiographic hallmarks). Asymmetric hypertrophy is supporting evidence. Myocardial mass increases with age and size. Continuous-wave Doppler echocardiography defines the degree of LV outflow-tract gradient.

HOLTER MONITORING

A 48-hour Holter monitor is necessary because a 24-hour study detects less than 50% runs of nonsustained VT. Repeated studies may be required.

Where facilities exist, a signal-averaged ECG is advisable, especially in younger patients. In this subgroup, an abnormal signal-averaged ECG appears to be a marker for sudden death. Further studies are necessary to confirm the role of the signal-averaged ECG in patients with HCM.

THERAPY

Management of the patient with HCM includes counseling and entails screening of all first-degree relatives of newly diagnosed cases. An ECG, chest x-ray, and echocardiogram should usually suffice to identify affected individuals but still cases can be missed.

Holter monitoring and/or examination of relatives is important

- Patients must be instructed to avoid strenuous competitive exercise because it can cause sudden death. A decrease in ventricular volume or increase in ventricular contractility increases the outflow gradient. Thus,

---

TABLE 14–2. ECHOCARDIOGRAPHIC HALLMARKS OF HYPERTROPHIC CARDIOMYOPATHY

1. Disproportionate septal thickness, septum to posterior wall ratio >1.5
2. Left ventricular myocardial segment >1.5 cm in thickness
3. Poor septal contraction, hypercontractile free posterior wall
4. Systolic anterior motion of the mitral valve when outflow tract gradient >30 mm Hg
5. Mid systolic aortic valve closure
6. Small left ventricular cavity, typically with virtual elimination in systole
7. Mitral regurgitation frequently present
8. Left ventricular outflow tract gradient at rest in about 35% of patients

TABLE 14–3. PHARMACOLOGIC AND SURGICAL INTERVENTIONS FOR THE
OBSTRUCTIVE AND END-STAGE PHASE OF HYPERTROPHIC CARDIOMYOPATHY

INTERVENTION	OBSTRUCTIVE PHASE	END STAGE
Negative inotropes		
Beta blockers	Yes (especially with latent obstruction)	Small dose considered
Verapamil	Yes	Contraindicated
Disopyramide	Yes	Contraindicated
Digoxin	Contraindicated	Needed & useful
Diuretics	Contraindicated	Needed & useful
Afterload-reducing agent:		
ACE Inhibitors	Contraindicated	Of some benefit in patients with ventricular dilatation and heart failure
Surgery	Myectomy	Transplant

dehydration and the use of preload-reducing agents, such as diuretics, nitrates, or ACE inhibitors, should be avoided
- Beta-agonists increase contractility and are contraindicated
- Digoxin increases contractility and its use should be avoided, except in the management of chronic atrial fibrillation, a fast ventricular response uncontrolled by amiodarone, beta blockers, or verapamil. Also useful in patients with end-stage disease with heart failure (see Table 14–3)
- Drugs that decrease myocardial contractility or produce myocardial relaxation, particularly beta blockers and calcium antagonists, play a major role in the control of symptoms
- Patients without significant obstruction with moderate mitral regurgitation and end-stage disease with heart failure and ventricular dilatation may benefit from the judicious use of ACE inhibitors (Table 14–3)

BETA-ADRENERGIC BLOCKING AGENTS

Clinical trials have documented the role of beta blockers in the management of HCM. Beta blockers and verapamil are equally effective for the management of symptoms, but beta blockers generally are safer and therefore are considered first-line therapy. Beneficial effects of beta-adrenergic blocking drugs include the following

- Decrease in myocardial contractility causes a decrease in "venturi" effect and therefore less obstruction
- Relief of dyspnea in about 40% of patients
- Significant relief of angina in 33 to 66% of patients
- The heart rate should be maintained between 55 and 60 beats per minute; this results in an improvement in coronary filling because of prolongation of the diastolic interval
- Improvement in diastolic dysfunction
- Partial control of supraventricular and ventricular arrhythmias

Angina, at times, may be caused by coincident atheromatous obstruction of major coronary arteries, but it is commonly a result of small vessel disease and decreased coronary flow reserve. Large doses of beta blockers are often required to produce adequate beta-adrenergic blockade. The therapeutic activity of beta blockers metabolized in the liver and calcium antagonists is blunted by cigarette smoking. It is important for patients with HCM to desist smoking because of other adverse effects, as well as the decrease in effectiveness of the two major pharmacologic interventions. Beta blockers do not appear to decrease the risk of sudden death in these cardiac patients. Because of the infrequent occurrence of HCM, clinical trials have included small numbers of patients, and a beta error is a possible reason for the lack of documentation of a decrease in the risk of sudden death with beta blocker therapy. These agents are particularly useful in patients with latent obstruction. Clinical experience has been mainly with propranolol; nonselective agents are preferred. Beta blockers with significant partial agonist activity, such as pindolol and acebutolol, are less desirable.

Contraindications to beta blocker therapy include

- Asthma
- Heart failure
- Severe peripheral vascular disease
- Sick sinus syndrome
- Marked bradycardia
- AV block (see Chapters 1 and 2)

Propranolol

Supplied: tablets; 40, 80, 120 mg (Inderal LA: 80, 120, 160 mg)

Dosage: 10 mg three times daily, increase slowly to 120 to 240 mg daily. A slow build-up of the dosage to 320 mg may be required or an equivalent dose of atenolol or metoprolol.

Sotalol

This is a nonselective hydrophilic, nonhepatic-metabolized beta blocker that, among the beta blockers, has a unique Class 3 antiarrhythmic activity and therefore may decrease the risk of sudden death. Where amiodarone is contraindicated or produces adverse effects, sotalol may be tried.

Supplied: tablets; 160 mg

Dosage: 80 to 240 mg daily. Start with 40 to 80 mg twice daily, and then increase, if needed, to a maximum of 240 mg daily. The drug can be given once daily, but it makes more sense to give smaller divided doses so that, in the event of adverse effects, the evening dose can be discontinued. Maintain a normal serum potassium and watch especially for precipitants of hypokalemia resulting from diuretic use and persistent diarrhea.

Caution. Do not use with potassium-losing diuretics. Care must be taken to maintain a normal serum potassium, to avoid the rare risk of torsades de pointes. Do not use in patients with renal failure.

Interactions. Beta blockers interact with amiodarone, diltiazem, verapamil, diuretics, quinidine, and Class 1A antiarrhythmics.

CALCIUM ANTAGONISTS

Verapamil

Verapamil enhances LV diastolic filling by improving ventricular relaxation, actions similar to those produced by beta-adrenergic blockade. Considerable experience with verapamil is now available, but the initial high expectations have not materialized and the drug has caused deaths. The verapamil decreases dyspnea and increases exercise capacity in some patients but does not appear to improve survival, and is contraindicated in patients with end stage disease associated with ventricular dilation and heart failure.

Supplied: tablets; 80, 120 mg, SR 240 mg (UK: 40 mg)

Dosage: 40 mg three times daily or 80 mg twice daily, increase slowly over weeks to 240 to 360 mg daily under close observation. Preferably, administration of the drug is begun in the hospital setting.

Adverse effects. High-grade AV block, asystole, sinus arrest, acute pulmonary edema, hypotension.

Contraindications
- Orthopnea or paroxysmal nocturnal dyspnea. Deaths have occurred in these patients as a result of verapamil use
- Heart failure and or end stage disease (Table 14–3)
- Sick sinus syndrome
- AV block and conduction defects

Interactions. The drug must not be combined with amiodarone and should not be used concomitantly with beta blockers, quinidine, or disopyramide (see Table 1–8).

Diltiazem

The actions of diltiazem are less intense than verapamil and midway between verapamil and nifedipine. Experience with the drug is limited. Adverse effects resemble those seen with verapamil. Importantly, the drug interacts with amiodarone, digoxin, and quinidine. Its use is questionable and perhaps not justifiable, except where beta blockers, verapamil, or a beta blocker–nifedipine combination is poorly tolerated. As with verapamil, diltiazem should not be used in patients with suspected high pulmonary capillary wedge pressures, because pulmonary edema may be precipitated.

Nifedipine

Nifedipine improves left ventricular filling. Some studies suggest that nifedipine can play a role in the amelioration of left ventricular diastolic dysfunction. The drug has virtually no electrophysiologic effects and thus is devoid of the serious sinus and AV nodal side effects of verapamil, diltiazem, and other benzothiazepine calcium antagonists.

Clinically, nifedipine has less negative inotropic effects than verapamil. Thus, heart failure is less likely to occur in patients at high risk for heart failure. In addition, interactions are not seen with amiodarone, beta blockers, digoxin, or disopyramide (Table 1–8).

Nifedipine causes peripheral vasodilatation, which may produce hypotension and an increase in outflow tract gradient, and thus must be used with care in patients with obstructive disease. The role of the drug when used with a beta blocker is logical, as the beta blocker will tend to reduce tachycardia caused by nifedipine. In selected patients without gradient, this combination provides symptomatic benefit.

Supplied: Adalat PA: tablets; 10, 20 mg. Nifedipine extended release, Procardia XL: 30, 60, 90 mg (Adalat XL in Canada). Adalat Retard: 10, 20 mg in the UK

Dosage: Begin with Adalat PA, 10 mg twice daily; increase over weeks to 20 mg twice daily or Procardia XL (nifedipine extended release) 30 mg once daily, increase slowly to a maximum of 60 mg daily, with concomitant beta blockade.

AMIODARONE

Amiodarone has gained widespread acceptance as a major advance in the management of patients with atrial fibrillation and, in others, to reduce the incidence of ventricular arrhythmias and sudden death where the risk is assessed to be high.

Indications
• Syncope resulting from ventricular arrhythmia is an indication, provided that sick sinus syndrome and AV block are excluded. In the latter subset of patients, pacing and amiodarone are advisable
• Atrial fibrillation: Prevention, conversion, and/or control of ventricular response. Amiodarone causes atrial fibrillation to convert to sinus rhythm in approximately 80% of patients and is especially effective in causing conversion to sinus rhythm when the duration of atrial fibrillation is short. Amiodarone also partially controls the ventricular response. The drug appears to be successful in preventing the progression of paroxysmal fibrillation that has been present for less than 1 week to chronic atrial fibrillation. Direct current cardioversion is indicated in pa-

tients with recent-onset atrial fibrillation who show hemodynamic deterioration: effective anticoagulation is essential and amiodarone cover facilitates conversion
• Suppression of potentially lethal arrhythmias

Electrophysiologic testing to select a drug that suppresses VT is generally not useful in these patients. Because amiodarone is the only drug that has been shown to decrease the risk of sudden death, it is used when indicated as the drug of first choice, regardless of testing. Electrophysiologic testing should be reserved for patients who have repeated syncope or uncontrollable arrhythmias and in whom amiodarone is unacceptable; the choice often lies between administration of sotalol and implantation of an anti-tachycardia device.

Supplied: tablets; 200 mg. ampules; 150 mg

Dosage: 200 mg three times daily for 5 to 7 days and 200 mg twice daily for 2 weeks, after which, if no major adverse effects and depending on effectiveness, the dose is reduced to 200 mg daily for 4 to 6 weeks and then 100 mg daily. The exact cutoff point for reduction is controlled by the results of 48-hour Holter monitoring. The aim is for 50 to 100 mg daily.

Administration of amiodarone by IV is reserved for patients with immediate life-threatening arrhythmias, including atrial fibrillation in some patients with HCM. The dosage is IV infusion 5 mg/kg, preferably via caval catheter over 1 to 2 hours (maximum 1.2 g in 24 hours).

Monitor. Because of the significant potential for adverse effects and drug interactions, monitor the following at 2 to 4 weeks for 3 months, then at least monthly or at appropriate intervals

• ECG for bradyarrhythmias, excessive QT prolongation, atrial fibrillation, or VT
• Serum potassium and magnesium levels
• Liver function tests, thyroid function tests
• Digoxin level, if concomitant use of digoxin with dosage halved
• Prothrombin time, international normalized ratio if on warfarin with dosage halved
• Chest x-rays at 3 and 6 months, and then every 6 months or annually thereafter or on occurrence of dyspnea, are also important for early detection of pulmonary infiltrates
• Lung function tests (see Chapter 6)
• Slit lamp examination for corneal deposits (Chapter 6)

Contraindications
• Sinus bradycardia
• Sick sinus syndrome and AV block require pacing if amiodarone is needed
• Clinical thyroid dysfunction is a relative contraindication
• Pregnancy and breastfeeding

Adverse effects. These include the following

- Severe bradyarrhythmias; asystole; rarely, torsades de pointes, especially in patients with bradycardia or a low serum potassium
- Hypothyroidism or, less often, hyperthyroidism occurs in about 5% of patients
- Corneal microdeposits are universal during chronic therapy but rarely become symptomatic
- Hepatitis with grossly elevated transaminase occurs in a small minority of patients and, because this condition has a propensity to progress to cirrhosis, immediate discontinuation of amiodarone is necessary (see Chapter 6)
- Nervous system manifestations are common with sleep disturbances, paraesthesias, or twitching that usually responds to dose reduction
- Photosensitivity, metallic taste, nausea, and vomiting
- Slate grey skin is related to high loading and maintenance doses. The skin must be protected from direct and indirect ultraviolet light
- Pulmonary infiltrates and alveolitis represent a life-threatening, usually late complication about which the patient should be warned; but this occurs in less than 1% of patients. The aforementioned adverse effects are uncommon with modern conservative dosing schedules. Severe side effects are rare if minimal effective doses are used and are usually reversible, except severe pulmonary infiltrates and skin pigmentation (see Chapter 6).

Interactions
- Amiodarone increases the activity of oral anticoagulants; both drugs may be required in patients with atrial fibrillation or in patients with embolization
- Verapamil and diltiazem may produce sinus arrest or AV block
- Digoxin levels increase markedly
- Quinidine levels increase and torsades de pointes may be precipitated
- Sotalol in combination may precipitate torsades
- Phenothiazines and tricyclics

Patients with cardiac arrest or sustained VT, in whom amiodarone therapy has failed, deserve consideration for an antitachycardia pacemaker defibrillator (see Chapter 18).

DISOPYRAMIDE

Disopyramide exerts a negative inotropic effect, and some studies indicate beneficial effects in some symptomatic patients during the obstructive phase, in whom beta blockers and/or amiodarone are contraindicated. The drug does not prolong life and is not effective for angina.

Dosage: 150 to 800 mg daily preferably as a once-daily long-acting preparation (see Table 6–8, Chapter 6).

Contraindications
- Sick sinus syndrome
- AV block
- Heart failure, end-stage disease with ventricular dilation (Table 14–3)

Interactions. Disopyramide must not be combined with verapamil, amiodarone, or a beta blocker.

DIGOXIN

Digoxin is contraindicated in HCM, except in patients with severe heart failure with end-stage disease unresponsive to very small doses of diuretics. If direct-current shock or amiodarone fails to convert atrial fibrillation to sinus rhythm and the ventricular response is more than 100 per minute, digoxin is advisable, especially if HF is present. If heart failure is not present, a beta blocker is advisable to decrease the ventricular response.

Interactions. These may occur with verapamil, diltiazem, and amiodarone.

ANTICOAGULANTS

Indications
- All patients with atrial fibrillation, to prevent embolism at the time of DC conversion, and when waiting for amiodarone to produce conversion
- Patients who remain in atrial fibrillation while on amiodarone should receive anticoagulants, but with careful monitoring of prothrombin time since amiodarone enhances the activity of coumarins and life-threatening bleeding can be precipitated

ANTIBIOTICS

Antibiotics should be given when needed to prevent bacterial endocarditis.

SURGERY/SEPTAL RESECTION, MITRAL VALVE SURGERY

Indications include the following
- Patients who have had adequate trials of beta blockers, verapamil, or amiodarone plus beta blocker and remain severely symptomatic with angina and dyspnea
- Outflow gradient greater than 50 mm Hg at rest
- Moderate or severe mitral regurgitation
- Very thick ventricular septum
- High LV end diastolic pressure

Surgery, which is only palliative, causes an 8% early and about 12% late mortality but depends on the expertise of the surgical team. When surgery is indicated, a septal myotomy/myectomy is performed. Surgery does not

reduce mortality, but a significant number of patients obtain symptomatic relief of anginal symptoms. The Düsseldorf experience shows an encouraging reduction in sudden death and syncope following successful myotomy/myectomy. Mitral valve replacement is indicated only for severe mitral regurgitation.
Transplantation may be considered for intractable symptoms.

APICAL HYPERTROPHIC CARDIOMYOPATHY

Apical HCM has a low risk of sudden death; an outflow tract gradient does not develop. ECG shows typical giant inverted T waves and high precordial QRS voltage. Angina, dyspnea, and arrhythmias may, however, occur. Syncope is uncommon. Management with beta blockers is appropriate. Digoxin is indicated if atrial fibrillation or heart failure supervenes. Amiodarone is indicated for paroxysmal atrial fibrillation with ventricular rates uncontrolled by digoxin and/or if VT or VF occurs. Prognosis appears relatively favorable in most patients with this form of HCM.

DILATED CARDIOMYOPATHY

A diagnosis of dilated cardiomyopathy (DCM) should be considered in a patient with right and left heart failure, documented global hypokinesis and dilatation of the left and/or right ventricles, and reduced systolic function in the absence of evidence of coronary heart disease, congenital, specific valvular, hypertensive, or specific heart muscle disease, and chronic excessive alcohol consumption. DCM is not due to alcohol but can be exaggerated by it.

CLINICAL HALLMARKS

- Progressive dyspnea on exertion over weeks or months, culminating in orthopnea, paroxysmal nocturnal dyspnea, and edema, which are common features. Physical signs of right and left heart failure are prominent in late cases. The extremities tend to be cool and pale due to vasoconstriction
- The apex beat is displaced downward and outward to the left due to LV dilatation
- Left lower parasternal lift or pulsation indicates RV dilatation
- The jugular venous pressure may be elevated and may show a systolic wave of tricuspid regurgitation
- A soft Grade I-II/VI systolic mitral murmur and a soft tricuspid systolic murmur are commonly present because of mitral and tricuspid regurgitation as a result of dilatation of the ventricles and valve rings as well as papillary muscle dysfunction
- S4 and S3 are constantly present, as well as sinus tachycardia; thus, a summation gallop is a frequent finding
- The loud S3 is present in virtually all cases and is often heard when heart failure is absent. This hallmark serves to differentiate dilated cardiomyopathy from a Class 4 ventricle due to coronary heart disease

where a soft S3 is heard during episodes of heart failure, but is frequently absent or quite soft when the individual is assessed not to be in heart failure, and in the absence of left ventricular aneurysm
- Blood pressure is frequently low, hypotension carries a poor prognosis

Aortic systolic or diastolic murmurs are conspicuously absent and serve to exclude specific valvular heart disease as a cause of the severe heart failure. These are signs of advanced disease. Echocardiographic diagnosis can be made before overt heart failure has developed.

INVESTIGATIONS

ELECTROCARDIOGRAM

Electrocardiographic features include

- Sinus tachycardia
- Flat or inverted T waves
- Modest LVH may be masked by low voltage
- Atrial fibrillation occurs in about 25%
- Left bundle branch block is observed in a significant minority
- Poor R wave progression (V2-V4) or Q waves of pseudo infarction may suggest an incorrect diagnosis of ischemic heart disease (Table 13–3)

CHEST X-RAY

The heart is enlarged and four-chamber enlargement is commonly present. There is usually evidence of a raised left atrial pressure in the pulmonary vascular pattern; pleural effusions may be present.

ECHOCARDIOGRAM

Echocardiographic features include

- Severe dilatation of both ventricles; there is global hypokinesis and commonly paradoxical movement of the septum
- Increased end systolic and end diastolic dimensions
- EF usually less than 35%; in the presence of heart failure, EF is usually 10 to 30%
- Atrial enlargement and ventricular thrombi are commonly seen
- A small pericardial effusion is frequent

ENDOMYOCARDIAL BIOPSY

Used as a research tool to exclude suspected known heart muscle disease and to detect evidence of myocarditis or viral particles.

HOLTER MONITORING

The results of Holter monitoring carried out for 48 hours help to define patients with potentially lethal ventricular arrhythmias.

ETIOLOGIC EVALUATION

Up to 50% of cases of myocarditis and dilated cardiomyopathy appear to be associated with enteroviral infections; however, causality has not been established with certainty. Molecular hybridization techniques have linked enteroviral infections to both human myocarditis and dilated cardiomyopathy.

Organ-specific cardiac autoantibodies have been detected in about 26% of patients with dilated cardiomyopathy, as opposed to less than 3% of patients with known cardiac disease. An immunologic process associated with a viral infection is observed in a minority of patients with dilated cardiomyopathy. The autoimmune process may have a genetic basis, and future studies are awaited to clarify and document the causes of dilated cardiomyopathy.

PROGNOSIS

• The 2-year mortality is approximately 50%
• Mortality after documented heart failure is about 50% in 1 year. The most important indication of prognosis is cardiac function. Patients with the lowest EF have the worst prognosis

Advice to patients and relatives regarding prognosis is fraught with difficulty because we have poor parameters from which to predict outcome. A patient presenting with severe heart failure with global hypokinesis and EF less than 20% and/or left bundle branch block with associated potentially lethal ventricular arrhythmias has a poor prognosis and is unlikely to survive beyond 6 to 12 months. However, patients with these diagnoses may survive for 2 years or more, and caution is necessary in discussions with both the patient and family. A few small-group studies suggest a trend toward a modest increased survival with the use of low-dose amiodarone to control arrhythmias, in addition to the usual measures for control of heart failure.

The prognosis of heart failure has been improved with the use of hydralazine combined with nitrate, and the VHeFT II study has shown ACE inhibitors to be superior to this combination (see Chapter 5).

THERAPY

The most important aspect of management of DCM is the prevention and control of heart failure, arrhythmias, and embolization.

The standard management for heart failure should be instituted

• Bed to chair rest for several days
• Oxygen and a sedative at night to allow restful sleep, which adds to the patient's comfort and reduces the workload of the failing myocardium
• Salt restriction
• Avoidance of alcohol is necessary in all patients with heart failure and especially in the patient with a Class 3 or 4 ventricle, because alcohol decreases the EF. Patients should be assessed for the presence of macro-

ovalocytes, decreased platelet counts, and increased levels of gamma glutamyltransferase, which may indicate alcohol damage

INOTROPES

Digoxin

Digoxin provides some benefit in heart failure patients in sinus rhythm and is indicated for atrial fibrillation with uncontrolled ventricular response (see Chapter 5). The dose should be adequate, but care is needed to avoid digitalis toxicity. In patients with refractory heart failure, IV dobutamine may cause temporary "improvement."

Milrinone has been shown in a multicenter study to increase mortality; oral positive inotropic agents other than digitalis are not advised.

DIURETICS

Diuretics play a vital role in the relief of symptoms and cannot be replaced by ACE inhibitors. The three groups of drugs, diuretics, digoxin, and ACE inhibitors, are complimentary.

Furosemide

Dosage: 40 to 80 mg daily. Increase only if shortness of breath and pulmonary congestion are not controlled by the addition of adequate doses of an ACE inhibitor; the use of ACE inhibitors is often limited by hypotension. Patients with poor systolic function often have low systolic pressures (less than 110 mm Hg), and it is sometimes necessary to discontinue diuretics for 24 to 48 hours to permit the selected ACE inhibitors to be commenced. Caution is needed to avoid hypokalemia and magnesium depletion. The latter can be treated with magnesium glycerophosphate (3 to 6 g daily).

ACE INHIBITORS

These agents have made a major contribution to survival of patients with heart failure; however, diastolic dysfunction in patients with dilated cardiomyopathy tend to worsen with ACE inhibitor therapy. The dosage and pharmacologic profile of ACE inhibitors are given in Table 1–5.

Captopril
(Capoten)

Dosage: 3 to 6.25 mg test dose; if hypotension is not precipitated, give 6.25 mg twice daily for 1 to 2 days and increase to 12.5 mg twice daily. Then over days to weeks, increase to 25 mg twice daily to a maximum of 50 mg daily. A dose in excess of 75 mg provides little added benefit for these patients and there is a risk of a lowered diastolic pressure with consequent poor coronary perfusion that may trigger an arrhythmic death.

The renin-angiotensin system is usually blocked by a daily captopril dosage of 25 mg and a daily maintenance dose of 37.5 to 75 mg is recommended. When the patient is stabilized on captopril 25 mg daily or an equivalent dose of the selected ACE inhibitor, the dose of furosemide can be increased as required to relieve congestion and shortness of breath.

Enalapril
(Vasotec, Innovace in the UK)

Dosage: 2.5 mg and observe for 4 hours. If there is no hypotension or other adverse effects, give 2.5 mg twice daily for 1 to 2 days, and then increase slowly over days or weeks to 5 to 10 mg once or twice daily. Increase dose interval or do not use in patients with renal failure, serum creatinine greater than 2.3 mg/dl (203 μmol/l).

Contraindications. ACE inhibitors are contraindicated in
- Renal artery stenosis of a solitary kidney or severe bilateral renal artery stenosis
- Aortic stenosis
- Restrictive cardiomyopathy, HCM with obstruction
- Severe carotid artery stenosis
- Severe anemia
- Pregnancy and during breastfeeding
- Relative contraindications include patients with collagen vascular diseases or concomitant use of immunosuppressive, because neutropenia and rare agranulocytosis observed with ACE inhibitors appear to occur in these patients

Adverse effects. These include the following
- Hypotension
- Hyperkalemia in patients with renal failure
- Pruritis and rash in about 10%
- Loss of taste appears to be specific for sulfhydryl compounds and occurs in approximately 7% of patients
- A very rare but important adverse effect is angioedema of the face, mouth, or larynx, which may occur in approximately 0.2% of treated patients and can be fatal
- Rarely, mouth ulcers, neurologic dysfunction, gastrointestinal disturbances, and proteinuria in about 1% of patients with pre-existing renal disease
- Neutropenia and agranulocytosis are rare and occur mainly in patients with serious intercurrent illness, particularly immunologic disturbances, altered immune response, or collagen vascular disease
- Cough occurs in about 10% of treated patients
- Occasionally, wheeze, myalgia, muscle cramps, hair loss, impotence or decreased libido, hepatitis or occurrence of antinuclear antibodies, and phemphigus may occur

Interactions. These may occur with allopurinol, acebutolol, hydralazine, NSAIDS, procainamide, pindolol, steroids, tocainide, immunosuppressives, and other drugs that alter immune response. Drugs that increase serum potassium levels have been emphasized.

BETA-ADRENERGIC BLOCKERS

Judicious use of beta blockers appears, however paradoxically, to benefit some patients with DCM, especially individuals with resting sinus tachycardia and/or diastolic dysfunction. Removal of sympathetic drive on myocytes and restoration toward normal of the downgrading of beta-adrenergic receptors in heart failure appear to provide benefits.

Reduction in heart rate decreases myocardial oxygen demand and also improves coronary blood flow. Prevention of arrhythmias, with even modest reduction in sudden deaths, is a potential benefit of careful beta-adrenergic blockade. Clinical trials have shown mixed results, however, and large-scale trials are underway.

Fortunately, all beta blockers are not alike, and two recent reports of studies using agents that have vasodilating properties (bucindolol and labetalol, an alpha beta blocker) indicate beneficial effects that must be assessed in large-scale trials.

Administration of bucindolol (25 to 200 mg daily) caused an increase in EF from 2.5 to 35% and improved functional class in 17% of 20 patients over 2 years.

A group in Hong Kong has shown that in an 8-week randomized, cross-over study of 12 patients with proven dilated cardiomyopathy, labetalol (50 to 200 mg twice daily over 8 weeks) produced salutary effects: 7 of 12 patients (58%) improved functional class. Also noted were 14% improvement in cardiac output on exercise, 22% improvement in treadmill exercise time, and 12% and 16% decreases in systemic vascular resistance at rest and at exercise, respectively. Pretreatment chest radiographs prior to and after 8-week dosage of labetalol (300 mg per day) showed a decrease of CT ratio from 71 to 58%.

All patients were maintained on digoxin, diuretics, and an ACE inhibitor throughout the study. This and other studies indicate that clinical deterioration may occur if beta blockers are withdrawn, especially after 2 or 3 months of therapy.

In the Hong Kong study, labetalol's beneficial effect was additive to that of ACE inhibitors. The alpha blocking property caused a decrease in systemic vascular resistance beyond that achieved by concomitant ACE inhibitor therapy and beta blockade resulted in salutary effects.

Labetalol

Supplied: 50, 100, 200 mg

Dosage: 25 mg daily, increase slowly over 2 to 3 weeks, 150 mg twice daily is worth a trial, provided that the systolic blood pressure remains greater than 100 mm Hg without a drop of 20 mm below the systolic blood pressure at commencement and with a pulse rate maintained above 60 beats per minute.

Metoprolol

Dosage: 2.5 mg twice daily, increase slowly to maximum of 25 mg with a careful watch for worsening of heart failure. Benefit may not be observed for several months and, at times, even following early deterioration.

Caution. Beta blocking agents should be used cautiously in properly selected patients until the results of a multicenter trial are available.

ORAL ANTICOAGULANTS

Warfarin is advisable in most patients to prevent embolization from atrial and ventricular thrombi: it is essential if there is atrial fibrillation. Pulmonary embolism and systemic embolization occur fairly frequently and worsen the dismal prognosis. In addition, immobilization during periods of heart failure predisposes deep vein thrombosis and pulmonary emboli (see anticoagulation control, Chapter 11).

ARRHYTHMIA CONTROL

Amiodarone

Neither significant clinical benefit nor improved survival has been documented with antiarrhythmic agents, except for a modest effect of amiodarone.

Dosage: 200 mg three times daily for 1 to 2 weeks, and then 100 to 200 mg daily, reducing to 5 or 6 days weekly. Consult the earlier discussion in this chapter as well as in Chapter 6 for advice on dosage, contraindications, and monitoring of adverse effects.

Sudden death in DCM is due to a combination of pump failure and potentially lethal arrhythmias. Amiodarone is advisable if repeated 48-hour Holter monitoring reveals nonsustained VT or frequent multiform ventricular ectopics and in patients with sustained VT or survivors of cardiac arrest. Survival appears to be improved after amiodarone therapy in this subset. These small group studies require support from further well-designed clinical trials that are presently being conducted. DCM has a 50% 2-year mortality rate and with heart failure, the mortality rate is 50% in 1 year. Therefore, significant bothersome amiodarone toxicity, which usually appears after about 3 or more years of low-dose therapy, is not a deterrent to the use of a drug that presently provides the only hope for improved survival.

In selected patients with malignant ventricular arrhythmias who fail to respond to amiodarone or require discontinuance of the drug because of adverse effects, consideration should be given to the use of a multiprogrammable pacemaker cardioverter defibrillator. Electrophysiologic testing in patients with dilated cardiomyopathy, as in other patients with severe left ventricular dysfunction, does not appear helpful. Also, the multiprogrammable cardioverter defibrillator is of little benefit to patients with severely impaired ventricular function. Consideration must be given to these patients for cardiac transplantation.

EXPERIMENTAL THERAPY

Other investigational therapy includes the use of an enzyme, coenzyme Q_{10}, a vitamin that has similarities to niacin and is believed to be an essential dietary component for the existence of human life. A recent clinical trial claims some improvement in survival.

CARDIAC TRANSPLANTATION FOR DCM

Young patients with refractory heart failure, Class IV ventricle, EF less than 12% and causing very poor quality of life, and without contraindications listed should be considered for cardiac transplantation. Patients who have been relatively stable may suddenly deteriorate markedly; if so, transplantation becomes urgent and life support by means of intra-aortic balloon pump or heart assist device may be needed.

Contraindications

• Noncardiac underlying diseases: Pulmonary, renal, hepatic, hematologic, neurologic, diabetic, psychiatric
• Alcoholism

RESTRICTIVE CARDIOMYOPATHY

The major abnormality is a restriction of ventricular filling, thus an increase in filling pressures. Restrictive cardiomyopathy (RCM) is a member of the group of diastolic heart failure in which diastolic function is impaired earlier and more severely than systolic function. The usual abnormality is impaired relaxation and compliance. Restrictive pathophysiology may occur at the pericardial, myocardial, or endomyocardial level.

The most common cause of RCM is endomyocardial fibrosis (EMF), especially in tropical regions. Myocardial involvement by amyloid, not associated with multiple organ involvement, is the most common cause of RCM in the Western world. Cardiac disease resulting from amyloid-associated multiple organ involvement, sarcoid, hemochromatosis, eosinophilic syndromes, scleroderma, adriamycin toxicity, and infectious agents, including tuberculosis, causing restrictive physiology is considered specific heart muscle disease. HCM may produce diastolic abnormalities similar to those in RCM.

CLINICAL HALLMARKS

- Intermittent fever, shortness of breath, cough, palpitations, edema, and tiredness
- Hypereosinophilia with abnormal eosinophil degranulation is seen in temperate climates (hypereosinophilic heart disease)
- Hypereosinophilia is less severe in tropical EMF
- Symptoms and signs of heart failure and of moderate to severe mitral and tricuspid regurgitation due to involvement of the papilliary muscles serve to differentiate RCM from constrictive pericarditis, as does the greater degree of cardiac enlargement on chest x-ray in the former condition (Table 13–3)
- During the early stages, EMF may mimic the hemodynamic and clinical features of constrictive pericarditis. Table 13–4 gives hemodynamic differences but significant overlap occurs
- The chest x-ray in patients with EMF may show calcification of the right or left ventricular apical myocardium
- Echocardiogram shows obliteration of the apices of the ventricles be echogenic masses, and Goodwin has likened this appearance to a boxing glove. Also, myocardial calcification may be detected, and in later stages, mitral and tricuspid regurgitation may require echocardiographic assessment
- The idiopathic endocardial fibrosis and associated thrombus may progressively obliterate the left or right ventricular cavities. Severe enlargement of the right atrium may occur

THERAPY

Medical therapy is unrewarding

- Steroids may be helpful in the early acute inflammatory phase associated with hypereosinophilia
- Anticoagulants are necessary because thromboembolism is common
- Restriction to filling does not respond to digoxin, diuretics, or vasodilators, and all three medications are relatively contraindicated. Arrhythmias may respond to small doses of beta blockers and potentially lethal arrhythmias may require amiodarone therapy
- Resection of masses of obliterating endocardial tissue with valve repair has produced apparent relief in some patients with EMF for a few years
- Cardiac transplantation may require consideration in intractable cases

SPECIFIC HEART MUSCLE DISEASE

Specific heart muscle disease (SHMD) usually produces a dilated form of cardiomyopathy with impaired systolic function.

Restrictive physiology is seen with amyloid, sarcoid, neoplasm, radiation, scleroderma, hemochromatosis, and eosinophilic endomyocardial disease, in which eosinophilia is usually present. Rarely, myocardial tuberculosis is present with restrictive features. Amyloid heart disease and

EMF are usually considered examples of RCM, but when cardiac involvement is associated with multiple organ disease, they qualify as SHMD. The findings of systemic disease of other organs, especially the liver, lymph nodes and skin, which can be easily submitted to biopsy, assist in defining the underlying cause. Endomyocardial biopsy is often required but may not be helpful in patchy disease such as sarcoid.

THERAPY

Treatment should be directed at the underlying disease. Occasionally, cardiac pacing is required for the management of complete heart block due to involvement of conduction tissue by sarcoid, scleroderma, or hemochromatosis.

Other heart muscle diseases include involvement due to infectious disease: Chagas due to Trypanosoma cruzi is transmitted by a triatoma bug. The disease is prevalent in South America but does occur in the southern United States.

The incidence of HIV is increasing, and myocarditis with pericardial effusion and cardiac tamponade is now surfacing in victims of AIDS. Myocardial involvement might be due to the HIV virus; although this is unproven, involvement by Kaposi, opportunistic infections, and effects of medications must also be excluded.

Rare involvement of cardiac muscle is seen with polymyositis, progressive muscular dystrophy, Friedreich's ataxia, and Fabry's disease.

Drugs, especially cocaine and toxins, may affect the myocardium; known toxins include cobalt (beer), chloroquine and emetine, phenothiazines, methysergide, and cancer chemotherapeutic agents (adriamycin, daunorubicin, doxorubicin, cyclophosphamide); also, methyldopa, and phenindione rarely cause a hypersensitivity myocarditis. Overdose with toxic doses of acetaminophen or cocaine may cause myocardial necrosis and arrhythmias, including torsades de pointes.

Treatment of these disorders involves removal and treatment of the infective agent or toxin where possible.

BIBLIOGRAPHY

Anderson JL, Gilbert M, O'Connell B: Long-term (2 year) beneficial effects of beta-adrenergic blockade with bucindolol in patients with idiopathic dilated cardiomyopathy. J Am Coll Cardiol, *17*:1373, 1991.

Baroldi G, Camerini F, Goodwin JF (eds.): Advances in cardiomyopathies. Berlin, Springer-Verlag, 1990.

Borggrefe M, Lösse B, Loogen F, et al.: The influence of myectomy/myotomy on arrhythmias in hypertrophic cardiomyopathy (Abstract). Circulation, *74*(Suppl II):II-227, 1986.

Chikamor R, Counihan PJ, Doi YL, et al.: Mechanisms of exercise limitation in hypertrophic cardiomyopathy. J Am Coll Cardiol, *19*:507, 1992.

Cox J, Krajden M: Cardiovascular manifestations of Lyme disease. Am Heart J, *122*:1449, 1991.

Camici P, Giampaolo C, Lorenzoni R, et al.: Coronary vasodilation is impaired in both hypertrophied and nonhypertrophied myocardium of patients with hypertrophic cardiomyopathy: A study with nitrogen-13 ammonia and positron emission tomography. J Am Coll Cardiol, *17*:879, 1991.

Chahine RA: Surgical versus medical therapy of hypertrophic cardiomyopathy: Is the perspective changing? J Am Coll Cardiol, *17*:643, 1991.

Deckers JW, Hare JM, Baughman KL: Complications of transvenous right ventricular endomyocardial biopsy in adult patients with cardiomyopathy: A seven-year survey of 546 consecutive diagnostic procedures in a tertiary referral center. J Am Coll Cardiol, *19*:43, 1992.

Gersony WM: The child with dilated cardiomyopathy: Prognostic considerations and management decisions. J Am Coll Cardiol, *18*:157, 1991.

Goodwin JF: Clinical decisions in the management of the cardiomyopathies. Drugs, *38*(6):988, 1989.

Goodwin JF: Congestive and hypertrophic cardiomyopathies. Lancet, *1*:731, 1970.

Goodwin JF (ed.): Heart muscle disease. Lancaster, England, MTP Press, 1985.

Goodwin JF: New serologic marker of cardiac autoimmunity in dilated cardiomyopathy. J Am Coll Cardiol, *15*:1535, 1990.

Greenspan AM: Hypertrophic cardiomyopathy and atrial fibrillation: A change of perspective. J Am Coll Cardiol, *15*:1286, 1990.

Grody WW, Cheng L, Lewis W: Infection of the heart by the human immunodeficiency virus. J Am Coll Cardiol, *66*:203, 1990.

Hejtmancik JF, Brink PA, Towbin J, et al.: Localization of gene for familial hypertrophic cardiomyopathy to chromosome 14q1 in a diverse US population. Circulation, *83*:1592, 1991.

Hirota Y, Shimizu G, Yoshio K, et al.: Spectrum of restrictive cardiomyopathy: Report of the national survey in Japan. Am Heart J, *120*:188, 1990.

Klues HG, Leuner C, Kuhn H: Left ventricular outflow tract obstruction in patients with hypertrophic cardiomyopathy: Increase in gradient after exercise. J Am Coll Cardiol, *19*: 527, 1992.

Kothari SS: Review: Pathogenesis of hypertrophic cardiomyopathy: another viewpoint. Int J Cardiol, *30*:9, 1991.

Langsjoen PH, Langsjoen Peter H, Folkers K: Long-term efficacy and safety of coenzyme Q_{10} therapy for idiopathic dilated cardiomyopathy. J Am Coll Cardiol, *65*:521, 1990.

Leung WH, Lau CP, Wong CK, et al.: Improvement in exercise performance and hemodynamics by labetalol in patients with idiopathic dilated cardiomyopathy. Am Heart J, *119*: 884, 1990.

Lewis JF, Maron BJ: Hypertrophic cardiomyopathy characterized by marked hypertrophy of the posterior left ventricular freewall: Significance and clinical implications. J Am Coll Cardiol, *18*:421, 1991.

Maron BJ: Q waves in hypertrophic cardiomyopathy: A reassessment. J Am Coll Cardiol, *16*: 375, 1990.

Maron BJ: The giant negative T wave revisited . . . in hypertrophic cardiomyopathy. J Am Coll Cardiol, *15*:972, 1990.

Maron BJ, Fananapazir L: Sudden cardiac death in hypertrophic cardiomyopathy. Circulation, *85*(suppl I):I-57, 1992.

McKenna WJ: Sudden death in hypertrophic cardiomyopathy: Identification of the "high risk" patient. *In* Cardiac arrhythmias: Where to go from here? Edited by P Burgada, HJJ Wellens. Mt. Kisco, Futura Publishing, 1987.

Olsen EGJ, Sekiguchi M (eds.): Restrictive cardiomyopathy and arrhythmias. Tokyo, University of Tokyo Press, 1990.

Panza JA, Maris TJ, Maron BJ: Development and determinants of dynamic obstruction to left ventricular outflow in young patients with hypertrophic cardiomyopathy. Circulation, *85*: 1398, 1992.

Robinson K, Frenneaux MP, Stockins B, et al.: Atrial fibrillation in hypertrophic cardiomyopathy: A longitudinal study. J Am Coll Cardiol, *15*:1279, 1990.

Rosenzweig A, Watkins H, Hwang D-S, et al.: Preclinical diagnosis of familial hypertrophic cardiomyopathy by genetic analysis of blood lymphocytes. New Eng J Med, *325*:1753, 1991.

Rossi MA: Editorial. Microvascular changes as a cause of chronic cardiomyopathy in Chagas' disease. Am Heart J, *120*:233, 1990.

Simson MB: Noninvasive identification of patients at high risk for sudden cardiac death. Circulation 85(suppl I):I-145, 1992.

Spirito P, Maron BJ: Relation between extent of left ventricular hypertropy and occurrence of sudden cardiac death in hypertrophic cardiomyopathy. J Am Coll Cardiol, *15*:1521, 1990.

Webb JG, Sasson Z, Rakowski H, et al.: Apical hypertrophic cardiomyopathy: Clinical follow-up and diagnostic correlates. J Am Coll Cardiol, *15*:83, 1990.

Woodley SL, Gilbert EM, Anderson JL: β-Blockade with bucindolol in heart failure caused by ischemic versus idiopathic dilated cardiomyopathy. Circulation, *84*:2426, 1991.

15

SYNCOPE

M. Gabriel Khan

Syncope, transient loss of consciousness as a result of inadequate cerebral blood flow, is a common problem representing up to 1% of medical admissions to general hospitals and up to 3% of emergency room diagnoses. Causes of syncope are often elusive, and the following points deserve attention

- An obvious cardiac cause can be defined by the history, physical examination, ECG, and Holter monitoring in approximately 10% of cases (see Fig. 15–1 and Table 15–1)
- Vasodepressor (vasovagal syncope), the common form of which is the simple faint, accounts for more than 35% of cases of syncope. It is therefore most important to exclude this benign problem
- Unexplained syncope constitutes a large group (35%), but in patients who have structural heart disease and unexplained syncope, electrophysiologic (EP) testing is rewarding in identifying a significant number of cardiac causes of syncope and increases the total cardiac cause of syncope to approximately 22%.
- In patients with unexplained syncope, if structural heart disease is not present, EP testing is rarely diagnostic and the head-up tilt test has proven useful in these patients (Fig. 15–1)
- Syncope may be the clue to possibly life-threatening underlying cardiac diseases
- Cardiac syncope carries a 24% incidence of sudden death in 1 year, as opposed to less than 2% sudden death per year in the remaining 78% of individuals. One-year mortality of patients with cardiac syncope ranges from 15 to 30%, versus less than 2% for individuals with unexplained syncope and without structural heart disease
- Figure 15–1 gives an algorithmic approach to the diagnosis of syncope
- Dizziness is often a feature of presyncope and has several causes that are difficult to determine. Figure 15–2 indicates steps to consider
- Postural hypotension is an important cause of syncope. It commonly occurs because of a decrease in preload and often occurs in patients on cardiac medications that cause venous pooling. Less often, syncope has a neurogenic cause, being a troublesome feature of autonomic neuropathy (Table 15–2)

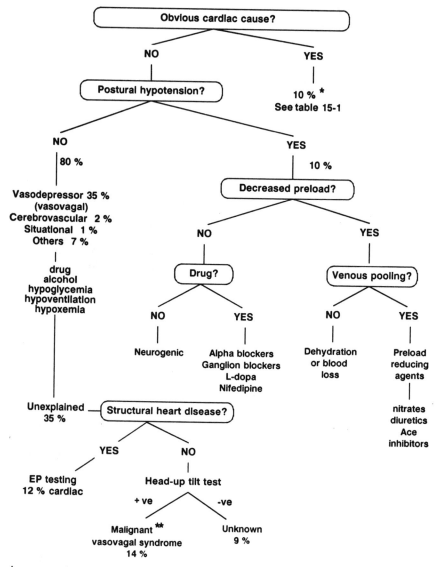

FIG. 15–1. Assessment of syncope.

TABLE 15-1. OBVIOUS CARDIAC CAUSES OF SYNCOPE AND APPROXIMATE INCIDENCE

CAUSES	APPROXIMATE INCIDENCE
Tachyarrhythmias	45%
Sustained and Nonsustained VT	
Torsades de pointes	
Atrial fibrillation	
Supraventricular tachycardia	
Long QT syndrome	
WPW syndrome	
Pacemaker mediated	
Bradyarrhythmias	35%
Sinus Node dysfunction	
(Sick sinus syndrome)	
AV block: second and third degree	
Drug induced	
Carotid sinus syncope	3%
Obstruction to stroke volume	10%
Aortic stenosis	
Hypertrophic cardiomyopathy	
Tight mitral stenosis	
Atrial myxoma or thrombus	
Cardiac tamponade	
Prosthetic valve dysfunction	
Pulmonary embolism	
Pulmonary hypertension	
Pulmonary stenosis	
Others	7%
Mitral valve prolapse	
Myocardial infarction	
Severe ischemic heart disease	
Coronary artery spasm	
Pacemaker syndrome	
Aortic dissection	
Fallot's tetralogy	

It must be reemphasized that head-up tilt testing has a role in defining the cause of unexplained syncope in patients without structural heart disease. The result may be expedited by the simultaneous administration of IV Edrophonium; in patients under age 50, isoproterenol is used in some centers, but a study by Kapoor, et al. questions the low specificity of this test.

These intensive investigations result in the prevention of some of the deaths associated with syncope, although syncope remains unexplained in a minority of patients.

PATIENT EVALUATION

The management of syncope entails the elucidation of the cause so that appropriate advice, medications, or corrective measures may be employed to prevent bodily injury or threat to life. Since most cardiac causes pose a

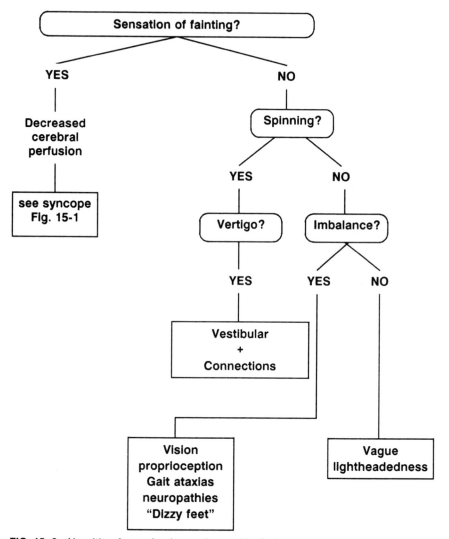

FIG. 15–2. Algorithm for evaluating patients with dizziness.

threat to life, it is important to use a methodical approach to solving the cause of syncope in a given individual. This medical solution calls for a sound knowledge of basic internal medicine and cardiology and should commence with a detailed history and physical examination.

Who should be admitted to a hospital

• Patients with suspected cardiac cause
• Patients with significant bodily injury
• The elderly patient in whom a readily identifiable cause is lacking
• Recurrent syncope of undetermined etiology
• Recurrence of syncope while awaiting investigation

TABLE 15–2. NONCARDIAC CAUSES OF SYNCOPE	
CAUSE	**APPROXIMATE INCIDENCE**
1. Vasodepressor (vasovagal)	35%
2. Postural hypotension	10%
A. Decrease preload	
a) Venous pooling, caused by extensive varicose veins, post-exercise vasodilation venous angioma in the leg. Drugs: nitrates, diuretics, ACE inhibitors	
b) Decreased blood volume: blood loss; dehydration: vomiting, diarrhea, excessive sweating, Addison's disease	
B. Drug induced	
a) Alpha blockers	
b) Ganglion blockers	
c) Bromocriptine	
d) L-dopa	
e) Nifedipine	
C. Neurogenic decrease autonomic activity	
a) Bedrest	
b) Neuropathies/diabetes	
c) Shy Drager syndrome	
d) Idiopathic	
D. Mastocytosis	
3. Cerebrovascular disease	2%
Transient ischemic attack	
Subclavian steal	
Basilar artery migraine	
Cervical arthritis, allanto-occipital dislocation compression vertebral artery	
4. Situational	1%
Cough, sneeze, micturition, defecation	
5. Others	7%
Drugs/alcohol	
Hypoglycemia	
Hypoxemia	
Hypoventilation	
Hysterical	
6. Unexplained	35%
Malignant vasovagal syndrome (Neurally mediated syncope) 30–60% of otherwise unexplained	

HISTORY AND PHYSICAL EXAMINATION

A detailed relevant history and physical examination are mandatory

- Check the blood pressure on the patient recumbent for more than 3 minutes and then on standing, to elicit postural hypotension
- Determine the blood pressure in the arms and legs
- Listen for bruits over the subclavian and carotid arteries
- Look for finger clubbing and cyanosis as signs of congenital cyanotic heart disease

- Perform a full cardiovascular examination. Check for left ventricular hypertrophy, presence of thrills, the murmur of aortic stenosis, hypertrophic cardiomyopathy, mitral stenosis, mitral valve prolapse, and the presence of prosthetic heart valve (see Table 15–1 and Chapter 12)
- Assess for tachyarrhythmias and bradyarrhythmias

The history should exclude the most common cause of faint, i.e., vasodepressor syncope. All known causes of syncope should be methodically excluded (see Fig. 15–1)

LABORATORY INVESTIGATIONS

After exclusion of postural hypotension, vasodepressor syncope, and cerebrovascular and situational causes, request the following

- Complete blood count, electrolytes, blood urea, serum creatinine, and serum calcium. These routine tests are not usually helpful
- Chest x-ray
- ECG
- Echocardiogram
- 24- or 48-hour Holter monitoring is advisable but has a low yield.

VASODEPRESSOR (VASOVAGAL) SYNCOPE

The simple faint is the most common cause of syncope and is easily recognized. Vasodepressor syncope virtually never occurs in a patient in the recumbent position. Precipitating circumstances are almost always present and typically occur in young individuals and occasionally in older patients in the setting of exhaustion, hunger, prolonged standing or sitting in a hot crowded room and sudden severe pain or trauma, venipuncture, fright, and sudden emotional stress.

The simple faint usually gives a warning of seconds to minutes: the feeling of weakness, nausea, vague upper abdominal discomfort, diaphoresis, yawn, sighing, hyperventilation, unsteadiness, blurring of vision, an unawareness prior to fainting. Importantly, vertigo is not a symptom associated with a simple faint. Thus, a good history identifies the faint and may save expensive and time-consuming investigations.

The constant findings in vasodepressor syncope are

- A sudden marked fall in total peripheral resistance, resulting in a drastic fall in blood pressure
- Decreased cerebral perfusion causing loss of consciousness
- Loss of consciousness usually occurs within 10 seconds of onset of diminished perfusion
- Return of consciousness in seconds to minutes if the individual remains flat with the legs elevated
- Injuries are most uncommon with vasodepressor syncope

The exclusion of epilepsy is relatively easy, but occasionally, syncope may be confused with akinetic seizures. Bradycardia in association with seizures has been described. The aura, if any, in epilepsy is transient but tells a story; convulsive movements occur before loss of consciousness. Injuries, including lip and tongue biting, and incontinence with a prolonged postictal state are not seen with vasodepressor syncope.

Because cardiac sympathetic overstimulation, vigorous left ventricular contraction, and stimulation of intramyocardial mechanoreceptors (C fibers) appear to be important underlying mechanisms in the genesis of unexplained syncope without structural heart disease, beta blockers have been given as rational therapy and have proven successful in some patients with this disabling form of syncope, known as malignant vasovagal syndrome, neurocardiogenic syncope, or neurally mediated syncope (Fig. 15–1). Atenolol (25 mg) or metoprolol (100 mg) daily may produce a salutary response. Esmolol IV may be used to predict the outcome of oral beta blocker therapy.

POSTURAL HYPOTENSION

Several cardiac medications may cause orthostatic hypotension, particularly in the elderly. Assess the following

- Check the blood pressure with the patient recumbent for at least 3 minutes and then on standing; a reduction in systolic pressure of 20 mm Hg or more represents orthostatic hypotension
- Check for evidence of decrease in preload, which may manifest itself by venous pooling that may occur on sudden standing after vigorous exercise or because of extensive varicose veins. Preload reducing agents, particularly, nitrates. ACE inhibitors or alpha$_1$ blockers may be implicated. Blood loss and dehydration are obvious causes, but an occult cause of the latter is Addison's disease
- If conditions causing a decrease in preload are not present, inquire about the use of medications that cause arterial dilatation, particularly alpha$_1$-adrenergic blockers such as prasozin and labetalol; ganglion-blocking drugs, L-dopa, bromocristine, and rarely nifedipine
- If drug use is excluded, postural hypotension may be caused by autonomic imbalance or neurologic diseases. Complete bed rest and a lack of leg exercise, plus a decrease in autonomic activity, commonly result in postural hypotension. Neuropathy, especially due to diabetes, Shy Drager, and other neurologic problems must be excluded

Standing from a recumbent or sitting position causes immediate pooling of blood in the lower limbs and a consequent fall in blood pressure that normally triggers a baroreceptor response and sympathetically mediated vasoconstriction and an increase in heart rate. As indicated above, conditions that impair baroreceptor function and decrease sympathetically mediated alpha$_1$ vasoconstriction may precipitate postural hypotension.

Orthostatic hypotension as a consequence of autonomic neuropathies and autonomic failure is difficult to treat successfully. It may respond to increased sodium intake or fludrocortisone (Florinef), 0.1 to 0.2 mg daily. The management of orthostatic hypotension caused by autonomic failure can be successfully managed in properly selected patients with midodrine (Amatine), a selective peripherally acting postsynaptic alpha$_1$ adrenergic agonist. Salutary effects are caused by an increase in arterial and venous tone; venous pooling is prevented. Initial dosage: 2.5 mg three times daily with monitoring of supine blood pressure, then increased in 2.5-mg increments at weekly intervals to a maximum of 10 mg three times daily. Caution is needed because the action of midodrine is identical to that of other alpha adrenergic receptor stimulants such as methoxamine or phenylephrine; an increase in total systemic resistance may cause supine hypertension that can precipitate heart failure, myocardial ischemia, infarction, or stroke in susceptible individuals. Supine hypertension is more common during the initiation of midodrine therapy; during the titration period, adverse effects include supine hypertension, which may cause headaches and pounding in the ears. Reflex bradycardia may occur, and caution is needed when the drug is combined with agents that cause bradycardia (digoxin, beta blockers, diltiazem, and verapamil). Urinary retention is an important adverse effect in elderly males. The drug is contraindicated in patients with significant coronary heart disease, heart failure, renal failure, urinary retention, thyrotoxicosis, and pheochromocytoma. Midodrine is renally excreted, and care is necessary to decrease the dose and increase the dosing interval in patients with renal dysfunction.

In patients who are not responsive to midodrine or fludrocortisone and have sustained injuries, atrial pacing with a heart rate of 100 per minute may afford some amelioration if combined with increased salt intake, fludrocortisone, elevation of the head of the bed during sleep, and full-length leotards to enhance venous return.

A release of histamine, prostaglandin D, and other vasodilators from mast cell proliferation mastocytosis causes vasodilatation is a rare cause of postural hypotension.

Instruct the patient to change posture slowly and to engage in calf muscle flexion prior to standing. Elevating the head of the bed and a gradual change in posture may provide a salutary response.

CEREBROVASCULAR DISEASE

SUBCLAVIAN STEAL

Occlusion of the subclavian artery proximal to its vertebral branch may produce symptoms when exercising the arm on the affected side. Blood is directed from the basilar system down the vertebral artery to the arm. The steal of blood may be sufficient to cause clouding of consciousness and syncope. A bruit maximal over the supraclavicular area near the origin of the vertebral artery may be heard. Subclavian steal is not common, and syncope is a rare occurrence.

TRANSIENT ISCHEMIC ATTACK (TIA)

Syncope occurs in approximately 7% of individuals with TIA and is more common with vertebral-basilar artery TIA. Associated symptoms include vertigo, diplopia, ataxia, and loss of postural tone in the legs. A drop attack without loss of consciousness is more common than syncope. Treatment with enteric-coated aspirin (30 to 165 mg once daily) is advisable. Patients who are unable to take aspirin should be tried on ticlopidine. Poor responders should be considered for balloon angioplasty or endarterectomy.

AORTIC ARCH SYNDROME

Pulseless disease (Takayasu's disease) is an arteritis-producing occlusion of the aortic arch vessels, and syncope may result. The blood pressure is lower in the arms than the legs.

CARDIAC CAUSES

The major determinant in cardiac syncope is a decrease in cardiac output due to reduced heart rate or ineffectual cardiac contractions secondary to arrhythmia. A diagnosis of cardiac syncope connotes a guarded prognosis with a mortality of up to 24% in one year, although this varies greatly according to the mechanism of the arrhythmia. Early diagnosis with appropriate therapy is lifesaving. Obvious causes of cardiac syncope are listed in Table 15–1.

TACHYARRHYTHMIAS

Sustained rapid ventricular tachycardia (VT), i.e., VT duration greater than 30 seconds, or symptomatic nonsustained VT commonly causes syncope. When VT is not apparent on the ECG rhythm strip or Holter monitoring, the underlying mechanism may be revealed by EP testing.

Atrial fibrillation or other supraventricular tachycardia with fast ventricular rates may cause syncope, especially in the elderly, or when rapid rates supervene in patients with Wolff-Parkinson-White Syndrome.

TORSADES DE POINTES

This arrhythmia is usually caused by Class IA agents (quinidine and procainamide) and Class 3 agents (sotalol causes syncope mainly in the presence of hypokalemia; amiodarone rarely causes torsades). Because torsades is a brady-dependent arrhythmia, acceleration of the heart rate utilizing isoproterenol or by pacing, constitutes effective modes of therapy. Magnesium sulphate IV will usually terminate the attacks pending initiation of more definitive therapy (see Chapter 6).

AORTIC STENOSIS, HYPERTROPHIC CARDIOMYOPATHY

Syncope in aortic stenosis is typically exertional and suggests significant disease with life expectancy of 1 to 3 years. With hypertrophic cardiomyopathy, syncope may be precipitated by exercise but can occur with normal activities or at rest (see Chapters 12 and 14).

ACUTE MYOCARDIAL INFARCTION

Syncope is an uncommon mode of onset of myocardial infarction (MI). However, approximately 64% of patients with acute inferior MI have significant bradycardia and hypotension that predispose syncope. Rarely, patients with extensive coronary artery disease present with exertional syncope.

SINUS NODE DYSFUNCTION, SICK SINUS SYNDROME

Severe bradycardia (30 to 40 per minute), sinus arrest, and brady- or tachyarrhythmias may cause lightheadedness, dizziness, confusion, memory loss, or presyncope. One or more of these associated symptoms usually produce a 1- to 10-second warning prior to syncope; however, syncope can occur without warning in this category of patients and injuries may occur.

The setting is usually ischemic heart disease with old infarction. The electrocardiogram may be normal or show evidence of old infarction, bradycardia, or sinus arrest. A 48-hour Holter gives about a 70% chance of detecting a significant arrhythmia, with symptoms noted in the patient's diary, as opposed to less than 48% with a single 24-hour Holter monitoring. Fairly often, repeat 48-hour Holter monitoring is necessary once or twice over a couple of weeks to identify a bradyarrhythmia that is symptomatic. Treatment of sinus node dysfunction is given in Chapter 18. Sinus node dysfunction and severe bradycardia causing presyncope or syncope may be due to drug therapy that inadvertently depresses sinus node function. Verapamil, diltiazem, digitalis, beta blockers, Class 1 antiarrhythmic agents, amiodarone, and especially their combinations may cause severe bradycardia, AV block, and asystole in susceptible individuals. Discontinuation of the causative agent or agents is unfortunately rarely practical and pacing is usually indicated.

AV BLOCK, STOKES-ADAMS ATTACKS

Patients with Mobitz Type II or third-degree AV block may suddenly have an occurrence of transient asystole or ventricular fibrillation with complete cessation of cerebral blood flow. Since VF is instantaneous, the cerebral circulation is suddenly deprived of perfusion, resulting in loss of consciousness usually without warning. Episodes can happen on sitting, lying, or walking. The unconscious patient appears very pale and, on arousal, becomes flushed as blood rushes to the head. When a patient is assessed hours or days later, ECG may show manifestations of Mobitz Type II or complete AV block, or right or left bundle branch block, or bilateral disease. Cardiac pacing should be instituted (see Chapter 18).

PROLONGED QT SYNDROME

Recurrent syncope in children and young adults with a positive family history may be due to the prolonged QT syndrome. Episodes of life-threatening arrhythmias appear to be precipitated by increased sympathetic stimulation. Thus, beta blockers have a role in management, despite a tendency for bradycardia in many of these patients. Propranolol in doses of 80 to 160 mg daily or a similar noncardioselective beta blocker without agonist activity is preferred.

When recurrent syncope is uncontrolled by beta blockers, combined pacing and beta blocker therapy may be required. In uncontrolled cases, excision of the left stellate ganglion may be a last resort.

CAROTID SINUS SYNCOPE

Carotid sinus syncope produces loss of consciousness most often by a cardioinhibitory bradycardic mechanism and rarely by vasodepressor effects. This uncommon condition represents less than 3% of patients with cardiac syncope and occurs mainly in men aged 61 to 76 years. Males outnumber females 4:1. The history of syncope occurring with sudden turning of the head, shaving, or a tight shirt collar should alert the physician. Episodes may occur in clusters or with dizzy spells. In some patients, attacks are rarely associated with any head movement or pressure on the neck. Right, left, or bilateral carotid sinus involvement occurs in approximately 60, 22, and 22%, respectively. In a 17-year follow-up of 89 patients, hypersensitivity of the right carotid sinus was 7:1 compared to the left. Because carotid sinus massage, even for 2 to 3 seconds, carries a risk in the elderly male, a provisional diagnosis is made by exclusion of other causes prior to attempting carotid sinus massage, which typically results in ventricular asystole for more than 3 seconds. Carotid sinus massage is best done in a hospital setting with resuscitative equipment standby, although if necessary, the transient asystole is usually easily terminated by asking the patient to cough or by giving one or more light chest thumps. Complications are TIA, rare hemiplegia, and asystole.

Because of the high spontaneous remission rate and good outcome in patients with carotid sinus syncope, only patients with recurrent syncope, particularly those with organic heart disease, should be considered for ventricular pacing and with programming the pacemaker rate well below the patients sinus rate. In a 2- to 8-year follow-up study by Brignole, et al., patients with carotid sinus syncope had an overall mortality rate that was not significantly different from control patients (5.8/100 person-years).

OTHER CAUSES OF CARDIAC SYNCOPE

- Obstruction of blood flow may occur with massive pulmonary embolism
- Myxoma and left atrial thrombosis may cause syncope precipitated by suddenly sitting up or leaning forward
- Syncope occurring in patients with a prosthetic heart valve presents a particularly life-threatening emergency requiring admission to exclude prosthetic valve malfunction or obstructing thrombus
- WPW syndrome or cardiac tamponade should present no problems in diagnosis

Fallot's tetralogy produces hypoxic spells that cause arterial vasodilatation. Beta blockers inhibit right ventricular contractility and decrease the right to left shunt; also, these agents produce peripheral vasoconstriction. Supraventricular tachycardia is controlled. These actions may ameliorate hypoxic syncope.

UNEXPLAINED SYNCOPE

Approximately 35% of syncopal attacks occur without a readily defined cause. From 10 to 25% of total electrophysiologic studies done in several large EP laboratories in the United States are for the resolution of the diagnosis of unexplained syncope.

ELECTROPHYSIOLOGIC STUDY

A provocative EP study is useful in revealing a cardiac cause in approximately 12% of patients with unexplained syncope. Approximately 21% of these patients with negative studies are subsequently diagnosed as having intermittent high-degree AV block or sinus node disease. Caution is therefore necessary because an EP study is not a sensitive test to expose symptomatic bradycardia.

EP studies have been shown to initiate sustained monomorphic VT in approximately 18% of patients and nonsustained VT in approximately 23%. Nonsustained VT, especially if only for a few seconds duration, carries a minimal risk in patients with syncope and requires no arrhythmia therapy. Patients with syncope and sustained monomorphic VT do not appear to benefit from antiarrhythmic therapy, and the incidence of syncope is not reduced except when amiodarone is used as therapy.

The exact incidence of sudden death is unknown but appears to be low in patients with syncope unresolved by extended Holter monitoring and EP testing.

In patients with structural heart disease, especially ischemic heart disease or cardiomyopathy, and severely impaired ventricular function, with Holter manifesting sustained monomorphic VT or EP-initiated sustained VT, amiodarone therapy is advisable. Holter monitor documentation of sustained VT is a strong predictor of EP-induced sustained monomorphic VT, but the use of EP testing is of dubious value in these patients.

Signal-averaged ECG in the absence of left bundle branch block and LV EF of less than 30% correlates well with the EP induction of sustained monomorphic VT, but this test is not advisable because regardless of results, EP studies are indicated in virtually all patients with structural heart disease and unexplained syncope.

EP studies appear to be justifiable in patients who have a high probability of induction of sustained monomorphic VT

- Post MI patients with unexplained syncope
- LV EF less than 30%
- Left ventricular aneurysm
- Complex ventricular ectopy on Holter

Patients who have undergone a detailed assessment, including a relevant history and physical investigations, who remain with syncope of unknown cause and a negative EP study, have a low (2%) incidence of sudden death. EP studies are falsely negative in over 20% of patients who continue to have syncope. Close follow-up with extended Holter monitoring or a second assessment of HV intervals and tests of sinus node function may reveal sinus node dysfunction or high-degree AV block.

HEAD-UP TILT TESTING

Head-up tilt testing has a role in delineating the pathophysiology, diagnosis, and management of patients with no detectable heart disease and unexplained syncope.

"Malignant" vasovagal syndrome or neurocardiogenic syncope, also termed neurally mediated syncope, occurs abruptly with no prodrome. Fitzpatrick and Sutton call this tilt-inducible syncope "malignant" vasovagal syndrome because of the history of trauma in association with abrupt syncope, which occurs without a prodrome. Over 50% of patients have been noted to have injured themselves prior to seeking medical attention. These patients have features that distinguish them from individuals who succumb to the simple faint; particularly prominent is the lack of warning and the occurrence of injuries.

From 40 to 70% of patients with unexplained syncope experience syncope on being tilted 60 degrees for 45 minutes. There is no standard protocol for the test, but current recommendations indicate the need for

- At least 60° tilt
- Duration of 45 minutes
- Use of foot plate support rather than saddle
- Isoproterenol infusion improves sensitivity with decreased tilt time of 10 minutes at 80 degrees tilt. The use of isoproterenol has the disadvantage of dosing difficulty and reduced specificity

Isoproterenol infusion increased the provocation of symptoms produced by head-up tilt from 2 to 87% in individuals with unexplained syncope over a 10-minute study period and from 0 to 73% in those with diagnosed cardiopressor syncope, during a 15-minute tilt at 60°. Isoproterenol is not recommended, however, in patients over age 50 because of cardiac adverse effects. Schienman, et al. prefer the use of edrophonium IV (10 mg). Where edrophonium results in a negative head-up tilt test, isoproterenol does not reveal a positive test. In a study by Kapoor, et al., isoproterenol infusion resulted in a nonsignificant difference in the rate of positive tests in 20 young patients with unexplained syncope and controls matched by age, sex, and absence of underlying heart disease.

Head-up tilt using 60° for 45 minutes does not appear to be useful in youthful subjects with typical vasovagal syncope, but in this group, the clinical diagnosis is usually apparent.

In unexplained syncope, both head-up tilt testing and EP evaluation are complimentary and can identify the underlying cause in approximately 74% of patients presenting with unexplained syncope.

BETA-ADRENERGIC BLOCKER

Patients without structural heart disease and neurocardiogenic syncope respond to beta-adrenergic blocking drugs. These agents have been shown to prevent neurocardiogenic syncope in 50 to 75% of patients. Atenolol (25 to maximum 50 mg), metoprolol sustained release (100 mg), or nadolol (20 mg) is effective. Propranolol is beneficial, but adverse effects are often bothersome. Sra, et al. have shown esmolol to be effective in predicting the outcome of head-up tilt response to oral metoprolol. All patients who had a negative head-up tilt test response with esmolol IV had a negative test during oral metoprolol therapy.

Like beta-adrenergic blockers, disopyramide has a negative inotropic effect and a tendency to increase peripheral vascular resistance and produces a salutary response in about 15% of patients in whom syncope is caused by a hypotensive bradycardic response. Disopyramide (100 to 150 mg) sustained release twice daily may be given a trial in patients in the absence of structural heart disease and in patients who have failed to respond to beta blockers.

BIBLIOGRAPHY

Aboud FM: Ventricular syncope. Is the heart a sensory organ? N Eng J Med, *320*:390, 1989.

Akhtar M, Jazayeri M, Sra J: Cardiovascular causes of syncope. Identifying and controlling trigger mechanisms. Postgraduate Medicine, *90*:87, 1991.

Almquist A, Goldenberg IF, Milstein S, et al.: Provocation of bradycardia and hypotension by isoproterenol and upright posture in patients with unexplained syncope. N Engl J Med, *320*:346, 1989.

Brignole M, Oddone D, Cogorno S, et al.: Long-term outcome in symptomatic carotid sinus hypersensitivity. Am Heart J, *123*:687, 1992.

Fitzpatrick A, Sutton R: Tilting towards a diagnosis in recurrent unexplained syncope. Lancet, *1*:658, 1989.

Fitzpatrick AP, Theodorakis G, Vardas P, et al.: Methodology of head-up tilt testing in patients with unexplained syncope. J Am Coll Cardiol, *17*:125, 1991.

Grubb BP, Temesy-Armos P, Hahn H, et al.: Utility of upright tilt-table testing in the evaluation and management of syncope of unknown origin. Am J Med, *90*:6, 1991.

Huang SKS, Ezri MD, Hauser RG, et al.: Carotid sinus hypersensitivity in patients with unexplained syncope: Clinical, electrophysiologic, and long-term follow-up observations. Am Heart J, *116*:989, 1988.

Igarashi Y, Yamazoe M, Suzuki K, et al.: Possible role of coronary artery spasm in unexplained syncope. Am J Cardiol, *65*:713, 1990.

Kapoor WN, Brant N: Evaluation of syncope by upright tilt testing with isoproterenol. A nonspecific test. Ann Intern Med, *116*:358, 1992.

Kapoor WN, Karp FM, Wiend S, et al.: A prospective evaluation and follow-up of patients with syncope. N Engl J Med, *309*:197, 1983.

Kenny RA, Bayliss J, Ingram A, et al.: Head-up tilt: A useful test for investigating unexplained syncope. Lancet, *1*:1352, 1986.

Kligfield P: Tilt table for the investigation of syncope: There is nothing simple about fainting. J Am Coll Cardiol, *17*:131, 1991.

Kushner JA, Kou WH, Kadish AH, et al.: Natural history of patients with unexplained syncope and a nondiagnostic electrophysiologic study. J Am Coll Cardiol, *14*:391, 1989.

Leitch JW, Klein GJ, Yee R, et al.: Syncope associated with supraventricular tachycardia. An expression of tachycardia rate or vasomotor response? Circulation, *85*:1064, 1992.

Moazez F, Peter T, Simonson J, et al.: Syncope of unknown origin: Clinical, noninvasive, and electrophysiologic determinants of arrhythmia induction and symptom recurrence during long-term follow-up. Am Heart J, *121*:81, 1991.

Milstein S, Buetikofer J, Dunnigan A, et al.: Usefulness of disopyramide for prevention of upright tilt-induced hypotension-bradycardia. Am J Cardiol, *65*:1339, 1990.

Paul T, Guccione P, Garson A: Relation of syncope in young patients with Wolff-Parkinson-White syndrome to rapid ventricular response during atrial fibrillation. Am J Cardiol, *65*: 318, 1990.

Pongiglione G, Fish FA, Strasburger JF: Heart rate and blood pressure response to upright tilt in young patients with unexplained syncope. J Am Coll Cardiol, *16*:165, 1990.

Ross BA, Hughes S, Anderson E, et al.: Abnormal responses to orthostatic testing in children and adolescents with recurrent unexplained syncope. Am Heart J, *122*:748, 1991.

Sheldon R, Killam S, et al.: Methodology of isoproterenol-tilt table testing in patients with syncope. J Am Coll Cardiol, *19*:773, 1992.

Sra JS, Anderson AJ, Sheikh SH, et al.: Unexplained syncope evaluated by electrophysiologic studies and head-up tilt testing. Ann Int Med, *114*:1013, 1991.

Sra JS, Murthy VS, Jazayeri MR, et al.: Use of intravenous esmolol to predict efficacy of oral beta-adrenergic blocker therapy in patients with neurocardiogenic syncope. J Am Coll Cardiol, *19*:402, 1992.

Strasberg B, Sagie A, Rechavia E, et al.: The noninvasive evaluation of syncope of suspected cardiovascular origin. Am Heart J, *117*:160, 1989.

16

CARDIOGENIC SHOCK

M. Gabriel Khan

Data from the Gruppo Italiano per lo Studio della Streptochinasi nell' Infarto Miocardico (GISSI)-1 trial and the Multicenter Investigation of Limitation of Infarct Size (MILIS) Study Group indicate that cardiogenic shock remains the major cause of death after hospitalization for acute myocardial infarction (MI). From 3 to 5% of patients with acute MI present with cardiogenic shock and 6 to 7% develop cardiogenic shock after hospital admission. Mortality rates have been reported to range from 65 to 80%.

PATHOPHYSIOLOGY OF SHOCK

Shock is a clinical state in which target tissue perfusion is inadequate to supply vital substrates and remove metabolic waste. Inadequate cellular oxygenation leads to marked generalized impairment of cellular function, multi-organ failure, and death.

Target tissue perfusion may be inadequate because of

• Marked reduction in cardiac output (CO)
• Maldistribution of blood flow or both (see Fig. 16–1)

Cardiogenic shock usually results from decreased systolic function secondary to catastrophic complications of cardiac disorders with marked lowering of CO (Table 16–1). Also, cardiac disorders, including massive MI, may cause acute alteration of ventricular compliance, which decreases preload and further decreases CO. Since arterial blood pressure equals CO multiplied by systemic vascular resistance (SVR), marked hypotension occurs, resulting in poor tissue perfusion.

Shock due to sepsis, anaphylaxis, and metabolic and toxic etiology produces marked vasodilatation, resulting in a large proportion of the vascular volume being distributed to the skin, splanchnic bed, muscles, and other nonvital areas, thus depriving the brain, heart, and kidneys of adequate perfusion. Maldistribution may also occur in some cases of cardiogenic shock. Marked vasodilation and maldistribution of blood flow that occurs in noncardiogenic shock causes hypovolemia and reduction in preload, which decreases cardiac output and leads to poor target tissue perfusion (Fig. 16–1). Preload reduction is most commonly due to the many causes of hypovolemia (Table 16–2).

444

NON-CARDIOGENIC SHOCK

CARDIOGENIC SHOCK

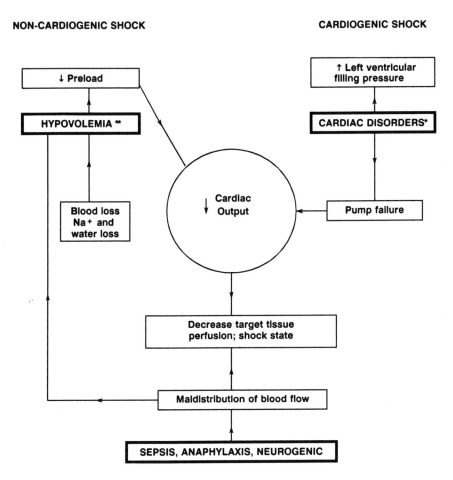

| * | See table 16-1 | ↑ Increase |
| ** | See table 16-2 | ↓ Decrease |

FIG. 16–1. Pathophysiology of shock.

Although the basic difficulty in the majority of patients with cardiogenic shock is a marked decrease in systolic function, a decrease in preload is also implicated. The end diastolic left ventricular volume, as measured by the left ventricular filling pressure, or PCWP reflects the effective preload, i.e., the load or stretch on a sarcomere immediately prior to contraction, but it must be emphasized that a high PCWP is not always an accurate measure of left ventricular preload. The PCWP is a relatively reliable index of left ventricular preload only when

• Ventricular compliance is normal or unchanging

TABLE 16–1. CAUSES OF CARDIOGENIC SHOCK

1. Mycocardial disorders
   a) Acute myocardial infarction and complications*
   b) Dilated and hypertrophic cardiomyopathy
2. Valvular
   a) Acute mitral regurgitation
   b) Acute aortic regurgitation
   c) Severe aortic stenosis
   d) Prosthetic valve dysfunction
3. Preload reduction
   A. Restriction to filling
      a) Cardiac tamponade
      b) Mitral stenosis, left atrial myxoma or thrombus
   B. Alteration of compliance
      a) Acute myocardial infarction, especially in the presence of right ventricular infarction
      b) Hypertrophic cardiomyopathy
   C. Decrease diastolic filling with tachyarrhythmias
4. Tachyarrhythmias, bradyarrhythmias
5. Other cardiovascular causes of shock
   a) Aortic dissection
   b) Pulmonary embolism
   c) Primary pulmonary hypertension

---

* See Chapter 4

TABLE 16–2. CAUSES OF NONCARDIOGENIC SHOCK

1. Hypovolemia
   a) blood loss
   b) effective plasma volume, dehydration, vomiting, diarrhea, burns acute pancreatitis, peritonitis, diabetic coma, adrenal failure
   c) iatrogenic: excessive diuresis in heart failure patients
2. Vasodilation and maldistribution of blood flow
   a) septicemia
   b) anaphylaxis
   c) renal failure
   d) hepatic failure
   e) acute pancreatitis
   f) malignant hyperthermia
   g) neurogenic shock: head or spinal cord injury (often bradycardic)

- Tight mitral stenosis, myxoma, or obstruction to pulmonary venous drainage are absent
- Severe mitral regurgitation is absent, because in this condition, the tall *V* wave in the left atrial pressure tracing elevates the mean pressure above left ventricular end diastolic pressure

Cardiac causes of preload reduction include

- Alteration of left or right ventricular compliance due to massive acute MI. Right ventricular infarction virtually always causes a decrease in

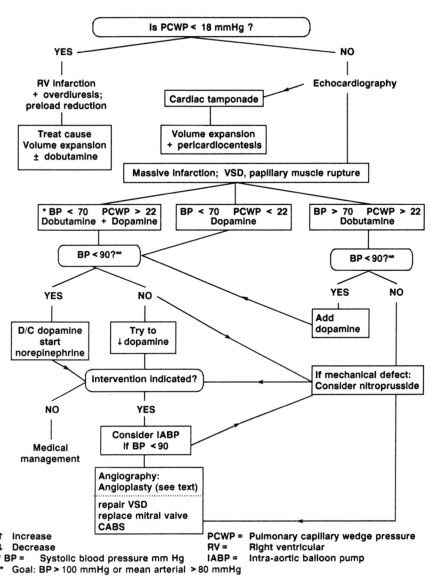

† Increase
↓ Decrease
* BP = Systolic blood pressure mm Hg
** Goal: BP > 100 mmHg or mean arterial > 80 mmHg

PCWP = Pulmonary capillary wedge pressure
RV = Right ventricular
IABP = Intra-aortic balloon pump

FIG. 16–2. Guidelines for the management of cardiogenic shock complicating myocardial infarction.

right ventricular preload; thus, volume loading has a role when combined with dobutamine (Fig. 16–2)
• Tight mitral stenosis, atrial myxoma
• Sudden loss of atrial function, especially important with right ventricular infarction, hypertrophic or restrictive cardiomyopathy
• Decreased diastolic filling time with tachyarrhythmias

- Increased intrapericardial pressure causing a high right atrial pressure yet decreased right ventricular preload, as with cardiac tamponade (Fig. 16–2)
- Shock complicating acute MI

Cardiogenic shock occurs in 5 to 15% of patients with acute MI that involves more than 35% of the myocardial mass or in patients with complications of myocardial rupture, ventricular septal defect (VSD) or severe mitral regurgitation, and mortality rate has remained high at approximately 80%.

In acute MI, early shock is aggravated by pain and arrhythmias, the correction of which can be salutary. Once shock develops, there is a vicious circle of increasing ischemia and decreasing CO. Early treatment with correction of aggravating factors is therefore of great importance. Table 16–3 gives cardiac medications that might worsen the shock state.

CLINICAL FEATURES

Marked decrease in cardiac output and poor target tissue perfusion give rise to the clinical findings

- Severe hypotension, systolic blood pressure generally less than 80 mm Hg without inotropes, systolic less than 90 mm Hg with inotropic support, or in previously hypertensive patients
- Cool peripheries, often with diaphoresis
- Clouding of consciousness, progressing to coma
- Cardiac index less than 2.2 L/min/m^2
- Pulmonary capillary wedge pressure (PCWP) greater than 18 mm Hg
- Oliguria, urine output less than 30 ml/hr
- A palpable radial pulse usually indicates a systolic blood pressure greater than 80 mm Hg
- A femoral pulse indicates a systolic blood pressure greater than 70 mm Hg
- A carotid pulse indicates a systolic blood pressure greater than 60 mm Hg

A very low CO decreases the intensity of murmurs, and it may be difficult to ascertain the degree of mitral regurgitation at the bedside. Echocardiography is a valuable tool to document the presence and significance of mechanical complications of infarction.

Right ventricular infarction is rare but must be excluded, since therapy is different from that given to patients with complications of left ventricular infarction. However, right ventricular infarction usually occurs in association with some degree of left ventricular infarction, and the PCWP may be less or greater than 18 mm Hg (Fig. 16–2).

Signs of right ventricular infarction are

- JVP elevated with absence of normal inspiratory fall, Kussmaul's sign
- Right ventricular gallop

- Clear lung fields on examination and on chest x-ray but interstitial pulmonary edema may be present caused by left ventricular failure as a result of commonly associated left ventricular infarction
- ECG evidence of inferoposterior infarction is usually present associated with ST segment depression (V_1, V_2, at times ST elevation V_1-V_4 and V_4R)
- Often the ratio of mean right atrial pressure to mean pulmonary capillary wedge pressure is greater than 0.8

THERAPY

Massive acute MI is the most common cause of cardiogenic shock. The prompt correction of aggravating factors and the use of thrombolytic agents within the first 2 hours of onset of anterior infarction carry the best hope of decreasing the incidence of cardiogenic shock. Since the in-hospital mortality for cardiogenic shock remains above 80%, even modest decrease in mortality must be pursued. Understandably, once cardiogenic shock is established, thrombolytic treatment with streptokinase or tPA does not significantly decrease mortality. However, the addition of hirudin or similar specific thrombin inhibitors to these agents may improve prolonged patency of the infarct-related artery. Randomized trials are necessary to document improvement in survival of patients with cardiogenic shock treated with streptokinase or tPA combined with hirudin, versus urgent coronary angioplasty.

Early recognition of the shock state and an immediate decision to pursue aggressive interventional therapy with coronary angioplasty are necessary in order to salvage lives.

Recent studies indicate that the very high mortality of patients with cardiogenic shock caused by massive evolving infarction is significantly reduced by urgent coronary angioplasty. Nothing is likely to be lost, and there is much to be gained from urgent angiography with a view to balloon angioplasty in these patients, as opposed to uncomplicated infarction, in which conservative initial management is recommended. Shock in patients with right ventricular infarction may be reversed by coronary angioplasty done up to 12 hours post onset of the shock state; this salutary effect may be related to a high incidence of reversible ischemia or stunned myocardium in these patients.

Surgical repair for acute severe mitral regurgitation or development of a large VSD may save a few lives, but a prognosis that depends critically on residual left ventricular function must remain guarded in this subset.

Cardiac tamponade caused by myocardial infarction and rupture requires immediate volume expansion to maintain an adequate preload and prompt pericardiocentesis, but successful surgical rescue is rare (see Chapter 4).

The conversion of acute atrial fibrillation to sinus rhythm in patients with acute MI, particularly right ventricular infarction, and in those with hypertrophic cardiomyopathy is advisable. Prompt electrical cardioversion is required for all arrhythmias if the patient is hemodynamically unstable (see Chapter 6). Even mild bradycardia is inappropriate for the patient in shock, and correction of this arrhythmia, too, may be beneficial.

SUPPORTIVE THERAPY

- In shock caused by MI, the shock state is aggravated by pain and arrhythmias, the correction of which can be salutary; morphine is used judiciously
- Ensure an adequate airway and maintain a PaO_2 of 75 to 120 mm Hg
- Utilize a well-fitted oxygen mask with a high flow rate of 10 to 15 liters per minute. Patients with clouding of consciousness or coma should be intubated if the decision is made to pursue interventional therapy
- Insert two large-bore 16 gauge catheters; one catheter is placed centrally under sterile conditions. Use a venous sheath with sidearm attachment and a balloon flotation catheter. Obtain duplicate blood samples from the superior vena cava, right atrium, and pulmonary artery for oximetric assessment
- Insert an indwelling arterial line, preferably femoral, for blood pressure and oximetric monitoring
- An indwelling catheter is necessary to monitor urinary output greater than 30 ml per hour
- Determine the PCWP. If less than 15 mm Hg, commence fluid challenge to bring the filling pressure of the left ventricle to 18 mm Hg (see Fig. 16–2)
- Obtain arterial blood gas analysis, electrolytes, BUN, creatinine, hemoglobin liver function tests, prothrombin time, and activated partial thromboplastin time (PTT) with creatine kinase (CK) and CK-MB
- Determine the CO by thermodilution technique and indirectly by assessment of arterial mixed venous oxygen content difference
- Monitor the cardiac rhythm and obtain rhythm strips every half hour
- Morphine is given in aliquots of 2 to 5 mg if the patient is in pain or is very uncomfortable
- Obtain right atrial, right ventricular, and pulmonary arterial pressures, and PCWP
- Check for elevated diastolic pressures and equalization of right atrial (greater than 10 mm Hg), pulmonary artery, and PCWP that would indicate cardiac tamponade
- Obtain reliable end-expiratory pressure tracings
- Determine the ratio of mean right atrial to mean PCWP; greater than 0.8 is often present in patients with right ventricular infarction
- Assess for large v waves with slow upslope in the wedge position that would indicate severe mitral regurgitation
- An oxygen step-up indicates intracardiac left-to-right shunt
- Transesophageal echocardiography (TEE) done urgently has proven very useful in the assessment of aortic dissection and is advisable in assessing patients with cardiogenic shock. TEE allows accurate assessment for dissection, cardiac tamponade, severe mitral regurgitation, interventricular septal rupture, and other lesions and assists with making a decision regarding aggressive therapy. The transthoracic technique may suffice in some patients or when TEE is not available
- Ensure an effective preload with an infusion of 0.9% saline, if needed to maintain left ventricular filling pressure 18 to 20 mm Hg and as high

as 24 mm Hg if necessary. It is advisable to err on the side of allowing some lung congestion to occur as left ventricular compliance is poor and requires increased preload to maintain cardiac output; see earlier discussion of preload. It is not advisable to give furosemide in an attempt to decrease mild pulmonary congestion because this may cause a decrease in preload and decreased CO; furosemide is required if pulmonary edema with a PCWP greater than 24 mm Hg is present

- Nitroprusside is indicated if there is documented acute severe mitral regurgitation and/or mechanical complications of infarction for which afterload reduction is considered necessary. Nitroprusside is commenced after stabilization of blood pressure with inotropes or IABP (Fig. 16–2)
- Captopril is useful when the patient improves and is being weaned from IV inotropes or nitroprusside

Figure 16–2 gives suggested guidelines for the management of cardiogenic shock. Patients with PCWP greater than 18 mm Hg and severely impaired stroke volume due to massive infarction comprise the largest group and urgent coronary angioplasty carries some hope for salvage. However, blood pressure and renal perfusion must be maintained during preparation for angioplasty. It must be reemphasized that a wait-and-see policy is not advisable and prompt angioplasty in selected patients with cardiogenic shock is strongly recommended with 18 hours of onset of infarction.

This recommendation will change with new information from ongoing prospective randomized trials. Pharmacologic agents do not improve survival in patients with cardiogenic shock and should be used mainly with an endeavor to support the patient through coronary angiography and angioplasty.

However, inotropes and vasopressors may have an increased role if thrombolytic therapy, which includes the addition of hirudin, proves useful in maintaining patency of the infarct-related artery.

TABLE 16–3. CARDIAC MEDICATIONS THAT MIGHT WORSEN THE SHOCK STATE

1. ACE INHIBITORS
   Renin angiotensin system vital to sustain blood pressure; agents decrease preload
2. BETA BLOCKERS
   Bradycardia, negative inotropic action, decrease cardiac output and blood pressure
3. ANTIARRHYTHMICS
   Negative inotropic action
4. CALCIUM ANTAGONISTS
   Negative inotropic action, bradycardia, decrease blood pressure
5. PRELOAD-REDUCING AGENTS
   Nitrates, ACE inhibitors, nitroprusside

INOTROPE/VASOCONSTRICTOR

The pharmacologic effects of vasoactive agents are given in Table 16–4. These pharmacologic agents are given by IV infusion, preferably using well-maintained infusion pumps and under strict supervision. It is necessary to titrate the dosages of these agents to correct severe hypotension, achieve improvement in CO, maintain an adequate LV filling pressure (18 to 20 mm Hg), and in some instances, to increase peripheral vascular resistance. In properly selected patients with mechanical defects after stabilization of blood pressure a reduction in afterload is essential (see Fig. 16–2).

Attempt to maintain a systolic blood pressure greater than 100 mm Hg or mean arterial pressure greater than 80 mm Hg and a urinary output greater than 30 ml/hour.

Dobutamine

Dosage: 2 to 10.0 μg/kg/min, titrated to achieve a desired inotropic effect directed by several measurements of CO, arteriovenous oxygen content difference, urine output and mentation (see Infusion Pump Chart, Table 16–5 and Fig. 16–2). Dobutamine should not be used alone in the severely hypotensive patient. Usually, if a dose in excess of 4 to 6 μg/kg/min is required and unacceptable hypotension exists, dopamine infusion is commenced at 5 μg/kg/min and dobutamine 4 to 6 μg/kg/min titrated up to a suggested maximum of 10 μg/kg/min of each agent. Occasionally, dobutamine titrated to a maximum of 20 μg/kg/min is necessary, especially if left ventricular filling pressure exceeds 24 mm Hg, a situation in which dopamine is relatively contraindicated. Thus, if the systolic blood pressure is less than 70 mm Hg and PCWP is greater than 24 mm Hg, a combination of dobutamine and norepinephrine is indicated.

Dopamine

Dosage: 2.5 to 10 μg/kg/min via a central line (see Infusion Pump Chart, Table 16–6). Dopamine at a dose of 0.5 to 4 μg/kg/min causes cardiac beta stimulation and also stimulates renal dopaminergic receptors producing renal arteriolar dilatation and an increase in urinary output. A dose of 4 to 6 μg/kg/min is initially advised if severe hypotension is present. At doses above 4 μg/kg/min, beneficial renal effects are lost, and mainly alpha-adrenergic vasoconstriction occurs with minimal beta stimulation that causes an increase in heart rate, CO, and blood pressure. A dose greater than 5 μg/kg/min is often required to raise systemic blood pressure in severely hypotensive patients. In patients with cardiogenic shock, a dose above 15 μg/kg/min without added dobutamine is seldom advisable, because at this dose, only marked alpha vasoconstriction occurs. It must be emphasized that while the combination of dopamine (6 to 10 μg/kg/min) and dobutamine (2 to 10 μg/kg/min) has several merits, dosages of either

TABLE 16–4. PHARMACOLOGIC EFFECTS OF VASOACTIVE DRUGS

RECEPTORS & PARAMETERS	DOBUTAMINE	DOPAMINE IBOPRAMINE	EPINEPHRINE	NOREPINEPHRINE	NITROPRUSSIDE	NITROGLYCERIN
Beta$_1$	+++	+ if dose < 5 μg/kg/min	+++	++++	Nil	Nil
Beta$_2$	+	Nil	++	Nil	Nil	Nil
Alpha	Nil	++ if >5 μg/kg/min +++ if >10 μg/kg/min Dopaminergic ++ if <5 μg/kg/min*	++	++++	Nil	Nil
Heart rate ↑	+	0/+	++	+	++	+
Inotropic effect	+++	+	++++	++	Nil	Nil
Arterial vasoconstriction SVR ↑	Nil	+++	++	++++	Nil	Nil
Arterial vasodilatation SVR ↓	0/+	Nil	++ (coronary)	Nil	++++	+
Venodilation preload →	Nil Nil	Nil Nil	Nil Nil	Nil Nil	+++ +++	+++ +++

+ = mild effect
++++ = strong effect
− = mild decrease
SVR = Systemic vascular resistance
* = Salutary renal effects

TABLE 16–5. DOBUTAMINE INFUSION PUMP CHART													
(dobutamine 2 amps (500 mg) in 500 ml (1000 μg/ml))													
WEIGHT (kg)	40	45	50	55	60	65	70	75	80	85	90	95	100	105
DOSAGE (μg/kg/min)	**RATE (ml/hr)**												
1.0	2	3	3	3	4	4	4	5	5	5	5	6	6	6
1.5	4	4	5	5	5	6	6	7	7	8	8	9	9	9
2.0	5	5	6	7	7	8	8	9	10	10	11	11	12	13
2.5	6	7	8	8	9	10	11	11	12	13	14	14	15	16
3.0	7	8	9	10	11	12	13	14	14	15	16	17	18	19
3.5	8	9	11	12	13	14	15	16	17	18	19	20	21	22
4.0	10	11	12	13	14	16	17	18	19	20	22	23	24	25
4.5	11	12	14	15	16	18	19	20	22	23	24	26	27	28
5.0	12	14	15	17	18	20	21	23	24	26	27	29	30	32
5.5	13	15	17	18	20	21	23	25	26	28	30	31	33	35
6.0	14	16	18	20	22	23	25	27	29	31	32	34	36	38
7.0	17	19	21	23	25	27	29	32	34	36	38	40	42	44
8.0	19	22	24	26	29	31	34	36	38	41	43	46	48	50
9.0	22	24	27	30	32	35	38	41	43	46	49	51	54	57
10.0	24	27	30	33	36	39	42	45	48	51	54	57	60	63
12.5	30	34	38	41	45	49	53	56	60	64	68	71	75	79
15.0	36	41	45	50	54	59	63	69	72	77	81	86	90	95
20.0	48	54	60	66	72	78	84	90	96	102	108	114	120	126

The above rates apply only for a 1000 mg/l concentration of dobutamine. If a different concentration must be used, appropriate adjustments in rates should be made. Usual dose range 2.5–10 μg/kg/min.
Fro:n: Khan M Gabriel: Cardiac Drug Therapy. 3rd Ed. London, W.B. Saunders, 1992.

drug in excess of 10 μg/kg/min have major disadvantages. If more than 15 μg/kg/min is required and the systolic or diastolic blood pressure remains very low, with a PCWP greater than 24 mm Hg, dopamine should be discontinued and norepinephrine should be tried in combination with dobutamine. Provided that filling pressures are adequate (greater than 18 mm Hg), failure of dopamine 15 μg/kg/min to raise systolic pressure to greater than 80 mm Hg, or diastolic greater than 60 mm Hg, or both necessitates the addition of norepinephrine; maximum suggested dose is 20 μg/kg/min. The IABP is preferred if the decision is made to proceed with interventional therapy (Fig. 16–2).

Norepinephrine

Dosage: Titrated 2 to 10 μg/min IV infusion to achieve desired hemodynamic effect, then wean the patient to dopamine plus or minus dobutamine. An increase in dosage in the range of 11 to 20 μg/minute is advised only after careful consideration. Care is also required to prevent extravasation, which causes necrosis.

Norepinephrine causes intense alpha-adrenergic vasoconstriction and has relatively modest beta-mediated myocardial chronotropic and inotropic

TABLE 16–6. DOPAMINE INFUSION CHART
DOPAMINE (800 MG) IN 500 ML 5% Dextrose/water
Use chart for: pump (ml/hour) *or*
  microdrip (drops/minute)

Example: 60 kg patient at 4.0 μg/kg/minute
—pump—set pump at 9 ml/hour
—microdrip—run solution at 9 drops/minute

WEIGHT (kg)	40	50	60	70	80	90	100
DOSAGE (μg/kg/min)	RATE: ml/hour (pump)						
1.0	1.5	1.9	2.3	2.6	3	3.4	3.8
2.0	3	3.8	4.5	5.3	6	6.8	7.5
3.0	4.5	5.6	6.8	7.9	9	10.1	11.3
4.0	6	7.5	9	10.5	12	13.5	15
5.0	7.5	9.4	11.3	13.1	15	16.9	18.8
6.0	9	11.3	13.5	15.8	18	20.3	22.5
7.0	10.5	13.1	15.8	18.4	21	23.6	26.3
8.0	12	15	18	21	24	27	30
9.0	13.5	16.9	20.3	23.6	27	30.4	33.8
10.0	15	18.8	22.5	26.3	30	33.8	37.5
12.0	18	22.5	27	31.5	36	40.5	45
15.0	22.5	28.1	33.8	39.4	45	50.6	56.3
20.0	30	37.5	45	52.5	60	67.5	75

effects. Alpha-mediated vasoconstriction produces an increase in systolic and diastolic pressures. Since the coronary arteries fill during diastole, it is imperative to maintain adequate diastolic blood pressures. However, since intense alpha vasoconstriction has adverse effects on renal and other tissues, norepinephrine should be considered a temporary maneuver until either the patient improves spontaneously or, as is more often the case, the decision is reached to proceed with aggressive therapy and insertion of the IABP prior to coronary angioplasty or surgery. It must be reemphasized that vasoactive drugs play a role in the temporary support of patients but do not themselves improve mortality.

Nitroprusside

Dosage: Begin with a very low dose (0.4 μg/kg/min) and titrate until a desired hemodynamic effect is achieved (see Infusion Pump Chart, Table 1–10).

Patients with severe mitral regurgitation or ventricular septal rupture require afterload reduction with nitroprusside and avoidance of vasocontrictor agents. Nitroprusside may cause a coronary steal; as well, diastolic blood pressure may be lowered. A Veterans Administration Study published in 1982 indicated that efficacy of nitroprusside in patients with acute MI was related to the time to treatment. Nitroprusside had a deleterious effect when administered to patients within 8 hours of onset of pain and a salutary effect in patients whose infusions were begun later. Mechanical complications of acute MI often occur more than 8 hours after the onset of pain, and nitroprusside, therefore, has a role in this category of patients (see Chapter 4). Tachycardia and thiocyanate toxicity should be anticipated (see Chapter 1). The combination of small dosages of dobutamine (2 to 6 µg/kg/min), dopamine (5 to 10 µg/kg/min), and nitroprusside is advisable when afterload reduction is necessary but without causing a fall in blood pressure. Afterload reduction by nitroprusside is indicated in patients with mechanical complications, ventricular septal defect, and severe mitral regurgitation after stabilization of arterial diastolic and coronary perfusion pressure by concomitant use of the IABP (Fig. 16–2). Captopril has been tried in these patients with some beneficial effects.

Nitroglycerin

Nitroglycerin infusion has a minor role in patients with mild cardiogenic shock, especially if there is ongoing ischemia, pulmonary congestion, and PCWP exceeding 22 mm Hg. Care is needed, however, to maintain systolic blood pressure greater than 100 mm Hg and an adequate preload. The PCWP should be maintained in the 18 to 20 mm Hg range and even as high as 22 mm Hg in some patients to achieve optimal cardiac output. Nitroglycerin is preferred to nitroprusside if ischemia is present or during the first 8 hours of infarction (see discussion of nitroprusside). IV nitroglycerin is contraindicated in patients with right ventricular infarction, hypovolemia, or PCWP less than 18 mm Hg. Also, caution is necessary in all patients with inferior infarction and cardiogenic shock because of the likely presence of right ventricular infarction. A marked fall in blood pressure due to decrease in preload with the commencement of oral or IV nitroglycerin should alert the physician to the presence of right ventricular infarction. Of course, this agent can be used for the treatment of ongoing ischemia if blood pressure has been stabilized by the use of dobutamine, dopamine, and/or IABP.

Amrinone

Amrinone IV is indicated for cardiogenic shock associated with severe pulmonary congestion, PCWP greater than 24 mm Hg if dobutamine and dopamine used alone or in combination are ineffective, and interventional therapy is not appropriate. However this agent may cause hypotension and is usually less effective than dobutamine.

Dosage: IV bolus 0.75 mg/kg over 2 to 5 minutes, then infusion of 5 to 10 µg/kg/min. An added bolus dose may be given 30 minutes later. The drug is not approved for oral use (see Chapter 5).

This phosphodiesterase inhibitor has both inotropic and vasodilating effects. The drug has an elimination half-life of 4 hours and excretion is renal, so caution is required in patients with renal failure and the dosage infused should be reduced. The plasma therapeutic level is approximately 3 µg/ml.

Amrinone may precipitate ventricular arrhythmias, rarely thrombocytopenia, hypotension, and hepatotoxicity. However, adverse effects are rare with short-term IV use.

Digoxin

Digoxin is an inotrope that is too weak to be of value in the acute setting of cardiogenic shock but is often required as maintenance therapy in patients with poor systolic function in the absence of mechanical complications and has a role, albeit small, during the withdrawal of dobutamine from dobutamine-dependent patients.

Withdrawal of dobutamine from dobutamine-dependent patients represents a major challenge. Binkley and others have successfully "weaned" dobutamine from more than 60% of these patients with hydralazine (25 mg administered orally every 6 hours). The dose is increased up to 50 to 200 mg every 6 hours as needed while the dobutamine infusion dose is gradually reduced over a 2- to 5-day period. These investigators have not found similar success in these situations with the administration of ACE inhibitors.

ACE inhibitors have a role in the longterm management. ACE inhibitors have also been used successfully in small-group studies during the acute phase of cardiogenic shock.

In addition, the correction of metabolic acidosis and/or alkalosis, hypoxemia, and control of arrhythmias are important in improving survival.

DEFINITIVE THERAPY

A firm decision concerning aggressive therapy, coronary angioplasty, or surgical repair with bypass surgery must be carefully weighed. The risks and tribulations of aggressive therapy must be discussed with the patient and family. The decision to proceed is usually not difficult in the less common situation when there is a structural problem such as a VSD or severe mitral regurgitation and left ventricular function is well preserved.

Contraindications to an aggressive approach include not only the patients wishes but also the presence of the following serious underlying diseases

- Pulmonary disease
- Cancer
- Cerebrovascular disease, stroke, TIA, severe carotid artery stenosis
- Intermittent claudication or known severe peripheral vascular disease
- Psychiatric disorders
- Renal failure (blood urea nitrogen and serum creatinine greater than 60 mg% and 3.5 mg/dl (300 μmol/l), respectively
- Neurologic disease
- Alcoholism with hepatic dysfunction, hematologic disease, or other contraindication to heparin therapy

Thus, only healthy individuals, preferably under age 70, in whom supportive therapy has been achieved within about 12 hours of onset of symptoms, should be considered for this heroic therapy.

Contraindications to IABP include

- Aortic regurgitation, if more than mild
- Aortic aneurysm, severe atherosclerosis of the aorta or iliofemoral arteries
- Contraindication to heparin therapy

If no contraindication exists, the IABP is placed from the femoral artery percutaneously over a guidewire and positioned in the thoracic aorta. The balloon is rapidly inflated with inert gas at the onset of diastole synchronized with the R wave of the ECG, and rapidly deflated just before the onset of systole. The IABP reduces afterload and increases diastolic pressure thus improving coronary perfusion pressure.

Complications of IABP occur in 10 to 30% of patients

- Death due to rupture of the balloon
- Aortic dissection
- Thrombus formation on the surface of the balloon with embolism
- Thrombus and cholesterol emboli to the kidneys or lower limbs
- Bleeding at puncture sites
- Trauma to the iliofemoral arteries and aorta may require surgery, including amputation of a leg
- Foot drop

Once the decision is made to pursue aggressive therapy, preparations should be made for urgent cardiac catheterization within an hour.

CORONARY ANGIOPLASTY

In four nonrandomized studies, in-hospital mortality was reduced from 77% to 30% with successful angioplasty reperfusion. A retrospective multicenter registry analysis of 69 patients indicated that the 2-year survival post urgent angioplasty recanalization of the related artery was 54%, as opposed to 11% without successful recanalization. Studies in patients with cardiogenic shock indicate about a 70% successful urgent angioplasty reperfusion of the infarct-related artery; in a study by Ghitis, et al., angioplasty was successful in up to 77% of patients who then experienced a hospital mortality rate of 19%, as opposed to mortality rates of 50% and 60% in patients in whom angioplasty was only partially successful or unsuccessful. Thus, there is much to be gained by attempting to rescue patients in this otherwise almost hopeless situation if adequate facilities and highly experienced staff are available.

SURGICAL INTERVENTION

The 2-year survival for patients after repair of ventricular septal rupture is about 80%, whereas for severe mitral regurgitation, survival is less than 40%. Thus, decision-making concerning surgical intervention should take into account the probable outcomes.

BIBLIOGRAPHY

Bates ER, Topol EJ: Limitations of thrombolytic therapy for acute myocardial infarction complicated by congestive heart failure and cardiogenic shock. J Am Coll Cardiol, 18:1077, 1991.

Binkley PF, Starling RC, Hammer DF, et al.: The dobutamine dependent patient: Successful withdrawal of positive inotropic support using hydralazine (Abstract). Clin Res, 38:878A, 1990.

Eltchaninoff H, Simpfendorfer C, Whitlow PL: Coronary angioplasty improves early and 1 year survival in acute myocardial infarction complicated by cardiogenic shock. J Am Coll Cardiol, 17:167A, 1991.

Francis GS: Vasodilators in the intensive care unit. Am Heart J, 121:1875, 1991.

Ghitis A, Flaker GC, Meinhardt S, et al.: Early angioplasty in patients with acute myocardial infarction complicated by hypotension. Am Heart J, 122:380, 1991.

Gruppo Italiano per lo Studio della Streptochinasi nell' Infarto Miocardico (GISSI). Effectiveness of intravenous thrombolytic treatment in acute myocardial infarction. Lancet, 1:397, 1986.

Hands ME, Rutherford JD, Muller JE, et al. and the MILIS Study Group: The in-hospital development of cardiogenic shock after myocardial infarction: Incidence, predictors of occurrence, outcome and prognostic factors. J Am Coll Cardiol, 14:40, 1989.

Killip T: Cardiogenic shock complicating myocardial infarction. J Am Coll Cardiol, 14:47, 1989.

Lee L, Erbel R, Brown T, et al.: Multicenter registry of angioplasty therapy of cardiogenic shock: Initial and long-term survival. J Am Coll Cardiol, 17:599, 1991.

Leier CV, Binkley PF: Acute positive inotropic intervention: The catecholamines. Am Heart J, 121:1866, 1991.

Miller L: Mechanical assist devices in intensive cardiac care. Am Heart J, 121:1887, 1991.

Moosvi AR, Khaja F, Villanueva L, et al.: Early revascularization improves survival in cardiogenic shock complicating acute myocardial infarction. J Am Coll Cardiol, 19:907, 1992.

Swan HJC, Ganz W, Forrester J, et al.: Catheterization of the heart in man with use of a flow directed balloon-tipped catheter. N Engl J Med, 283:447, 1970.

17
PREOPERATIVE MANAGEMENT OF CARDIAC PATIENTS UNDERGOING NONCARDIAC SURGERY

M. Gabriel Khan

Cardiovascular complications account for approximately 50% of deaths in patients submitted to major noncardiac surgery and more than 90% of these occur in patients with coronary heart disease (CHD). Cardiac patients with a high risk of postoperative infarction and cardiac death can be identified by careful elucidation of the history and a physical examination, followed by ECG, chest x-ray, and where needed, Holter monitoring, echocardiogram, and stress test either by exercise or utilizing dipyridamole-thallium scintigraphy.

In patients with CHD, it is necessary to carefully evaluate

- Left ventricular reserve
- Coronary reserve or ischemic burden

These findings and an understanding of the complications that may occur in patients with CHD, when submitted to the intensive stress of catecholamines, hypotension, decreased preload or hypervolemia, myocardial depressant effect, and interactions of cardiac medications, are vital for the formulation of a rational plan of management.

PATHOPHYSIOLOGY OF CARDIOLOGIC COMPLICATIONS FROM SURGERY

Activation of the sympathetic nervous system and sensitization of the ischemic myocardium to increase catecholamines appear to play a major role in initiating ischemic complications. Poorly perfused myocardium is in jeopardy during the increased demands imposed by the cardiac response to intense sympathetic/catecholamine stimulation, which occurs perioperatively and maximally in the postoperative period.

The 12- to 72-hour postoperative hypermetabolic state imposes considerable demands that require adequate left ventricular (LV) function and coronary flow reserve. Holter monitoring indicates an increased incidence of painless ischemia prior to adverse cardiac outcomes during the 2- to 5-day postoperative period. Importantly, the inadvertent withdrawal of antianginal or antihypertensive medications may predispose intraoperative and postoperative complications. Also, surgical trauma promotes activation of new platelets, which with added stasis, are linked to the initiation of venous thromboembolism.

RISK STRATIFICATION AND PLAN OF MANAGEMENT

Minor surgery, (opthalmologic, transurethral resection of the prostate, herniorrhaphy, hysterectomy, and orthopedic surgery), usually cause no complications in cardiac patients, provided that these individuals are hemodynamically stable and do not have major contraindications to elective surgery (Table 17–1).

Major surgery is tolerated relatively well by cardiac patients, except in those with myocardial infarction (MI) less than 6 months previously, unstable angina, overt heart failure, severe aortic stenosis, and angina Class 2-3 in association with peripheral vascular disease and a strongly positive stress test or abnormal dipyridamole-thallium scan.

Patients undergoing vascular surgery are at highest risk for cardiac events. Patients with aortic abdominal aneurysms pose a considerable risk because of the magnitude of myocardial stress imposed during aortic cross clamping. Virtually all patients with abdominal aortic aneurysms have at least one of the following: significant CHD, hypertension, or renovascular disease.

Further estimation of risk requires consideration of the following

- Emergency surgery for life-threatening conditions must be done regardless of risk and is performed under hemodynamic monitoring, with rapid optimization of medical therapy that must not delay surgical intervention
- In patients where surgery is elective but promptly required, the consultant's major task is quickly to optimize medical therapy, assess risks, and determine, if necessary, how long surgery should be deferred

---

TABLE 17–1. CARDIAC CONTRAINDICATIONS TO ELECTIVE NONCARDIAC SURGERY

1. Myocardial infarction <6 months*
2. Overt heart failure
3. Severe aortic stenosis
4. Unstable angina
5. Mobitz Type II, complete AV block, sick sinus syndrome

* Elective but promptly needed surgery justifiable after three months post myocardial infarction with full hemodynamic monitoring (see Table 17–2); emergency surgery can be done earlier

---

The Goldman Cardiac Risk Index does not take into consideration vital information that may be gleaned from echocardiography, ejection fraction (EF), exercise stress testing, dipyridamole thallium scintigraphy, and Holter monitoring for silent ischemia. The Goldman classification was devised in the 1970s in cardiac and noncardiac patients and underestimates risks in Class 4 patients.

Estimation of risk is an academic exercise in patients requiring emergency surgery for conditions that pose an immediate serious threat to life, such as aortic dissection, perforated viscus, ruptured spleen, or continued massive hemorrhage with marked hemodynamic deterioration. In these patients, the risks are well known to the surgeon and anesthesiologist and should be communicated to the patient or next of kin and the role of the consultant cardiologist in this setting is to assist with prompt hemodynamic stabilization of the patient. Mortality is clearly related to the following

- Age over 70 years: Mortality is up to 10 times higher than in patients under age 65
- Type of major surgery
- Previous MI
- Unstable or Class 3 and 4 angina (see Chapter 2)
- Cardiac failure, present or past
- Severity of aortic stenosis

Studies in the 1970s indicated that post MI patients less than 3 months have a postoperative reinfarction rate of about 24%. Recent studies indicate that intensive hemodynamic monitoring can reduce postoperative infarction rates to less than 6% at 3 months and to approximately 3% at 3 to 6 months (Table 17–2). A 10 to 15% incidence of postoperative infarction was observed in patients with stable angina Class 2 or 3 and peripheral vascular disease with an abnormal dipyridamole thallium scan. A high mortality is to be expected in patients less than 3 months post MI, unstable angina, overt heart failure, and moderate/severe aortic stenosis. Elective surgery should be postponed or cancelled in these subgroups.

Patients with Class 2 to 3 angina with peripheral vascular disease and a positive stress test if at low workload, heart rate less than 120/minute, or an abnormal dipyridamole-thallium scan have a very high risk of postoperative infarction (15 to 30%).

Up to 60% of intraoperative and postoperative infarcts occur silently and with a high mortality. About 90% of postoperative cardiac events occur in

TABLE 17–2. APPROXIMATE INCIDENCE OF POSTOPERATIVE MYOCARDIAL INFARCTION

STUDIES	NO MI	MI >6 MONTHS	3–6 MONTHS	<3 MONTHS
1970s	0.5%	5%	15%	30%
1980s*		<1%	3%	6%
Angina Class 2–3 + PVD and abnormal dipyridamole-thallium scan (15–30%)				

* Full hemodynamic monitoring

TABLE 17–3. HIGH RISK CARDIAC PATIENTS FOR ELECTIVE NONCARDIAC SURGERY*

1. Angina Class 3 + PVD
2. Angina Class 3, no PVD, strongly positive stress test
3. Angina Class 2, no PVD, strongly positive stress test
4. Angina Class 2 + PVD normal dipyridamole-thallium scan
5. >6 months post MI and any of the above categories
6. >6 months post MI moderate hypertension and/or diabetes
7. Holter evidence of silent ischemia in above categories of patients
8. Episodes of VT or frequent multiform ventricular ectopy
9. Bradyarrhythmias
10. Heart failure: more than one episode
11. Heart failure: one episode necessitating triple therapy**
12. Ejection fraction <35%
13. Aortic stenosis: moderate
14. Hypertrophic or dilated cardiomyopathy
15. Tight mitral stenosis

PVD = Peripheral vascular disease
* Excluding causes contraindicating surgery (Table 17–1)
** Digoxin, diuretic, and ACE inhibitor

patients with apparent or occult CHD, whereas valvular, hypertensive, and other heart disease account for the remaining patients with a low incidence of serious events.

Cardiac patients at high risk for elective noncardiac surgery are listed in Table 17–3. Most of the remaining large pool of cardiac patients undergo elective major surgery without significant risk, and it makes no sense to label them as low or good risk patients.

PATIENT ASSESSMENT

HISTORY

A careful relevant history backed up, if needed, by a spouse or relative is vital. The assessment of the patient should result in a clear knowledge of the

- Left ventricular reserve, taking into account information gleaned from the history, physical, chest x-ray, and echocardiography with evaluation of the LV function (Fig. 17–1)
- Coronary reserve, as derived from assessment of effort tolerance, exercise stress testing (see Chapter 2), and/or dipyridamole-thallium scintigraphy and occasionally coronary angiography
- Extent of hypertension, if present
- Significance of a detectable aortic systolic murmur or mitral stenosis

In addition, the assessment should include a meticulous review of all drugs the patient is taking. The number and usage of cardiac medications may give clues to the extent of underlying disease and continuation of

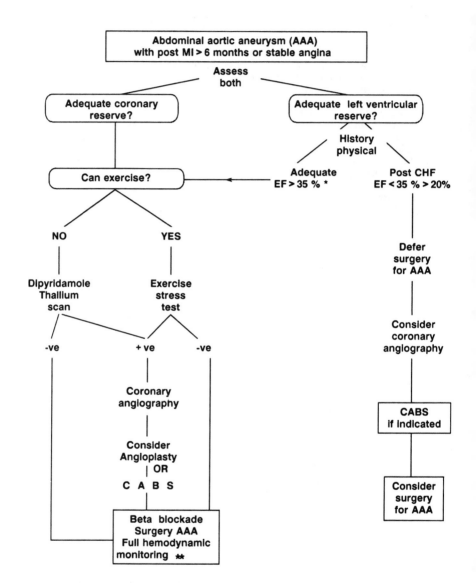

MI =   myocardial infarction; CABS = Coronary artery bypass surgery

*   Absence of mitral regurgitation

**   Arterial line, balloon flotation catheter, cardiac monitor 4 days

FIG. 17–1. Preoperative assessment of the very high risk surgical patient.

some but discontinuation of others may be necessary to assure salutary effects.

- Aspirin is a commonly used drug in cardiac patients. In most patients, aspirin should be discontinued 2 days prior to most surgical procedures and 5 days prior to ophthalmologic or urologic surgery
- Oral anticoagulants and NSAIDS must be discontinued days prior to surgery
- Calcium antagonists tend to decrease blood pressure, which may be further lowered by anesthetic agents and sedatives. Calcium antagonist dosage may be decreased slightly if angina is stable, and to a greater extent if LV EF is less than 40% and systolic blood pressure is in the 95 to 110 mm Hg range
- Beta blockers must not be stopped prior to surgery, however, because they prevent tachycardia during intubation and may be beneficial in preventing perioperative and postoperative ischemic events (see Chapter 2 for IV and oral dosages)
- If nitrates are not being taken by the patient, they may have to be added with care, but not to cause a decrease in blood pressure
- IV nitroglycerin infusion may be required perioperatively
- Antihypertensive agents, digoxin, and diuretics are discussed later in this chapter

PHYSICAL EXAMINATION

- Examine the chest for abnormal precordial movement indicating LV wall motion abnormalities
- Look for cardiomegaly and/or S3 gallop, which indicates LV dysfunction
- Determine whether an aortic systolic murmur exists. Verify if aortic stenosis is significant: symptoms of shortness of breath on moderate effort, chest pain or presyncope, LV thrust, delayed carotid upstroke, decreased intensity or absence of the aortic second sound in the second right interspace or over the right carotid. If any one of these symptoms or signs is present, defer elective surgery pending results of Doppler echocardiography (see Chapter 12)
- Carefully evaluate internal jugular pulsations for prominent waves and pressure exceeding 2 cm above the sternal angle indicative of heart failure with or without the presence of crepitations over the lung bases.
- Assess cardiac rhythm disturbances: atrial fibrillation with a fast ventricular response must be controlled
- Assess hypertension, hypotension, and for postural hypotension
- Deeply palpate the abdomen for the presence of abdominal aortic aneurysm and assess the carotid and peripheral circulation. Patients with peripheral vascular disease have a higher incidence of complications indicative of widespread occlusive atheromatous vascular disease

INVESTIGATIONS

ELECTROCARDIOGRAM

It is customary for all patients over age 35 to have a resting ECG performed within a few days prior to surgery, and consideration should be given to the following

- This control tracing makes changes that may appear postoperatively more meaningful, e.g., the sudden occurrence of P pulmonale, ST depression V_1 to V_3, and/or right bundle branch block may suggest acute cor pulmonale caused by pulmonary embolism
- If the resting ECG is abnormal, it should be compared to previous tracings to exclude recent or ongoing ischemia. If acute ischemia is confirmed, further investigations are necessary: request an exercise test if surgery is elective and the coronary reserve is questionable (see Chapters 2 and 4). If the patient is unable to exercise, then dipyridamole-thallium scintigraphy has a role
- Multifocal ventricular premature beats (VPCs) or other ventricular arrhythmias may require temporary control, but unifocal VPCs in the absence of ongoing ischemia or electrolyte abnormality are not of concern
- The fast ventricular response with atrial fibrillation should alert the physician to the need for digoxin
- ECG evidence of old infarction is particularly important in confirming the patient's history of old infarctions. An extensive infarct (see criteria given in Chapter 3) or anterior infarction carries a much higher surgical risk than inferior infarction
- ST elevation present months after infarction strongly suggests LV aneurysm and increases surgical risk as well as an increased incidence of LV systemic embolization. Left bundle branch block or other intraventricular conduction delay or left ventricular hypertrophy are indicative of an increased risk of perioperative infarction and/or death
- Left atrial enlargement is an important finding in keeping with left ventricular hypertrophy or LV dysfunction overt LV failure or significant mitral stenosis and/or regurgitation

DIPYRIDAMOLE-THALLIUM SCINTIGRAPHY

This is a clinically useful and relatively safe test in detecting ischemic myocardial segments and has been shown to give prognostic information concerning the risk of cardiac event up to 2 years following surgery for peripheral vascular disease. A reversible thallium defect and late redistribution after dipyridamole-thallium imaging are significant predictors of future cardiac events in patients with peripheral vascular disease. These patients benefit from coronary angiography and coronary angioplasty or bypass surgery if these are indicated. Following bypass surgery, the incidence of cardiac events in these patients is decreased by 95%.

The dipyridamole-thallium scan is contraindicated in patients with

- Unstable angina

TABLE 17–4. ADVERSE EFFECTS OF DIPYRIDAMOLE-THALLIUM SCINTIGRAPHY	
ADVERSE EFFECT	PERCENTAGE
Chest pain*	19
Death**	0.05
Non fatal MI	2
Headache	12
Dizziness	20
Hypotension*	5
*Wheezing in patients with asthma of COPD	>20

* Quickly relieved by stopping dipyridamole infusion and giving IV aminophylline (5 mg/kg over 20 minutes)
** Represents patients with unstable angina

- Angina at low level effort or at rest, stable Class 3 or 4 angina
- Patients with asthma or wheezing

Adverse effects of dipyridamole-thallium scintigraphy are given in Table 17–4.

HOLTER MONITORING

Preoperative Holter monitoring for 24 to 48 hours is helpful in detecting silent ischemia and is especially useful in patients with aortic aneurysms requiring surgery and in patients at high risk as listed in Table 17–3. This investigation is not cost effective, however, and reliability is critically dependent on details of the technique employed at individual centers.

Studies using postoperative Holter monitoring indicate that at 1 to 4 days postoperative, 40 to 60% of patients with CHD develop "ischemic" changes that may herald an incidence of fatal or nonfatal infarction of 1 to 2%. It is probably not cost justifiable, however, to monitor 100 cardiac patients in an attempt to save one fatal infarct or four nonfatal infarctions. Importantly, MI is usually caused by occlusion of a coronary artery by thrombus overlying a fissured plaque of atheroma, the occurrence of which does not usually correlate with the presence of silent ischemia observed more than 12 hours prior to the events. However, where arrhythmias are suspected, Holter monitoring is certainly relevant in the preoperative assessment of patients complaining of syncope or presyncope. Significant bradyarrhythmias that may require pacing or frequent multiform or other wide complex ventricular ectopics may be uncovered in these patients.

ECHOCARDIOGRAPHY

Echocardiography is a most valuable tool, especially in patients such as those listed in Table 17–3. Patients with suspected LV dysfunction, valvular heart disease, or cardiomyopathy should have echocardiographic assessment. The detection of regional wall motion abnormalities will greatly heighten the suspicion that significant coronary artery disease is present. LV systolic function is assessed, and an EF is reported by some echocardiographers if mitral regurgitation is absent. The echocardiographic EF in patients with CHD is subjective to some errors in interpretation but is a useful guide for comparative studies and echocardiography is necessary for evaluating the degree of aortic stenosis or other structural abnormalities. The radionuclide ECG gated study cannot be used in patients with atrial fibrillation. Both studies give falsely high EF in patients with mitral regurgitation; echocardiography is a more cost-effective test.

CARDIAC DISEASES, ASSESSMENTS, AND THERAPY OPTIMIZATION

ISCHEMIC HEART DISEASE

If the patient suffers from angina pectoris, assess if it is stable or unstable angina

- Class 1: Chest pain on extraordinary effort (see Chapter 2)
- Class 2: Chest pain on normal activities that require moderate exertion, such as walking 0.5 to 1 mile briskly, with pain occurring mainly up hills and against a cold wind. Absence of rest angina except if emotionally precipitated
- Class 3: Chest pain on mild activities, such as walking 2 blocks or approximately 200 yards
- Class 4: Angina at rest
- Unstable angina: New onset angina, a change in pattern and frequency, progressive angina (see Chapter 2)

Do not be lulled into satisfaction with the history of low pain frequency or low nitroglycerin consumption. Inactivity due to intermittent claudication and peripheral vascular disease can decrease the frequency of chest pain and nitro consumption, such that severe obstructive CHD may be present with the patient only experiencing "mild" angina. Importantly, silent ischemia may occur, especially in patients with angina who have diabetes and in patients with unstable syndromes. A history of increasing angina, change in pattern, or angina at rest indicates severe CHD with limited coronary reserve. It must be reemphasized that rare or completely absent pain in an inactive patient is of little help in decision-making.

Patients with stable Class 2 angina without compromised LV function should undergo exercise stress testing before major elective surgery. The ability to complete more than 6 minutes of a Bruce or similar protocol without experiencing chest pain, ischemic changes, or an inappropriate fall in blood pressure is evidence of adequate coronary reserve (see Chapter 2) and suffices for most major surgery. In patients with Class 3 angina (Tables 17–3 and 17–5) and in those with EF < 35%, elective surgery should be deferred until coronary angiography and revascularization are achieved. Both CABS and angioplasty in patients with severe CHD have reduced the mortality that can be caused by noncardiac surgery (Table

TABLE 17–5. FACTORS THAT DECREASE RISK OF ELECTIVE NONCARDIAC SURGERY

1. Coronary artery bypass surgery
2. *Role of angioplasty in patients with impaired coronary reserve, EF >40%
3. Exercise stress test negative for ischemia
4. Absence of silent ischemia or frequent multiform ventricular ectopics on Holter
5. Ejection fraction >40%
6. Pre-, peri-, and postoperative use of beta blockade if not contraindicated
7. Nitrates commencing 6 hours preoperative and for 48 to 96 hours postoperative: transdermal nitrate q 6h × 24 to 96 hours, then wean off
8. Adequate control of heart failure for a few months prior to surgery
9. Low dose aspirin (80 to 162.5 mg daily from day 2) to prevent fatal or nonfatal MI or thromboembolism

* Strongly advised (role to be defined by clinical trials)

17–5). Patients with Class 3 angina and those with MI within the previous 3 to 6 months constitute a high-risk group. If emergency surgery is necessary in this category of patients and in others considered at high risk, full hemodynamic monitoring should be instituted with arterial line, Swan-Ganz catheter, and continuous cardiac monitoring carried out during surgery and for about 4 days following. Decision-making steps in the preoperative assessment of the very high-risk surgical patient are given in Figure 17–1.

Progress in anesthesia and surgery allows surgical procedures to be performed successfully in patients who, in the 1960s and 1970s, would have been considered prohibitive surgical risks.

HEART FAILURE

Overt or minor heart failure is not an uncommon preoperative problem for which a cardiology consultation is required. Consideration must be given to the following

- Document effort tolerance, degree of dyspnea, orthopnea, paroxysmal nocturnal dyspnea, and signs of heart failure
- The presence of LV enlargement, S3 gallop, and the history of two or more episodes of heart failure add to the risk and in these patients, optimization of medical therapy with the combination of ACE inhibitor, digoxin at correct dosage, and titrated use of furosemide, should result in reduction in the risk of heart failure due to surgery. These patients require preoperative hemodynamic monitoring, and particular attention to the avoidance of fluid overload is required
- It is important to recognize that heart failure may be present without clinical signs of congestion. Echocardiographic evaluation of LV systolic function is a useful assessment (Chapter 5)
- Overt heart failure is a contraindication to elective surgery. If emergency surgery is required, the use of IV nitroglycerin, digoxin, and diuretics, as well as ACE inhibitors, may cause some amelioration in 24 hours to

enable urgent surgery, but intensive hemodynamic monitoring is essential

- If heart failure occurred more than 1 year prior and an S3 or marked cardiomegaly is absent with the patient stabilized on digoxin, a diuretic, and/or ACE inhibitor, elective surgery can proceed
- For patients in the above groups, an echocardiogram is necessary to determine chamber size, ventricular contractility, presence or absence of aortic stenosis, degree of mitral regurgitation, as well as EF. It must be reemphasized that the EF is not accurate in the presence of significant mitral regurgitation
- Patients with EF less than 30% are at higher risk for the development of pulmonary edema in the postoperative phase. If surgery is mandatory, intensive hemodynamic monitoring is essential
- Chest x-ray should be evaluated for the degree of cardiomegaly. Mild cardiomegaly is acceptable, but moderate to severe cardiomegaly requires echocardiographic evaluation correlated with the history and physical findings. Patients with severe CHD commonly exhibit no significant radiographic cardiomegaly, and the radiograph cannot be relied upon in the assessment of cardiomegaly in patients with CHD (the largest subset of cardiac patients). Thus, echocardiography has an increasing role

Digoxin is indicated in cardiac patients with atrial fibrillation and an uncontrolled ventricular response. The drug is also indicated in patients with signs or symptoms of heart failure and in those with a history of heart failure (see Chapter 5). The use of digoxin, when indicated, does not increase the risk of a cardiac event, and studies that have tried to demonstrate this point fail to recognize that in these patients, mortality and morbidity are high, regardless of the use of digoxin. A digoxin level is not an essential requirement if one follows the rule that in patients under age 70 with a normal creatinine level, the maintenance dose should be 0.25 mg daily and in patients over age 70 with normal serum creatinine, the dose is usually 0.125 mg daily.

Exception to the above guidelines: Atrial fibrillation with a fast ventricular response requires higher titrated dosage. If the dosage is not in accordance with the schedule given above or digoxin toxicity is in question, the level should be estimated (see Chapter 5).

HYPOTENSION AND HYPERTENSION

Hypotension caused by hemorrhage or medications must be promptly corrected. In the management of hypotension, consider the following

- Anesthesiologists correctly detest written advice to "avoid hypotension"
- Patients with CHD are commonly prescribed a combination of beta blockers, calcium antagonists, and nitrates; interaction with anesthetic agents and mild sedatives may cause a significant fall in blood pressure
- If the patient's systolic blood pressure is in the range of 95 to 105 mm Hg on the aforementioned cardiac medications, it is wise to write an appropriate phrase: "Propensity to develop hypotension in view of rel-

atively low blood pressure and medications that predispose blood pressure lowering." The doses of the relevant agents particularly calcium antagonists, which are not lifesaving agents may then be reduced to permit the systolic pressure to increase to the range of 120 to 130 mm Hg

- When hypotension occurs in the operating room, an increase in IV saline is usually given to elevate blood pressure. At times, this may precipitate subtle heart failure, which may go undetected because, in practice, not all cardiac patients are monitored with balloon flotation catheters
- Caution is necessary to avoid over prescribing transdermal nitrates for use during surgery in patients with borderline hypotension. Also, the nitrate patch should not be applied to the chest because a defibrillator paddle placed in contact with the nitrate patch may cause an explosion

Systolic pressure greater than 240 mm Hg and diastolic greater than 110 mm Hg that does not respond to nifedipine (10 mg orally repeated in 2 hours if needed, plus or minus nitropaste, is considered a contraindication to elective surgery and requires investigation and control prior to elective surgery. If emergency surgery is needed, blood pressure control can be obtained with the use of IV nitroglycerin, labetalol, or nitroprusside. For dosage information, see Table 2–9 (nitroglycerin), Table 1–10 (nitroprusside), and Chapter 1 (labetalol). IV nitroglycerin is superior to nitroprusside in patients with CHD, because the latter agent may cause a coronary steal. If tachycardia is provoked by these agents, a short-acting beta blocker such as esmolol IV or metoprolol should be given (see Table 2–8 or 3–4); propranolol has a longer duration of action at beta-adrenergic receptors, and the negative inotropic action of this agent may persist for 12 to 16 hours and negative chronotropic effects may last up to 36 hours. However, propranolol is commonly the only IV preparation available in some countries; 1 mg IV is equivalent to the oral 20 mg, and 1 mg IV can be given over 2 minutes and repeated if needed every 1 to 6 hours. Caution is necessary to avoid a beta blocker, including the alpha$_1$ beta blocker labetalol, in patients who have asthma, heart failure, or in those who have moderate LV dysfunction. Also, calcium antagonists are not all alike (see Chapters 1 and 2), and while verapamil and diltiazem are contraindicated in patients with EF less than 40%, nifedipine may be permissible in some.

Antihypertensive agents should not be discontinued prior to surgery, except when drug treatment is inappropriate, causing unduly low blood pressure or postural hypotension. Many patients with mild hypertension require no drug therapy. On admission, if a diuretic has been used, this can be discontinued until a few days prior to discharge. If a beta blocker is being given, this should be continued because of its salutary effects during induction of anesthesia and their cardioprotective effects in the peri- and post-operative periods.

The following antihypertensive agents must not be discontinued suddenly because rebound may occur

- Clonidine
- Guanfacine
- Methyldopa

- Bethanidine
- Beta blockers or calcium antagonists

Patients with mild to moderate hypertension that is not completely controlled, with systolic blood pressure in the 180 to 210 range and diastolic pressure between 95 and 105, will benefit from an increase in medications and/or from the addition of transdermal nitroglycerin, and surgery should not be delayed.

High blood pressure is usually well tolerated since premedication and anesthetic agents lower blood pressure levels. The serum potassium should be maintained at a normal level greater than 4.0 mEq(mmol)/L and metabolic alkalosis should be avoided since these conditions may increase the risk of cardiac events.

ABDOMINAL AORTIC ANEURYSM

Patients with abdominal aortic aneurysms (AAA) are at high risk because they often have concomitant severe coronary artery disease and require extensive preoperative evaluation. Figure 17–1 gives suggested steps in how to manage patients undergoing surgery for abdominal aortic aneurysm and similar high risk patients. These patients commonly have moderately severe hypertension that must be controlled. Also, CHD is nearly always present but may not be manifest, because the patient's exercise capacity usually is reduced because of intermittent claudication.

Evaluations include

- Echocardiographic assessment of LV function
- Holter monitoring to document arrhythmias and/or silent ischemia
- Historic details of effort tolerance and an exercise stress test evaluate coronary reserve. If the latter cannot be done, dipyridamole-thallium scintigraphy or similar noninvasive study should be considered
- Baseline renal function

Surgery is necessary when the AAA exceeds 6 cm. If the renal arteries are in proximity and require revascularization, the risk of precipitating severe irreversible renal failure may be prohibitive and the decision to proceed with surgery must be carefully considered. Also, the duration of surgery increases the incidence of cardiac death in patients with concomitant CHD. Coronary artery revascularization, therefore, is preferred in some patients prior to surgery for AAA.

VALVULAR HEART DISEASE

AORTIC STENOSIS

Severe aortic stenosis is a contraindication to elective surgery. It is usually not difficult to determine whether the murmur indicates severe aortic stenosis. In patients over age 50, more than 90% of aortic systolic murmurs are due to calcific aortic sclerosis, less than 2% are due to significant stenosis, and less than 1% are due to severe stenosis. When stenosis occurs in this category of patients, however, the progression can be quite rapid over months (see Chapter 12). Severe stenosis due to bicuspid and rheumatic valvular disease, and rarely aortic sclerosis, nearly always causes one or more of the following cardinal symptoms or signs

- Dyspnea on moderate activity
- Exertional presyncope or syncope
- Chest pain
- A loud harsh ejection systolic murmur over the aortic area that radiates into the neck, except when cardiac output is low
- Delayed carotid upstroke, a useful sign in patients under age 65
- Decrease or loss of the second heart sound in the second left interspace or over the right carotid artery
- Clinical and/or electrocardiographic LV hypertrophy

If two of these cardinal features are present, surgery should be postponed pending the result of Doppler flow echocardiography. The mean Doppler gradient correlates well with the mean gradient obtained by catheterization; some laboratories report the maximal instantaneous gradient, which tends to be slightly higher than the aortic peak gradient obtained at catheterization.

Symptomatic patients with severe aortic stenosis, valve area less than $0.7 \text{ cm}^2/\text{m}^2$, should undergo valve replacement prior to elective noncardiac surgery. In patients with moderate stenosis, valve area 0.8 to $1.2 \text{ cm}^2/\text{m}^2$, the type of surgery and risks must be individualized (see Chapter 12).

The vast majority of patients with aortic sclerosis and mild aortic stenosis present no problems during surgery. Antibiotic prophylaxis is advised for patients with aortic valve disease.

AORTIC PROSTHETIC HEART VALVE

Discontinue anticoagulants 3 days prior so that the prothrombin time reaches 20% of control, or reverse the prothrombin time with fresh frozen plasma and vitamin K. Anticoagulants can be recommenced on the second postoperative day. The discontinuation of anticoagulants for surgery carries a risk of thromboembolism and coverage with heparin may be required depending on the extent of the delay in the resumption of oral anticoagulants. Antibiotic coverage is necessary for all procedures (see Chapter 9).

MITRAL VALVE DISEASE

Critical mitral stenosis is fortunately rare, and elective surgery is postponed until valvotomy has been performed. Symptoms and signs are detailed in Chapter 12. Mitral regurgitation of all grades is usually well tolerated, except if heart failure is present.

Following discontinuation of oral anticoagulants, vitamin K is given 36 hours prior to surgery if the atrial size is greater than 5 cm and if there is a previous history of thromboembolism. It is advisable to switch to IV heparin, and when the prothrombin time is less than 1.25 times the control, oral anticoagulants can be discontinued. Heparin is discontinued 6 hours preoperatively and cautiously recommenced 12 to 24 hours postoperatively, followed by oral anticoagulation. A 2-day overlap with heparin, until the prothrombin time or INR is at the desired range for 2 days, is advisable (see Chapter 11 for anticoagulant control). Patients with mitral valve disease and atrial fibrillation are at high risk for systemic embolism during the postoperative period.

HYPERTROPHIC CARDIOMYOPATHY

Approximately 33% of patients with hypertrophic cardiomyopathy (HCM) have a significant resting outflow tract gradient and an additional 33% obtain a gradient on provocation (see Chapter 14).

More than 80% of the stroke output occurs before the mitral valve impinges on the hypertrophied septum, producing a pressure gradient. This gradient is increased by hypovolemia or hypotension as well as by preload-reducing agents such as nitrates which should be avoided. General anesthesia is safe in most patients with HCM. Spinal anesthesia appears to increase the operative risk because of associated hypotension.

ANTIBIOTIC PROPHYLAXIS FOR VALVULAR HEART DISEASE

Patients with prosthetic heart valves require antibiotic coverage for all procedures. All patients with valvular heart disease should receive coverage for dental and surgical procedures (except for a few procedures listed in Chapter 9). Mitral valve prolapse manifested by a murmur or click needs coverage because the murmur may be intermittent.

ARRHYTHMIAS

SUPRAVENTRICULAR

Patients with atrial fibrillation should be digitalized to control the ventricular response. The apical rate should remain between 70 to 90 and should not exceed 110 if the patient is walked down a 200-foot corridor or one flight of stairs.

PSVT is managed with digoxin or beta blockers. If SVT occurs during surgery, it can be controlled with short-acting esmolol, metoprolol, or with IV propranolol 1 mg given over 2 minutes. The IV dosage of beta-adrenergic blockers is given in Tables 2–8 and 3–4. Verapamil should be avoided because of its negative inotropic effect, but it can be used in patients with good LV function. Adenosine, which has a half-life of less than 10 seconds, is as effective as verapamil, does not depress cardiac contractility, and is preferred in patients with LV dysfunction but must be avoided in patients with active ischemia (see Chapter 6).

VENTRICULAR

Frequent multiform VPCs or ventricular tachycardia should be managed with lidocaine IV bolus (50 to 100 mg) and IV infusion (2 to 3 mg/min) (see Tables 3–8 and 3–9). Procainamide is rarely required for VT (see Fig. 6–4).

PACEMAKERS

Mobitz Type 1 AV block does not require pacing. Right bundle branch block with left anterior hemiblock or Mobitz Type 1 AV block does not require temporary pacing. An external transthoracic pacer should be available (see Chapter 18).

Mobitz Type 2, complete AV block, or significant sinus pauses require temporary pacing prior to emergency or elective surgery.

Electrocautery interference may transiently inhibit the output of implanted pulse generators despite electric shielding of the pacemaker. This is rare with the bipolar connections of newer pulse generators, however. A magnet should be available in the operating room to convert the pacing system, if necessary. The surgeon is advised to use the cautery in short 2- to 3-second bursts and to keep the equipment as far from the thorax as possible. The carotid and radial pulses must be monitored, because electrosurgery interferes with the ECG.

COR PULMONALE

Cor pulmonale carries a major risk since these patients have significant hypoxemia, with PaO_2 less than 55 mm Hg $PaCO_2$ greater than 45 mm Hg; the FEV_1 is commonly less than 30 (Chapter 19). These findings contraindicate elective surgery under general anesthesia and pose problems for emergency life-threatening conditions. If emergency surgery is absolutely necessary, hemodynamic monitoring, optimization of respiratory medications, and ventilatory support in the ICU setting is often necessary for days to weeks (see Chapters 22 and 29).

STRATEGIES FOR PREVENTION

There are no formulated strategies directed at prevention of postoperative fatal or nonfatal infarction. Some of the following steps are of proven value and some, although rational, must be tested by properly designed clinical trials. Table 17–5 gives factors that decrease the risk of cardiac events in high-risk patients undergoing elective surgery.

Consider the following

- CABS helps reduce morbidity and mortality in categories 1 to 5 given in Table 17–3 but does carry its own risks, so individual decisions must be made. There is adequate proof from clinical trials that CABS patients usually undergo noncardiac surgery without significant complications. Coronary balloon angioplasty may provide similar protection but requires documentation in clinical trials
- Exercise stress test or dipyridamole-thallium scintigraphy is of proven value in selecting patients for coronary angiography with a view to coronary angioplasty or CABS
- The preoperative and perioperative use of a beta-blocking agent (and for at least 1 week postoperative) may decrease morbidity and mortality, especially because the ischemic complications largely are mediated by

sympathetic stimulation and catecholamines. Beta blockade is known to have a salutary effect and lifesaving potential in patients with CHD where ischemia is provoked by catecholamines (see Fig. 2-7 and Chapter 2).

- Nitrates administered 1 hour preoperative and postoperative for 4 to 5 days, although unproven to decrease postoperative cardiac events, are advisable in patients at high risk. Transdermal nitroglycerin is used continuously for 2 or 3 days. It is then advisable to skip 10 to 12 hours daily to avoid tolerance unless, in doing so, ischemic symptoms appear (see Chapter 2, Unstable Angina).

Detection and prevention of silent ischemia is still in its infancy in terms of management. Silent ischemia is observed in the pre-, peri-, and postoperative period in approximately 70 and 84% of cardiac patients undergoing noncardiac surgery. In two reported studies indicating a high incidence of silent ischemia during the second to fourth postoperative days, however, the incidence of cardiac events was low (1 to 1.4% fatal infarction, 3 and 1.5% nonfatal infarction, 4 and 6.6% heart failure). Holter monitoring up to 4 days postoperative as well as being technically difficult for ST segment monitoring, therefore, is not cost effective.

The following steps may prove rewarding

- The combination of low-dose aspirin and a beta blocking drug carries the best chance of preventing fatal or nonfatal reinfarction during the postoperative period
- Aspirin (80 mg) or half of a regular aspirin given a few hours preoperative or 12 to 24 hours postoperative then 160 mg daily for 2 weeks is advisable in patients at high risk for fatal or nonfatal infarction. As well, the incidence of thromboembolism is moderately reduced by postoperative aspirin therapy in some categories of surgical patients. It is unlikely that a small dose of 80 mg of aspirin will significantly increase postoperative bleeding, but this agent must be avoided in opthalmic surgery
- Allopurinol has been shown to have a beneficial effect in the prevention of perioperative infarction in patients undergoing CABS
- Importantly, since acute MI in the postoperative phase is silent in over 60% of cases, no therapy can be given for unrecognized silent disease. Thus, aspirin plus a beta blocker seems advisable for high-risk patients undergoing surgery
- If MI is detected postoperatively, thrombolytic agents are contraindicated
- Aspirin (80 to 162 mg) and allopurinol, however, must be tested in randomized clinical trials before recommendation concerning widespread use can be endorsed

BIBLIOGRAPHY

Deron SJ, Kotler MN: Noncardiac surgery in the cardiac patient. Am Heart J, *116*:831, 1988.
Erbel R: Transesophageal echocardiography. Circulation, *83*:339, 1991.
Johnson WD, Kayser KL, Brenowitz JB, et al.: A randomized controlled trial of allopurinol in coronary bypass surgery. Am Heart J, *121*:20, 1991.

Mangano DT, Browner WS, Hollenberg M, et al.: Association of perioperative myocardial ischemia with cardiac morbidity and mortality in men underoing noncardiac surgery. N Engl J Med, 323:1781, 1990.

Mangano DT, Hollenberg M, Fegert G, et al.: Perioperative myocardial ischemia in patients underoing noncardiac surgery - I: Incidence and severity during the 4 day perioperative period. J Am Coll Cardiol, 17:843, 1991.

Prohost GM: Dipyridamole thallium test. Circulation, 84:931, 1991.

Ranhosky A, Kempthorne-Rawson J, et al.: The safety of intravenous dipyridamole thallium myocardial perfusion imaging. Circulation, 81:1205, 1990.

Shaw L, Chaitman BR, Hilton TC, et al.: Prognostic value of dipyridamole thallium-201 imaging in elderly patients. J Am Coll Cardiol, 19:1390, 1992.

Younis LT, Aguirre F, Byers S, et al.: Perioperative and long-term prognostic value of intravenous dipyridamole thallium scintigraphy in patients with peripheral vascular disease. Am Heart J, 119:1287, 1990.

18

NONPHARMACOLOGIC THERAPY FOR CARDIAC ARRHYTHMIAS: CARDIAC PACING, IMPLANTABLE CARDIOVERTER-DEFIBRILLATORS, CATHETER AND SURGICAL ABLATION

Davendra Mehta
Sanjeev Saksena

Cardiac pacing is used for the treatment of bradyarrhythmias both on a temporary and a permanent basis. Nonpharmacologic methods of management of tachyarrhythmias include catheter and surgical ablation and implantation of devices. In the following sections, management of various brady- and tachyarrhythmias using device and ablation therapy is discussed.

TEMPORARY CARDIAC PACING

INDICATIONS

The use of a temporary cardiac pacemaker is an important procedure for establishing an adequate heart rate and, secondarily, cardiac output in patients with symptoms of bradyarrhythmia. It is usually an emergent procedure and, thus, is an important therapy available to emergency room physicians and cardiologists. The subsequent need for permanent pacing in a particular patient is based on whether the rhythm disturbance is a) temporary or permanent and b) on the severity of associated symptoms. Temporary pacing is indicated in a variety of clinical circumstances in which a symptomatic bradycardia is present or is likely to occur. These can include the following

• Acute myocardial infarction (MI)
• Drug-induced bradyarrhythmias
• During cardiac catheterization
• Immediate treatment of tachyarrhythmia

ACUTE MYOCARDIAL INFARCTION

The use of temporary cardiac pacemakers in patients with acute MI is best understood when the basis of vascular supply of the conduction system of the heart is considered.

The sinoatrial node, which is located near the junction of the right atrium and the superior vena cava, is supplied by the sinoatrial nodal artery. This is a branch of the right coronary artery in 55% of individuals and of the circumflex artery in the remainder. The atrioventricular (AV) node is supplied by the AV nodal branch of the right coronary artery in approximately 90% of individuals, and by the left circumflex coronary artery in the remaining 10%. There is very little collateral blood supply for these structures. In contrast, the His bundle and proximal portions of both the left and right bundles have a dual blood supply from the AV nodal artery and the septal branch of the left anterior descending coronary artery. This anastomosis can allow retrograde flow into the His bundle and the AV node when the AV nodal artery is blocked. The right bundle branch, however, is a compact structure and receives blood supply from the left anterior descending artery. The left bundle branch is anatomically less discrete. The left anterior fascicle receives blood supply from the branches of the left anterior descending artery and the left posterior fascicle receives blood from the AV nodal and posterior descending arteries.

Conduction disturbances associated with right coronary artery occlusion depend on the site of occlusion. Occlusion proximal to the sinoatrial nodal artery can result in sinus node dysfunction, while occlusion more distally can result in AV block at the level of AV node. Therefore, AV block might result from occlusion of the AV nodal branch of the right coronary artery alone and is not necessarily associated with a sizable MI. Since the bundle branches are more diffuse, bundle branch block is usually associated with extensive anterior MI.

The decision to insert a temporary pacemaker in patients with acute MI is dependent on the location of the block, the extent of MI, and the presence of preexisting conduction system presence. Inferior infarction is usually associated with conduction disturbances proximal to the His bundle. Escape rhythms usually have a narrow QRS complex, tend to be fast and stable, and respond well to atropine. AV block in these situations is usually transient. Indications for temporary pacing in these patients include a heart rate of less than 40 beats/minute and symptoms of low cardiac output or bradycardia associated with angina or ventricular irritability. In asymptomatic patients with a stable escape rhythm despite complete AV block, temporary pacemakers need not be inserted. However, the longterm prognosis of patients with inferior MI and high-degree AV block is worse than in patients without AV block.

New abnormalities of the conduction system distal to the AV node are usually seen with anterior MI. Both high-degree AV block and bundle branch blocks can be observed. In these cases, the escape rhythms are associated with a wide QRS complex, are slower and less stable, and usually do not respond to atropine. Frequently, they progress to complete AV block. These patients also have extensive MI and often have signs of pump failure. As progression to complete AV block contributes independently to morbidity and mortality, temporary cardiac pacing is performed more promptly than for inferior wall infarction. Pacing is recommended in patients who are at risk of complete AV block and include

- Type II second-degree AV block
- New bifascicular block (right bundle branch block with left anterior or left posterior block) or complete left bundle branch block
- Left or right bundle branch block with first- or second-degree AV block
- Alternating left or right bundle branch block
- Preexisting right bundle branch block with new left fascicular block or first-degree AV block

DRUG-INDUCED BRADYARRHYTHMIAS

Antiarrhythmic drugs, beta blocking agents, clonidine, calcium channel blocking agents, digoxin, methyldopa, reserpine, and parasympathomimetic agents can lead to bradycardia as a result of sinus node dysfunction, sinus arrest, sinus exit block, and AV nodal block at toxic levels. These arrhythmias may occur even at low or therapeutic levels as a result of idiosyncratic reaction or if the conduction system is previously diseased. Temporary cardiac pacing is indicated in these conditions for the duration of drug effects or until the drug effects are counteracted. If longterm therapy with these agents is needed, as in the case of some antiarrhythmic agents for ventricular arrhythmias, permanent cardiac pacing is indicated.

Temporary cardiac pacing is also indicated for immediate management of torsades de pointes or arrhythmias related to prolonged QT interval, which can be drug induced or drug exacerbated. Pacing has been demonstrated to reduce temporal dispersion of repolarization in this situation. Temporary overdrive pacing is used until reversible factors such as electrolyte imbalance or toxic drug levels have been corrected or permanent pacemaker insertion has been carried out. Overdrive pacing of the atrium or the ventricle has been shown to be effective and is the treatment of choice for management of these patients.

DURING CARDIAC CATHETERIZATION

Temporary cardiac pacing is used prophylactically in the cardiac catheterization laboratory when there is a risk of complete AV block during the procedure. In patients with preexisting left bundle branch block, right heart catheterization can result in transient complete AV block. Thus, it is advisable to insert a temporary pacemaker prior to the procedure. Significant bradycardia and asystole can occur during injection of radiopaque dye into the right coronary artery. This risk is small in patients with a normal conduction system but may be higher in patients with preexisting sinoatrial or conduction system disease. Thus, prophylactic temporary pacing is recommended in the latter group. Prophylactic temporary cardiac pacemakers are inserted in all patients undergoing coronary angioplasty, because there is a significant risk of symptomatic bradycardia during balloon inflation in the right or circumflex coronary arteries.

MANAGEMENT OF TACHYCARDIAS

The use of temporary cardiac pacing in patients with tachyarrhythmias can be diagnostic or therapeutic. Simultaneous recording of the surface electrocardiogram and the atrial activity using a temporary pacing electrode is useful in studying AV relationships. Such recordings are also useful in diagnosing broad complex tachycardia. Ventriculoatrial (VA) dissociation suggests the diagnosis of ventricular tachycardia (Fig. 18-1). One-to-one VA relationship suggests the diagnosis of supraventricular arrhythmia with aberration or pre-excitation but might also be seen in ventricular tachycardia when associated with 1:1 retrograde conduction. Recording of atrial activity is also helpful in patients with other supraventricular arrhythmias, e.g., recording atrial rates of 250 to 300 beats/minute, establishes diagnosis of atrial flutter, and in atrial fibrillation, fibrillating activity can be identified.

Electrical stimulation using temporary pacemakers might be helpful in terminating a wide range of tachycardias, including atrial flutter, sinoatrial,

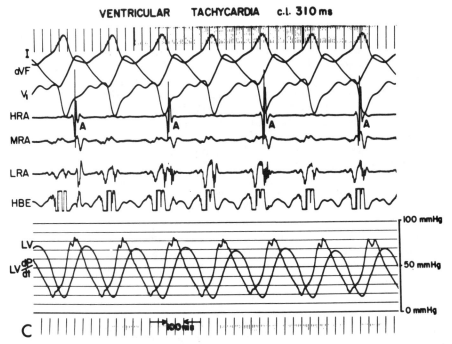

FIG. 18–1. Three lead surface electrocardiogram, atrial and ventricular electrograms, and blood pressure recordings in a patient with broad complex tachycardia. There is complete dissociation between atrial (HRA = high right atrial; MRA = mid right atrial) and ventricular electrogram as seen on His-bundle recording (HBE). This confirms the diagnosis as ventricular tachycardia. Reproduced with permission from: Saksena S, Ciccone J, Craelius W, et al.: Studies on left ventricular function during sustained ventricular tachycardia. J Am Coll Cardiol, 4:501–508, 1984.

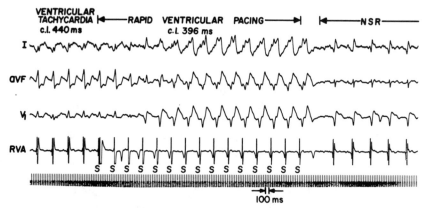

FIG. 18–2. Termination of ventricular tachycardia (cycle length 440 ms) by overdrive ventricular pacing (cycle length 396 ms). First four complexes of the illustration represent ventricular tachycardia, followed by 15 beats of overdrive pacing at the right ventricular apex. Sinus rhythm ensues after termination of overdrive pacing. RVA = electrogram from the right ventricular apex. Reproduced with permission from: Saksena S, Chandran P, Shah Y, et al.: Comparative efficacy of transvenous cardioversion and pacing in patients with sustained ventricular tachycardia. Circulation, 772:153–160, 1985.

AV nodal, and AV reentrant tachycardias, and at times, sustained ventricular tachycardias (Fig. 18-2). Atrial or ventricular fibrillation cannot be terminated by pacing. Pacing is used if the catheter is already in place or if drug therapy is ineffective and recurrent cardioversions are necessary due to frequent arrhythmia recurrence. Pacing at a rate slightly faster than the tachycardia (overdrive pacing) can terminate atrial flutter, AV reentry, and ventricular tachycardias. Timed premature beats or pacing at rates slower than the tachycardia (underdrive pacing) can terminate reciprocating AV reentrant and ventricular tachycardias.

In addition to terminating tachyarrhythmias, pacing can prevent tachyarrhythmias that are bradycardia dependent or those associated with prolonged QT interval (Fig. 18-3). In patients with frequent ventricular premature beats associated with sinus bradycardia, pacing at a rate 10 to 25% faster than the spontaneous rate can help reduce the frequency of ventricular premature beats. Atrial pacing can be used to convert a hemodynamically unstable atrial tachyarrhythmia such as atrial flutter to a hemodynamically more favorable arrhythmia such as atrial fibrillation, in which concealed conduction results in a better control of the ventricular response.

Although in most instances temporary cardiac pacing is performed in the right ventricle, atrial and dual chamber temporary cardiac pacemakers can be indicated in the following situations.

Temporary Atrial Pacemakers

Atrial pacing can prove to be a better choice in the following conditions
• Sinus node dysfunction without AV block
• Overdrive pacing for atrial and junctional tachycardias

L.D.
69
MVP

1. CONTROL

VENTRICULAR TACHYCARDIA : c.l.- 520 msec.

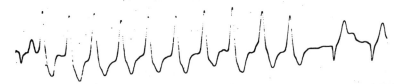

2. ORAL VERAPAMIL

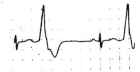

3. ATRIAL PACING

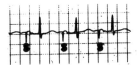

FIG. 18-3. Suppression of frequent ventricular premature beats and nonsustained ventricular tachycardia by overdrive atrial pacing. 1 and 2) Runs of nonsustained ventricular tachycardia (cycle length 520 ms) that are partially suppressed by oral verapamil leading to ventricular bigemeny. 3) Atrial pacing at 72 beats per minute leads to total suppression of ventricular arrhythmia. Reproduced with permission from: Goldschlager N, Saksena S: Hemodynamic effects of cardiac pacing. *In* Electrical Therapy for Cardiac Arrhythmias: Pacing Anti-Tachycardia Devices, Catheter Ablation. Edited by: Saksena S, Goldschlager N. Philadelphia, W.B. Saunders, 1990, p 168.

- Differential diagnosis of broad complex tachycardia
- Drug-induced sinus bradycardia
- Spontaneous or drug-induced prolonged QT interval and ventricular arrhythmias

Temporary Dual Chamber Pacing

- Patients with noncompliant ventricles who need temporary pacing
- Sizable acute MI (especially right ventricular infarction) and AV block
- To assess the efficacy of a permanent dual chamber pacemaker, in a trial by measuring blood pressure and cardiac output in ventricular and dual chamber pacing modes
- In patients who need temporary pacemakers for bradycardia or poor hemodynamic status in the immediate postoperative period

METHODS OF TEMPORARY CARDIAC PACING

Temporary cardiac pacing can be established by transvenous, transthoracic, transesophageal, and epicardial approaches. The choice of a specific route is dependent on factors such as availability of the device, indications for pacing, expertise of the physician, and the clinical situation. The transvenous approach is the most often used method.

TRANSVENOUS

External or internal jugular, subclavian, antecubital, and femoral venous approaches are most often used for introduction of pacing catheter electrodes. Under radiographic control, the electrode tip is positioned in the right atrial appendage or the right ventricular apex for stable atrial and ventricular pacing, respectively. In an emergency or in the absence of radiological facilities, a balloon-tipped flotation electrode catheter can be used to enter the right ventricle. A pacing threshold of < 1 V is usually satisfactory. It increases over the following few days, probably due to tissue edema around the electrode tip. Although invasive when compared to transthoracic and transesophageal approaches, transvenous pacing is rapidly accomplished and is reliable when instituted. Atrial, ventricular, and dual chamber pacing can be achieved, and atrial and ventricular electrocardiograms can be selectively recorded for diagnostic purposes. Once initiated, it causes little patient discomfort and is thus ideal for prolonged use. Complications include ventricular arrhythmias, especially in patients with acute MI, pericarditis, ventricular perforation, bleeding, pulmonary embolism, air embolism, pneumothorax when the subclavian vein is used for lead introduction, and local and systemic infections.

TRANSTHORACIC

This was the first modality to be used for temporary pacing. Gel patches are applied on the chest, one over the anterior precordium and the other over the lower part of the left scapula. These are connected to an external stimulator. It can be rapidly instituted but causes significant discomfort to conscious patients and is thus not ideal for prolonged use. Furthermore, it cannot be used for atrial pacing. This mode is only used in an emergency situation before a temporary transvenous pacemaker can be inserted.

TRANSESOPHAGEAL

The pacing electrode, often mounted within a soluble capsule, is swallowed by the patient. It is positioned such that atrial capture is obtained. The pulse generator used for transvenous pacing cannot be used for esophageal pacing, because longer pulse duration stimuli (up to 10 ms) with output ranging from 10 to 30 mA are required for capture. This method does allow for an easy and noninvasive approach for atrial pacing. Selective ventricular capture can be obtained in only 5 to 6% of cases. Thus, it is not recommended for pacing in patients with AV block. Its current use is mainly in the diagnosis and treatment of cardiac arrhythmias, particularly in the pediatric age group, for the following purposes

- Record atrial activity for diagnosis of broad complex tachycardia
- Diagnose sinus tachycardia and atrial flutter
- Diagnose accessory bypass tracts by unmasking pre-excitation
- Test sinoatrial and AV nodal function
- Initiate and terminate supraventricular tachycardias and serially test the efficacy of antiarrhythmic drugs
- Document ventriculoatrial (VA) conduction in patients with permanent pacemakers and symptoms suggestive of pacemaker syndrome

Complications are uncommon, although most patients experience some epigastic or substernal discomfort during pacing. Because of its instability and discomfort, transesophageal pacing is not reliable for bradycardia support.

EPICARDIAL

Temporary epicardial atrial and ventricular pacing is used during and after cardiac surgery. Teflon-coated stainless steel wires with bared tips are sutured to the epicardium and brought to the surface to be used for sensing and pacing. In the postoperative period, these can be removed by gentle traction. They are very useful in the diagnosis and management of postoperative arrhythmias. The use of atrial electrodes in addition to the ventricular wires has been increasingly stressed, because the atrial electrodes are helpful in the diagnosis of supraventricular tachycardia and in differentiation of sinus tachycardia, atrial flutter, ectopic atrial tachycardia, and ventricular tachycardias. Epicardial AV sequential pacing can be used to improve hemodynamic status in patients with poor cardiac output and "relative bradycardia," i.e., heart rate not slow enough to be defined as bradycardia by classical definitions but inappropriately low to maintain cardiac output for increased postoperative needs. These leads can also be used for tachycardia termination. Atrial flutter can be terminated by rapid pacing by continuous or burst pacing 10 to 40 beats/minute faster than the flutter rate. Similarly, ventricular tachycardia can be terminated by bursts of rapid ventricular pacing. Postoperative electrophysiologic testing can be performed using these leads and largely replicates the endocardial approach.

PERMANENT CARDIAC PACING

INDICATIONS

Permanent cardiac pacemakers have undergone a rapid technologic evolution since they were first introduced in the 1960s for the treatment of Stokes–Adams attacks due to AV block. Many options in pacemaker therapy are now available and, consequently, the indications for their use have greatly expanded. The type of pacemaker used for a particular patient can be chosen with regard to the specific indication for cardiac pacing, including the underlying rhythm disturbance and the heart disease. Current indications for permanent pacemakers have been divided into specific widely accepted categories

- Class 1 indications: Conditions in which a permanent pacemaker must be implanted, provided the condition is chronic or recurrent and not due to transient causes such as acute MI, electrolyte imbalance, or drug toxicity
- Class 2 indications: Conditions in which pacemakers are frequently used, but there may be differences in opinion among experts with respect to their use for these conditions
- Class 3 indications: Conditions for which there is general agreement that pacemaker therapy is not indicated

The specific conditions included in these classes are further elucidated below.

CLASS 1

- Acquired, symptomatic, chronic, or intermittent complete AV block
- Congenital complete AV block with significant bradycardia or symptoms due to bradycardia
- Symptomatic advanced (type II) second-degree AV block
- Bifascicular or trifascicular block with intermittent type II second-degree AV block, even without symptoms directly attributable to the AV block
- Symptomatic (syncope, seizures, heart failure, dizziness, or confusion) sinus bradycardia. It must be documented that the symptoms are directly related to bradycardia
- Drug-induced symptomatic sinus bradycardia, when there is no acceptable alternative to longterm use of drug therapy
- Sinus node dysfunction: This category includes tachycardia–bradycardia syndrome, sinoatrial block, and sinus arrest
- Potentially life-threatening ventricular arrhythmias secondary to bradycardia with or without symptoms
- Carotid sinus hypersensitivity with recurrent syncope associated with spontaneous events (like neck movements) provoking carotid sinus stimulation, or if carotid sinus pressure induces asystole of > 3 seconds duration in the absence of any mediation that depresses the sinus or AV node

CLASS 2

- Asymptomatic acquired complete AV block (permanent or intermittent) with ventricular rate of ≥ 40 beats/minute
- Asymptomatic type II second-degree AV block
- Bifascicular or trifascicular block with syncope that is not proven to be due to intermittent complete AV block, but other causes of syncope have been excluded
- Congenital complete AV block with bradycardia but no symptoms

- Sinus node dysfunction with a heart rate of < 40 beats/minute, but there is no clearly documented association between symptoms consistent with bradycardia and the actual occurrence of bradycardia
- Recurrent syncope without clear, provocative events and a hypersensitive cardioinhibitory carotid sinus response
- Overdrive pacing to prevent ventricular arrhythmias in patients with recurrent ventricular tachycardia

CLASS 3

- First-degree or asymptomatic type I second-degree AV block
- Fascicular block with first-degree AV block without symptoms suggestive of intermittent high-degree AV block
- Sinus bradycardia or sinoatrial block without significant symptoms
- Asymptomatic sinus bradycardia, including those in whom substantial sinus bradycardia (heart rate < 40 beats/minute) is a consequence of long-term drug treatment, which can be withdrawn or modified
- Hypersensitive cardioinhibitory response to carotid sinus stimulation in the absence of symptoms
- Recurrent syncope of undetermined cause, in the absence of a cardioinhibitory response

SPECIFIC CONDITIONS

DISORDERS OF ATRIOVENTRICULAR CONDUCTION

First-Degree Atrioventricular Block

The PR interval comprises the sinoatrial, intra-atrial, AV nodal, His Bundle, and His-Purkinje conduction intervals. The clinical significance of solitary prolongation of the PR interval is dependent on the site of conduction delay and on the underlying cardiac condition. Isolated prolongation of PR interval, in most instances, is due to delayed conduction at the level of AV node as a result of enhanced vagal tone or drug therapy (digitalis, beta blockers, or calcium antagonists). It is generally a benign condition and is not an indication for permanent pacemaker therapy because it usually does not progress to symptomatic advanced AV block. However, first-degree AV block associated with either left or right bundle branch block, particularly of recent onset, usually reflects the presence of infra-His conduction delay. This is an indication for implantation of a permanent pacemaker, especially when associated with symptoms or intermittent complete AV block.

Second-Degree Atrioventricular Block

Type I second-degree AV block is most often observed in the setting of acute MI, after drug therapy (digitalis, beta blockers, and calcium blockers), or when high vagal tone is present, as in trained athletes (Fig. 18-4A). It has also been reported in hypervagotonia related to specific maneuvers

488

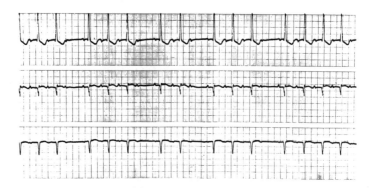

A. TYPE I SYNCOPE 2ND DEGREE AV BLOCK

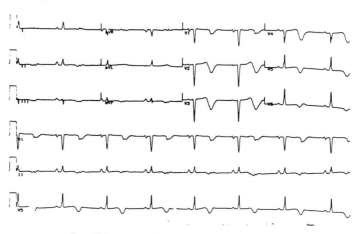

B. TYPE II 2ND DEGREE AV BLOCK

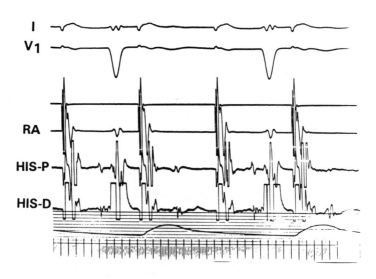

C. INFRA-HIS BLOCK DURING ATRIAL PACING

such as swallowing, deglutition, yawning, and micturition. Its prognostic significance is dependent on coexisting symptoms and heart disease. It is, most often, benign in nature. Isolated asymptomatic type I second-degree AV block does not warrant insertion of a permanent cardiac pacemaker. When associated with drug refractory hypervagotonia and resulting in serious symptoms such as syncope, permanent cardiac pacing is indicated.

Type II second-degree AV block usually indicates the presence of conduction system disease beyond the AV node (Figs. 18-4B and 18-4C). It is often due to isolated degenerative conduction system diseases but can be seen with regional or diffuse myocardial disease or acute MI. During acute MI, it may precede complete AV block. Type II second-degree AV block unrelated to antiarrhythmic drug therapy is considered an indication for permanent cardiac pacing. The natural history of this bradyarrhythmia, even in initially asymptomatic individuals, is progression to severe bradycardia and related symptoms.

Complete (Third-Degree) Atrioventricular Block

Symptomatic advanced or complete AV block is considered an indication for implantation of a permanent pacemaker, particularly when due to infranodal disease. Third-degree AV nodal block can, at times, be asymptomatic, transient, or due to reversible factors. If stable or obviously reversible, permanent pacing can be deferred unless symptoms develop. There is a continuing debate about timing of pacemaker implantation in asymptomatic individuals with chronic stable complete AV block. The nature of escape rhythm is often helpful in making a decision. Junctional escape rhythms, which are associated with a relatively narrow QRS complex, are often stable over time and responsive to physiological demands (Fig. 18-5). Escape rhythms originating in Purkinje or ventricular tissues are identified by wide QRS complexes, are less stable, and tend to have slow attenuated rate responsiveness to catecholamine stimulation, hence, permanent pacing is recommended.

FIG. 18–4. Second-degree AV block. Panel A: Three lead electrocardiogram illustrating Type I second-degree/Wenckebach AV block. In an asymptomatic individual with this arrhythmia, permanent pacemaker is not indicated and a reversible cause should be eliminated. The level of block is usually above the His bundle. Panel B: Twelve lead electrocardiogram and a 3 lead (V_1, II, V5) rhythm strip of 2:1 Type II second-degree AV block. Alternate P waves superimpose T waves and are best seen in leads II and V_1. Permanent pacing is indicated as AV block in these patients and is usually below the level of His bundle. Panel C: Intracardiac recordings from the same patient with Type II second-degree AV block seen in Panel B illustrating 2:1 infra-His block during atrial pacing. I and V_1 = electrocardiographic leads; RA = right atrial electrogram with atrial pacing; HIS-P and HIS-D = proximal and distal His bundle electrograms, respectively. His bundle recording show all atrial, His, and ventricular electrograms. First paced atrial beat is followed by an His complex and a ventricular electrogram while the second is followed only by an His bundle deflection and no ventricular electrogram illustrating an infra-His block.

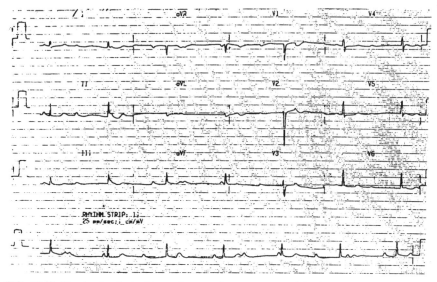

FIG. 18–5. Twelve lead electrocardiogram from a young girl with congenital complete heart (AV) block. The escape rhythm is high junctional and the QRS complexes are narrow. In this condition, permanent cardiac pacing is indicated only if the patient develops severe bradycardia or related symptoms.

Fascicular Blocks

There is considerable controversy concerning the rationale for permanent pacemaker therapy in patients with documented bifascicular and trifascicular block. Patients with advanced fascicular block and symptoms believed to be due to AV block have a high mortality largely due to a significant incidence of sudden death. It has also been shown that although pacing relieves transient symptoms like presyncope and syncope, it may not reduce the frequency of sudden death. One predictor of progression of advanced fascicular block to complete AV block is prolonged His to ventricular (HV) conduction interval. Patients with bifascicular block with a prolonged HV interval (> 80 ms) develop AV block more readily than patients who have a normal HV interval. In one study, the incidence of progression to second- and third-degree AV block over 30 months was 12% and 25% for those with HV intervals > 70 ms and 100 ms, respectively. In comparison, the patients with normal HV interval had a 3.5% incidence of AV block. HV prolongation usually accompanies advanced cardiac disease and is associated with increased sudden death rate, which may be related to the underlying heart disease. Implantation of permanent pacemakers has also not reduced mortality in symptomatic individuals with bundle branch block and electrophysiologic evidence of infranodal conduction delay. In patients with normal HV interval and bundle branch block, evaluating AV conduction after intravenous disopyramide or procainamide infusion has been suggested as a means to predict patients prone to subsequent AV block.

SINUS NODE DYSFUNCTION/SICK SINUS SYNDROME

The symptom complex of sinus bradycardia, sinus arrest, sinoatrial exit block, and/or paroxysmal atrial tachyarrhythmias is often referred to as "sick sinus syndrome." One or more types of sinus nodal bradyarrhythmias and atrial flutter, atrial fibrillation, or atrial tachycardia can be present in the same patient. Symptoms in these patients can be related to the tachycardia, the bradycardia, or both, but are most often due to the sudden changes in heart rate involved in conversion from one rhythm to another. These patients usually present with palpitations, weakness, dizziness, and syncope. About one-third of patients with sick sinus syndrome have conduction abnormalities involving the AV node and the bundle branches.

Permanent pacemakers in patients with sick sinus syndrome are indicated in the presence of symptoms. Correlation of symptoms with a specific arrhythmia is essential, although this may be difficult in view of the intermittent nature of arrhythmias. Asymptomatic sinoatrial exit block, sinus bradycardia, and sinus pauses do not constitute an indication for permanent pacemaker therapy. There is disagreement about the absolute duration of the asystolic period that requires pacing. Sinus pauses of 3 seconds or sustained symptomatic sinus rates < 40 beats/minute in the awake patient are usually accepted as indications for permanent pacing. In such individuals prior to pacemaker implantation, it is essential to determine that symptoms are related to bradycardias before proceeding to pacemaker implantation. Electrophysiological evaluation of sinus node function is performed in patients who are asymptomatic during detailed noninvasive monitoring but has a low sensitivity. In North America, sick sinus syndrome accounts for 46% of all pacemaker implantations. Demand ventricular pacing has been performed widely for this condition. Demand atrial pacemakers are indicated for those patients with sick sinus syndrome who do not have any evidence of AV conduction abnormality. Peripheral embolization, atrial fibrillation, and congestive heart failure occur less frequently in patients with demand atrial pacemakers, as compared to those with demand ventricular pacemakers.

CAROTID SINUS HYPERSENSITIVITY

Mechanical stimulation of the carotid sinus region results in vagal stimulation with secondary sinus bradycardia and PR interval prolongation. In some patients, these responses are exaggerated. Hyperactive carotid sinus responses result in excessive bradycardia (cardioinhibitory response) (Fig. 18-6) and/or hypotension (vasodepressor response). Ventricular asystole of 3 seconds or a decrease in blood pressure to 30 to 50 mm Hg without heart rate changes, especially when associated with symptoms, is considered abnormal. The incidence of the cardioinhibitory type of carotid sinus hypersensitivity is substantially higher than that of the vasodepressor type. Clinically, symptoms of dizziness, presyncope, and syncope are often precipitated by a tight neck collar, neck rotation, or neck extension. In patients with symptomatic cardioinhibitory carotid sinus hypersensitivity, implantation of a permanent pacemaker is indicated. Permanent demand ven-

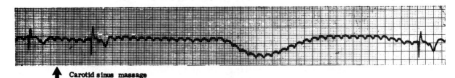

Atrial Flutter with Carotid Hypersensitivity:Pause of 8.2 seconds

↑ Carotid sinus massage

FIG. 18–6. Electrocardiographic lead V₁ demonstrating carotid sinus hypersensitivity in a patient with atrial flutter. Right carotid sinus massage resulted in ventricular asystole with a pause of 8.2 seconds.

tricular pacing usually eliminates symptoms in patients with cardioinhibitory carotid sinus hypersensitivity but does not often benefit vasodepressor carotid sinus hypersensitivity. The type of pacemaker recommended depends on frequency of symptoms. Occasional symptoms are best treated by demand ventricular pacemaker systems. Even in patients who show profound sinus bradycardia during carotid sinus massage, demand atrial pacemakers should not be used because of the high incidence of concomitant or late AV block. Dual chamber pacemakers are preferred for patients with frequent symptoms; this pacing mode has been shown to be associated with a lesser degree of decline in blood pressure and has been used as adjunctive therapy.

Mineralocorticoid therapy, denervation of the carotid sinus, and ephedrine administration have also been shown to be effective in selected patients with vasodepressor carotid sinus hypersensitivity.

PERMANENT PACING IN ACUTE MYOCARDIAL INFARCTION

The management of bradyarrhythmias related to conduction disturbances in acute MI is determined by the site of the culprit MI, hemodynamic consequences of the arrhythmia, and arrhythmia duration after acute MI. The requirement for temporary pacing does not, by itself, constitute an indication for permanent pacing.

Inferior Myocardial Infarction

Conduction disturbances are often seen in patients with acute inferior wall MI. These are due to ischemia of the AV node or the perinodal regions. Sinus node dysfunction may also occur. First-degree AV block and Mobitz I second-degree AV block, if present, are usually transient, unassociated with hemodynamic disturbances, and do not require pacing therapy. A minority of patients will develop higher degree or symptomatic AV block. Temporary pacing is indicated, particularly if the patient is hemodynamically unstable. If symptomatic second- or third-degree AV block persists beyond 2 to 3 weeks after MI, permanent pacemaking may be indicated.

Anterior Myocardial Infarction

Conduction disturbances in anterior MI are usually related to ischemic necrosis of conduction tissue distal to the AV node, with involvement of the His-Purkinje system and bundle branches. These arrhythmias most often accompany a relatively large anteroseptal MI. Permanent pacing is generally indicated for

• New onset bifascicular block
• Persistent Mobitz type II second-degree or complete AV block
• Transient Mobitz type II second-degree or complete AV block when associated bundle branch block (trifascicular block) is present

This is because of the substantial potential of these conduction disturbances for the development of complete AV block. Patients with anterior wall MI who have AV conduction and intraventricular conduction disturbances, except left anterior hemiblock, have a poor short- and longterm prognosis and an increased incidence of sudden death. The poor prognosis is primarily related to the extent of MI rather than to the AV block itself. Mortality is high even with pacemaker therapy due to myocardial failure.

TYPES OF PACEMAKERS

Permanent pacemakers can be classified on the basis of five characteristics

• The cardiac chamber paced by the device
• The chamber sensed by the device
• Device response to sensing
• Device programmability
• Additional functions

A five-position North American Society of Pacing and Electrophysiology/ British Pacing and Electrophysiology Group generic pacemaker code is used to describe pacemakers on the basis of the above features

• Position 1 in the code designates the chamber or chambers paced. (Symbols used in this position are O = none, A = atrium, V = ventricle, D = dual atrium and ventricle, S = single chamber for pacemakers that can be used in atrium or ventricle)
• Position 2 in the code designates the chamber sensed by the device. (Symbols O, A, V, and D are used, as in position 1)
• Position 3 in the code designates response to a sensed event. (Symbols used are O = none, T = triggered, I = inhibited, D = dual, i.e., triggered and inhibited)
• Position 4 in the code designates the degree of programmability and the presence of a rate modulation mechanism. (Symbols used are O = none, P = rate and output programmability, M = multiprogrammability, C = communicating, i.e., devices with telemetry, R = rate responsiveness)
• Position 5 in the code designates an antitachycardia function. (Symbols used indicate the mode of pacing used to terminate tachycardia and include B = burst, N = normal rate competition, S = scanning, E = external)

Generally, the first three or four positions are used, e.g., a VVIR pacemaker implies a pacemaker that paces and senses the ventricle, is inhibited by a sensed event, and has rate response function.

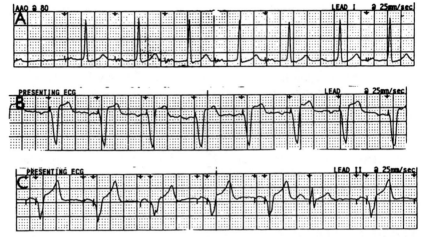

FIG. 18–7. Different modes of pacemaker function are shown. A) AOO–fixed rate atrial pacing. Note narrow paced QRS complexes in response to paced atrial beats. B) VDD–the pacemaker senses the atrium and the ventricle and paces the ventricle. Each spontaneous P wave is followed by a paced ventricular complex. C) DDD pacing–the pacemaker senses and paces in the atrium and the ventricle. The sixth complex of this strip represents a spontaneous P wave that conducts to the ventricle, resulting in a narrow QRS complex with the pacing spike occurring in the ventricular refractory period. Arrows indicate pacing stimulus artefacts.

The following pacing modes are currently used in different clinical situations.

AOO: Fixed rate (asynchronous) atrial pacing (Fig. 18-7A)

AAT: Triggered atrial pacing: output pulse delivered into P wave; paces atrium at a preset interval

AAI: Demand atrial pacing: output inhibited by sensed atrial signals

AAIR: AAI pacing with variable atrial pacing rate based on changes in metabolic demand

VOO: Fixed rate (asynchronous) ventricular pacing

VVT: Triggered ventricular pacing: output pulse delivered into R waves; paces ventricle at a preset escape interval

VVI: Demand ventricular pacing: output inhibited by sensed ventricular signal

VVIR: VVI pacing with sensor-based changes in pacing rates based on metabolic demand

DVI: Pacing in both atrium and ventricle; senses R waves only

DDI: AAI + VVI pacing; tracking of atrial rate by ventricular sensing does not occur

VDD: Paces in ventricle; senses both atrium and ventricle; synchronizes with atrial activity and paces ventricle after a preset AV interval (Fig. 18-7B)

DOO: Fixed rate (asynchronous) atrial and ventricular pacing at specific AV interval

DDD: Paces and senses both atrium and ventricle; synchronizes with atrial activity and paces ventricle after preset AV interval (Fig. 18-7C)

DDDR: DDD pacing with sensor-based increase or decrease in paced atrial and ventricular rates in response to changes in metabolic demand

Appropriate choice of the pacing mode in a particular rhythm disturbance is dependent on the underlying heart disease. A good knowledge of the physiology of the individual pacing modes and underlying heart disease helps in permitting knowledgeable selection of the pacemaker.

SPECIAL FUNCTIONS

Dual Chamber Pacemakers

A dual chamber pacemaker system utilizes both an atrial and a ventricular lead and maintains AV synchrony (Fig. 18-8). Since ventricular pacing results in loss of AV synchrony and can produce a lower cardiac output than sinus rhythm or atrial pacing at similar rates, dual chamber pacemakers are generally considered a more physiologic choice. They produce improved cardiac performance, which manifests as better exercise tolerance and improved subjective sense of well-being. Patients with reduced systolic function, impaired ventricular diastolic compliance, mitral or tricuspid valvular insufficiency, or congestive heart failure have a significantly higher cardiac output, with the maintenance of AV synchrony resulting from dual chamber pacing.

Dual chamber pacing is clinically indicated in conditions when preservation of AV synchrony is important for patient management. These include

• Occurrence of pacemaker syndrome following implantation of a ventricular pacemaker
• Anticipation of pacemaker syndrome after documentation of VA conduction and hypotension during ventricular pacing
• Vasopressor type of carotid sinus hypersensitivity
• Patients with impaired left ventricular function and cardiac failure, in whom dual chamber pacing is associated with a demonstrable higher cardiac output
• In patients with marked restriction of left ventricular filling due to left ventricular hypertrophy (including restrictive cardiomyopathies). In these conditions, the atrial contribution to left ventricular filling is substantial and essential to maintain cardiac output. Ventricular pacing can lead to congestive heart failure or hypotension

Pacemaker Syndrome

Some patients with or without normal ventricular function may experience symptoms with ventricular pacing. This includes dyspnea, cough, chest discomfort, abdominal or neck pulsations, abdominal distention, nausea,

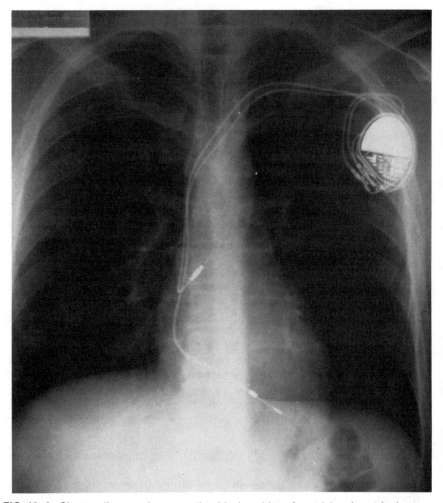

FIG. 18–8. Chest radiogram demonstrating ideal positions for atrial and ventricular cardiac leads in a patient with dual chamber pacemaker. Both atrial and ventricular leads are bipolar.

poor appetite, fatigue, poor stress tolerance, dizziness, and near syncope or frank syncope during ventricular pacing. This syndrome is referred to as "pacemaker syndrome" and is a result of loss of AV synchrony and/or retrograde VA conduction. It can be electrocardiographically documented by the presence of a retrograde P wave in the ST segment or T of the surface electrocardiographic leads II, III and a VF. This condition is often seen in patients with sinus node dysfunction who are treated with a ventricular pacemaker. At times, even patients with complete antegrade AV block can have preserved VA conduction. Diagnosis of pacemaker syndrome should always be considered when persistent or new symptoms suggestive of low cardiac output or heart failure occur after satisfactory implantation of a permanent ventricular pacemaker. Symptoms may be directly induced or exacerbated by pacing. A dual chamber pacemaker is the treatment of choice in patients with pacemaker syndrome. Maintenance of AV synchrony is important in these patients, as VA conduction causes hemodynamic derangements that raise atrial pressures and decreases cardiac output with associated symptoms (Figs. 18-9A and 18-9B).

Single chamber ventricular pacing is appropriate for patients with bradycardia associated with chronic atrial arrhythmias. However, in patients with paroxysmal atrial arrhythmias (atrial tachycardia, atrial flutter, and fibrillation), maintaining AV synchrony and preventing VA conduction have been shown to reduce the recurrence rate of atrial tachyarrhythmias.

Single chamber atrial pacing is indicated in patients with predominant sinus bradycardia and normal AV conduction. A normal resting PR interval and 1:1 AV conduction with an atrial pacing rate of 120 beats/minute are generally considered acceptable AV nodal conduction for this pacing mode. This mode is particularly useful in patients with bradycardias when the pacemaker is being implanted to prevent ventricular tachycardias, as in long QT syndrome.

Bipolar Pacemakers

In a unipolar pacemaker system, the pacemaker lead tip electrode is used as the cathode for the pacing stimulus, and the outer surface of the pulse generator casing is used as the anode. Bipolar pacemaker systems use leads carrying both the anodal and the cathodal electrodes in its distal end. These leads are thicker and stiffer than unipolar pacing leads. The outer casing of a bipolar pacemaker pulse generator is thus not a part of the pacing circuit. In a unipolar pacemaker system, the electric circuit includes the entire lead as well as the surface of the pacemaker unit and intervening tissue, which results in increased sensitivity to electromagnetic and physiologic signals originating from noncardiac sources, e.g., electrical cautery during surgery and thoracic muscle potentials. These signals can result in inappropriate inhibition or triggering of the pacemaker output, depending on the type of pulse generator. The large electrical circuit in unipolar systems produces a markedly larger stimulus artefact in the electrocardiogram when compared to bipolar pacemaker systems (Fig. 18-10). In addition, unipolar pacemakers, when in contact with thoracic muscles, can result in anodal stimulation and muscle twitching with each pacemaker impulse. This problem is not seen with bipolar pulse generators unless there is a disruption in lead insulation. Thus, bipolar pacemakers have distinct advantages over the unipolar units and, in due course of time, are likely to replace them in clinical practice.

Programmable Pacemakers

Programmable pacemakers have multiple parameters that can be reset noninvasively after surgical implantation with the use of an external programming device and a telemetric link with a wand. The majority of the pacemakers manufactured today have some degree of programmability.

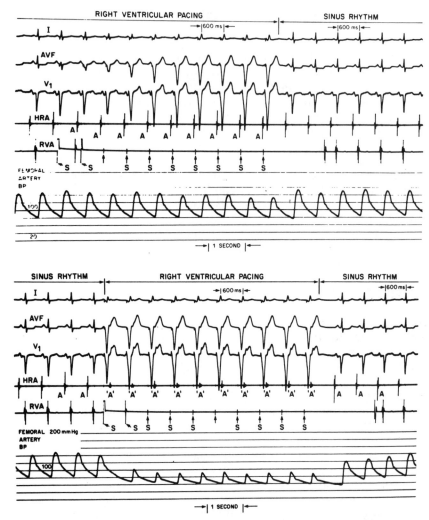

FIG. 18–9. Simultaneous electrocardiographic (leads I, AVF, and V₁), intracardiac (HRA = high right atrial; RVA = right ventricular apex) and femoral artery blood pressure recordings during ventricular pacing illustrating etiology of "pacemaker syndrome." A = the atrial electrogram in sinus rhythm; A′ = the retrograde atrial electrogram during ventricular pacing; S = the stimulus artefact. Panel A: Each ventricular paced beat is preceded by an atrial contraction, thus maintaining an antegrade and relatively normal AV relationship, and is associated with a near normal femoral artery blood pressure. Panel B: In this strip, atrial contraction is simultaneous with or immediately follows ventricular paced beats, as would occur in a patient with ventricular pacing and intact VA conduction. This altered relationship is associated with a marked fall in blood pressure as seen on femoral artery blood pressure recordings. Reproduced with permission from: Goldschlager N, Saksena S: Hemodynamic effects of cardiac pacing. *In* Electrical Therapy for Cardiac Arrhythmias: Pacing Anti-Tachycardia Devices, Catheter Ablation. Edited by: Saksena S, Goldschlager N. Philadelphia, W.B. Saunders, 1990, pp 169, 170.

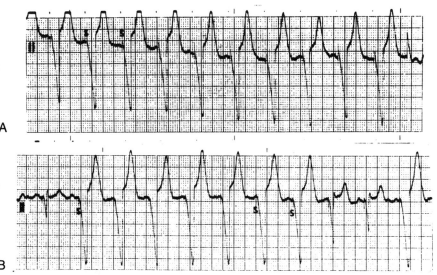

FIG. 18-10. Ventricular pacing during exercise in a patient with rate responsive pacemaker (VVIR). A) Pacemaker is programmed to unipolar pacing mode and is associated with a large stimulus artefact. B) In the same patient, programming the pacemaker to bipolar pacing mode and recording the same electrocardiographic lead results in a much smaller stimulus artefact.

Parameters that are commonly programmable include lower and upper rates of pacing (in dual chamber and rate responsive units), energy output, refractory period, sensitivity, mode of function (VVI, AAI, DDD, etc.), and delay between atrial and ventricular outputs. Optimal programming of pacemaker parameters based on lead thresholds and sensed electrogram can help in prolonging battery longevity, correcting sensing and pacing problems, and improving the functional capacity of the patient. Most pacemaker problems during follow-up can be treated by noninvasive reprogramming of device parameters. This reduces the need for surgical intervention during device follow-up, excepting for pulse generator replacement at the end of battery life.

Rate Responsive Pacemakers

A major limitation of single chamber demand pacemakers is the lack of ability to increase rate with exercise or increased metabolic demand. By tracking the atrial rate, dual chamber pacing systems are capable of providing changes in the heart rate as determined by the sinus node. However, a large proportion of patients requiring pacemakers have sinus node dysfunction or inadequate heart rate response to exercise or increased metabolic demand. Even in patients with AV block, the prevalence of sinus node dysfunction is high. Dual chamber devices are also unsuitable for patients with frequent atrial arrhythmias, which may then result in in-

TABLE 18–1. SENSORS FOR RATE RESPONSIVE PACEMAKERS (CLINICALLY RELEASED OR UNDER INVESTIGATION)

SENSOR	DEVICE
Ventricular repolarization Evoked QT interval (Stimulus T interval)*	Quintech (Vitatron)
Ventricular depolarization gradient	Prism (Telectronics)
Movement—Activity sensing Piezo-electric crystal*	Elite, Legend, Activitrax. (Medtronic)
Respiration Respiratory rate Minute ventilation*	Meta MV (Telectronics)
Central venous temperature*	Kelvin 500 (Cook)
Mixed venous oxygen gradient	
Myocardial contractility Rate of change of right ventricular pressure Right ventricular stroke volume Right ventricular pre-ejection period	Precept (CPI)
* Indicated the sensors in clinical use at present	

appropriate pacemaker-related tachycardias. Thus, in these patients, single chamber pacemakers that increase pacing rate in response to activity or increased metabolic demand (body movement, respiratory rate, temperature, oxygen saturation) are indicated (Fig. 18-10). A variety of sensors that modulate the pacing rate are being used clinically or are under evaluation (Table 18-1). Single chamber ventricular rate responsive pacemakers are usually indicated in patients with chronic atrial arrhythmias and sinus bradycardia, while atrial rate responsive pacemakers are used for patients with sinus node dysfunction and preserved AV conduction.

MANAGEMENT OF PACEMAKER MALFUNCTION

Systematic analysis of pacemaker problems is essential for appropriate management and is usually performed by personnel familiar with individual device function. Specialized pacemaker clinics are often required for complex device malfunction analysis. Most problems can often be diagnosed noninvasively using electrocardiograms (including Holter monitoring), radiological examination, and device telemetry. They can be treated using the programmable features of the device if there is ample understanding of the device capabilities and its lead system. While this is feasible in most instances, a small proportion of patient problems could be related to hardware failure (lead or device), in which case operative intervention is necessary. For better understanding, problems associated with permanent pacemakers can be classified into sensing malfunction, pacing malfunction, lead complications, generator malfunction, and pacemaker infection.

SENSING MALFUNCTION

UNDERSENSING

Appropriate sensing of the cardiac event, i.e., intracardiac electrogram in demand pacemakers, inhibits the pacemaker; in the absence of such an event, the pacemaker emits an electrical impulse at a preprogrammed rate. Undersensing of cardiac events can thus result in inappropriate pacing. This is diagnosed on an electrocardiogram by a pacemaker spike at an inappropriately short interval after a spontaneous event, e.g., if it occurs earlier than 0.86 second when the programmed rate is 70 bpm (Fig. 18-11). Rarely, undersensing can lead to pacing on T waves and can trigger a ventricular arrhythmia. Undersensing is often accompanied by a change in pacing threshold.

In the immediate period after pacemaker insertion, undersensing can be related to lead dislodgement or edema. Later, it is often related to fibrosis at the lead tip–myocardium interface or lead fracture. Gross lead dislodgements are easily diagnosed by x-ray examination, while microdislodgements can manifest as intermittent failure to pace and/or sense. Improved lead designs with the use of active fixation mechanisms have made these complications unusual. However, if lead dislodgement occurs, lead repositioning under fluoroscopic control is necessary. Fibrosis at the lead–myocardial tissue interface can lead to late undersensing. Use of steroid-eluting electrodes decreases tissue reaction. Undersensing can generally be managed by reprogramming the pacemaker and making it more sen-

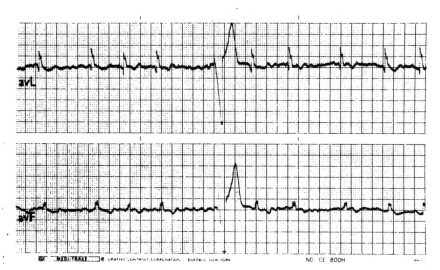

FIG. 18–11. Electrocardiographic recording from a patient in atrial fibrillation who has a VVI pacemaker, demonstrating normal sensing function. The demand pacemaker has been programmed to a rate of 60 beats per minute. Following the fourth QRS complex, an escape interval of 1.0 sec before the paced beat indicates accurate sensing.

sitive to electrogram amplitude. Lead fractures usually occur late, i.e., after months to years, and present as failure to both sense and pace.

OVERSENSING

Atrial and ventricular events are sensed and assumed to occur when signal amplitude equals or exceeds the programmed sensing threshold in an implanted cardiac pacemaker. However, any electrical signal of this magnitude that is transmitted via the lead may be identified as a cardiac event, thus inhibiting pacemaker output. Such signals can be other intracardiac signals such as repolarization waves (T waves) and distant depolarizations, e.g., atrial repolarization for ventricular leads and ventricular repolarization in the case of atrial leads, or noncardiac potentials such as myopotentials and extraneous electromagnetic signals. Diagnosis of oversensing is made by electrocardiographic documentation of inappropriate inhibition of pacemaker output in the absence of a spontaneous cardiac event. Commonly, this occurs as a result of arm exercises caused by myopotential interference or exposure to an electromagnetic field.

Oversensing is predominantly seen with unipolar cardiac pacemakers because of a large open circuit that extends from the electrode tip (cathode) to the generator casing across the intervening body tissue (anode). It is more often seen with atrial and dual-chamber pacemakers because of relatively small atrial electrograms requiring a low sensitivity threshold setting for detection. In unipolar devices, oversensing can often be resolved by making the devices less sensitive, i.e., programming the amplitude of minimum sensed electrogram to a higher value.

The use of bipolar pacing leads has substantially eliminated the problem of oversensing. In these leads, both the anodal and cathodal electrodes are at the lead tip, thereby eliminating a large pacing circuit. Oversensing of near field signals (T waves) can occur with bipolar leads but can usually be managed by increasing the sensitivity setting and/or prolonging the postventricular blanking period (the programmed interval after the QRS complex when no signals are sensed). Oversensing can also result from a loose set screw, insulation breaks, conductor fracture, and current leaks. These conditions should be considered if other causes for inappropriate inhibition of the pacemaker output are not found.

PACING MALFUNCTION

Pacing malfunction can present either as failure to capture or failure of pacemaker output. In the former situation, a pacing stimulus will be seen on the electrocardiographic recording. This stimulus is absent in the latter instance. Failure to capture can be due to

- Lead displacement or dislodgement
- Rise in pacing threshold due to fibrosis, infarction at the electrode site, effect of drugs, or electrolyte imbalance
- Increased resistance in the lead system due to lead fracture
- Pacemaker component failure

The minimum voltage output required to produce a consistent contraction of the heart muscle at a given pulse duration is the stimulation threshold. A stimulation threshold $\leq$ 1 V at 0.5 ms stimulus pulse width is satisfactory at initial implant. It rises acutely 2–4 times) within 2 weeks and gradually declines and stabilizes after 6 to 12 weeks. The final threshold may or may not exceed the implant values. Thus, the pacemaker output is initially programmed 3 to 5 times the stimulation threshold to allow an adequate safety margin for this transient rise. Immediately after implantation, the pacing threshold is dependent on the electrode position, and even microdisplacement can lead to a failure to consistently pace the heart. Long term pacing threshold is dependent on the electrode tissue interface, maturity polarity of the pacing electrode, conductor insulation integrity, myocardial injury (infarction or myocarditis), and concomitant drug therapy or electrolyte imbalance.

Noninvasive analysis of the pacemaker impulse helps determine whether pacing failure is related to lead malfunction or device malfunction. The magnet rate of the device and evaluation of the stimulus pulse width can help identify the likelihood of component failure secondary to battery depletion. If present, the device has to be replaced. When related to changes at the tissue-electrode interface, programming the pacing output to a higher level is attempted. At times, it is difficult to diagnose the cause of pacing failure noninvasively and it might be necessary to expose the electrode at surgery to test the lead and pulse generator individually. Absence of pacing stimulus output can be due to the following three causes

• Inhibition of pacemaker due to oversensing
• Lead fracture
• Component failure or battery depletion

Placing the generator in asynchronous mode by magnet application over the generator pocket helps differentiate these causes. When related to oversensing, magnet application over the pocket results in pacemaker output and capture (if the stimulus is beyond the refractory period of the preceeding QRS complex). There is no pacemaker output despite magnet application in component failure or lead fracture. An overpenetrated chest x-ray may help detect a lead fracture. Operative intervention is necessary to replace either the fractured lead or the depleted pulse generator.

LEAD COMPLICATIONS

LEAD FRACTURE

A lead fracture with complete lack of electrical conductivity presents with a total absence of pacing stimulus artefacts. However, in most instances, lead fractures present with intermittent electrical discontinuity so that the artefact is intermittently present. Radiological examination can confirm the fracture. Another lead problem is insulation fracture, which is often due to a technical error at the implant or the use of certain polyurethane-insulated leads that have shown a high incidence of polyurethane degradation. This can result in inappropriate sensing due to oversensing (see above). A large insulation leak also results in lack of capture due to shunting of current into the tissue at the site of fracture. This can also result in muscle stimulation at the site of the leak. Muscle twitching in patients with unipolar pacemakers early after implantation is often related to a high pacing output. This is seen with a deep-seated generator pocket when the device touches a muscle. Twitching that starts late after implant is usually related to lead insulation fracture. The diagnosis of an insulation leak in an implanted lead is confirmed at the time of reoperation by direct measurement of lead impedance, which can be very low or infinite. In some devices, this may be accomplished noninvasively by telemetry of lead impedance via the device.

PULSE GENERATOR MALFUNCTION

Pulse generator failure can result from battery depletion or malfunction of a device circuit. The following criteria can be used for differentiation of these two conditions:

Power Source Depletion
Spontaneous decline in pacing rate
Decline in magnet rate
Loss of sensing (late manifestation)
Erratic pacing

Circuit Malfunction
Erratic stimulation
Erratic or absent sensing
Programming problems
Telemetry failure/errors
Absent or erratic magnetic mode
No output without any lead fracture

The presence of one or more of these observations raises the suspicion of generator malfunction. Generator replacement is the treatment of choice. At the time of reoperation, lead function and integrity should be carefully checked to establish any contribution of lead malfunction to the premature pulse generator depletion.

PACEMAKER INFECTION

Infection of the implanted pacemaker system is one of the most serious and potentially fatal complications associated with cardiac pacemakers. Local infection of the pocket usually occurs shortly after implantation and is often due to Staphylococcus aureus. Late infection is rare and is associated with Staphylococcus epidermidis, particularly in immunocompromised patients. Infection of the pacemaker system should be suspected in any patient with an implanted device manifesting a persistent febrile illness. It can be clinically obvious with signs of inflammation at the pacemaker pocket (erythema, tenderness, warmth) and effusion in the region leading to abscess formation and a hectic toxic febrile course. More often, pacemaker infection is subtle, masquerading as fever of unknown origin, weight loss, failure to thrive, and other signs consistent with subacute bacterial endocarditis. Untreated, it can result in acute or subacute bacterial endocarditis, suppurative myocarditis, and pancarditis and can be fatal.

Pacemaker infections warrant culture-guided antibiotic therapy, total removal of the pulse generator and the lead system, local pocket drainage with secondary drainage, and implantation of a new pacemaker system at a different site. Such therapy should be undertaken at an experienced pacemaker surgical center.

Compared to infection, erosion of the pacemaker pocket is a late complication and often occurs in excessively lateral implants in thin individuals. As the unit erodes, it tends to get infected. If not infected, referred to as "dry erosion" with sterile wound, reimplantation of the device in a deeper pocket can be successful. Most often, explanation of the system and reimplantation of a new system at an alternate location is required.

NONPHARMACOLOGIC THERAPY FOR TACHYCARDIAS

ABLATION

Ablation applies to destruction of substrate either during surgery or using energy applied via a percutaneous catheter.

Catheter ablation is the treatment of choice for symptomatic patients with atrial flutter/fibrillation, AV nodal tachycardia, and supraventricular tachycardia due to accessory bypass tracts who need nonpharmacological therapy. The procedure is successful in 70 to 95% of these patients. Its efficacy is dependent on precise localization of the AV conduction system or bypass tract as ascertained by a prior electrophysiologic study using multiple electrode catheters in the right atrium, AV junction, right ventricle, and coronary sinus.

Catheter ablation procedures involve delivery of DC current or radiofrequency current (same as used for electrocautery) at the target site in the AV conduction system or accessory pathway. For the accessory pathways related to right AV groove, catheters are placed in the right atrium, and for posteroseptal accessory pathways, electrodes at the coronary sinus orifice are used to deliver the ablative energy. For left-side freewall accessory pathways, electrode catheters are introduced retrogradely from the femoral artery into the left ventricle or transseptally from the right atrium and positioned across the left AV groove at a previously localized site to deliver ablation energy.

When direct current is used, a shock of 160 to 250 J is delivered from a standard external defibrillator under general anesthesia, with the catheter electrode as the cathode and an interscapular plate as the anode. It generates energy in excess of 2,000 V and produces a combination of light, heat, barotrauma, and an intense electrical gradient, which causes tissue damage with catheter ablation. The lesions produced by direct current are relatively large, and delivery of uncontrolled energy can result in serious complications. The use of DC shock has declined due to the risk of potentially fatal complications such as rupture of the coronary sinus, cardiac rupture, hypotension, congestive heart failure, thromboembolic complications, and septicemia. Thus, the use of DC shock for the ablation of the AV conduction system or accessory pathways is often relegated as a second choice.

Radiofrequency current and low-energy modified DC shocks have proven to be more safe and very effective alternate energy sources. Radiofrequency is an alternating current with frequency in the range of 100 to 5,000 kHz. Energy can be delivered using an electrical catheter, and general anesthesia is not needed. However, use of specially designed catheters with a larger surface area of the delivery tip and with steerable distal ends has significantly increased the efficacy of radiofrequency ablation. With precise localization of the AV pathway by electrophysiologic study and in trained hands, up to 98% of accessory pathways can now be ablated using percutaneous catheter techniques with radiofrequency energy. Loss of pre-excitation with normalization of the PR interval and noninducibility of reentrant tachycardia are taken as markers of successful ablation. Incidence of complications with the use of radiofrequency ablation is low; complications include pericardial tamponade and occasional injury to the circumflex artery, as it lies in the AV groove. Radiofrequency ablation is the preferred method of treatment for all AV accessory pathways, irrespective of the location.

Catheter and surgical ablation both offer definitive treatment of tachyarrhythmias. However, these methods may only be applied when the substrate for the arrhythmia can be carefully defined. This substrate could encompass either an automatic focus or a reentrant pathway. Ablation or excision of the automatic focus or part or all of the reentrant pathway can lead to permanent cure of the tachycardia but necessitates precise localization. The development of catheter and operative cardiac mapping techniques has made this feasible, with markedly improved efficacy of the above techniques in many reentrant supraventricular and ventricular arrhythmias. In this section, indications, methodology, and efficacy of catheter ablation and surgery in the management of supraventricular and ventricular arrhythmias are discussed.

SUPRAVENTRICULAR ARRHYTHMIAS

Underlying mechanisms for supraventricular arrhythmias have been previously discussed (Chapter 6). For the purpose of nonpharmacologic therapy, they can be classified into

- Atrial tachycardias (including automatic atrial tachycardia, atrial flutter and fibrillation)
- Paroxysmal supraventricular tachycardias due to dual AV nodal pathways
- Paroxysmal supraventricular tachycardias due to one or more accessory AV bypass tracts

With the growing availability and use of definitive means of treatment for supraventricular tachycardias, pharmacologic therapy is often a temporary alternative until a decision to undertake catheter ablation or surgery is made. When compared to pharmacologic therapy and implantable devices, catheter ablation and surgery offer permanent therapeutic options and are preferred by the patient and physician in many clinical circumstances. Due to the highly invasive nature of surgical ablation and the associated small but definite mortality, this method is generally considered after catheter ablation has been unsuccessful.

Surgical ablation is currently restricted to patients who fail or refuse catheter ablation or are undergoing surgery for a different reason. To some extent, the choice of therapy is also governed by the expertise available at the treating center in delivering nonpharmacologic therapy.

Current Indications for Catheter Ablation

- Supraventricular tachycardias associated with severe symptoms or leading to life-threatening electrical or hemodynamic consequences such as syncope, ventricular failure, cardiomyopathy, and cardiac arrest (ventricular fibrillation). Ventricular tachycardia and fibrillation are special risks for patients with Wolff-Parkinson-White (WPW) Syndrome and short antegrade refractory period of the pathway (< 250 ms)
- Symptomatic patients without life-threatening problems who are refractory to multiple antiarrhythmic drugs
- Patients intolerant to antiarrhythmic drugs, despite their effective control of the arrhythmia
- Patient preference for nonpharmacologic therapy as an alternative to prolonged pharmacological treatment. This is particularly important in young patients, due to employment implications, and in female patients contemplating pregnancy

Atrial Tachycardias Including Atrial Flutter and Fibrillation

In atrial fibrillation, as well as most cases of atrial flutter and atrial tachycardias, control of symptoms can be achieved by ablation of the AV junction (i.e., AV node-His bundle) resulting in therapeutic complete AV or modification of AV conduction. Insertion of a permanent pacemaker is necessary, especially when heart block is induced. Modification of AV conduction is attempted but can culminate into complete AV block (Fig. 18-12). In some patients with atrial flutter and atrial tachycardia, it is possible to map the focus of atrial arrhythmia and selectively ablate it, thus leaving AV conduction intact and precluding the need for a permanent pacemaker.

Catheter ablation of the AV junction is performed using a standard bipolar catheter electrode, which is positioned across the His bundle to record an His bundle electrogram with an atrial and a ventricular electrogram. Initially, DC shock of 200 to 400 J was used for ablation, and general anesthesia was required. The original technique has now undergone considerable refinement. Steerable catheters provide more precise localization

POST-ABLATION EPS (7 DAYS)

SINUS RHYTHM WITH ATRIOVENTRICULAR BLOCK

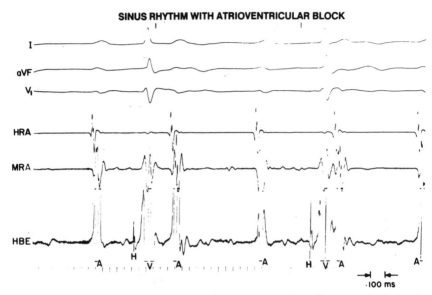

FIG. 18–12. Electrocardiographic and intracardiac recordings from a patient who had radiofrequency catheter ablation of AV node. Atrial electrograms show regular atrial activity. His-bundle electrograms show 2:1 AV block above the level of His as alternate atrial complexes and are not nonconducted or followed by an His electrogram. Reproduced with permission from: Tullo NG, An H, Saksena S: Ablation using radiofrequency current and low energy direct current shocks. *In* Electrical Therapy for Cardiac Arrhythmias: Pacing Anti-Tachycardia Devices, Catheter Ablation. Edited by: Saksena S, Goldschlager N. Philadelphia, W.B. Saunders, 1990, p 692.

of the AV node. Radiofrequency energy is used instead of DC shocks. The efficacy of catheter technique is high; graded or complete AV block is achieved in 85 to 90% of patients. In patients who fail to develop AV block with radiofrequency or DC electrode catheter ablation, chemical ablation of the AV node by injecting 95% ethyl alcohol into the AV nodal artery has been reported to be successful. This technique remains investigational and its use is restricted as a last resort when standard methods have failed.

Intraoperative resection of the AV conduction system continues to decline in frequency and is used only when a surgical procedure is performed for another indication in a patient with atrial tachycardia. There are now attempts at surgical correction of atrial flutter and fibrillation by electrically isolating fibrillating atrial tissue. However, these procedures, termed the "corridor" and "maze" operations, are complicated and still in the experimental stages of development. While these operations may restore sinus nodal rhythm with physiological rate response, they may not restore hemodynamically significant atrial function.

Dual Atrioventricular Nodal Pathways

Refractory tachycardias associated with dual AV nodal pathways were treated by AV junctional ablation, leading to complete heart block and implantation of a pacemaker. It has recently become possible, based on better understanding of a dual AV nodal pathway anatomy, to modify the AV node by catheter ablation or surgery and to eliminate one of the pathways without producing complete AV block. Reentry is related to the presence of dual AV nodal pathways. It is unclear if one of the pathways is an atrionodal tract or a partial extranodal circuit. If the area adjacent to the AV node is carefully mapped, the extranodal/nodal circuit components are identified by the activation of the adjoining atrial segment during tachycardia or ventricular pacing. Radiofrequency energy application in this area results in modification of one of the AV node pathways noninducibility of arrhythmia, and preserved AV conduction via the alternate pathway. Success of this procedure is high, but there is always a risk of complete heart block. Selective ablation of the slow pathway is reported to have lower risk of heart block.

Surgery has also been used to cure AV nodal reentry. Dissection of the AV node to cause denervation or cryoablation of the perinodal tissues has been successfully attempted. However, catheter ablation to modify the AV node has now superceded all previous procedures and should be attempted in all patients with AV nodal tachycardias refractory to multiple antiarrhythmic drugs.

Atrioventricular Bypass Tract and Pre-Excitation Syndromes

There has been a dramatic change in the management of tachycardias associated with AV bypass tracts over the last two decades with the development of very effective and safe surgical and subsequently catheter ablative techniques. Ablation procedures are more widely used when supraventricular tachycardias are associated with WPW Syndrome. They are also used in the uncommon varieties of pre-excitation syndromes such as Lown-Ganong-Levine Syndrome, tachycardias associated with Mahaim fibers or James fibers, and nonparoxysmal junctional tachycardias. This is largely related to a better definition of anatomic substrate in the classical variety of WPW Syndrome. The macroreentry circuit in patients with classical variety of WPW Syndrome comprises the atrium, AV node, His-Purkinje system, ventricle, and accessory bypass tract. In general, interruption at any level can lead to control of arrhythmia. However, interruption of the accessory pathway is the procedure of choice because it maintains the physiologic transmission of the sinus impulse and eliminates the risk of atrial fibrillation leading to a fast ventricular rate as a result of ventricular pre-excitation (Figs. 18-13A and 18-13B).

Surgical Resection of Atrioventricular Bypass Tract

Intraoperative ablation of the bypass tract is reserved for patients who have failed repeated percutaneous ablation or when another cardiac surgical procedure is being undertaken in a patient with WPW Syndrome. Mapping

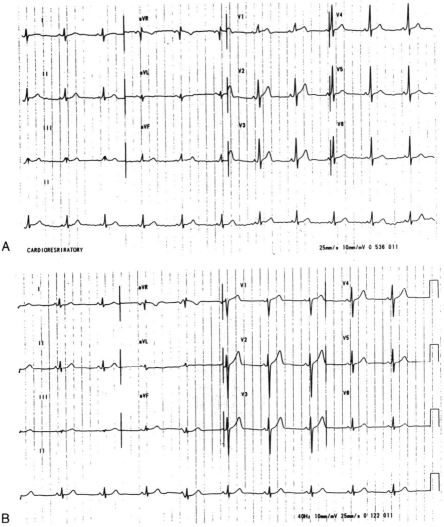

FIG. 18–13. Twelve lead electrocardiograms of a patient with Wolff-Parkinson-White syndrome prior to and following catheter ablation of the bypass tract. Panel A: This was recorded prior to ablation and shows a short PR interval and prominent delta waves. Panel B: After catheter ablation of the bypass tract, the electrocardiogram is normal with no delta waves.

for the accessory pathway is repeated during surgery, after the heart has been exposed and orthodromic tachycardia has been initiated, when a simultaneous recording of the entire AV groove can be easily obtained.

After the heart has been exposed, a multipolar strip electrode or a band electrode is placed just above the AV groove and orthodromic tachycardia is induced. Electrodes showing the earliest atrial activation during orthodromic tachycardia or during ventricular pacing identify the site of the accessory pathway. Endocardial and epicardial approaches have been used for resection. The epicardial approach may be superior, because it avoids the need for prolonged cardiopulmonary bypass. In each case, the AV groove is dissected at the location of the pathway as identified by prior mapping techniques. Adjunctive ablation methods such as cryothermia have been shown to improve results with each of the above approaches. After completion of the ablative procedure, programmed AV stimulation is repeated to reevaluate bypass tract conduction, inducibility of tachycardia, and evidence of additional pathways. Loss of delta wave and absence of inducible arrhythmia indicate surgical success (Figs. 18-14A and 18-14B). Map-guided ablation of the accessory pathways has resulted in high efficacy and low surgical mortality (< 2%). Although accessory pathways in all locations are amenable to surgery, results are better with single freewall accessory pathways than with septal or multiple accessory tracts. Septal accessory tracts remain problematic with conventional surgical methods, resulting in a persistent low incidence of postoperative heart block due to the proximity of the normal conduction system.

VENTRICULAR TACHYARRHYTHMIAS

Therapeutic modalities for the management of ventricular tachyarrhythmias include antiarrhythmic drugs, implantable devices, catheter ablation, and surgery. The majority of ventricular arrhythmias are related to ischemic heart disease, with or without myocardial scarring, and are reentrant in nature, as they can be initiated and terminated by programmed electrical stimulation of the heart.

Surgery for Ventricular Tachycardia

Map-guided surgical ablation also offers a potential cure for ventricular tachycardia and is presently the first line of nonpharmacologic treatment. It involves resection or removal of the arrhythmia substrate. This procedure is most often used in patients with coronary artery disease, and the substrate is usually the scar from a prior MI or surrounding regions. Patients with drug refractory ventricular tachycardias, in whom tachycardias can be induced and terminated by programmed electrical stimulation (reentrant tachycardia) and who have reasonably preserved left ventricular function (left ventricular ejection fraction > 20 to 25%), are considered for surgical ablation. Sustained monomorphic ventricular tachycardia that is hemodynamically stable with localized regional wall motion abnormality (scar or aneurysm) is ideal for map-guided surgical ablation. Nonsustained and polymorphic ventricular tachycardias and primary ventricular fibrillation are not suitable for surgical ablation.

Initially, visually guided standard resection techniques were used. These successfully suppressed the arrhythmia in 30 to 40% of patients. Development of electrophysiologic techniques and map-guided resection procedures allows more accurate resection of arrhythmia substrate, thus in-

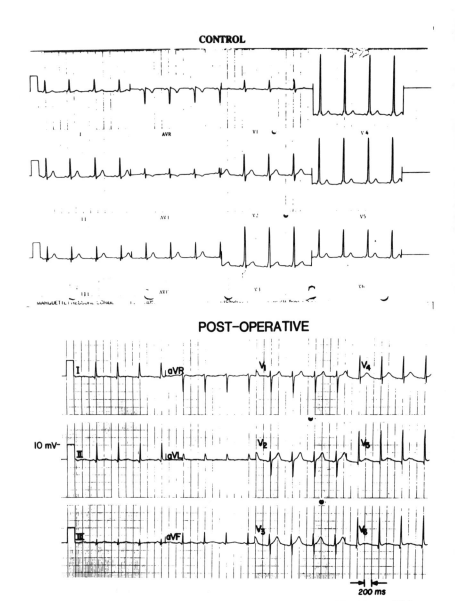

FIG. 18–14. Twelve lead electrocardiograms of a patient with Wolff-Parkinson-White syndrome prior to and following surgical resection of the bypass tract. Panel A: This was recorded prior to ablation and shows a short PR interval and obvious delta waves. Panel B: After surgery, there is a normal PR interval and no delta waves. Reproduced with permission from: Saksena S: Laser ablation of tachycardias: Experimental basis and preliminary clinical application. *In* Nonpharmacological Therapy for Tachyarrhythmias. Edited By: Breithardt G, Borggrefe M, Zipes DP. Mt. Kisco, Futura Publishing Company, 1987, p 172.

creasing the success rate to between 80 and 90%. Resection of a precisely localized focus also preserves left ventricular function.

Mapping during surgery is performed using high-density electrode systems. Epicardial recording is performed with a sock that fits the outside of the heart and has up to 56 recording electrodes. Left ventricular endocardial electrical activity is recorded with a latex balloon that has 56 electrodes on its surface. These allow simultaneous recordings from multiple sites in sinus rhythm and in ventricular tachycardia, thus giving an instantaneous beat-to-beat activation map. The sequence of activation is plotted, and the area of earliest activity is identified by the computer within 2 to 4 minutes. During tachycardia, the site of earliest activation is considered as the site of origin of ventricular tachycardia. In sinus rhythm, these areas can be identified by mid diastolic, fragmented, or continuous electrical activity. Sinus rhythm mapping is sometimes useful in patients in whom ventricular tachycardia cannot be induced at the time of surgery.

Surgical techniques used for tissue ablation have also undergone continuous evolution. Two surgical techniques are now generally used for resection. In encircling endocardial ventriculotomy, a transmural ventriculotomy is performed perpendicular to the endocardium in order to anatomically and electrically isolate the areas of endocardial fibrosis that have been visually and electrophysiologically identified. Epicardium and coronary vessels are spared. The more extensively used operation is endocardial resection, which is based on the fact that arrhythmias arise in the subendocardium, usually at the border territory of an infarction. At the site identified by mapping, endocardium is peeled, particularly at the rim of the infarction or aneurysm. Compared to encircling endocardial ventriculotomy, this operation preserves left ventricular function to a greater extent. Cryoablation has been used as an adjuvant to the above procedures and is especially useful when identified areas of ventricular tachycardia origin such as the papillary muscle cannot be resected. Laser energy has also been successfully used to surgically ablate sites of origin of ventricular tachycardia with good longterm results. This approach permits direct ablation with the tachycardia in progress in the operating room.

Surgery, in selected patients, thus offers the best means of treating recurrent sustained ventricular tachycardia. Improved short- and longterm results are seen in patients with well-preserved left ventricular function, fewer than three morphologies of documented ventricular tachycardia, and no inducible ventricular tachycardia after surgery. Five-year survival after surgery ranges from 40 to 70% in different series.

Catheter Ablation

Catheter ablation is a secondary choice in ablative therapy of ventricular tachyarrhythmias. It is considered in patients with drug-resistant ventricular tachycardias or other special circumstances. These include

- Failure of surgical ablation
- Poor candidate for surgical ablation due to anatomic or physiologic factors
- Markedly increased risk of surgical ablation due to concomitant organ system diseases, e.g., advanced renal or pulmonary disease

• Incessant tachycardia that cannot be terminated by pacing or DC cardioversion

The use of ablative techniques in the treatment of ventricular tachycardias is based on the principal of destroying a limited area of ventricular muscle that is involved in the generation or propagation of tachycardia. This area is localized by simultaneously recording ventricular activation from multiple sites in the ventricle during tachycardia. The site that shows earliest activation is ablated.

Catheter electrodes are used to deliver DC shocks using a conventional defibrillator or radiofrequency energy at the localized site. Ablation of multiple sites is required for patients in whom ventricular tachycardias of different morphologies are present. In general, catheter ablation is not advisable if more than three morphologies of spontaneous or induced ventricular tachycardias have been documented. In more than 50% of patients, ventricular tachycardia is still inducible after delivery of adequate energy at an appropriate site. Longterm control of arrhythmia is achieved in only 10 to 20% of patients. Complications include myocardial perforation, thrombus formation, hypotension, and rarely, induction and precipitation of previously unknown ventricular arrhythmias. Radiofrequency ablation seems to provide some advantages in the form of lower complication rates and easy applicability but has not been associated with an increased success rate. Thus, the therapeutic role of catheter ablation of ventricular tachycardias remains a secondary one, awaiting further evolution.

IMPLANTABLE CARDIOVERTER-DEFIBRILLATORS

The clinical use of implantable cardioverter-defibrillators has added a new dimension to the management of patients with dangerous ventricular arrhythmias. These devices automatically detect ventricular tachyarrhythmias and deliver a shock via epicardial patch electrodes or endocardial lead electrodes, usually within 30 seconds or arrhythmia onset. For ventricular tachycardia, the shock is synchronized, but the shock is asynchronous for ventricular fibrillation. As the shock is directly delivered to the heart, energy required for internal cardioversion/defibrillation is 15 to 40 J, compared to 200 to 350 J required for external cardioversion. The new generation of implantable cardioverter-defibrillators, in addition, have antibradycardia pacing and algorithms for pace termination of ventricular tachycardias (Fig. 18-15).

INDICATIONS FOR IMPLANTABLE CARDIOVERTER-DEFIBRILLATOR DEVICES

Implantable cardioverter-defibrillators are indicated in any patient with hemodynamically unstable ventricular tachyarrhythmia that is unrelated to acute MI, electrolyte imbalance, or drug toxicity. Concerning the use of cardiac pacemakers, specific indications for cardioverter-defibrillator implantation can be divided into three categories. The current recommen-

THIRD GENERATION ICD

VT: Pacing & Shock Rx

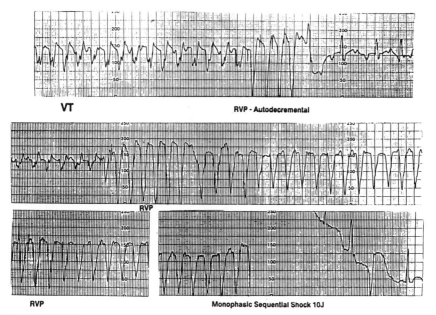

FIG. 18–15. Holter recordings demonstrating termination of ventricular tachycardia by third-generation implantable cardioverter-defibrillator. Top tracing illustrations termination of ventricular tachycardia by a burst of overdrive ventricular pacing. Middle trace shows failure to terminate another similar episode of ventricular tachycardia by overdrive pacing with an increase in rate of tachycardia, which is finally terminated by a synchronized shock of 10 J delivered by the implanted device (bottom trace).

dations from the North American Society of Pacing and Electrophysiology are as follows:

Class I
(Should be implanted)

• One or more documented episodes of hemodynamically significant ventricular tachycardia or fibrillation in a patient in whom electrophysiologic testing and ambulatory monitoring cannot be used to accurately predict efficacy of therapy
• One or more documented episodes of hemodynamically significant ventricular tachycardia or fibrillation in a patient for whom no drug is found to be effective or no drug is currently available and appropriately tolerated
• Continued inducibility at electrophysiologic study of hemodynamically significant ventricular tachycardia or fibrillation despite best available

drug therapy or despite surgery or catheter ablation if drug therapy has failed

Class II
(Cardioverter-defibrillator can be used)

• One or more documented episodes of hemodynamically significant ventricular tachycardia or fibrillation in a patient for whom drug efficacy testing is possible
• Recurrent syncope of undetermined origin in a patient with hemodynamically significant ventricular tachycardia or fibrillation induced at electrophysiologic study, for whom no effective or tolerated drug is available or appropriate

Class III
(Cardioverter-defibrillator should not be used)

• Recurrent syncope of undetermined cause in a patient without inducible tachycardias
• Arrhythmias not due to hemodynamically significant ventricular tachycardia or fibrillation
• Incessant ventricular tachycardia or fibrillation

An implantable cardioverter-defibrillator system is composed of two sensing electrodes, two shocking (cardioversion/defibrillation) electrodes, and the device. Defibrillation leads can be epicardial patches or endocardial lead electrodes. Implantation of epicardial patch electrodes requires thoracotomy, and two or three patch electrodes are placed on the heart. Sensing/pacing leads can be epicardial or endocardial in location. Epicardial screw-in electrodes are used for sensing ventricular signals. Endocardial electrodes are usually inserted via the subclavian or cephalic veins into the right ventricle. Before the leads are connected to the device, adequacy of lead function is tested. The minimal amount of energy required to reproducibly terminate induced ventricular fibrillation is referred to as the "defibrillation threshold." A safety margin of ≥ 10 J between the defibrillation threshold and output of the device is desirable. The efficacy of the device in terminating ventricular arrhythmias is established before it is implanted in the abdominal pocket. Its efficacy is again confirmed by electrophysiologic study prior to discharge. Perioperative mortality associated with cardioverter-defibrillator implantation using epicardial leads is 1 to 5%. This mortality rate is likely to decrease with the use of transvenous defibrillation lead systems.

Following hospital discharge, patients are monitored every 2 months for appropriate device use and device status. Frequent use of shock therapy often indicates recurrent ventricular or uncontrolled supraventricular arrhythmias and the need for concomitant drug therapy. Appropriate device use for ventricular tachycardia/ventricular fibrillation is reported to occur in 50 to 75% of all implanted patients. This rate increases along with the length of follow-up. Initial shocks occurring more than 1 year after implant are common. Patients with implantable cardioverter-defibrillators can have a fairly normal lifestyle but are advised to refrain from driving due to the risk of syncopal ventricular tachycardia/ventricular fibrillation. Pulse generator longevity is currently 3 to 4 years. Replacement is usually necessary but can be based on device use; it is a debatable issue in patients who do not experience shocks for more than 5 years after implant. Another frequently encountered problem in the management of these patients is the occurrence of spurious discharges. These are shocks delivered by the device, usually in the absence of symptoms or during exercise. In most instances, these are related to supraventricular arrhythmias such as atrial fibrillation with a fast ventricular rate, sinus tachycardia, or recurrent nonsustained ventricular tachycardia. They can usually be managed by device reprogramming and/or appropriate concomitant pharmacologic therapy. Less frequently, spurious shocks can result from lead fracture of the sensing electrodes, myopotential sensing, or the use of electrocautery. It is recommended to disconnect the implantable cardioverter-defibrillator device during surgery if clinically feasible.

Since their availability for clinical use in 1984, over 15,000 cardioverter-defibrillators have been implanted throughout the world. Their use has been shown to be associated with low recurrent sudden death rates in survivors of cardiac arrest related to ventricular tachycardia and ventricular fibrillation. With the availability of antitachycardia pacing and better algorithms for antitachycardia pacing, the use of cardioverter-defibrillators is gradually expanding. High cost, however, remains an important limiting factor in their more extensive use. These devices can be anticipated to replace extensive drug testing procedures or high-risk surgical ablative procedures in patients with recurrent ventricular tachycardia/ventricular fibrillation.

CLINICAL RESULTS WITH PROGRAMMABLE CARDIOVERTER-DEFIBRILLATORS AND NONTHORACOTOMY LEAD SYSTEMS

Recent developments in device technology have made possible the availability of demand ventricular pacing, programmable tachycardia detection, and programmable tachycardia therapies in implantable cardioverter-defibrillator devices. A major advance has been the availability of nonthoracotomy defibrillation lead systems, which have obviated the need for thoracotomy in most patients. In a clinical report of 200 patients implanted with programmable pacemaker-cardioverter-defibrillators, device function permitted demand ventricular pacing for bradyarrhythmias, long Q-T interval or tachycardia suppression, as well as programmable (3 to 30 joules) energy shocks for treatment of ventricular tachycardia and ventricular fibrillation. Ventricular tachycardia or ventricular fibrillation recognition is based on electrogram rate and required reconfirmation prior to shock delivery. The patients in this study were followed for up to 23 months. The incidence of sudden death during follow-up was 1% with a total cardiac mortality of 6.5%. Perioperative mortality in this study, which used epicardial lead systems with a thoracotomy, was 5.5%. In another study, the longterm results of epicardial and endocardial lead systems were compared; 660 patients were implanted with a programmable pacemaker-cardioverter-defibrillator with either endocardial leads (226 patients) or epicardial leads. The perioperative mortality was 5.5% for epicardial leads and 0.4% for endocardial leads. This difference was statistically significant. Life table analysis showed improved total 1-year survival of 96.4% for endocardial leads versus 85.4% for epicardial leads (p < 0.001).

Future devices are likely to have multiprogrammable parameters for pacing for tachycardias and bradycardias, shock therapy for tachycardias, and implantation using nonthoracotomy approaches.

SUGGESTED READING

Bergfeldt L, Rosenquist M, Vallin H, Edhag O: Disopyramide-induced second and third degree atrioventricular block in patients with bifascicular block. An acute stress test to predict atrioventricular block progression. Br Heart J, 53:328, 1985.

Benditt DG, Gornick CC, Dunbar D, et al.: Indication for electrophysiological testing in the diagnosis and assessment of sinus node dysfunction. Circulation, 75(Suppl III):II-93, 1987.

Bexton RS, Camm AJ: First degree atrioventricular block. Eur Heart J, 5(Suppl A):107, 1984.

Calkins H, Sousa J, El-Atassi R, et al.: Diagnosis and cure of the Wolff-Parkinson-White syndrome or paroxysmal supraventricular tachycardias during a single electrophysiology test. N Engl J Med, 324:1612, 1991.

Camm AJ, Ward DE, Spurrell RAJ, Reis GM: Cryothermal mapping and cryoablation in the treatment of refractory cardiac arrhythmias. Circulation, 62:67, 1980.

Dreifus LS, Gillette PC, Fisch C, et al.: Guidelines for implantation of cardiac pacemakers and antiarrhythmia devices: A report of the American College of Cardiology/American Heart Association Task Force on Assessment of Diagnostic and Therapeutic Cardiovascular Procedures (Committee on Pacemaker Implantation). J Am Coll Cardiol, 18:1, 1991.

Cox JL: The status of surgery for cardiac arrhythmias. Circulation, 71:413, 1985.

Echt DS, Armstrong K, Schmidt P, et al.: Clinical experience, complications, and survival in 70 patients with automatic implantable cardioverter/defibrillator. Circulation, 71:289, 1985.

Frink JR, James TN: Normal blood supply to the human His bundle and the proximal bundle branches. Circulation, 47:8, 1973.

Furman S, Hayes D, Holmes DR: A Practice of Cardiac Pacing. Mt Kisco, New York, Futura Publishing Co, Inc., 1989.

Gabry MD, Behrens M, Andrews C, et al.: Comparison of myopotential interference in unipolar-bipolar programmable DDD pacemakers. PACE, 10:1322, 1987.

Gallagher JJ, Smith WM, Kerr CR, et al.: Esophageal pacing. A diagnostic and therapeutic tool. Circulation, 65:336, 1982.

Gallagher JJ, Svenson RH, Kassell JH, et al.: Catheter technique for closed chest ablation of the atrioventricular conduction system. N Engl J Med, 306:194, 1982.

Gann D, Tolentino A, Samet P: Electrophysiological evaluation of elderly patients with sinus bradycardia: A long-term follow-up study. Ann Intern Med, 90:24, 1979.

Gomes JAC, El-Sherif N: Atrioventricular block: Mechanism, clinical presentation, and therapy. Med Clin North Am, 68:955, 1984.

Josephson ME, Wellens HJJ: Tachycardias: Mechanisms, diagnosis Treatment. Philadelphia, Lea & Febiger, 1984.

Hindman MC, Wagner GS, Ja Ro M, et al.: The clinical significance of bundle branch block complicating acute myocardial infarction. 2. Indication for temporary and permanent pacemaker insertion. Circulation, 58:689, 1978.

Jackman WM, Wang X, Friday KJ, et al.: Catheter ablation of accessory atrioventricular pathways (Wolff-Parkinson-White syndrome) by radiofrequency current. N Engl J Med, 324:1605, 1991.

Keren A, Tzivoni D, Gavish D, et al.: Etiology warning signs and therapy of torsades de pointes. A study of 10 patients. Circulation, *64*:1167, 1981.

Kastor JA: Atrioventricular block. N Engl J Med, *292*:462, 572, 1975.

Luderitz B, Saksena S (eds.): Interventional Electrophysiology. Mount Kisco, New York, Futura Publishing Company Inc., 1991.

Madigan NP, Flaker GC, Curtis JJ, et al.: Carotid sinus hypersensitivity: beneficial effects of dual-chamber pacing. Am J Cardiol, *53*:1034, 1984.

McAnulty JH, Rahimotolla SH, Murphy E: Natural history of "high risk" bundle branch block: Final report of a prospective study. N Engl J Med, *307*:137, 1982.

Mirowski M, Reid PR, Mower MM, et al.: Termination of malignant ventricular arrhythmias with an implantable automatic defibrillator in human beings. N Engl J Med, *303*:322, 1980.

Phibbs B, Freifman HS, Garaboys TB, et al.: Indications for permanent pacing in the treatment of bradyarrhythmias: Report of an independent study group. JAMA, *252*:1307, 1984.

Reinhart S, McAnulty JH, Dobbs J: Type and timing of permanent pacemaker failure Chest, *82*:443, 1982.

Rosenqvist M, Brandt J, Schuller H: Atrial versus ventricular pacing in sinus node disease. A treatment comparison study. Am Heart J, *111*:450, 1969.

Rubin IL, Jagendorf B, Goldberg AL: The esophageal lead in the diagnosis of tachycardias associated with aberrant ventricular conduction. Am Heart J, *57*:19, 1959.

Scheinman MM, Morady F, Hess DS, et al.: Catheter-induced ablation of the atrioventricular junction to control refractory supraventricular arrhythmias. J Am Med Assoc, *248*:851, 1982.

Scheinman MM, Peters RW, Morady F, et al.: Electrophysiology studies in patients with bundle branch block. PACE, *6*:1157, 1983.

Sealy WC, Halter BF Jr., Blumenchein SD, et al.: Surgical treatment of Wolff-Parkinson-White syndrome. Ann Thorac Surg, *8*:1, 1969.

Saksena S, Goldschlager N (eds.): Electrical therapy for cardiac arrhythmias. Philadelphia, W.B. Saunders, 1990.

Saksena S, Hussain SM, Gielchinsky I, et al.: Intraoperative mapping-guided argon laser ablation of malignant ventricular tachycardia. Am J Cardiol, *59*:78, 1989.

Saksena S, Mehta D, the PCD investigators: Long-term results of implantable cardioverter-defibrillators using endocardial and epicardial lead systems: A worldwide experience. PACE, *15*:505, 1992.

Saksena S, Parsonnet V: Implantation of a cardioverter/defibrillator without thoracotomy using a triple electrode system. JAMA, *259*:69, 1988.

Saksena S, Poczobutt-Johanos M, Castle L, et al.: Long-term multicenter experience with a second-generation implantable pacemaker-defibrillator in patients with malignant ventricular tachyarrhythmias. J Am Coll Cardiol, *19*:490, 1992.

Saksena S, Tullo NG, Krol RB, Mauro AM: Initial clinical experience with endocardial defibrillation using an implantable cardioverter-defibrillator with a triple electrode system. Arch Int Med, *149*:2333, 1989.

Smith WM, Gallaher JJ: "Les torsades de pointes:" An unusual ventricular arrhythmia. Ann Inter Med, *93*:578, 1980.

Stein PD, Mathur VS, Herman MV, Levine HD: Complete heart block induced during cardiac catheterization of patients with pre-existing bundle branch block: The hazard of bilateral bundle branch block. Circulation, *34*:783, 1966.

Tchou PJ, Kadri N, Anderson J, et al.: Automatic implantable cardioverter-defibrillators and the survival of patients with left ventricular dysfunction and malignant ventricular arrhythmias. Ann Int Med, *109*:529, 1988.

Waldo AL, Wells JL, Cooper TB, MacLean WAH: Temporary cardiac pacing: Application and techniques in the treatment of cardiac arrhythmias. Prog Cardiovasc Dis, *23*:451, 1981.

Waldo AL, MacLean WAH, Cooper TB, et al.: Use of temporarily placed epicardial atrial wire electrodes for the diagnosis and treatment of cardiac arrhythmias following open-heart surgery. J Thorac Cardiovasc Surg, *76*:500, 1978.

Walter PF, Crawley IS, Dorney ER: Carotid sinus hypersensitivity and syncope. Am J Cardiol, 42:396, 1978.

Weber H, Schmitz L: Catheter technique for closed-chest ablation of an accessory atrio-ventricular pathway. N Engl J Med, *308*:653, 1983.

Wohl AJ, Laborde NJ, Atkins JM, et al.: Prognosis of patients permanently paced for sick sinus syndrome. Arch Intern Med, *136*:406, 1976.

Zoll PM: Resuscitation of heart in ventricular standstill by external electric stimulation. N Engl J Med, *247*:768, 1952.

Zoll PM, Zoll RH, Falk RH, et al.: External non-invasive cardiac pacing: Clinical trials. Circulation, *71*:937, 1985.

19

PULMONARY HYPERTENSION AND COR PULMONALE

M. Gabriel Khan

PULMONARY HYPERTENSION

Because primary pulmonary hypertension (PPH) is rare, accounting for less than 0.1% of all cases of pulmonary hypertension, it will be discussed after considering the more important causes of secondary pulmonary hypertension (see Fig. 19–1).

PATHOPHYSIOLOGY

Normal resting peak systolic pulmonary artery pressure at sea level ranges from 20 to 25; the mean is 12 to 16 mm Hg, and the end diastolic ranges from 6 to 10 mm Hg. The pulmonary circulation is a low-resistance circuit. Normally, an arteriovenous pressure gradient of only 2 to 10 mm Hg exists to circulate the cardiac output through the low-resistance pulmonary vascular channels. Pulmonary hypertension exists when pulmonary vascular resistance increases and the pulmonary artery systolic and mean pressures at rest are consistently above 30 and 20 mm Hg, respectively.

CAUSES OF PULMONARY HYPERTENSION

Pulmonary hypertension may be caused by several disease states, including the following

- Physiologic from all causes of hypoxemia
- Diseases, primarily of the lung parenchyma, that also affect the pulmonary vascular bed
- Vascular improvement in Pulmonary thromboembolism and systemic disease
- Left ventricular failure, mitral stenosis or regurgitation, rarely left atrial myxoma or pulmonary veno-occlusive disease
- Congenital heart disease, left-to-right shunts

Figure 19–1 presents an algorithmic approach derived from considering the parts of the pulmonary circulation in which increased resistance to

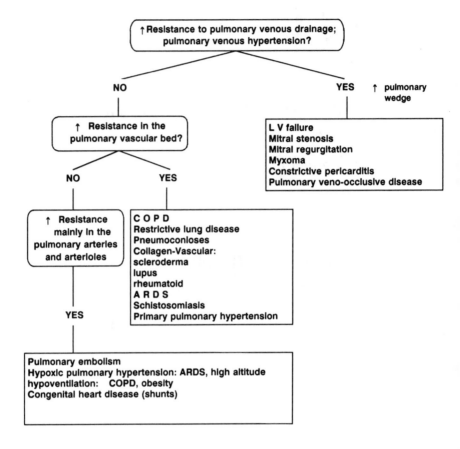

↑ Increase
↓ Decrease

FIG. 19–1. Common causes of pulmonary hypertension.

blood flow actuates pulmonary hypertension. Except when the diagnosis is clinically obvious, it is advisable to first exclude pulmonary venous hypertension that results in an increase in pulmonary wedge pressure.

CLINICAL FEATURES

Mild pulmonary hypertension (pulmonary artery pressure 40/20, mean greater than 25 mm Hg) is usually asymptomatic. Moderate pulmonary hypertension with pulmonary artery pressure of 50 to 60 (systolic) and 25 to 30 (diastolic) (mean greater than 40 mm Hg) may cause dyspnea on exertion and easy fatigability. These symptoms occur more commonly with severe pulmonary hypertension (pulmonary artery pressure greater than

80/35, mean greater than 55 mm Hg). Tachypnea and occasional chest pain, presyncope, syncope, and rarely sudden death may also occur.

Symptoms and signs may be caused by underlying diseases listed in Figure 19–1. Common findings include the following

- A giant A wave in the jugular venous pulse
- A left parasternal lift or heave due to right ventricular hypertrophy
- A parasternal, palpable systolic pulsation in the left intercostal space
- An accentuated, pulmonary component of the second heart sound
- An ejection click due to dilatation of the main pulmonary artery
- A fourth heart sound at the lower left sternal border, and with severe pulmonary hypertension or cor pulmonale, a right-sided S3 that increases on inspiration
- An early decrescendo diastolic murmur maximal in the second left intercostal space caused by pulmonary regurgitation
- A murmur of tricuspid regurgitation with prominent V waves if the tricuspid valve annulus is dilated
- Finally, signs of right heart failure

INVESTIGATIONS

CHEST X-RAY AND ELECTROCARDIOGRAM

- X-ray evidence of dilatation of the main, right, and left pulmonary arteries with attenuation of peripheral branches
- Electrocardiogram (ECG): peaked P waves in Leads II, III and AVF due to right atrial enlargement; $S_1 Q_3$, $S_1 S_2 S_3$, S wave in V_5, or an R to S ratio in V_5 of less than 3.5; right axis deviation, right ventricular hypertrophy, and ST segment depression with T wave inversion in leads V_1 to V_3

ECHOCARDIOGRAPHY

Echocardiographic evaluation is extremely useful in detecting causes of left heart failure, left atrial enlargement, mitral stenosis, myxoma, elevation of the pulmonary artery pressure, right ventricular hypertrophy, tricuspid regurgitation, enlargement of cardiac chambers, or shunts.

LUNG SCAN

The lung scan is not diagnostic and must be analyzed in conjunction with a probability clinical assessment (see Chapter 30 and Fig. 30–1).

In the absence of chronic obstructive lung disease, lung scan, helps in differentiating pulmonary embolism from PPH

- Normal lung scan or diffuse mottling, salt and pepper pattern, and no segmental defects strongly suggest PPH if other causes of secondary pulmonary hypertension are excluded
- One or more segmental or larger defects suggest pulmonary embolism (Fig. 30–1)

PULMONARY ANGIOGRAPHY

If pulmonary embolism versus PPH cannot be resolved by the aforementioned systematic clinical approach and investigations outlined, pulmonary angiogram is advisable to exclude chronic pulmonary embolism. Also, fiberoptic angioscopy can verify the presence of thrombi in the pulmonary arteries and evaluate their accessibility for removal.

LUNG BIOPSY

- In patients with moderate to severe pulmonary hypertension, transbronchial biopsy may cause significant bleeding and is contraindicated
- Sampling errors are common
- May be useful to confirm the type of interstitial lung disease causing pulmonary hypertension

THERAPY

Treatment of secondary pulmonary hypertension entails adequate management of the underlying disease. Hypoxemia must be corrected. If the PaO_2 is less than 55 mm Hg at rest, oxygen is advisable for at least 15 hours daily (see Chapter 22).

NIFEDIPINE
(Procardia XL, Nifedipine Extended Release)

Nifedipine may cause a decrease in pulmonary artery pressure, especially in patients with collagen vascular disease. The response to calcium antagonists is variable; large doses of nifedipine (90 to 180 mg daily) may be required. Some patients respond, while others do not. If an acute response occurs with a reduction in pulmonary artery pressure, then a salutary long-term response usually can be expected.

DIGOXIN

Digoxin is indicated only for the management of atrial fibrillation with a ventricular response greater than 80/minute at rest or greater than 100/minute on mild activities such as walking 100 feet or more.

FUROSEMIDE

Patients with right heart failure due to pulmonary hypertension triggered by increased resistance in the vascular bed or pulmonary arteries benefit from small doses of furosemide (20 to 40 mg daily). In these patients, larger doses of diuretics have a propensity to precipitate electrolyte imbalance, especially hypochloremic metabolic alkalosis. Occasionally, acetazolamide may be given 3 days weekly, if needed, for correction of this electrolyte abnormality. Caution is necessary, because this combination may cause hypokalemia (see Chapter 5).

Pulmonary thromboembolism is a major cause of pulmonary hypertension and is discussed in Chapter 30.

PRIMARY PULMONARY HYPERTENSION

PPH is extremely rare. The diagnosis is entertained only after exclusion of all causes of secondary pulmonary hypertension, particularly recurrent pulmonary embolism.

ETIOLOGY

PPH occurs most often in children and young adults. A marked frequency has been observed in the Indian subcontinent. A national registry report of 187 patients indicated that 63% of patients were women, (mean age 36 ± 15). In the Mayo Clinic follow-up study of 120 patients, 73% were female, the mean age was 34 years, and in two families, PPH occurred in two brothers.

The etiology of PPH is unknown, but the following associations have been noted as possible factors or aggravating mechanisms

- Thromboembolism and amniotic fluid embolism. Occult thromboembolism may cause slow progressive pulmonary hypertension with clinical manifestations only in the terminal stage of illness and is difficult to exclude as a cause of clinically diagnosed PPH. In some studies, up to 50% of patients diagnosed as PPH were found to have thromboembolism. Occult thromboembolism is not the underlying process, however, in the majority of patients with PPH
- Most patients with PPH have plexogenic arteriopathy similar to that observed in the Eisenmenger syndrome and in cases in which severe pulmonary hypertension and death were caused by appetite suppressants. Most children in the Indian subcontinent present in the late teenage years and die within 5 years with an aggressive plexiform arteriopathy, arteritis, and fibrinoid necrosis affecting the small muscular pulmonary arteries of undetermined cause
- Familial cases have been reported with autosomal dominant inheritance
- Toxic cooking oil syndrome
- The anorexigenic agent (aminorex fumarate). In Europe, PPH occurred in 0.2% of individuals ingesting this agent, which is no longer available
- Raynaud's phenomenon was reported in 8.2% of cases in the 1991 National Registry and in 10% of cases in the Mayo Clinic study. In families of patients with PPH, Raynaud's phenomenon may occur in members not affected by PPH. This suggests that vasospasm in pulmonary arteries may be a factor. This association deserves investigative exploration. However, the association may be related to the presence of undetected collagen-vascular or autoimmune disease
- A defect in the nitric oxide synthase system may be implicated and deserves intensive study. Vascular endothelial cells synthesize nitric oxide from L-arginine. Nitric oxide is a potent vasodilator now known to be the endothelium-derived relaxing factor (EDRF). The circulatory system

is believed to be in a state of active vasodilation under the influence of many factors, including prostacyclin and nitric oxide. Thus, systemic and pulmonary hypertension may be envisaged as a state of hypovasodilation. In patients with PPH, this pathophysiologic mechanism may be confined, perhaps genetically, to the pulmonary arterioles
• Prolonged intense pulmonary vasoconstriction causes pulmonary hypertension and pathologic changes, including plexogenic pulmonary arteriopathy and fibrinoid necrosis. It is of interest that inhaled nitric oxide administered to patients with PPH resulted in a marked decrease in pulmonary vascular resistance, equal to that achieved with IV prostacyclin

CLINICAL FEATURES

The most common clinical findings derived from the Mayo Clinic study and the National Registry include the following

• Progressive dyspnea (66%); decreased exercise tolerance may be incapacitating
• Fatigue and weakness (20%)
• Presyncope, syncope, or dizziness (22%)
• Raynaud's phenomenon (10%)
• Exertional chest pain (10%) caused by right ventricular myocardial ischemia and/or distension of the major pulmonary arteries
• A left parasternal heave due to right ventricular hypertrophy
• A palpable systolic pulsation caused by a dilated pulmonary artery
• A large A wave in the jugular venous pulse
• A loud pulmonic component of the second heart sound (98%), and a closely split second heart sound
• A pulmonary ejection click

Prognosis in the Mayo Clinic study was poor; only 21% of patients survived 5 years. The results from the National Prospective Registry recruitment and follow-up of 194 patients indicated survival rate at 1 year (68%), 3 years (48%), and 5 years (34%). Mortality was closely associated with three variables

• Mean pulmonary artery pressure
• Mean right atrial pressure
• Mean cardiac index as shown in Table 19–1

INVESTIGATIONS

Because the clinical features, ECG, chest x-ray, echocardiography, and lung scan do not serve to distinguish all cases of PPH of secondary pulmonary hypertension, right heart catheterization and pulmonary angiogram are virtually always required prior to labeling the patient as having PPH. In addition, the pathologic lesions of PPH appear to be indistinguishable from those found in patients with secondary pulmonary hypertension caused by congenital heart disease, appetite-suppressing agents, and/or scleroderma.

TABLE 19–1. MEDIAN SURVIVAL FOR PATIENTS WITH PRIMARY PULMONARY HYPERTENSION COMPARED WITH THREE HEMODYNAMIC VARIABLES*

HEMODYNAMIC VARIABLE		MEDIAN SURVIVAL TIME IN MONTHS
Mean pulmonary artery pressure	≥85 mm HG	12
	<55 mm Hg	48
Mean right atrial pressure	≥20 mm Hg	1
	<10 mm Hg	46
Mean cardiac index	<2 l/min/m²	17
	≥4 l/min/m²	43

* Modified from Ann Intern Med, *115*:343, 1991.

Indications for right heart catheterization and pulmonary angiography include the following

- If the history, physical, and chest x-ray are not in keeping with secondary pulmonary hypertension
- Echocardiographic assessment shows the absence of left heart disease and the presence of unexplained moderate to severe pulmonary hypertension
- The presence of normal arterial blood gases
- A normal lung scan or salt and pepper pattern
- Exclusion of chronic pulmonary embolism, which is a conflicting diagnosis requiring pulmonary angiography

THERAPY

Symptomatic patients with moderate to severe pulmonary hypertension may show a partial response to calcium antagonists. Nifedipine has advantages over verapamil, because the latter drug may cause a worsening of right heart failure.

Titrated high doses of nifedipine extended release (180 to 240 mg daily) and diltiazem (up to 720 mg daily) have been shown to cause substantial reduction in pulmonary artery pressure in some patients with PPH but diltiazem may worsen right heart failure. Reduction in pulmonary artery pressure and pulmonary vascular resistance persisted at 1 year in at least four of 13 patients treated with nifedipine. Five of the 13 individuals failed to respond to massive doses of these agents. This variability in response has been documented in other small studies.

Nifedipine has been shown to partially prevent acute pulmonary vasoconstriction caused by hypoxemia. Calcium antagonists are known to cause ventilation perfusion derangements, however, and may provide hypoxemia in some patients.

Prostacyclin is an expensive mode of therapy administered as a continuous infusion. This agent is effective and has a small role in controlling elevated pulmonary hemodynamics for weeks to months in properly selected patients considered for lung transplantation. In a study of 22 patients, hemodynamic and clinical benefits were maintained up to 18 months with continuous prostacyclin infusion.

In a recent study, Pepke-Zaba, et al. observed the acute effects of inhaled nitric oxide compared with continuous IV prostacyclin in eight patients with severe pulmonary hypertension. Prostacyclin caused significant reduction in pulmonary and systemic vascular resistance. Inhaled nitric oxide showed a similar decrease in pulmonary vascular resistance but, as expected, had no effect on systemic vascular resistance as a result of rapid inactivation of nitric oxide by hemoglobin.

Further developments are anticipated in the research of phenomena that involve vasoconstriction and hypovasodilatation, which appear to have escaped homeostatic control.

Anticoagulants are recommended in all patients with PPH. In the Mayo Clinic study, survival was shown to be improved in some patients with this form of therapy.

Heart-lung, double-lung, or single-lung transplantation has a role in properly selected patients. Obliterative bronchiolitis remains a major problem in more than 33% of patients, the majority of whom require high-dose corticosteroids. In a study of single-lung transplant carried out in 12 patients for pulmonary hypertension, 11 patients survived up to 22 months. The 3-month hemodynamic report indicated a reduction of pulmonary artery systolic pressure from 92 ± 7 mm Hg to 29 ± 6 mm Hg (p = 0.001). In specialized centers, these procedures continue with hope for improved survival and relief of suffering for some patients.

COR PULMONALE

Heart disease secondary to lung disease is classified as cor pulmonale. Right ventricular hypertrophy or right heart failure may occur as a result of severe pulmonary hypertension caused by a number of diseases affecting the pulmonary vascular bed or arteries as outlined earlier in this chapter. The most common causes of cor pulmonale are longstanding chronic bronchitis and emphysema; patients in this category usually show PaO_2 less than 55 mm Hg when they are free from an exacerbation of the disease. Pulmonary hypertension and right ventricular hypertrophy develop in up to 25% of patients, and right heart failure is manifest in about 10% of these individuals.

Notable findings include

- Increased shortness of breath on minimal exertion
- Easy fatigability at rest
- Tachypnea
- Pursed lip expiration
- Parodoxical abdominal breathing and constant use of accessory muscles of respiration
- Asterixis, chemosis, and engorgement of blood vessels in the fundi caused by hypercapnia
- Central cyanosis with warm peripheries is the usual finding; the occurrence of added peripheral cyanosis with cold peripheries indicates that heart failure has supervened

In patients with cor pulmonale, cardiac murmurs may be difficult to detect. In particular, it is easy to miss the murmur of significant mitral regurgitation. Echocardiography is recommended to exclude significant mitral regurgitation if doubt exists in a patient with right heart failure and COPD. Bothersome shortness of breath may be improved with the addition of ACE inhibitors in patients in whom valve repair or replacement is not feasible. Surgery may be contraindicated because of the terminal respiratory status.

ECG commonly shows

• Poor R wave progression in V_2-V_3 that may mimic anteroseptal infarction
• P Pulmonale and right ventricular hypertrophy with "strain pattern"

THERAPY

The treatment of exacerbation of chronic bronchitis with bronchodilators, albuterol (salbutamol), ipratropium, and pulsed corticosteroid therapy may produce temporary symptomatic relief (see Chapter 22). Cessation of smoking, breathing exercises, efficient physiotherapy, and advice on nutrition are necessary.

Correction of hypoxemia with continuous oxygen administration (minimum 15 hours daily) to keep the PaO_2 greater than 60 mm Hg may provide a modest improvement in survival.

Monitor blood gases to maintain the pH in the normal range and adequate oxygenation without increasing the $PaCO_2$. Digoxin is advisable in the management of atrial fibrillation with uncontrolled ventricular response, but it has little effect in the absence of atrial fibrillation.

FUROSEMIDE

At low doses, furosemide is given for bothersome bilateral pitting edema.

Dosage: 20 to 40 mg daily for a few days, then alternate day therapy is preferred. Edema should be allowed to subside gradually over weeks. The edema improves with the slow correction of hypoxemia. It must be reemphasized that diuretics commonly precipitate hypochloremic metabolic alkalosis in these patients, and acetazolamide (250 mg three times daily) given 3 days weekly once or twice monthly may be required. Alkalosis causes hypoventilation, and this complication must be avoided.

Pneumococcal vaccine and influenza immunization should be utilized. Acute cor pulmonale is usually precipitated by massive pulmonary embolization; the further discussion of this topic appears in Chapter 30.

BIBLIOGRAPHY

D'Alonzo GE, Barst RJ, Ayres SM, et al.: Survival in patients with primary pulmonary hypertension. Results from a National Prospective Registry. Ann Intern Med, *115*:343, 1991.
Fuster V, Steele PM, Edwards WD, et al.: Primary pulmonary hypertension national history and the importance of thrombosis. Circulation, *70*:580, 1984.

Pasque MK, Trulock EP, Kaiser LR, et al.: Single-lung transplantation for pulmonary hypertension. Three-month hemodynamic follow-up. Circulation, *84*:2275, 1991.

Pietra GG, Edwards WD, Kay JM, et al.: Histopathology of primary pulmonary hypertension. A qualitative and quantitative study of pulmonary blood vessels from 58 patients in the National Heart, Lung and Blood Institute Primary Pulmonary Hypertension Registry. Circulation, *80*:1198, 1989.

Pepke-Zaba J, Higenbottam TW, Dinh-Xuan AT, et al.: Inhaled nitric oxide as a cause of selective pulmonary vasodilatation in pulmonary hypertension. Lancet, *338*:1173, 1991.

Rich S, Dantker DR, Ayres SM, et al.: Primary pulmonary hypertension. A national prospective study. Ann Intern Med, *107*:216, 1987.

Rich S, Kaufman E: High dose titration of calcium channel blocking agents for primary pulmonary hypertension: Guidelines for short-term drug testing. J Am Coll Cardiol, *18*:1323, 1991.

Part II
RESPIRATORY SYSTEM

20

BRONCHODILATORS IN LUNG DISEASE

Susan K. Pingleton
Michael E. Nelson
Diana S. Dark

Bronchodilators, one of the most common treatment modalities, are widely used in the treatment of many types of acute and chronic lung disease. Originally, many bronchodilator preparations were available without prescription. However, as the nature of the physiologic responses and the side effects of the agents became known, their use became more carefully regulated. Most bronchodilators now require a physician's consultation and prescription prior to dispensing.

Despite the development of numerous pharmacologic therapies for controlling the inflammatory component of obstructive airway disease, bronchodilators have remained the first line of therapy in both acute and chronic disease. It has also become apparent that these agents have beneficial physiologic effects in addition to their bronchodilatory effects. Knowledge of the effects of each class of bronchodilators is imperative in choosing an agent for the appropriate clinical circumstances.

AEROSAL GENERATION, CHARACTERISTICS, AND DELIVERY

- Bronchodilators are available in several different dosage forms: Aerosol, oral, and intravenous
- Currently, there are three types of systems used to generate aerosols for clinical use: jet nebulizers, ultrasonic nebulizers, and metered-dose inhalers

A jet nebulizer (or atomizer) produces a high-velocity air stream, either by compressed gas or by a squeeze bulb, which creates a pressure drop across a liquid feeding tube. Fluid is forced upward through the tube as a result of the pressure difference and is then vaporized into a mist and dispersed by the air stream. A jet nebulizer is commonly used in hospitals and for home care to deliver medication in solution.

An ultrasonic nebulizer uses a piezoelectric crystal that, when exposed to an electrical field, transforms high-frequency electric oscillations into

rapid mechanical vibrations that are coupled with the liquid to be nebulized. As the crystal vibrates, creating turbulence in the solution, aerosol
droplets are formed. The droplets are then removed from the generation
chamber by a stream of air. Ultrasonic nebulizers have high outputs and
are commonly used to induce cough and sputum production or for bron-
choprovocational challenges. While they are rarely used to administer
bronchodilators therapeutically, ultrasonic nebulizers are used to deliver
selected other medications.

The most widely used nebulizer is the metered-dose inhaler (MDI)

- These pressurized canisters dispense a single bolus of an aerosol, either
a suspension or a solution
- In a suspension system, fine crystals of medications are embedded in a
propellant and released when the device is actuated
- In solution systems, the formulation consists of a homogeneous mixture
of medications and co-solvents in propellants

In addition to pressurized canisters, several types of powder metered-
dose inhalers also exist. The two most common are the Spinhaler and
Rotahaler

- The Spinhaler mechanism consists of a capsule that is inserted into a
propeller-driven turbine. After the capsule is punctured, inhaling
through the canister causes the propeller to rotate and the capsule to
vibrate, thus releasing the contents in a turbulent airstream. Usually, one
single inspiration at high speed will dispense all of the drug
- The Rotahaler uses a slight variation of this technique. Inspiration causes
the chamber to spin, and a cutting block opens the capsule and releases
the powdered drug in a spiral airstream

Both the Spinhaler and Rotahaler dispense relatively large quantities of
drug and can be used by patients who have difficulty mastering the techniques required to use a pressurized device. Once an aerosol is generated,
if it is to be effective, it must be inhaled into the lungs and deposited on
the airway surfaces

- The main factors that control the rate at which this occurs are the size of
the particles and the manner in which they are inhaled
- Most therapeutic aerosols contain a wide range of particle sizes; the
smaller ones are the most important therapeutically. Most studies indicate
that the optimum size for intrapulmonic deposition ranges between 1 and
5 microns
- Larger particles tend to impact the upper airways, smaller particles tend
not to sediment and are exhaled

Increasing flow rates during inspiration increase the linear velocities of
the particles and thereby enhance their tendency to impact on the airway
walls. This is particularly prevalent at airway branch points and bends,
where the particles are unable to follow the airstream

- Sedimentation is facilitated by increasing the residence time of the particles by slowing the frequency of respiration and by breath-holding

AEROSOL TECHNIQUE

It is important for as much medication to enter and remain within the airways as possible. Inspiratory flow rate is the most critical variable and should be kept low (approximately 1 l/sec), inhaling over approximately 5 seconds, and inspiration should be followed by a 5- to 10-second period of breath-holding. This low inspiratory flow rate reduces unwanted impaction in the oropharynx; breath-holding facilitates deposition by gravity.

PATIENT INSTRUCTION

Proper aerosol technique is most important (Table 20–1).

- Remove cap from inhaler and shake for a few seconds
- Place inhaler between lips or 2 to 30 cm in front of open mouth for best results
- Take a deep breath and exhale completely
- Begin inhalation and immediately actuate the device to deliver medication
- Finish inhalation slowly, and then hold breath for 5 to 10 seconds
- Wait 2 to 3 minutes and repeat

Inhalation with an open mouth can deliver twice as much medication to the lower respiratory tract as inhalation with the lips closed around the end of the device

- Even with the best techniques, only about 10 to 15% of the aerosol cloud from a metered-dose inhaler will reach the intrathoracic airways. The remainder is deposited on the walls of the mouth and pharynx and is then swallowed
- Therapeutic benefits are derived from the drug that is applied topically in the lung, not from the quantity that ends up in the gut
- Bronchodilatation begins within minutes, while plasma levels of the drug are not yet measurable or are at extremely low levels. With noninhalational routes of administration, bronchodilatation is delayed, and it tends

---

TABLE 20–1. PATIENT INSTRUCTION FOR OPTIMAL MDI USE

- Remove cap from inhaler
- Shake inhaler for a few seconds
- Hold inhaler upright and tilt head back slightly
- Place inhaler between lips* or approximately 2 cm in front of open mouth. Alternatively, a spacer device can be used
- Take a deep breath and exhale completely
- Begin inhaling slowly and immediately press down on top of inhaler to deliver aerosol medicine
- Complete inhalation and hold breath for 5 to 10 seconds
- Wait at least 2 to 3 minutes then repeat above for subsequent puffs

---

* Recommended for anticholinergic drug, ipratropium bromide, to avoid contact with eyes, or use a spacing device

to be found in association with blood levels of the drug that are three to five times those seen with the inhaled route

The main advantage of inhalational therapy is that it minimizes systemic side effects, thereby increasing the safety margin of the drug employed

• The inhaled route delivers a much smaller dose directly to the airways, which produces maximum bronchodilatation with minimum blood levels
• Microgram quantities of inhaled beta$_2$ adrenergic agonists produce maximum dilatation of the airway, whereas milligram quantities of the same agent must be given orally to achieve the same therapeutic effect

BRONCHODILATORS

The bronchodilators discussed in this chapter will be grouped according to the following classifications

• Beta adrenergic agonists
• Anticholinergic agents
• Methylxanthines

Other drugs thought to have some bronchodilator effects (cromolyn sodium, nedocromil sodium, steroids) is covered in Chapter 21.

A comparison of various bronchodilators is presented in Table 20–2.

TABLE 20–2. COMPARISON OF BRONCHODILATORS			
	BETA ADRENERGIC AGONISTS	ANTICHOLIN-ERGICS*	METHYL-XANTHINES#
ETIOLOGY OF ASTHMA			
Allergic	+ + + +	+ +/−	+ +/−
Emotional	+ +	+ + + +	+/−
Exercise-induced	+ + + +	+/−	+ +/−
Intrinsic	+ + +	+ +/−	+ +/−
Irritant-induced	+ + + +	+ + +	+ +/−
CHRONIC OBSTRUCTIVE PULMONARY DISEASE			
Emphysema	+/−	+ + +	+ +/−
Bronchitis	+ + +	+ + +	+ +/−
ACTION			
Onset	Fast (5 min)	Slow (1–2 hrs)	Variable
Duration	Variable	Variable	Long
ADVERSE EFFECTS			
Arrhythmia-potential	+ + +	+/−	+ + + +
Hypokalemia	+ +	−	+/−
Nausea	+ +	−	+ + + +
Tachycardia	+ + + +	+/−	+ +
Tremor	+ + +	−	+ + +

* Ipratropium bromide will be compared as it is the safest and most frequently prescribed.
# Oral preparations will be compared

BETA$_2$ ADRENERGIC AGONISTS

Beta agonists provide the foundation for acute reversal therapy of obstructive airway disease. The rapidity with which they work make them the first choice of physicians and patients. The beneficial effects of epinephrine in the treatment of asthma were described early in the 20th century. Subsequently, numerous other agents similar in structure but more beta$_2$ selective have been developed and tried by several routes with variable degrees of success. The greatest benefit of the beta$_2$ selective agonists may not be in the bronchodilatory capabilities but rather in the diminution of the adverse cardiac side effects. With the advent of beta$_2$ selective agonists, the use of nonselective beta agonists such as isoproterenol, metaproterenol, and isoetharine has become inadvisable.

Pharmacology and Mechanisms of Action
- Beta agonists are structural analogs of norepinephrine
- Substitutions generally involve the terminal amine and/or the hydroxyl groups on the benzene ring
- Modification of the ring constituents generally results in prolongation of action, while modification of the terminal amine confers beta selectivity
- Aerosolized beta$_2$ agonists have a relatively short time to onset of action, generally within 15 minutes. Oral formulations have an onset of action in the range of 30 minutes to 1 hour, which depends on gastrointestinal absorption. The duration of action depends on the formulation of the ring constituent and varies with each compound. In general, the oral formulations of beta agonists have a longer duration of action when compared to their aerosol counterparts as a result of gradual absorption through the GI tract
- Beta$_2$ agonist stimulation of bronchial smooth muscle results in relaxation and, consequently, bronchodilatation. This effect is believed to be mediated by increased intracellular cyclic AMP levels. Increased cyclic cAMP leads to a reduction in cytosolic calcium and smooth muscle relaxation. Virtually all beta receptors in the bronchial smooth muscles are of the beta$_2$ subtype

In addition to the smooth muscle relaxation effects, beta$_2$ agonists are known to exert other effects in the airways

- Both beta$_1$ and beta$_2$ agonists increase mucus secretion from submucosal glands. Beta$_2$ agonist stimulation increases ion transport in epithelial cells which, in turn, leads to increased water secretion. Beta receptor stimulation may thereby improve mucociliary clearance
- The secretion of histamine and other mast cell mediators appears to be modulated by beta$_2$ adrenergic stimulation, as is pulmonary vasoconstriction
- Lastly, beta adrenergic receptors are found throughout the alveolar walls. Approximately two-thirds are of the beta$_2$ subtype. While stimulation of these alveolar beta receptors results partly in stimulation of surfactant secretion by Type II pneumocytes, the function of beta receptors in other cell populations is not yet clearly defined

Adverse effects. While oral and even systemic forms of some beta agonists are available, the preferred method of drug delivery is topically via metered-dose inhaler, passive inhalation device, or aerosol generator. Studies have failed to demonstrate a significant advantage for one route of administration in regard to pharmacologic efficacy. However, the variable absorption of the oral formulations makes them less predictable. In addition, the side effects associated with oral or systemically delivered beta agonists are much greater than with topically delivered medication. These side effects are the result of stimulation of nonpulmonary beta$_1$ receptors. Therefore, they are much more prevalent when nonspecific beta agonists are used

- Common beta$_1$ side effects include tachycardia, palpitations, and muscle tremors. In practice, these three side effects limit the frequency of dosing of beta agonists in obstructive airway disease
- Hypokalemia may also result from beta agonist use. This appears to be mediated by beta$_2$ receptor stimulation of a membrane-bound Na/K ATPase. This hypokalemic response has been implicated in the development of cardiac arrhythmias and is speculated to have a role in sudden death in patients with asthma. Hypokalemia and alterations in the electrocardiogram are documented with the use of a beta$_2$ agonist. These effects are potentiated by concomitant use of diuretics. It would be prudent, therefore, to closely monitor serum potassium in those patients given frequent high dose beta$_2$ agonists concomitantly with potassium-losing diuretics. This would be especially true of patients at risk for cardiac arrhythmias, such as those with congestive heart failure or ischemic heart disease
- Ironically, hypoxemia due to increased ventilation/perfusion mismatching may occur. This is generally not an indication to discontinue the use of the beta agonist, as the hypoxemia is usually mild

Dosage. The dosage and recommended dosing frequency of some of the currently available beta$_2$ selective agonists are given in Table 20–3. While by no means a complete list of available beta$_2$ agonists, this table serves as a guide for selection of agents. The recommendations in Table 20–3 are intended for use in mild to moderate obstructive airway disease. It must be remembered that dosing frequency must be tailored to the clinical situation. More frequent dosing intervals of the shorter acting beta$_2$ selective agonists (salbutamol, terbutaline) have been reported in more severe obstructive disease, specifically status asthmaticus. In this case, the dosing intervals may be decreased to every 30 to 60 minutes, although this should be done only in hospitalized, monitored patients. Lastly, some clinical situations require reductions in dosage and dosing interval, most notably in patients with heart disease or those receiving monoamine oxidase inhibitors and/or tricyclic antidepressants.

Clinical Applications. The aforementioned pharmacologic and cellular response also have clinical merit. Beta adrenergic stimulation, either topically or systemically, results in improved airflow and enhanced clearance of secretions. These effects translate into symptomatic improvement in

TABLE 20–3. BETA$_2$ AGONIST PREPARATIONS		
BETA$_2$ AGONIST	**FORMULATION**	**DOSAGE**
Albuterol (USA)	Tablet; 2 mg	Up to 4 mg qid
Salbutamol (Canada, UK)	Tablet; 24 mg	Up to 4 mg qid
Ventolin (USA, Can, UK)	Syrup; 2 mg/5 ml	Up to 4 mg qid
Proventil (USA)	Repetabs; 4 mg (ext.	Up to 16 mg bid
Aerolin (UK)	release)	
Salbulin (UK)	MDI; 90 mcg/puff	2 puffs q 4–6 hrs
	Solution; 0.25%	2.5 mg/3 ml q 4–6 hrs
	Solution; 0.5%	2.5 mg/3 ml q 4–6 hrs
	Rotocaps; 200 μg	200 mcg q 4–6 hrs
Bitolterol	MDI 350 μg/puff	2–3 puffs q 4–6 hrs
Tornalate (USA)		
Fenoterol	MDI; 180–360 μg/puff	1–2 puffs q 6–8 hrs
Berotec (Canada, UK)		
Pirbuterol	MDI; 200–400 μg/puff	1–2 puffs q 6 hrs
Maxair (USA)		
Exirel (UK)		
Reproterol	MDI; 500 μg/puff	1 puff q 6 hrs
Bronchodil (UK)		
Rimiterol	MDI; 400–600 μg/puff	1 puff q 6 hrs
Plumadil (UK)		
Terbutaline	Tablet; 2.5 mg	2.5–5 mg q 6–8 hrs not
Brethaire (USA)	Tablet; 5 mg	>15 mg/day
Brethine (USA)	Solution; 1 mg/ml	Nebulizer 1–2 mg q 4–6
Bricanyl (USA, Can, UK)		hrs
		Subcutaneous – 0.25 mg
		repeated in 15–30 min
		Not >0.5 mg q 4 hrs
		IV – Not
		recommended
	MDI; 200 μg/puff	2 puffs q 4–6 hrs

patients with both reversible (asthma) and nonreversible (chronic bronchitis and emphysema) obstructive airway disease.

Beta$_2$ agonist therapy is most effective in the treatment of asthma and in the prevention of exercise-induced (and other forms) bronchospasm. Numerous clinical studies have documented spirometric improvement and improvements in mobilization of secretions as well as subjective improvement in patient-scored performance scales following the use of beta agonist bronchodilator therapy. Beta$_2$ agonists are the cornerstone of emergent therapy for the management of acute asthma and exacerbations of other forms of reversible obstruction airway disease (some patients with chronic obstructive pulmonary disease).

However, a recent report noted worsening of control of asthma symptoms following scheduled use of a long-acting beta$_2$ agonist. Possible explanations for these results included further airway narrowing, resulting from stimulation of secretions by the beta agonist, and a heightened late phase response due to tolerance of higher exposure to allergens. These data deserve further investigation, but in light of the wealth of data supporting beta$_2$ agonist use, it would seem imprudent to abandon this therapy solely on the basis of this report.

While the effects of beta$_2$ agonists are most pronounced in patients with reversible obstructive airway disease, there is also data suggesting beneficial effects in chronic airflow obstruction with less reversibility. These beneficial effects include improvements in objective measurements of airway function, improvements in exercise capacity, and improvements in overall subjective quality of life measurements. However, while beta$_2$ agonists are clearly superior to anticholinergics in asthma, anticholinergics have equivalent, if not greater, effects in most patients with chronic bronchitis and emphysema. This is particularly true for patients with "fixed" obstructive airway disease.

ANTICHOLINERGICS

Anticholinergics alkaloids have been used for a variety of purposes for thousands of years. Their use in the treatment of respiratory illness can be dated back at least three centuries, and their use was widespread by the mid-1800s. The anticholinergic agents lost favor with the advent of adrenaline in the early 20th century. Despite the major role that the parasympathetic nervous system plays in the regulation of airway diameter, the development of cholinergic antagonists has lagged behind beta adrenergic agonists. Currently, two forms of anticholinergic bronchodilators are most commonly used: atropine (as SO_4 and methonitrate salts) and ipratropium bromide (Atrovent, Iprafen). While other agents are also available, such as glycopyrrolate (Rubinol), Triazinamium (Multergan), and oxitropium bromide, limited clinical study data are available to allow for recommendations regarding the use of these agents as bronchodilators. Other quaternary ammonium derivatives of atropine, however, will likely be released in the future.

Pharmacology and Mechanism of Action

- Anticholinergic bronchodilators act through antagonism of the muscarinic receptor
- Stimulation of these receptors is believed to be responsible for "resting" bronchomotor tone
- Muscarinic receptors are found predominantly in the larger, central airways, and the anticholinergics are believed to exert their greatest bronchodilatory effects on these airways
- Anticholinergics appear to mediate the bronchoconstrictive effects of certain stimuli, including cholinergics (carbachol and metacholine), cold air, and psychogenic stimuli
- Anticholinergic bronchodilators have little or no effect on those bronchoconstrictive effects believed to be the result of inflammatory mediators, e.g., histamine. This makes them theoretically less effective for antigen-induced bronchoconstriction, as is frequently seen in asthma
- Compared to beta agonists, the anticholinergics have a delayed onset of action with maximal response occurring in 1 to 2 hours. However, the

duration of action is longer with the effects being maintained for up to 6 hours

Adverse effects. The adverse effects of anticholinergic alkaloids are easily predicted and result from their antagonism of the muscarinic receptor

- Inhalation of atropine may result in mouth dryness, dry skin, mydriasis, tachycardia, urinary retention, flushing, gastrointestinal disturbances, and visual blurring. These symptoms are dosage dependent. Higher doses (> 5 mg) result in CNS excitement, fever, headache, weakness, slurred speech, bowel and bladder dysfunction, delirium, and eventually coma
- There have also been reports of decreased mucociliary clearance secondary to the use of atropine. The mechanism of this effect is multifactorial

Adverse effects do not seem to be a problem with ipratropium bromide. The use of ipratropium bromide is much less frequently associated with side effects, even in large doses. It has been estimated that dosages 100 times greater than currently used for bronchodilatory effects would be necessary to produce significant side effects

- The most common complaints associated with ipratropium bromide use are a bitter taste, mouth dryness, and throat or tracheal irritation. These are usually well tolerated, and the incidence is significantly decreased when a spacer device is used
- One adverse effect that is clinically significant is mydriasis after inadvertent aerosol delivery to the eyes. This can result in acute angle closure glaucoma, in addition to unnecessary diagnostic evaluation by individuals not aware of this side effect

The difference in the side effect profiles of the two anticholinergics is the result of structural differences. Atropine is a tertiary ammonium compound with a neutral charge, while ipratropium bromide is a quaternary ammonium compound with a positive charge. The charge difference makes ipratropium bromide relatively lipid insoluble, resulting in markedly decreased systemic absorption of ipratropium bromide as compared to atropine.

Dosage. As stated previously, only two anticholinergic agents are available for inhalation, (ipratropium bromide and the SO_4 salt of atropine). With the advent of ipratropium bromide in most markets, the use of atropine salts has waned. The enhanced toxic effects after systemic and oral administration make inhalation the preferred route for delivery. The usual dose of ipratropium bromide is two to four puffs via metered dose inhaler every 6 hours. Each actuation of the metered-dose inhaler contains 40 μg of ipratropium. Higher doses have been shown to be beneficial in patients with chronic obstructive pulmonary disease with essentially no increase in adverse effects. An inhalant solution (250 μg/ml) is available in Europe and Canada for use as a wet aerosol with a recommended dose of 100 to 500 μg every 4 hours. This agent is often given in combination (salbutamol

0.5 ml in 2 ml ipratropium every 4 to 6 hours). The dose of atropine (which is not available for administration via metered dose inhaler) is 0.025 to 0.05 mg/kg/dose, usually 2 to 3 mgs/dose administered four times daily. Doses between 0.075 and 0.1 mg/kg have been used but are poorly tolerated. Children tend to tolerate larger doses better than adults.

Clinical Applications. Despite mechanisms that suggest significant clinical utility in asthma, anticholinergic alkaloids have shown greatest benefit in other forms of obstructive lung disease, i.e., chronic bronchitis and emphysema. Because ipratropium bromide is the safest and most commonly used anticholinergic agent, the following discussion of the clinical applications will focus on its use

- In diseases such as chronic bronchitis and emphysema, the use of ipratropium bromide may result in therapeutic effects comparable to or even greater than those of the beta adrenergic agonists
- In addition, the combined effect of ipratropium bromide and beta$_2$ agonists appears to be better than either drug alone. This synergistic effect appears to be active in asthma as well. Ipratropium bromide also appears to act synergistically with methylxanthines. The three agents together have also been shown, in some instances, to be more effective than any single agent or combination of agents
- While studies have occasionally documented an actual decrease in pO_2 following beta agonist therapy for acute exacerbation of obstructive airway disease, this does not occur with ipratropium
- In patients with fixed obstructive pulmonary disease unresponsive to beta agonist therapy (specifically emphysema), ipratropium use may not show an improvement in FEV_1 but it results in an increase in vital capacity with subsequent decreased work of breathing and hence symptomatic improvement
- Tachyphylaxis does not appear to develop with ipratropium therapy in contrast to beta agonist therapy
- Older patients with obstructive airway disease appear to have a better clinical response to ipratropium than to beta agonists
- The effects of ipratropium bromide have a longer duration of action when compared to the presently available beta$_2$ agonists, although longer acting beta$_2$ agonists are currently undergoing trial (see Table 20–2)

While the effects of ipratropium bromide in asthma are less clear, there currently exists a considerable amount of data to support its use in asthmatic patients. Specifically, in those patients whose symptoms are not controlled by beta$_2$ agonist or theophylline therapy, a trial of ipratropium bromide is indicated as an adjunct to these therapies.

THEOPHYLLINE

Theophylline is a methylxanthine and has been in use in obstructive airway disease since the early 20th century. Its use has decreased since its time of greatest popularity in the 1970s and 1980s. As a drug with a narrow therapeutic range, significant potential side effects, and requiring monitoring of serum levels, theophylline is a less desirable agent when compared to other bronchodilators.

Pharmacology and mechanisms of action. The precise mechanism of action of bronchodilatation by methylxanthines is not well defined, but the primary effect appears to be relaxation of smooth muscle in the bronchial walls

- Initial research was concentrated on the inhibition of phosphodiesterase. However, other phosphodiesterase inhibitors currently in use in clinical medicine (e.g., dipyridamole) do not result in bronchodilatory effects similar to those of theophylline
- Other proposed mechanisms of bronchodilatory action have included antagonism of adenosine receptors, prostaglandin antagonism, altered metabolism of smooth muscle, and stimulation of catecholamine release

While evidence exists supporting each of these mechanisms, none is completely able to explain the entire range of the effects of theophylline at this time. The bronchodilatory mechanism of theophylline is multifactorial and may involve other pathways as well

- In addition to its bronchodilatory effects, theophylline may increase diaphragmatic contractility and reduce diaphragmatic fatigue
- There is evidence of improved biventricular cardiac performance as well
- Theophylline may stimulate hypoxic ventilatory drive, enhance mucociliary clearance, inhibit mast cell mediator release, and decrease pulmonary artery vasoconstriction
- There are data to suggest an anti-inflammatory mechanism of theophylline in the therapy of asthma. It appears to be effective in blunting the late asthmatic response to bronchial challenge. This action of theophylline requires further definition

While these mechanisms have scientific support from in vitro studies, their clinical utility or relevance has yet to be adequately determined.

Most theophylline preparations are primarily hepatically metabolized, with the exception of dihydroxypropyl theophylline, which is excreted unchanged in the urine. Unlike other bronchodilators, theophylline use is best guided by serum concentrations

- Multiple studies have shown that the bronchodilatory effects are relatively insignificant in most patients at a serum level of less than 10 μg/ml (10 mg/l or 55 μmol/l)
- At levels greater than 20 μg/ml (20 mg/l or 110 μmol/l), toxic effects often emerge
- Thus, it is recommended that serum concentrations between 10 and 20 μg/ml (10 to 20 mg/l or 55 to 110 μmol/l) define the therapeutic endpoints
- Benefit may be observed in some patients at lower serum theophylline concentrations, in the range of 6 to 10 μg/ml (6 to 10 mg/l or 35 to 55 μmol/l). This is seen predominantly in patients who receive theophylline in addition to beta agonist therapy. The benefits deal primarily with sub-

jective measures of improvement, such as patient's perception of disease activity, quality of life, and decreased hospital admissions

Adverse effects. The use of methylxanthines in pulmonary disease is limited by side effects. These effects are generally dose related and are much more prevalent at plasma concentrations greater than 20 µg/ml (20 mg/l or 110 µmol/l).

- The most common side effects include abdominal discomfort, nausea, vomiting, diarrhea, headaches, tremor, and restlessness
- A mild diuretic effect and increased gastric acid secretion may also occur
- Insomnia and other disturbances of sleep pattern have been reported
- While these symptoms are bothersome to patients and may result in non-compliance, they are rarely life-threatening
- However, theophylline, even at therapeutic concentrations, has been associated with cardiac dysrhythmia, including atrial and ventricular premature contractions, atrial fibrillation, and perhaps most commonly, multifocal atrial tachycardia. At higher concentrations, seizures and more malignant cardiac arrhythmias may occur, which can be lethal, albeit rare.

Side effects can be evident in some patients at any serum concentration but are distinctly more common with levels greater than 30 µg/ml (30 mg/l or 165 µmol/l). Adequate monitoring and maintenance of theophylline levels in the therapeutic range lessens these adverse drug manifestations.

Dosage. Theophylline is available via a variety of routes and in a variety of forms. The oral and intravenous (IV) routes are by far the most common means of administration

- Rectal, intramuscular, and inhaled routes are unreliable, painful, and ineffectual, respectively, and each should be avoided
- Theophylline and aminophylline (ethylenediamine salt of theophylline) are the most widely used IV formulations
- Multiple substituted derivatives are available in oral formulations. While some are longer acting, better tolerated, or better absorbed than others, there is really no clear advantage of one form or another in bronchodilatory effects

A partial list of available oral formulations is shown in Table 20–4. While dosage must be individualized for the patient and the underlying illness, rough estimates of oral dosing are as follows

- Oral loading dose—5 mg/kg ideal body weight
- Oral maintenance dose—10 mg/kg ideal body weight per day, divided into one of three doses, depending upon formulation

Oral dosage must be adjusted to maintain serum level of 10 to 20 µg/ml (10 to 20 mg/l or 55 to 110 µmol/l).

IV dosing estimates are as follows

- Loading dose—5 to 6 mg/kg ideal body weight over 20 to 30 minutes
- Maintenance dose—0.4 to 0.6 mg/kg ideal body weight per hour

TABLE 20–4. COMMON ORAL THEOPHYLLINE PREPARATIONS	
PRODUCT NAME	**FORMULATION**
ANHYDROUS THEOPHYLLINE COMPOUNDS	
Bronchodyl	Capsule; 100 and 200 mg
Aerolate	Liquid; 150 mg/15 ml
Aerolate III	Capsule; 65 mg
Aerolate Jr	Capsule; 130 mg
Aerolate SR	Capsule; 260 mg
Constant-T	Tablet; 200 and 300 mg
Elixophyllin	Capsule; 100 and 200 mg
	Elixir; 80 mg/15 ml
Elixophyllin SR	Capsule; 125 and 250 mg
Quibron-T	Tablet; 300 mg
Quibron-T/SR	Tablet; 300 mg
Resbid	Tablet; 250 and 500 mg
Slo-bid	Capsule; 50, 75, 100, 125, 200, and 300 mg
Slo-Phyllin	Capsule; 60, 125, 250 mg
	Tablet; 100 and 200 mg
	Syrup; 80 mg/15 ml
T-PHYL	Tablet; 200 mg
Theo-24	Capsule; 100, 200, 300 mg
Theochron	Tablets; 100, 200, 300 mg
Theoclear L.A.	Capsule; 130, 260 mg
Theoclear 80	Syrup; 80 mg/15 ml
Theo-Dur	Tablets; 100, 200, 300, 450 mg
Theo-Dur Sprinkle	Capsule; 50, 75, 125, 250 mg
Theolair	Tablet; 125 and 250 mg
	Liquid; 80 mg/15 ml
Theolair-SR	Tablets; 200, 250, 300, 500 mg
Theostat	Syrup; 80 mg/15 ml
Uniphyl	Tablet; 400 mg
DIHYDROXYPROPYL THEOPHYLLINE COMPOUNDS	
Dilor	Tablet; 200 and 400 mg
	Syrup; 100 mg/15 ml
	Injectable; 250 mg/ml
Lufyllin	Tablet; 200 and 400 mg
	Syrup; 100 mg/15 ml
	Injectable; 250 mg/ml
ETHYLENEDIAMINE THEOPHYLLINE COMPOUNDS	
Aminophyllin	Tablet; 100 and 200 mg
Somophyllin	Liquid; 105 mg/5 ml

As with the oral dosage, IV dosage requires adjustment based upon serum concentrations. It must be remembered that most theophylline preparations are metabolized hepatically and dosage adjustment is necessary for patients with hepatic insufficiency. In addition, geriatric patients and patients with congestive heart failure or cor pulmonale also require lowered dosing. Cigarette smokers require increased dosage. Children frequently require higher doses than adults. A dosing guideline and common

---

TABLE 20–5. DOSING GUIDELINES FOR INTRAVENOUS THEOPHYLLINE

INTRAVENOUS DOSAGE

5–6 mg/kg ideal body weight given over 20–30 minutes if no theophylline preparation used in the last 24 hours

2–3 mg/kg ideal body weight given over 20–30 minutes if a theophylline preparation used in the last 24 hours

Maintain an infusion rate of **0.4–0.6 mg/kg** ideal body weight per hour with the following adjustments in dosing due to other clinical circumstances:

INCREASE DOSAGE	DECREASE DOSAGE
0.6–0.8 mg/kg/hr	**0.3–0.4 mg/kg/hr**
Children	Elderly
Cigarette Smoker	Hepatic Insufficiency
Hyperthyroidism	Hypothyroidism
Marijuana Use	Congestive Heart Failure
High Protein Diet	Febrile Illness
Medications (Table 20–6)	Medications (Table 20–6)

Serum theophylline concentration should be determined approximately 6 hours after initial infusion and dosage adjusted accordingly. A general rule is adjustment of dose by 25% to achieve an increment or decrement of 5 μg/ml (5 mg/l or 27.5 μmol/l) in serum theophylline concentration.

---

clinical scenarios requiring dosage adjustment are given in Table 20–5. Theophylline drug interactions are listed in Table 20–6.

Clinical indications. Theophylline and other methylxanthines are seen in patients with asthma

- Although it has little effect on the airways of normal individuals, theophylline ameliorates bronchoconstriction in individuals with asthma
- The bronchodilatory effects add to those of beta agonists and anticholinergics but theophylline is a less effective bronchodilator than either agent alone

There is a subset of patients with asthma who experience symptoms during the nocturnal hours and have disrupted sleep secondary to these symptoms. In these patients, there has been some improvement in symptoms and sleep with bedtime dosing of a 24-hour theophylline preparation.

The beneficial effects of theophylline in patients with chronic bronchitis and emphysema are less clear. There does appear to be subjective symptomatic improvement in patients with chronic bronchitis, but objective improvement in airflow is lacking. Theophylline should be considered for use in patients with asthma and chronic bronchitis who have failed optimal inhalation therapy prior to the initiation of systemic steroids. However, the decision to begin theophylline therapy versus steroid therapy should include a knowledge of possible drug interactions and underlying disease states that alter theophylline pharmacokinetics. In some cases, the toxicity of short-term systemic steroids will be less than the toxicity of theophylline and may therefore be the preferred alternative.

TABLE 20–6. THEOPHYLLINE INTERACTIONS

DRUG	EFFECT	RESPONSE
Allopurinol	Decrease theophylline clearance	Decrease dose of theophylline
Barbiturates	Increase theophylline clearance	Increase dose of theophylline
Carbamazepine	Increase theophylline clearance	Increase dose of theophylline
Corticosteroids	Variable metabolic effects	Monitor theophylline levels
Coumarins	Interferes with assay method for serum level resulting in falsely low values	No adjustment in dose necessary
Diltiazem	Slight decrease in theophylline clearance	Possible decrease in theophylline dose
Erythromycin	Decrease theophylline clearance	Decrease dose of theophylline
Estrogens	Decrease theophylline clearance	Decrease dose of theophylline
H_2 Blockers		
Cimetidine	Decrease theophylline clearance	Decrease dose of theophylline
Ranitidine	No effect	No adjustment
Famotidine	No effect	No adjustment
Influenza Vaccine	Decrease theophylline clearance	Decrease dose of theophylline
Interferon	Decrease theophylline clearance	Decrease dose of theophylline
Isoniazid	Decrease theophylline clearance	Decrease dose of theophylline
Isoproterenol	Increase theophylline clearance	Increase dose of theophylline
Lithium	Increase lithium clearance	Increase dose of lithium
Mexiletine	Decrease theophylline clearance	Decrease dose of theophylline
Nicorette	No effect	No response
Oral contraceptives	Decrease theophylline clearance	Decrease dose of theophylline
Pancuronium	Decrease pancuronium responsiveness	Increase dose of pancuronium
Phenytoin	Increase theophylline clearance	Increase dose of theophylline
Quinolones	Decrease theophylline clearance	Decrease dose of theophylline
Tobacco smoking	Increase theophylline clearance	Increase dose of theophylline
Troleandomycin	Decrease theophylline clearance	Decrease dose of theophylline
Verapamil	Decrease theophylline clearance	Decrease dose of theophylline
Vidarabine	Decrease theophylline clearance	Decrease dose of theophylline

BIBLIOGRAPHY

AEROSOL THERAPY

Dolovich MB, Ruffin RE, Roberts R, Newhouse MT: Optimal delivery of aerosols for metered dose inhalers. Chest, *80*(6 Suppl):911, 1981.

Newhouse MT, Dolovich MB: Control of asthma by aerosols. N Engl J Med, *315*:870, 1986.

BRONCHODILATORS IN GENERAL

Guyatt GH, Townsend M, Pugsley SO, et al.: Bronchodilators in chronic air-flow limitation: Effects on airway function, exercise capacity, and quality of life. Am Rev Respir Dis, *135*:1069, 1987.

National Asthma Education Program/Expert Panel Report: Guidelines for the Diagnosis and Management of Asthma. US Dept of Health and Human Services, Publication No. 91-3042, 1991.

Torphy TJ: Action of mediators on airway smooth muscle: Functional antagonism as a mechanism for bronchodilator drugs. Agents and Actions, *23*(Suppl):37, 1988.

Ziment I: Pharmacologic therapy of obstructive airway disease. Clin Chest Med, *11*:461, 1990.

BETA AGONISTS

Clifton GD, Hunt BA, Patel RC, Burki NK: Effects of sequential doses of parenteral terbutaline on plasma levels of potassium and related cardiopulmonary responses. Am Rev Respir Dis, *141*:575, 1990.

Colacone A, Wolkove N, Stern E, et al.: Continuous nebulization of albuterol (salbutamol) in acute asthma. Chest, *97*:693, 1990.

Haahtela T, Jarvinen M, Tuomo K, et al.: Comparison of a beta$_2$-agonist, terbutaline, with an inhaled corticosteroid budesonide, in newly detected asthma. N Engl J Med, *325*:388, 1991.

Higgins BG, Powell RM, Cooper S, Tattersfield AC: Effect of salbutamol and ipratropium bromide on airway calibre and bronchial reactivity in asthma and chronic bronchitis. Eur Respir J, *4*:415, 1991.

Lipworth BJ, McDevitt DG, Struthers AD: Hypokalemic and ECG sequelae of combined beta-agonist/diuretic therapy: Protection by conventional doses of spironolactone but not triamterene. Chest, *98*:811, 1990.

Nelson HS: Adrenergic therapy of bronchial asthma. J Allergy Clin Immunol, *77*:771, 1986.

Ramsdale EH, Otis J, Kline PA, et al.: Prolonged protection against methacholine-induced bronchoconstriction by the inhaled β$_2$ agonist formoterol. Am Rev Respir Dis, *143*:998, 1991.

Sears MR, Taylor DR, Print CG, et al.: Regular inhaled beta-agonist treatment in bronchial asthma. Lancet, *336*:1391, 1990.

Sly RM, et al.: Position Statement: Adverse effects and complications of treatment with beta-adrenergic agonist drugs. J Allergy Clin Immunol, *75*:443, 1985.

van Schayck CP, Folgering H, Harbers H, et al.: Effects of allergy and age on response to salbutamol and ipratropium bromide in moderate asthma and chronic bronchitis. Thorax, *46*:355, 1991.

Waldeck B, Olsson OA, Svensson LA: New possibilities for the beta-adrenoreceptor agonist bronchodilator drugs. Agents and Actions, *23*(Suppl):55, 1988.

ANTICHOLINERGICS

Braun SR, McKenzie WN, Copeland C, et al.: A comparison of the effects of ipratropium and albuterol in the treatment of chronic obstructive pulmonary disease. Arch Intern Med, *149*:544, 1989.

Chapman KR: The role of anticholinergic bronchodilators in adult asthma and chronic obstructive pulmonary disease. Lung, *168*(S):295, 1990.

Chervinsky P: Concomitant bronchodilator therapy and ipratropium bromide: A clinical review. Am J Med, *81*(5A):67, 1986.

Gilman MJ, Meyer L, Carter J, Slovis C: Comparison of aerosolized glycopyrrolate and metaproterenol in acute asthma. Chest, *98*:1095, 1990.

Gong H, Brik A, Tashkin DP, Dauphinee B: Effects of inhaled thiazinamium chloride on histamine-induced and exercise-induced bronchoconstriction. Ann Allergy, *62*:230, 1989.

Gross NJ: Ipratropium bromide. N Engl J Med, *319*:486, 1988.

Gross NJ, Bankwala Z: Effects of an anticholinergic bronchodilator on arterial blood gases of hypoxemic patients with chronic obstructive pulmonary disease. Am Rev Respir Dis, *136*: 1091, 1987.

Gross NJ, Petty TL, Friedman M, et al.: Dose response of ipratropium as a nebulized solution in patients with chronic obstructive pulmonary disease. Am Rev Respir Dis, *139*:1188, 1989.

Gross NJ, Skorodin MS: Anticholinergic, antimuscarinic bronchodilators. Am Rev Respir Dis, *129*:856, 1984.

Jannun DR, Mickel SF: Anisocoria and aerosolized anticholinergics. Chest, *90*:148, 1986.

Karpel JP: Bronchodilator responses to anticholinergic and beta-adrenergic agents in acute and stable COPD. Chest, *99*:871, 1991.

Karpel JP, Pesin J, Greenberg D, Gentry E: A comparison of the effects of ipratropium bromide and metaproterenol sulfate in acute exacerbations of COPD. Chest, *98*:835, 1990.

Malani JT, Robinson GM, Scheviratne EL: Ipratropium bromide induced angle closure glaucoma. NZ Med J, *95*:749, 1982.

Ziment I, Au JP: Anticholinergic agents. Clin Chest Med, *7*:355, 1986.

METHYLXANTHINES

Arkinstall WW, Atkins ME, Harrison D, Stewart JH: Once-daily sustained-release theophylline reduces diurnal variation in spirometry and symptomatology in adult asthmatics. Am Rev Respir Dis, *135*:316, 1987.

Bukowsky M, Nakatsu K: The bronchodilator effect of caffeine in adult asthmatics. Am Rev Respir Dis, *135*:173, 1987.

Crea F, Pupita G, Galassi AR, et al.: Effect of theophylline on exercise-induced myocardial ischemia. Lancet, *1*;683, 1989.

Hendeles L, Massanari M, Weinberger M: Update on the pharmacodynamics and pharmacokinetics of theophylline. Chest, *88*:103S, 1985.

Murciano D, Auclair M-H, Pariente R, Aubier M: A randomized controlled trial of theophylline in patients with severe chronic obstructive pulmonary disease. N Engl J Med, *320*:1521, 1989.

Pauwels RA: New aspects of the therapeutic potential of theophylline in asthma. J Allergy Clin Immunol, *83*:548, 1989.

Peake MD, Chrystyn J, Mulley BA: Response to oral theophylline in severe chronic obstructive airways disease. Br J Med, *298*:523, 1989.

Taylor DR, Buick B, Kinney C, et al.: The efficacy of orally administered theophylline, inhaled salbutamol, and a combination of the two as chronic therapy in the management of chronic bronchitis with reversible air-flow obstruction. Am Rev Respir Dis, *131*:747, 1985.

Wrenn K, Slovis CM, Murphy F, Greenberg RS: Aminophylline therapy for acute bronchoplastic disease in the emergency room. Ann Int Med, *115*(4):241, 1991.

21

ASTHMA

Susan K. Pingleton
Steven W. Stites
Lewis Wesselius

Asthma is a disease of the airways characterized by increased responsiveness of the trachea and bronchi to a wide range of stimuli. Intermittent symptoms of cough, chest tightness, and wheezing usually alter in severity, either due to treatment or spontaneously. The widespread airway narrowing results from a combination of smooth muscle contraction, inflammation, edema, and mucous secretion. This working definition of asthma is incomplete due to the difficulty in describing the precise nature of this disease. Importantly, airway inflammation is present in virtually all patients with asthma and, with widespread mucous plugging of airways, is a constant finding in patients who have died of status asthmaticus.

MAJOR CLASSIFICATIONS

EXTRINSIC ASTHMA

Extrinsic asthma occurs in atopic patients, that is, those with production of IgE antibodies to allergens. These allergens may be of a wide variety.

INTRINSIC ASTHMA

Intrinsic asthma occurs in patients without evidence of atopy, usually adults.

OCCUPATIONAL ASTHMA

Symptoms of occupational asthma occur with exposure to provoking allergens at a work place and often improve when the patient is removed from that environment. Unfortunately, many patients exhibit features of several categories, making classification difficult.

EPIDEMIOLOGY

PREVALENCE

Lack of uniform diagnostic criteria and reporting make exact estimations difficult

- Asthma has been reported worldwide, although there are large differences in prevalence. This ranges from less than 1% (Tokelau islanders) to 17% or more (New Zealand)
- Prevalence in the United States is estimated at 7 to 10% of children and 5% of adults
- Prevalence rates in developed countries are higher than those in underdeveloped countries
- Incidence of asthma appears to be increasing in the United States and worldwide
- Role of heredity is unclear; while studies have been unable to define the precise role of genetic factors, there appear to be a familial predisposition and occurrence in asthma

AGE/SEX

- Asthma may occur at any age
- One-half of all cases develop before the age of 10, another one-third by the age of 40
- There is a 2 to 1 male predominance in childhood, which equalizes by the age of 40

MORTALITY

- About 0.4 deaths per 100,000 cases in the United States; around 2.0 in New Zealand
- Mortality rates have been steady or increasing despite treatment advances

PATHOPHYSIOLOGY OF ASTHMA

The cardinal feature of asthma is hyperresponsiveness of the tracheobronchial tree. This can be familial or acquired and is influenced by inflammation in the airways. The pathophysiology of asthma suggests that patients with asthma have abnormalities of the bronchial smooth muscle, the autonomic nervous system, and the cells present in the airways.

BRONCHIAL SMOOTH MUSCLE

Bronchial smooth muscle lines the bronchi and small airways. In asthma, this muscle is hypertrophied and hyperplastic. While normal muscle cells contract about 20% in length, these cells contract further in asthma. Bronchial smooth muscle is under a complex system of controls that are not well understood

- Bronchodilation is achieved by stimulating beta$_2$ adrenergic receptors
- Histamine, acetylcholine, (leukotrienes), and prostaglandins F2a and D2 cause narrowing
- Adenosine, dopamine, and other factors may also influence bronchial smooth muscle contraction

THE AUTONOMIC NERVOUS SYSTEM

Four major components of the autonomic nervous system aid in regulation.
The beta-adrenergic system is found on bronchial smooth muscle, epithelial, and alveolar cells. Stimulation causes smooth muscle relaxation, possibly via adenyl cyclase and cyclic adenosine monophosphate (AMP)

- Function of these receptors is deranged in asthma
- Bronchodilators stimulate these receptors and cause bronchial relaxation
- Circulating levels of catecholamines stimulate the beta-adrenergic system; lower levels of catecholamines at night cause an increase in nocturnal symptoms

The alpha-adrenergic system includes airway receptors, but their role in asthma is unclear

- Stimulation may cause airway narrowing
- There may be a role in releasing mast cell mediators

The cholinergic system supplies nerves to bronchial smooth muscle throughout the length of the airway and controls mucous gland secretion

- Impact on bronchial hyperresponsiveness is unclear
- Cholinergic blocking drugs can cause some dilatation and decrease mucus production

The nonadrenergic inhibitory nervous system maintains airway patency

- Major peptide may be the neurotransmitter vasoactive intestinal peptide
- Other neuropeptides, such as substance P, have roles that are not well defined

CELLS PRESENT IN THE AIRWAY

Numerous cells have been found to have a role in bronchial hyperresponsiveness. This is an area of intense investigation. While specific mediators and pathways are being described, the general picture is not clear. The following is a brief review of some cells that may contribute to the pathogenesis of asthma

- Mast cells, which are present in increased numbers throughout the airways in asthmatics, release a number of mediators, including histamine, that can cause smooth muscle contraction and increase vascular permeability and mucus production. Several prostaglandins and leukotrienes are also produced and may have key roles in bronchoconstriction

- Basophils may be active in the late phase of mediator release and may also release histamine
- Bronchial epithelial cells produce several mediators, including PGE_2, and are frequently shed in increased numbers in asthmatics
- Eosinophils infiltrate the airways and can release tissue-damaging substances such as peroxidase and major basic protein
- Alveolar macrophages may induce mast cell mediator release and contribute to bronchoconstriction
- Lymphocytes produce IgE, interleukins, lymphokines, and other substances that may increase bronchial hyperresponsiveness
- Vascular endothelial cells become leaky and result in increased airway edema
- Mucus-secreting cells in the airway are increased in number and size in patients with asthma and contribute to mucous plugging

AIRWAY PATHOLOGY

The complex forces that combine to cause asthma result in certain macroscopic and microscopic features that are common to those who have died from this disease. At autopsy, macroscopic features in fatal attacks include

- Overinflated lungs that do not deflate upon opening the thoracic cavity
- Widespread airway plugging with thick mucus
- Airway wall thickening
- Upper lobe bronchiectasis (sometimes)
- Little evidence of emphysema

Microscopically, there are four major findings in fatal cases

- Infiltration of airway walls by inflammatory cells, particularly eosinophilic infiltration
- Epithelial desquamation
- Smooth muscle hypertrophy
- Basement membrane thickening; subepithelial deposition of collagen

Other features of asthma include mucus gland hyperplasia and increased goblet cell numbers. Patients with asthma who are asymptomatic appear to have varying degrees of the abnormalities noted above.

BRONCHIAL HYPERRESPONSIVENESS

Bronchial hyperresponsiveness is a key feature of asthma. The precise mechanism for its occurrence is unknown. In humans, it can be characterized by

- Increased severity of bronchoconstriction in response to low doses of histamine and methacholine
- Wide variability in the level of bronchial hyperresponsiveness, even in patients with clinical asthma
- Inability to always demonstrate bronchial hyperresponsiveness in response to provocation testing during complete remission

TRIGGERS OF ASTHMA

The actual mechanism by which specific agents cause asthmatic symptoms is not completely elucidated. However, there are certain triggers that can increase bronchial hyperresponsiveness in known asthmatics.

ALLERGENS

Allergic asthma depends upon IgE response modulated by B and T cell lymphocytes and the interaction of mast-cell-bound IgE with antigen. Small amounts of antigen reach distal airways, where mast cells interdigitate with epithelial cells. There is usually an immediate response, resulting in bronchoconstriction, followed in some patients by a late-phase response 6 to 10 hours later. Once contracted, the mast cells and other cells release mediators that cause constriction, edema, and vascular congestion

- Major airborne allergens include house dust, mites, and pollens
- Asthmatics who respond to allergens usually have a fair number of antigens that can trigger their disease
- The role of different foods (cow's milk, monosodium glutamate, preservatives, food coloring agents, etc.) are not clearly defined, although some individuals may react strongly
- Symptoms can be continual or seasonal, depending on the antigen

PHARMACOLOGIC AGENTS

Pharmacologic agents triggering asthma include drugs such as aspirin, tartrazine dye, beta blockers, and sulfating agents

- Nasal polyps, rhinorrhea, and asthma comprise a syndrome that has been associated with aspirin use in some patients
- Sulfating agents such as potassium and sodium bisulfite, sulphur dioxide, and others are widely used in the fresh food industry and may cause symptoms in some

ENVIRONMENTAL AND AIR POLLUTION

Climatic conditions can increase the concentration of allergens and cause exacerbation of asthma. Occupational asthma refers to patients who develop symptoms while in the work place in response to some specific trigger. These symptoms will often improve when the patient is out of the offending environment, but chronic problems can also occur. Specific agents include

- Wood and vegetable dusts, such as western red cedar
- Metal salts, such as platinum, chrome, and nickel
- Pharmaceutical agents, including antibiotics, piperazine, and cimetidine
- Industrial chemicals and plastics, such as toluene, isocyanate, phthalic acid, ethylenediamine, and others

- Biologic enzymes, including detergents
- Animal and insect dusts, serums, and secretions

The underlying mechanisms for airway obstruction in occupational asthma include the formation of specific IgE, the direct release of factors causing bronchoconstriction by the offending agent, and direct airway stimulation.

INFECTIONS

Respiratory infections by viruses and bacteria are the most common causes of asthma exacerbation. Respiratory syncytial and parainfluenza virus are major offenders in children, while rhinovirus and influenza virus are most common in adults. The reason that viruses induce asthma is unclear, but bronchial hyperresponsiveness may last up to 8 weeks. Bacteria are less common than viruses as triggers of asthmatic exacerbation but can super-infect a prior viral process.

EXERCISE

Physical exertion can worsen asthma and the first episode often occurs with exercise in children. This acute process may be due to thermal changes in the intrathoracic airways as heat and water are transferred from tracheal mucosa to the inspired air. High ventilation may lower airway temperature farther, especially in colder, dryer air, and worsen symptoms. Hence, ambient temperatures and the level of exertion may correlate with the degree of obstruction. Activities such as cross-country skiing or ice skating usually produce more symptoms than swimming.

STRESS

Objective evidence suggests that psychological features play a role in asthmatic symptoms. These interactions are complex but may be related to vagal efferent activity mediating airway caliber. The extent of the influence of psychological factors on asthma is unclear.

CLINICAL HALLMARKS OF ASTHMA

MEDICAL HISTORY

- Dyspnea
- Chest tightness
- Wheezing
- Cough
- Exercise intolerance
- Rhinitis
- Sinusitis
- Nasal polyposis
- Atopic dermatitis

The hallmark of asthma is the variable nature of respiratory symptoms that are caused by the changing degree of airway obstruction. The marked variability in degree of airway obstruction is the main factor distinguishing asthma from other forms of chronic obstructive lung disease. Typically, symptoms in asthma are episodic.

In some cases, the patient's clinical history may be so characteristic of asthma that a presumptive diagnosis of asthma can be comfortably made on the history alone. It is important to remember, however, that "not all that wheezes is asthma" and, in most cases, it will be necessary to have objective data to support a clinical diagnosis.

Other features of medical history include

- Positive family history for allergies/asthma (50%)
- Aspirin sensitivity (5 to 10%)
- Frequent association with sinusitis

Pertinent findings of the physical examination include

- Head and neck: Nasal polyps may be present
- Chest: Scattered or diffuse wheezes, prolonged expiration

DIFFERENTIAL DIAGNOSIS OF ASTHMA

- Emphysema
- Bronchitis
- Congestive heart failure
- Pulmonary emboli
- Foreign body in airway
- Aspiration
- Carcinoid syndrome
- Bronchiectasis
- Laryngeal edema
- Hyperventilation syndrome
- Factitious wheezing
- Cystic fibrosis

USEFUL TESTS IN DIAGNOSING ASTHMA

PULMONARY FUNCTION TESTING

Patients with asthma may have normal routine pulmonary function studies if they are in remission at the time of testing. When patients are symptomatic, however, abnormalities in pulmonary function should be present.

Spirometry

- FEV_1: Decreased
- FEV_1/FVC: Decreased
- Typically, a 20% or greater increase in FEV_1 is noted after administration of an inhaled bronchodilator

TABLE 21–1. CHANGES IN THE ARTERIAL BLOOD GASES				
SEVERITY OF ATTACK	MILD	MODERATE	SEVERE	VERY SEVERE
pH	↑	↑	normal	↓
PaO_2	normal	↓	↓	↓
$PaCO_2$	↓	↓	normal	↑

Lung Volumes

- Total lung capacity: Normal or increased
- Residual volume: Increased

Diffusion Capacity (Transfer Factor)

- Normal or increased

ARTERIAL BLOOD GASES

Arterial blood gases may be normal if the patient is in remission at the time of testing. If the patient is symptomatic, however, arterial blood gases will demonstrate abnormalities, the pattern of abnormalities indicates the disease severity. The arterial blood gases may be useful, therefore, in determining the aggressiveness of treatment and the need for close monitoring of patients in the hospital or in the intensive care unit (see Table 21–1).

CHEST X-RAY

The chest x-ray is generally of little value in making a diagnosis of asthma. In asthmatics presenting with an acute attack, the chest x-ray generally appears normal or demonstrates hyperinflation. The main value of the chest x-ray is to rule out densities and/or atelectasis secondary to mucus plugging and other diagnostic possibilities, such as pneumothorax or pneumonia.

LABORATORY TESTS THAT MAY HAVE DIAGNOSTIC UTILITY

- Blood leukocytes: Asthmatics frequently demonstrate moderate eosinophilia (5 to 15% of polymorph neutrophils)
- Sputum exam: May demonstrate eosinophils, Curschmann's spirals
- Serum IgE: Elevated in some patients with asthma, but many will have normal levels, so clinical value is limited
- Radioallergosorbent test (RAST): Identifies specific IgE antibodies in the serum, although it is less sensitive than skin testing

BRONCHOPROVOCATION TESTING

It has been postulated that all patients with asthma demonstrate exaggerated bronchial reactivity to a variety of stimuli. These stimuli may include natural triggers such as exercise or cold air or may be a result of artificial pharmacologic stimulation of airways with methacholine or histamine. The evaluation of airway responsiveness to challenge with aerosolized methacholine or histamine has become part of the diagnostic armamentarium in evaluating patients with atypical asthma. Bronchoprovocation testing generally determines the concentration of aerosolized methacholine or histamine that causes a 20% decrease in FEV_1 (PD20 FEV_1). A normal bronchoprovocation study is considered by some investigators to be strong evidence against a diagnosis of asthma. Some studies in children and patients with occupational asthma suggest, however, that bronchial hyperresponsiveness may not be present universally in subjects that appear clinically to have asthma. In addition, bronchial hyperresponsiveness can be demonstrated in many patients with chronic bronchitis as well as in some patients with allergic rhinitis and some apparently normal subjects after viral infections.

Bronchoprovocation testing

- Is positive in a high percentage of patients with asthma; the test is not necessary if typical asthmatic symptoms and signs have been documented
- May also be positive in patients with other pulmonary disorders and in some normal patients
- Does not correlate well with symptoms
- A normal methacholine study in the setting of typical asthmatic symptoms, however, suggests the need for further investigation for another possible diagnosis

THERAPY OF ASTHMA

An array of pharmacologic agents are available for the treatment of asthma. The available agents can be classified as bronchodilators, functioning primarily to directly reduce bronchoconstriction (see Chapter 20), or as anti-inflammatory agents (corticosteroids or cromolyn), decreasing airway inflammation, which is the primary stimulus for bronchoconstriction and bronchial hyperresponsiveness. Inhaled corticosteroids are listed in Table 21-2.

Some patients with chronic, stable asthma have symptoms even with multi-drug treatment (inhaled steroids, beta₂ agonists, theophylline, cromolyn, or ipratropium). In these patients, oral corticosteroids have a role (see Table 21-3).

Another drug potentially useful in management of chronic, stable asthma is Ketotifen

- Antihistamine with anti-asthma properties
- Unclear role in management of asthma
- Not available in the United States

TABLE 21–2. INHALED CORTICOSTEROIDS*: AEROSOL METERED DOSE INHALER

PRODUCT	SUPPLIED	DOSAGE†
Beclomethasone		
Beclovent	50 µg/puff	2 puffs 2–4 times daily
Vanceril	100–200 µg/Rotacap	
Becloforte	250 µg/puff	1–2 puffs 2 times daily
Becotide (UK)	50 µg/puff	2 puffs 2–4 times daily
	200 µg/puff	1–2 puffs 2–4 times daily
	100–200 µg Rotacaps	2–4 times daily
Budesonide		
Pulmicort Turbuhaler‡	100–400 µg/puff	1–2 puffs 2–3 times daily
Flunisolide	250 µg/puff	1–2 puffs 2 times daily
Bronalide		
Bronkolid		
Aerobid		
Triamcinolone acetate§	100 or 200 µg/puff	2–4 puffs 2 times daily

* Not recommended for acute attacks
† Dose inhaled 10–20 minutes after beta$_2$ agonist inhalation. Dose > 1500 µg/daily: risk adrenal suppression and osteoporosis
‡ Pulmicort chlorofluorocarbon-based inhaler replaced by Pulmicort Turbuhaler (non-chlorofluorocarbon) in some countries
§ High dosage of fluorinated agents may rarely cause myopathy

TABLE 21–3. TREATMENT OF CHRONIC, STABLE ASTHMA

PATIENT TYPE	AGENTS RECOMMENDED
1. Only occasional dyspnea, such as with exercise	Beta$_2$ agonist inhaled as needed
2. Chronic cough without airway obstruction	Inhaled steroid regularly
3. Frequent or prolonged episodes of dyspnea	Inhaled steroid regularly and beta$_2$ agonist as needed
4. Asthma not controlled by inhaled steroids and beta$_2$ agonists	Consider cromolyn and adding ipratropium

Methotrexate may be useful in treating chronic, stable asthma

- Controversial if it has a steroid-sparing effect in patients with severe asthma
- Should be used in low doses (15 mg weekly)
- Beneficial effects in patients with asthma are still uncertain, and this agent must be used with extreme care due to significant side effects (neutropenia, liver injury, restrictive lung disease)

CLINICAL DATA INDICATING SEVERE ASTHMA

MEDICAL HISTORY

- Previous ICU admission, frequent emergency room visits, or hospital stay beyond 4 days for treatment of documented severe asthma
- Recent oral corticosteroid use for exacerbation
- Brittle asthma

PHYSICAL EXAM

- Extreme dyspnea with inability to speak more than a few words.
- Pulsus paradoxus > 18 mm Hg
- Use of accessory muscles and paradoxical thoracoabdominal motion
- Diaphoresis
- Inability to lie supine
- Heart rate > 120 beats/minute
- Respiratory rate > 30
- Absence of audible wheezing in a patient with severe exacerbation of asthma

ARTERIAL BLOOD GASES

- PaO_2 < 60 mm Hg
- $PaCO_2$ ≥ 40 mm Hg

EXPIRATORY FLOW

- PEFR or FEV_1 < 30% of predicted for adults
- Failure of PEFR to improve at least 10% after initial treatment

STATUS ASTHMATICUS

Status asthmaticus refers to an asthmatic episode that does not respond to usual initial therapy and is severe enough to threaten life. This form of asthma is a medical emergency and requires intensive treatment and monitoring. The history is usually one of poorly controlled asthma that progresses over days or weeks, although in some cases there will be a more abrupt onset (see Chapter 28).

TREATMENT OF ACUTE, SEVERE ASTHMA

Initial treatment in the emergency room for patients with acute, severe asthma should include inhaled beta₂ agonists and intravenous corticosteroids.

BETA₂ AGONISTS

Beta₂ selective agents should be given frequently by inhalation, e.g., every 20 minutes over the first hour.

- Inhaled beta₂ agonists (see Chapter 20): Albuterol (Salbutamol) 2.5 to 5 mg (0.5 to 1 ml of 0.5% solution)
- Subcutaneous beta agonists: Epinephrine (1:1000) 0.3 to 0.5 ml, avoid in older asthmatics (>40) and anyone with a history of heart disease; Terbutaline 0.24 to 0.50 mg

CORTICOSTEROIDS

In patients with severe asthma, early use of intravenous (IV) corticosteroids is warranted. The optimal dose of corticosteroids is not known, but doses of 80 to 125 mg of methylprednisolone repeated every 6 to 8 hours have been recommended. Patients who have responded to IV steroids can be safely switched to comparable doses of oral steroids. Because oral doses of steroids are frequently significantly lower than IV doses, however, it is wise to carefully monitor the clinical response of the patient during the switch from IV to oral steroids. Following discharge from the hospital, oral steroids should be tapered carefully with frequent determination of PEFR to monitor for any deterioration in pulmonary function (see oral dosages, Chapter 22). Inhaled steroids are not useful in the treatment of acute, severe asthma, but should be used to aid in the weaning process of oral steroids. Inhaled steroids have a role in patients with asthma requiring beta₂ agonists more than three times daily for control.

Corticosteroids increase the effectiveness of beta₂ agonists and have been demonstrated to induce the formation of new beta₂ receptors in the human lung.

ANTICHOLINERGICS

Several studies have demonstrated some benefit from adding nebulized ipratropium bromide to treatment with inhaled beta₂ agonists in acute, severe asthma. The nebulized form of ipratropium is presently not available in the United States, and it is not known whether the metered-dose inhaler would be of comparable benefit. Given the safety and lack of significant side effects associated with the use of ipratropium, it is a reasonable adjunct to treatment in patients who have demonstrated a limited clinical response to beta₂ agonists and corticosteroids (see Chapter 20).

Dosage: Ipratropium (via nebulizer) 500 μg/2 ml unit; administer 2 ml every 4 hours; in severe asthma, give every 2 hours for four doses then 4 to 6 hours under supervision. When the patient has been stabilized, a metered-dose inhaler (20 μg puff, one to four puffs three to six times daily) may be required.

METHYLXANTHINES

There is little objective evidence that addition of methylxanthine therapy adds any significant benefit to patients treated with beta₂, agonists and IV or oral corticosteroids. Some studies have demonstrated that although there was no therapeutic benefit, a significant increase in treatment toxicity (including nausea and palpitations) was associated with the addition of methylxanthine therapy. There appears to still be a role for methylxanthines in chronic treatment of asthma, but it appears that these agents do not have a clear role in the treatment of acute, severe asthma. In patients who are being treated chronically with methylxanthines and present with acute, severe asthma, it is reasonable to obtain a serum theophylline level and, if subtherapeutic, administer aminophylline or theophylline to bring serum levels to a safe therapeutic range (10 to 15 μg/ml, United States; 10 to 20 mg/l, UK; 55 to 110 μmol/l, Canada). See Chapter 20 and Tables 20–5, 20–6, for dosage and factors that alter theophylline levels.

ADDITIONAL MEASURES

SUPPLEMENTAL OXYGEN

Supplemental oxygen should generally be provided by nasal cannula to these patients. Oxygenation should be monitored by pulse oximetry; oxygen flow rates can then be titrated to maintain oxygen saturation above 90%. In some cases, a higher inspired concentration of oxygen provided by a high-flow face mask may be required. In severely obstructed patients, it is important to obtain frequent arterial blood gases, in addition to following oximetry, to determine whether there are progressive increases in arterial CO_2 that would indicate impending ventilatory failure.

MECHANICAL VENTILATION

Endotracheal intubation and mechanical ventilation of patients in status asthmaticus are last-resort treatments indicated in patients with impending ventilatory failure. Indications for intubation include

- Inability to maintain airway control resulting in progressive increase in arterial CO_2 tension to elevated levels (particularly > 50 mm Hg)
- Altered mental status
- Clinical evidence of respiratory muscle fatigue (paradoxical movement of diaphragm)
- Refractory hypoxemia, acidemia or seizures

Mechanical ventilation of asthma patients may be complicated by very high airway pressures, which may lead to barotrauma. Mortality associated with mechanical ventilation for status asthmaticus has been reported to be relatively high (i.e., 5 to 23%). Controlled hypoventilation, which uses lower tidal volumes and a lower respiratory rate and tolerates some hypercarbia while maintaining oxygenation, may result in a lower mortality. In general, the tidal volume and respiratory rate should be adjusted to maintain peak airway pressures to <50 cm H_2O (see Chapter 29).

OUTPATIENT MANAGEMENT OF THE SEVERE ASTHMATIC

Optimal outpatient management of patients with severe asthma should include routine assessment of PEFR, as the presence or absence of symptoms may not accurately reflect lung function. Appropriate adjustments in inhaled medications or in oral corticosteroids should be made if the PEFR falls significantly. Patients should be instructed to obtain emergency medical assistance if the PEFR falls dramatically (<150 L/min). Monitoring PEFR on a regular basis will help limit any delay in initiating treatment for bronchospasm. This approach may help reduce mortality that may result from delayed initiation of treatment for bronchospasm in some asthmatics.

MORTALITY FROM ASTHMA

Features that characterize patients at increased risk for asthma-associated death include

- Age over 55 years
- Prior history of ICU admission, intubation, or respiratory acidosis
- Hospitalization for asthma in last year
- Recent withdrawal from systemic steroids
- Psychological or psychosocial problems
- Lack of access to health care
- Inadequate medical management

In spite of new pharmacologic agents and a better understanding of the pathologic mechanisms of asthma, mortality rates for asthma have increased recently in a number of countries, including the United States, Canada, Australia, New Zealand, and the UK, as well as other European countries. The reason for this increase is unclear. One apparent factor in many deaths, however, is delay in initiating appropriate treatment for worsening asthma. Mortality in asthmatics is generally associated with a history of worsening over several days. However, in some patients, death may occur very abruptly, following rapid decompensation over a period of several hours or less.

BIBLIOGRAPHY

Barnes PJ: A new approach to the treatment of asthma. N Engl J Med, *321*:1517, 1989.

Beasley R, Cushley M, Holgate ST: A self management plan in the treatment of adult asthma. Thorax, *44*:200, 1989.

Darioli R, Perret C: Mechanical controlled hypoventilation in status asthmaticus. Am Rev Respir Dis, *129*:385, 1984.

Larsen GL: Asthma in children. N Engl J Med, *326*:1540, 1992.

Littenberg B, Gluck EH: A controlled trial of methylprednisolone in the emergency treatment of acute asthma. N Engl J Med, *314*:150, 1986.

Littenberg G: Aminophylline treatment in severe, acute asthma. A meta-analysis. JAMA, *259*: 1678, 1988.

National Asthma Education Program, Expert Panel Report Guidelines for the Diagnosis and Management of Asthma. National Institutes of Health, Bethesda, MD

Ratto D, Alfaro C, Sipsey J, et al.: Are intravenous corticosteroids required in status asthmaticus? JAMA, *260*:527, 1988.

Rebuck AS, Chapman KR, Abboud R, et al.: Nebulized anticholinergic and sympathomimetic treatment of asthma and chronic obstructive airways disease in the emergency room. Am J Med, *82*:59, 1987.

Siegel D, Shepard D, Gelb A, Weinberg PF: Aminophylline increases the toxicity but not the efficacy of an inhaled beta-adrenergic agonist in the treatment of acute exacerbations of asthma. Am Rev Respir Dis, *132*:283, 1985.

Wasserfallen JB, Schaller MD, Feihl F, Perret CH: Sudden asphyxic asthma: a distinct entity? Am Rev Respir Dis, *142*:108, 1990.

22

CHRONIC OBSTRUCTIVE PULMONARY DISEASE

Susan K. Pingleton
Randy G. Dotson
Gerald R. Kerby

Chronic obstructive pulmonary disease (COPD) is a generic term used to describe the condition in patients with expiratory airflow obstruction. The diseases usually included under the heading COPD are chronic bronchitis and emphysema, which both have varying degrees of expiratory airflow obstruction.

CHRONIC BRONCHITIS

The definition of chronic bronchitis is based on a clinical symptom complex: Cough with sputum production for 3 months of the year over 2 consecutive years in the absence of other causes with or without expiratory airflow obstruction.

The pathophysiology is described as chronic excessive secretion of mucus with hypertrophy of the subepithelial tracheobronchial mucous glands. The goblet cells are another source of excessive mucous secretion. Studies have demonstrated that the mucous glands are increased in size. The Reid Index, or ratio of gland to bronchial wall thickness, is the most common means of measuring mucous gland enlargement.

- The increased bronchial smooth muscle present in chronic bronchitis has been determined to result from smooth muscle hyperplasia. A correlation has been demonstrated between decreased FEV_1 and increased amounts of smooth muscle in the major airways. Increased amounts of smooth muscle are related neither to bronchodilator response nor to methacholine responsiveness in surgically resected lung
- Bronchoscopy and bronchoalveolar lavage performed on patients with chronic bronchitis demonstrated increased inflammation of the tracheobronchial tree compared to that of asymptomatic smokers or normal individuals. Bronchial samples of the lavage demonstrated increased neutrophils. Airway netrophilia was associated with sputum production, airway obstruction, and cigarette smoking

- Bronchial walls are thickened with encroachment on the airway lumen. Patients with severe obstruction had double the bronchial wall width internal to the cartilage/lumenal diameter of that in patients without obstruction. Most series have reported that the increase in bronchial wall thickness resulting from mucous gland hypertrophy is minimal

EMPHYSEMA

Emphysema is defined as the abnormal, permanent enlargement of the airspace distal to the terminal (nonrespiratory) bronchioles with concomitant destruction of their walls without obvious fibrosis. Emphysema can be classified as follows

- Centriacinar emphysema: This form of emphysema involves the respiratory bronchioles with scarring and focal dilatation of the bronchiole and adjacent alveoli, and exists as centrilobular and focal emphysema. Centrilobular emphysema is most frequently associated with prolonged cigarette smoking. It usually involves the posterior upper lobes and is the most common clinically expressed form of emphysema. Focal emphysema is associated with exposure to biologically inactive dust and is uniformly distributed throughout the lung
- Panacinar emphysema: This form of emphysema involves dilatation of all the respiratory airspaces and of the secondary lung lobule with either diffuse or focal involvement. The diffuse form may be associated with deficiency of protease inhibitors (alpha$_1$ antitrypsin deficiency), and the lung bases are involved more often than the upper lobes

RISK FACTORS

Risk factors include

- Cigarette smoking: Smoking is by far the most important single factor associated with the development of COPD. Only a portion of chronic smokers, however, show an accelerated decline in FEV_1. Chronic cough and sputum occur independent of the development of airflow obstruction
- Air pollution: Exposure to particulate matter is related to symptoms of chronic bronchitis and reduction in pulmonary function. Exposure to irritants can lead to cellular changes and acute respiratory infection or may enhance allergic response
- Occupational exposure: Exposures to both organic and inorganic dust may lead to symptoms of chronic bronchitis. Any effect that such exposure may have on the development of airflow obstruction has been difficult to demonstrate in cross-sectional studies; however, most longitudinal studies show the accelerated decline in indices typical of an airflow associated with chronic dust exposure. The effect is more pronounced in smokers
- Atopy: The role of immunologic response and airway hyperresponsiveness in the development of COPD is important. The immunologic precursors to COPD are in part genetically determined. Bronchial reactivity

may be a precursor to obstructive airway disease. A relationship exists between COPD prevalence and serum IgE levels
- Heredity: Hereditary factors, such as deficiency of protease inhibitors (alpha$_1$-antitrypsin deficiency), have been related to the development of emphysema. Prevalence of this deficiency has been shown by blood donor studies to be 350 per 1,000,000. Nonsmoking patients may remain asymptomatic with little abnormality of lung function through their 6th to 7th decades of life; however, smokers with protease inhibitor deficiencies may experience severely limited respiratory function by age 40
- Socioeconomic factors: The lower the socioeconomic status, the higher the prevalence rate of COPD. Occupational status was found to be weakly related to respiratory symptoms and disease

CLINICAL HALLMARKS

HISTORY

- Dyspnea or acute chest illness with cough, sputum production, chest tightness, and wheezing may be of sufficient magnitude to bring the patient to seek medical attention. This condition usually occurs in the 6th to 7th decade of life. Chronic bronchitis and emphysema often coexist and are reviewed together in the remaining sections
- The dyspnea is usually of insidious onset
- Smoking of more than 20 cigarettes per day for 25 or more years is often present. Hemoptysis may occur and, if so, is usually associated with the development of purulent sputum in a lower respiratory tract infection. Recurrent symptoms of cough, increased and/or purulent sputum, wheeze, and dyspnea are common

PHYSICAL SIGNS

- Active accessory muscles (scalenes and sternomastoids) are a consistent finding with significant airflow obstruction because of the inability of the diaphragm to produce the force required for inspiration
- Pursed lip expiration is a common feature in patients with severe airflow obstruction
- Examination of patients with emphysema often demonstrates a barrel chest, caused by air trapping, and thus a prominent sternal angle, horizontal ribs, and an increased anteroposterior diameter. Also seen is a low diaphragm with limited motion or decreased excursion. Normal diaphragmatic excursion is approximately 5 to 6 cm
- Indrawing of the intercostal space is a sign of hyperinflation of the chest
- Paradoxical abdominal and diaphragmatic movement during respiration indicates diaphragmatic fatigue or weakness. Patients with exacerbations of COPD who manifest this sign are more likely to require ventilator assistance
- Hoover's sign, paradoxical inward movement of the lateral costal margin, may be observed and is caused by horizontal rather than vertical

(downward) diaphragmatic contraction that results from the flat position of the diaphragm. Hoover's sign is not a sign of diaphragmatic fatigue
- Tracheal tug, the downward movement of the thyroid cartilage and trachea with each inspiration, may be observed
- Wheezes (rhonchi), which are musical sounds produced by the rapid passage of air through a bronchus that is narrowed to the point of closure, may be heard. The walls of the bronchus oscillate between closed and barely open positions and generate audible sound. Wheezes are typically expiratory but may occur in both inspiration and expiration. Although wheezes vary in pitch, inferences as to the size of the airways involved cannot be made from the pitch
- Cardiac dullness is decreased
- Reduction in breath sounds is marked
- Central cyanosis and signs of cor pulmonale—jugular venous distension, hepatojugular reflux, hepatomegaly, and pedal edema (see Chapter 19)—are apparent
- Signs of hypercapnia (asterixis, chemosis, and fundal vessel dilatation), usually without papilledema, are important indicators of elevated Pa_{CO_2}
- A forced expiratory time of greater than 6 seconds indicates airflow limitation. This maneuver is performed by placing the stethoscope over the trachea and requesting the patient to expire from full inspiration to full expiration. Normally the patient should be able to expire completely in less than 6 seconds
- Finger clubbing is not a feature of COPD and, if present, should alert the physician to other possible causes, such as bronchiectasis and carcinoma

INVESTIGATIONS

CHEST RADIOGRAPHY

The chest x-ray may reveal the marked and persistent overdistension of the lungs that is strongly suggestive of emphysema; however, the sensitivity of chest radiography for the detection of emphysema is poor. The diaphragms are often low and flattened in emphysema. An enlarged retrosternal airspace (greater than 3.5 cm) and a deep anteroposterior diameter of the chest may be present.

- Hyperinflated, hypertransradiant lungs, as well as a large and small bullae, are seen
- Excessively rapid tapering of the vascular shadows with narrow-angle branching and general oligemia resulting from loss of pulmonary vessels is apparent
- A narrow, seemingly elongated heart is not uncommon
- The chest x-ray of the patient with chronic bronchitis may be normal or may demonstrate accentuation of the normal bronchovascular markings
- Heart size is not a sensitive indicator of cor pulmonale

- The chest x-ray may be suggestive of emphysema if air trapping, hyperinflation, vascular deficiency, and bullae are present, but these findings are often not present until late in the course of the disease

PULMONARY FUNCTION TESTING

- Forced expiratory volume in 1 second (FEV_1) is reduced. An FEV_1 below 70% of that predicted for age-, sex-, and height-matched controls is abnormal and indicates airflow obstruction
- The ratio of FEV_1 to forced vital capacity (FVC) of less than 70% with incomplete reversibility indicates an airflow obstruction. Moderate airflow obstruction is evidenced as an FEV_1/FVC ratio of less than 65%, whereas severe airflow obstruction is evidenced as an FEV_1/FVC ratio of less than 60% with a markedly reduced FEV_1 (less than 0.75 L)
- The FVC may be normal or may decrease in proportion to any increase in the residual volume
- The diffusing capacity for carbon monoxide (D_{LCO}) is usually reduced in emphysema and often remains near normal in chronic bronchitis
- Arterial blood gas values may be normal or may show varying degrees of hypoxemia or hypercapnia, depending on the type of disease and the point in its natural course. Patients with predominant chronic bronchitis typically develop hypoxemia and hypercapnia earlier in the progression of airflow obstruction than do patients with predominant emphysema, who may have normal or near-normal blood gas values despite severe airflow obstruction ($FEV_1 < 0.75$ L). In such patients, development of hypercapnia is often a preterminal sign

THERAPY

Therapy should be directed at

- Improvement of reversible airflow obstruction
- Treatment of complications in COPD
- Oxygen therapy
- Pulmonary rehabilitation
- Prevention
- Home care

Improvement of reversible airflow obstruction involves treatment of bronchospasm, mucosal inflammation, and infection and control of abnormal and excessive mucoid or mucopurulent secretions that occur with varying degrees of clinical significance at different times in the same patient. A careful clinical assessment of the patient and examination of the sputum often provide hints as to which of these components of airway obstruction is contributing most to the current exacerbation.

PHARMACOLOGIC THERAPY

Salutary effects are obtained in most patients with the use of bronchodilators. Occasionally pulsed corticosteroids are used in combination with antibiotics during exacerbations when bacterial infection is deemed present. The main classes of compounds used in the treatment of COPD are

- Beta$_2$ adrenergic agonist (Table 20–3)
- Anticholinergic agents (Table 20–1, see Chapter 20)
- Methylxanthines (discussed in detail in Chapter 20; see Tables 20–4, 20–5, 20–6)
- Corticosteroids (Table 22–1)

ANTIBIOTICS

- The use of antibiotics in an exacerbation of COPD has been demonstrated in various studies to be both beneficial and of little benefit. The initial infection in most patients with an acute exacerbation of COPD is most commonly viral. Because of impaired mucociliary clearance, bacterial superinfection occurs in a substantial proportion of patients. Accurately differentiating those patients whose course will be improved by antibiotics from those who will receive no benefit is difficult or impossible. The administration of a broad-spectrum antimicrobial agent to a patient who is producing purulent, copious sputum during an exacerbation is a reasonable addition to therapy. Current recommended antibiotics include trimethoprim/sulfa, amoxicillin, or tetracycline
- Sputum culture is not helpful or necessary in most exacerbations. If the patient fails to improve with first-line therapy, culture should be obtained because the emergence of drug-resistant organisms, especially Pseudomonas, may occur after repeated courses of antibiotics. Choice of antibiotics when drug-resistant organisms are present should be guided by sensitivity testing

CORTICOSTEROIDS

As potent anti-inflammatory drugs, corticosteroids may be useful in the treatment of active bronchial inflammation. Judicious use is mandatory because of the well-known deleterious side effects of long-term, high-dose corticosteroids.

- Hospitalized patients with acute exacerbations causing respiratory failure should receive high-dose IV methylprednisolone, 250 to 500 mg/24 hr. (Supplied: vials, 40 or 125 mg; convenient to give 80 to 125 mg every 6 hours.) After 48 hours, the dose may be halved daily until a dose of 40 to 60 mg is reached. The patient is then changed to oral prednisone, and the dosage is tapered.
- Outpatients with exacerbations associated with acute, purulent bronchitis often benefit from a short, pulsed dose of oral prednisone. A dose of 40 to 60 mg/day for 5 days without tapering is frequently successful in accelerating improvement in airflow obstruction. If obstruction flares when corticosteroids are stopped, a tapering schedule may be needed.
- Patients with severe airflow obstruction (FEV$_1$ < 1 L) deserve 1 controlled trial of corticosteroids to determine whether they are 1 of the approximately 20% who show substantial improvement in airway obstruction. Prednisone administered 40 to 60 mg/day for 2 to 4 weeks is an adequate trial (Table 22–1). The trial *must* be controlled by baseline

TABLE 22–1. CORTICOSTEROIDS AND BRONCHODILATORS

NAME	PREPARATION	ROUTE OF ADMINISTRATION
Methylprednisolone (Solu-Medrol)	80 to 125 mg q 6 hrs	Intravenous
Prednisolone (Medrol)	Variable (initial 20–40 mg qd)	Oral
Dexamethasone (Decadron)	4–10 mg qd to qid	Intravenous, oral
Prednisone	Variable (40–60 mg qd to bid)	Oral
ANTICHOLINERGIC AGENTS:		
Atropine	1–3 mg q 6 hrs	Nebulized aerosol
Ipratropium bromide (Atrovent)	2–4 puffs qid	Metered dose inhaler
BETA$_2$ AGONISTS:		
(See Table 20–3, Chapter 20)		
METHYLXANTHINES:		
(See Chapter 20 for detailed description of methylxanthines)		

and post-therapy measurements of FEV_1. A response is determined by improvement in airflow obstruction. Most patients show subjective improvement because of the euphoric effect of the drug. Maintenance of a therapeutic response requires chronic corticosteroid therapy.

- Inhaled corticosteroids are commonly ineffective in patients with COPD, even in those who improve with systemic therapy. The lack of effect is probably caused by poor peripheral aerosol distribution.
- Patients requiring chronic corticosteroid therapy to maintain improved airway function should be tapered to the lowest possible single daily dose or tried on alternate-day administration (1 dose every 48 hours) to minimize side effects. Measures to prevent weight gain, hyperglycemia, and osteoporosis are important.

TREATMENT OF COMPLICATIONS

ACUTE EXACERBATIONS

Acute exacerbations consist of increased dyspnea, chest tightness, and wheezing usually accompanied by increased cough and sputum production. The most common cause is acute lower respiratory infection, usually viral. Exposure to respiratory irritants may also cause an exacerbation. Treatment depends on the severity of the baseline disease and of the exacerbation. Severity is best judged by peak flow measurement, spirometry, and/or arterial blood gas measurement in addition to symptoms. An increasing order of intensity of therapy involves

- Increased frequency of inhaled bronchodilators
- Antibiotic administration

- Use of pulsed corticosteroids
- Oxygen if Pa_{O_2} less than 55 mm Hg
- Mechanical ventilation for ventilatory failure with consideration of the patient's and the family's wishes

PULMONARY THROMBOEMBOLISM

An estimated 20 to 40% of patients with exacerbation of COPD experience acute pulmonary thromboembolism. Risk factors for pulmonary thromboembolism in this group of patients include inactivity and cor pulmonale. The symptoms and signs of pulmonary embolism are associated with those of deep venous thrombosis and include leg swelling and pain. Findings in the chest include pleuritic chest pain, hemoptysis, dyspnea, and possibly a pleural friction rub. The ventilation perfusion lung scan is often equivocal because of the already present ventilation and perfusion mismatching secondary to underlying lung pathology from COPD (see Chapters 19 and 30).

PNEUMOTHORAX

Spontaneous pneumothorax rarely causes the exacerbation of COPD and is most often secondary to the rupture of a bulla or bleb. Identification of a pneumothorax can be lifesaving. The chest examination often reveals decreased breath sounds on the side of the pneumothorax. The affected side of the chest is often more hyperresonant than the contralateral side, but this finding is difficult to ascertain clinically. If tension is involved, the trachea may be shifted to the opposite side of the pneumothorax and hemodynamic deterioration may arise emergently.

NEUROMUSCULAR ABNORMALITIES (RESPIRATORY DRIVE DEPRESSION)

- Sedative/hypnotic medication
- Narcotic analgesics
- Metabolic alkalosis, which may be caused by diuretics that induce hypochloremia and elevated bicarbonate levels
- Hypocalcemia
- Hypomagnesemia
- Hypophosphatemia

OXYGEN THERAPY

The predominant pathophysiologic mechanism leading to hypoxemia and hypercapnia in COPD is ventilation/perfusion mismatching leading to increased numbers of gas exchanging units with low $\dot{V}/\dot{Q}$ ratios. In addition, when the work of breathing exceeds respiratory muscle capacity for work, generalized hypoventilation occurs, either acutely or chronically, thus further worsening both hypoxemia and hypercapnia. Hypoxemia may be

TABLE 22–2. F_{IO_2}/FLOW RATE EQUIVALENTS	
NASAL CANNULA FLOW RATE (L/MIN)	**APPROXIMATE F_{IO_2} (%)**
1	23
2	27
3	30
4	33
5	36
6	40

acutely lethal. Chronic hypoxemia leads to pulmonary hypertension, polycythemia, cognitive impairment, and premature death.

TYPES

- Nasal cannula: The most comfortable, generally most suitable means for oxygen therapy in COPD (Table 22–2). Less likely to be removed by patients
- Oxygen masks: Venturi masks achieve the most accurate control of F_{IO_2}. Rebreather and nonrebreather masks can achieve F_{IO_2} between 40 and 80%. All masks are somewhat uncomfortable and more likely to be removed
- Endotracheal intubation with mechanical ventilation: Can achieve F_{IO_2} of 100%. Necessary when adequate oxygenation cannot be achieved without hypercapnia with respiratory acidosis severe enough to cause somnolence or coma
- Oxygen conservation devices: Pulsed flow devices and reservoir devices both conserve oxygen by avoiding the wasted oxygen that does not reach the alveolar level or is delivered during expiration

ACUTE EXACERBATIONS

Oxygen therapy is indicated during acute exacerbations when the room air Pa_{O_2} is less than 60 mm Hg or the Sa_{O_2} is less than 90%. The dose of oxygen required is generally low unless pneumonia or pulmonary embolism is present.

- In the absence of hypercapnia, the dose of oxygen is not critical. A $Pa_{O_2} > 65$ mm Hg or $Sa_{O_2} > 90\%$ is adequate
- Hypercapnic patients may depend on their hypoxic drive to stimulate respiration. Oxygen therapy may result in worsening hypercapnia and respiratory acidosis. Many such patients can be successfully treated with carefully controlled F_{IO_2} achieving a Pa_{O_2} between 55 and 65 mm Hg without producing clinically significant respiratory acidosis. A Venturi mask or pediatric oxygen flowmeter may be used to achieve a more precise F_{IO_2}
- If a Pa_{O_2} of 55 mg Hg cannot be achieved without clinically significant

respiratory acidosis, mechanical ventilation may be required. Clinically significant respiratory acidosis is best judged by cerebral effects (somnolence, coma, inability to cooperate with therapy) rather than by any arbitrary level of Pa_{CO_2} or pH
- Hypoxemia can be rapidly lethal or deleterious. Respiratory acidosis can be tolerated for several hours. Oxygen should *never* be discontinued in a patient with respiratory failure who has a rising Pa_{CO_2}
- The duration of oxygen therapy for acute exacerbation is unpredictable. Some patients require several weeks of oxygen therapy to restore their previous level of Pa_{O_2}. If the Pa_{O_2} is below 55 mm Hg at the time of discharge, home administration of oxygen should be arranged with a repeat blood gas measurement taken in 2 to 4 weeks to determine when or whether oxygen therapy can be discontinued

CHRONIC

Stable patients with COPD who remain hypoxemic despite optimal medical therapy benefit from long-term oxygen therapy. Documented benefits are improved survival, decreased pulmonary artery pressure and polycythemia, improved cognitive function, improved exercise tolerance, decreased dyspnea, and fewer hospitalizations. Oxygen is usually delivered via nasal cannula. Oxygen conservation devices may decrease the cost of oxygen and extend the duration of use for a portable oxygen system.

GUIDELINES FOR LONGTERM OXYGEN THERAPY

- $Pa_{O_2} \leq 55$ mm Hg or $Sa_{O_2} < 88\%$ at rest breathing air
- $Pa_{O_2} < 60$ mm Hg or $Sa_{O_2} < 90\%$ at rest breathing air in patients with either cor pulmonale, pulmonary hypertension, or polycythemia
- $Pa_{O_2} \leq 55$ mm Hg or $Sa_{O_2} < 88\%$ during exercise or sleep
- Dose: Oxygen flow sufficient to raise Pa_{O_2} to 65 mm Hg or $Sa_{O_2} \geq 90\%$
- Duration: At least 15 h/day unless only needed during exercise or sleep

OXYGEN DELIVERY SYSTEMS

- Cylinders: Bulky, high-pressure regulators, frequent change required, moderately expensive, short duration for portable use, unsuitable for flow rates > 2 L/min
- Liquid: Most portable, most expensive, requires replenishment every 1 to 2 weeks, excellent when high flows are required
- Concentrators: Least expensive with flows > 2 L/min, require electricity, not portable

PULMONARY REHABILITATION

The objectives of pulmonary rehabilitation are to control and alleviate symptoms and complications and to achieve optimal ability to carry out activities of daily living. Optimal medical control of the disease should be achieved prior to attempts at rehabilitation. Patient education concerning the disease, symptoms of complications, medications, and respiratory therapy is an important component of optimal medical management, as well as part of a pulmonary rehabilitation program. The most important factor in pulmonary rehabilitation is patient motivation.

PATIENT SELECTION

Screening should include spirometry, arterial blood gas measurements, and exercise evaluation. A standard 6- or 12-minute walk, cycle, or treadmill test can be used. Ventilatory limit can be predicted from the FEV_1 ($FEV_1 \times 40$). Exercise-induced oxygen desaturation should be evaluated during exercise by oximetry or blood gas measurements because patients with exercise-induced oxygen desaturation should receive oxygen during exercise if it increases exercise performance.

COMPONENTS OF REHABILITATION

- Exercise reconditioning: Exercise training can improve exercise tolerance and performance. The type of exercise (stair climbing, walking, treadmill, ergometer) is unimportant. Most patients with COPD are too limited by ventilatory capacity to achieve improved cardiovascular fitness. The improvement in performance is likely related to improved musculoskeletal efficiency and "desensitization" to the sensation of dyspnea. Performance usually improves with 20 to 30 minutes of exercise, 3 to 5 times per week
- Inspiratory muscle training: Measures to specifically increase inspiratory muscle strength, such as inspiratory resistance breathing, may improve diaphragmatic strength, but the improvement in clinical symptoms is questionable
- Breathing retraining: Several maneuvers (pursed-lip breathing, expiratory abdominal augmentation, synchronization of movement of abdomen and thorax, relaxation techniques for accessory respiratory muscles), as well as psychologic assurance, appear to allow patients to recover more rapidly from dyspnea induced by exercise
- Energy conservation: Instruction in work simplification and the use of energy conservation devices (wheelchair, electric cart) allow patients more independence and greater participation in activities of daily living
- Nutrition: Advanced COPD is frequently associated with loss of weight and muscle mass. Patients need to maintain sufficient protein/calorie intake to prevent malnutrition. Frequent small meals or use of liquid formula diets may help
- Psychosocial management: Patients with COPD often suffer from anxiety, depression, and problems related to cognitive, perceptual, and motor activity. Education, counseling, supervised exercise, and supportive therapy can be useful. Psychiatric consultation and the use of antianxiety and/or antidepressive medications are indicated in selected patients

PREVENTION

SMOKING

Educational and psychosocial measures that lead to a choice not to smoke are the most cost-effective in approaching the problem of COPD. The accelerated rate of decline in FEV_1 that occurs in susceptible smokers appears to return to a normal rate once smoking has stopped, even when early airflow obstruction is present. Surveys of ex-smokers suggest that a physician's advice is the singlemost important factor leading to smoking cessation. Other adjunctive measures, such as self-help, group counseling, hypnosis, and nicotine substitution, may benefit selected patients.

OCCUPATIONAL AND ENVIRONMENTAL POLLUTION

Although far less important than smoking, inhaled irritants and dusts accelerate the normal aging decline in FEV_1, especially in patients who smoke. Measures to control atmospheric and occupational pollution and protection of workers need to be taken.

VACCINATION

Patients with COPD should receive an annual vaccination against influenza. Unvaccinated patients may benefit from amantadine during an influenza epidemic. Vaccination with a multivalent pneumoccocal vaccine is recommended.

ALPHA₁-ANTITRYPSIN REPLACEMENT THERAPY

In the rare patient with COPD caused by alpha$_1$-antitrypsin deficiency (at 1%), replacement therapy should be considered. When therapy should be started is uncertain, but most clinicians advise beginning when the patient shows early signs of emphysema. Whether the progression of far-advanced disease is affected by replacement is uncertain.

HOME CARE

The goals of home care are to

- Improve the quality of life by allowing patients with advanced disease to remain in a home environment
- Minimize or prevent complications that would require hospitalization
- Detect changes in physical or psychosocial status that indicate need for changes in management
- Provide treatment for the patient and improve adherence to the therapeutic program
- Foster a positive and independent attitude

Home care programs may be

- Hospital based

- Community based: Visiting nurse association, community or public health agency, proprietary nursing agent, durable medical equipment company

BIBLIOGRAPHY

American Thoracic Society: Standards for the diagnosis and care of patients with chronic obstructive pulmonary disease (COPD) and asthma. Am Rev Respir Dis, *136*:225, 1987.

Bates B: A Guide To Physical Examination. Third Edition. Philadelphia, JB Lippincott, 1983.

Burrows B: Airways obstructive diseases: pathogenic mechanisms and natural histories of the disorders. Med Clin North Am, *74*:547, 1990.

Clausen JL: The diagnosis of emphysema, chronic bronchitis and asthma. Clin Chest Med, *11*:405, 1990.

Gross, NJ: Chronic obstructive pulmonary disease. Current concepts and therapeutic approaches. Chest, *97*:19S, 1990.

Hodgkin JE: Pulmonary rehabilitation. Clin Chest Med, *11*:447, 1990.

Hudson LD, Monti CM: Rationale and the use of corticosteroids in chronic obstructive pulmonary disease. Med Clin North Am, *74*:661, 1990.

Make BJ: Introduction to pulmonary rehabilitation. Clin Chest Med, *7*:519, 1986.

Petty T: Definitions in chronic pulmonary disease. Clin Chest Med, *11*:363, 1990.

Simon G: Principles of the Chest X-Ray Diagnosis. Third Edition. London, Butterworth, 1971.

Stockley RA: Alpha$_1$ antitrypsin and the pathogenesis of emphysema. Lung, *165*:61, 1987.

Thurlbeck WM: Pathophysiology of chronic obstructive pulmonary disease. Clin Chest Med, *11*:389, 1990.

Ziment I: Pharmacologic therapy of obstructive airways disease. Clin Chest Med, *11*:461, 1990.

23

RESTRICTIVE LUNG DISEASE
David R. Moller

The term "restrictive lung disease" encompasses a large, diverse group of diffuse lung diseases characterized by filling of the alveoli and/or infiltration of the pulmonary interstitium, which results in a characteristic pattern of restrictive lung impairment with reduction in lung volumes and decrease in the compliance of the lung.

CLASSIFICATION

A classification based on the known cause or symptom complex of this group of disorders is given in Table 23–1.

PATHOPHYSIOLOGY

Disorders involving the pulmonary interstitium are associated with inflammation and/or fibrosis of the alveolar structures. The inflammatory component may be dominated by mononuclear cells, neutrophils, eosinophils, or lymphocytes and is termed an "alveolitis." The inflammatory process may be associated with various degrees of fibrosis; both processes result in restrictive physiologic disturbances

- Forced vital capacity (FVC) and 1-second forced expiratory volume (FEV_1) are reduced proportionately in the absence of associated obstructive airway disease; thus, the FEV_1/FVC is commonly normal or supernormal
- Lung volumes (total lung capacity [TLC], vital capacity [VC], and residual volume [RV]) are reduced
- Lung compliance is reduced
- Diffusing capacity for carbon monoxide (D_{LCO}) and the difference between the alveolar and arterial oxygen tensions are frequently reduced
- Hypoxemia results from mismatching of ventilation and perfusion. Chronic respiratory alkalosis occurs, and respiratory acidosis may supervene with advanced disease
- Gas exchange is typically disturbed during exercise and often correlates well with the severity of the disease

---

TABLE 23–1. CLASSIFICATION OF RESTRICTIVE LUNG DISEASE

1. Familial or Congenital
   Familial pulmonary fibrosis
   Gaucher's disease
   Niemann-Pick disease
   Hermansky-Pudlak syndrome
   Familial hypercaciuric hypercalcemia and interstitial lung disease
   Neurofibromatosis and tuberous sclerosis
2. Environmental Lung Disease
   Inorganic Dust Diseases (Pneumoconiosis)
   Asbestosis
   Silicosis
   Coal worker's pneumoconiosis
   Siderosis
   Talcosis
   Hard metal disease
   Hypersensitivity Pneumonitis
   Organic dusts
   Chemicals
   Granulomatous Diseases
   Beryllium disease
   Diffuse Lung Injury
   NO_2 (silo-filler's disease)
   Irritant chemicals
3. Infections
   Viral
   Bacterial
   Mycobacterial
   Fungal
   Parasitic
4. Drug Reactions
   Chemotherapeutic agents
   Antiarrhythmic agents
   Antibiotics
   Illicit drugs
   Miscellaneous
5. Physical Reagents
   Radiation lung disease
6. Rejection-Associated Pulmonary Fibrosis
7. Primary Eosinophilic Pneumonias
   Löffler's syndrome
   Chronic eosinophilic pneumonia
   Allergic bronchopulmonary aspergillosis
   Tropical pulmonary eosinophilia
   Pulmonary vasculitis—
   Churg-Strauss syndrome
   Hypereosinophilic syndromes
8. Disorders of Unknown Cause
   Sarcoidosis
   Idiopathic pulmonary fibrosis
   Collagen vascular lung disease
   Bronchiolitis obliterans organizing pneumonia
   Eosinophilic granuloma
   Pulmonary vasculitis
   Wegener's granulomatosis
   Goodpasture's syndrome
   Systemic necrotizing vasculitis
   Hypersensitivity vasculitis
   Lymphomatoid granulomatosis
   Lymphocytic infiltrative disorders
   Idiopathic pulmonary hemosiderosis
   Lymphangioleiomyomatosis
   Amyloidosis
   Pulmonary alveolar proteinosis
   Pulmonary alveolar microlithiasis
   Lipid pneumonia

- Similar physiologic changes are noted with airspace involvement except that hypoxemia may be more severe because of greater shunt fractions compared to disorders with predominant interstitial involvement

APPROACH TO THE DIAGNOSIS

Management of the patient with restrictive lung disease begins by establishing a definitive diagnosis whenever possible. Most patients have progressive dyspnea and/or diffuse pulmonary infiltration on chest x-ray. Review of the clinical history, physical examination, and all previous and current films give important clues to the diagnosis and chronicity of the disease.

The initial diagnostic sequence starts by excluding multiple other possible causes of progressive dyspnea and/or diffuse pulmonary infiltration.

Left ventricular failure, primary pulmonary hypertension, and pulmonary embolism must be considered. All patients should be evaluated for known causes of interstitial lung disease, such as occupational and environmental agents, drugs, connective tissue diseases, and infectious pneumonias, by performing a detailed history, a physical examination, and serum studies.

HISTORY

- Rapid changes in symptoms and radiologic pattern are unusual except in pulmonary edema, hemorrhage, or pneumonia
- The importance of a careful occupational, environmental, and drug histories cannot be overemphasized because it can lead to a specific diagnosis
- Fever suggests an infectious process, collagen vascular disorder, malignancy, hypersensitivity pneumonitis, sarcoidosis, or drug reaction
- Hemoptysis is commonly seen in advanced fibrocystic sarcoidosis, pulmonary vasculitis (e.g., Wegener's granulomatosis, Goodpasture's syndrome), blood dyscrasias, or infections

PHYSICAL EXAMINATION

- Interstitial pulmonary fibrosis is frequently associated with end inspiratory, "Velcro" crepitations (crackles)
- Bronchiolitis obliterans organizing pneumonia and, uncommonly, hypersensitivity pneumonitis or idiopathic pulmonary fibrosis may demonstrate high-pitched, musical, mid inspiratory squeaks
- Digital clubbing is found in 10 to 15% of patients with pulmonary fibrosis, usually as a late manifestation of the disease

CHEST X-RAY

The chest x-ray often provides considerable help in narrowing the differential diagnosis when combined with the history and physical examination.

Traditionally, diseases causing diffuse infiltration on chest x-ray are divided into "interstitial" or "alveolar" disorders based on their typical radiographic presentation (Table 23–2). Alveolar-filling diseases are associated with small, nodular, ill-defined infiltrates reflecting material in the distal airspaces. Confluence of these opacities may lead to large areas of consolidation associated with air bronchograms and silhouetting of normal structures. Interstitial disease processes are associated with reticular, reticulonodular, or nodular patterns or a ground-glass appearance

- Many restrictive diseases have involvement of both alveolar and interstitial components on pathologic examination, and the radiographic pattern is mixed
- As many as 10% of symptomatic individuals with diffuse lung disease initially have a normal chest x-ray
- Mediastinal adenopathy is common in sarcoidosis, lymphoma, granulomatous infections, lymphangitic carcinomatosis, silicosis, beryllium

---

TABLE 23–2. RADIOGRAPHIC FEATURES OF RESTRICTIVE LUNG DISEASE

PREDOMINANTLY ALVEOLAR PATTERN
Diffuse pulmonary hemorrhage
  Goodpasture's syndrome
  Idiopathic pulmonary hemosiderosis
  Vasculitis
  Bleeding diathesis
  Drugs
Pulmonary exudates
  Infectious pneumonias
  Eosinophilic pneumonias
  Pulmonary alveolar proteinosis
  Lipoid pneumonia
  Sarcoidosis
  Idiopathic pulmonary fibrosis (desquamative phase)
Neoplasms
  Bronchioalveolar cell carcinoma
  Lymphoma
  Metastatic carcinoma
PREDOMINANTLY INTERSTITIAL PATTERN
Inflammatory disorders
  Sarcoidosis
  Pneumoconiosis
  Eosinophilic granuloma
  Hypersensitivity pneumonitis
  Idiopathic pulmonary fibrosis
  Interstitial pneumonitis associated with collagen vascular disorders
  Familial pulmonary fibrosis
  Bronchiolitis obliterans organizing pneumonia (mixed pattern)
Infections
Neoplasms
  Lymphangitic carcinomatosis
  Metastatic carcinoma
  Lymphoma

---

disease, and amyloidosis and is uncommon in Wegener's granulomatosis
- Pleural effusions associated with interstitial lung disease are commonly seen with tuberculosis and other infections, collagen vascular diseases, asbestos-related diseases, and lymphangitic carcinomatosis, and are uncommon in lymphangioleiomyomatosis (chylous effusions) and drug reactions (e.g., nitrofurantoin)
- Diffuse pulmonary infiltration in immunocompromised patients alters the diagnostic possibilities strongly in favor of opportunistic infections, diffuse pulmonary hemorrhage or edema, malignancy, or drug reactions

COMPUTED TOMOGRAPHY (CT)

CT of the lungs is an important tool in the evaluation of patients with restrictive lung disease, and is best performed using high-resolution, thin-section (1- to 2-mm-thick slices) techniques (HRCT). Several studies have demonstrated the greater accuracy of HRCT over conventional radiography in the diagnosis of diffuse infiltrative lung diseases.

LABORATORY STUDIES

Often a specific diagnosis can be confirmed by conventional tests. Microbiology cultures, sputum cytology, and serum studies (e.g., antinuclear antibody, rheumatoid factor, antineutrophil cytoplasmic antibody, viral titers) provide evidence for specific disease processes. Superficial lymph node or skin biopsies are often helpful in the diagnosis of malignancy, sarcoidosis, tuberculosis, or fungal diseases.

FIBEROPTIC BRONCHOSCOPY

In the absence of a specific diagnosis, most individuals with diffuse pulmonary infiltration undergo lung biopsy via fiberoptic bronchoscopy. Multiple transbronchial biopsy specimens obtained from different sites are sent for histologic and microbiologic analysis and culture. Needle aspiration biopsy of enlarged paratracheal, subcarinal, or hilar nodes can increase the likelihood of making a specific diagnosis of a granulomatous or neoplastic process

- Bronchoscopic biopsy has proved effective in diagnosing infectious diseases (tuberculosis, fungal, pneumocystis), sarcoidosis, and lymphangitic carcinomatosis. The technique may also yield a specific diagnosis in Wegener's granulomatosis, Goodpasture's syndrome, eosinophilic granuloma, pulmonary alveolar proteinosis, and eosinophilic pneumonia
- Bronchoalveolar lavage (BAL) may provide diagnostic information with appropriate microbiologic and cytologic analysis of the fluid. Although the role of BAL in the diagnosis and staging of noninfectious, nonmalignant interstitial diseases is unproven, the differential cell counts often show characteristic profiles in many interstitial lung diseases that may provide evidence for a specific disorder. The risk of these procedures when performed by an experienced bronchoscopist is small, with < 3% incidence of pneumothorax with transbronchial biopsy. Serious bleeding is unusual; however, patients with a bleeding diathesis should be excluded from biopsy procedures

OPEN LUNG BIOPSY

An open lung biopsy is occasionally necessary for definitive histologic diagnosis of a diffuse lung disease if prior investigations do not establish a diagnosis with reasonable certainty

- Open lung biopsy should not be performed if the findings will not alter the approach to treatment
- The risk of open lung biopsy is low in younger patients without significant heart disease

TABLE 23–3. THERAPY OF SOME TREATABLE RESTRICTIVE LUNG DISEASES		
DISORDER	**PRIMARY THERAPY**	**SECONDARY THERAPY**
Known Etiology		
Infections	Antimicrobials	
Pneumoconiosis	Removal from exposure	
Hypersensitivity pneumonitis	Removal from exposure	Corticosteroids
Drug reactions	Discontinue drugs	Corticosteroids
Unknown Etiology		
Sarcoidosis	Corticosteroids	
Idiopathic pulmonary fibrosis	Corticosteroids	Cytotoxic Agent*
Interstitial pneumonitis associated with collagen vascular disorders	Corticosteroids	Cytotoxic Agents*
Bronchiolitis obliterans organizing pneumonia	Corticosteroids	
Wegener's granulomatosis	Cytotoxic agents* plus corticosteroids	? Co-trimoxazole
Goodpasture's syndrome	Plasmapheresis, corticosteroids	Cytotoxic agents*
Pulmonary vasculitis	Corticosteroids	Cytotoxic agents*
Eosinophilic granuloma (histiocytosis X)	Quit smoking	Corticosteroids
Chronic eosinophilic pneumonia	Corticosteroids	
Tropical pulmonary eosinophilia	Diethylcarbamazine citrate	
Pulmonary alveolar proteinosis	Lung lavage	

* Cyclophosphamide, azathioprine are most commonly used.

THERAPY

Management involves specific therapy for treatable disease (Table 23–3) and general supportive care for all.

Supportive care includes

- Compassionate health care professionals
- Exercise and diet programs
- Supplemental oxygen for exercise-associated or resting hypoxemia
- Bronchodilators for symptomatic airway disease resulting from bronchial hyperresponsiveness associated with many restrictive lung disorders
- Infection prophylaxis with influenza vaccine and possibly pneumococcal vaccine
- Antibiotic therapy begun promptly at the first sign of an upper respiratory tract infection or exacerbation of cough and sputum production
- Diuretic therapy with the appearance of cor pulmonale

HYPERSENSITIVITY PNEUMONITIS

This group of diseases is characterized by an immunologic reaction to repeated inhalation of one of a variety of organic dusts or inorganic chemicals resulting in granulomatous inflammation of the pulmonary interstitium (Table 23–4). The occupational origin of many of these agents has led to descriptive names for each clinical syndrome. The prototype is "farmer's lung" caused by inhalation of thermophilic actinomycetes spores from moldy hay. Though the agents differ widely, the clinical presentations are similar.

PATHOPHYSIOLOGY

A heightened immunologic response to inhaled antigens results in a characteristic lymphocytic-mononuclear interstitial inflammation with poorly formed noncaseating granulomas. This result is typically mirrored by bronchoalveolar lavage with findings of a marked increase in the proportion of CD8+ T-cytotoxic lymphocytes. The inflammatory process may lead to progressive fibrosis and end-stage respiratory failure if unchecked.

CLINICAL HALLMARKS

Two clinical presentations occur

- Acute form: Fever, chills, dyspnea, cough, and fine crackles with transient leukocytosis, pulmonary infiltrates, and restrictive impairment noted 4 to 12 hours following exposure; recovery occurs in 24 to 48 hours with no further exposure. With repeated acute exposures, symptoms become less clearly defined to a specific exposure. Example—cleaning bird cages by a sensitized individual
- Chronic form: Insidious progression of dyspnea, cough, anorexia, weight loss (can be profound), and progressive interstitial lung disease

TABLE 23–4. ETIOLOGIC AGENTS IN HYPERSENSITIVITY PNEUMONITIS

OCCUPATION	DUST EXPOSURE	ANTIGEN
Farmer	Moldy compost (hay, sugar cane, mushrooms)	Thermophilic actinomycetes
Home/office worker	Contaminated ventilation system	Thermophilic actinomycetes, amebae
Bird breeder	Avian dust	Avian proteins
Animal handler	Rodent dander	Rodent proteins
Detergent worker	Bacterial enzymes	Bacillus subtilis proteins
Woodworker	Moldy wood dust	Fungi—Aspergillus, Alternaria, Pullularia sp.
Malt/cheese worker	Malt or cheese mold	Fungi—Penicillium sp.
Wheat worker	Infested wheat	Wheat weevil protein
Plastics worker	Plastic components	Isocyanates, anhydrides
Painters	Paint hardeners	Isocyanates

with hypoxemia and restrictive impairment. A diffuse reticulonodular pattern or fibrosis is seen on chest x-ray. Example—farmer with chronic low-level exposure to moldy hay

- Airway obstruction is uncommon but may be a manifestation of non-specific bronchial hyperresponsiveness. The presence of significant air-way obstruction should always raise the possibility of occupational asthma, because many of these occupations involve exposures to dusts known to result in IgE-mediated and non–IgE-mediated asthma

DIAGNOSIS

A careful occupational and environmental history remains the key to a diagnosis. In the acute form, correlation of symptoms to exposure may be highly suggestive of the diagnosis. The diagnosis may be difficult to es-tablish in the chronic form and relies heavily on identifying possible ex-posure to putative disease-causing agents

- Positive serum precipitating antibodies to the organic dust document exposure, but a positive test does not by itself establish a diagnosis of disease
- Inhalation challenge testing under controlled conditions can often es-tablish a diagnosis in individuals with acute or subacute disease, but such testing entails considerable risk in those with significant respiratory impairment
- Bronchoscopic biopsy or, occasionally, open lung biopsy may be needed if a diagnosis remains uncertain

THERAPY

Avoidance of the offending agent is the mainstay of treatment

- Clean humidifiers and change humidifier water frequently
- Reduce occupational exposure to organic dusts whenever possible by improved industrial hygiene, ventilation, and air purification engineer-ing
- Discourage dependence on personal dust respirators because they are difficult to use properly and are not effective in excluding all respirable dust. The remaining fraction can cause new attacks in a sensitized person
- Avoid work place or avocational exposure if environmental control mea-sures are ineffective in preventing continued disease. Unfortunately, many individuals refuse to restrict their exposures and return to their work (e.g., farmers) or avocation (e.g., bird breeders). The patient should be advised of the significant risk for progressive interstitial fi-brosis with continued exposure

CORTICOSTEROIDS

Corticosteroids are effective in alleviating acute symptoms. Data support the benefit of steroids in diminishing the risk of developing fibrotic lung changes on chest x-rays, although a benefit in lung function is unproved.

Acute Disease

- Respiratory symptoms are self-limiting, and usually therapy is not necessary
- For the ill patient with significant radiographic infiltration and hypoxemia, oral corticosteroids (rarely, IV steroids) are indicated with oxygen and antipyretics

Suggested Regimen: Prednisone 40 to 60 mg/day in divided doses for 2 to 3 days, then as a single morning dose until significant clinical, radiologic, and physiologic improvement occurs. Taper dose over 4 to 6 weeks.

Subacute Disease (repeated acute exposures)

- Reduce exposure
- Longterm corticosteroid therapy

Suggested Regimen: Prednisone 40 to 60 mg/day for 2 weeks. Taper slowly over 3 to 4 months until a dose of 15 to 30 mg/day is reached. Slowly taper to find lowest possible effective dose. Alternate-day therapy may be tried to minimize longterm complications.

Chronic Disease

- Decrease exposure
- Trial of corticosteroids as outlined for subacute disease. Evaluate response at 6 months using clinical, radiologic, and pulmonary function tests. Continue therapy only if a positive response can be objectively documented

DRUG-INDUCED INTERSTITIAL LUNG DISEASE

Many drugs can induce pathophysiologic reactions that can be classified into one of the following syndromes

- Chronic interstitial pneumonitis and fibrosis
- Hypersensitivity reactions
- Pulmonary infiltrates with eosinophilia
- Drug-induced lupus syndrome
- Diffuse alveolar hemorrhage

CHRONIC INTERSTITIAL PNEUMONITIS AND FIBROSIS

The patient with this form of chronic drug-induced interstitial lung disease typically appears with the insidious onset of cough, dyspnea, and fatigue, with bibasilar crackles, interstitial pulmonary infiltrates most prominent in the lower lobes, restrictive lung impairment, and hypoxemia. The most commonly implicated drugs include bleomycin, busulfan, nitrosourea compounds, amiodarone, nitrofurantoin, and hexamethonium (Table 23–5).

TABLE 23–5. DRUG-INDUCED INTERSTITIAL LUNG DISEASE (SELECTED DRUGS)

DRUG	PRESENTATION	FREQUENCY	RELATIONSHIP TO DOSE	FEATURES	STEROIDS	PROGNOSIS
Bleomycin	HR*	Uncommon	—	—	Good	Good
	CIPF†	5–10%	> 300 mg total	Synergistic toxicity with O_2, age	Poor	Variable
Busulfan	CIPF	Common	> 500 mg total	Dysplastic—appearing type II pneumocytes	Poor	Poor
Nitrosoureas (BCNU, CCNU, methyl CCNU)	CIPF	1%	> 1,000 mg/M^2	Synergistic with other alkylating agents	Variable	Poor
Methotrexate	HR	Uncommon	> 20 mg/week	Granulomatous inflammation	Good	Good
Cyclophosphamide	CIPF	Rare	None	—	Variable	Variable
Azathioprine	HR	Rare	None	—	Good	Good
Amiodarone	HR	Uncommon	—	—	Good	Good
	CIPF	Common	> 400–800 mg/day for months	Foamy macrophages multilamellar inclusions	Variable	Variable
Nitrofurantoin	HR	Common	—	Eosinophilia in 30%, + ANA in 60%	Good	Good
	CIPF	Uncommon	—		Variable	Variable
Gold Salts	HR	Uncommon	—	—	Good	Good

* Hypersensitivity reaction.
† Chronic interstitial pneumonitis and fibrosis.

The pathogenesis is thought to involve drug-induced lung injury and fibrosis as a result of both direct toxic effects and indirect toxicity from associated inflammatory and immune processes. Considerable evidence shows that toxic O_2-derived radicals mediate the lung toxicity in bleomycin, busulfan, and nitrofurantoin drug reactions

- A relationship to dose is seen with bleomycin, busulfan, the nitrosoureas, amiodarone, and methotrexate (Table 23–5)
- The prognosis is variable even when the drug is discontinued. Improvement, stabilization, or progressive fibrosis may be seen. Corticosteroids are generally not helpful, although beneficial effects have been reported in case reports of toxicity from amiodarone, nitrofurantoin, and mitomycin

HYPERSENSITIVITY REACTIONS

Hypersensitivity reactions have been reported with numerous drugs, most commonly nitrofurantoin, sulfonamides, amiodarone, methotrexate, gold salts, salicylates, and nonsteroidal anti-inflammatory agents.

Clinical hallmarks include acute onset of cough, dyspnea, fever, myalgias, arthralgias, and occasional urticaria, pleuritis, and peripheral eosinophilia. Chest x-ray commonly shows alveolar and/or interstitial infiltrates, occasionally with pleural effusions

- BAL frequently demonstrates an increase in the number and proportion of lymphocytes as a result of specific increases in the CD8 + T-cytotoxic cell population. Similar findings are seen in classic hypersensitivity pneumonitis, thus suggesting that similar immunopathogenic mechanisms are operative. BAL may be diagnostically useful, therefore, as a marker of a hypersensitivity drug reaction
- Discontinuation of the drug usually leads to complete resolution. A short course of corticosteroids may be indicated to hasten improvement and alleviate symptoms in individuals who are particularly ill

PULMONARY INFILTRATES WITH EOSINOPHILIA

Many drugs cause a clinical syndrome similar to Löffler's syndrome; the most common are methotrexate, salicylates, nitrofurantoin, sulfa drugs, penicillins, amiodarone, gold compounds, and procarbazine. The process is self-limiting with discontinuation of the drug. Corticosteroids are usually unnecessary but provide prompt symptomatic relief.

DRUG-INDUCED LUPUS SYNDROME

This drug-induced syndrome resembles spontaneous lupus except that renal and neurologic involvement is rare. Fever, pleuritis, arthralgia, and occasionally, pulmonary infiltrates are seen. Drugs most commonly implicated in this syndrome include procainamide, hydralazine, diphenylhydantoin, and isoniazid

- Antinuclear antibody (ANA) and antihistone antibody are positive but anti–double-stranded DNA antibody is characteristically negative. Discontinuing the drug usually produces a prompt response
- Corticosteroids are often beneficial and hasten symptomatic recovery

DIFFUSE ALVEOLAR HEMORRHAGE

Intrapulmonary hemorrhage may occur with anticoagulant or thrombolytic therapy and suggests the possibility of an underlying intrapulmonary lesion. Isolated case reports of diffuse alveolar hemorrhage have been reported in association with penicillamine and occupational exposure to trimellitic anhydride.

PRIMARY EOSINOPHILIC PNEUMONIAS

The primary eosinophilic pneumonias are characterized by pulmonary infiltration by eosinophils with or without peripheral blood eosinophilia (see Table 23–1). Eosinophils possess a wide array of pro-inflammatory substances, such as major basic protein, lysosomal hydrolases, cytokines, and arachadonic acid metabolites, capable of causing direct tissue injury, as well as of mediating antiparasitic and antimicrobial effects. Persistent eosinophilic lung inflammation may be associated with fibrosis and restrictive impairment.

LÖFFLER'S SYNDROME

Löffler's syndrome can be defined as migratory pulmonary infiltrates and peripheral eosinophilia with absent or mild symptoms that last less than 1 month and whose cause is unknown. Many cases are probably caused by unrecognized drug reactions, parasitic infestations, or allergic bronchopulmonary aspergillosis. Asthma is an uncommon feature seen late in the course of the disease. The disease is self-limiting and generally requires no therapy.

CHRONIC EOSINOPHILIC PNEUMONIA

When eosinophilic infiltration of the lung is prolonged or recurrent and of unknown cause, the process is termed chronic eosinophilic pneumonia.

CLINICAL HALLMARKS

- Most common in middle-aged women
- Dyspnea, productive cough, fevers, night sweats, weight loss, and wheezing (50% of individuals) are predominant symptoms
- Chest x-ray typically shows peripheral alveolar infiltrates in a pattern termed the "photographic negative of pulmonary edema"
- Peripheral eosinophilia is found in only two thirds of individuals
- BAL findings of > 40% eosinophils (normal < 1%) are highly suggestive of the diagnosis in the proper clinical and radiologic context

- Restrictive lung impairment, often with superimposed airflow limitation, low diffusing capacity, and hypoxemia, is characteristic
- Severe cases of eosinophilic pneumonia may progress to acute respiratory failure
- A diagnosis is usually made on the basis of symptoms, a characteristic radiographic pattern, and the exclusion of other causes of pulmonary eosinophilia

THERAPY

Corticosteroids are the treatment of choice to alleviate symptoms and prevent irreversible fibrosis. Typically, the response to steroids is dramatic with symptomatic improvement in hours and clearing of the chest x-ray within days.

Suggested Regimen: Prednisone 40 to 60 mg/day for 2 weeks; with clinical improvement, taper to 20 to 30 mg/day for 2 months. Further slow tapering can be tried using daily or alternate-day administration of steroids. Often small doses of steroids (equivalent to ≤ 10 mg/day) are sufficient to prevent symptomatic and/or radiologic relapse. Treatment is usually given for a minimum of 8 to 12 months. Relapse is common even after a year, and treatment may be necessary for several years. Concomitant obstructive airway disease should be treated with bronchodilators.

TROPICAL PULMONARY EOSINOPHILIA

Tropical pulmonary eosinophilia is caused by a local hypersensitivity response to microfilaria of Wuchereria bancrofti or Brugia malayi introduced by mosquito bite and traveling through the lungs during its life cycle.
Suspect in individuals from or traveling from India, Sri Lanka, Southeast Asia, Pakistan, or Indonesia.

CLINICAL HALLMARKS

- New-onset asthma, severe cough, chest pain, and hemoptysis are characteristically worse at night; fevers, fatigue, and weight loss are also common
- Wheezing and/or crackles may be present
- Restrictive lung impairment more common than airway obstruction
- Chest x-ray may be normal or show mixed alveolar and reticulonodular infiltrates; cavitation, pleural effusions, and consolidation rarely are present
- Marked peripheral eosinophilia ($> 2,000/\text{mm}^3$), elevated IgE levels, and high titers of antifilarial antibodies are present

THERAPY

Tropical eosinophilia is treated with the antifilarial drug diethylcarbamazine citrate.

Supplied: tablets; 50 mg.

Dosage: 5 mg/kg/day for 7 to 10 days. Treatment causes a rapid disappearance of symptoms. Patients may relapse and respond again to treatment. Longstanding disease, however, is less likely to respond to therapy.

Adverse Effects: Headache, nausea, vomiting, and arthralgias.

CHURG-STRAUSS SYNDROME

This rare syndrome, also known as allergic angiitis and granulomatosis, is a life-threatening multisystem vasculitis associated with asthma, allergic rhinitis, fever, and hypereosinophilia (peripheral blood eosinophilia with eosinophilic tissue infiltrates). Asthma or allergic rhinitis symptoms may predate diagnosis for as many as 30 years. Neurologic involvement (particularly mononeuritis multiplex) may presage a widespread vasculitic phase that is commonly associated with granulomatous inflammation of the heart, gastrointestinal tract, skin, and musculoskeletal system. Abnormal chest x-rays usually showing localized infiltrates are found in more than 25% of patients. A diagnosis of Löffler's syndrome or chronic eosinophilic pneumonia commonly precedes the diagnosis of Churg-Strauss syndrome.

Corticosteroids are the mainstay of treatment. Pulsed methylprednisolone or cytotoxic agents are indicated in severe cases. The prognosis is favorable in many patients, with a median survival of about 9 years.

SARCOIDOSIS

Sarcoidosis is a multisystem disorder of unknown cause characterized by noncaseating granulomata in affected organs. The disease is found worldwide, although geographic and racial differences in the frequency of the disease are striking. In the United States, sarcoidosis is more common in the African-American population, particularly among women.

PATHOPHYSIOLOGY

Although the inciting stimulus is unknown, active immunologic processes are likely responsible for the accumulation of activated macrophages and CD4+ T-helper lymphocytes in discrete granulomas at sites of active disease. These granulomas affect tissue function by distortion of parenchymal architecture and by involvement in inflammatory processes that can result in tissue fibrosis.

CLINICAL HALLMARKS

- Most commonly affects young adults
- Patient most frequently presents with hilar adenopathy, pulmonary infiltrates, eye or skin lesions
- May be asymptomatic
- Acute-onset disease frequently involves bilateral hilar adenopathy (BHA) and erythema nodosum or uveitis

- The lungs are the most commonly affected organ
- Common respiratory symptoms include cough, dyspnea, and chest discomfort; the onset may be insidious. Sputum production and hemoptysis are often seen in advanced disease
- Other clinical manifestations result from involvement of specific organ systems, such as the peripheral lymphatics, skin, eye, liver, spleen, heart, bone, joints, and adrenals; pathologic involvement in many organs occurs much more frequently than clinical symptoms
- Cutaneous anergy to recall antigens, such as tuberculin, Candida, mumps, and Trichophyton, is characteristic

INVESTIGATIONS

- Chest x-rays are classified by international convention as type I (BHA only), type II (BHA and pulmonary infiltrates), and type III (parenchymal infiltrates alone, fibrosis or local honeycombing)
- Pulmonary function tests can be normal or may demonstrate restrictive impairment and/or reduction in the diffusion capacity. Advanced fibrocystic sarcoid can demonstrate obstructive impairment caused by distortion of the airways from progressive scarring and by bullous and cystic changes superimposed upon restrictive lung volumes
- Arterial blood gases may be normal or show hypoxemia at rest or with exercise

DIAGNOSIS

A diagnosis is based on a compatible clinical picture with histologic confirmation of noncaseating granulomas and absence of other known causes of granulomas. Tuberculosis, fungal diseases, lymphoma, beryllium disease, drug reactions, and local sarcoid reactions must be excluded

- Biopsy specimens of superficial abnormalities, such as skin, palpable lymph node, lip, or conjunctivae, should be attained whenever possible; yield of these procedures significantly decreases in absence of visible abnormality
- Transbronchial biopsies or bronchoscopic needle biopsies of mediastinal nodes frequently can confirm a diagnosis of intrathoracic sarcoidosis
- Mediastinoscopy is occasionally indicated if lymphoma or cancer is suspected, e.g., because of asymmetric mediastinal or hilar adenopathy

PROGNOSIS

Most individuals with BHA alone or as a presentation of acute sarcoidosis undergo remission of the disease. The presence of pulmonary infiltrates worsens the prognosis, particularly in the absence of BHA.

Individuals with sarcoidosis who undergo a remission usually do so in the first 1 to 2 years.

THERAPY

Management of the patient with sarcoidosis starts with an assessment of involvement of vital organ systems. All patients should have a chest x-ray, pulmonary function tests (FVC, FEV_1, diffusing capacity), liver function tests [alkaline phosphatase, aspartate aminotransferase (AST), alanine aminotransferase (ALT)], serum calcium, complete blood count (CBC), urinalysis, and complete ophthalmologic examination. Clinical evidence of involvement of other organ systems dictates additional testing, e.g., sinus films, ECG, bone/joint x-rays, and neurologic testing

- Clinical evaluations with repeated measurements of chest x-ray, pulmonary function tests, or abnormal serologic studies suffice to monitor patients and determine the need for treatment. Newer tests, such as angiotensin converting enzyme, gallium scans, and BAL, are nonspecific and have no proven benefit in monitoring the patient
- Observation for spontaneous remission is indicated for asymptomatic individuals with BHA, or with BHA and pulmonary infiltrates and normal lung function
- Acute sarcoidosis with fever, malaise, erythema nodosum, and BHA can usually be managed with nonsteroidal anti-inflammatory agents, such as ibuprofen
- Corticosteroids are the mainstay of treatment for sarcoidosis with serious vital organ involvement
- Chloroquine or hydroxychloroquine may be more effective than corticosteroids in the management of skin and mucosal disease
- Immunosuppressive agents, e.g., methotrexate, are occasionally used for disfiguring skin lesions, such as lupus pernio, but have unproven benefit in treating pulmonary sarcoidosis and entail serious potential risks in young individuals

CORTICOSTEROIDS

Corticosteroids are the drugs of choice for pulmonary sarcoidosis. Although their benefit has been unproved by long-term studies, agreement is widespread that corticosteroids can reduce or eliminate symptoms, improve pulmonary function, and suppress disease activity. Many investigators also believe that longterm steroid treatment can prevent or delay progressive fibrosis in individuals with chronic active pulmonary sarcoidosis.

Indications

- Corticosteroids should be *promptly* instituted with evidence of serious vital organ involvement, e.g., active ocular, myocardial or neurosarcoid involvement, hypercalcemia, or significant hepatic, renal, or muscle dysfunction
- Use of corticosteroids is indicated for persistent or progressive symptomatic pulmonary sarcoidosis

- Minimally symptomatic individuals with near-normal lung function and stable pulmonary infiltrates that have persisted for 1 to 2 years are often given a short trial (2 to 3 months) with steroids to determine any potential for improvement in lung function
- Topical corticosteroids are indicated for anterior uveitis; systemic steroids are indicated for posterior eye disease

A suggested regimen for the treatment of sarcoidosis with corticosteroids is given in Figure 23–1. Prednisone 5-mg tablets are used to facilitate tapering of the dose. Starting doses of prednisone higher than 30 to 40 mg daily are rarely needed (e.g., ocular, neurosarcoid). Alternate-day administration of steroids is advocated by some authors, though experience is limited and compliance may be more difficult than with daily administration of low-dose corticosteroids. Inhaled steroids do not appear to be effective for pulmonary sarcoidosis and are not recommended

- Exacerbations of pulmonary sarcoidosis can occur at doses of < 15 mg/day; the vast majority of individuals can be controlled with doses of between 5 to 15 mg/day

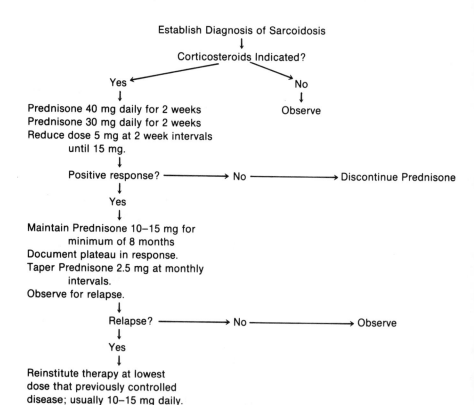

FIG. 23–1. Suggested initial regimen for corticosteroid treatment of sarcoidosis.

TABLE 23–6. COMPLICATIONS OF CORTICOSTEROID THERAPY	
ADVERSE EFFECTS	**SURVEILLANCE/INTERVENTION**
Endocrine: Increased appetite, weight gain, cushingoid habitus, hyperglycemia, adrenal axis suppression	Monitor weight, blood, urine sugar; diet and insulin if needed; steroid replacement during stress
Neurologic: Emotional liability, depression, psychosis, pseudotumor cerebri	Mental status exam; use lowest possible dose
Cardiac: Sodium and fluid retention, hypertension	Monitor weight and blood pressure; 4 g sodium restriction; treat sustained hypertension
Ocular: Glaucoma, cataracts	Ophthalmologic exam
Musculoskeletal: Osteopenia, osteoporosis, aseptic necrosis of bone, compression fractures, myopathy	Exercise program; possibly supplemental calcium and vitamin D for women
Gastrointestinal: Peptic ulcer, pancreatitis	Antacids or sucralfate for history of peptic ulcers
Cutaneous: Striae, ecchymosis, easy bruisability, acne	

• Relapse of pulmonary sarcoidosis is unlikely on a maintenance dose of steroids. Acute respiratory infections, often bacterial, are the most common cause of respiratory exacerbations and should be treated promptly with antibiotics while maintaining low-dose steroids. Other causes of respiratory exacerbations include congestive heart failure and pulmonary emboli

Adverse Effects (Table 23–6): Low-dose corticosteroid therapy as used for maintenance therapy in sarcoidosis is usually well tolerated. Weight gain, hypertension, and diabetes (in susceptible individuals) are the most common adverse effects encountered.

Caution: Check for diabetes, especially in individuals with sarcoid liver disease because these patients may be particularly susceptible to serious hyperglycemia.

CHLOROQUINE AND HYDROXYCHLOROQUINE

Indications*

• Use of first-line drugs in the treatment of skin and mucosal sarcoidosis if corticosteroids are not required for pulmonary or systemic sarcoidosis
• May be particularly useful in severe nasal, sinus, and laryngeal sarcoid, conditions that are often not controlled with corticosteroids alone. Oc-

---

* Not currently approved by the FDA for these indications.

casionally, chloroquine is used with low-dose steroids needed for treatment of pulmonary sarcoidosis
- These drugs do not appear to be effective in pulmonary sarcoidosis

Chloroquine phosphate
(Aralen)

Dosage: 500 mg daily for 2 weeks, then 250 mg daily for 5½ months. Use no longer than 6 months at a time, followed by a 6-month rest period. This regimen may be repeated as needed. Major concern is ocular toxicity with long-term administration. Ophthalmologic examinations should be performed prior to administration and at 3- and 6-month intervals.

Adverse Effects
- Retinopathy
- Gastrointestinal upset (mild); transient headache
- Discoloration of nailbeds and mucous membranes
- Dermatitis, reversible

Caution
High daily doses of chloroquine (> 250 mg) may cause retinopathy, toxic cardiomyopathy, and neuropathy. Do not exceed 250 mg daily after first 2 weeks.

Hydroxychloroquine sulfate
(Plaquenil)

Anecdotal evidence suggests that hydroxychloroquine is not as effective as chloroquine in the treatment of mucocutaneous sarcoidosis. The pharmacologic characteristics of hydroxychloroquine are similar to those of chloroquine, although ocular toxicity may be somewhat less.

Dosage: 400 mg daily for 2 weeks, then 200 mg daily for 5½ months; 400 mg hydroxychloroquine is equivalent to 500 mg chloroquine.

MANAGEMENT PROBLEMS IN PULMONARY SARCOIDOSIS

HEMOPTYSIS

Hemoptysis is a frequent problem in advanced fibrocystic sarcoidosis and is frequently associated with mycetomas. The usual precipitating cause is respiratory infection in areas of bronchitis and bronchiectasis.

Treatment is initiated with broad-spectrum antibiotics, bed rest, and cough suppression. Hospitalization for observation and management is indicated for serious hemoptysis. For recurrent disabling hemoptysis, elective arteriography and embolotherapy can be considered following localization of the bleeding site by bronchoscopic examination.

MYCETOMAS (FUNGUS BALLS)

Mycetomas are a complication of fibrocystic sarcoidosis. The most frequent causative organism is Aspergillus fumigatus, which colonizes a fibrobullous or fibrocystic space. Invasive aspergillus infection is rare, even in the presence of low-dose corticosteroids. Bacterial infection of the surrounding bronchitic and bronchiectatic areas is common and leads to chronic sputum production and hemoptysis.

Treatment should be conservative with broad-spectrum antibiotics. An occasional patient may benefit from daily antibiotics, rotated at 2- to 4-week intervals, to suppress recurrent infections and hemoptysis

- Antifungal agents are not beneficial because they do not penetrate the fungus ball
- Surgical resection is rarely feasible because of the presence of severe bilateral restrictive lung disease superimposed upon fibrocystic disease

IDIOPATHIC PULMONARY FIBROSIS

Idiopathic pulmonary fibrosis (IPF), also known as cryptogenic fibrosing alveolitis, is a disease of unknown cause that produces diffuse interstitial inflammation and fibrosis. Although the clinical course is highly variable, most cases progress to severe respiratory impairment and death within 2 to 10 years of diagnosis.

PATHOPHYSIOLOGY

- A chronic active immunologic and inflammatory reaction of the lung interstitium leads to destruction and distortion of alveoli, with fibrosis and progressive disorganization of pulmonary architecture. The physiologic consequences are stiff, noncompliant lungs that increase the work of breathing and impair gas exchange
- Although the inciting cause is unknown, activated macrophages, neutrophils, lymphocytes, and eosinophils are present in the lower respiratory tract and likely modulate the fibrotic, destructive changes in the interstitium
- A classification proposed in the 1960s described several distinct pathologic processes of interstitial pneumonitis based on the dominant cell type and architecture. Most investigators believe that two of the entities, desquamative interstitial pneumonitis and usual interstitial pneumonitis, are not clinically distinct, but are part of the pathologic spectrum seen in IPF

CLINICAL HALLMARKS

- Onset is usually at 40 to 70 years of age
- Gradual, progressive dyspnea on exertion and nonproductive cough are characteristic, with progressive restrictive lung impairment and impaired gas exchange, particularly with exercise

- Constitutional symptoms of weight loss, fever, fatigue, myalgia, and arthralgia may be present, but are more common with pulmonary fibrosis associated with collagen vascular disease
- Chest auscultation commonly reveals bibasilar, late inspiratory, "Velcro" crackles
- Clubbing of the fingers may be found late in the course of the disease
- Cardiac examination is normal except in advanced stages of the disease when signs of pulmonary hypertension are present, see Chapter 19.

INVESTIGATIONS

- Chest x-ray: Plain films reveal reticular or reticulonodular interstitial infiltrates usually most prominent in the lower lung fields. Occasionally, an alveolar filling pattern is seen. "Honeycomb" lung is a late radiographic finding that is nonspecific. Of individuals with biopsy-proven IPF, 5 to 10% may have a normal chest x-ray on presentation.
- Pulmonary function tests: Restrictive impairment with reduced lung volumes (FVC, TLC, and RV) and low $D_{L_{CO}}$ is characteristic. Mild hypoxemia with respiratory alkalosis is typical early in the disease; hypercarbia is a late manifestation of IPF. An exercise-associated oxygen desaturation level of less than 60 mm Hg is common when the $D_{L_{CO}}$ is decreased to less than 40 to 50% of the predicted value

DIAGNOSIS

Prior to initiating specific therapy for IPF, the clinician must establish the diagnosis with reasonable certainty because the only treatments recognized to impact favorably on the natural progression of the disease are corticosteroids and/or cytotoxic agents.

SERUM STUDIES

Antinuclear antibodies and rheumatoid factor may be present in low titer, but overlap exists with pulmonary fibrosis associated with connective tissue diseases.

CT

High-resolution, thin section CT scans demonstrate a characteristic peripheral predominance of interstitial opacities with patchy areas intermingled with small cystic spaces. In contrast, sarcoidosis, silicosis, hypersensitivity pneumonitis, and lymphangitic carcinomatosis demonstrate nodular opacities.

FIBEROPTIC BRONCHOSCOPY

In the absence of a specific diagnosis, bronchoscopy with transbronchial biopsy and BAL are indicated to exclude (with reasonable certainty) infection, sarcoidosis, lymphangitic carcinomatosis, pulmonary alveolar proteinosis, and eosinophilic granuloma

- The presence of patchy fibrosis in transbronchial biopsy specimens is nonspecific, but may be sufficient to establish a reasonable diagnosis of IPF after exclusion of likely alternatives
- BAL is an important research tool, but has a limited role in the diagnosis and management of IPF. Analysis of BAL cells typically reveals an increase in total numbers of cells, as well as increased proportions of neutrophils and eosinophils. A subset of patients may demonstrate increased proportions of BAL lymphocytes; these patients may be more responsive to corticosteroids. An increase in BAL eosinophils has been associated with a poor therapeutic response

OPEN LUNG BIOPSY

A definitive diagnosis of IPF requires an open lung biopsy to provide sufficient tissue for pathologic analysis. If the diagnosis is uncertain or absolute verification of the diagnosis is necessary, an open lung biopsy may be justified. Some investigators recommend an open lung biopsy in almost all patients with suspected IPF unless the patient is elderly or major operative risks exist.

THERAPY

Management of the patient with IPF involves supportive care and, in most instances, specific drug therapy.

Specific drug therapy for IPF involves the longterm use of corticosteroids, cytotoxic agents, or both. The decision to treat individuals with IPF is difficult because the agents have considerable potential toxicities, they are effective in only a minority of patients, and the natural history of the disease is highly variable with no accurate predictors of its eventual course or responsiveness to therapy

- Important factors in the decision to treat are the age of the patient, the rate of disease progression, the degree of respiratory impairment, and the presence of serious complicating diseases
- As many as 20% of individuals with IPF demonstrate no evidence of disease progression. These individuals tend to be minimally symptomatic, with normal or near-normal pulmonary function and lung biopsy results that show minimal fibrosis without inflammatory changes. Treatment is unnecessary in this subgroup of patients with IPF. Follow-up examinations at 3-month intervals for at least 1 to 2 years are recommended to assess stability of the disease
- Individuals with severe pulmonary impairment or incapacitating complicating diseases may not be candidates for therapy
- Factors that presage a favorable response to therapy include a younger age at presentation, mild pulmonary function abnormalities, a cellular lung biopsy specimen, and, perhaps, an elevated proportion of lymphocytes in BAL fluid. A tendency for an unfavorable response to therapy is seen with an older age at presentation, the presence of severe pulmonary impairment, widespread honeycomb pattern on chest x-ray,

a fibrotic lung biopsy specimen, and, perhaps, increased proportions of neutrophils or eosinophils in BAL fluid

- The response to therapy cannot be accurately predicted by any combination of factors; thus, therapy should not be withheld solely because of the presence of an unfavorable factor
- Evaluation for progression of the disease includes clinical assessment, chest x-ray, pulmonary function tests (FVC, FEV_1, D_{LCO}), and resting or exercise arterial blood gas determinations. Gallium scan and BAL findings are of unproven benefit in monitoring disease activity and should be reserved for research studies

CORTICOSTEROIDS

Corticosteroids are the standard drugs used to initiate therapy for IPF. Their effectiveness is based on clinical experience and limited retrospective studies. An optimal drug regimen has not been determined by the available studies

- Approximately 10 to 30% of patients experience improvement or stabilization of pulmonary function on steroid therapy alone
- Higher doses of ($\geq$ 1 mg/kg/day prednisone) appear to be more effective than lower doses
- Patients who respond to steroids usually demonstrate a positive response within 2 to 3 weeks with a maximum response by 2 to 3 months

Suggested Regimen: Prednisone 60 to 80 mg/day (i.e. 1 mg/kg/day) for 6 to 8 weeks. If response is positive, continue for another 6 to 8 weeks, then slowly taper to 30 to 40 mg/day (0.5 mg/kg/day) over 3 to 4 months (i.e. 5 mg q 2 weeks)

- Progression of disease is common at doses of < 30 mg/day prednisone, and may necessitate longterm therapy (years)
- Some investigators recommend a higher starting dose, i.e. prednisone 1.5 mg/kg/day not to exceed 100 mg for the first 3 to 6 weeks
- Alternate-day therapy is recommended for maintenance therapy by some authors, although the schedule is of unproven benefit

Adverse Effects (Table 23–6): Adverse effects are common with chronic administration of corticosteroids in the dose range typically used for IPF. Because of the considerable toxicity of long-term administration of corticosteroids in IPF and the low frequency of positive responders, cyclophosphamide has been used increasingly either alone or, more commonly, with lower doses of steroids in the initial treatment of IPF.

CYTOTOXIC AGENTS

Cyclophosphamide
(Cytoxan)

Recent clinical trials have substantiated the effectiveness of cyclophosphamide when combined with low-dose corticosteroids in treatment of IPF. Cyclophosphamide alone may be effective in the initial treatment of IPF. The comparative effectiveness of these regimens is unknown.

TABLE 23–7. PHARMACOLOGY OF CYTOTOXIC AGENTS USED IN THE TREATMENT OF INTERSTITIAL LUNG DISEASE

	CYCLOPHOSPHAMIDE	AZATHIOPRINE
Trade name	Cytoxan	Imuran
Oral form	25, 50 mg tablets	50 mg tablets
Route of administration	Oral, IV	Oral
Mechanism of action	Cytotoxicity; immunosuppression	Immunosuppression; cytotoxicity
Active metabolites	Phosphoramide mustard, acrolein	6-mercaptopurine
Metabolism	Hepatic, renal	Hepatic, renal
Dosage range	1–2 mg/kg/day	1–3 mg/kg/day
Approved indications	Many neoplastic disorders	Adjunctive therapy in transplant rejection; severe rheumatoid arthritis
Complications	Leukopenia	Leukopenia
	Hemorrhagic cystitis	Toxic hepatitis (rare)
	Anorexia, nausea, vomiting*	Dermatitis (rare)
	Alopecia*†	Anorexia, nausea, vomiting*
	Gonadal dysfunction (common)	Gonadal dysfunction (uncommon)
	Pulmonary fibrosis (rare)	Pulmonary fibrosis (rare)
	Bladder fibrosis	Potential carcinogenesis
	Potential carcinogenesis	
Interactions	—	Allopurinol (inhibits metabolism of 6-mercaptopurine; reduce to 25% of usual dose)

* Uncommon with doses usually employed for IPF
† Reversible with discontinuing drug

Cyclophosphamide is an alkylating agent that is absorbed orally, is activated in the liver to form several cytotoxic derivatives, and causes immunosuppression of both T- and B-cell function (Table 23–7).

Dosage: 1.5 mg/kg/day in a single morning dose. Adjust dose (range 1 to 2 mg/kg/day) as tolerated with the goal of maintaining the peripheral white blood cell (WBC) count between 3,500 and 5,000 cells/mm^3 (absolute neutrophil count > 1,000 cells/mm^3), a level that minimizes the risk of opportunistic infections.

Assess clinical effectiveness no sooner than 3 months into treatment, which should be continued for at least 1 year in patients who are improved or have stabilized. Steroids can be tapered over 3 to 4 months and cyclophosphamide continued alone. Patients who do not respond should discontinue cyclophosphamide and taper off steroids.

Adverse Effects (see Table 23–5): The leukopenic effects of a given dose of cyclophosphamide lag 1 to 2 weeks; adjust dosage when WBC count first begins to decline to avoid significant neutropenia. Cyclophosphamide is associated with hemorrhagic cystitis; patients should be instructed to force fluids and to void frequently to minimize the local toxicity of the drug in the bladder. Hematuria may result from hemorrhagic cystitis or glomerulonephritis.

Monitor: Monitor toxicity with frequent patient visits. Weekly CBC and urinalysis until a stable dosage is obtained; then every 2 to 3 weeks. With careful monitoring, cyclophosphamide in these modest doses is often tolerated better than high doses of corticosteroids.

Azathioprine

Limited studies of a few patients and anecdotal experience suggest that azathioprine can be useful in the treatment of IPF. The drug is not believed to be as effective as cyclophosphamide but the side effects tend to be less severe. A patient who does not respond to combined steroid and cyclophosphamide treatment is unlikely to respond to azathioprine.

Indications: Individuals with IPF unable to tolerate cyclophosphamide but who are candidates for cytotoxic therapy.

Dosage: 2 mg/kg/day in a single dose (range 1 to 3 mg/kg/day) not to exceed 200 mg/day.

LUNG TRANSPLANTATION

Early results show great promise in treating patients with end-stage restrictive lung disease with lung transplantation. Single lung transplant appears to be the procedure of choice for restrictive lung disease resulting in pulmonary fibrosis.

Individuals with severe, progressive IPF unresponsive to therapy may be candidates for single lung transplantation.

COLLAGEN VASCULAR LUNG DISEASE

The collagen vascular disorders are systemic, multiorgan diseases that are grouped together because of their common association with inflammation of blood vessels, connective tissues, and serosal surfaces. Each disorder is associated with a spectrum of lung diseases (Table 23–8).

DIFFUSE INTERSTITIAL LUNG DISEASE

Chronic interstitial lung disease may be seen in each of the collagen vascular disorders, most commonly in rheumatoid arthritis and scleroderma. These disorders resemble IPF both clinically and histopathologically

- The interstitial process exhibits a nonspecific pattern with varying degrees of interstitial mononuclear cell and/or neutrophilic inflammation and fibrosis

TABLE 23–8. PULMONARY MANIFESTATIONS OF SOME COLLAGEN VASCULAR DISEASES

Rheumatoid Arthritis
  pleural disease (effusions)
  diffuse interstitial pneumonitis
  necrobiotic nodules
  Caplan's syndrome
  pulmonary hypertension (arteritis)
  apical fibrobullous disease
  bronchiolitis obliterans with and without organizing pneumonia
  cricoarytenoid arthritis
Systemic Lupus Erythematosus
  pleural disease (pleuritis, effusions)
  atelectasis
  acute lupus pneumonitis
  diffuse interstitial lung disease
  pulmonary hemorrhage
  respiratory muscle dysfunction
Progressive Systemic Sclerosis
  diffuse interstitial fibrosis
  pulmonary vascular disease
  aspiration pneumonia
  chest wall restriction secondary to thoracic skin sclerosis
  pleural disease

Polymyositis—Dermatomyositis
  interstitial pneumonitis
  aspiration pneumonia
  respiratory myositis
  pulmonary hypertension
  bronchiolitis obliterans organizing pneumonia
Mixed Connective Tissue Disease
  diffuse interstitial lung disease
  pulmonary hypertension (vasculitis)
  pleural disease
  diaphramatic muscle dysfunction
Sjögren's Syndrome
  respiratory mucosal dryness
  pleurisy
  chronic airway disease
  lymphocytic interstitial pneumonia
  pseudolymphoma
  lymphoma
  amyloid
  pulmonary hypertension (vasculitis)

- Restrictive lung impairment with reduced lung volumes, low diffusing capacity, and hypoxemia at rest or with exercise is characteristic
- Dyspnea, cough, and sputum production are common
- Chest x-rays demonstrate bibasilar interstitial infiltrates usually predominant in the lower lung fields
- Fiberoptic bronchoscopy with biopsy may be employed to exclude other causes of interstitial lung disease, such as infection or malignancy, if the diagnosis is uncertain
- Open lung biopsy is occasionally indicated to exclude pulmonary vasculitis or other treatable cause of aggressive interstitial lung disease in this patient group

RHEUMATOID LUNG

- Diffuse interstitial disease in rheumatoid arthritis, termed "rheumatoid lung," is often associated with systemic symptoms, pleural effusions, and/or necrobiotic nodules
- The course of the disease varies greatly but, in general, is not as aggressive as IPF and is not as responsive to treatment

Careful observation is indicated to objectively document progression of the disease before consideration of treatment. A decision to treat must be tempered by the generally poor response to therapy.

Corticosteroids are considered to be the initial treatment of choice. Prednisone 1 mg/kg/day for 6 to 8 weeks is recommended. The dose is then slowly tapered to 20 to 30 mg/day for 6 months. If no improvement is documented, steroids should be tapered off. Alternatively, in an appropriate candidate for aggressive therapy, cyclophosphamide or azathioprine can be added in a schedule similar to that outlined for the treatment of IPF.

SYSTEMIC LUPUS ERYTHEMATOSUS

ACUTE LUPUS PNEUMONITIS

Clinical hallmarks include high fever, cough, tachypnea, hypoxemia, and pulmonary infiltrates; occasionally, the process may rapidly progress to respiratory failure.

Management requires aggressive treatment with corticosteroids and, often, cytotoxic agents. Because the presentation can mimic a pneumonia/sepsis syndrome, broad-spectrum antibiotics are used until infection is excluded.

> **Suggested Regimen:** Methylprednisolone succinate (Solu-Medrol) 60 mg IV every 6 hours for 3 to 4 days. If not improved, add cyclophosphamide 2 mg/kg/day IV (alternatively, azathioprine 3 mg/kg/day). Taper to oral doses when clinical picture has stabilized.

A more chronic interstitial pneumonitis with features similar to IPF can occur, but tends to be more indolent. Management is similar to that for rheumatoid interstitial lung disease, although response to treatment is often better than the response for rheumatoid arthritis.

PROGRESSIVE SYSTEMIC SCLEROSIS

Diffuse interstitial lung disease, termed "scleroderma lung," is seen in about 90% of patients with scleroderma. Biopsy results typically show fibrosis with little active inflammatory change. The course is usually indolent.

Medical therapy is unrewarding, with evidence of efficacy of corticosteroids or cytotoxic agents only in rare, isolated case reports.

Aspiration pneumonitis as a result of esophageal disease may lead to recurrent episodes of respiratory distress and should be treated preventively with elevation of the head of the bed and delay of bedtime for 3 to 4 hours after meals.

POLYMYOSITIS—DERMATOMYOSITIS

Interstitial lung disease resulting in fibrosis is found in about 5% of patients with polymyositis or dermatomyositis and is associated with serum anti-Jo-1 antibody.

Progressive disease should be treated with corticosteroids, because many individuals respond favorably. Cyclophosphamide has also been reported to be effective.

Aspiration pneumonitis, respiratory myositis, and malignancy may complicate the picture.

MIXED CONNECTIVE TISSUE DISEASE

Interstitial lung disease similar to that found in systemic lupus erythematosus or polymyositis can occur. The natural course is variable but often responds well to steroids. A rapidly progressive interstitial pneumonitis unresponsive to steroids has also been described; cytotoxic drugs may be effective if used early in the course of disease.

SJÖGREN'S SYNDROME

A wide spectrum of interstitial lung diseases can occur in primary Sjögren's syndrome

- Lymphocytic interstitial pneumonitis (LIP) is a clinical and histopathologic entity that can be idiopathic; it may be associated with autoimmune disorders, hypogammaglobulinemia, acquired immunodeficiency syndrome, bone marrow transplantation, or T- and B-cell malignancies. Pseudolymphoma may be a localized form of LIP appearing as single or multiple well-circumscribed masses without adenopathy. Both LIP and pseudolymphoma may evolve to frank lymphoma
- Diffuse interstitial fibrosis
- Bronchiolitis obliterans organizing pneumonia

Although not confirmed by controlled studies, the response of many patients with LIP to corticosteroid therapy has been excellent. Cytotoxic agents may also be effective. A subset of patients may progress to end-stage fibrosis despite treatment; no distinguishing features can predict this lack of response.

BRONCHIOLITIS OBLITERANS ORGANIZING PNEUMONIA (BOOP)

This disorder usually appears as a poorly resolving pneumonia or occasionally is confused with IPF. The distinction from IPF is important because most patients with BOOP respond favorably to corticosteroid therapy in contrast to the low response rate in IPF. This clinical entity is usually idiopathic but occasionally is seen in association with a collagen vascular disease, following inhalation of a toxic fume, or following infection (viral, Mycoplasma, Legionella).

PATHOPHYSIOLOGY

Injury to the bronchioles leads to reparative processes involving granulation tissue that extends in the form of polyps into the alveolar ducts and alveoli, thereby resulting pathologically in organizing pneumonia. Unlike bronchiolitis obliterans (without organizing pneumonia), restrictive changes are characteristic.

CLINICAL HALLMARKS

- Most patients are 40 to 60 years old
- Flu-like illness with fever, malaise, persistent nonproductive cough, dyspnea, and fatigue of short duration (several weeks to months) often dates onset of symptoms
- Midinspiratory squeaks are characteristic; paninspiratory crackles or occasionally wheezing may also be found on physical examination
- Chest x-ray demonstrates variable bilateral, patchy ground-glass opacities typically in the lower lung fields; rarely a miliary pattern is seen
- Pulmonary function tests characteristically show restrictive impairment with low diffusing capacity and hypoxemia
- CT scan often demonstrates a distinctive picture with patchy, subpleural areas of hazy, ground-glass opacities juxtaposed to normal or hyperlucent areas
- Transbronchial biopsy specimens may show organizing pneumonia, but rarely demonstrate bronchiolitis obliterans. Although not diagnostic, the histopathologic findings, combined with a typical clinical and radiologic picture, are frequently suggestive enough to establish the diagnosis. If the diagnosis remains in doubt, an open lung biopsy should be considered

THERAPY

Corticosteroid therapy is effective in most cases of BOOP; frequently the response is dramatic, within days of institution of therapy. In untreated patients, clinical improvement is rare. A few patients have aggressive disease despite therapy.

Suggested Regimen: Prednisone 1 mg/kg/day (e.g. 60 to 80 mg/day) for 2 months; taper to 20 to 40 mg/day over next 2 to 4 months. Subsequently, slow taper can be tried, eventually switching to alternate-day dosage sufficient to control symptoms and radiographic/functional evidence of disease. Aim to treat for a minimum of 8 to 12 months. Relapse is common with doses lower than 20 to 30 mg/day or with early cessation of treatment.

EOSINOPHILIC GRANULOMA OF THE LUNG

Eosinophilic granuloma of the lung is the form of histiocytosis X that primarily affects the lungs of adults (also called primary pulmonary histiocytosis X). Like Letterer-Siwe disease and Hand-Schüller-Christian disease in children, eosinophilic granuloma shares in common an abnormal accumulation of atypical histiocytes in stellate-shaped granulomatous inflammatory lesions in affected tissues

- Atypical histiocytes have been identified as Langerhans'-type macrophages because of the presence of X-bodies (Birbeck granules) seen with electron microscopy or by staining for the S-100 protein or OKT_6 surface antigen

- Eosinophils are not a constant feature of the inflammatory lesions
- The inflammatory process involves primarily the pulmonary interstitium and can lead to fibrocystic changes and pathologic honeycombing
- Although the cause is unknown, more than 90% of individuals have a history of smoking, which leads to the hypothesis that exposure to an unknown antigen in the smoke incites an immunologic reaction associated with recruitment of Langerhans'-type macrophages (and eosinophils) into the lung

CLINICAL HALLMARKS

- Most patients are 20 to 40 years old
- Racial predominance is in Caucasians; the disease is rare in African-Americans
- Symptoms include cough, dyspnea, fever, weight loss, and bone pain, but patient may be asymptomatic
- Pneumothorax is common
- Diabetes insipidus is seen in about 5% of individuals
- Chest x-rays show nodular or reticulonodular infiltrates that may have an upper lobe predominance and spare the costophrenic angles; honeycomb lung and fibrocystic changes and are seen in more advanced disease
- Pulmonary function tests may be normal or show mixed restrictive and obstructive impairment with low diffusing capacity; hypoxemia is common, particularly with exercise
- Bronchoscopic biopsy procedures are often not diagnostic because of the small amount of tissue sampled but are useful in excluding other interstitial disorders
- BAL typically shows a marked increase ($> 10\%$; normal $< 1\%$) in the proportions of OKT_6-staining mononuclear cells. This finding may not be seen in more advanced disease
- If the diagnosis is uncertain, open lung biopsy with electron microscopic analysis of the inflammatory lesions, in addition to S-100 and OKT_6 staining, may be required for definitive diagnosis

THERAPY

Management is tempered by the fact that the course of the disease is unpredictable, but often self-limiting. Less than 5% of individuals progress to end-stage respiratory failure

- Primary therapy begins by counseling the patient to quit smoking
- Anecdotal evidence suggests that corticosteroids improve symptoms and promote radiographic resolution. Although their beneficial effect on the natural course of the disease has not been proved, corticosteroids are recommended for progressive disease
- Isolated, symptomatic bony lesions can be treated with curettage or local radiotherapy

- For progressive, widespread disease unresponsive to corticosteroids, one of the Vinca alkaloids, vincristine or vinblastine, is recommended

WEGENER'S GRANULOMATOSIS

Classic Wegener's granulomatosis is a systemic, necrotizing granulomatous vasculitis of the upper and lower respiratory tracts associated with necrotizing glomerulonephritis and disseminated vasculitis of the small vessels. When untreated, < 10% of affected individuals survive 2 years. A limited form of the disease without renal involvement has a much better prognosis.

PATHOPHYSIOLOGY

The pathogenesis likely involves a hypersensitivity response by T-cells to an unknown antigen with the development of necrotizing granulomas and vasculitis and subsequent tissue injury. Recent studies suggest that antineutrophil cytoplasmic autoantibodies directed against myeloid lysosomal enzymes are a marker for the disease and may play a pathogenic role.

CLINICAL HALLMARKS

- The clinical presentation is quite variable, but most commonly reveals upper respiratory tract symptoms of sinusitis, rhinitis, and otitis media
- Cough, dyspnea, and hemoptysis are manifestations of lower respiratory tract disease. Hemoptysis may be massive and mimic Goodpasture's syndrome
- Renal involvement results in azotemia, proteinuria, and hematuria, and can progress to end-stage renal failure
- Systemic vasculitis frequently involves several organ systems, e.g., the joints, eyes, skin, central nervous system, heart

INVESTIGATIONS

- Chest X-Ray: Nodular infiltrates are common, may be asymptomatic, and often cavitate. Simultaneous clearing and worsening of different areas of the lung may be seen. Progressive, diffuse interstitial lung disease is uncommon. Pleural effusions are seen in a minority of patients. Mediastinal adenopathy is rare
- Pulmonary Function Tests: Reduced lung volumes and diffusing capacity are characteristic. Obstructive impairment caused by upper airway (e.g., tracheal stenosis) or endobronchial disease is common
- Serum Studies: The erythrocyte sedimentation rate (ESR) and C-reactive protein are elevated, rheumatoid factor may be seen in 50% of patients. Both are nonspecific
- Antineutrophil Cytoplasmic Antibodies (ANCA): Elevated titers of ANCA are frequently present in patients with classic Wegener's granulomatosis, but may not be seen in individuals with more limited dis-

ease. Initial reports of high specificity must be confirmed before their role in the diagnosis of Wegener's granulomatosis can be established

DIAGNOSIS

A diagnosis of Wegener's granulomatosis requires biopsy confirmation. A nasal mucosal biopsy is easy to perform but usually shows nonspecific inflammation. Bronchoscopic biopsies (transbronchial, bronchial) are also usually nondiagnostic but help to exclude infection and malignancy. If the diagnosis is in doubt, an open lung biopsy is often needed to establish a definitive diagnosis.

THERAPY

Prospective and retrospective clinical studies have shown that cyclophosphamide is effective in inducing longterm remissions in patients with Wegener's granulomatosis. The initial dose of cyclophosphamide depends on the severity and rapidity of progression of the disease. Corticosteroids are initiated at the same time for their more immediate anti-inflammatory effects and then are tapered slowly as cyclophosphamide takes effect. Most investigators use a schedule similar to that used in protocol studies from the National Institutes of Health.*

COMBINED CYCLOPHOSPHAMIDE AND CORTICOSTEROID THERAPY

Cyclophosphamide Dosage: 2 mg/kg/day as a single morning oral dose. Adjust the dosage to keep WBC > 3,500; maintain for at least 1 year after complete remission has been achieved, then taper by 25-mg increments every 2 to 3 months

- Expect 2 to 4 weeks for maximum response to cyclophosphamide
- For stable or slowly progressing disease, begin cyclophosphamide 1 mg/kg/day, increasing by 25 mg every 2 weeks until improvement is noted or toxicity occurs

Corticosteroid Dosage: Prednisone 1 mg/kg/day in divided doses for 2 weeks, then as single daily morning dose for 1 month. Switch to alternate-day therapy over the next month, then taper slowly over 6 to 12 months.

Adverse Effects (see Tables 23–6 and 23–7)

- Azathioprine may be given if cyclophosphamide is contraindicated; however, most investigators suggest that azathioprine is not as effective as cyclophosphamide
- Case reports suggest that co-trimoxazole (Bactrim, Septra) may be successful in a subset of patients with indolent disease or those who did not respond to conventional therapy. Further studies are underway to

---

* See Leavitt and Fauci listing in Bibliography.

assess the effectiveness of this drug in treatment of nonfulminant Wegener's granulomatosis

OTHER THERAPIES

- Infections of the sinuses (usually staphylococcal) and lungs are common and warrant aggressive antibiotic therapy. Surgical drainage of the sinuses may be needed to treat persistent sinusitis
- Upper airway obstruction secondary to tracheal stenosis may require surgical dilatation or tracheostomy
- Renal transplantation has been successfully tried in individuals with end-stage renal failure who are in remission

FULMINANT WEGENER'S GRANULOMATOSIS

- Rapidly progressive glomerulonephritis
- Severe hemoptysis
- Threatened organ failure

THERAPY

Cyclophosphamide Dosage: 4 mg/kg/day IV for 3 days, then reduce to 2 mg/kg/day and adjust as previously described.

Corticosteroid Dosage: Prednisone 1 mg/kg/day in divided doses similar to the schedule previously described.

PULMONARY ALVEOLAR PROTEINOSIS

This rare disorder of unknown cause is characterized by the accumulation of lipoprotein-rich material similar in composition to surfactant in alveoli. This material stains positive with periodic acid-Schiff (PAS) and contains many lamellar bodies, similar to inclusions within surfactant synthesizing type II pneumocytes.

CLINICAL HALLMARKS

- Most commonly appears insidiously with dyspnea, cough, and occasional sputum production
- Crackles are often present on chest auscultation
- Serum lactate dehydrogenase is frequently elevated
- Chest x-ray demonstrates diffuse, bilateral "alveolar" infiltrates, often in a perihilar distribution; pleural effusion and hilar adenopathy are uncommon
- Often a marked disparity is seen between mild clinical symptoms and extensive radiographic infiltrates
- Diagnostic approach usually begins with fiberoptic bronchoscopy with transbronchial biopsies and BAL to demonstrate PAS-staining intra-al-

veolar material; if this approach is nondiagnostic, an open lung biopsy may be needed

THERAPY

* Whole lung lavage is the treatment of choice. The procedure involves placement of a double lumen tube to ventilate one lung while the other side is lavaged with 10 to 20 L of saline. This procedure is best performed by medical teams experienced in the procedure
* Infections are a frequent complication of the disease and require aggressive therapy

BIBLIOGRAPHY

Basset, F, Soler P, Jaurand MC, Bigron J: Ultrastructural examination of bronchoalveolar lavage for diagnosis of pulmonary histiocytosis X. Thorax, *32*:303, 1977.

Carette S, Macher AM, Nussbaum A, Plotz PH: Severe acute pulmonary disease in patients with systemic lupus erythematosus: Ten years of experience at the National Institutes of Health. Semin Arthritis Rheum, *14*:52, 1984.

Claypool WD: Proceedings of the fourth annual Chicago lung conference. Chest, *100*:230, 1991.

Claypool WD, Rogers R, Matuschak G: Update on the clinical diagnosis, management, and pathogenesis of pulmonary alveolar proteinosis (phospholipidosis). Chest, *85*:550, 1984.

Cooper AD Jr., White DA, Matthay RA: Drug-induced pulmonary disease. Part 1: Cytotoxic drugs. Am Rev Respir Dis, *133*:321, 1986. Part 2: Noncytotoxic drugs. Am Rev Respir Dis, *133*:488, 1986.

Costabel U: The alveolitis of hypersensitivity pneumonitis. Eur Respir J, *1*:5, 1988.

Crystal RG, Bitterman PB, Rennard SI, et al.: Interstitial lung disease of unknown cause. Disorders characterized by chronic inflammation of the lower respiratory tract. N Engl J Med, *310*:154, 1984.

Daniele PR, Elias JA, Epstein PE, Rossman MD: Bronchoalveolar lavage: Role in the pathogenesis, diagnosis and management of interstitial lung disease. Ann Intern Med, *102*:93, 1985.

DeRemee R, McDonald T, Weiland L: Wegener's granulomatosis: Observations on treatment with antimicrobial agents. Mayo Clin Proc, *60*:27, 1985.

Dickey BF, Myers AR: Pulmonary disease in polymyositis/dermatomyositis. Semin Arthritis Rheum, *14*:60, 1984.

Epler GR, Colby TV, McLoud TC, et al.: Bronchiolitis obliterans organizing pneumonia. N Engl J Med, *312*:152, 1985.

Friedman PJ, Liebow AA, Sokoloff J: Eosinophilic granuloma of lung. Clinical aspects of primary pulmonary histiocytosis in the adult. Medicine, *60*:385, 1981.

Gilman WJ, Wang KP: Transbronchial lung biopsy in sarcoidosis. An approach to determine the optimal number of biopsies. Am Rev Respir Dis, *122*:742, 1980.

Greenwald GI, Tashkin DP, Gong H, et al.: Longitudinal changes in lung function and respiratory symptoms in progressive systemic sclerosis. Prospective study. Am J Med, *83*:83, 1987.

Hance AJ, Basset F, Saumon G, et al.: Smoking and interstitial lung disease: The effect of cigarette smoking on the incidence of pulmonary histiocytosis X and sarcoidosis. Ann NY Acad Sci, *465*:643, 1986.

Hunninghake GW, Fauci AS: Pulmonary involvement in collagen-vascular diseases. Am Rev Respir Dis, *119*:471, 1979.

Johns CJ, Scott PP, Schonfeld SA: Sarcoidosis. Annu Rev Med, *40*:353, 1989.

Johns CJ, Zachary JB, Ball WC Jr.: A ten year study of corticosteroid treatment of pulmonary sarcoidosis. Johns Hopkins Med J, *134*:271, 1974.

Johnson MA, Kwan S, Snell NJC, et al.: Randomised controlled trial comparing prednisolone alone with cyclophosphamide and low dose prednisolone in combination in cryptogenic fibrosing alveolitis. Thorax, *44*:280, 1989.

Leavitt R, Fauci A: State of the art: Pulmonary vasculitis. Am Rev Respir Dis, *134*:149, 1986.

Liebow AA, Carrington CB: The eosinophilic pneumonias. Medicine, *48*:251, 1969.

Martin RJ, Rogers RM, Myers NM: Pulmonary alveolar proteinosis: Shunt fraction and lactic acid dehydrogenase concentration as aids to diagnosis. Am Rev Respir Dis, *117*:1059, 1978.

Martin WJ II, Rosenow EC III: Amiodarone pulmonary toxicity: Recognition and pathogenesis—part I and part II. Chest, *93*:1067;1242, 1988.

Matthay RA, Schwartz MI, Petty TL, et al.: Pulmonary manifestations of systemic lupus erythematosus: Review of twelve cases of acute lupus pneumonitis. Medicine, *54*:397, 1974.

Mossman B, Gee B: Asbestos-related disease. N Engl J Med, *321*:1721, 1989.

Muller NL, Miller RR: Computed tomography of chronic diffuse infiltrative lung diseases. Am Rev Respir Dis, *142*:1206;1440, 1990.

Prakash UBS, Barham SS, Carpenter HA, et al.: Pulmonary alveolar phospholipoproteinosis: Experience with 34 cases and a review. Mayo Clin Proc, *62*:499, 1987.

Prophet D: Primary pulmonary histiocytosis X. Clin Chest Med, *3*:643, 1982.

Reynolds HY: Bronchoalveolar lavage. Am Rev Respir Dis, *135*:250, 1987.

Reynolds HY, Fulmer JD, Kazmierowski JA, et al.: Analysis of cellular and protein content of bronchoalveolar lavage fluid from patients with idiopathic pulmonary fibrosis and chronic hypersensitivity pneumonitis. J Clin Invest, *59*:165, 1977.

Rossi GA, Bitterman PB, Rennard SI, et al.: Evidence for chronic inflammation as a component of the interstitial lung disease associated with progressive systemic sclerosis. Am Rev Respir Dis, *131*:612, 1985.

Schmidt CD, Jensen RL, Christensen LT, et al.: Longitudinal pulmonary function changes in pigeon breeders. Chest, *93*:359, 1988.

Schneider EL, Epstein CJ, Kaback MJ, Brandes D: Severe pulmonary involvement in adult Gaucher's disease. Am J Med, *63*:475, 1977.

Schwartz MI, King TE: Interstitial Lung Disease. Philadelphia, B.C. Decker Inc. 1988.

Schwartz MI, Matthay RA, Sahn SA: Interstitial lung disease in polymyositis and dermatomyositis: Analysis of six cases and review of the literature. Medicine, *55*:89, 1976.

Shure D: Bronchoscopy-Transbronchial biopsy and needle aspiration. Chest, *95*:5, 1989.

Siltzbach LE: Sarcoidosis: Clinical features and management. Med Clin North Am, *51*:483, 1967.

Specks U, Wheatley CL, McDonald TJ, et al.: Anticytoplasmic autoantibodies in the diagnosis and follow-up of Wegener's granulomatosis. Mayo Clin Proc, *64*:28, 1989.

Sullivan WD, Hurst DJ, Harman CE, et al.: A prospective evaluation emphasizing pulmonary involvement in patients with mixed connective tissue disease. Medicine, *63*:92, 1984.

Thomas PD, Hunninghake GW: Current concepts of the pathogenesis of sarcoidosis. Am Rev Respir Dis, *135*:747, 1987.

Turner-Warwick M, Burrows B, Johnson A: Cryptogenic fibrosing alveolitis: Clinical features and their influence on survival. Thorax, *35*:171, 1980.

Turner-Warwick M, Haslam PL: The value of serial bronchoalveolar lavages in assessing the clinical progress of patients with cryptogenic fibrosing alveolitis. Am Rev Respir Dis, *135*: 26, 1987.

Van der Woude F, Lobatto S, Permin H, et al.: Autoantibodies against neutrophils and monocytes: Tool for diagnosis and marker of disease activity in Wegener's granulomatosis. Lancet, *1*:425, 1985.

Watters LC, Schwarz MI, Cherniack RM, et al.: Idiopathic pulmonary fibrosis: Pretreatment bronchoalveolar lavage cellular constituents and their relationships with lung histopathology and clinical response to therapy. Am Rev Respir Dis, *135*:696, 1987.

Wiener-Kronish JP, Sollinger AM, Warnock ML, et al.: Severe pulmonary involvement in mixed connective tissue disease. Am Rev Respir Dis, *124*:499, 1981.

Winterbauer RH: The treatment of idiopathic pulmonary fibrosis. Chest, *100*(1):233, 1991.

Yoshida S, Akizuki M, Mimori T: The precipitating antibody to an acidic nuclear protein antigen, the Jo-1, in connective tissue disease: A marker for a subset of polymyositis with interstitial pulmonary fibrosis. Arthritis Rheum, *26*:604, 1983.

24

BACTERIAL PNEUMONIA

Joseph P. Lynch, III
Galen B. Toews

Despite the proliferation of a vast array of potent, broad-spectrum anti-microbials within the past decade, mortality from bacterial pneumonia remains high. Pneumonia is the 4th leading cause of death among elderly patients (6th overall), and is the leading cause of death resulting from nosocomial infections. The past decade has been marked by increasingly resistant microorganisms capable of generating more sophisticated enzymes that inactivate even the most advanced antimicrobial drugs. This chapter reviews the specific organisms involved in bacterial pneumonia, and the appropriate use of antimicrobials for the treatment of this complication in both community and hospital settings. The clinical features, prognosis, relevant pathogens, and therapeutic strategies differ markedly between these disparate patient populations. Certain pathogens, such as Pseudomonas aeruginosa and Acinetobacter calcoaceticus, are virtually only seen as opportunists in nosocomial settings in critically ill, mechanically ventilated patients. By contrast, Streptococcus pneumoniae and Mycoplasma pneumoniae, common pathogens in the community setting, are rarely implicated in nosocomial pneumonias. Recognition of the differences between pneumonia arising in these settings is critical to arrive at curative yet cost-effective treatment strategies. Community-acquired pneumonia and the salient pathogens involved (some of which overlap with nosocomial pneumonia) are reviewed initially. Nosocomial pneumonia is then covered, emphasizing the importance of gram-negative bacilli in this setting, the pathogenic mechanisms responsible for acquisition of gram-negative bacilli in the lower respiratory tract, and recent concepts of prophylactic antibiotics aimed at eradicating gut flora and reducing gram-negative colonization. Also described are new techniques (bronchoscopy, bronchoalveolar lavage) designed to define more clearly the microbiology of pneumonias, the specific pathogens involved in both community and nosocomial pneumonias, and controversies and strategies of antibiotic use.

614

COMMUNITY-ACQUIRED PNEUMONIA

EPIDEMIOLOGY

Despite substantial advances in the development of new antimicrobials, community-acquired pneumonia (CAP) remains an important cause of morbidity and mortality. In the United States, more than 900,000 cases of CAP occur annually, incurring costs in excess of $1.5 billion and resulting in more than 50,000 deaths. Only 20 to 30% of cases of CAP occur in young, previously healthy adults; in the remaining cases, a predisposing risk factor can be identified (e.g. old age, a history of cigarette smoking, chronic ethanol abuse, chronic obstructive lung disease, malignancy, cardiac disease, diabetes mellitus, previous strokes, debilitation, liver disease, renal insufficiency, corticosteroid/immunosuppressive therapy, residence in a nursing home, or any serious pre-existing disease). While fatalities may occur in all populations, pneumonia is particularly lethal in elderly patients or in patients with significant associated conditions. Mortality is low (<5%) in young, previously healthy adults, and many such patients can be treated with antibiotics on an outpatient basis. Several recent prospective investigations of CAP in adults, however, have cited mortality rates ranging from 5 to 13% among patients requiring hospitalization; even higher fatality rates (from 15 to 30%) have been noted in the presence of serious associated diseases, multilobar involvement, bacteremia, or an age greater than 60. Progression of CAP to respiratory failure requiring mechanical support may occur in as many as 10 to 20% of patients; in this context, Streptococcus pneumoniae and Legionella pneumophila are the most likely pathogens. Unfortunately, by the time patients with CAP develop respiratory failure of sufficient severity to warrant mechanical ventilation, mortality rates exceeding 20 to 40% are characteristic. Prognostic factors at the time of presentation that have been associated with a higher mortality rate include tachypnea (>30/min), diastolic hypotension, renal failure, serious associated diseases, shock, and age older than 60 years. In light of the life-threatening nature of CAP, an aggressive therapeutic approach is warranted. Broad-spectrum parenteral antimicrobials are appropriate for most cases of CAP; oral agents may be appropriate for younger adults without serious associated conditions who are not acutely ill. Antimicrobial agents must be modified according to clinical and host factors, including age, presence or absence of underlying disease, prior use of antimicrobials, extent of radiographic changes, and severity of the disease process. Recognition of the important pathogens involved in CAP (and antimicrobial susceptibility patterns) is critical to the effective design of therapeutic strategies.

MICROBIOLOGIC CAUSE

The most important pathogens implicated in CAP have been well delineated in multiple, elegant epidemiologic studies that have applied both cultural and serologic data. In individual cases, however, a specific microbiologic cause can be demonstrated in only 30 to 60% of patients. Nevertheless, an awareness of the likely pathogens (based on what is known from epidemiologic studies), may guide therapy even when a precise microbiologic diagnosis is not possible. Streptococcus pneumoniae (pneumococcus) is the single most important pathogen in all age groups, accounting for 30 to 70% of cases. Mycoplasma pneumoniae has been implicated as the causative agent in 20 to 30% of CAP in young adults (younger than age 35), but accounts for only 1 to 9% of CAP in older adults. Legionella and Chlamydia spp each account or 2 to 6% of CAP, but the incidence of these pathogens has been variable among geographic regions. The prevalence of microorganisms not previously appreciated as community-acquired pathogens, such as Hemophilus influenzae, Staphylococcus aureus, and enteric gram-negative bacilli (GNB), appears to have increased during the past 2 decades.

- In several recent studies, Hemophilus influenzae has been the second- or third-most common pathogen, accounting for 5 to 18% of CAP in adults
- GNB (predominantly Enterobacteriaeceae) have been implicated in 3 to 8% of cases in recent series; even higher prevalence rates have been noted in elderly patients, residents of chronic care facilities, or patients with significant underlying diseases
- Staphylococcus aureus accounts for 3 to 8% of CAP in adults, usually in patients with risk factors for staphylococcal carriage, such as nursing home residence, advanced age, intravenous drug abuse, chronic dialysis, or in association with epidemics of influenza
- Moraxella (Branhamella) catarrhalis, which has only recently been recognized as an important pathogen in exacerbations of bronchitis, accounts for 1 to 2% of CAP
- Viruses, particularly influenza, parainfluenza, and adenovirus have been implicated in as many as 5 to 15% of CAP; most cases occur during the winter months

CLINICAL AND RADIOGRAPHIC FEATURES

- Clinical and radiographic features of CAP may suggest certain pathogens, but are not specific. An abrupt onset associated with high fever, a shaking chill, pleuritic chest pain, and lobar consolidation on physical examination and chest x-ray is highly characteristic of bacteremic infections caused by Streptococcus pneumoniae. Identical features, however, may be observed with other bacteria, such as Hemophilus influenzae, Escherichia coli, Klebsiella, or Legionella spp; admittedly, this type of presentation is rare with Mycoplasma or Chlamydia
- Many of the "classic" features of acute bacillary pneumonia may be absent, particularly in elderly or debilitated patients. Nearly 25% of patients older than 65 years with pneumonia are afebrile; leukocytosis is present in only 50 to 70%. Clinical features of pneumonia in this context may be subtle; lethargy, fatigue, nausea, anorexia, or deterioration in overall condition may be the predominant features. Unfortunately, delay in recognition and treatment of pneumonia may be disastrous. Mortality associated with CAP in the elderly population ranges from 10 to 25%

Chest radiographic changes in CAP are variable. Patchy bronchopneumonic infiltrates are most common

- Dense lobar consolidation with air bronchograms occurs in fewer than 33% of patients
- Pleural effusions complicate CAP in 10 to 25% of patients, and are not etiologically specific
- Cavitation, rare with Streptococcus pneumoniae, Mycoplasma, or Chlamydia, suggests such pathogens as Staphylococcus aureus, Klebsiella (or other GNB), anaerobes, or nonbacterial causes, such as mycobacteria, fungi, neoplasm
- An air fluid level is most characteristic of an anaerobic or mixed aerobic/anaerobic lung abscess
- Basilar interstitial or reticulonodular infiltrates suggest Mycoplasma spp; however, frank lobar pneumonia indistinguishable from bacillary pneumonias may also be seen in as many as one third of the cases of Mycoplasma spp. Small (2 to 3 cm) patchy bronchopneumonic infiltrates have been stated to be characteristic of Moraxella catarrhalis, but also may be observed with a wide range of pathogens
- Radiographic features may favor certain pathogens, but significant overlap exists. Thus, smears and cultures of sputum, blood, or pleural fluid (when present) are important to substantiate a specific microbiologic diagnosis

ETIOLOGIC (CULTURAL) DIAGNOSIS

Despite a relatively low sensitivity and specificity, sputum smears and cultures should be obtained in all cases of suspected or proven pneumonia. The sputum gram stain is most useful to distinguish predominantly gram-negative from gram-positive organisms, but is not specific for a unique organism.

- Sputa demonstrating numerous leukocytes, rare or absent contaminating epithelial cells, uniform morphologic and staining characteristics of microorganisms, and many intracellular organisms within leukocytes may guide therapy. For example, lancet-shaped diplococci in pairs suggest Streptococcus pneumoniae, clumps of gram-positive cocci suggest Staphylococcus aureus, gram-negative coccobacillary forms in a smoker may suggest Hemophilus influenzae, and gram-negative rods are characteristic of Klebsiella spp or other Enterobacteriaceae
- In most instances, however, mixed gram-negative and gram-positive organisms are observed. Even when a dominant pathogen is noted, the reliability of sputum smears is inexact
- Caution should be taken when basing initial therapy solely on a sputum gram stain
- In bacteremic cases of pneumonia, the pathogen can be isolated in only 40 to 60% of sputum cultures. Higher rates of isolation can be expected if a "good quality" sputum is obtained, but in clinical practice, a pathogen can be isolated from sputum cultures in only 25 to 50% of cases of pneumonia (including nonbacteremic cases)

- Identification of the microorganisms on sputum cultures may take 2 or 3 days; even longer delays can be expected for antimicrobial susceptibility profiles
- The value of sputum cultures is further confounded because potential pathogens, such as Streptococcus pneumoniae and Hemophilus influenzae, may be part of normal oral flora. Thus, the isolation of a potential pathogen from sputum does not prove that the isolated pathogen is responsible for pneumonia. This inconclusiveness may be particularly true in pneumonia caused by atypical pathogens, Legionella spp, or anaerobes; in such instances, only normal oral flora may be isolated on routine sputum cultures.

In summary, Gram's stain and cultural results may be useful as guides to the diagnosis in some cases, but are frequently nondiagnostic and may even be misleading.

More aggressive techniques, such as bronchoscopy with bronchoalveolar lavage (BAL) and protected brush for quantitative cultures, are more accurate than sputa cultures in establishing a precise microbiologic diagnosis. Bronchoscopy, however, is invasive, associated with mild discomfort, and expensive (cost exceeds $500 in most centers); thus, bronchoscopic procedures are inappropriate for the routine diagnosis of CAP. Other techniques, such as blood cultures and thoracentesis, may establish a specific microbiologic diagnosis in some cases. Blood culture studies should always be performed in instances of CAP, because a positive blood culture is highly specific for the responsible pathogen and may allow redirection of therapy once cultural results become available. Only 5 to 15% of blood cultures, however, are positive in CAP; higher rates of bacteremia have been noted in the presence of lobar pneumonia with consolidation and rigors. Thoracentesis should be done when a substantial pleural effusion is present, but this development occurs in fewer than 15% of patients. Isolation of a pathogen from pleural fluid is highly specific. Serologic tests (IgG and IgM antibodies) for Mycoplasma, Legionella, or Chlamydia spp may be useful in large epidemiologic investigations, but are of no value in the initial management of individual patients.

SPECIFIC PATHOGENS ENCOUNTERED IN CAP

Prior to reviewing approaches to therapy, the salient features of the most important pathogens involved in community-acquired pneumonia will be reviewed.

TYPICAL PNEUMONIAS

Streptococcus Pneumoniae

Epidemiology

- Streptococcus pneumoniae (pneumococcus) remains the most common cause of CAP (accounting for 30 to 60% of cases) and, with Legionella spp, has been associated with the most fatalities resulting from CAP.

Streptococcus pneumoniae has been implicated in only 15 to 30% of CAP in most recent series, but these data underestimate its true frequency, because no causative pathogen was identified in 50 to 70% of cases. Pneumococcal pneumonia has a predilection for the elderly patient and for patients with pre-existing disease, such as ethanol abuse and chronic obstructive pulmonary disease (COPD). It can also affect previously healthy individuals in all age groups

- S. pneumoniae and Mycoplasma pneumoniae are the two most common causes of CAP in adults under age 35
- Streptococcus pneumoniae is the leading cause of pneumonia in all age groups (including the elderly). Thus, therapy for CAP (irrespective of age and presence or absence of underlying disease) should always include coverage for S. pneumoniae

Clinical Features:

- Classic features include a temperature of greater than 103°F, drenching sweats, chills, purulent sputum, pleuritic chest pain, and lobar consolidation. These features occur in 50 to 70% of persons with bacteremic pneumonia caused by S. pneumoniae, but do not distinguish pneumococcal pneumonia from other bacillary pneumonias
- Many of these manifestations are absent in non-bacteremic forms, in the elderly population, or in patients with serious associated diseases
- A single shaking chill, often stated to be a hallmark for pneumococcal pneumonia, occurs in fewer than 10% of patients; recurrent chills are more common
- Blood-tinged sputum occurs in as many as 15% of patients
- Constitutional symptoms, myalgias, nausea, vomiting, and prostration may be prominent. Headache is a common early feature; stiff neck may reflect meningeal spread. Diarrhea, seen in 20 to 30% of cases of legionellosis, occurs in fewer than 10% of cases of pneumococcal pneumonia
- Bacteremia occurs in 15 to 30% of patients; higher rates have been noted among patients with dense lobar consolidation and rigors
  The course of pneumococcal pneumonia is highly variable, but may be fulminant. Mortality in bacteremic cases of pneumococcal pneumonia ranges from 15 to 30%, and has not changed significantly over the past 3 decades. Multilobar involvement, respiratory failure requiring mechanical ventilatory support, extrapulmonary spread (endocarditis, meningitis) leukopenia, age older than 60 years, and certain serotypes (e.g., type 3 strains) have been associated with even higher mortality rates.

Laboratory Studies: The demonstration of lancet-shaped, gram-positive diplococci on sputum gram stain supports the diagnosis, particularly when intracellular forms are present within leukocytes. Sputum cultures are positive in only 40 to 60% of bacteremic cases. Counterimmunoelectrophoresis (CIE) can be done in cerebrospinal fluid or pleural fluid, but we have not employed this diagnostic modality in tracheobronchial secretions. Peripheral blood leukocytosis or left shift on differential count occurs in greater than 80% of patients; leukopenia has been noted in as many as 33% of alcoholic or debilitated patients, and has been associated with a worse prognosis. Chest x-rays demonstrate lobar consolidation with air bronchograms in 30 to 60% of patients; patchy bronchopneumonic infiltrates occur as commonly. Pleural effusions have been noted in as many as 20% of patients; empyema occurs in less than 5%.

Preferred Therapy

- Penicillin G, 4.8 to 10 million units IV until clinical improvement and defervescence have been achieved
- Penicillin VK, 500 mg qid orally, then can be substituted for a full 10- to 14-day course

Alternative Agents

- Erythromycin, 500 mg q6h, or doxycycline, 100 mg bid, IV or oral
- Virtually all beta-lactams, clindamycin, and trimethoprim/sulfamethoxazole (TMP/SMX) are active against S. pneumoniae

Note: Penicillin G has an exceptionally low minimal inhibitory concentration (MIC) and is less expensive and less toxic than most alternative agents.

Antimicrobial Resistance: Decreased susceptibility to penicillin and resistance to multiple antimicrobials (including tetracycline and erythromycin) have been increasing worldwide. This increasing resistance has been most evident in Spain, where the prevalence of pneumococci resistant to penicillin rose from 6% in 1979 to 44% by 1989. High rates of resistance to other antimicrobials have also been noted in Spain; over the decade from 1979 to 1989, 56% and 43% of isolates of S. pneumoniae were resistant to tetracycline and chloramphenicol, respectively; 5% were resistant to erythromycin. In South Africa, where penicillin-resistant pneumococci were first described, 15% of penicillin-resistant isolates were noted over the period from 1979 to 1986. These strains remain highly susceptible to third-generation cephalosporins. In most countries (including the United States), however, less than 5% of isolates exhibit even moderate resistance (increased MIC) to penicillin. Resistance to erythromycin also has been highly variable; in the United States, less than 0.7% of S. pneumoniae are resistant to erythromycin, whereas rates as high as 22% have been noted in France. Penicillin and erythromycin remain highly efficacious for the treatment of pneumococcal pneumonia; however, antimicrobial resistance trends must be monitored carefully over time to assess changes in susceptibility among different geographic regions.

Pneumococcal Vaccination: The efficacy and indications for pneumococcal vaccine (Pneumovax) remain controversial. Early studies published in the 1970s confirmed that pneumococcal vaccination was effective in reducing pneumococcal infections in closed populations at high risk (e.g. South African gold miners, New Guinea highlanders, immunocompetent Air Force recruits) and in children with sickle cell anemia. Despite the widespread use of the 14-valent vaccine for more than 10 years, however, the efficacy of this vaccine in preventing pneumococcal infections in high-risk patients is far from clear. Studies assessing the 14-valent vaccine have yielded discrepant results; this vaccine failed to influence the rate of pneumococcal infections in a large Veterans Cooperative Study. In some studies, failure rates have been associated with a serotype not encompassed by the vaccine. Because the 14-valent vaccine covered only 75 to 80% of serotypical strains, a 23-valent vaccine (currently in clinical use) was developed to cover more than 90% of strains implicated in pneumococcal infections. The superiority of this 23-valent vaccine over the previous 14-valent vaccine has not been fully established, and failures may occur among vaccinated patients. Failure may be attributable to inability to mount an antibody response (among debilitated individuals with impaired immune systems) or failure to cover serotypes not present in the vaccine. Despite the lack of firm data supporting efficacy, vaccination with the 23-valent vaccination should be administered to patients at risk for S. pneumoniae. Revaccination should not be done.

Hemophilus Influenzae

Epidemiology

- Hemophilus influenzae is a pleomorphic gram-negative rod that accounts for 5 to 15% of pneumonias, both community acquired and hospital acquired. Both typeable (encapsulated, primarily type B) and nontypeable (nonencapsulated) strains are capable of causing disease
- H. influenzae is a common commensal and may be part of normal oral flora; 20 to 40% of healthy individuals harbor H. influenzae in the oropharynx, and colonization rates of 50 to 70% have been demonstrated among smokers with COPD. H. influenzae was unappreciated as a pulmonary pathogen until the late 1970s, when a series of bacteremic and nonbacteremic reports of pneumonia caused by this organism were described
- H. influenzae characteristically affects smokers, or elderly debilitated patients, but may also affect previously normal hosts

Clinical Features: Clinical features of H. influenzae pneumonia are indistinguishable from those of other bacillary pathogens. Lobar or segmental bronchopneumonic infiltrates are characteristic. Mortality rates of 10 to 20% have been reported with bacteremic pneumonia caused by H. influenzae; higher rates have been noted in immunosuppressed or debilitated individuals.

Diagnosis: Pleomorphic gram-negative rods are characteristic on Gram's stain. Because H. influenzae is often part of normal oral flora, however, distinguishing infection from colonization may be difficult. The diagnosis of lower respiratory tract infection caused by H. influenzae may be further confounded by the fastidious growth requirements of the organism, and other bacteria may overgrow the culture plates. Thus, even in bacteremic cases of H. influenzae pneumonia, sputum cultures have been positive for the organism in only 40 to 60% of patients.

Preferred Therapy

- Ampicillin/sulbactam, cefuroxime, ceftriaxone
- Oral agents (amoxicillin/clavulanate, cefuroxime axetil, TMP/SMX) may be acceptable for mild infections in young, otherwise healthy individuals or following initial parenteral therapy

Alternative Agents

- TMP/SMX, fluoroquinolones, newer macrolides (azithromycin, chlarithromycin
- Ampicillin, only for beta–lactamase-negative strains, and activity of erythromycin is marginal

Antimicrobial Resistance: Antimicrobial resistance has developed to what previously had been a highly susceptible pathogen. In the early 1970s, more than 99% of strains were susceptible to ampicillin. By the early 1980s, beta–lactamase-producing (ampicillin-resistant) strains of H. influenzae emerged. By 1990, 10 to 20% of strains exhibited resistance to ampicillin; virtually all isolates are susceptible to ampicillin/sulbactam, cefuroxime, third-generation cephalosporins, antipseudomonal penicillins, imipenem, and fluoroquinolones. First-generation cephalosporins are not reliable (only 40 to 50% of strains are susceptible); fewer than 50% of isolates are susceptible to erythromycin. The activity of tetracyclines is modest. More than 90% of strains are susceptible to TMP/SMX.

Moraxella (Branhamella) Catarrhalis

Epidemiology

- Moraxella catarrhalis (formerly termed Neisseria catarrhalis or Branhamella catarrhalis) has long been recognized as part of the normal bacterial flora of the upper respiratory tract and as an important pathogen in otitis media and sinusitis (particularly in children). Its role in lower respiratory tract infections has been appreciated only recently. In the early 1970s, Moraxella catarrhalis was implicated in acute exacerbations of bronchitis in patients with COPD. Subsequent investigations have suggested that M. catarrhalis may account for 1 to 3% of CAP (most frequently in the winter months)
- More than 80% of lower respiratory tract infections caused by M. catarrhalis in patients with COPD or underlying diseases. Its role as a nosocomial pathogen is controversial

In addition to direct pathogenicity, the presence of beta–lactamase-secreting M. catarrhalis as commensals in the upper respiratory tract may confer antimicrobial resistance among co-infecting pathogens, such as Hemophilus influenzae or Streptococcus pneumoniae. This phenomenon, known as indirect pathogenicity, may result in clinical resistance of organisms ordinarily susceptible to beta-lactam antibiotics. In such cases, antibiotics effective against both Moraxella catarrhalis (to eradicate beta-lactamase production) and the co-infecting pathogen are required.

Clinical Features: M. catarrhalis is of low virulence, and respiratory tract infections caused by M. catarrhalis are typically mild, manifesting as exacerbations of chronic bronchitis or purulent tracheobronchitis. Pneumonia occurs in only 5 to 20% of cases of M. catarrhalis infections and is usually mild. Cough, purulent sputum, and dyspnea are characteristic. Rhinorrhea, headache, and myalgias are rare. Fever occurs in fewer than 50% of patients, even when pneumonia is present. Chest x-rays typically are normal (in bronchitis) or show patchy bronchopneumonic infiltrates; lobar consolidation is less common. Empyema, necrotizing pneumonia, and cavitation do not occur. Bacteremia occurs in fewer than 1% of patients. Fatalities have been rare and usually reflect serious pre-existing underlying diseases.

Diagnosis: Morphologically, M. catarrhalis resembles other Neisseria species; kidney–bean-shaped gram-negative diplococci are characteristic on Gram's stain. Pleuritic chest pain, dense lobar consolidation, and extreme prostration rarely occur with pneumonia caused by M. catarrhalis; such signs and symptoms suggest an alternative pathogen.

Preferred Therapy

• Cefuroxime (oral or IV), ampicillin/sulbactam, amoxicillin/clavulanate

Alternative Therapy

• TMP/SMX, erythromycin, tetracycline, quinolones

Antimicrobial Resistance: Antimicrobial resistance of M. catarrhalis to penicillins has increased dramatically over the past decade. Beta–lactamase (penicillinase)-producing strains of M. catarrhalis were first described in 1977; now, 50 to 85% of isolates produce beta-lactamase. Thus, most isolates are resistant to penicillins; however, penicillins with beta-lactamase inhibitors (e.g. Augmentin, Unasyn, Timentin), second- or third-generation cephalosporins, TMP/SMX, tetracycline, erythromycin, azalides, and the fluoroquinolones are efficacious against both beta–lactamase-positive and beta–lactamase-negative strains. Virtually all beta–lactamase-negative strains are susceptible to penicillin, ampicillin, and most beta-lactams.

ATYPICAL PNEUMONIAS

Pneumonia caused by Mycoplasma pneumoniae, Chlamydia pneumoniae (TWAR), and viruses may be grouped under the term "atypical pneumonias." These pathogens are considered atypical because many of the cardinal features of acute bacterial pneumonia, such as leukocytosis, pleuritic chest pain, rigors, and consolidation findings, are usually lacking. Cough is often nonproductive, and extrapulmonary features, such as sore throat, arthritis, myalgias, gastrointestinal symptoms, headache, and viral prodromal symptoms, may dominate the clinical picture. Mycoplasma pneumoniae has a predilection for previously healthy young individuals; Chlamydia-TWAR and viruses affect all age groups. Mycoplasma and Chlamydia spp are usually mild and self-limited; fatalities are rare. The spectrum of viral pneumonitis is varied, and is covered in a separate chapter. Bibasilar interstitial infiltrates or small, patchy, subsegmental infiltrates are characteristic findings on chest x-ray of pneumonia caused by Mycoplasma pneumoniae or Chlamydia-TWAR; however, classic lobar pneumonia indistinguishable from bacillary pneumonias may occur in as many as 20% of patients. Although characteristic clinical and radiographic features exist, none reliably discriminates between atypical and typical bacillary pathogens.

Mycoplasma Pneumoniae

Epidemiology

- Mycoplasma pneumoniae, a cell–wall-deficient microbe within the class Mollicutes, is a pathogen of low virulence that accounts for 2 to 14% of CAP. Mycoplasma pneumoniae has a striking predilection for younger patients and often spares older individuals, thereby suggesting that pre-existing antibody or prior exposure may confer lasting protection
- M. pneumoniae has been implicated in 20 to 30% of pneumonias in adolescents and adults younger than age 35. By contrast, Mycoplasma accounts for only 2 to 9% of pneumonias among adults between the ages of 40 and 60 and for only 1 to 3% of pneumonias among adults over age 60. Mycoplasma has rarely been implicated as a nosocomial pathogen
- Epidemics of Mycoplasma have been described in university dormitories, military institutions, schools, and families; prolonged close contact is usually necessary for transmission of infection. Pneumonia caused by M. pneumoniae occurs in only 3 to 10% of exposed individuals

Clinical Features

- Despite the frequency of M. pneumoniae in certain populations, its importance as a serious pulmonary pathogen is overrated, because pneumonia caused by M. pneumoniae is usually mild and rarely life threatening. Bronchitis and upper airway symptoms are the predominant features of infections from M. pneumoniae. Radiographically evident pneumonia can be demonstrated in only 5 to 15% of infected individuals and rarely warrants hospitalization
- The onset of mycoplasmal pneumonia may be insidious, however, and the course may be protracted. Typical features include fever, malaise, headache, and an intractable, hacking cough, which may be productive or nonproductive. Features commonly observed in acute bacillary pneu-

monia, such as pleuritic chest pain, rigors, and lobar consolidation, are uncommon. Rhinorrhea, sore throat, earache, and hoarseness occur in 25 to 50% of mycoplasmal infections. On physical examination, erythema of the oropharynx and tender cervical lymphadenopathy can be appreciated in 30 to 50% of patients. Rhonchi and a few scattered crackles may be detected on auscultation; frank consolidation findings are rare. Bullous myringitis, a frequently emphasized feature of mycoplasmal pneumonia, occurs in 3 to 7% of patients. Nausea, vomiting, diarrhea, myalgias, and arthralgias occur in 20 to 45% of patients, but do not distinguish mycoplasmal pneumonia from pneumonias caused by bacteria, Legionella, or Chlamydia spp. Skin rashes occur in 10 to 15% of patients with mycoplasmal pneumonia; diffuse maculopapular rash, petechiae, urticaria, erythema nodosum, and erythema multiforme have been described
- Rare complications of mycoplasmal infections include encephalitis, neurologic symptoms, myocarditis, pericarditis, and hemolytic anemia, which occur in 1 to 3% of patients

Ancillary Laboratory Features: Chest x-ray findings are variable. Diffuse or patchy interstitial infiltrates or patchy bronchopneumonia are most characteristic. Frank lobar consolidation with air bronchograms is evident in fewer than 15% of patients. Cavitation does not occur. Small pleural effusions have been noted in 5 to 15% of patients. Peripheral blood leukocyte counts are usually normal, but neutrophilia or a left shift in the differential count occurs in 60 to 80% of patients. Cold agglutinin IgM antibodies have been demonstrated in 40 to 70% of patients. Cold agglutinins, however, may be positive in 10 to 15% of viral or bacterial pneumonias and, thus, are of limited diagnostic value.

Diagnosis: Definitive diagnosis of Mycoplasma is difficult in the early phases of the disease. Cultures of sputum or pharyngeal washings may demonstrate the organism, but specialized cultural techniques are required. Growth may be slow, and 2 to 3 weeks may be required to isolate the organism. More recently, cDNA probes specific for Mycoplasma spp have been developed, with sensitivities and specificities of up to 89%. In most cases, the diagnosis has been substantiated by serologic techniques *after* the disease has run its course. Serum complement fixation (CF) antibody directed against Mycoplasma spp is the preferred test because of its high specificity and sensitivity. A fourfold titer rise from acute to convalescent sera or single titers of greater than 1:128 are considered diagnostic of recent or active infection. More recently, indirect fluorescent antibody and enzyme-linked immunosorbent assay (ELISA) methods have been applied to detect IgM antibodies against M. pneumoniae; neither technique has been shown to be superior to CF titers.

Preferred Therapy

- Erythromycin, 250 to 500 mg qid oral or IV
- Doxycycline, 100 mg bid oral or IV; tetracycline, 250 mg qid

Erythromycin has slightly superior activity in vitro, but therapeutic results in vivo are probably equivalent to those of erythromycin or tetracycline derivatives. Progression to respiratory failure is rare with or without treatment. The course, however, appears to be shortened with therapy. Complete resolution of symptoms may be delayed; cough, malaise, and fatigue may persist for 4 to 6 weeks. Therapy should be continued for 14 to 21 days to prevent recrudescent illness and clinical relapse.

Alternative Agents

- Fluoroquinolones (e.g. ciprofloxacin, ofloxacin)
- Azalides (e.g. azithromycin)
- Chlarithromycin (Biaxin)

Note: Because Mycoplasma spp lack a cell wall, beta-lactams and other cell–wall-active antibiotics have no significant activity against Mycoplasma.

Chlamydia Pneumoniae (TWAR)

Epidemiology: Chlamydia pneumoniae (strain TWAR) is a newly described obligate intracellular bacteria capable of causing respiratory tract infections, including rhinitis, sinusitis, pharyngitis, tonsillitis, bronchitis, and pneumonia. C. pneumoniae (TWAR) is one of three recognized species within the genus Chlamydia; the other species are C. trachomatis and C. psittaci. Grayston and co-workers first described Chlamydia-TWAR as a causative agent of pneumonia in 1986, when a serologic assay implicated Chlamydia-TWAR in 9 of 76 (12%) pneumonias at the Student Health Service at the University of Washington. The prevalence of Chlamydia-TWAR as a cause of pneumonia has not been delineated, as few prospective studies have been performed. In one prospective study at the University of Washington in Seattle, 20 cases of pneumonia caused by Chlamydia-TWAR were identified from 1983 to 1988; Chlamydia-TWAR accounted for 10% of cases of CAP and 4% of cases of bronchitis over the 5-year study period. By 1988, Chlamydia-TWAR had been implicated by serologic techniques as the cause of epidemic outbreaks of pneumonia in Finland, Denmark, Norway, and England, and was shown to be an endemic cause of CAP in the United States, Canada, and Europe. Recent prospective studies in the United States, Nova Scotia, and Europe suggest that Chlamydia-TWAR may account for as much as 6 to 12% of CAP in some regions. Chlamydia-TWAR has also been implicated as a rare cause of nosocomial pneumonia in Veterans and large municipal hospitals. Worldwide, the prevalence of TWAR antibody in sera has ranged from 25 to 50%. Rates of circulating antibody are low in young children, increase from adolescence to middle age, and remain elevated even in the elderly person. The mode of transmission has not been clarified, but man-to-man transmission is most likely.

Clinical Features

- Clinical features of Chlamydia-TWAR pneumonia are similar to those of Mycoplasma pneumoniae; fever and cough occur in 50 to 80% of

patients. Severe sore throat, often with hoarseness, has been noted in more than 33% of patients, and may be the presenting feature
- Chest x-rays typically demonstrate small (2 to 3 cm), patchy bronchopneumonic infiltrates; dense lobar consolidation is rare. Pleural effusions are rare in young adults, but may be observed in as many as 20% of older adults (many of whom may have coexisting organisms). Peripheral blood leukocyte and differential counts are usually normal
- The illness is usually mild (albeit often protracted); hospitalization is rarely necessary. Tetracyclines or erythromycin may shorten the duration of illness. Fatalities have been rare, and occur virtually only in patients with serious, coexisting disease(s)

Diagnosis: Diagnosis of Chlamydia-TWAR pneumonia may be made by culture, direct fluorescent antibody (DFA) staining of sputum, or by serologic methods. The organism is difficult to culture, and specialized culture methods (HeLa 229 or yolk sac of embryonic chicken eggs) are required; even with these techniques, sensitivity has been low. DFA staining of expectorated sputum or tracheal secretions may demonstrate the organism; data affirming its sensitivity and specificity are limited. In most cases the diagnosis has been confirmed by serologic studies, which have been performed in a few reference laboratories. Two serologic studies are used. The microimmunofluorescence test (micro-IF) measures an antigen specific for Chlamydia-TWAR, whereas the complement fixation (CF) test measures Chlamydia genus antibodies that cross-react with other Chlamydia spp. The micro-IF assay measures both IgM and IgG titers and is the most accurate serologic test. IgM antibody titers greater than 16 or IgG titers greater than 512 suggest recent or active infection; lower titers of IgG antibody suggest previous infection. The micro-IF test has been positive in more than 90% of culturally confirmed cases and is more than 95% specific. Antibodies do not appear until 10 or more days after the onset of illness, however, and titers may peak at 6 to 12 weeks. CF studies are less sensitive; as many as 30% of patients with culturally confirmed infections have nondetectable CF antibodies. A fourfold rise in CF titer or single antibody titers exceeding 64 are considered evidence of recent infection. Primary infection, which is most characteristic of adolescents or young adults, has been associated with a striking rise in IgM titer within the first 3 weeks, followed by a rise in IgG titer at the convalescent serum assay at 8 weeks. Reinfection with Chlamydia-TWAR may also occur, particularly in older adults; in this context, striking increases in IgG titers are observed without elevation in IgM. Because circulating Chlamydia-TWAR antibodies may require 3 or more weeks to become detectable, serologic studies are of greatest value for epidemiologic studies but have little role in the management of individual patients. An aggressive search for Chlamydia-TWAR in individual patients is not cost effective. Empiric therapy with tetracyclines should be considered for patients with persistent, protracted lower respiratory tract illness (bronchitis, pneumonia) refractory to prior antimicrobials with beta-lactams or erythromycin, even if a definitive diagnosis has not yet been corroborated.

Preferred Therapy

- Doxycycline or tetracycline orally for 14 to 21 days

Alternative Agents

- Erythromycin, 500 mg qid (less effective than tetracyclines)
- Fluoroquinolones, azalides (highly active in vitro, but limited data in vivo)

Note: Beta-lactams and aminoglycosides have no significant activity.

Legionella spp

Epidemiology

Pneumonia caused by Legionella pneumophila (legionnaire's disease) was first described in Philadelphia in 1976. Since that sentinel observation, several outbreaks of legionellosis have been noted in both community and nosocomial settings. Several species and strains of Legionella exist, but more than 95% of such infections are caused by L. pneumophila

- Legionella spp are endemic in the community, and account for 2 to 10% of CAP; the prevalence of nosocomial legionellosis appears to be lower, but has been implicated in as many as 10% of pneumonias in some centers
- Nosocomial acquisition has been linked to contamination by L. pneumoniae of the hospital water distribution system. Environmental control measures aimed at eradicating Legionella spp from hospital water supplies have been highly efficacious in limiting nosocomial legionellosis. Advanced age, renal failure, cigarette smoking, ethanol abuse, organ transplantation, and serious underlying disease have been associated with a higher prevalence of legionellosis and a predilection for more severe disease (including respiratory failure and fatalities)

Clinical Features

- Legionella spp have been associated with severe respiratory failure in 20 to 40% of patients and with fatality rates of 10 to 30%
- Clinically, pneumonia caused by Legionella spp may be indistinguishable from other bacterial pneumonias; diffuse alveolar infiltrates, patchy bronchopneumonic infiltrates, or lobar consolidation may occur. Pleural effusions occur in fewer than 10 percent of patients, cavitation has been described, but is rare

Several features that occur more commonly with pneumonia caused by Legionella spp than with pneumonia caused by other pathogens may provide clues to the diagnosis. These include

- Progression of pneumonia while taking antimicrobials (particularly penicillins or cephalosporins)
- Hyponatremia in 20 to 50% of patients

- Neurologic symptoms (confusion, lethargy, headache) in 20 to 30% of patients
- Gastrointestinal symptoms (principally nausea, vomiting, diarrhea) in 20 to 40% of patients
- Elevations in serum transaminases in 20 to 40% of patients

Although characteristic, these features do not distinguish legionellosis from other types of pneumonia.

Diagnosis: Legionella spp are gram-negative rods but are difficult to visualize on conventional Gram's stains. In addition, Legionella spp have fastidious growth requirements; thus, specialized media are required for culture. The diagnosis requires demonstration of the Legionella organisms by DFA or cultures of expectorated sputum, tracheal secretions, or BAL. The organisms can be identified also in tissue by using *Dieterle* silver stains or DFA. Newer diagnostic techniques, such as ELISA or radioimmunoassay for urinary antigen or gen-probe detection of L. pneumophila in respiratory secretions, have been developed, but the role of these adjunctive techniques has not been established. Measurements of serum antibodies against Legionella spp by the indirect fluorescent technique are invaluable to determine the prevalence of legionellosis in prospective epidemiologic surveys, but are of no value in individual patients, because results may not be available for at least 2 to 4 weeks. A single titer of 1:256 or a fourfold or greater rise in specific antibody titer is considered diagnostic of acute infection.

Preferred Therapy

- Erythromycin, 1 g q6h IV; 500 mg qid orally may be substituted once clinical improvement and defervescence have occurred; 21 days of therapy are optimal
- Rifampin, synergistic in vitro; consider combining with erythromycin in seriously ill or immunocompromised host

Alternative Therapy

- Doxycycline, 100 mg bid IV followed by oral administration once patient's condition has improved
- Ciprofloxacin, ofloxacin, azalides, TMP/SMX (highly active in vitro; limited data in man)

Note: Beta-lactams and aminoglycosides are not active against Legionellae spp.

VIRUSES

Pneumonia caused by viruses (e.g. influenza A and B, parainfluenza, respiratory syncytial virus, and adenovirus) may account for 5 to 15% of CAP and may be indistinguishable from bacterial or atypical pneumonias. Viral pneumonias are reviewed in chapter 25.

EMPIRIC (INITIAL) THERAPY

In most cases of pneumonia, therapy is empiric, based on the probability of certain pathogens being involved. Initial treatment for CAP (undertaken while waiting for cultural confirmation) should be sufficiently broad to cover most likely pathogens while avoiding polypharmacy or excessively expensive or toxic antimicrobials. Choice of empiric therapy must be modified based on such clinical features as age, the presence or absence of underlying disease, radiographic appearance, prior use of antimicrobials, and severity of the pneumonic process.

YOUNG PREVIOUSLY HEALTHY ADULTS

Pneumonia in previously healthy young adults (< age 35) can be successfully treated with a variety of agents, including penicillin G, ampicillin, ampicillin/sulbactam, erythromycin, doxycycline, or cefuroxime. Mycoplasma pneumoniae has been implicated in 20 to 30% of CAP in this population; Streptococcus pneumoniae has been implicated in 30 to 60%. Chlamydia, Legionella spp, and Hemophilus influenzae each account for 2 to 6% of cases, viruses for 5 to 15%, and Enterobacteriaceae or Staphylococcus aureus for fewer than 2% of CAP in previously healthy young adults. In view of the limited spectrum of microbes involved in this patient population, relatively narrow spectrum (and less expensive) agents can be considered. The choice of agent depends in part on the clinical and radiographic presentation

- If a lobar process is evident and a sputum Gram's stain demonstrates predominantly gram-positive cocci within leukocytes, treatment with penicillin G or ampicillin may be adequate
- These agents fail to cover atypical pneumonias (e.g. those caused by Mycoplasma, Legionella and Chlamydia spp), but have excellent activity against Streptococcus pneumoniae and other streptococci (see Fig. 24–1)
- When a sputum Gram's stain or clinical course is nonspecific, however, treatment with erythromycin or doxycycline to provide coverage against atypical pathogens may be appropriate. These agents are also active against S. pneumoniae, but provide marginal coverage against Hemophilus influenzae
- When atypical pneumonia is unlikely based on clinical grounds and Gram's stain is nondiagnostic, the use of broader-spectrum agents, such as ampicillin/sulbactam or cefuroxime, is reasonable, because these antimicrobials are highly active against Streptococcus pneumoniae, Hemophilus influenzae, Staphylococcus aureus, and certain Enterobacteriaceae

Exceptionally-broad-spectrum agents, such as ticarcillin/clavulanate, piperacillin, ceftazidime, or imipenem/cilastatin (excellent choices for empiric treatment of nosocomial pneumonia), have no role for CAP. Less expensive agents are equally efficacious in a community-acquired setting. Ciproflox-

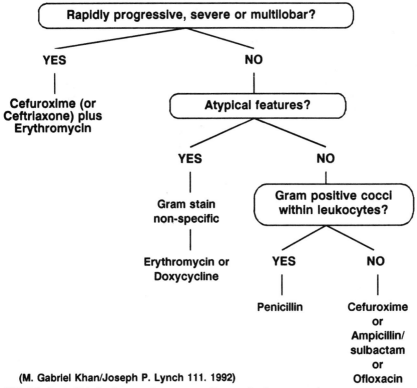

(M. Gabriel Khan/Joseph P. Lynch 111. 1992)

FIG. 24–1. Antibiotic therapy for community-acquired pneumonia.

acin has marginal activity against Streptococcus pneumoniae and is inappropriate for CAP in young, previously healthy adults.

In summary, penicillins (penicillin G, ampicillin, ampicillin/sulbactam), erythromycin, or doxycycline are acceptable as first-line agents for the empiric treatment of CAP in young, previously healthy adults. Regardless of the specific antimicrobial agent utilized, IV therapy is recommended for patients who are acutely ill, toxic, or exhibit multilobar involvement. Oral therapy can be substituted once clinical improvement and defervescence have occurred. Combination therapy with a penicillin plus erythromycin is warranted for patients exhibiting a deteriorating course or fulminant disease. Therapeutic strategies and appropriate antimicrobials for specific pathogens that may be implicated in CAP are described in detail in the sections that follow.

ELDERLY PATIENTS OR THOSE WITH UNDERLYING DISEASE

The pathogens responsible for causing CAP in elderly patients or adults with pre-existing disease differ considerably from those observed in young, healthy adults. Old age, residence in chronic care facilities, ethanol abuse, diabetes mellitus, chronic obstructive lung disease, congestive heart failure, renal failure, malnutrition, or any serious underlying disease may impair local or systemic immune defenses, and may lead to colonization of the oropharynx and lower respiratory tract with enteric GNB. This proclivity for colonization with GNB may lead to infections with these same organisms. Although Streptococcus pneumoniae remains the most common single cause of pneumonia (accounting for 30 to 50% of cases), enteric GNB, Hemophilus influenzae, and Moraxella catarrhalis emerge as important pathogens in this older compromised group. Klebsiella, Escherichia coli, and Proteus spp (pathogens that rarely affect young, previously healthy adults) occur with increasing frequency in the elderly patient or in adults of any age with underlying disease.

In several recent studies, 3 to 10% of community-acquired pneumonias in this context were caused by enteric gram-negative rods. Hemophilus influenzae has been implicated in as many as 10 to 20% of pneumonias in smokers or patients with COPD; Moraxella catarrhalis has been implicated in 1 to 2% of such patients

- In the elderly patient or debilitated patient of any age, enteric GNB and Hemophilus influenzae may account for 20% or more of pneumonias. Taken together, GNB, H. influenzae, and Staphylococcus aureus equal or exceed the prevalence of Streptococcus pneumoniae as causes of CAP in this patient population
- In these "at-risk" patient populations, treatment strategies must encompass these pathogens.
- Broader-spectrum agents are needed to encompass S. pneumoniae, Hemophilus influenzae, Moraxella catarrhalis, and Enterobacteriaceae (principally Escherichia coli, Klebsiella, and Proteus spp).
- Penicillin G and ampicillin do not provide adequate coverage against GNB or Hemophilus influenzae and are not recommended
- Ampicillin/sulbactam (Unasyn) provides increased activity against H. influenzae, Escherichia coli, and Klebsiella spp, but has limited activity against other GNB.
- Cefuroxime (a second-generation cephalosporin) and ceftriaxone (a third-generation cephalosporin) are advisable empiric treatment of pneumonia for these "at-risk" patients
- Exceptionally-broad-spectrum agents, such as antipseudomonal penicillins or imipenem, are efficacious, but are too expensive to justify as first-line therapy
- Ciprofloxacin has broad-spectrum activity against GNB and Hemophilus influenzae and has been used with success in community-acquired and nursing—home-acquired pneumonias. The activity of ciprofloxacin against Streptococcus pneumoniae and anaerobes is marginal, however; thus, this agent should be restricted to patients in whom the presence of these pathogens is unlikely. Specific therapy against Mycoplasma pneumoniae (e.g. erythromycin or doxycycline) is usually not warranted for elderly patients, because fewer than 2% of CAP in this age group are caused by Mycoplasma spp

- For rapidly progressive, multilobar, or severe pneumonias, however, combination therapy with a broad-spectrum beta-lactam, such as cefuroxime or ceftriaxone, to cover Hemophilus influenzae, Staphylococcus aureus and Enterobacteriaceae together with erythromycin to cover Legionella and Mycoplasma is appropriate (see Fig. 24–1)

ORAL VERSUS INTRAVENOUS ADMINISTRATION

Given the high mortality (10 to 20%) of CAP in elderly adults or patients with serious associated diseases, parenteral (IV/intramuscular) antibiotics are preferable as initial therapy in these patient populations. Parenteral therapy is preferred for patients with multilobar pneumonia, a setting that has been associated with a two- to fourfold increase in mortality. With few exceptions, parenteral administration achieves higher serum and tissue levels compared to those reached with oral therapy and more effectively reduces the bacterial burden. Oral therapy should be reserved for patients meeting all the following criteria

- Age under 55 years
- No prior underlying disease
- Pneumonia confined to a segment or lobe
- Clinically not toxic, hypotensive, or severely ill
- No nausea, vomiting, or gastrointestinal symptoms that preclude predictable oral absorption
- Reliable patient, committed to taking the antibiotic and assuring outpatient follow-up examination

Unless the conditions are met, therapy should be initiated with a broad-spectrum parenteral agent. In most cases, such therapy requires hospitalization. In addition to assuring adequate administration of antimicrobials, hospitalization allows closer scrutiny of the patient and prompt response to any complications (e.g. shock, empyema) that may develop. The duration of hospitalization must be individualized. Parenteral therapy is advised until clinical improvement and defervescence have been achieved. Oral agents may be substituted within 2 to 4 days in patients exhibiting prompt responses to therapy. A total course of 10 to 14 days (parenteral plus oral) is recommended.

Outpatient therapy with intramuscular ceftriaxone, 1 g/day, is a reasonable alternative for ambulatory patients at risk for gram-negative infection but for whom hospitalization may not be essential. An initial dose can be administered in the outpatient clinic or physician's office, with additional daily doses given for 1 to 2 days. Once a favorable response has been documented, an oral agent may be substituted.

OPTIONS FOR PENICILLIN-ALLERGIC PATIENTS

- For young, healthy individuals in whom the risk of gram-negative infections is low, doxycycline or erythromycin should provide adequate coverage as single agents

- Older patients or patients with underlying diseases require broader-spectrum agents with activity against Hemophilus influenzae, enteric GNB, and gram-positive bacilli. In this context, ciprofloxacin (despite its marginal activity against Streptococcus pneumoniae) or ofloxacin or TMP/SMX may be used
- For severe, life-threatening pneumonias, combined therapy with agents active against Legionella (erythromycin or doxycycline) and broad-spectrum agents should be given. The combination of clindamycin, which has excellent gram-positive and anaerobic coverage, plus aztreonam, which has exclusively gram-negative activity, can also be used for serious infections; neither agent is adequate alone because of their limited spectra

ANTIMICROBIAL RESISTANCE

Antimicrobial resistance has increased at an alarming rate in both community and nosocomial settings; in fact, the use of certain broad-spectrum antimicrobials, such as third-generation cephalosporins and ciprofloxacin, may select out isolates displaying high-grade resistance to multiple antimicrobials. Bacteria acquire resistance by multiple mechanisms including

- Enzymatic inactivation of the antibiotic (e.g. beta-lactamases, aminoglycoside-modifying enzymes)
- Alteration of target sites (e.g. penicillin-binding proteins, DNA gyrases, ribosomes, RNA polymerase)
- Decreased antibiotic permeability through the bacterial cell wall (e.g. resistance to imipenem or quinolones)
- Active efflux of antibiotic from the bacteria

Production of beta-lactamases is the most important mechanism of bacterial resistance to beta-lactam antibiotics. Beta-lactamases differ in selectivity for the target (e.g. penicillinases, cephalosporinases) and stability. Antimicrobial resistance increases dramatically concomitant with widespread use of specific classes of antibiotics. In this context, mostly staphylococci in the 1940s (in the earliest days of penicillin use) were susceptible to penicillin. By the late 1950s, most staphylococci produced penicillinase (a beta-lactamase) and were resistant. These isolates remained susceptible to antistaphylococcal penicillins, such as methicillin. Alterations in penicillin-binding proteins (PBPs), however, led to methicillin-resistant staphylococci and penicillin-resistant Streptococcus pneumoniae. In some countries, more than 5% of strains of S. pneumoniae are resistant to penicillin and erythromycin by this mechanism; fortunately, this high level of antimicrobial resistance has not yet been encountered in the United States.

Emergence of resistance has been dramatic with other pathogens. Beta-lactamase-producing (ampicillin-resistant) strains of Escherichia coli were rare in the 1960s; now only 60 to 70% of isolates are susceptible to ampicillin. In 1974, the first beta-lactamase-producing strain of Hemophilus influenzae was identified; 15 to 20% of isolates are now resistant to ampicillin. Similarly, beta-lactamase-positive strains of Moraxella catarrhalis constituted fewer than 1% of isolates in 1977; now, 40 to 80% that produce beta-lactamase are resistant to penicillin.

In most gram-negative organisms, beta-lactam resistance results from plasmid-mediated beta-lactamases. Over the past decade, a striking increase in plasmid-mediated beta-lactamases and novel enzymes produced by Enterobacteriaceae have been observed. Several of these newer beta-lactamases inactivate third-generation cephalosporins, antipseudomonal penicillins, and aztreonam, but do not affect imipenem. Of concern is the conference of resistance from some of these plasmid-mediated beta-lactamases to multiple agents of a different antibiotic class (e.g. chloramphenicol, gentamicin, tetracycline). These highly resistant, transferable isolates suggest caution in the unrestricted, widespread use of some of the newer broad-spectrum antimicrobials.

In addition, some bacteria (e.g. Pseudomonas aeruginosa, Enterobacter, Citrobacter, and Serratia spp) produce inducible chromosomally mediated beta-lactamases; in this class, exposure to beta-lactams may augment beta-lactamase production by derepressing enzymes controlling production. Use of the fluoroquinolones or imipenem has been associated with rapid emergence of resistant Pseudomonas aeruginosa, caused by changes in permeability of the outer membrane of the bacterial cell wall. This mutational change may also result in cross-resistance to antibiotics of unrelated classes. For example, quinolones have been associated with the emergence of resistant Enterobacteriaceae, which were also less susceptible to beta-lactams, aminoglycosides, chloramphenicol, and tetracyclines.

These resistance trends bode poorly for the future; the pharmaceutic industry will have to meet the challenge to keep ahead of these "smart organisms." Antimicrobial susceptibility profiles will undoubtedly change radically in the next decade, and some antibiotics currently in use may become obsolete or distinctly less effective. In this context, antimicrobials that were efficacious only 2 decades ago for CAP, such as ampicillin, are no longer adequate for empiric treatment of CAP. Since 1983, strains of Enterobacteriaceae producing novel beta-lactamases, such as Klebsiella spp, Escherichia coli, and Proteus spp, have markedly reduced the effectiveness of first-generation cephalosporins and penicillins. Thus, an awareness of the relevant pathogens involved in community and nosocomial infections, and of the changing patterns of antimicrobial resistance, is required to develop rational treatment strategies.

NOSOCOMIAL PNEUMONIA

MICROBIOLOGY AND EPIDEMIOLOGY

Pneumonia develops in 0.5 to 2% of hospitalized patients and has been associated with a mortality rate of 30 to 60%. The economic impact is enormous; nosocomial pneumonia may accrue costs in excess of $3 billion in the United States annually. The microbiologic characteristics of nosocomial pneumonia have been well characterized in several careful epidemiologic studies. In striking contrast to CAP, such pathogens as Streptococcus pneumoniae and Mycoplasma pneumoniae account for only 3 to 8% of pneumonias in hospitalized patients. Enteric GNB are responsible for 70 to 85% of nosocomial pneumonias. Enterobacteriaceae (predominantly Klebsiella and Enterobacter spp) have been implicated in 30 to 50% of nosocomial pneumonias; 15 to 20% are caused by Pseudomonas aeruginosa. Hemophilus influenzae is responsible for 3 to 8% of nosocomial pneumonias. A host of other aerobic enteric GNB, such as Providencia, Citrobacter, Morganella, and Acinetobacter spp, may each account for an additional 2 to 5% of cases. Aerobic gram-positive organisms, such as Staphylococcus spp (S. aureus and S. epidermidis) and streptococci account for 10 to 25% of nosocomial pneumonias. A disproportionate amount of gram-positive infections, however, occurs in patients with intravascular devices, such as Hickman catheters, atrioventricular shunts, and hemodialysis shunts, and in neurosurgical patients or patients receiving hyperalimentation via indwelling central lines. Group D streptococci (enterococcus spp) may be isolated frequently in sputum or tracheal secretions and often are admixed with other organisms, particularly in patients who have previously received cephalosporins (agents to which enterococci are invariably resistant). Enterococci (either as the sole pathogen in respiratory secretions or in blood cultures) account for no more than 1 or 2% of nosocomial pneumonias, however.

The importance of anaerobes in the pathogenesis of nosocomial pneumonia is controversial. Some studies have isolated anaerobes in only 2 to 5% of cases of ventilator-associated pneumonia, whereas others have found a prevalence of as many as 20 to 30% of cases by using meticulous culture techniques. This disparity may reflect a difference in vigilance when looking for anaerobes and culture techniques. In many cases in which anaerobes have been implicated, additional pathogenic organisms have been isolated concomitantly. Anaerobes are probably less important as primary pathogens in nosocomial pneumonia, but may play an important contributory role in polymicrobial infections, which may account for as many as 15 to 40% of nosocomial pneumonias.

The microbiologic features of nosocomial pneumonia and antimicrobial resistance patterns are constantly changing, and outbreaks of nosocomial infection caused by bacteria exhibiting multiple antibiotic resistances, such as Enterobacter, Klebsiella, and Aceinetobacter spp, have been reported with increasing frequency over the past decade. Sporadic cases and epidemic outbreaks of nosocomial pneumonia caused by Legionella spp, viruses, Mycoplasma, Chlamydia-TWAR, and Moraxella (Branhamella) catarrhalis have been described, but in the aggregate, they account for no more than 5 to 10% of cases in most institutions.

Fungi, notably Aspergillus spp, may cause nosocomial pneumonia in immunocompromised hosts, particularly in granulocytopenic patients with hematologic malignancies or in organ transplant recipients. Fungal pneumonias rarely occur in other settings. Pulmonary infections caused by Candida spp are unusual and virtually only occur in the context of hematogenous dissemination. When such involvement does occur, the patient is usually terminally ill from multiple other factors. Because nonbacterial pathogens are infrequently the cause of nosocomial pneumonia, except in specific high-risk groups, these pathogens are not further addressed here.

VIRULENCE OF PATHOGENS

Both host factors and difference in virulence among infecting organisms are important in dictating prognosis and mortality of nosocomial pneumonia. Mortality is significantly increased in the presence of serious concurrent diseases, such as renal or hepatic insufficiency, coma, multiorgan failure, hypotension, old age, debilitation, malnutrition, prior treatment with corticosteroids/chemotherapy, or any disorder that may impair immune defenses. Nevertheless, mortality rates for aerobic gram-negative bacillary pneumonia (30 to 50%) are consistently higher than mortality rates associated with gram-positive bacilli (5 to 25%). For certain pathogens, such as Pseudomonas aeruginosa and Acinetobacter spp, mortality may be even higher, approaching 60 to 80%. Several factors may contribute to this higher mortality

- Pseudomonas aeruginosa may release virulence factors and exotoxins that may inactivate host defenses and cause necrosis of lung parenchyma
- Nosocomially acquired gram-negative pathogens are often highly resistant to antibiotics
- Infected patients are often already debilitated when they acquire the organism

PATHOGENESIS

Both environmental and host factors contribute to the high prevalence of pneumonia. The risk of nosocomial pneumonia is increased in the elderly patient, in patients with serious associated diseases, and with increasing duration of hospital stay. The incidence is particularly high (10 to 40%) in critically ill patients requiring mechanical ventilatory support for more than 48 hours. A much lower prevalence of pneumonia has been reported in patients not requiring ventilatory support in the intensive care unit (ICU) or in coronary care units. Several studies have demonstrated an incremental risk of nosocomial pneumonia associated with increased duration of mechanical ventilation. These data suggest that mechanical ventilation may operate as an independent risk factor for pneumonia, but also undoubtedly identify a population of patients who are debilitated and have more serious concurrent illnesses.

Invasive devices, such as central venous catheters, arterial lines, indwelling bladder catheters, and endotracheal, nasotracheal, or tracheostomy tubes, have been associated with a higher prevalence of nosocomial infections and pneumonia. Inadequate hand-washing techniques by medical personnel may be a source of spread of potentially pathogenic bacteria, particularly in the ICU. Blood-borne seeding to the lung from extrapulmonary sites, such as the postoperative wound, soft tissue, or urinary tract, may also occur, resulting in pneumonia.

The dominant mechanism by which nosocomial pneumonia occurs, however, is via aspiration of endogenous oropharyngeal bacilli into the tracheobronchial tree. Oropharyngeal and tracheal colonization with enteric GNB is markedly increased in hospitalized patients and in patients with serious underlying diseases and is an important precursor of infection. Once oropharyngeal or tracheal colonization with GNB has occurred, aspiration of oropharyngeal contents and bacteria, an event that occurs commonly, may precipitate lower respiratory tract infection in critically ill patients with impaired host defenses.

Several investigations suggest that the gastrointestinal (GI) tract may serve as a reservoir for proliferation of GNB, thereby resulting in the colonization of the airway and lower respiratory tract. Agents that increase gastric pH, such as cimetidine or antacids, have been associated with higher rates of nosocomial pneumonia in critically ill, mechanically ventilated patients in both retrospective and prospective studies. In this context, prophylactic regimens for stress ulcer that employ sucralfate (an agent that does not affect gastric pH) have been associated with a lower rate of bronchopulmonary colonization and pneumonia in mechanically ventilated patients compared to the rate in patients receiving antacids alone or in combination with H2 antagonists. Few studies, however, have directly compared H2 antagonists (used alone) with sucralfate, and the independent risk of nosocomial pneumonia with H2 antagonists alone is not clear. Although this area remains controversial, the recognition that alkalinization of the stomach may facilitate proliferation of enteric GNB within the GI tracts has led to prophylactic antimicrobial strategies aimed at reducing the bacillary burden in the gut.

SELECTIVE GI TRACT DECONTAMINATION

Several investigators recently employed aggressive prophylactic regimens that selectively reduce enteric aerobic gram-negative rods while preserving anaerobic flora in an attempt to reduce colonization and infection with GNB. This concept, known as selective digestive tract decontamination (SDD), employs nonabsorbable antibiotics (polymyxin E, tobramycin, and amphotericin B) given orally and as an adhesive paste applied to the oral mucosa every 6 hours. This regimen is combined with a 4-day course of intravenous cefotaxime and is administered to patients at high risk for developing nosocomial pneumonia.

Pioneering investigations by Stoutenbeek, van Saene, and co-workers in the Netherlands, and by Unertl and co-workers in Germany, noted striking reductions in nosocomial pneumonia in critically ill, mechanically ventilated trauma patients treated prophylactically with SDD; however, overall mortality was unaffected. Ledingham and co-workers in Scotland randomized 163 ICU patients to SDD or no therapy and noted a substantial reduction in gram-negative tracheal colonization and nosocomial pneumonias among the patients who received SDD. No impact on mortality or length of stay was achieved.

In light of these initial studies demonstrating a reduced incidence of nosocomial pneumonia, several other groups in the Netherlands and in Europe have employed SDD in high-risk mechanically ventilated patients. In virtually all studies, SDD prophylaxis has been associated with a marked reduction in tracheal colonization with enteric bacteria and in the rate of nosocomial pneumonias; however, no convincing impact on overall mortality or length of stay has been demonstrated. Recently, Aerdts and co-workers used a novel regimen of SDD (norfloxacin was given in place of tobramycin and a lower dose of IV cefotaxime was used) in patients receiving prolonged mechanical ventilation. Use of this regimen resulted in lower rates of colonization of the oropharynx and stomach, and rates of pneumonia were lower with this regimen than with untreated controls. To date, the widespread use of SDD in several centers in Europe has not been associated with an increase in antimicrobial resistance.

Data employing SDD in the United States are limited. Flaherty and Weinstein at the Michael Reese Hospital in Chicago randomly selected patients in a cardiac surgical ICU to receive sucralfate (without SDD) or SDD employing oral and topical administration of polymyxin E, gentamycin, and nystatin. Cefotaxime, a fixture of most of the European regimens, was not given, but most patients did receive surgical prophylaxis with first-generation cephalosporins. Patients receiving SDD also were treated with H2 blockers or antacids, which have been associated in previous studies with a higher risk of nosocomial pneumonia. The overall rates of infection and pneumonia were lower in patients treated with SDD than in patients receiving sucralfate without SDD. No differences in mortality or length of stay were noted in either group. Studies to determine whether even lower rates of nosocomial pneumonia could be achieved in prophylactic regimens employing sucralfate (rather than H2 blockers or antacids) in combination with SDD would be of interest. Although the emergence of resistant organisms has not been noted among patients receiving SDD, the concern that unrestricted application of SDD may promote development of highly resistant organisms is real. Additional prospective studies that vigilantly search for resistant organisms must be done before SDD can be endorsed as standard or recommended therapy.

DIAGNOSIS

The diagnosis of nosocomial pneumonia may be difficult, particularly in patients in the ICU or in postoperative surgical patients, because infiltrates on the chest x-ray may be seen with other concurrent disorders, such as congestive heart failure, atelectasis, pulmonary embolism, or adult respiratory distress syndrome (ARDS). Pneumonia complicates ARDS in 50 to 75% of patients; persistence or progression of respiratory failure in ARDS may reflect concomitant pulmonary suppuration, which may not be evident clinically. The hallmarks of bacterial infection may be lacking in critically ill or debilitated patients unable to mount an adequate host response. Pleuritic chest pain, high fever, and chills are usually lacking; chest x-rays often demonstrate only minimal, patchy infiltrates that mimic fluid overload or congestive heart failure. Frank consolidation with air bronchograms or cavitation, the cardinal findings of suppurative infection, is present in a distinct minority of patients. Thus, a high index of suspicion is required to make a diagnosis of lower respiratory tract infection in a timely fashion.

The development of unexplained leukocytosis (or left shift), worsening dyspnea, purulent tracheobronchial secretions, or new infiltrates on chest x-ray warrants an aggressive approach.

A Gram's stain of expectorated sputum or tracheal secretions should be done to assess a predominant organism, but one should avoid over-reliance on sputum/tracheal aspirates, smears, and cultures in dictating therapeutic strategy. Potential pathogens may be demonstrated on culture of tracheal aspirates in 60 to 100% of pneumonias, but cultures are also positive in most patients without clinical evidence of infection. Thus, specificity is low (< 20%).

Blood cultures should be done, even though only 5 to 10% of cases of nosocomial pneumonias are bacteremic. Unfortunately, in many cases, a precise microbiologic diagnosis is never established despite appropriate cultures.

INVASIVE TECHNIQUES

Recently, invasive diagnostic techniques, such as fiberoptic bronchoscopy (FB) with a sheathed catheter (protected brush [PB]) and BAL and quantitative cultures have been employed to define more accurately the microbacteriologic aspect of nosocomial pneumonia. In one prospective study, Fagon and co-workers performed FB with PB and quantitative cultures in 147 mechanically ventilated patients who, within 12 hours, had developed a new pulmonary infiltrate and purulent tracheal secretions. PB culture colony counts exceeded 10^3 cfu/ml (the threshold level, based on previous data by these investigators) in 56 patients, 52 of whom were subsequently believed to have pneumonia based on clinical or necropsy criteria. By contrast, among patients with colony counts less than 10^3 cfu/ml, no cases of pneumonia were proved.

Despite these impressive results, several limitations of the study are apparent: 59 patients judged not to have pneumonia were already receiving antibiotics at the time of inclusion into the study; antibiotics were maintained or added for nonpulmonary indications in nearly one half of these patients; and necropsies were not performed in many patients in the negative culture group. Thus, the implication of a "negative bronchoscopic culture" is not clear, because a significant proportion of patients in the negative culture group may have had pneumonia.

Several other groups have reported sensitivities of 65 to 95% with FB and PB for the diagnosis of bacterial pneumonia; false-positive rates have consistently been less than 10%. Quantitative cultures of BAL fluid combined with cytocentrifuged BAL Gram's stains may also corroborate a specific etiologic diagnosis. With BAL, upper airway contamination must be excluded by demonstrating fewer than 1% squamous epithelial cells (SECs) on BAL Gram's stain, and different threshold criteria (10^5 cfu/ml) are applied. Using these criteria, pathogens have been recovered by BAL (colony counts > 10^5 cfu/ml) in 70 to 95% of patients with bacterial pneumonia, with false-positive rates of less than 10%.

Results of PB and BAL in the diagnosis of ventilator-associated pneumonia have been comparable in some studies; others have suggested that BAL cultures are less accurate than PB cultures. Gram's stains and analysis of intracellular organisms on BAL fluid may be helpful in confirming or refuting a diagnosis of (infectious) pneumonia. In some studies, pathogens were demonstrated on Gram's stain of cytocentrifuged BAL fluid in 50 to 75% of patients with bacterial pneumonia; numerous intracellular organisms with polymorphonuclear leukocytes (PMNs) or more than 25% PMNs containing intracellular organisms were highly predictive of infection (> 90% specificity). Although these data are impressive, other investigators have found an unacceptably high rate of false-negative PB and BAL cultures in the diagnosis of pneumonia, both in humans and in animal models. In some studies, cultures of PB were sterile in 30 to 47% of pneumonias; further, microorganisms were present on Gram's stain in fewer than 30% of patients when PB cultures were positive. False-negative results may be even higher when samples are obtained while patients already are receiving antibiotics.

Thus, we do not believe that "negative" studies reliably exclude pneumonia. This inconclusiveness underscores the importance of performing PB *prior to* initiation of antimicrobial therapy to obtain reliable data. Unfortunately, doing so is often impractical. Further, as yet no evidence shows that the routine application of FB with PB or BAL in suspected nosocomial pneumonia and the modification of therapy according to these results have reduced either morbidity or mortality. These various techniques have great promise, and may be particularly useful in severely immunocompromised hosts, such as in patients with granulocytopenia or in patients taking corticosteroids or immunosuppressive agents in whom unusual opportunistic pathogens are a concern, or in patients with failing regimens who are experiencing complications. In nonimmunocompromised hosts with nosocomial pneumonia, however, the role of invasive bronchoscopic techniques must be better defined. In view of the additional time, expense (which usually exceeds $500), and discomfort associated with these invasive procedures, bronchoscopy is not recommended in patients who have nosocomial pneumonia without complications. Additional studies are warranted to better define the impact of these techniques on prognosis in *selected* populations of patients and thereby better determine the appropriate indications for their use.

SPECIFIC PATHOGENS

In the following sections, the epidemiologic characteristics, clinical features, and antimicrobial susceptibility of specific pathogens are reviewed. Some of the pathogens, such as Acinetobacter spp, Pseudomonas cepacia, and Xanthomonas maltophilia, are rare causes of nosocomial pneumonia, but are included in part to review antimicrobial susceptibility profiles.

ENTERIC GRAM-NEGATIVE BACTERIA

Acinetobacter Calcoaceticus

Epidemiology: Acinetobacter calcoaceticus (formerly classified as Mima and Herellea species) is an aerobic gram-negative coccobacillus of relatively low virulence that often exhibits resistance to multiple antimicrobials and may emerge by selection pressure in critically ill, debilitated patients. A. calcoaceticus is almost universally found in water and soil, and is a common commensal in humans; colonization rates of 7% for throat and 25% for skin have been reported. The lung is the most common site of primary infection, followed by urinary tract, surgical wounds, and skin; secondary bacteremia occurs in 4 to 8% of patients. Acinetobacter has accounted for only 1 to 2% of nosocomial pneumonias in recent series, but higher rates (approaching 10%) have been reported by some centers in mechanically ventilated patients in ICUs who have received previous antimicrobials. Risk factors associated with the acquisition of Acinetobacter include tracheostomy or endotracheal intubation, surgery, residence in an ICU, prolonged mechanical ventilatory support, and recent use of antibiotics. Transient hand colonization by hospital personnel has been associated with outbreaks of pneumonia in critically ill, mechanically ventilated patients in an ICU; other environmental sources of Acinetobacter infections include contaminated nebulizers, dialysis baths, and hospital equipment. Acinetobacter is a rare cause of CAP; the largest series of community-acquired Acinetobacter pneumonia included only 6 patients diagnosed over a 5-year period from 3 teaching hospitals in the United States.

Preferred Therapy

- TMP/SMX, antipseudomonal penicillins, imipenem/cilastin, ceftazidime, aminoglycosides, and the fluoroquinolones are usually highly active (choice of agent depends on results of susceptibility testing)
- Combine with an aminoglycoside to confer synergistic killing

Note: Acinetobacter spp are often highly resistant to multiple antibiotics. Most isolates are resistant to ampicillin and first- and second-generation cephalosporins; activity of third-generation cephalosporins is variable. Multiply resistant strains displaying high-level resistance to aminoglycosides have recently been described. Risk factors for acquisition of aminoglycoside-resistant Acinetobacter spp include prior therapy with cephalosporins and aminoglycoside, extended ICU care, and prolonged respiratory therapy.

Enterobacteriaceae

Several species of Enterobacteriaceae (e.g. Enterobacter, Serratia, Proteus, Providentia, Citrobacter freundii) possess inducible, chromosomally mediated beta-lactamases (cephalosporinases) that inactive all cephalosporins, and may affect antipseudomonal penicillins and monobactams. By contrast, other Enterobacteriaceae, such as Escherichia coli and Klebsiella pneumoniae, rarely produce cephalosporinases, and thus, monotherapy with cephalosporins may be appropriate for these latter organisms. Serious infections caused by organisms producing inducible beta-lactamases, however, may warrant combination therapy (e.g. an antipseudomonal penicillin plus an aminoglycoside). Alternatively, monotherapy with imipenem or ciprofloxacin may be adequate because most isolates (including beta-lactamase-producing strains) are highly susceptible to these agents. Double beta-lactam combinations are not appropriate for beta-lactamase-producing organisms because both agents may be inactivated by the bacterial enzyme.

Enterobacter Species

Epidemiology: Infections caused by species of the genus Enterobacter (formerly Aerobacter) have increased dramatically in recent years as a cause of nosocomial or community-acquired infections among debilitated patients who have received previous antimicrobials. Enterobacter spp (predominantly E. cloacae and E. aerogenes) accounted for 6% of nosocomial infections in the Nosocomial Infections Surveillance Survey in 1984, but continue to increase in frequency. Enterobacter spp are now the third most common cause of nosocomial pneumonia (behind Pseudomonas aeruginosa and Staphylococcus aureus), accounting for 7 to 12% of nosocomial pneumonias. The emergence of Enterobacter spp has in part been the result of selection pressure from the widespread use of antimicrobials to which these organisms are resistant; in recent studies, 20 to 35% of Enterobacter isolates were multiply resistant to most beta-lactams; in addition, resistance may emerge rapidly during antibiotic therapy.

Preferred Therapy

- Imipenem (combine with aminoglycoside)
- Antipseudomonal penicillin (combine with aminoglycoside)

Alternative Agents

- Ciprofloxacin, TMP/SMX, aztreonam

Note:

- Third-generation cephalosporins should not be used; may induce resistance
- Sulbactam and clavulanate do not affect beta-lactamases produced by Enterobacter spp

Antimicrobial Resistance: Virtually all isolates of Enterobacter spp are resistant to penicillin, ampicillin, and first-generation cephalosporins. Resistance to cephalosporins via chromosomally mediated inducible beta-lactamases continues to increase; fewer than 50% of isolates are susceptible to second-generation cephalosporins, and 20 to 30% of isolates are now resistant to third-generation cephalosporins. The activity of antipseudomonal penicillins is variable; approximately 70 to 80% of isolates are susceptible in nosocomial settings. Imipenem is usually active even in strains broadly resistant to other beta-lactams. Other agents that may be active even against highly resistant isolates include TMP/SMX, ciprofloxacin, and aminoglycosides. Aminoglycoside resistance, however, has also increased in recent years; amikacin may be active against strains resistant to gentamicin/tobramycin. The use of third-generation cephalosporins has been associated with an increased rate of Enterobacter infections, as well as with multiresistant strains. Multiresistant Enterobacter spp have been associated with a high mortality rate as compared to that of sensitive strains. Chow and colleagues, in a multicenter prospective study of Enterobacter bacteremia, noted that emergence of resistance during therapy occurred in 19% of patients receiving third-generation cephalosporins, but in none of 50 patients receiving other beta-lactams (antipseudomonal penicillins, aztreonam, imipenem) and in only 1 of 89 patients receiving aminoglycosides. Chromosomally mediated inducible cephalosporinases (beta-lactamases) capable of inactivating all cephalosporins are not normally expressed, but may be triggered on exposure of the organism to cephalosporins (particularly agents known to induce beta-lactamase, such as cefoxitin and ceftazidime). Once the cephalosporinase has been induced and expressed, resistance to multiple beta-lactam antibiotics (including penicillins) may result. Unfortunately, neither clavulanate nor sulbactam inhibit the beta-lactamases produced by Enterobacter spp. The potential for third-generation cephalosporins to induce antimicrobial resistance has major therapeutic implications; third-generation cephalosporins should not be used for Enterobacter infections, regardless of in vitro susceptibility. Imipenem (in combination with an aminoglycoside) may be preferred as empiric therapy for serious pneumonia caused by Enterobacter spp pending susceptibility results; antipseudomonal penicillins, aztreonam, or ciprofloxacin can be substituted for imipenem for susceptible strains. Prospective controlled studies have not been performed, but best results have been achieved when two antibiotics have been used: a beta-lactam (or quinolone) with an aminoglycoside to confer synergy and limit the emergence of antimicrobial resistance; however, there is no proof that combination therapy either is more efficacious or more greatly reduces the emergence of resistant isolates as compared to monotherapy.

Escherichia Coli

Epidemiology: Escherichia coli remains an important pathogen in both community- and hospital-acquired bacteremias and infections. Urinary tract and gastrointestinal sites are the most common sources of infection; however, E. coli accounts for 6 to 8% of nosocomial pneumonias and as much as 1 to 3% of CAP, particularly in debilitated patients with significant underlying disease(s). Mortality resulting from E. coli pneumonia has been 20 to 30% in most series; most deaths have been in elderly, debilitated patients, and may reflect severe impairments in host defenses rather than failure of antimicrobial therapy.

Preferred Therapy

- Ampicillin/sulbactam, cefuroxime, or cefotetan (these agents are highly effective and less expensive than third-generation cephalosporins, imipenem, or aztreonam)
- Ampicillin (only for beta–lactamase-negative strains)

Alternative Agents

- TMP/SMX, ciprofloxacin, aztreonam, imipenem

Antimicrobial Resistance: In the 1970s, ampicillin was the preferred agent for infection caused by E. coli. Beta–lactamase-producing strains of E. coli have increased dramatically within the past decade, however; 30 to 50% of isolates are now resistant to ampicillin. Nearly 100% of beta–lactamase-positive and -negative strains are susceptible to ampicillin/sulbactam (Unasyn), cefuroxime, cephamycins (cefoxitin, cefotetan), and third-generation cephalosporins. Antipseudomonal penicillins (ticarcillin/clavulanate, piperacillin) are less consistently active (85 to 95% of strains are susceptible). Other antimicrobial agents with excellent activity against E. coli include imipenem, aztreonam, TMP/SMX, ciprofloxacin, and aminoglycosides. Most cases of pneumonia caused by E. coli respond to monotherapy with less expensive agents, such as ampicillin (only for susceptible strains), ampicillin/sulbactam, or second-generation cephalosporins (e.g., cefuroxime or cefotetan); the addition of an aminoglycoside could be considered for serious, life-threatening cases.

Klebsiella Pneumoniae

Epidemiology: Klebsiella pneumoniae, an aerobic gram-negative rod within the family Enterobacteriaceae, is a well-recognized cause of community-acquired pneumonia in patients with underlying diseases (e.g. ethanol abuse, diabetes mellitus, old age, debilitation) and accounts for 5 to 9% of nosocomial pneumonias. K. pneumoniae is the most common enteric GNB colonizing elderly or debilitated individuals in nursing homes or chronic care facilities, and has been implicated in 1 to 3% of CAP occurring in this context. Clinical features are indistinguishable from other bacillary pneumonias. A high rate of bacteremia and suppurative complications, such as lung abscesses and empyema, has been noted, however.

Preferred Therapy

• Second- or third-generation cephalosporins (monotherapy is adequate)

Alternative Agents

• Imipenem, ciprofloxacin, aztreonam, TMP/SMX

Antimicrobial Resistance: K. pneumoniae is resistant to penicillin and ampicillin, but is highly susceptible to cefuroxime, all third-generation cephalosporins, imipenem, aztreonam, fluoroquinolones, TMP/SMX, and aminoglycosides. Most strains are susceptible to first-generation cephalosporins, but the MIC may be marginal. The activity of the antipseudomonal penicillins is variable; more than 90% of isolates are susceptible to piperacillin, whereas fewer than 30% are susceptible to ticarcillin or azlocillin. More than 95% of strains are susceptible to ticarcillin/clavulanate (Timentin). Monotherapy with IV cefuroxime (for susceptible strains) is usually efficacious and less expensive than such therapy with other extended-spectrum agents. Combination therapy with an aminoglycoside may confer synergy, but is usually not necessary except in fulminant or refractory cases. Intravenous TMP/SMX or ciprofloxacin is an acceptable alternative for patients allergic to beta-lactams.

Serratia Marcescens

Epidemiology: Serratia spp (primarily S. marcescens, but S. liquefaciens and other species may account for as many as 15% of isolates) account for 3 to 5% of nosocomial pneumonias, with even higher rates in mechanically ventilated patients in ICUs. Rare cases of CAP have been described among patients with risk factors for gram-negative infections (e.g. ethanol abuse, nursing home residence, diabetes mellitus, and intravenous drug abuse). Clinical features are similar to other gram-negative bacillary pneumonias; a necrotizing pneumonia with frequent cavitation is characteristic. Pseudohemoptysis may result from the red pigment produced by S. marcescens. The prognosis for pneumonia caused by Serratia spp has been poor; mortality rates exceed 60% in some studies.

Preferred Therapy

- Third-generation cephalosporin (combine with aminoglycoside)

Alternative Agents

- Imipenem, aztreonam, ciprofloxacin, TMP/SMX

Antimicrobial Resistance: Serratia spp are resistant to penicillin, ampicillin, ampicillin/sulbactam, and most first-generation cephalosporins. Most isolates are highly susceptible to aminoglycosides, third-generation cephalosporins, aztreonam, ciprofloxacin, and imipenem. Antipseudomonal penicillins are less consistently effective. In view of the high mortality associated with Serratia pneumonia, we recommend combination therapy with a beta-lactam to which the organism is susceptible plus an aminoglycoside.

Pseudomonas Aeruginosa

Epidemiology: Pseudomonas aeruginosa is the most common GNB implicated in nosocomial pneumonias. P. aeruginosa accounts for 15 to 20% of nosocomial pneumonias, with even higher rates (20 to 30%) among mechanically ventilated patients in ICUs. P. aeruginosa is rare as a community-acquired pathogen, except among patients with known risk factors for acquisition of pseudomonads, such as bronchiectasis, cystic fibrosis, immunosuppressive/corticosteroid therapy, intravenous drug abuse, or granulocytopenia. P. aeruginosa accounts for less than 3% of pneumonias even in nursing home or elderly patients; in this context, Enterobacteriaceae (e.g. Klebsiella, Escherichia coli, Proteus spp), staphylococci, and Hemophilus influenzae are more common. The overall mortality from Pseudomonas pneumonia is high (50 to 70%), which in part reflects the debilitated state of patients infected with this pathogen, as well as the high virulence of these organisms.

Preferred Therapy

- Piperacillin or ceftazidime (combine with aminoglycoside)
- Imipenem (reserve for resistant strains; combine with aminoglycoside)

Alternative Agents

- Ciprofloxacin, aztreonam

Antimicrobial Resistance: P. aeruginosa is resistant to most antimicrobials; the antipseudomonal penicillins are active against 80 to 95% of strains. Activity of piperacillin in vitro is 2 to 8 times greater than that of the other antipseudomonal penicillins; whether this enhanced activity in vitro is clinically significant in vivo is not known. Among the cephalosporins, only ceftazidime and cefoperazone can be considered active (80 to 95% of isolates are susceptible). Other agents with excellent antipseudomonal activity (> 90% of isolates susceptible) include imipenem, aztreonam, aminoglycosides, and ciprofloxacin. Piperacillin and ceftazidime (in combination with an aminoglycoside) are excellent first-line agents for infections caused by P. aeruginosa. Imipenem/cilastin and ciprofloxacin have exceptional activity against P. aeruginosa, but these agents should be reserved for infections in which resistance to more conventional beta-lactams is documented or suspected. Rapid development of resistance has been noted when imipenem or ciprofloxacin has been used as monotherapy; thus, combination therapy (with an aminoglycoside) is also recommended. Oral ciprofloxacin may dramatically reduce antimicrobial drug costs; provided the isolate is susceptible, this agent is administered after 7 to 10 days of parenteral therapy. Aminoglycosides are inadequate as single agents, but may be important in providing synergistic killing. In most centers, differences between the aminoglycosides are slight; thus gentamicin is preferred because of its lower cost. Tobramycin or amikacin should be reserved for gentamicin-resistant strains (or strains exhibiting a high MIC). Because of the high mortality associated with P. aeruginosa pneumonia, combination therapy with an aminoglycoside and an antipseudomonal beta-lactam (or quinolone) for a minimum of 14 to 21 days is recommended. Panresistant Pseudomonas have been noted with increasing frequency among patients with cystic fibrosis and patients who have received multiple courses of antimicrobials.

Pseudomonas Cepacia

Epidemiology: Pseudomonas cepacia, a member of the Pseudomallei group of pseudomonads, is an aerobic gram-negative rod of low virulence that is virtually nonpathogenic in normal, healthy individuals. P. cepacia, however, is a rare cause of pneumonia in mechanically ventilated patients in ICUs, in debilitated patients who have received multiple courses of antimicrobials (particularly imipenem), and in patients with cystic fibrosis. P. cepacia is ubiquitous in the environment and is able to thrive and proliferate in tap water, antiseptic solutions, disinfectants, and medications. Sporadic outbreaks of local colonization or infection with P. cepacia have been noted in burn units, surgical wounds, indwelling catheters, and drug abusers. Lower respiratory tract colonization with P. cepacia in patients with cystic fibrosis has been associated with increasing severity of disease, the prior use of aminoglycosides, a deteriorating course, and shortened survival. P. cepacia virtually never causes infection in previously healthy individuals, but cutaneous infections have been observed in troops following prolonged immersion in water.

Preferred Therapy

- TMP/SMX, ciprofloxacin, aztreonam (depending on susceptibility)
- Aminoglycosides may confer synergistic killing in some strains

Alternative Agents

- Ceftazidime, chloramphenicol

Note: Virtually all isolates are resistant to imipenem.

Antimicrobial Resistance: P. cepacia exhibits high-grade resistance to multiple antimicrobials; unique inducible beta-lactamases and altered membrane permeability may confer resistance to beta-lactams, aminoglycosides, and structurally unrelated antibiotics. Virtually all isolates are resistant to first- and second-generation aminoglycosides, penicillin, ampicillin, and imipenem. The use of imipenem may predispose to colonization or superinfection with P. cepacia. Susceptibility to antipseudomonal penicillins and ceftazidime is variable. TMP/SMX, chloramphenicol, ciprofloxacin, and aztreonam are the most active agents; however, more than 50% of isolates are resistant to these antimicrobials.

Xanthomonas Maltophilia

Epidemiology: Xanthomonas (formerly Pseudomonas) maltophilia is a rare nosocomial opportunistic pathogen that has been increasingly seen as a nosocomial pathogen, particularly in debilitated patients with tracheostomies or indwelling catheters. Predisposing risk factors for nosocomial infections caused by X. maltophilia include prior use of antimicrobials (particularly imipenem, to which this organism is invariably resistant), residence in an ICU, indwelling central venous lines, tracheostomies, neutropenia, diabetes mellitus, malignant neoplasms, and intravenous drug abuse. Community-acquired lower respiratory tract infections resulting from Xanthomonas are rare, but have been well recognized in patients with cystic fibrosis receiving multiple previous courses of antimicrobials. Mortality rates associated with pneumonia caused by this pathogen have exceeded 50% in most series. This rate not only reflects the debilitated state of patients who acquire this organism, but also the high-grade resistance that X. maltophilia exhibits to most antimicrobial agents.

Preferred Therapy

- TMP/SMX (ciprofloxacin also acceptable)

Alternative Agents

• Antipseudomonal penicillins, ceftazidime (only a minority are susceptible)

Note: Addition of aminoglycosides does not confer synergy, although some antibiotic combinations (e.g. ciprofloxacin plus ceftazidime) may.

Antimicrobial Resistance: X. maltophilia is highly resistant to most beta-lactams; isolates are uniformly resistant to ampicillin, first- and second-generation cephalosporins, aztreonam, and imipenem. Fewer than 40% of isolates are susceptible to the antipseudomonal penicillins or aminoglycosides; 30 to 70% are susceptible to ceftazidime or cefoperazone. Most strains are sensitive to TMP/SMX, chloramphenicol, fluoroquinolones, and minocycline. Intravenous TMP/SMX is preferred as initial therapy (pending susceptibility results), *ciprofloxacin* is an acceptable alternative. Combinations of agents may be considered in refractory cases, but clinical data are lacking. Synergy has been achieved in vitro with TMP/SMX in combination with antipseudomonal penicillins or rifampin. Ciprofloxacin may also confer additive or synergistic killing in combination with ceftazidime or antipseudomonal penicillins. By contrast, the addition of aminoglycosides usually does not enhance antimicrobial activity.

GRAM-POSITIVE COCCI

Streptococci (Strains Other Than Enterococcus)

Epidemiology: Streptococcus spp other than Streptococcus pneumoniae (e.g. hemolytic and viridans streptococci) account for 1 to 4% of CAP; facultative anaerobic and anaerobic Streptococcus spp also may play a contributory role in aspiration pneumonias or lung abscess in the community. Streptococci have been isolated in 1 to 5% of nosocomial pneumonias; in this context, streptococci are usually part of mixed (polymicrobial) infections. Classification of streptococci is confusing, because nomenclature has been developed based on hemolytic reaction on blood agar, biochemical characteristics, and Lancefield classification (e.g. groups A through G). Streptococci are speciated according to biochemical characteristics; some strains of streptococci within the same species may exhibit hemolysis (i.e. "hemolytic streptococci"), whereas others do not (i.e. "viridans streptococci"). S. milleri is the most common of the viridans streptococci, which also include S. mutans, S. sanguis, S. mitis, S. bovis, and other species. Hemolytic strains include group B streptococci and a host of species (including S. milleri). Taxonomic classification of streptococci is confusing; e.g. group F streptococci (of the Lancefield classification) comprise at least 5 species (predominantly S. milleri and S. anginosus). Many strains are simply submitted as "microaerophilic" or "anaerobic" streptococci. Because streptococci constitute part of normal oral flora, isolation of streptococci from tracheobronchial secretions must be interpreted with caution.

Clinical Features: As a group, streptococci exhibit a striking proclivity for necrosis, abscess formation, and empyema. Although severe pneumonia caused by streptococci may occur even in previously healthy young adults, most infections occur in patients with serious underlying disease(s). Dementia, esophageal disease, prior strokes, old age, and neurologic impairment are predisposing factors. Aspiration pneumonitis progressing to a necrotizing pneumonitis, with or without abscess formation, is characteristic. Coinfection with other pathogens is common.

Preferred Therapy

- Penicillin G or ampicillin
- Combine with aminoglycoside for life-threatening infections

Alternative Agents

- Third-generation cephalosporins, imipenem (highly active but expensive)
- Erythromycin, clindamycin, vancomycin for patients allergic to penicillin

Antimicrobial Resistance: Penicillin G and ampicillin are highly active against most streptococci, except group D streptococci (enterococcis), and are the preferred agents. The activity of antipseudomonal penicillins is no greater than that of penicillin G or ampicillin. The activity of cephalosporins (including third-generation agents) is excellent. Imipenem has outstanding activity against most isolates. Aztreonam is inactive; the activity of ciprofloxacin is modest. Erythromycin, clindamycin, and vancomycin are acceptable for patients allergic to beta-lactams. Aminoglycosides may confer synergistic activity; thus, for fulminant, life-threatening infections, combination therapy with penicillin and an aminoglycoside is reasonable. Response of beta-hemolytic streptococcal disease to therapy may be slow and does not preclude curative outcome.

Group D Streptococci (Enterococci)

Epidemiology: Group D streptococci (enterococci) include S. faecalis (85 to 90%), S. faecium (5 to 15%), and S. durans (< 1%). Enterococci are a frequent cause of urinary tract, pelvic, and intra-abdominal infections, but their role in pneumonia is controversial; enterococcus pneumonia is rare (< 1%) in either nosocomial or community-settings. Risk factors for acquisition of enterococci include instrumentation of the gastrointestinal or genitourinary tract, immunosuppression, diabetes, cancer, debilitation, prolonged hospitalization, and the use of broad-spectrum agents, such as cephalosporins, to which enterococci are uniformly resistant.

Preferred Therapy

- Ampicillin (or vancomycin) combined with an aminoglycoside

Note: Cephalosporins are uniformly resistant.

Antimicrobial Resistance: Enterococci are uniformly susceptible to vancomycin and ampicillin, but these agents are bacteriostatic; thus, an aminoglycoside (typically gentamicin) should be added to confer synergy. Activity of penicillin is slightly less than that of ampicillin. Gentamicin is the most reliable aminoglycoside. Susceptibility to erythromycin is variable. Enterococci are resistant to all cephalosporins and most beta-lactams because of altered PBPs with low affinity for beta-lactams. Plasmid mediated, aminoglycoside-modifying enzymes may confer high-grade resistance to aminoglycosides. Beta-lactamase production is a rare mechanism of resistance against enterococci.

Staphylococcus Aureus

Epidemiology: Staphylococci, both coagulase positive (S. aureus) and coagulase negative (S. epidermidis), account for 10 to 15% of nosocomial pneumonias and are often polymicrobial. Primary staphylococcal pneumonia in the community is rare in the absence of risk factors. Staphylococcus spp, however, are responsible for 3 to 8% of CAP; even higher rates may be observed in patients with risk factors for acquisition of staphylococci, such as diabetes mellitus, IV drug abuse, debilitation, intravenous lines, Hickman catheters, residence in an ICU (particularly neurosurgical), and recent surgery.

Clinical Features: Staphylococcal pneumonia may be associated with a lobar process with air bronchograms indistinguishable from pneumococcal or other bacillary pneumonias; however, staphylococci exhibit a propensity for empyema formation and necrosis of lung parenchyma. Hematogenous seeding may give rise to multiple nodular or fluffy infiltrates, often with cavitation; this pattern is often observed in drug addicts or patients with endocarditis. Gram's stain of expectorated sputum or tracheal secretions demonstrates gram-positive cocci in clusters.

Preferred Therapy

- Oxacillin or cloxacillin (only for methicillin-susceptible strains)
- Vancomycin (uniformly active for both methicillin-susceptible and methicillin-resistant strains)

Alternative Agents

- Erythromycin, clindamycin, imipenem

Antimicrobial Resistance: Most S. aureus isolates produce beta-lactamases and are resistant to penicillin G and ampicillin; however, many are susceptible to antistaphylococcal penicillins (oxacillin, nafcillin, and cloxacillin). Cefazolin is usually highly active against methicillin-sensitive strains. Third-generation cephalosporins, particularly ceftazidime, have only modest activity against staphylococci, whereas the antipseudomonal penicillins and imipenem/cilastin are usually adequate for methicillin-sensitive S. aureus. These agents are suboptimal for methicillin-resistant S. aureus (MRSA).

Methicillin-resistant Staphylococcus Aureus (MRSA)

Epidemiology: Within the past two decades, the emergence of MRSA has become recognized as an important problem in hospitalized patients and IV drug abusers. Isolates have also been described within the community, in nursing homes, and in chronic care facilities.

Preferred Therapy

• Vancomycin

Alternative Agents

• TMP/SMX, clindamycin, imipenem

Antimicrobial Resistance: Methicillin resistance results from alteration of PBPs, which also confers resistance to cephalosporins. Resistance to other classes of antibiotics (e.g. erythromycin, aminoglycosides, tetracycline, clindamycin) is common among MRSA strains and has been noted with increasing frequency. Strains resistant to both aminoglycosides and methicillin were noted in Australia in the late 1970s; these isolates also displayed striking resistance to other antibiotics and were markedly different from MRSA detected in 1961. These aminoglycoside–methicillin-resistant strains were often resistant to all beta-lactams; imipenem was often active against these strains but less so than methicillin-sensitive strains. In 1989, Maple and colleagues reported antimicrobial resistance patterns for 106 MRSA from 21 countries. More than 90% of strains exhibited resistance to aminoglycosides. Other agents to which resistance was exhibited included tetracycline (86%), trimethoprim (69%), clindamycin (66%), rifampicin (26%), and ciprofloxacin (17%). Patterns of resistance differed among geographic regions, e.g. strains of MRSA isolated from the United Kingdom and Australia were resistant to trimethoprim, whereas ciprofloxacin-resistant strains were noted from France and Germany. Vancomycin is highly active against even these resistant strains and is the drug of choice. Alternative agents that have been successfully used for the treatment of MRSA include clindamycin, TMP/SMX, and the quinolones. Resistance to these other agents may occur, however, and they therefore cannot be considered consistently effective. The fluoroquinolones (ofloxacin, ciprofloxacin, perfloxacin) are active against both methicillin-sensitive and methicillin-resistant S. aureus. Quinolone-resistant MRSA have been noted with increasing frequency, however; selection of quinolone-resistant strains may occur in vitro with increasing concentrations of ciprofloxacin. Resistant isolates may emerge in as many as 10 to 20% of patients during a course of therapy. These data raise questions regarding the future utility of quinolones for S. aureus infections and suggest that caution be exercised in using quinolones for mild or moderate staphylococcal infections. Teicoplanin, a novel glycopeptide antibiotic related to vancomycin with less toxicity and a longer half-life, is not yet available in the United States.

Coagulase-negative Staphylococci (Staphylococcus epidermidis)

Epidemiology: Coagulase-negative staphylococci (Staphylococcus epidermidis) have been increasingly isolated as causative agents implicated in bacteremia in granulocytopenic patients and in infection of Hickman catheters, central venous catheters, neurosurgical and arteriovenous shunts, and prosthetic heart values. The importance in pulmonary infections is less clear.

Preferred Therapy

- Vancomycin
- Nafcillin (only for susceptible strains)

Antimicrobial Resistance: By the late 1980s, 35 to 70% of coagulase-negative staphylococci exhibited resistance to methicillin; virtually all such isolates are susceptible to vancomycin. Most hospital isolates of S. epidermidis are resistant to all beta-lactams as a result of alterations in penicillin-binding proteins. Many community-acquired strains of S. epidermidis are inhibited by beta-lactams. Despite widespread use of vancomycin worldwide for gram-positive infections, resistant strains have been rare.

THERAPY

Because the diagnostic techniques used to ascertain the microbiologic cause of pneumonia remain inexact, treatment of nosocomial pneumonia often remains empiric. In view of the potentially lethal nature of nosocomial pneumonia, it is advisable to initiate therapy with broad-spectrum parenteral antibiotics pending identification of the responsible organism(s). Selection of antibiotics in this context should take into account findings on sputum Gram's stain, host and environmental factors that may point to specific pathogens, the known frequency of specific isolates in the hospital or ICU setting, and antimicrobial susceptibility patterns within institutions (and individual ICUs). Antimicrobial therapy can be switched to a narrower-spectrum agent once a definitive microbiologic diagnosis has been established.

Patients who had recently received parenteral antimicrobial agents are at risk of acquiring highly resistant organisms, such as Pseudomonas aeruginosa, Acinetobacter, Serratia spp, and methicillin-resistant staphylococci. Antibiotic resistance patterns may vary widely within hospitals or even within ICUs within hospitals, depending on previous trends of antibiotic use. For example, at the University of Michigan, sweeping changes in antimicrobial resistance have been noted over the past decade. In 1981, fewer than 1% of Staphylococcus aureus isolates were resistant to methicillin; by 1989, 17% of strains were methicillin resistant.

Similarly, the prevalence of gentamicin-resistant Pseudomonas aeruginosa increased from 3% in 1982 to 12% in 1989. During the same time frame, high-level gentamicin-resistant enterococci climbed from fewer than 1% of isolates to 20%, and Enterobacter cloacae isolates resistant to cefotaxime increased from 7 to 24%. Similar disturbing trends have been noted in other institutions. An awareness of existing (or recent) antimicrobial susceptibility data within institutions (or individual ICUs) may guide therapy. Selection pressure from prior antimicrobials administered either for prophylaxis or for treatment of infections in individual patients may also predispose to highly resistant pathogens (e.g. Enterobacter spp among patients receiving third-generation cephalosporins; Pseudomonas cepacia following the use of imipenem). When nosocomial pneumonia develops (or progresses) in a patient receiving antibiotics, we usually switch to a different class of antimicrobials or to agents with a differing spectrum.

TREATMENT REGIMENS FOR SERIOUS NOSOCOMIAL PNEUMONIA

Various treatment strategies have been proposed as initial therapy for nosocomial pneumonia. These include single-agent therapy (monotherapy) with a broad-spectrum beta-lactam, such as a third-generation cephalosporin, extended spectrum penicillin, or imipenem/cilastin; double beta-lactam therapy; or combination therapy with a beta-lactam antibiotic and an aminoglycoside. Alternative strategies employing combinations of antimicrobials (e.g. fluoroquinolones plus aminoglycosides, vancomycin plus aztreonam) have been proposed.

Monotherapy with Broad-Spectrum Beta-Lactams

Several studies have noted high success rates treating serious nosocomial infections with third-generation cephalosporins, ticarcillin/clavulanate, or imipenem/cilastin (agents that possess exceptional gram-negative activity). The potential advantages of monotherapy are obvious; the toxicities and expense of additional agents are avoided. Most studies of monotherapy, however, have been in granulocytopenic patients with fever and sepsis. In this context, pneumonia has accounted for fewer than 10% of cases, and no pathogen was isolated in more than one half of the "septic" episodes. Thus, data derived from these trials may not necessarily pertain to nosocomial pulmonary infections.

In a landmark study in 1986, Pizzo and co-workers reported that monotherapy with ceftazidime was as effective as combination therapy with cephalothin, carbenicillin, and gentamicin in 550 episodes of fever and presumed sepsis in neutropenic patients with malignancies. Fewer than 7% of these patients had pneumonia. Further, ceftazidime (as a single agent) was curative in only 30% of documented infections; 59% of ceftazidime-treated patients were cured following the addition of antimicrobials or change in therapy. Overall failure rates with *documented* infections were comparable with ceftazidime and combination therapy (11% and 9%, respectively); lower failure rates were noted among patients with "suspected" infections in whom no organism was isolated.

More recently, Liang and associates prospectively evaluated 100 febrile episodes in 89 neutropenic patients with malignancy who were randomized to either ceftazidime (2 g q8h) or imipenem/cilastin (500 mg q6h) as initial monotherapy. Monotherapy with imipenem had a higher rate of favorable responses (77%) than did monotherapy with ceftazidime (56% response); the advantage of imipenem was even greater among those with microbiologically documented infections (81% response with imipenem vs 33% response with ceftazidime). An additional 21% with imipenem and 23% with ceftazidime responded to the addition of cloxacillin and amikacin following failure of monotherapy. Mortality was low in both groups; (0 of 48 [0%] for imipenem; 2 of 52 [4%] for ceftazidime). Only 12 patients, however, had documented pneumonia, 6 of whom failed on monotherapy. Meunier and co-workers reported that monotherapy with IV ciprofloxacin had a lower success rate (65%) than did combination therapy with piperacillin plus amikacin (91%). Other investigators have noted high rates of clinical failures and high rates of antimicrobial resistance when ciprofloxacin is used as monotherapy for serious infections caused by Staphylococcus aureus or Pseudomonas aeruginosa. Together, these data suggest that monotherapy (with beta-lactams or quinolones) may be associated with a significant rate of failures in granulocytopenic patients, particularly in the context of lower respiratory tract infections.

Other investigators have failed to observe differences between combination or single-agent therapy. For example, Bru and co-workers prospectively evaluated 87 infectious episodes in febrile neutropenic patients randomized to ticarcillin/clavulanate alone or to combination therapy with ticarcillin/clavulanate and amikacin. Response rates were comparable (83% with single-agent and 85% with combination therapy). Mangi and associates noted that monotherapy with cefoperazone was as effective as an aminoglycoside (gentamicin) in combination with either clindamycin or cefazolin in 139 patients with hospital-acquired pneumonia. Cures were achieved in 45 of 52 patients (87%) with cefoperazone and in 44 of 61 (72%) patients with combination therapy. Only 8 cases of pneumonia caused by P. aeruginosa were documented, however, 3 of whom failed therapy. Further, clindamycin has no significant activity against gram-negative organisms, and cefazolin (a first-generation cephalosporin) has a limited gram-negative spectrum when compared to that of third-generation cephalosporins. Unfortunately, few studies have specifically addressed whether *incremental* benefit is achieved by the addition of an aminoglycoside to a broad-spectrum agent, such as ceftazidime or imipenem/cilastin. Monotherapy may be as effective as combination therapy in some circumstances, but the efficacy of monotherapy for nosocomial gram-negative pneumonia (particularly when P. aeruginosa has been implicated) has not been convincingly established. This area remains controversial.

Double Beta-Lactam Therapy

Nephrotoxicity may complicate aminoglycoside use in as many as 10 to 25% of patients, particularly when concomitant illnesses or risk factors are present. Thus, alternative strategies employing combinations of agents but without using aminoglycosides have been considered. In this context, some investigators advocate combining two beta-lactam agents with overlapping spectra of microbiologic activity (double beta-lactam therapy). The concept of beta-lactam therapy offers little over single-agent therapy unless synergistic killing can be achieved. In this context, some combinations, such as ceftazidime and piperacillin or aztreonam plus beta-lactams, are frequently synergistic in vitro, whereas other double beta-lactam combinations, such as imipenem/cilastin plus other beta-lactams, may be antagonistic. Overall response rates achieved in granulocytopenic patients treated with double beta-lactam combinations have generally been comparable to those attained with aminoglycoside-containing regimens. In addition, the emergence of antimicrobial resistance with double beta-lactam therapy is a concern, because emergence of beta–lactamase-producing isolates may confer resistance to both beta-lactams. By contrast, the use of an aminoglycoside, which acts via a different mechanism, would not be affected by beta-lactamases.

Combination Therapy with a Beta-Lactam and an Aminoglycoside

Although monotherapy with a beta-lactam (to which the organism is susceptible) is probably adequate for most gram-negative bacillary pneumonias caused by Escherichia coli, Klebsiella, and Proteus spp, several conceptual reasons support the use of combination therapy in critically ill patients with gram-negative pneumonia, especially with highly resistant or virulent pathogens, such as Pseudomonas aeruginosa, Acinetobacter, and Serratia spp. The *theoretic* advantages of combination therapy over monotherapy include

- Synergistic microbiocidal activity against many bacteria can be achieved
- Combination therapy markedly improves survival in animal models of Pseudomonas infection compared to survival with monotherapy
- In humans, reduced survival of patients with gram-negative pneumonia has been noted in patients with subtherapeutic peak aminoglycoside levels
- Improved survival was demonstrated in patients with granulocytopenic cancer when gram-negative bacteremia was treated with ceftazidime plus long-course (10 days) amikacin compared to survival with ceftazidime plus short-course (5 days) amikacin (multicenter European Oncology trial)
- Improved survival has been noted in some studies in immunocompromised patients when the infecting organism is susceptible to both the beta-lactam and the aminoglycoside
- In a recent study by Hilf and associates of 200 patients with Pseudomonas aeruginosa bacteremia, mortality was lower with combination therapy employing an antipseudomonal beta-lactam plus an aminoglycoside (27% mortality) as compared to mortality with monotherapy (47% mortality). The survival advantage was even greater among patients with pneumonia or in the ICU
- Combining an aminoglycoside with a beta-lactam may limit or prevent the emergence of antimicrobial resistance because mechanisms of resistance differ; this conceptual advantage has not yet been verified in clinical trials

Novel Therapeutic Strategies

Additional strategies employing antibiotic combinations have been tried. Viscoli and associates prospectively randomized febrile, neutropenic children with malignancy to ceftazidime plus vancomycin or ceftazidime plus amikacin. Response rates and mortality were comparable with both regimens. Colardyn and co-workers noted a higher response rate and improved survival with azotreonam combined with either cloxacillin or oxacillin as compared to tobramycin combined with either cefuroxime or cefotaxime in one randomized, prospective study of mechanically ventilated patients with pneumonia. Superinfection was substantially higher in the aminoglycoside group, thus suggesting that aztreonam plus an agent conferring gram-positive activity (e.g. vancomycin) may be a valuable alternative to beta-lactam combinations employing aminoglycosides.

EMPIRIC THERAPY (PRIOR TO IDENTIFICATION OF A SPECIFIC ORGANISM)

In view of the relatively high prevalence of Pseudomonas aeruginosa as a cause of nosocomial pneumonia in mechanically ventilated patients, *initial empiric* therapy in this context should include coverage against P. aeruginosa

- Combination therapy with an antipseudomonal broad-spectrum beta-lactam, such as ceftazidime, piperacillin, ticarcillin/clavulanate, or imipenem/cilastatin, and an aminoglycoside (typically gentamicin because of its lower cost) is preferred as initial therapy. If contraindications to aminoglycosides exist, monotherapy with ceftazidime or imipenem may be adequate
- Ciprofloxacin can be substituted for the beta-lactam when the patient is allergic to penicillin
- Agents with broad-spectrum gram-negative activity but without antipseudomonal activity, such as ceftriaxone, cefotaxime, and ceftizoxime, may be adequate in noncritically ill, nonventilated patients in whom the risk of infections caused by Pseudomonas spp is lower. First- or second-generation cephalosporins, ampicillin, or ampicillin/sulbactam are not adequate for the *initial empiric* treatment of nosocomial pneumonia. Aminoglycosides *alone* are not adequate for the treatment of gram-negative bacterial pneumonia.

Modification of Antimicrobial Therapy

The initial (empiric) antimicrobial therapy should be reassessed once cultural results are available (usually by 48 to 72 hours) and the clinical course has been clarified. The appropriate agent(s) depends on the suspected (or confirmed) organism(s) and the microbiologic susceptibility results for each individual patient. For infections caused by P. aeruginosa, combination therapy with an extended-spectrum penicillin (e.g. piperacillin or ticarcillin), ceftazidime, or imipenem/cilastin plus an aminoglycoside is warranted. Other third-generation cephalosporins, such as cefotaxime, ceftizoxime, and ceftriaxone, extended-spectrum penicillins, or imipenem/ cilastin provide excellent activity against most other enteric GNB. First- or second-generation cephalosporins may be substituted for more expensive agents if a specific organism has been isolated and has been shown to be susceptible. If highly susceptible pathogens, such as Escherichia coli, Klebsiella, and Proetus spp, are isolated and the patient is improving, the aminoglycoside may be discontinued. For highly virulent strains, such as Pseudomonas aeruginosa, Serratia, Acinetobacter, and Enterobacter spp, the synergistic microbiocidal activity achieved with combination therapy is important to maintain for the duration of therapy.

DURATION

Irrespective of the agent(s) utilized, duration of therapy for nosocomial pneumonia must be adequate to avoid recrudescent infection. Although the duration of therapy must be individualized according to clinical response and severity of the disease process, treatment is usually necessary for a *minimum* of 10 days; a more prolonged course (extending for as long as 21 or more days) may be appropriate for more virulent pathogens, such as Pseudomonas aeruginosa, or for complicated, severe, or protracted cases.

ANAEROBIC PLEUROPULMONARY INFECTIONS

EPIDEMIOLOGY

Aspiration of many oropharyngeal bacilli may lead to a spectrum of pleuropulmonary manifestations, including acute pneumonitis, necrotizing pneumonia with cavitation, lung abscess, and empyema. Anaerobes constitute the dominant flora of the upper respiratory tract and may have a primary role (often admixed with other pathogens) in all these pleuropulmonary syndromes. The predominant oropharyngeal anaerobes include Bacteroides melaninogenicus, Fusobacterium nucleatum, peptococcus, peptostreptococcus, and microaerophilic streptococci. Bacteroides fragilis and species within the B. fragilis group (e.g. B. ovatus, B. vulgatus, and B. thetaiotaomicron) account for 10 to 15% of isolates. Anaerobes have been implicated as either sole or concomitant pathogens in 60 to 97% of aspiration pneumonias or primary lung abscesses and in 6 to 15% of pneumonias in the community. The importance of anaerobes in nosocomial pulmonary infections remains controversial; enteric GNB are more virulent and likely of greater importance than are anaerobes in nosocomial pneumonias. Nevertheless, anaerobes may be important pathogens in circumstances fostering massive aspiration of oropharyngeal contents or in the context of primary lung abscess or empyema.

CLINICAL FEATURES

Aspiration pneumonia should be considered in patients with primary neurologic or esophageal disease; common associated conditions include reduced level of consciousness, alcohol or drug abuse, general anesthesia, previous strokes, seizures, periodontal disease, and the presence of nasogastric, endotracheal, and tracheostomy tubes. Aspiration pneumonia preferentially involves the dependent segments of the lung (posterior segments of the upper lobes and superior segments of the lower lobes) as a result of gravitational forces; however, basilar infiltrates may also occur. Community-acquired aspiration pneumonia often exhibits an indolent course, evolving over 1 to 3 weeks. Cough, sputum production, and low-grade fever are characteristic. The hallmarks of acute bacillary pneumonias, such as chills, rigors, pleuritic chest pain, consolidation findings, are usually lacking. In fact, constitutional signs, such as weight loss, anemia, and generalized weakness, may be the presenting features. The course of aspiration pneumonitis may be more fulminant, however, particularly when Staphylococcus aureus or enteric GNB are present concomitantly. Chest x-rays typically demonstrate patchy infiltrates without clear evidence for consolidation; persistence of the pneumonic infiltrate may lead to necrosis and cavitation. An air-fluid level indicates a lung abscess.

MICROBIOLOGY

The microbiologic aspects of aspiration pneumonitis/lung abscess differ depending on the host and risk factors for the acquisition of GNB. Normal oral flora consist largely of anaerobes and aerobic gram-positive cocci; aerobic enteric GNB are absent. By contrast, aerobic GNB, such as Klebsiella, Enterobacter spp, and Pseudomonas aeruginosa, frequently colonize the oropharynx and lower respiratory tract of hospitalized patients and may also be present in large numbers among debilitated or immunosuppressed individuals living in the community. These differences mandate differing treatment strategies for aspiration pneumonia/lung abscess acquired in the community or in the hospital setting.

When aspiration occurs in the community, common respiratory pathogens, such as streptococci and gram-positive aerobes, may be mixed with anaerobes. By contrast, in nosocomial infections, aerobic GNB may predominate and the importance of anaerobes is less clear. Aspiration pneumonia in patients in nursing homes or chronic care facilities, or in patients with risk factors for gram-negative oropharyngeal and lower respiratory tract colonization (e.g. history of ethanol abuse, heart failure, diabetes mellitus, liver failure, old age, and debilitation), may include an admixture of anaerobes and aerobic GNB.

Clarification of the microbiologic cause of aspiration pneumonia (or lung abscess) is usually difficult. Expectorated sputum cultures often grow only normal oral flora, because concomitant upper respiratory tract flora usually overgrow any anaerobes that may be present. Foul-smelling, putrid sputum is a clue to the presence of anaerobes but is only present in one third of patients. Gram's stain of expectorated sputum or empyema fluid may demonstrate a mixture of both gram-negative (e.g. Bacteroides spp, Fusobacterium nucleatum) and gram-positive (e.g. streptococci, peptococci) organisms; however, these findings are nonspecific and of limited value. Only percutaneous needle aspiration, transtracheal aspirates, or thoracenteses can be considered reliable sources for anaerobic cultures. Because of the invasive nature of percutaneous needle aspiration or transtracheal aspiration, however, these procedures are not recommended for the microbiologic diagnosis of aspiration pneumonia or lung abscess. Pioneering studies in the early 1970s by Gorbach, Finegold, and Bartlett (using transtracheal aspirates) elegantly delineated the organism(s) responsible for aspiration pneumonia or primary lung abscess in the community. Of primary lung abscesses, 50% were caused by pure anaerobes; 47% by a mixture of anaerobes and aerobes, and 3% by predominantly aerobes.

THERAPY

Antibiotic therapy is almost always sufficient for management of anaerobic pneumonitis or lung abscess; drainage of abscess cavities usually can be accomplished by expectoration of sputum and local percussion and drainage. Progression of the infection to the pleural space may result in empyema; in such cases, aggressive drainage (employing a surgical empyema tube) in addition to antibiotics is required.

Community-acquired aspiration pneumonitis in patients without serious associated diseases usually can be treated with limited-spectrum agents directed primarily against anaerobes. Penicillin G (8 to 12 million U daily) may be adequate for uncomplicated aspiration pneumonia or lung abscess acquired in the community. The marginal activity of penicillin G against Bacteroides fragilis, however, has raised doubts about its role as primary therapy for anaerobic pulmonary infections. Clindamycin has superior activity against anaerobes (including B. fragilis) compared to penicillin G and has been advocated by some clinicians as preferred therapy for community-acquired aspiration pneumonitis/lung abscess. Clindamycin may be efficacious even in patients in whom therapy with penicillin G previously failed, and was superior to penicillin G in one multicenter, prospective study of community-acquired lung abscess. In that study, patients treated with IV clindamycin (600 mg q 8h) exhibited more rapid clinical improvement and defervescence, and had a lower rate of short-term and late relapses compared to patients who received penicillin (6 million U daily). Given the historical success with penicillin over many decades for the treatment of lung abscess and aspiration pneumonia, however, many authors still advocate penicillin G as primary therapy for uncomplicated lung abscess/aspiration pneumonia because of its lower cost. The decision as to initial therapy must be individualized. In view of its lower cost, penicillin G is a reasonable first-line agent for patients with mild disease. Clindamycin is preferred for seriously ill patients with lung abscess or for patients who have failed initial therapy with penicillin.

Metronidazole (Flagyl) has exquisite activity against anaerobes (including B. fragilis) in vitro, but has been associated with a high failure rate when used as monotherapy for pulmonary anaerobic infections and is not recommended. The poor results achieved with metronidazole may reflect its poor activity against aerobic and microaerophilic streptococci, which are often present concomitantly. Alternative agents with excellent anaerobic activity include ampicillin, cefotetan, imipenem, and chloramphenicol.

Neither penicillin G nor clindamycin has significant activity against GNB. Thus, when aspiration pneumonia occurs in patients residing in chronic care facilities or with serious associated disease(s), a broader-spectrum agent (to cover concomitant GNB) is required. In this context, antipseudomonal penicillins or ceftotetan (2 g q12h) are reasonable agents for empiric therapy; routine addition of an aminoglycoside in this context is not recommended, except in fulminant or severe cases. For clinically significant aspiration pneumonia occurring in the hospital setting, ticarcillin/clavulanate or piperacillin, combined with an aminoglycoside, are reasonable choices; cefotetan is less desirable because it lacks activity against Pseudomonas aeruginosa. Imipenem has outstanding activity, and should be considered for complicated polymicrobial pneumonias when resistance to less expensive agents is suspected. Ciprofloxacin TMP/SMX, and cephalosporins lack activity against many anaerobes (particularly Bacteroides fragilis) and are not recommended for polymicrobial anaerobic infections.

PREFERRED THERAPY FOR COMMUNITY ACQUIRED LUNG ABSCESS

- Penicillin G for uncomplicated lung abscess in community (because of low cost)
- Clindamycin (for complicated lung abscess or penicillin failure)

Note: Metronidazole has been associated with a high failure rate for anaerobic infections above the diaphragm and therefore is not recommended.

ALTERNATIVE AGENTS

- Cefotetan, antipseudomonal penicillins, imipenem (these agents may be particularly useful when infection with enteric GNB coexists)

CLINICAL FEATURES

Clinical response to antimicrobial therapy is variable, depending on antibiotic susceptibility, host defenses, extent and severity of the infection, and presence or absence of parenchymal necrosis, empyema and other such conditions. Defervescence with acute anaerobic pneumonitis may be rapid; lysis of fever occurs within 48 hours in most patients, and within 5 days in 80% of patients. A prolonged course of therapy is recommended, however, because relapses may occur with short-term (7 to 10 days) antibiotic therapy. A more prolonged febrile pattern (even with appropriate antimicrobials) is typical of lung abscess or empyema. In such cases, fever may persist for 5 to 10 days or more despite adequate antimicrobial therapy. When a frank lung abscess (cavitation with an air-fluid level) is present, resolution may be delayed, and 2 to 4 months of therapy may be necessary to prevent recrudescence of infection. In this context, initial parenteral therapy for 7 to 10 days, followed by an oral antibiotic (e.g. penicillin V potassium, ampicillin, or clindamycin), is reasonable.

ANTIMICROBIAL RESISTANCE

Virtually all anaerobes (including those of the B. fragilis group) are invariably susceptible to imipenem, chloramphenicol, and metronidazole. Penicillin G and ampicillin have exquisite activity against normal oral anaerobes; however, more than 90% of B. fragilis spp are resistant to penicillins. Beta–lactamase-producing strains of B. melaninogenicus are increasing, thus suggesting that further increases in penicillin-resistant isolates can be expected in the future. Antipseudomonal penicillins have moderate activity against anaerobes (including B. fragilis spp); however, recent studies have shown resistance rates to piperacillin/mezlocillin of 5 to 20%. Clavulanic acid and sulbactam are active against many beta–lactamase-producing Bacteroides spp; fewer than 1% of isolates are resistant to ticarcillin/clavulanate.

The activity of cephalosporins against anaerobes is variable. The activity of the cephamycins (cefoxitin, cefotetan) against anaerobes is excellent, which in part reflects the ability of these molecules to resist beta-lactamases. Ceftazidime and cefoperazone have poor activity; other cephalosporins have only modest activity. Aztreonam, TMP/SMX, and the fluoroquinoles have poor activity against anaerobes.

Clindamycin has been the cornerstone of therapy for anaerobic infections for nearly 2 decades. Since 1980, however, antimicrobial resistance to the penicillins, cephamycins, and clindamycin has been increasing. Studies from France, Spain, and the United States have demonstrated resistance to clindamycin in 2 to 8% of strains of B. fragilis and in 16 to 22% of isolates among the non-fragilis species of the B. fragilis group. Even higher rates of resistance to cefoxitin and cefotetan (5 to 30%) have been described.

SPECIFIC ANTIMICROBIAL AGENTS

This section is a review of specific antimicrobial agents used in the treatment of pneumonia. Some of the antibiotics, such as chloramphenicol, are discussed more for historical interest. Disproportionate attention is given to some of the newer agents, such as the azalides and quinolones, because data in this regard have only recently emerged. This increased attention, however, does not imply that these agents are more important or effective than traditional antimicrobials, such as penicillins and cephalosporins.

BETA-LACTAMS

This class of agents includes penicillins, cephalosporins, carbapenems, and monobactams; the four-membered beta-lactam ring (usually fused to a second ring) is integral to the structure. Modifications or substitutions of the beta-lactam ring may alter antimicrobial activity, or resistance to beta-lactamases.

PENICILLINS

Since the introduction of penicillin for clinical use in 1941, the penicillin group of antibiotics has remained key to the treatment of pulmonary infections. Penicillins have excellent bactericidal activity and relatively low toxicity. The basic structure of the penicillin group of antimicrobials consists of a beta-lactam ring fused to a 5-membered thiazolidine ring; modification of the side chains attached to the beta-lactam ring may alter the antimicrobial spectrum, beta-lactamase, stability, and pharmacokinetics. Many of the newer penicillins are modifications of ampicillin. Substitution of a carboxy group for an amino group on ampicillin produced the carboxy-penicillins, carbenicillin and ticarcillin. Substitution of a ureido group for the carboxy group produced the ureidopenicillins (piperacillin, mezlocillin, azlocillin).

Mechanism of Action: Penicillins interfere with bacterial cell wall (peptidoglycan) synthesis and activate endogenous autolytic enzymes, inducing cell lysis. Killing of GNB requires that penicillins penetrate outer portions of the bacterial cell wall and combine with key PBPs on the inner membrane of the bacteria. Penicillins fail to activate autolytic enzymes in enterococci and some streptococci; thus, in these cases, addition of a second antimicrobial, such as rifampin or aminoglycoside, is recommended to achieve bactericidal activity.

Antimicrobial Resistance: The most common mechanism of resistance to penicillins is via beta-lactamases. Beta-lactamases are produced by both gram-negative and gram-positive bacilli and hydrolyze the beta-lactam ring, thereby inactivating penicillin. Additional mechanisms of resistance to penicillin can result from alterations in PBPs (resulting in decreasing affinity for penicillins) or changes in bacterial cell wall permeability. MRSA is an example of the former mechanism; multiresistant Pseudomonas aeruginosa may be mediated by the latter mechanism.

Toxicity: Adverse effects include maculopapular rash, eosinophilia, drug fever (particularly with ampicillin and methicillin), bleeding disorders with high doses of carbenicillin and ticarcillin, and seizures when in high doses (particularly in presence of renal failure).

Benzyl-penicillin
(penicillin G)

Benzyl-penicillin, or penicillin G, was the first of the penicillins available for clinical use (introduced in 1941) and is the parent drug of this family. Penicillin G has outstanding activity against Streptococcus pneumoniae and most streptococci, and remains the preferred agent, with few exceptions, for infections caused by these pathogens. Because of its limited spectrum, however, penicillin G is rarely employed as empiric therapy for CAP and has no role in nosocomial settings.

Antimicrobial Spectrum: Outstanding activity against S. pneumoniae (pneumococci), S. pyogenes (group A), all other beta-hemolytic streptococci, most S. viridans, and group D streptococci (enterococcus spp). More than 80% of staphylococci are resistant. Anaerobes (with exception of beta-lactamase [+] strains of Bacteroides fragilis) are exquisitely sensitive. Active against gram-negative cocci, such as Neisseria meningitidis and N. gonorrhoeae. No significant activity against Hemophilus influenzae or enteric GNB. No activity against Mycoplasma, Chlamydia, Legionella spp; most Moraxella catarrhalis are now resistant.

Toxicity: Low incidence of side effects, but hypersensitivity reactions (anaphylaxis, rash) may occur with all penicillins. Less toxic than other penicillins; gastrointestinal side effects and diarrhea much less common than with extended-spectrum penicillins. No significant phlebitis.

Dosage: 4.8 to 10 million U of aqueous crystalline penicillin G IV daily in 4 to 6 divided doses; oral penicillin (the potassium salt of phenoxymethyl penicillin [Penicillin VK]) can be substituted in a dose of 500 mg qid once clinical response and defervescence have occurred.

Indications: Drug of choice for pneumonia caused by Streptococcus pneumoniae and most other streptococci

- One of the choices for empiric therapy for suspected lung abscess (clindamycin may be superior)
- Therapeutic for infections caused by enterococci (Streptococcus faecalis and S. faecium); however, these streptococci are inhibited but not killed by penicillins alone. Thus, must be combined with either rifampin or an aminoglycoside

Because of its limited spectrum penicillin G is not suitable as empiric therapy for CAP except when S. pneumoniae is strongly suspected from a compatible clinical picture and confirmatory Gram's stain. Penicillin G has no therapeutic role for nosocomial pneumonia.

Antistaphylococcal Penicillins

The semisynthetic penicillins were developed for treatment of beta–lactamase-producing staphylococci resistant to penicillin G; the addition of an acyl side chain prevented disruption of the beta-lactam ring by beta-lactamases. The three semisynthetic penicillins available for parenteral use are methicillin (Staphcillin, Celbenin), nafcillin (Nafcil, Unipen), and oxacillin (Prostaphlin).

Antimicrobial Spectrum: Active against most staphylococci including beta–lactamase-producing strains. Not active against methicillin-resistant staphylococci. Less active than penicillin G against streptococci and other penicillin-susceptible organisms. No significant activity against anaerobes. No activity against GNB, Chlamydia, Mycoplasma, or Legionella spp.

Toxicity: Similar to that of penicillin, but also includes interstitial nephritis. Intensely irritating to veins (phlebitis).

Dosage: 1 to 2 g IV q4-6h; oral antistaphylococcal penicillins (cloxacillin or dicloxacillin) can be substituted in some patients when clinical response has occurred (dose, 250 to 500 mg qid).

Indications: In view of their limited spectrum of activity, the antistaphylococcal penicillins should be reserved for patients with pneumonia caused by susceptible strains of staphylococci. Other agents are preferred for other pathogens. Nafcillin, oxacillin, and methicillin are equivalent in efficacy, but side effects (particularly interstitial nephritis) are most frequent with methicillin. Thus, nafcillin and oxacillin are preferred agents.

Aminopenicillins

The aminopenicillins (ampicillin, amoxicillin) were the first of the penicillins to have activity against GNB. Ampicillin (the first of the aminopenicillins) was developed by adding an amino group to the benzylpenicillin molecule; other agents (amoxicillin, bacampicillin) were later developed. These agents have significant activity against Hemophilus influenzae and selected enteric GNB. Ampicillin and amoxicillin were widely used in the early 1970s as empiric therapy for CAP because they extended the spectrum of penicillin G. Within the past 2 decades, second- and third-generation cephalosporins and newer agents with superior gram-negative activity have been developed. Ampicillin and amoxicillin have no activity against Klebsiella pneumoniae and indole-positive Proteus spp, and can no longer be considered reliable against Hemophilus influenzae or Escherichia coli. Antimicrobial resistance to these agents has increased dramatically over the past decade, even among isolates that previously were highly susceptible, such as Hemophilus influenzae, Moraxella catarrhalis, and Escherichia coli). These factors have relegated ampicillin and amoxicillin to secondary roles in the treatment of pneumonia.

Antimicrobial Spectrum: Excellent activity against gram-positive cocci (including Streptococcus pneumoniae, other streptococci, enterococci) and anaerobes (comparable to penicillin G). Active against Neisseria spp, beta–lactamase-negative strains of Hemophilus spp (not against beta–lactamase-producing H. influenzae, which comprise 10 to 20% of isolates), 60 to 70% of Escherichia coli, and Proteus mirabilis. Fails to cover beta–lactamase-producing strains of Moraxella catarrhalis. No significant activity against Klebsiella, Enterobacter, Serratia, indole-positive Proteus, or Pseudomonas spp. No activity against Chlamydia, Mycoplasma pneumoniae, or Legionella spp.

Toxicity: Similar to that of penicillin G except higher incidence of diarrhea and gastrointestinal symptoms (10 to 15%) and skin rash (3 to 5%).

Dosage: Ampicillin 1 to 2 g IV q6h; in some patients, oral ampicillin 500 mg qid (or amoxicillin 500 mg tid) can be substituted once a clinical response to IV therapy has been demonstrated.

Indications:

- Choice for pneumonia caused by a susceptible strain of Hemophilus influenzae, Escherichia coli, or Proteus mirabilis
- Infections caused by enterococci (combine with an aminoglycoside)

Because of the limited spectrum of ampicillin and amoxicillin, other agents are preferred for empiric therapy of CAP or nosocomial pneumonia.

BETA-LACTAMASE INHIBITORS

Clavulanate and sulbactam inhibit beta-lactamases produced by certain gram-positive and gram-negative bacteria (e.g. Hemophilus influenzae, Klebsiella pneumoniae, staphylococci), but lack intrinsic antibacterial activity. The addition of these beta-lactamase inhibitors to the parent compound (ticarcillin, ampicillin, amoxicillin) extends the spectrum of activity of these agents to include beta–lactamase-producing strains resistant to the parent compound alone. Clavulanate and sulbactam do not improve the activity of the parent compound for beta–lactamase-negative strains or bacteria that are resistant by mechanisms other than beta-lactamase production. In addition, neither clavulanate nor sulbactam affects beta-lactamases of the type 1 Richmond-Sykes classification produced by Pseudomonas aeruginosa, Enterobacter, Morganella, and Serratia spp. These agents are not adequate for infections caused by MRSA.

Ampicillin/Sulbactam
(Unasyn)

The addition of sulbactam to ampicillin extended the spectrum of ampicillin to include beta–lactamase-producing strains of Staphylococcus aureus, Moraxella catarrhalis, Hemophilus influenzae, Bacteroides fragilis, Klebsiella, Escherichia coli, Proteus, and Acinetobacter spp. Ampicillin/sulbactam (Unasyn) is less active than third-generation cephalosporins against Enterobacteriaceae.

Antimicrobial Spectrum: Excellent activity against gram-positive bacteria (including Staphylococcus aureus, streptococci, and enterococci) and anaerobes (inhibiting more than 95% of strains, including Bacteroides fragilis). Active against Moraxella catarrhalis, Neisseria spp, Hemophilus influenzae, Escherichia coli, Klebsiella spp, and Proteus mirabilis. Not active against Pseudomonas aeruginosa, Serratia, Enterobacter spp, or difficult-to-treat gram-negative infections.

Dosage: Supplied as 3-g or 1.5-g vials for IV use in fixed 2:1 ratio of ampicillin to sulbactam); dose, 1.5 to 3 g q6h (pharmacokinetics similar to those of ampicillin).

Indications:

- Ampicillin/sulbactam (Unasyn) is most useful for polymicrobial infections including anaerobes
- Reasonable as empiric therapy for CAP in nonimmunocompromised hosts. Less useful for nosocomial pneumonia because of its lack of activity against Pseudomonas aeruginosa and limited spectrum of activity against gram-negative bacteria
- Excellent for pelvic and abdominal infections

Amoxicillin/Clavulanate
(Augmentin)

The combination of amoxicillin/clavulanate (Augmentin) was the first of the penicillin/beta-lactamase inhibitors available for clinical use (marketed in the United States in 1984). This agent is available only in oral form.

Antimicrobial Spectrum: Spectrum of ampicillin/amoxicillin plus beta–lactamase-producing strains of Hemophilus influenzae, Escherichia coli, Proteus, Klebsiella, Moraxella catarrhalis, and Staphylococcus aureus. No activity against Pseudomonas aeruginosa, Serratia, Enterobacter, Citrobacter, and MRSA.

Toxicity: Similar to that of ampicillin or amoxicillin.

<u>Dosage:</u> 250 to 500 mg tid.

Indications:

- Amoxicillin/clavulanate (Augmentin) is useful as oral empiric therapy for mild CAP (in patients at low risk for more resistant gram-negative bacteria) or following initial therapy with a parenteral agent

Antipseudomonal Penicillins

Carbenicillin (Geopen, Pyopen), a carboxypenicillin produced by substituting a carboxyl group for the amino group on ampicillin, extended the gram-negative spectrum of ampicillin and was the first of the penicillins with significant activity against Pseudomonas aeruginosa. Substitutions on carbenicillin resulted in ticarcillin (Ticar), which had even broader gram-negative activity. Attachment of ureido groups to the acyl side chain of ampicillin led to the "ureidopenicillins," which include piperacillin (Pipracil), mezlocillin (Mezlin), and azlocillin (Azlin). Antipseudomonal penicillins are effective in the treatment of CAP, nosocomial pneumonias, and serious nosocomial sepsis, and as empiric treatment of sepsis in immunocompromised, granulocytopenic hosts.

Antimicrobial Spectrum: Antipseudomonal penicillins are broad-spectrum agents active against most GNB, including beta–lactamase-negative Hemophilus influenzae, most Enterobacteriaceae, indole-positive Proteus, Providencia, Morganella, and Pseudomonas aeruginosa. The activity of antipseudomonal penicillins against Escherichia coli is less predictable (only 80 to 90% of isolates susceptible) than that of third-generation cephalosporins. As many as 20 to 40% Enterobacter spp are resistant. The carboxypenicillins (ticarcillin, carbenicillin) are not reliable against Klebsiella, Serratia spp, or enterococci; the ureidopenicillins, particularly piperacillin, have generally good activity against these pathogens. Piperacillin and mezlocillin have excellent activity against Klebsiella spp (> 80% of isolates susceptible), whereas only 10 to 30% of Klebsiella spp are susceptible to carbenicillin, azlocillin, and ticarcillin. Compared to the other penicillins, piperacillin has slightly greater activity (lower MIC) in vitro, and is the most active agent against Pseudomonas aeruginosa. Whether these in vitro differences result in improved efficacy in vivo has not been established. Timentin represents a fixed combination of 3 g of ticarcillin and 100 mg of clavulanate potassium (a beta-lactamase inhibitor). The clavulanate binds to beta-lactamases secreted by staphylococci, Bacteroides fragilis, Moraxella catarrhalis, Hemophilus influenzae, Klebsiella spp, Proteus spp, and certain enteric GNB and thus extends the spectrum of activity of ticarcillin to include these beta–lactamase-producing organisms. Clavulanate, however, does not affect type 1 beta-lactamases, such as those released by certain strains of Pseudomonas, Serratia, Citrobacter, and Enterobacter spp. Thus, clavulanate does not improve (and may actually reduce) the activity of ticarcillin against these strains. In addition, clavulanate does not improve the activity of ticarcillin against strains of bacteria resistant by mechanisms other than beta-lactamase production (e.g. changes in the permeability of the cell wall). The activity of ticarcillin/clavulanate is no greater than that of ticarcillin alone against susceptible, beta–lactamase-negative strains. Thus, for susceptible organisms, ticarcillin alone is preferable and is less expensive than ticarcillin/clavulanate (Timentin). Ticarcillin/clavulanate exhibits good activity against staphylococci in vitro (including MRSA), but treatment failures in vivo suggest that ticarcillin/clavulanate (Timentin) is not adequate for proven infections caused by MRSA (irrespective of in vitro susceptibility data). Ticarcillin/clavulanate (Timentin) has only modest activity against enterococci. Activity of the antipseudomonal penicillins against streptococci and most gram-positive bacteria is good, but less effective than that afforded by penicillin G or ampicillin. None of these agents (except for ticarcillin/clavulanate [Timentin]) is effective against beta–lactamase-producing strains of staphylococci. MRSA are invariably resistant. Anaerobic activity is generally excellent, but is less than the anaerobic activity of metronidazole or clindamycin; beta–lactamase-producing strains of Bacteroides fragilis may be susceptible only to ticarcillin/clavulanate (Timentin). The major "holes" in coverage are Escherichia coli, Enterobacter spp (resistance rates in nosocomial settings of 15 to 30%), and staphylococci (beta-lactamase producing and MRSA).

Toxicity: Adverse effects include skin rash, hypokalemia and sodium load (particularly with disodium salts carbenicillin and ticarcillin; 4.7 mEq of sodium/g for carbenicillin and ticarcillin; only 1.8 mEq/g for mezlocillin and piperacillin). Prolonged bleeding time and abnormalities in coagulation tests, especially in uremic patients, noted with carbenicillin, which is no longer used.

<u>Dosage:</u> 3 to 4 g IV q4-6h (3.1 g q4-6h for ticarcillin/clavulanate).

Indications:

- Piperacillin or ticarcillin/clavulanate (Timentin) may be used as first-line agents for empiric therapy of nosocomial pneumonia, serious nosocomial sepsis, or when Pseudomonas aeruginosa is a consideration (e.g. cystic fibrosis, mechanical ventilation, previous antimicrobials, granulocytopenia, immunocompromised hosts). Ticarcillin/clavulanate has superior gram-positive activity, but slightly less gram-negative activity compared to piperacillin; overall, these agents are therapeutically equivalent for serious nosocomial infections. Both agents are superior to mezlocillin or azlocillin in this context. Combination therapy with an aminoglycoside may provide synergy and is recommended. Antipseudomonal penicillins are not recommended for CAP. P. aeruginosa is rarely a consideration in this context, and less expensive agents (e.g. cefuroxime, ceftriaxone, ampicillin/sulbactam) provide adequate coverage against community-acquired respiratory pathogens, including most Enterobacteriaceae.

CEPHALOSPORINS

Since the first cephalosporin, cephalothin (Keflin), became available in the United States in 1964, the proliferation of newer-generation agents, with differing spectra, beta-lactamase stability, and properties, has been remarkable. Cephalosporins are the most widely prescribed antibiotic as a class, accounting for more than 50% of antibiotic sales. All cephalosporins have the four-membered beta-lactam ring bound to a six-membered dihydrothiazine ring. The cephalosporin nucleus is inherently more resistant to beta-lactamases than is the penicillin nucleus. Modification of position 7 of the beta-lactam ring alters beta-lactamase stability and antimicrobial activity. For example, the presence of an iminomethoxy group (e.g. cefuroxime, cefotaxime, ceftizoxime, ceftriaxone) confers enhanced beta-lactamase stability but loss of gram-positive activity. Ceftazidime has a prophylcarboxyl group at position 7, which results in superior activity against Pseudomonas aeruginosa but reduces antimicrobial activity against gram-positive agents. Cefoxitin and cefotetan (in which a methoxy group is substituted at position 7) are considered cephamycins rather than cephalosporins; the methoxy group confers resistance to gram-negative beta-lactamases (by steric hindrance) but also results in less affinity for PBPs. Substitutions at position 3 alter the pharmacokinetics without influencing antimicrobial activity; substitution at this position explains the long half-life of ceftriaxone.

Mechanism of Action: Cephalosporins bind to PBPs and interfere with bacterial cell wall (peptidoglycan) synthesis.

Antimicrobial Spectrum: Cephalosporins have broad-spectrum activity against both gram-negative and gram-positive bacteria. Gram-positive activity (particularly against staphylococci) is best with cefazolin and modest with succeeding generations; ceftazidime has poor activity. Adequate against most streptococci (including Streptococcus pneumoniae), but generally less active than penicillins; ceftazidime is least active. Anaerobic activity is modest (only cefoxitin, cefotetan, and moxalactam) and less than that of penicillins. Cephalosporins are active against beta–lactamase-producing Bacteroides fragilis. First-generation cephalosporins have marginal activity against Hemophilus influenzae; the second-generation cephalosporins (cefoxitin and cefotetan) have modest activity. Cefamandole is active only against ampicillin-susceptible strains. Cefuroxime and all third-generation agents are highly active. Activity against enteric GNB improves with each succeeding generation (particularly against Enterobacteriaceae). First-generation cephalosporins are active against most strains of Escherichia coli, Proteus mirabilis, and Klebsiella pneumoniae, but do not typically cover Enterobacter, Citrobacter, Serratia, Providencia, Proteus vulgaris, and Morganella spp. These species are variably sensitive to cefuroxime, cefotetan, and cefoxitin; most are inhibited by third-generation agents. Only ceftazidime and cefoperazone have significant activity against Pseudomonas aeruginosa. Acinetobacter calcoaceticus is usually resistant to all cephalosporins, although some strains are susceptible to ceftazidime. None of the cephalosporins is active against enterococci, MRSA, chlamydia, mycoplasma, or Legionella spp.

Toxicity: Adverse effects include hypersensitivity reactions, fever, rash (1 to 5%), nonspecific gastrointestinal symptoms (5 to 10%). The presence of methylthiotetrazole group in position 3 with cefamandole, cefotetan, cefoperazone, and moxalactam is associated with hypoprothrombinemia. Only moxalactam has been associated with significant risk of clinical bleeding.

First-Generation Cephalosporins

The first-generation cephalosporins for parenteral use include cephalothin (Keflin), cephapirin (Cefadyl), Cephradine (Velosef), and cefazolin (Ancef, Kefzol). Only cefazolin is currently used. Cefazolin has limited activity against Hemophilus influenzae, and its activity against Enterobacteriaceae (including Klebsiella pneumoniae and Escherichia coli) is inconsistent. The spectrum of oral cephalexin (Keflex) is similarly narrow. First-generation cephalosporins are not recommended for empiric treatment of either community- or hospital-acquired pneumonia. Cefazolin should be restricted to uncomplicated pneumonias caused by an organism that is highly susceptible to this agent.

Dosage: 1 g q 8 h.

Second-Generation Cephalosporins

These agents include cefuroxime (Zinacef, Cefurox), cefamandole (Mandol), cefonicid (Monocid), cefoxitin (Mefoxin), and cefotetan (Cefotan) for parenteral use; cefaclor (Ceclor) and cefuroxime axetil (Ceftin) are available for oral administration. Cefamandole is no longer used, and cefoxitin has largely been replaced by cefotetan, except for antimicrobial surgical prophylaxis.

Antimicrobial Spectrum: Second-generation cephalosporins have broader activity against gram-negative bacteria (including most Escherichia coli, Klebsiella, Proteus spp, and Hemophilus influenzae) compared to that of first-generation agents. Activity against staphylococci is modest, but is excellent against Streptococcus pneumoniae and most streptococci (other than enterococci).

Cefuroxime
(Zinacef, Cefurox)

Cefuroxime, a broad-spectrum agent with excellent activity against common respiratory pathogens, has supplanted cefamandole as the cephalosporin of choice for empiric treatment of CAP. Several features favor the use of cefuroxime over cefamandole: greater beta-lactamase stability; the lack of the methylthiotetrazole side chain, which has been associated with prolongation of prothrombin time and risk of bleeding; superior central nervous system (CNS) penetration; slightly longer half-life (q8h vs q6h dosing).

Antimicrobial Spectrum: Active against Streptococcus pneumoniae, Staphylococcus aureus, Hemophilus influenzae, Klebsiella pneumoniae, and oral anaerobes.

Dosage: 0.75 to 1.5 g IV q8h; can switch to oral formulation, cefuroxime axetil (Ceftin) after an initial response to parenteral cefuroxime.

Indications: Cefuroxime is excellent for empiric therapy of CAP in adults, including in elderly patients and patients with underlying disease. Cefuroxime has excellent CNS penetration. Cefuroxime is not recommended for nosocomial pneumonia (unless a susceptible pathogen is identified) because alternative agents (third-generation cephalosporins, antipseudomonal penicillins, imipenem) have broader activity against gram-negative bacteria.

Cefuroxime axetil (Ceftin) for oral use is more active than cefaclor against Moraxella catarrhalis and Hemophilus influenzae and is an ideal agent for completing a course of therapy after an initial brief course of IV cefuroxime (dose of cefuroxime axetil is 500 mg bid).

Cefonicid
(Monocid)

Cefonicid may be comparable to cefuroxime but has been used sparingly for the treatment of lower respiratory tract infections. Few studies have evaluated cefonicid in this context. The antimicrobial activity of cefonicid is no greater than that of cefuroxime. Ceftriaxone (a third-generation cephalosporin that has greater gram-negative activity) can also be dosed once daily. Thus, there is little advantage of cefonicid over cefuroxime or ceftriaxone, agents that have been widely used for empiric therapy of CAP. Neither cefuroxime nor cefonicid has any role in nosocomial pneumonias.

Antimicrobial Spectrum: Similar to that of cefuroxime, but slightly less active than cefuroxime against staphylococci, Hemophilus influenzae, and Enterobacteriaceae.

Dosage: 1 to 2 g IV/IM q24h.

Cefotetan
(Cefotan)

Cefotetan, a cephamycin, has superior anaerobic activity as compared to that of other cephalosporins, but has less activity against Hemophilus influenzae. Cefotetan is particularly suited for aspiration pneumonias or polymicrobial infections involving anaerobes and enteric GNB.

Antimicrobial Spectrum: Superior anaerobic activity (including beta–lactamase-producing Bacteroides fragilis); less activity against Hemophilus influenzae as compared to that of cefuroxime.

Toxicity: Has methylthiotetrazole side chain; theoretic risk for bleeding (low).

Dosage: 1 to 2 g q12h.

Indications:

• Empiric therapy of community-acquired or nursing–home-acquired pneumonias in alcoholic patients, patients with esophageal disease, or patients in whom aspiration is suspected (particularly when polymicrobial anaerobic/gram-negative bacillary infections are a consideration)

Third-Generation Cephalosporins

Within this group, cefotaxime (Claforan), ceftizoxime (Cefizox), and ceftriaxone (Rochephin) have similar antimicrobial spectra and may be therapeutically equivalent. The activity of cefotaxime may be slightly greater against Staphylococcus aureus as compared to that of the other agents; none is active against Pseudomonas aeruginosa. Ceftazidime (Fortaz, Tazidime, Tazicef) and cefoperazone (Cefobid) are the only cephalosporins with significant activity against P. aeruginosa; however, these agents have inferior activity against anaerobes, Staphylococcus aureus, and gram-positive bacteria compared to that of cefotaxime, ceftizoxime, and ceftriaxone. Moxalactum is no longer used because of bleeding complications associated with its use.

Antimicrobial Spectrum: Third-generation cephalosporins extend the gram-negative spectrum of second-generation agents to include Serratia, Morganella morganii, Providencia spp, and Citrobacter spp in addition to Escherichia coli, Klebsiella spp, and Proteus mirabilis. Despite widespread use over the past decade, the activity of third-generation cephalosporins against Escherichia coli, Klebsiella spp (K. pneumoniae, K. oxytoca), Proteus spp, Serratia, Hemophilus spp, Neisseria, and Providencia has remained excellent (> 95% susceptible). All the third-generation agents are extremely active against Hemophilus influenzae and other Hemophilus spp, such as H. parainfluenzae, including beta–lactamase-producing isolates. Some strains (10 to 20%) of Citrobacter freundi are resistant. Enterobacter spp (E. cloacae, E. aerogenes) are a major weakness; 20 to 40% of strains produce beta-lactamases that hydrolyze cephalosporins. The prevalence of resistant strains of Enterobacter spp has increased dramatically within the past decade, particularly in centers in which use of third-generation cephalosporins is high. Among the cephalosporins, only ceftazidime and cefoperazone have significant activity against Pseudomonas aeruginosa. Activity against Pseudomonas cepacia is variable; some strains are inhibited by ceftazidime, but most are resistant to other agents. Xanthomonas maltophilia is generally resistant. Activity against Acinetobacter spp is variable; usually certizoxime, ceftriaxone, and cefoperazone exhibit poor activity; some strains are susceptible to cefotaxime or ceftazidime. Third-generation cephalosporins are highly active against Moraxella catarrhalis. Gram-positive activity is variable; cefotaxime (and its diacetyl metabolite) is the most active; ceftazidime is the least active. Cefotaxime, certozoxime, and ceftriaxone are highly active against streptococci, including Streptococcus pneumoniae, S. pyogens, hemolytic streptococci, S. mutans, S. milleri, S. sanguis, S. mitis, S. bovis, and the viridans group of streptococci). These agents are also moderately active against methicillin-sensitive Staphylococcus aureus; ceftazidime and moxalactum exhibit fair to poor activity. MRSA and enterococci (Streptococcus faecalis, S. faecium) are invariably resistant to cephalosporins (irrespective of in vitro susceptibility testing). Anaerobic activity of third-generation cephalosporins is fair. The activity is modest against mouth anaerobes (peptococci, peptostreptococci, Bacteroides melaninogenicus), but is fair to poor against the B. fragilis group. Moxalactum and ceftizoxime are the most active agents in this class; ceftazidime is the least active.

Cefotaxime
(Claforan)

Cefotaxime is an excellent agent for empiric therapy of nosocomial pneumonias because of its broad-spectrum activity, low toxicity, and relatively low cost compared to that of other third-generation cephalosporins. Its lack of activity against Pseudomonas aeruginosa makes it less than ideal for treatment of ICU-acquired pneumonias unless this pathogen has been excluded.

Antimicrobial Spectrum: Broad-spectrum antimicrobial activity comparable to that of ceftriaxone and ceftizoxime; cefotaxime's activity against Staphylococcus aureus may be superior to that of these agents.

Distinguishing Features: The desacetyl metabolite of cefotaxime (desaccetylcefotaxime) has excellent antimicrobial activity similar to that of the parent compound, but has a longer half-life and confers improved activity against staphylococci (including Staphylococcus epidermidis). It is synergistic with cefotaxime against susceptible strains of Enterobacteriaceae. Cefotaxime, ceftriaxone, and ceftizoxime penetrate well into the cerebrospinal fluid (CSF) and can be used to treat meningitis.

Dosage: 1 to 2 g IV q8h.

Indications:

- Cefotaxime, however, is an excellent empiric agent for nosocomial pneumonia arising outside the ICU when Pseudomonas aeruginosa is not a major consideration and is acceptable treatment for documented pneumonia caused by Escherichia coli, Klebsiella, Proteus, Serratia, Hemophilus influenzae, and other susceptible organisms

Because of its inadequate activity against P. aeruginosa, cefotaxime (or ceftriaxone or ceftizoxime) are not recommended for empiric treatment of pneumonia in mechanically ventilated patients suffering from complications and residing in ICUs.

Ceftriaxone
(Rocephin)

Because of its broad-spectrum antimicrobial activity and prolonged half-life, which permits once-daily dosing, ceftriaxone is one of the most widely used antibiotics, both in the community and nosocomial setting.

Antimicrobial Spectrum: Similar to that of cefotaxime and ceftizoxime.

Toxicity: Ceftriaxone is primarily eliminated by the biliary system. Compared to other cephalosporins, ceftriaxone causes slightly increased gastrointestinal symptoms and diarrhea. High concentrations in bile may lead to biliary sludge (biliary pseudolithiasis) and symptoms resembling cholelithiasis.

Dosage: 1 to 2 g q24h (q12h dosing is not recommended, because any cost advantage achieved with once-daily dosing is negated by more frequent administration; cefotaxime or ceftizoxime is less expensive when administered in a comparable dose q8h).

Distinguishing Features: The prolonged half-life of ceftriaxone allows once-daily dosing; 90% protein binding as compared to 15 to 35% for ceftizoxime and cefotaxime. Ceftriaxone has excellent penetration into the CSF, as does cefotaxime and ceftizoxime.

Indications:

- The antimicrobial spectrum of ceftriaxone is exceptionally broad, and thus, this agent may be useful in the empiric therapy of community- or hospital-acquired pneumonias. Because of its prolonged half-life, which permits once-daily dosing, ceftriaxone may be used as initial therapy for CAP in nursing homes or in patients with underlying diseases because coverage is excellent against Streptococcus pneumoniae, most Enterobacteriaceae, and Hemophilus influenzae. Intramuscularly administered ceftriaxone (1 g q24 h) may permit outpatient administration in the clinic or emergency department, with follow-up doses at 24 hr. Subsequent therapy can be converted to an oral agent once clinical improvement has occurred. This strategy may limit the need for hospitalization among patients deemed to require parenteral antibiotic therapy

- Ceftriaxone may be useful in the nosocomial setting as well, but its lack of significant activity against Pseudomonas aeruginosa makes this agent less appropriate for treatment of ICU-acquired pneumonia

Cefoperazone
(Cefobid)

Cefoperazone has broad-spectrum antimicrobial activity and is the only cephalosporin other than ceftazidime to have excellent activity against Pseudomonas aeruginosa. Cefoperazone has been successfully used as empiric therapy for nosocomial pneumonia. Significant gaps in the spectrum exist, however. Cefoperazone is less consistently active against common GNB, such as Escherichia coli and Klebsiella, as compared to cefotaxime, ceftriaxone, and ceftizoxime, and its activity against Pseudomonas aeruginosa is less than that of ceftazidime. Thus, we rarely use cefoperazone, and prefer these other agents (the specific choice depends on suspected or confirmed organisms).

Antimicrobial Spectrum: Excellent activity against P. aeruginosa (greater than that of either ceftriaxone or ceftizoxime but less than that of ceftazidime); less consistent activity against some Enterobacteriaceae, including Escherichia coli and Klebsiella spp, and less beta-lactamase stability compared to that of other third-generation cephalosporins. Modest activity against anaerobes and gram-positive bacilli (less than that of cefotaxime).

Toxicity: Contains methylthiotetrazole chain, and thus has potential for bleeding resulting from prothrombin deficiency.

Dosage: 1 to 2 g q8-12 h.

Distinguishing Features: Excreted primarily via biliary route (75%); 90% protein bound.

Ceftazidime
(Fortaz, Tazidime, Tazicef)

Ceftazidime is the most active cephalosporin against Pseudomonas aeruginosa and has excellent activity against most GNB. Its activity against gram-positive bacilli and anaerobes is less than that of other cephalosporins. This agent is most appropriate when P. aeruginosa is a consideration.

Antimicrobial Spectrum: Excellent activity against P. aeruginosa; comparable to other third-generation cephalosporins against Enterobacteriaceae and aerobic GNBs; least active of the cephalosporins against staphylococci, gram-positive cocci, and anaerobes.

Dosage: 1 to 2 g IV q8h.

Indications:

• Cornerstone of therapy for pneumonia when Pseudomonas aeruginosa is suspected or documented (e.g. in mechanically ventilated patients, patients in ICU, patients with cystic fibrosis or neutropenia)

When P. aeruginosa is not a prime consideration, less expensive third-generation cephalosporins (e.g. cefotaxime, ceftizoxime, or ceftriaxone) that have better gram-positive and anaerobic activity are preferable to ceftazidime. Ceftazidime has no role in the treatment of CAP (except in patients at risk for P. aeruginosa, such as patients with cystic fibrosis).

Moxalactum
(Moxam)

Moxalactum has an excellent antimicrobial spectrum and outstanding anaerobic activity; however, the presence of a thiomethyltetrazole group and carboxyl group may cause aberrations in prothrombin synthesis and platelet adhesiveness. Because severe bleeding diathesis may complicate its use, moxalactum is no longer used.

Cefixime
(Suprax)

Cefixime is the only third-generation cephalosporin that can be administered orally. Cefixime is more active than second-generation agents against enteric GNB, but has poor activity against staphylococci and anaerobes and fails to cover Pseudomonas spp. The role of this agent in the treatment of community-acquired and nosocomial pneumonias has not yet been established.

CARBAPENEMS

The carbapenems represent a new class of beta-lactams that differ from the penicillins by the substitution of a carbon atom for sulphur at position 1 and an unsaturated bond between carbon atoms 2 and 3 in the 5-membered ring. Carbapenems also have unique side chains that confer remarkable resistance to a variety of beta-lactamases and provide antipseudomonal activity.

Imipenem/Cilastatin
(Primaxin)

The only carbapenem currently in clinical use is the N-formimidoly derivative of thienamycin (imipenem). Because imipenem is not stable to renal dedrogenases and its degradation products may be nephrotoxic, imipenem is administered with a fixed combination of the dehydropeptidase inhibitor, cilastin.

Antimicrobial Spectrum: Imipenem has the broadest spectrum of activity among all beta-lactams. Imipenem is active against most GNB, including multiply resistant Pseudomonas aeruginosa, Serratia spp, and Acinetobacter spp, but Pseudomonas cepacia and Xanthomonas maltophilia are nearly invariably resistant. Imipenem is highly active against gram-positive cocci (including both methicillin-sensitive and MRSA strains); however, the MIC90 for MRSA isolates may be 8 to 400 times the MIC90 for susceptible strains, and vancomycin is preferred for MRSA. The activity of imipenem against Streptococcus faecium and methicillin-resistant Staphylococcus epidermidis is inconsistent; anaerobic activity (including Bacteroides fragilis species) is outstanding.

Toxicity: Imipenem may induce seizures. Although the risk of seizures is low ($<$ 0.5%) among patients with normal renal function and no underlying neurologic disease, considerably higher rates of seizures (10 to 20%) have been noted among patients with renal failure who are receiving conventional dosages or who have underlying CNS disease. In this context, imipenem is not recommended. Superinfection or colonization with Xanthomonas maltophilia or Pseudomonas cepacia may complicate therapy.

Dosage: 0.5 to 1.0 IV q8h. In view of the exquisite sensitivity of most organisms to imipenem. Initiate therapy at 500 mg q8h, and reserve higher doses (to a maximum of 1,000 mg q6h) for serious infections caused by Pseudomonas aeruginosa or pathogens with a relatively high MIC.

Distinguishing Features: The extraordinarily broad antimicrobial spectrum of imipenem may relate to its ability to penetrate well through the outer cell envelope of GNB, its high affinity for PBP targets, and its resistance to a wide variety of beta-lactamases. Imipenem is not hydrolyzed by penicillinases or cephalosporinases, which degrade penicillins, third-generation cephalosporins, and aztreonam. Concerns have been raised about the unrestricted use of imipenem/cilastin. Imipenem is a powerful inducer of chromosomally mediated beta-lactamases in Enterobacter, Pseudomonas aeruginosa, and other strains, which interestingly do not alter the activity of imipenem against these bacteria; these may, however, hydrolyze other beta-lactams. Although resistant Enterobacteriaceae have been infrequent, even with extensive use of imipenem, resistance to Pseudomonas aeruginosa developed in as many as 25% of patients when imipenem was used as monotherapy.

Indications:

- Because of its remarkably broad antimicrobial spectrum, imipenem may be useful as empiric therapy for severe nosocomial pneumonias
- Particular utility in patients with pneumonias and complications in whom regimens have failed or in patients in whom antimicrobial resistance to more conventional beta-lactams is likely

Because of its expense, CNS toxicity, and potential for selection of resistant organisms, imipenem is not indicated for CAP or uncomplicated nosocomial infections susceptible to other beta-lactams.

Meropenem

Meropenem is a new carbapenem currently being evaluated in clinical trials in the United States, and has an extraordinarily broad spectrum of activity. Meropenem appears to be slightly less active than imipenem against gram-positive organisms but may be slightly more active against gram-negative organisms; anaerobic activity is comparable. As with imipenem, Xanthomonas maltophilia is usually resistant. Meropenem may have some advantages over imipenem, e.g. meropenem carries no definite risk of seizures, induction of beta-lactamases is less with meropenem; and meropenem is stable to human renal dehydropeptidases and thus does not require the concomitant administration of an enzyme inhibitor.

MONOBACTAMS

Aztreonam
(Azactam)

Aztreonam is the first of a generation of monobactams within the beta-lactam group. Elimination of the second carbon ring leaves the beta-lactam ring as a monocyclic compound. Although aztreonam is a beta-lactam, the cleavage of the second member of the beta-lactam ring makes this agent structurally dissimilar from other beta-lactams, such as penicillin, cephalosporins, and imipenem/cilastin. Thus, aztreonam may be used safely in patients who are allergic to penicillins or cephalosporins because cross-reactivity with these agents does not occur.

Antimicrobial Spectrum: Aztreonam is highly active against aerobic GNB, including most strains of P. aeruginosa, and is stable against beta-lactamases; however, aztreonam has no significant activity against gram-positive organisms or anaerobes. Aztreonam may provide synergy with aminoglycosides; also, synergy may be achieved with aztreonam and other beta-lactams in more than 40% of isolates.

Toxicity: Uncommon (< 1% rash, < 2% serious diarrhea).

Dosage: 1 to 2 g q8h (lower doses of 1 g q12h may be adequate provided the organism is susceptible with a low MIC (< 1 µg/L). Dosage must be reduced in the presence of impaired renal function.

Indications: Aztreonam has a greater role in nosocomial infections in which aerobic GNB are suspected or documented, and, in combination with agents with gram-positive activity, such as clindamycin, vancomycin, or a beta-lactam, provides exceptional broad-spectrum activity, however, as empiric therapy for serious nosocomial pneumonia. The use of aztreonam may eliminate the need for an aminoglycoside in this context. Aztreonam has minimal activity against common pathogens implicated in bronchitis and CAP, such as Streptococcus pneumoniae and Moraxella catarrhalis, and should not be used as empiric therapy in these conditions. Because of its narrow spectrum and high rate of superinfections with gram-positive organisms, aztreonam is not recommended as monotherapy for pneumonia.

AMINOGLYCOSIDES

Aminoglycosides currently used in the United States include gentamicin (Garamycin), tobramycin (Nebcin), and amikacin (Amikin). The use of aminoglycosides in the treatment of pneumonia is controversial. Several factors argue against the use of these agents: their high toxicity (nephrotoxicity/ototoxicity); their low penetration into bronchial secretions and lung tissue; their inactivation at low pH (conditions that may prevail in infected lung parenchyma); and the availability of alternative broad-spectrum agents with gram-negative activity and less toxicity (e.g. beta-lactams, quinolones). Despite these arguments, aminoglycosides may be useful as adjunctive therapy (combined with a broad-spectrum antimicrobial agent, such as beta-lactams or quinolones), primarily to achieve synergistic killing.

Antimicrobial Spectrum: Exceptionally broad spectrum against aerobic GNB; no significant activity against anaerobes. May confer synergistic killing against certain gram-positive organisms, such as enterococci and staphylococci, in combination with beta-lactams.

Toxicity: Nephrotoxicity and ototoxicity are most important. Synergistic toxicity may occur when aminoglycoside is combined with other nephrotoxic agents, such as vancomycin. Risk factors associated with enhanced nephrotoxicity include old age, prior aminoglycoside use, and pre-existing renal disease. The toxicity of tobramycin and gentamicin are comparable; both agents may be slightly more nephrotoxic than amikacin and netilmicin. Netilmicin shows the least ototoxicity. Peak and trough serum levels are mandatory to limit toxicity. Peak levels exceeding 6 μg/ml are required for optimal microbiocidal activity; however, trough levels greater than 2 μg/ml (2 mg/l) correlate with excessive toxicity.

Dosage: 3 to 5 mg/kg/day IV, or IM in divided doses q8h for gentamicin/tobramycin; 15 mg/kg/day for amikacin. (Two- to three-fold higher doses are required in patients with cystic fibrosis because of the rapid clearance of aminoglycosides in this patient population.) Dose adjustment may be required (need peak and trough serum levels).

Novel dosing regimens of aminoglycosides have recently been suggested. In animals, a single large daily dose of aminoglycoside has been associated with comparable or improved clinical efficacy and less nephrotoxicity and ototoxicity as compared to equivalent dosages given in multiple doses throughout the day. Higher serum levels are achieved with single daily dosing, thus suggesting that bactericidal activity may be enhanced.

Single dosing would be cost-saving, because less pharmacy and nursing time would be required. Single-dose regimens, however, have not been studied in humans; thus, the safety and efficacy of this practice have not been established.

Nebulized Administration: Klastersky, et al. in Europe have suggested that nebulized or intratracheal aminoglycosides may improve outcome for the therapy of gram-negative lower respiratory infections. Despite extensive use of nebulized aminoglycosides for Pseudomonas infections in patients with cystic fibrosis and for nosocomial gram-negative pneumonia, no solid data affirm the efficacy of this practice. In 1990, Brown and colleagues reported the results of a double-blind randomized trial of intratracheal tobramycin (40 mg q8h) versus placebo in the treatment of gram-negative bacillary pneumonia; conventional parenteral antibiotics with beta-lactam and aminoglycoside were administered concomitantly. Despite a higher rate of eradication of gram-negative organisms from sputum in the group receiving intratracheal tobramycin, no differences in clinical improvement or survival were found between groups. Thus, we do not believe that nebulized or intratracheal aminoglycosides offer any significant advantages for the treatment of gram-negative lower respiratory tract infections.

Special Considerations: Gentamicin is considerably less expensive than other agents in this class, yet is generally comparable in efficacy and toxicity. Thus, gentamicin is the preferred aminoglycoside for empiric treatment, unless high rates of gentamicin resistance are suspected or confirmed in the institution. Tobramycin and gentamicin are equivalent for most bacteria; MICs may be slightly lower for tobramycin than for gentamicin for Pseudomonas aeruginosa. Gentamicin provides superior killing against enterococci and Staphylococcus aureus when compared to that of tobramycin. The clinical importance of these in vitro differences is not clear. The cost savings associated with gentamicin (approximately $20/day less than tobramycin, $100/day less than amikacin) is substantial. Amikacin is exceptionally expensive and should be reserved for cases in which resistance to tobramycin/gentamicin has been demonstrated or strongly suspected.

Indications: Aminoglycosides are inadequate as single agents for pulmonary infections. The addition of an aminoglycoside to a broad-spectrum antimicrobial should be considered in the following circumstances to provide synergistic killing:

- As initial empiric therapy for serious sepsis or nosocomial pneumonias caused by suspected or proven gram-negative enteric bacteria
- Pneumonia caused by highly virulent pathogens, such as Pseudomonas spp, Enterobacter spp, Serratia, and Acinetobacter spp; continue aminoglycoside for duration of therapy
- Infections caused by enterococci (combine with penicillin or vancomycin)

MACROLIDES

The macrolides represent a class of antimicrobials characterized by sub-stituted 14-, 15-, or 16-member rings; macrolides penetrate into tissues better than do beta-lactams. Erythromycin (a 14-member macrolide) has been the only antibiotic of this class in clinical use in the United States for the past 2 decades. Several newer 14-member macrolides with a spectrum of activity similar to that of erythromycin but with more resistance to acid hydrolysis have been synthesized; these include roxithromycin, chlarith-romycin, dirithromycin, erythromycylamine, and flurithromycin. Chlar-ithromycin (Biaxin) is the only one of these newer macrolides currently available in the United States.

ERYTHROMYCIN

Erythromycin, a macrolide antibiotic first isolated in 1952, is active against Streptococcus pneumoniae, Moraxella catarrhalis, mycoplasma, and Le-gionella spp, and has been used extensively for community-acquired bron-chitis and pneumonia. Penicillins and cephalosporins, however, have a much broader spectrum of activity and are the preferred agents for most CAP. Erythromycin is not consistently reliable against Hemophilus in-fluenzae, has no significant activity against GNB, and is less active than penicillins against streptococci, staphylococci, and anaerobes. Thus, eryth-romycin should be reserved primarily for CAP in young healthy adults who are at low risk for resistant pathogens or in patients in whom My-coplasma, Chlamydia, or Legionella spp are suspected.

Mechanism of Action: Interferes with microbial protein synthesis at the ribosomal level (binds to 50S ribosome subunit).

Antimicrobial Spectrum: Effective against Streptococcus pneumoniae, other streptococci (except enterococcus), and Moraxella catarrhalis; not re-liable against Staphylococcus aureus or S. epidermidis (10 to 40% of strains are resistant). Only 40 to 70% of Hemophilus influenzae are susceptible. Anaerobic coverage is modest (10 to 20% of oral anaerobes and 30 to 40% of Bacteroides fragilis are resistant). No significant gram-negative activity. Excellent against Legionella and Mycoplasma spp; less active than tetra-cyclines against Chlamydia spp.

Toxicity: Gastrointestinal side effects (principally nausea, epigastric distress, diarrhea, and vomiting) are common (> 20%) and limit its use-fulness. IV erythromycin is intensely irritating to veins and may cause phlebitis. Hepatotoxicity (cholestatic hepatitis) is a rare complication (pri-marily with the estolate form) that usually resolves with cessation of ther-apy.

Dosage: 500 to 1,000 mg q6h IV; 250 to 500 mg q6h orally. The active component is the erythromycin base. Oral forms include an acid-resistant enteric coated tablet, erythromycin stearate (a salt), erythromycin ethylsuccinate (an ester), and erythromycin estolate (an ester salt). These salts and esters confer more stability against gastric acids than does the parent compound. Erythromycin lactobionate and erythromycin gluceptate are available for IV use. Oral absorption is not consistently reliable. IV administration is recommended as initial therapy for serious infections (e.g. Legionella spp); oral therapy may be substituted once a clinical response has occurred.

Indications: Erythromycin provides excellent coverage against common pathogens acquired in the community, including Streptococcus pneumoniae, Legionella, Chlamydia, and Mycoplasma spp and may be used as first-line therapy among young, previously healthy adults with CAP in whom potentially resistant pathogens, such as Staphylococcus aureus and enteric GNB, are rarely problematic. In view of its limited spectrum of activity against GNB and marginal activity against Hemophilus influenzae, however, erythromycin is not adequate as monotherapy for CAP in patients at risk for infections with these pathogens (e.g. age over 55, ethanol abuse, cigarette smoking, or any pre-existing underlying disease). Erythromycin has no role in the treatment of nosocomial pneumonias, except as adjunctive therapy when Legionella spp are suspected.

NEWER MACROLIDES

CHLARITHROMYCIN
(Biaxin)

Chlarithromycin (Biaxin) is the first of the newer macrolides to be introduced into the United States. Chlarithromycin retains the antimicrobial activity of erythromycin, but also extends its spectrum to include Hemophilus influenzae and some Enterobacteriaceae. Chlarithromycin is as effective as cefaclor (Ceclor), cefuroxime axetil (Ceftin), and cefixime (Suprax) for mild to moderate lower respiratory tract infections (bronchitis, pneumonia).

Toxicity: Much less than erythromycin; significant gastrointestinal symptoms complicate its use in only 3 to 6% of cases.

Dosage: 250 to 500 mg b.i.d. for 7 to 14 days.

AZALIDES

The addition of a nitrogen atom to the macrolide ring (resulting in a 15-member ring) results in compounds (azalides) that are far more resistant to acid hydrolysis than is erythromycin (or other macrolides). Azalides have greater penetration into tissues, a larger volume of distribution, and a longer half-life (> 2 days) compared to such characteristics of macrolides, beta-lactams, or quinolone antibiotics. Azithromycin is the first azalide to be developed for clinical use, although several other agents are currently being studied.

Azithromycin
(Zithromax)

Azithromycin is a promising agent that extends the spectrum of erythromycin to cover Hemophilus influenzae and some Enterobacteriaceae and has few side effects. Azithromycin has only recently become available in the United States and additional studies are required to determine its position for empiric therapy of CAP.

Mechanism of Action: Inhibits protein synthesis at 50S ribosomal level.

Antimicrobial Spectrum: Azithromycin is highly active (comparable to erythromycin) against Chlamydia, Mycoplasma, and Legionella spp. It is bactericidal against Streptococcus pneumoniae and erythromycin-sensitive strains of streptococci and staphylococci, but is less active than erythromycin against these organisms. Azithromycin has no activity against erythromycin-resistant strains of streptococci or staphylococci; MRSA and enterococci are usually resistant. Activity against anaerobes is slightly superior to that of erythromycin. Most oral anaerobes, such as peptococci, peptostreptococci, and Bacteroides melaninogenicus, are readily inhibited; activity against Bacteroides fragilis is marginal. Azithromycin is much more active against GNB than are the 14–member-ring macrolides. Azithromycin is bactericidal against Hemophilus influenzae, Neisseria spp, and Moraxella catarrhalis. Activity against Enterobacteriaceae is inconsistent, but some strains of Escherichia coli, Klebsiella, Enterobacter, and Citrobacter spp are susceptible. Most isolates of Serratia or Acinetobacter spp are resistant; activity is insignificant against Pseudomonas spp or Xanthomonas maltophilia.

Toxicity: Minor, primarily gastrointestinal.

Dosage: 500 mg initial dose, then 250 mg once daily for 2 to 5 days.

Distinguishing Features: Azithromycin is more acid stable, and better absorbed following oral administration than is erythromycin. It also has a much longer biologic half-life. A unique property of azithromycin is its ability to be concentrated in phagocytes and within tissues; phagocytes continue to concentrate azithromycin intracellularly for as many as 24 hours. The preferential distribution of the drug in tissues and its slow release result in high concentrations of active drug at sites of infection for prolonged periods despite low serum concentrations. Levels of azithromycin in sputum, bronchial mucosa, and alveolar macrophages may exceed the MIC for most common respiratory pathogens for 2 to 4 days following a single 500-mg oral dose.

Indications:

- In view of its excellent activity against common respiratory pathogens (Streptococcus pneumoniae, Hemophilus influenzae, Moraxella catarrhalis, chlamydia, mycoplasma, legionella), prolonged half-life (permitting once-daily dosing), and low incidence of side effects, azithromycin may be a logical agent for CAP among nonimmunocompromised hosts in whom the risk of serious gram-negative pathogens is low. Data evaluating azithromycin for moderately severe or severe pneumonias are limited. Studies in Europe and the United States, however, have shown oral azithromycin to be superior or equivalent to amoxicillin or cefaclor for the treatment of sinus and lower respiratory tract (primarily bronchitis) infections

The role of azithromycin as empiric therapy for CAP in moderately ill patients at risk for gram-negative pathogens (e.g. patients with ethanol abuse, diabetes mellitus, age > 65 years, residence in chronic care facility, COPD, and serious underlying diseases) needs to be studied. Currently, cefuroxime or ceftriaxone are preferred in this context. Azithromycin is not appropriate treatment for nosocomial pneumonia.

TETRACYCLINES

Tetracyclines, derived from Streptomyces spp, were isolated in the early 1950s. Substitutions on the hydronaphthacene four-ringed nucleus differentiate the derivatives tetracycline hydrochloride, oxytetracycline, chlortetracycline, doxycycline, and minocycline. Tetracyclines (particularly doxycycline) are inexpensive and relatively effective agents for uncomplicated bronchitis, but have a limited role as therapeutic agents for pneumonia.

Mechanism of Action: Bind to 30S subunit of bacterial ribosomes.

Antimicrobial Spectrum: Tetracyclines are active against Streptococcus pneumoniae; modest against other Streptococcus spp; generally not adequate for Staphylococcus aureus or enterococci. Anaerobic activity is modest (Bacteroides fragilis spp are resistant); marginal against Hemophilus influenzae; not active against most enteric GNB; drug of choice for Chlamydia and Rickettsiae spp; acceptable for Mycoplasma and Legionella spp.

Toxicity: Gastrointestinal (nausea, emesis, GI distress) common; photosensitivity (doxycycline or minocycline); discoloration of teeth or depression of bone growth in infants and children; vertigo. Outdated tetracyclines may cause renal tubular acidosis. Fatal hepatotoxicity has been described, but is rare.

Dosage: 250 to 500 mg orally qid for tetracycline, oxytetracycline, and chlortetracycline; doxycycline and minocycline 100 mg bid (oral or IV). Food binds the drug and impairs absorption; tetracyclines need to be taken on empty stomach. This effect is less problematic with doxycycline and minocycline.

Distinguishing Features: Doxycycline (Vibramycin) has a prolonged half-life (permitting twice-daily dosing) and is less affected by food; activity is as good as that of other tetracyclines, and is the preferred agent.

Indications: Tetracyclines are the drug of choice for pulmonary infections caused by Chlamydia and Mycoplasma spp and are acceptable alternatives to erythromycin for legionella infections.

Tetracyclines are active against Streptococcus pneumoniae, but significant gaps in the spectrum (including inconsistent activity against Hemophilus influenzae) make these agents unsuitable for CAP except in young, previously healthy adults in whom atypical pneumonia is a major consideration. Except for nosocomial legionellosis, tetracyclines have no role for nosocomial pneumonia.

FLUOROQUINOLONES

Fluoroquinolones are derivatives of nalidixic acid and include enoxacin, perfloxacin, ofloxacin, ciprofloxacin, and norfloxacin. Currently, only four fluoroquinolones are available in the United States: ciprofloxacin (Cipro); norfloxacin (Noroxin), ofloxacin (Floxin) and temafloxacin (Omniflox). Norfloxacin is recommended only for urinary sepsis, whereas both ciprofloxacin and ofloxacin may have important roles in the treatment of lower respiratory tract infections, including serious gram-negative bacillary pneumonias. Temafloxacin (Omniflox) has less consistent activity against P. aeruginosa than ciprofloxacin or ofloxacin but has enhanced activity against anaerobes and S. pneumoniae.

Antimicrobial Spectrum: Excellent potency against aerobic GNB, including most Enterobacteriaceae, Hemophilus influenzae, Neisseria spp, Moraxella catarrhalis, and Pseudomonas aeruginosa; less active against P. cepacia or Xanthomonas maltophilia. Good activity against Staphylococcus aureus and S. epidermidis, but less active against streptococci (including Streptococcus pneumoniae). Minimal activity against anaerobes. (Note: Temafloxacin has good activity against anaerobes).

Distinguishing Features: These fluoroquinolones (with the exception of norfloxacin) exceed most other antibiotics in their ability to penetrate into the lower respiratory tract. Ciprofloxacin, ofloxacin, and temafloxacin penetrate into the bronchial lining and achieve high concentrations in the lung, bronchial mucosa, and sputum; concentrations in the lung typically exceed serum concentrations. The concentration of quinolones in macrophages and polymorphonuclear leukocytes may enhance clinical efficacy.

Mechanism of Action of Quinolones: Antagonizes bacterial DNA gyrase (interferes with DNA replication).

Antimicrobial Resistance: Resistance to quinolones can be mediated by mutations affecting DNA gyrase or drug permeability, or both; plasmid-mediated resistance has not been observed. Spontaneous single-step mutations to quinolones are rare, but high-level resistance may develop by serial exposure of bacteria to increasing drug concentrations. Chromosomal mutations that alter DNA gyrase confer resistance to quinolones alone; a change in the bacterial outer membrane proteins confers resistance to multiple agents (including beta-lactams). Resistance to Pseudomonas aeruginosa may require multiple mutations, whereas a single-step mutation may be sufficient to induce resistance against Staphylococcus aureus. Importantly, alterations in outer membrane proteins (an important cause of resistance to quinolones) may confer resistance to structurally unrelated antibiotics, such as beta-lactams, aminoglycosides, and chloramphenicol. Cross-resistance to antibiotics outside the quinolone class, such as beta-lactams and aminoglycosides, has been associated with changes in outer membrane proteins of the mutated bacteria. This type of resistance is not unique to quinolones, however, because multiple drug resistances may occur in beta–lactam- or aminoglycoside-selected mutants.

CIPROFLOXACIN
(Cipro)

Ciprofloxacin was released in the United States in 1987 as the first oral antibiotic with activity against Pseudomonas aeruginosa. Ciprofloxacin immediately gained widespread popularity and by 1989 was the fourth most commonly prescribed antibiotic (more than 5 million prescriptions at a cost of $248 million). Ciprofloxacin has excellent activity against common respiratory pathogens implicated in CAP, such as Hemophilus influenzae, Moraxella catarrhalis, chlamydia, and legionella. Oral or IV ciprofloxacin has been associated with cure rates exceeding 80% in community-, nursing–home-, and hospital-acquired pneumonias. Significant gaps in the spectrum of ciprofloxacin exist however. Despite its excellent gram-negative activity, ciprofloxacin has only modest activity against Streptococcus pneumoniae, other gram-positive organisms, and anaerobes. Ciprofloxacin is less than optimal therapy for infections caused by S. pneumoniae. Thus, ciprofloxacin is not generally recommended as first-line therapy for CAP nor should ciprofloxacin be used for anaerobic or aspiration pneumonias. Intravenous ciprofloxacin appears comparable to broad-spectrum beta-lactams, including ceftazidime, for hospital-acquired pneumonias or sepsis in neutropenic patients, and may be suitable for suspected or documented gram-negative bacillary infections. Unrestricted use of ciprofloxacin, however, may lead to increasing antimicrobial resistance; thus, alternative agents (penicillins and cephalosporins) are preferred as first-line therapy.

Antimicrobial Spectrum: Exceptionally broad activity against aerobic gram negative organisms (including Pseudomonas aeruginosa, Hemophilus influenzae, and Enterobacteriaceae. Excellent against Staphylococcus aureus including MRSA. Marginal activity against Streptococcus pneumoniae and group A streptococci. Poor anaerobic activity. Excellent against chlamydia, Legionella spp, and Moraxella catarrhalis.

Toxicity: Uncommon; GI symptoms most common (3 to 6%); colitis rare. CNS effects (headache, dizziness, sleep disturbance) occur in 1 to 2%; rash, in 0.5 to 2%. Do not use in pregnancy, because fetal deaths and skeletal abnormalities have been noted in animals in utero.

Dosage: 200 to 400 mg IV q12h; oral, 500 to 750 mg bid.

Indications:

- Because oral bioavailability is excellent, oral ciprofloxacin may be adequate for nursing—home-acquired or hospital-acquired pneumonias provided the pathogen is susceptible and when S. pneumoniae has been reasonably excluded. More importantly, oral ciprofloxacin may be substituted in hospitalized patients receiving more expensive parenteral agents, such as beta-lactams, for documented infections caused by susceptible pathogens. The substitution of an effective oral agent may markedly reduce drug costs and shorten the hospital stay
- Intravenous ciprofloxacin IV (400 mg q12h) combined with an aminoglycoside is a reasonable option for the treatment of nosocomial pneumonia in patients unable to tolerate beta-lactams or with organisms resistant to beta-lactams. Antimicrobial resistance, particularly among Staphylococcus aureus and Pseudomonas aeruginosa, may develop quickly when ciprofloxacin is used alone. Thus, when ciprofloxacin is used for serious nosocomial pneumonias, P. aeruginosa infections, or sepsis in neutropenic patients, it is advisable to combine this agent with an aminoglycoside. Ciprofloxacin is not recommended as first-line empiric therapy for nosocomial pneumonia, because beta-lactams are usually efficacious

Ciprofloxacin is not suitable for infections caused by streptococci or anaerobes.

Antimicrobial Resistance: Although ciprofloxacin remains highly active against aerobic GNB, and has broad-spectrum activity, data from Europe suggest that increasing drug-resistant strains of Pseudomonas aeruginosa and Staphylococcus aureus have been associated with the liberal use of ciprofloxacin. Emergence of resistance may be particularly common for infections in which many organisms are present, such as in cystic fibrosis, or for infections in sequestered areas where tissue penetration of the antibiotic may be inadequate, such as osteomyelitis. Within 3 years of the introduction of the drug to the United States, 4 to 6% of strains of Pseudomonas aeruginosa and Staphylococcus aureus were resistant; higher rates of resistance (10 to 15%) have been observed in some institutions. In Japan, resistance to other GNB, including Serratia marcescens, has increased since the introduction of ciprofloxacin. This potential for rapid induction of antimicrobial resistance has led to concerns about using ciprofloxacin as first-line therapy. Whether combining ciprofloxacin with an additional antibiotic limits or reduces the emergence of resistance is not known; however, combination therapy appears ineffective in limiting resistance against Pseudomonas aeruginosa in patients with cystic fibrosis. Notwithstanding these concerns, ciprofloxacin remains an excellent drug, particularly for the treatment of gram-negative pneumonia with pathogens displaying broad resistance to other antimicrobials.

Ofloxacin
(Floxin)

Although limited data are available, ofloxacin represents an attractive agent for empiric treatment of CAP because its spectrum covers most common respiratory pathogens, including streptococci, staphylococci, Hemophilus influenzae, Enterobacteriaceae, Chlamydia, Mycoplasma, and Legionella. In a recent multicenter trial, Sanders and associates reported that oral ofloxacin (400 mg q12h) was as effective as parenteral antibiotic therapy (specific antimicrobial agents were selected by individual investigators) for patients hospitalized for CAP. Among 69 patients receiving oral ofloxacin, 56 were cured and 13 were improved. In that study, patients with neutropenia, rapidly fatal illnesses, or severe renal failure were excluded.

Antimicrobial Spectrum: Similar to that of ciprofloxacin. Excellent activity against Hemophilus influenzae (both ampicillin-sensitive and ampicillin-resistant strains), Neisseria, Escherichia coli, Moraxella catarrhalis, and most Enterobacteriaceae. Less active in vitro against Pseudomonas aeruginosa as compared to ciprofloxacin; studies in vivo in cystic fibrosis exacerbations suggest both agents may be comparable. Modest gram-positive activity; less active than penicillins against streptococci. Moderate activity against staphylococci (including Staphylococcus epidermidis and MRSA). Anaerobic activity fair to poor. Active against Chlamydia, Mycoplasma, and Legionella spp.

Toxicity: Similar to that of ciprofloxacin; few serious adverse effects. Unlike ciprofloxacin, no effect on theophylline.

Dosage: Oral 400 mg q12h (98% bioavailability); IV 400 mg q12h.

Antimicrobial Resistance: As with other fluoroquinolones, development of resistance, particularly by Pseudomonas aeruginosa and Staphylococcus aureus, may be problematic with ofloxacin. Susceptibility to ofloxacin, however, has been demonstrated in some strains exhibiting high-grade resistance to ciprofloxacin.

TEMAFLOXACIN
(Omniflox)

Temafloxacin (Omniflox), released for use in the United States in 1992, has been shown to be as effective as amoxicillin for lower respiratory tract infections and may be superior to the other fluoroquinolones for respiratory infections due to gram-positive or anaerobic organisms. Oral temafloxacin is almost completely absorbed, with greater than 90% bioavailability. A parenteral form is not available.

Antimicrobial Spectrum: Similar to ciprofloxacin and ofloxacin, but temafloxacin has less consistent activity against Pseudomonas aeruginosa and other GNB as compared to these agents. However, temafloxacin has superior activity against anaerobes and Streptococcus pneumoniae.

Toxicity: Similar to the other fluoroquinolones.

Dosage: 400 mg b.i.d. for bronchitis; 600 mg b.i.d. for pneumonia.

Indications: Because of its activity against anaerobes and S. pneumoniae, temafloxacin can be used for the treatment of mild to moderate community-acquired lower respiratory tract infections (pneumonia or bronchitis). Because the other fluoroquinolones have superior activity against P. aeruginosa, ciprofloxacin and ofloxacin are preferred in nosocomial settings.

OTHER AGENTS
CHLORAMPHENICOL
(Chloromycetin)

Chloramphenicol was an enormously popular antibiotic in the 1950s because of its broad-spectrum activity against anaerobes, gram-positive cocci, and selected GNB. The recognition, however, that aplastic anemia and the "grey baby syndrome" were complications arising from its use led to a dramatic decline in prescriptions for this agent in the 1960s. Currently, chloramphenicol should be restricted to infections resistant to alternative agents.

Mechanism of Action: Binds to 50S subunit of the 70S bacterial ribosome (blocks the attachment of aminotransfer RNA to the ribosomes).

Antimicrobial Spectrum: Broad-spectrum agent, but other antimicrobials preferred for common pathogens. Excellent activity against unusual pathogens that exhibit resistance to most antimicrobials (e.g. Rickettsieae, Pseudomonas pseudomallei, P. cepacia, and Salmonella typhi).

Toxicity: Aplastic anemia ($< 1:20,000$ cases); dose-related myelosuppression; hemolytic anemia; grey baby syndrome in infants; reversible neurologic dysfunction.

Dosage: 100 mg/kg orally or IV.

Indications: Chloramphenicol is rarely used unless alternative agents are contraindicated because of allergies or antimicrobial resistance (e.g. rickettsieae, Salmonella typhi, Pseudomonas cepacia, and some strains of P. pseudomallei).

TRIMETHOPRIM/SULFAMETHOXAZOLE
(Bactrim, Septra; Co-trimoxazole)

Trimethoprim/sulfamethoxazole (TMP/SMZ), formulated as a fixed ratio of 1:5 TMP/SMZ, was first introduced in the United States in 1973. TMP/SMZ has primarily been used for the treatment of opportunistic organisms (principally Pneumocystis carinii and Nocardia spp), but also has a wide spectrum of activity against gram-positive and gram-negative organisms. TMP/SMZ is equal to or superior to ampicillin for the treatment of acute and chronic bronchitis; even with prolonged use, emergence of resistance has been uncommon. Few studies have assessed TMP/SMZ as primary therapy for bacterial pneumonia.

Mechanism of Action: TMP and SMZ interfere with bacterial cell replication by inhibiting sequential enzymes involved in the formation of tetrahydrofolic acid. TMP inhibits dihydrofolate reductase; SMZ competitively inhibits synthesis of dihydrofolic acid from paraaminobenzoic acid. The inhibition of differing enzyme steps improves antimicrobial activity and confers synergistic killing.

Antimicrobial Spectrum: Active against more than 99% of Streptococcus pneumoniae and Moraxella catarrhalis; excellent activity against most gram-positive organisms, including streptococci and staphylococci (including MRSA); not adequate against group A streptococci or enterococci. Active against more than 80% of strains of Hemophilus influenzae (including ampicillin-resistant strains). Anaerobic activity is limited; most isolates, including Bacteroides spp, are susceptible in vitro, but clinical efficacy has not been established. TMP/SMX has excellent activity against Enterobacteriaceae, and emergence of resistance has been rare. Consistently high activity against Escherichia coli, Proteus mirabilis; active against most strains of P. vulgaris, Klebsiella, and Serratia spp; Pseudomonas aeruginosa is usually resistant. TMP/SMX is usually active against P. cepacia, P. pseudomallei, Xanthomonas maltophilia, Citrobacter, Enterobacter cloacae, and Acinetobacter spp (pathogens that are often resistant to third-generation cephalosporins). Excellent activity against Legionella spp in vitro and in animal models of legionellosis; data in man are lacking, however.

Toxicity: Skin rash (3%) (usually minor); exfoliative dermatitis (Stevens-Johnson syndrome) or erythema multiforme rare ($< 1:10,000$); excessive fluid when administered intravenously in high doses; nausea, GI distress (3 to 10%); diarrhea ($< 1\%$); may contribute to marrow toxicity in patients with hematologic neoplasia or underlying marrow disorder; substantial increase in incidence and severity of side effects in patients with the acquired immunodeficiency syndrome (AIDS).

Dosage: Regular strength tablets (80 mg TMP; 400 mg SMZ) or double strength (160/800); for parenteral use, 1 ampoule (5 ml) contains 80 mg TMP and 400 mg SMX/ml. Doses of 20 mg/kg/day for TMP component in 4 divided doses for Pneumocystis carinii; lower doses q8-12h may be adequate for bacterial infections.

Indications:

• TMP/SMZ is a reasonable option for both CAP and nosocomial pneumonias in patients with hypersensitivity reactions to penicillins or beta-lactams. TMP/SMZ is less expensive than third-generation cephalosporins or antipseudomonal penicillins, and may be given orally following a favorable response to parenteral therapy (60 to 75% bioavailable). Despite an excellent in vitro susceptibility profile, clinical experience with TMP/SMX in the treatment of pneumonia has been limited. TMP/SMX, however, has been successfully used in nosocomial infections caused by staphylococci (including MRSA) and in serious gram-negative infections caused by Enterobacteriaceae, Serratia marcescens, and Acinetobacter spp

CLINDAMYCIN
(Cleocin)

Clindamycin is a derivative of lincomycin, which has outstanding anaerobic activity and excellent activity against most aerobic gram-positive cocci (with the exception of MRSA). Because of its lack of activity against GNB, clindamycin has no role as monotherapy for empiric therapy of polymicrobial or nosocomial pneumonia. Alternative agents are preferred for CAP.

Mechanism of Action: Binds to 50S subunit of bacterial ribosomes and suppresses intracellular protein synthesis. Clindamycin, erythromycin, and chloramphenicol act at the same site and thus antagonize each other.

Antimicrobial Spectrum: Highly active against anaerobes, including Fusobacterium spp, peptostreptococci, peptococci, clostridia, and Bacteroides spp (including B. fragilis); excellent activity against Streptococcus pneumoniae, most streptococci, and methicillin-sensitive Staphylococcus aureus; enterococci, and MRSA are resistant. No significant activity against aerobic gram-negative rods. Does not cover Mycoplasma, Chlamydia, or Legionella spp.

Toxicity: Skin rash (5 to 10%); diarrhea (2 to 10%); pseudomembranous colitis no more common with clindamycin than with many other antibiotics commonly prescribed; metallic taste in mouth with parenteral administration (4%).

Dosage: 150 to 450 mg tid (orally); maximal IV dose 900 mg q8h, but 600 mg q8h is probably adequate even for serious infections; dose must be reduced in renal failure.

Indications:

- Primary therapy for community-acquired anaerobic lung abscess or aspiration pneumonia (penicillin G is an alternative, but clindamycin may be more efficacious
- Combination of clindamycin with aztreonam may provide outstanding empiric therapy for nosocomial pneumonia in patients allergic to beta-lactams in whom penicillins, cephalosporins, and imipenem are contraindicated

Not recommended for most CAP; beta-lactams or erythromycin preferred. In view of its lack of activity against GNB, clindamycin is not recommended for nosocomial pulmonary infections because other agents, such as antipseudomonal penicillins, imipenem, or cefotetan, may have adequate anaerobic activity while also providing superior activity against enteric GNB.

METRONIDAZOLE
(Flagyl)

Metronidazole is a nitroimidazole introduced in 1957 for the treatment of parasitic diseases; anecdotal clinical successes as therapy for anaerobic bacterial infections were reported in 1962. By the late 1970s, with the increased prevalence of beta–lactamase-producing strains of Bacteroides fragilis and other anaerobes, clindamycin and metronidazole replaced penicillins as the preferred agents for anaerobic infections. Resistance to clindamycin has now emerged in 3 to 9% of strains within the B. fragilis group, but no significant resistance has developed to metronidazole. Metronidazole has the best bactericidal activity of all antimicrobials against anaerobes and has been successfully used for anaerobic infections in abdominal, pelvic, and extrapulmonary sites; its role in pulmonary infections is controversial. Failures have been observed with metronidazole as monotherapy for primary lung abscess or aspiration pneumonia, thereby suggesting that the lack of activity against aerobes and GNB may limit its utility in pleuropulmonary infections.

Mechanism of Action: Enters bacterial cell; reduction of the nitro group of the drug releases toxic intermediates and free radicals that damage (bacterial) DNA and other macromolecules.

Antimicrobial Spectrum: Almost exclusively limited to obligate anaerobes; no significant activity against GNB or aerobic gram positive organisms.

Toxicity: Minor; GI effects; CNS toxicity or peripheral neuropathy (rare); disulfiram-like effects in patients ingesting alcohol.

Dosage: Loading dose of 15 mg/kg (or 1,000 mg) IV, then 7.5 mg/kg IV q6h; oral dose is 500 mg tid.

Indications: Despite its excellent anaerobic activity, high failure rates have been noted when metronidazole has been used as monotherapy for respiratory tract infections (including aspiration pneumonia and lung abscess). This high failure rate may relate to its lack of activity against some Streptococcus spp and other aerobes that are often involved in polymicrobial respiratory infections.

VANCOMYCIN
(Vancocin)

Vancomycin, a complex glycopeptide initially isolated from Streptomyces orientales, has been in use since 1956, primarily for treatment of staphylococcal infections. The use of vancomycin declined following the introduction of methicillin, but interest in this agent has surged over the past decade concomitant with an increased incidence of awareness of methicillin-resistant staphylococci, the increasing prevalence of gram-positive infections among patients with granulocytopenic cancer, and its efficacy against Clostridium difficile colitis.

Mechanism of Action: Multiple mechanisms of action include inhibition of bacterial cell wall synthesis (interferes with glycopeptide synthesis); occurs at an earlier step than penicillins; interferes with RNA synthesis; alters permeability of bacterial cell membrane.

Antimicrobial Spectrum: Vancomycin is exceptionally active against aerobic gram-positive cocci but has a narrow spectrum. Vancomycin is bactericidal against aerobic gram positive organisms (Staphylococcus epidermidis and S. aureus, including MRSA), diphtheroids (e.g. Corynebacteria), streptococci, pneumococci, and clostridia but is only bacteriostatic against enterococci. No significant activity against gram-negative organisms, anaerobes, Mycoplasma, Chlamydia, or Legionella spp.

Toxicity: Phlebitis ($> 10\%$ in some series); maculopapular or erythematous rash (4 to 5%); hearing loss, particularly with high serum levels; "red man's syndrome" (erythematous flushing of the torso, neck, and face associated with pruritus, hypotension, and rarely cardiac arrest caused by histamine release). Nephrotoxicity rare, but may occur when administered concomitantly with aminoglycoside.

Dosage: Loading dose 15 mg/kg; then 500 to 1,000 mg IV q12h; administer slowly over 60 minutes; more rapid infusion rates may be associated with red man's syndrome, pain, or hypotension. Substantial dose reductions required in presence of renal failure; in this situation, serum levels are required to assure therapeutic levels and reduce toxicity (peak levels: aim for serum concentrations of 20 to 40 µg/ml 2 hours post completion of infusion; trough levels, 5 to 10 µg/ml). Intramuscular route not available; oral administration does not provide adequate tissue or serum levels.

Indications:

- Vancomycin should be restricted to proven or suspected infections caused by gram-positive organisms resistant to more conventional agents, such as penicillins. Because of its narrow spectrum, vancomycin is not adequate as single-agent empiric therapy for pneumonia. Vancomycin is bactericidal against MRSA and other gram-positive organisms that exhibit resistance to penicillins (e.g. pathogenic Corynebacterium

spp, Staphylococcus epidermidis) and is the drug of choice for these pathogens
- Effective against infections caused by enterococci but need to combine with gentamicin for bactericidal activity

Special Considerations: Antimicrobial resistance to vancomycin rarely (if ever) develops during therapy; no cross-resistance occurs between vancomycin and unrelated antibiotics. Thus, vancomycin remains exceptionally reliable against traditionally susceptible organisms (gram-positive cocci) even with widespread use.

REFERENCES

COMMUNITY-ACQUIRED PNEUMONIA

Epidemiology

1. Berntsson E, Blomberg J, Lagergard T, Trollfers B: Etiology of community-acquired pneumonia in patients requiring hospitalization. Eur J Clin Microbiol, 4:268, 1988.
2. Fang GD, Fine M, Orloff J, et al.: New and emerging etiologies for community-acquired pneumonia with implications for therapy. A prospective multicenter study of 359 cases. Medicine, *69*:307, 1990.
3. Farr BM, Kaiser DL, Harrison BDW, Connolly CK: Prediction of microbial etiology at admission to hospital for pneumonia from the presenting clinical features. Thorax, *44*: 1031, 1989.
4. Farr BM, Sloman AJ, Fisch MJ: Predicting death in patients hospitalized for community-acquired pneumonia. Ann Intern Med, *115*:428, 1991.
5. Fine MJ, Smith DN, Singer DE: Hospitalization decision in patients with community-acquired pneumonia: a prospective cohart study. Am J Med, *89*:713, 1990.
6. Marrie TJ, Durant H, Yates L: Community-acquired pneumonia requiring hospitalization: 5-year prospective study. Rev Infect Dis, *11*:586, 1989.
7. Research Committee of the British Thoracic Society and the Public Health Laboratory Service: Community-acquired pneumonia in adults in British Hospitals in 1982–1983: A survey of aetiology, mortality, prognostic factors and outcome. Q J Med, *239*:195, 1987.
8. Woodhead MA, MacFarlane JT, McCracken JS, et al.: Prospective study of the aetiology and outcome of pneumonia in the community. Lancet, *1*:671, 1987.

Severe Community-Acquired Pneumonia Requiring Mechanical Ventilatory Support or ICU

9. Feldman C, Kallenbach JM, Levy H, et al.: Community-acquired pneumonia of diverse aetiology: prognosis features in patients admitted to an intensive care unit and a "severity of illness." Intensive Care Med, *15*:302, 1989.
10. Hook EW, Horton CA, Schaberg DR: Failure of intensive care unit support to influence mortality from pneumococcal pneumonia. JAMA, *249*:1055, 1983.
11. Ortqvist A, Sterner G, Nilsson AJ: Severe community-acquired pneumonia: factors influencing need of intensive care treatment and prognosis. Scand J Infect Dis, *17*:377, 1985.
12. Pachon J, Prados MD, Capote F, et al.: Severe community-acquired pneumonia. Etiology, prognosis, and treatment. Am Rev Respir Dis, *142*:369, 1990.
13. Torres A, Serra-Batlles J, Ferrer A, et al.: Severe community-acquired pneumonia. Epidemiologic and prognostic factors. Am Rev Respir Dis, *144*:312, 1991.

Elderly

14. Crossley KB, Thurn JR: Nursing–home-acquired pneumonia. Semin Respir Infect, *4*:64, 1989.
15. Fine MJ: Pneumonia in the elderly: the hospital admission and discharge decisions. Semin Respir Infect, *5*:303, 1990.
16. Gray J: Treatment of pneumonia in the elderly: pharmacological considerations. Semin Respir Infect, *5*:295, 1990.
17. Hanson LC, Weber DJ, Rula WA, Samsa GP: Risk factors for nosocomial pneumonia in the elderly. Am J Med, *92*:161, 1992.
18. Marrie TJ: Epidemiology of community-acquired pneumonia in the elderly. Semin Respir Infect, *5*:260, 1990.
19. Venkatesan P, Gladman J, Macfarlane JT, et al.: A hospital study of community-acquired pneumonia in the elderly. Thorax, *45*:254, 1990.
20. Verghese A, Berk SL: Bacterial pneumonia in the elderly. Medicine, *62*:271, 1983.

NOSOCOMIAL PNEUMONIA

Overview and Epidemiology

21. Bartlett JG, O'Keefe P, Tally F, et al.: Bacteriology of hospital-acquired pneumonia. Arch Intern Med, *146*:868, 1986.
22. Bryan CS, Reynolds KL: Bacteremic nosocomial pneumonia: analysis of 172 episodes from a single metropolitan area. Am Rev Respir Dis, *129*:668, 1984.
23. Craven DE, Barber TW, Steger KA, Montecalvo MA: Nosocomial pneumonia in the 1990s: Update of epidemiology and risk factors. Semin Respir Infect, *5*:157, 1990.
24. Craven DE, Kunches LM, Lichtenberg DA, et al.: Nosocomial infection and fatality in medical and surgical intensive care unit patients. Arch Intern Med, *148*:1161, 1988.
25. Fagon J, Chastre J, Domart Y, et al.: Nosocomial pneumonia in patients receiving continuous mechanical ventilation. Prospective analysis of 52 episodes with use of a protected specimen brush and quantitative culture techniques. Am Rev Respir Dis, *139*:877, 1989.
26. Horan TC, White JW, Jarvis WR, et al.: Nosocomial infection surveillance 1984. CDC Surveillance Summaries, MMWR, *35*(1SS):17SS, 1986.
27. Jarvis WR, Edwards JR, Culver DC, et al.: Nosocomial infections in adult and pediatric intensive care units in the United States, 1986–1990. Am J Med, *91*(Suppl 3B):185, 1991.
28. Saviteer SM, Samsa GP, Rutala WA, et al.: Nosocomial infections in the elderly. Increased risk per hospital day. Am J Med, *84*:661, 1988.
29. Weinstein RA: Epidemiology and control of nosocomial infections in adult intensive care units. Am J Med, *91*(Suppl 3B):179, 1991.

Pathogenesis—Role of H2 Antagonists/Antacids

30. Cook DJ, Laine LA, Guyatt GH, Raffin TA: Nosocomial pneumonia and the role of gastric pH. A meta-analysis. Chest, *100*:7, 1991.
31. Driks MR, Craven DE, Celli BR, et al.: Nosocomial pneumonia in intubated patients given sucralfate as compared with antacids or histamine type 2 blockers. N Engl J Med, *317*:1376, 1987.
32. Kappstein I, Friedrich TH, Hellinger P, et al.: Incidence of pneumonia in mechanically ventilated patients treated with sucralfate or cimetidine as prophylaxis for stress bleeding. Am J Med (in press).
33. Tryba M: Risk of acute stress bleeding and nosocomial pneumonia in ventilated intensive care unit patients: sucralfate versus antacids. Am J Med, *43*:117, 1987.

34. Tryba M: Sucralfate versus antacids or H2-antagonists for stress ulcer prophylaxis: a meta-analysis on efficacy and pneumonia rate. Crit Care Med, 19:942, 1991.

Prevention

35. Aerdts SJ, Clasener HA, van Dalen R, et al.: Prevention of bacterial colonization of the respiratory tract and stomach of mechanically ventilated patients by a novel regimen of selective decontamination in combination with initial cefotaxime. J Antimicrob Chemother, 26(*Suppl A*):59, 1990.
36. Aerdts SJ, van Dalen R, Clasener HA, et al.: Antibiotic prophylaxis of respiratory tract infection in mechanically ventilated patients. A prospective, blinded, randomized trial of the effect of a novel regimen. Chest, *100*:783, 1991.
37. Brun-Bruisson C, Legrand P, Rauss A, et al.: Intestinal decontamination for control of nosocomial multiresistant gram-negative bacilli: Study of an outbreak in an intensive care unit. Ann Intern Med, *110*:873, 1989.
38. Cerra FB, Maddaus MA, Dunn DL, et al.: Selective gut decontamination reduces nosocomial infections and length of stay but not mortality or organ failure in surgical intensive care unit patients. Arch Surg, *127*:163, 1992.
39. Craven DE, Steger KA, Barber TW: Preventing nosocomial pneumonia: state of the art and perspectives for the 1990s. Am J Med, *91*(*Suppl 3B*):44, 1991.
40. Flaherty JP, Weinstein RA: Infection control and pneumonia prophylaxis strategies in the intensive care unit. Semin Respir Infect, *5*:191, 1990.
41. Gastinne H, Wolff M, Delatour F, et al.: A controlled trial in intensive care units of selective decontamination of the digestive tract with nonabsorbable antibiotics. N Engl J Med, *326*:594, 1992.
42. Ledingham IM, Eastaway AT, McKay IC, et al.: Triple regimen of selective decontamination of the digestive tract, systemic cefotaxime, and microbiological surveillance for prevention of acquired infection in intensive care. Lancet, *1*:785, 1988.
43. Stoutenbeek CP, van Saene HKF, Miranda DR, et al.: The effect of oropharyngeal decontamination using topical nonabsorbable antibiotics on the incidence of nosocomial respiratory tract infections in multiple trauma patients. J Trauma, *27*:1, 1987.
44. Unertl K, Ruckdeschel G, Selbmann HK, et al.: Prevention of colonization and respiratory infections in long-term ventilated patients by local antimicrobial prophylaxis. Intensive Care Med, *13*:106, 1987.

DIAGNOSTIC TECHNIQUES FOR PNEUMONIA

Sputum

45. Lentino JR, Lucks DA: Nonvalue of sputum culture in the management of lower respiratory tract infections. J Clin Microbiol, *25*:758, 1987.
46. Levy M, Dromer F, Brion N, et al.: Community-acquired pneumonia: importance of initial noninvasive bacteriologic and radiographic investigations. Chest, *92*:43, 1988.

Bronchoscopy with Protected Brush

47. Chauncey JB, Lynch JP III, Hyzy RC, Toews GB: Invasive techniques in the diagnosis of bacterial pneumonia in the intensive care unit. Semin Respir Infect, *5*:215, 1990.
48. Mediur GU: Ventilator-associated pneumonia in patients with respiratory failure. A diagnostic approach. Chest, *97*:1208, 1990.
49. Ortqvist A, Kalin M, Lejdebron L, Lundberg B: Diagnostic fiberoptic bronchoscopy and protected brush culture in patients with community-acquired pneumonia. Chest, *97*:576, 1990.

50. Pham LH, Brun-Buisson C, Legrand P, et al.: Diagnosis of nosocomial pneumonia in mechanically-ventilated patients: comparison of a plugged telescoping catheter with the protected specimen brush. Am Rev Respir Dis, *143*:1055, 1991.

Bronchoalveolar Lavage

51. Chastre J, Gagon JY, Soler P, et al.: Quantification of BAL cells containing intracellular bacteria rapidly identifies ventilated patients with nosocomial pneumonia. Chest, *95*: 190S, 1989.
52. Guerra LF, Baughman RP: Use of bronchoalveolar lavage to diagnose bacterial pneumonia in mechanically ventilated patients. Crit Care Med, *18*:169, 1990.
53. Meduri GU, Baselski V: The role of bronchoalveolar lavage in diagnosing nonopportunistic bacterial pneumonia. Chest, *100*:179, 1991.
54. Meduri GU, Wunderink RG, Leeper KV, Beals DH: Management of bacterial pneumonia in ventilated patients. Protected bronchoalveolar lavage as a diagnostic tool. Chest, *101*: 500, 1992.
55. Pugin J, Auckenthaler R, Mili N, et al.: Diagnosis of ventilator-associated pneumonia by bacteriologic analysis of bronchoscopic and nonbronchoscopic "blind" bronchoalveolar lavage fluid. Am Rev Respir Dis, *143*:1121, 1991.
56. Torres A, Bellacasa JP, Xaubert A, et al.: Diagnostic value of quantitative cultures of bronchoalveolar lavage and telescoping plugged catheters in mechanically ventilated patients with bacterial pneumonia. Am Rev Respir Dis, *140*:306, 1989.

SPECIFIC PATHOGENS

Acinetobacter

57. Barnes DJ, Naraqi S, Igo JD: Community-acquired Acinetobacter pneumonia in adults in Papua New Guinea. Rev Infect Dis, *10*:636, 1988.
58. Buxton AE, Anderson RL, Werdegar D, et al.: Nosocomial respiratory tract infection and colonization with Acinetobacter calcoaceticus. Epidemiologic characteristics. Am J Med, *65*:507, 1978.
59. Glew RH, Moellering RC Jr, Kunz LJ: Infections with Acinetobacter calcoaceticus (Herrellea vaginicola): clinical and laboratory studies. Medicine (Baltimore), *56*:79, 1977.
60. Peacock JE Jr, Sorrell LA, Sottile FD, et al.: Nosocomial respiratory tract colonization and infection with aminoglycoside-resistant Acinetobacter calcoaceticus var anitratus: Epidemiologic characteristics and clinical significance. Infect Control Hosp Epidemiol, *9*(7):302, 1988.
61. Smego RA Jr.: Endemic nosocomial Acinetobacter calcoaceticus bacteremia. Clinical significance, treatment, and prognosis. Arch Intern Med, *145*:2174, 1985.

Anaerobes

62. Appleman MD, Heseltine PNR, Cherubin CE: Epidemiology, antimicrobial susceptibility, pathogenicity, and significance of Bacteroides fragilis group organisms isolated at Los Angeles County-University of Southern California Medical Center. Rev Infect Dis, *13*:12, 1991.
63. Bartlett JG: Anaerobic infections of the lung. Chest, *91*:901, 1987.
64. Bartlett JG: Bacterial infections of the pleural space. Semin Respir Infect, *3*:308, 1988.
65. Breuil J, Burnat C, Patey O, Dublanchet A: Survey of Bacteroides fragilis susceptibility patterns in France. J Antimicrob Chemother, *24*:69, 1989.
66. Cuchural CJ Jr, Tally FP, Jacobus NV, et al.: Susceptibility of the Bacteroides fragilis group in the United States: analysis by site of isolation. Antimicrob Agents Chemother, *21*:717, 1988.

67. Finegold SM: Anaerobes: problems and controversies in bacteriology, infections, and susceptibility testing. Rev Infect Dis, 12(*Suppl 2*):S223, 1990.
68. Finegold SM: Aspiration pneumonia. Rev Infect Dis, 13(*Suppl 9*):S737, 1991.
69. Garcia-Rodriquez JE, Garcia-Sanchez JE: Evolution of antimicrobial susceptibility in isolates of the Bacteroides fragilis group in Spain. Rev Infect Dis, 12:S142, 1990.
70. Levinson ME, Mangura CT, Lorber B, et al.: Clindamycin compared with penicillin for the treatment of anaerobic lung abscess. Ann Intern Med, 98:466, 1983.

Moraxella (Branhamella) Catarrhalis

71. Hager H, Verghese A, Alvarez S, et al.: Branhamella catarrhalis respiratory infections. Rev Infect Dis, 9:1140, 1987.
72. Nicotra B, Ribera M, Lumen JI, Wallace RJ Jr.: Branhamella catarrhalis as a lower respiratory tract pathogen in patients with chronic lung disease. Arch Intern Med, 146:890, 1988.
73. Wright PW, Wallace RJ, Jr.: Pneumonia due to Moraxella (Branhamella) catarrhalis. Semin Respir Infect, 4:40, 1989.

Enterobacter

74. Bodey GP, Elting SL, Rodriquez S: Bacteremia caused by Enterobacter: 15 years of experience in a cancer hospital. Rev Infect Dis, 13:550, 1991.
75. Chow JW, Fine MJ, Shlaes DM, et al.: Enterobacter bacteremia: clinical features and emergence of antibiotic resistance during therapy. Ann Intern Med, 115:585, 1991.
76. Gaston MA: Enterobacter: an emerging nosocomial pathogen. J Hosp Infect, 11:197, 1988.
77. Weinstein RA: Endemic emergence of cephalosporin-resistant enterobacter: relation to prior therapy. Infect Control 7(*Suppl*):120, 1986.

Escherichia Coli

78. Berk SL, Neumann P, Holtsclaw S, Smith JK: Escherichia coli pneumonia in the elderly: with reference to the role of E. coli K1 capsular polysaccharide antigen. Am J Med, 72:899, 1982.
79. Gransden WR, Eykyn SJ, Phillips I, Rowe B: Bacteremia due to Escherichia coli: a study of 861 episodes. Rev Infect Dis, 12:1008, 1990.
80. Jonas M, Cunha BA: Bacteremic Escherichia coli pneumonia. Arch Intern Med, 142:2157, 1982.

Hemophilus Influenzae

81. Berk SI, Holtsclaw SA, Wiener SL, Smith JK: Nontypeable Haemophilus influenzae in the elderly. Arch Intern Med, 142:537, 1982.
82. Doern GV, Jorgensen JH, Thornsberry C: National collaborative study of the prevalence of antimicrobial resistance among clinical isolate of Haemophilus influenzae. Antimicrob Agents Chemother, 32:180, 1988.
83. Musher DM, Kubitshek KIR, Crennan J, et al.: Pneumonia and acute febrile tracheobronchitis due to Haemophilus influenzae. Ann Intern Med, 99:444, 1983.
84. Powell M, Koustia-Coudzou C, Voutsinas D, et al.: Resistance of clinical isolates of Haemophilus influenzae in United Kingdom 1986. Br Med J, 295:176, 1987.
85. Quinones CA, Memon MA, Sarosa GA: Bacteremic Hemophilus influenzae pneumonia in the adult. Semin Respir Infect, 4:12, 1990.
86. Slater LN, Guarnaccia J, Makintubee S, Istre GR: Bacteremic disease due to Haemophilus influenzae capsular type f in adults: report of five cases and review. Rev Infect Dis, 12:628, 1990.

87. Wallace RJ, Musher DM, Septimus EJ, et al.: Hemophilus influenzae infections in adults: Characterization of strains by serotypes, bioptyes, and beta-lactamase production. J Infect Dis, *144*:101, 1981.
88. Wallace RJ, Steele LC, Brooks DL, et al.: Ampicillin, tetracycline, and chloramphenicol resistant Haemophilus influenzae in adults with chronic lung disease—relationship of resistance to prior antimicrobial therapy. Am Rev Respir Dis, *137*:695, 1988.

Klebsiella Pneumoniae

89. Carpenter JL: Klebsiella pulmonary infections: occurrence at one medical center and review. Rev Infect Dis, *12*:672, 1990.

Pseudomonas Aeruginosa

90. Bisbe J, Gatell JM, Puig J, et al.: Pseudomonas aeruginosa bacteremia; univariate and multivariate analyses of factors influencing the prognosis in 133 episodes. Rev Infect Dis, *10*:629, 1988.
91. Gallagher PG, Watanakunakorn C: Pseudomonas bacteremia in a community teaching hospital, 1980–1984. Rev Infect Dis, *11*:846, 1989.
92. Pennington, JE, Ehrie MG, Hickey WF: Host defense mechanisms against pneumonia due to Pseudomonas aeruginosa. Rev Infect Dis, *6*:(Suppl 3):S657, 1984.
93. Roston KVI, Anaissie EA, Bodey GP: In vitro susceptibility of Pseudomonas species to 15 antimicrobial agents. J Antimicrob Chemother, *19*:193, 1987.

Pseudomonas Cepacia

94. Conly JM, Klass L, Larson J, et al.: Pseudomonas cepacia colonization and infection in intensive care units. Can Med Assoc J, *134*:363, 1986.
95. Goldman DA, Klinger JD: Pseudomonas cepacia: Biology, mechanisms of virulence, epidemiology. J Pediatr, *108*:806, 1986.
96. Martone WJ, Tablen OC, Jarvis WR: The epidemiology of nosocomial epidemic Pseudomonas cepacia infections. Eur J Epidemiol, *3*:222, 1987.
97. Tomashefski JF, Thomassen MJ, Bruce MC, et al.: Pseudomonas cepacia-associated pneumonia in cystic fibrosis. Relation of clinical features to the histologic pattern of pneumonia. Arch Pathol Lab Med, *12*:166, 1988.

Serratia Marcescens

98. Siato H, Elting L, Bodey GP, Berkey P: Serratia bacteramia: review of 118 cases. Rev Infect Dis, *11*:912, 1989.
99. Yu VL: Serratia marcescens: historical perspective and clinical review. N Engl J Med, *300*:887, 1979.

Staphylococcus Aureus

100. Brumfitt W, Hamilton-Miller J: Methicillin-resistant Staphylococcus aureus. N Engl J Med, *320*:1188, 1989.
101. Cohen SH, Morita MM, Bradford M: A seven-year experience with methicillin-resistant Staphylococcus aureus. Am J Med, *91*(Suppl 3B):233, 1991.
102. Linnemann CC, Moore P, Staneck JL, Pfaller MA: Reemergence of epidemic methicillin-resistant Staphylococcus aureus in a general hospital associated with changing staphylococcal strains. Am J Med, *91*(Suppl 3B):238, 1991.
103. Maple PAC, Hamilton-Miller JMT, Brumfitt W: World-wide antibiotic resistance in methicillin-resistant Staphylococcus aureus. Lancet, *1*:537, 1989.

104. Mylotte JM, McDermott C, Spooner JA: Prospective study of 114 consecutive episodes of Staphylococcus aureus bacteramia. Rev Infect Dis, *9*:891, 1987.
105. Rello J, Quintana E, Ausina V, et al.: Risk factors for Staphylococcus aureus nosocomial pneumonia in critically ill patients. Am Rev Respir Dis, *142*:1320, 1990.
106. Watanakunakorn C: Bacteremic Staphylococcus aureus pneumonia. Scand J Infect Dis, *19*:623, 1987.
107. Wenzel RP, Nettleman MD, Jones RN, Pfaller MA: Methicillin-resistant Staphylococcus aureus: implications for the 1990s and effective control measures. Am J Med, *91*:(*Suppl 3B*):221, 1991.

Staphylococcus Epidermidis

108. Fidalgo S, Vazquez F, Mendoza MC, et al.: Bacteremia due to Staphylococcus epidermidis: Microbiologic, epidemiologic, clinical, and prognostic features. Rev Infect Dis, *12*: 520, 1990.
109. Hamory BH, Parisi JT: Staphylococcus epidermidis: a significant nosocomial pathogen. Am J Infect Control, *15*:59, 1987.
110. Martin MA, Pfaller MA, Wenzel RP: Coagulase-negative staphylococcal bacteremia. Mortality and hospital stay. Ann Intern Med, *110*:9, 1989.

Streptococcus Pneumoniae

111. Austrian R, Gold J: Pneumococcal bacteremia with especial reference to bacteremic pneumonoccal pneumonia. Ann Intern Med, *60*:759, 1964.
112. Coonrod JD: Pneumococcal pneumonia. Semin Respir Infect, *4*:4, 1989.
113. Esposito AL: Community-acquired bacteremic pneumococcal pneumonia. Effect of age on manifestations and outcome. Arch Intern Med, *144*:945, 1984.
114. Finkelstein MS, Petkun WM, Freedman ML, Antopol SC: Pneumococcal bacteremia in adults: age-dependent differences in presentation and in outcome. J Am Geriatr Soc, *31*: 19, 1983.
115. Hager HL, Woolley TW, Berk SL: Review of recent pneumococcal infections with attention to vaccine and nonvaccine serotypes. Rev Infect Dis, *12*:267, 1990.
116. Orf S, Ryan JL, Barden G, et al.: Pneumococcal pneumonia in hospitalized patients: clinical and radiological presentations. JAMA, *249*:214, 1983.
117. Pallares R, Gudiol F, Linares J, et al.: Risk factors and response to antibiotic therapy in adults with bacteremic pneumonia caused by penicillin-resistant pneumococci. N Engl J Med, *317*:18, 1987.

Other Streptococci

118. Basiliere JL, Bistron HW, Spence WF: Streptococcal pneumonia: Recent outbreaks in military recruit populations. Am J Med, *44*:580, 1968.
119. Bradley SF, Gordon JJ, Baumgartner DD, et al.: Group C streptococcal bacteremia: analysis of 88 cases. Rev Infect Dis, *13*:270, 1991.
120. Braunstein H: Characteristics of Group A streptococcal bacteremia in patients at the San Bernardino County Medical Center. Rev Infect Dis, *13*:8, 1991.
121. Salata RA, Lerner PI, Shales DM, et al.: Infections due to Lancefield group C streptococci. Medicine (Baltimore), *68*:225, 1989.
122. Stamm AM, Cobbs CG: Group C streptococcal pneumonia: report of a fatal case and review of the literature. Rev Infect Dis, *2*:889, 1980.
123. Verhese A, Berk SL, Boelen LJ, Smith JK, et al.: Group B streptococcal pneumonia in the elderly. Arch Intern Med, *142*:1642, 1982.

Group D Streptococcus (Enterococcus)

124. Berk SL, Verghese A, Holtsclaw SA, Smith JK: Enterococcal pneumonia: occurrence in patients receiving broad-spectrum antibiotic regimens and enteral feeding. Am J Med, 74:153, 1983.
125. Gullberg RM, Homann SR, Phair JP: Enterococcal bacteremia: analysis of 75 episodes. Rev Infect Dis, 11:74, 1989.
126. Magnussen CP, Cave J: Nosocomial enterococcal infections: association with use of third-generation cephalosporins. Am J Infect Control, 16:241, 1988.
127. Patterson JE, Zervos MJ: High level gentamicin resistance in Enterococcus: microbiology, genetic basis, and epidemiology. Rev Infect Dis, 12:644, 1990.
128. Zervos MJ, Kauggman CA, Therasse PM, et al.: Nosocomial infection by gentamicin resistant Streptococcus faecalis: an epidemiologic study. Ann Intern Med, 106:687, 1987.

Xanthomonas Maltophilia

129. Chow AW, Wong J, Bartlett KH: Synergistic interactions of ciprofloxacin and extended-spectrum beta-lactams or aminoglycosides against multiply drug-resistant Pseudomonas maltophilia. Antimicrob Agents Chemother, 32:782, 1988.
130. Elting LS, Bodey GP: Septicemia due to Xanthomas species and non-aeruginosa Pseudomonas species: increasing incidence of catheter-related infections. Medicine, 69:296, 1990.
131. Elting LS, Khardori N, Bodey GP, Fainstein V: Nosocomial infection caused by Xanthomonas maltophilia: a case-control study of predisposing factors. Infect Control Hosp Epidemiol, 11:134, 1990.
132. Khardori N, Elting L, Wong E, et al.: Nosocomial Xanthomonas maltophilia infections in cancer patients. Rev Infect Dis, 12:997, 1990.
133. Marshall WF, Keating MR, Anhalt JP, Steckerberg JM: Xanthomonas maltophilia: An emerging nosocomial pathogen. Mayo Clin Proc, 64:1097, 1989.
134. Muder RR, Yu VL, Dummer JS, et al.: Infection caused by Pseudomonas maltophilia: Expanding clinical spectrum. Arch Intern Med, 147:1672, 1987.
135. Yu VL, Felegie TP, Yee RB, et al.: Synergistic interaction in vitro with use of three antibiotics simultaneously against Pseudomonas maltophilia. J Infect Dis, 142:602, 1980.

ATYPICAL PNEUMONIAS (mycoplasma, chlamydia, legionella)

Atypical Pneumonias (General)

136. Cotton EM, Strampfer MJ, Cunha BA, et al.: Legionella and mycoplasma pneumoniae: a community hospital experience with atypical pneumonias. Clin Chest Med, 8:441, 1987.
137. Woodhead MA, MacFarlane JT: Comparative clinical and laboratory features of legionella with pneumococcal and mycoplasma pneumonias. Br J Dis Chest, 81:133, 1987.

Legionella

138. Falco V, de Sevilla TF, Alegre J, et al.: Legionella pneumophila. A cause of severe community-acquired pneumonia. Chest, 100:1007, 1991.
139. Granados A, Podzamczer D, Gudiol F, Manresa F: Pneumonia due to Legionella pneumophila and pneumococcal pneumonias: similarities and differences of presentation. Eur Respir J, 2:130, 1989.
140. Korvick JA, Yu VL, Fang G: Legionella species as hospital-acquired respiratory pathogens. Semin Respir Infect 2:34, 1987.
141. Muder RR, Yu VL, Fang GD: Community-acquired Legionnaire's disease. Semin Respir Infect, 4:32, 1989.

142. Reingold AL: Role of legionellae in acute infections of the lower respiratory tract. Rev Infect Dis, *10*:1018, 1988.
143. Roig J, Aguilar X, Ruiz J, et al.: Comparative study of Legionella pneumophilia and other nosocomial-acquired pneumonias. Chest, *99*:344, 1991.
144. Yu VL, Kroboth FJ, Shonnard J, et al.: Legionnaire's diseases: new clinical perspective from a prospective pneumonia study. Am J Med, *73*:357, 1982.

Mycoplasma

145. Ali NJ, Sillis M, Andres BE, et al.: The clinical spectrum and diagnosis of Mycoplasma pneumoniae infection. Q J Med, *58*:241, 1986.
146. Foy HM, Kenny GE, Cooney MK, et al.: Long-term epidemiology of infections with Mycoplasma pneumoniae. J Infect Dis, *139*:681, 1979.
147. Murray HW, Masur H, Senterfit LB, et al.: The protein manifestations of Mycoplasma pneumoniae infections in adults. Am J Med, *58*:229, 1975.

Chlamydia-TWAR

148. Atmar RL, Greenberg SB: Pneumonia caused by Mycoplasma pneumoniae and the TWAR agent. Semin Respir Infect, *4*:19, 1989.
149. Grayston JT, Diwan VK, Cooney M, Wang S: Community- and hospital-acquired pneumonia associated with Chlamydia TWAR infection documented serologically. Arch Intern Med, *149*:169, 1989.
150. Grayston JT, Kuo CC, Wang SP, Altman J: A new Chlamydia psittaci strain called TWAR from acute respiratory tract infections. N Engl J Med, *315*:161, 1986.
151. Grayston JT, Campbell LA, Kuo CC, et al.: A new respiratory tract pathogen: Chlamydia pneumoniae strain TWAR. J Infect Dis, *161*:618, 1990.
152. Kleemola M, Saikku P, Visakorpi R, et al.: Epidemics of pneumonia caused by TWAR, a new Chlamydia organism, in military trainees in Finland. J Infect Dis, *157*:230, 1988.
153. Marrie TJ, Grayston JT, Wang SP, Kuo CC: Pneumonia associated with the TWAR strain of Chlamydia. Ann Intern Med, *106*:507, 1987.

SPECIFIC ANTIBIOTICS

Antibiotics (reviews)

154. Donowitz GR, Mandell GL: Beta-lactam antibiotics. N Engl J Med, *318*:420, 490, 1988.
155. McGehee JL, Podnos SD, Pierce AK, Weissler JC: Treatment of pneumonia in patients at risk of infection with gram-negative bacilli. Am J Med, *84*:597, 1988.
156. Pennington JE: Approach to therapy of respiratory infections in the critical care setting. Semin Respir Infect, *5*:226, 1990.

Penicillins

157. Parry MF: The penicillins. Med Clin North Am, *71*:1093, 1987.
158. Wright AJ, Wilkowske CJ: The penicillins. Mayo Clin Proc, *66*:1047, 1991.

Cephalosporins

159. Fekety FR: Safety of parenteral third-generation cephalosporins. Am J Med, *88(Suppl 4A)*:38S, 1990.
160. Gustaferro CA, Steckelberg JM: Cephalosporin antimicrobial agents and related compounds. Mayo Clin Proc, *66*:1064, 1991.

161. Neu HC: Pathophysiologic basis for the use of third-generation cephalosporins. Am J Med, *88(Suppl 4A)*:3S, 1990.
162. Quenzer RW: A perspective of cephalosporins in pneumonia. Chest, *92*:531–535, 1987.

Cefonicid

163. Geckler RW, McCormack GD, Goodman JS: Comparison of cefonicid and cefamandole for the treatment of community-acquired infections of the lower respiratory tract. Rev Infect Dis, *6*:S847, 1984.

Cefuroxime

164. Pines A, Raaat H, Khorasani M, Mullinger BM: Cefuroxime and ampicillin compared in a double-blind study in the treatment of lower respiratory tract infections. Chemotherapy, *27*:459, 1981.

Cefotetan

165. Wexler HM, Finegold SM: In vitro activity of cefotetan compared with that of other antimicrobial agents against anaerobic bacteria. Antimicrob Agents Chemother, *32*:601, 1988.

Cefoperazone

166. Gardner WG: Multicentered clinical evaluation of cefoperazone for the treatment of lower respiratory tract infections. Rev Infect Dis, *5*:SA137, 1983.
167. Mangi RJ, Greco T, Ryan J, et al.: Cefoperazone versus combination antibiotic therapy of hospital-acquired pneumonia. Am J Med, *84*:68, 1988.
168. Mangi RJ, Ryan J, Berenson C, et al.: Cefoperazone versus ceftazidime monotherapy of nosocomial pneumonia. Am J Med, *85(Suppl 1A)*:44, 1988.

Ceftazidime

169. Quinn JP, DiVencenzo CA, Foster J: Emergence of resistance to ceftazidime during therapy for Enterobacter cloacae infections. J Infect Dis, *155*:942, 1987
170. Trenholme GM, Pottage JC Jr, Karakusis PH: Use of ceftazidime in the treatment of nosocomial lower respiratory tract infections. Am J Med, *79S(Suppl 2A)*:32, 1985.

Cefotaxime

171. Maslow MJ, Simberkoff MS, Rahal JJ: Clinical efficacy of a synergistic combination of cefotaxime and amikacin against multiresistant pseudomonas and serratia infections. J Antimicrob Chemother, *16*:227, 1985.
172. Perkins RL: Clinical trials of cefotaxime for treatment of bacterial infections of the lower respiratory tract. Rev Infect Dis, *4(Suppl)*:S421, 1982.
173. Quintiliani R, Nightingale CH, Tilton R: Comparative pharmacokinetics of cefotaxime and ceftizoxime and the role of desacetylcefotaxime in the antibacterial activity of cefotaxime. Diagn Microbiol Infect Dis, *2*:63S, 1984.
174. Reeves JH, Russell GM, Cade JF, McDonald M: Comparison of ceftriaxone with cefotaxime in serious chest infections. Chest, *96*:1292, 1989.

Ceftriaxone

175. Baumgartner JD, Glauser HP: Single daily dose treatment of severe refractory infections with ceftiraxone. Cost savings and possible parenteral outpatient treatment. Arch Intern Med, *143*:1868, 1983.
176. Baumgartner JD, Glauser HP: Tolerance study of ceftriaxone compared with amoxicillin in patients with pneumonia. Am J Med, *77*:54, 1984.
177. Bittner MJ, Pugsley M, Horowitz EA, et al.: Randomized comparison of ceftriaxone and cefamandole therapy in lower respiratory tract infections in an elderly population. J Antimicrob Chemother, *18*:621, 1986.
178. Park HZ, Lee SP, Schy AL: Ceftriaxone-associated gallbladder sludge. Identification of calcium-ceftriaxone salt as a major component of gallbladder precipitate. Gastroenterology, *100*:1665, 1991.

Beta-lactamase Inhibitors

179. Graninger W, Leitha T, Griffin K, et al.: Activity of clavulanate-potentiated penicillins against methicillin-resistant Staphylococcus aureus. J Antimicrob Chemother, *24(Suppl B)*:49, 1989.
180. Livermore DM, Akova M, Wu P, Yang Y: Clavulanate and beta-lactamase induction. J Antimicrob Chemother, *24(Suppl B)*:23, 1989.
181. Rolinson GN: Evolution of beta-lactamase inhibitors. Rev Infect Dis, *13(Suppl 9)*:S727, 1991.
182. Roy C, Segura C, Torrellas A, et al.: Activity of amoxicillin/clavulanate against beta–lactamase-producing Escherichia coli and Klebsiella spp. J Antimicrob Chemother *24(Suppl B)*:41, 1989.
183. Wiedemann B, Kliebe C, Kresken M: The epidemiology of beta-lactamases. J Antimicrob Chemother, *24(Suppl B)*:1, 1989.

Ampicillin/sulbactam (Unasyn)

184. Greenwood D, Eley A: In vitro evaluation of sulbactam, a penicillinic acid sulphone with beta-lactamase inhibitory properties. J Antimicrob Chemother, *10*:117, 1982.
185. Wexler HM, Harrix B, Carter RWT, Finegold SM: In vitro activity efficacy of sulbatam combined with ampicillin against anaerobic bacteria. Antimicrob Agents Chemother, *27*:876, 1985.

Ticarcillin/clavulanate (Timentin)

186. Rosell GA, Bode R, Hamilton B, et al.: Clinical trial of the efficacy and safety of ticarcillin and clavulanic acid. Antimicrob Agents Chemother, *27*:291, 1985.
187. Schwigon CD, Hulla FW, Schulze B, et al.: Timentin in the treatment of nosocomial bronchopulmonary infections in intensive care units. J Antimirob Chemother, *17(Suppl C)*:115, 1986.
188. Shenep JL, Hughes JT, Roberson PK, et al.: Vancomycin, ticarcillin, and amikacin compared with ticarcillin-clavulanate and amikacin in the empirical treatment of febrile, neutropenic children with cancer. N Engl J Med, *319*:1053, 1988.

Monobactams (Aztreonam)

189. Brewer NS, Hellinger WC: The monobactams. Mayo Clin Proc, *66*;1152, 1991.
190. Clergeot A, Steru D, Rosset MA, Carbon C: Efficacy and safety of low-dose aztreonam in the treatment of moderate to severe infections due to gram-negative bacilli. Rev Infect Dis, *13(Suppl 7)*:S648, 1991.

191. Colardyn F, Gala JL, Veschraegen G, et al.: Infections in intensive care units: can the combination of a monobactam and a penicillin replace the classic combination of a beta-lactam agent and an aminoglycoside? Rev Infect Dis, *13*(*Suppl 7*):S640, 1991.
192. Cook JL: Gram-negative bacillary pneumonia in the nosocomial setting. Role of aztreonam. Am J Med, *88*(*Suppl 3C*):34S, 1990.
193. Davies BI, Maesen FP, Teengs J: Aztreonam in patients with acute exacerbations of chronic bronchitis: failure to prevent an emergence of pneumonoccal infections. J Antimicrob Chemother, *15*:375, 1985.

Carbapenems (Imipenem/cilastin)

194. Acar JF: Therapy for lower respiratory tract infections with imipenem/cilastin: a review of worldwide experience. Rev Infect Dis, *7*(*Suppl 3*):S513, 1985.
195. Calandra G, Lydick E, Corrigan J, et al.: Factors predisposing to seizures in seriously ill infected patients receiving antibiotics: experience with imipenem/cilastin. Am J Med, *84*: 911, 1988.
196. Fan W, del Busto R, Love M, et al.: Imipenem-cilastin in the treatment of methicillin-sensitive and methicillin-resistant Staphylococcus aureus infections. Antimicrob Agents Chemother, *29*:26, 1986.
197. Hartenauer U, Weilemann LS, Bodmann KF, et al.: Comparative clinical trial of ceftzidime and imipenem/cilastin in patients with severe nosocomial pneumonias and septicaemias. J Hosp Infect, *15*(*Suppl A*):61, 1990.
198. Hellinger WC, Brewer NS: Imipenem. Mayo Clin Proc, *66*:1074, 1991.
199. Margaret BS, Drusano GL, Standiford HC: Emergence of resistance to carbapenem antibiotics in Pseudomonas aeruginosa. J Antimicrob Chemother, *24*(*Suppl A*):161, 1989.
200. Moellering RC Jr., Eliopoulos GM, Sentochnick DE: The carbapenems: New broad spectrum beta-lactam antibiotics. J Antimicrob Chemother, *24*(*Suppl A*):1, 1989.
201. Quinn J, Studemeister AE, DiVencenzo CA: Resistance to imipenem in Pseudomonas aeruginosa: Clinical experience and biochemical mechanisms. Rev Infect Dis, *10*:892, 1988.
202. Sobel JD: Imipenem and aztreonam. Infect Dis Clin North Am, *3*:613, 1989.

Aminoglycosides

203. Bodem CR, Lampton LM, Miller DP, et al.: Endobronchial pH. Relevance of aminoglycoside activity in gram-negative bacillary pneumonia. Am Rev Respir Dis, *127*:39, 1983.
204. Edson S, Terrell CL: The aminoglycosides. Mayo Clin Proc, *66*:1158, 1991.
205. Eisenberg JM, Koffer H, Glick HA, Connell ML: What is the cost of nephrotoxicity associated with aminoglycosides? Ann Intern Med, *107*:900, 1987.
206. Kapusnik JE, Hackbarth CJ, Chambers HF, et al.: Single, large, daily dosing versus intermittent dosing of tobramycin for treating experimental pseudomonas pneumonia. J Infect Dis, *158*:7, 1988.
207. Moore RD, Smith CR, Leitman PS: Association of aminoglycoside plasma levels with therapeutic outcome in gram-negative pneumonia. Am J Med, *77*:657, 1984.

Inhaled Aminoglycosides

208. Brown RB, Kruse JA, Counts GW, et al.: Double-blind study of endotracheal tobramycin in the treatment of gram-negative bacterial pneumonia. Antimicrob Agents Chemother, *34*:269, 1990.
209. John JF Jr.: What price success? The continuing saga of the toxic:therapeutic ratio in the use of aminoglycoside antibiotics. J Infect Dis, *158*:1, 1988.

210. Sculie JP, Coppens L, Klastersky J: Effectiveness of mezlocillin and endotracheally administered sisomicin with or without parenteral sisomicin in the treatment of gram-negative bronchopneumonia. J Antimicrob Chemother, 9:63, 1982.

Clindamycin

211. Buchwald D, Soumerai SB, Vandevanter N, et al.: Effect of hospitalwide change in clindamycin dosing schedule on clinical outcome. Rev Infect Dis, 11:619, 1989.
212. Klainer ASA: Clindamycin. Med Clin North Am, 71:1169, 1987.
213. Smilack JD, Wilson WR, Cockerill FR III: Tetracyclines, chloramphenicol, erythromycin, clindamycin, and metronidazole. Mayo Clin Proc, 66:1270, 1991.
214. Smith SM, Mangia A, Eng RH, et al.: Clindamycin for colonization and infection by methicillin-resistant Staphylococcus aureus. Infection, 16:95, 1988.
215. Brittain DC: Erythromycin. Med Clin North Am, 71:1147, 1987.
216. Eady EA, Ross JI, Cove JH: Multiple mechanisms of erythromycin resistance. J Antimicrob Chemother, 26:461, 1990.
217. Washinton JA, Wilson WR: Erythromycin: a microbiological and clinical perspective after 30 years of clinical use. Mayo Clin Proc, 60:189, 271, 1985.
218. Karma P, Pukander J, Pentila M, et al.: The comparative efficacy and safety of chlarithromycin and amoxicillin in the treatment of outpatients with acute maxillary sinusitis. J Antimicrob Chemother 27(Suppl A):83, 1991.

Azalides (Azithromycin)

219. Balmes R, Clerk G, Dupont B, et al.: A comparative study of azithromycin and amoxicillin in the treatment of lower respiratory tract infections. Eur J Clin Microbiol Infect Dis, 10: 437, 1991.
220. Chirgwin K, Roblin PM, Hammerschlag MR: In vitro susceptibilities of Chlamydia pneumonia (Chlamydia sp. strain TWAR). Antimicrob Agents Chemother, 33:1634, 1989.
221. Dark D: Multicenter evaluation of azithromycin and cefaclor in acute lower respiratory tract infections. Am J Med, 91(Suppl 3A):31S, 1991.
222. Kitzis MD, Goldstein FW, Miegi M, Acar JF: In vitro activity of azithromycin against various gram-negative bacilli and anaerobic bacteria. J Antimicrob Chemother, Jan 25 Suppl A:15, 1990.
223. Maslell JP, Sefton AM, Williams JD: Comparative in vitro activity of azithromycin and erythromycin against gram-positive cocci, Haemophilus influenzae, and anaerobes. J Antimirob Chemother, Jan 25 Suppl A:19, 1990.
224. Neu HC: Clinical microbiology of azithromycin. Am J Med, 91(Suppl 3A):12S, 1991.
225. Schondwald S, Gunjaca M, Klacny Babic L, et al.: Comparison of azithromycin and erythromycin in the treatment of atypical pneumonias. J Antimicrob Chemother, Jan 25 Suppl A:123, 1990.

Metronidazole

226 Brogden RN, Heel RC, Speight TM, Avery GS: Metronidazole in anaerobic infections: a review of its activity, pharmacokinetics, and therapeutic use. Drugs, 16:387, 1978.
227. Perlino CA: Metronidazole vs clindamycin treatment of anaerobic pulmonary infection. Failure of metronidazole therapy. Arch Intern Med, 141:1424, 1981.

Tetracyclines

228. Francke EL, Neu HC: Chloramphenicol and tetracyclines. Med Clin North Am, 71:1155, 1987.

Trimethoprim/sulfa

229. Cockerill FR III, Edson RS: Trimethoprim-sulfamethoxazole. Mayo Clin Proc, *66*:1260, 1991.
230. Elwell LP, Wilson HR, Knick VB, Keith BR: In vitro and in vivo efficacy of the combination trimethoprim/sulfamethoxazole against clinical isolates of methicillin-resistant Staphylococcus aureus. Antimicrob Agents Chemother, *29*:1092, 1986.
231. Foltzer MA, Reese RE: Trimethoprim-sulfamethoxazole and other sulfonamides. Med Clin North Am, *71*:1177, 1987.
232. Huovinen P: Trimethoprim resistance. Antimicrob Agents Chemother, *31*:1451, 1987.
233. Quintiliani R, Levitz RE, Nightingale CH: Potential role of trimethoprim-sulfamethoxazole in the treatment of serious hospital-acquired bacterial infections. Rev Infect Dis, *9*:S160, 1987.
234. Sattler FR, Remington JS: Intravenous sulfamethoxazoe and trimethoprim for serious gram negative bacillary infection. Arch Intern Med, *143*:1709, 1983.

Vancomycin

235. Leclercq R, Delot E, Duval J, et al.: Plasmid-mediated resistance to vancomycin and teicoplanin in Enterococcus faceium. N Engl J Med, *319*:157, 1988.
236. Levine JF: Vancomycin: a review. Med Clin North Am, *71*:1135, 1987.
237. Rubin M, Hathorn JW, Marshall D, et al.: Gram-positive infections and the use of vancomycin in 550 episodes of fever and neutropenia. Ann Intern Med, *108*:30, 1988.
238. Schwalbe RS, Stapleton JT, Gilligan PH: Emergence of vancomycin resistance in coagulase-negative staphylococci. N Engl J Med, *316*:927, 1987.
239. Sorrell TC, Packham DR, Shanker S, et al.: Vancomycin therapy for methicillin-resistant Staphylococcus aureus. Ann Intern Med, *97*:344, 1982.
240. Wilhelm MP: Vancomycin. Mayo Clin Proc, *66*:1165, 1991.

Fluoroquinolones

241. Hooper DC, Wolfson JS: Fluoroquinolone antimicrobial agents. N Engl J Med, *324*:383, 1991.
242. Thys JP: Quinolones in the treatment of bronchopulmonary infections. Rev Infect Dis, *10(Suppl 1)*:S212, 1988.
243. Trucksis M, Hooper DC, Wolfson JS: Emerging resistance to fluoroquinolones in staphylococci: an alert. Ann Intern Med, *114*:424, 1991.

Ciprofloxacin

244. Ball P: Emergent resistance to ciprofloxacin amongst Pseudomonas aeruginosa and Staphylococcus aureus: clinical significance and therapeutic approaches. J Antimicrob Chemother, *26(Suppl F)*:1650, 1990.
245. Cooper B, Lawlor M: Pneumococcal bacteremia during ciprofloxacin therapy for pneumococcal pneumonia. Am J Med, *87*:475, 1989.
246. Frieden TR, Mangi RJ: Inappropriate use of oral ciprofloxacin. JAMA, *264*:1438, 1990.
247. Lode H, Wiley R, Hooken G, et al.: Prospective randomized controlled study of ciprofloxacin versus imipenem/cilastin in severe clinical infections. Antimicrob Agents Chemother, *31*:1491, 1987.
248. Haddow A, Heinz G, Wantuck D: Ciprofloxacin (intravenous/oral) versus ceftazidime in lower respiratory tract infections. Am J Med, *87(Suppl 5A)*:113S, 1989.
249. Khan FA, Basir R: Sequential intravenous-oral administration of ciprofloxacin vs ceftazidime in serious bacterial respiratory tract infections. Chest, *96*:528, 1989.

250. Mehon L, Ernst JA, Sy ER, et al.: Sequential intravenous/oral ciprofloxacin compared with intravenous ceftazidime in the treatment of serious lower respiratory tract infections. Am J Med, *87(Suppl 5A)*:119, 1989.
251. Paladino JA, Sperry HE, Backes JM, et al.: Clinical and economic evaluation of oral ciprofloxacin after an abbreviated course of intravenous antibiotics. Am J Med, *91*:462, 1991.
252. Peterson PK, Stein D, Guay DRP, et al.: Prospective study of lower respiratory tract infections in an extended care nursing home program: potential role of oral ciprofloxacin. Am J Med, *85*:164, 1988.
253. Piercy EA, Barbara D, Luby JP, Mackowiak PA: Ciprofloxacin for methicillin-resistant Staphylococcus aureus infections. Antimicrob Agents Chemother, *33*:128, 1989.
254. Shalit I, Berger SA, Gorea A, Frimerman H: Widespread quinolone resistance among methicillin-resistant Staphylococcus aureus isolates in a general hospital. Antimicrob Agents Chemother, *33*:593, 1989.
255. Trenholme GN, Schmitt BA, Spear J, et al.: Randomized study of intravenous/oral ciprofloxacin versus ceftazidime in the treatment of hospital and nursing home patients with lower respiratory tract infections. Am J Med, *87(Suppl 5A)*:116, 1989.
256. Unertl KE, Lenhart FP, Forst H, et al.: Brief report: ciprofloxacin in the treatment of legionellosis in critically ill patients including those cases unresponsive to erythromycin. Am J Med, *87(Suppl 5A)*:128S, 1989.

Ofloxacin

257. Chidiak C, Leroy O, Beuscart C, et al.: Efficacy and safety of oral ofloxacin for treatment of pneumonia. Rev Infect Dis, *11(Suppl 5)*:1223, 1989.
258. Gentry LO, Rodriguez-Gomez G, Kohler RB, et al.: Ofloxacin, parenteral followed by oral, for nosocomial pneumonia and community-acquired pneumonia requiring hospitalization. Am Rev Respir Dis, *145*:31–35, 1992.
259. Lipsky BA, Tack KJ, Kuo C, et al.: Ofloxacin treatment of Chlamydia pneumoniae (Strain TWAR) lower respiratory tract infections. Am J Med, *89*:722, 1990.
260. Sanders WE, Morris JF, Alessi PK, et al.: Oral ofloxacin for the treatment of acute bacterial pneumonia: use of a nontraditional protocol to compare experimental therapy with usual care in a multicenter clinical trial. Am J Med, *91*:261, 1991.
261. Stocks JM, Wallace RJ Jr., Griffith DE, et al.: Ofloxacin in community-acquired lower respiratory tract infections: a comparison with amoxicillin or erythromycin. Am J Med, *87(6C)*:52S, 1989.

Perfloxacin

262. Martin C, Gouin F, Fourrier F, et al.: Perfloxacin in the treatment of nosocomial lower respiratory tract infections in intensive care patients. J Antimicrob Chemother, *21*:795, 1988.
263. Davey PG: Efficacy of temafloxacin versus ciprofloxacin or amoxicillin for lower respiratory tract infections in smokers and the elderly. Am J Med, *91(Suppl 6A)*:101S, 1991.
264. Hardy DJ: Activity of temafloxacin and other fluoroquinolones against typical and atypical community-acquired respiratory tract pathogens. Am J Med, *91(Suppl 6A)*:12S, 1991.
265. Pankey GA: Temafloxacin: an overview. Am J Med, *91(Suppl 6A)*:166S, 1991.

Combination Therapy (Aminoglycoside plus Beta-lactam)

266. Bru JP, Michallet M, Legrand C, Swierz P et al.: A prospective randomized study comparing the efficacy of Timentin alone or in combination with amikacin in the treatment of febrile neutropenic patients. J Antimicrobial Chemother *17(Suppl C)*:203–209, 1986.

267. EORTC International Antimicrobial Therapy Cooperative Group: Ceftazidime combined with a short or long course of amikacin for empirical therapy of gram-negative bacteremia in cancer patients with granulocytopenia. N Engl J Med, *317*:1692, 1987.

268. Hilf M, Yu VL, Sharp JA, et al.: Antibiotic therapy for Pseudomonas aeruginosa bacteremia: outcome correlations in a prospective study of 200 patients. Am J Med, *87*:540, 1989.

269. LaForce FM: Systemic antimicrobial therapy of nosocomial pneumonia: monotherapy versus combination therapy. Eur J Clin Microbiol Infect Dis, *8*:61, 1989.

270. Liang R, Yung R, Chiu E, et al.: Ceftazidime versus imipenem-cilastin as initial monotherapy for febrile neutropenic patients. Antimicrob Agents Chemother, *34*:1336, 1990.

271. Meunier F, Zinner SH, Gaya H, et al.: Prospective randomized evaluation of ciprofloxacin versus piperacillin plus amikacin for empiric antibiotic therapy of febrile granulocytopenic cancer patients with lymphomas and solid tumors. Antimicrob Agents Chemother, *35*:873, 1991.

272. Pizzo PA, Hathorn JW, Hiemenz J, et al.: A randomized trial comparing ceftazidime alone with combination antibiotic therapy in cancer patients with fever and neutropenia. N Engl J Med, *315*:552, 1986.

273. Rusnak MG, Drake TA, Hackbarth CJ, et al.: Single versus combination antibiotic therapy for pneumonia due to Pseudomonas aeruginosa in neutropenic guinea pigs. J Infect Dis, *149*:980, 1984.

Double Beta-lactam Therapy

274. DeJohngh CA, Joshi JH, Thompson BW, et al.: A double beta-lactam combination versus an aminoglycoside-containing regimen as empiric therapy for febrile granulocytopenic cancer patients. Am J Med, *80(Suppl 5C)*:101, 1986.

275. Winston DJ, Ho WG, Bruckner DA, Champlin RE: Beta-lactam antibiotic therapy in febrile granulocytopenic patients. A randomized trial comparing cefoperazone plus piperacillin, ceftazidime plus piperacillin, and imipenem alone. Ann Intern Med, *115*:849, 1991.

276. Winston DJ, Ho WG, Champtlin RE, et al.: Ureidopenicillins, aztreonam, and thienamycin: efficacy as single drug therapy of severe infections and potential as components of combined therapy. J Antimicrob Chemother, *17(Suppl A)*:55, 1986.

Other Combinations

277. Rodriguez JR, Ramirez-Ronda CH, Nevarez M: Efficacy and safety of aztreonam-clindamycin versus tobramycin-clindamycin in the treatment of lower respiratory tract infections caused by aerobic gram negative bacilli. Antimicrob Agents Chemother, *27*:246, 1985.

278. Viscoli C, Moroni C, Boni L, et al.: Ceftazidime plus amikacin versus ceftazidime plus vancomycin as empiric therapy in febrile neutropenic children with cancer. Rev Infect Dis, *13*:393, 1991.

Antimicrobial Resistance

279. Grayson ML, Eliopoulos GM: Antimicrobial resistance in the intensive care unit. Semin Respir Infect, *5*:204, 1990.

280. Michea-Hamzehpour M, Pecheve JC, Marchou B, et al.: Combination therapy: A way to limit emergence of resistance? Am J Med, *80(Suppl 6B)*:138, 1986.

281. Patterson JE, Zervos MS: High-level gentamicin resistance in Enterococcus: microbiology, genetic, basis, and epidemiology. Rev Infect Dis, *12*:644, 1990.

282. Sanders CC, Sanders WE Jr., Goering RV, et al.: Selection of multiple antibiotic resistance by quinolones, beta-lactams and aminoglycosides with special reference to cross-resistance between unrelated drug classes. Antimicrob Agents Chemother, *26*:797, 1984.

283. Sanders WE, Sanders CC: Inducible beta-lactamases: clinical and epidemiological implications for use of newer cephalosporins. Rev Infect Dis, *10*:830, 1988.
284. Schaberg DR, Culver D, Gaynes RP: Major trends in the microbial etiology of nosocomial infections. Am J Med, *91(Suppl 3B)*:725–755, 1991.
285. Tenover FC: Novel and emerging mechanisms of antimicrobial resistance in nosocomial pneumonia. Am J Med, *91(Suppl 3B)*:373, 1991.

Oral Antibiotics

286. Cooper TJ, Ladusans E, Williams PE, et al.: A comparison of oral cefuroxime axetil and oral amoxicillin in lower respiratory tract infections. J Antimicrob Chemother, *16*:373, 1985.
287. Schmidt EW, Zimmerman I, Ritzerfeld W, et al.: Controlled prospective study of oral amoxicillin/clavulanate vs ciprofloxacin in acute exacerbations of chronic bronchitis. J Antimicrob Chemother, *24(Suppl B)*:185, 1989.

25

FUNGAL, MYCOBACTERIAL, AND VIRAL PULMONARY INFECTIONS

Galen B. Toews
Joseph P. Lynch, III

PNEUMOCYSTIS CARINII

ORGANISM

Pneumocystis was first described in 1909 by Chagas, who thought he had discovered a developmental stage of the trypanosome. Carini, who identified the organism in the alveoli of a rat that had concomitant trypanosomal infection, made the same mistake. Delanoe recognized the organism as a distinct species in 1912 and named it Pneumocystis carinii.

P. carinii is a unicellular eucaryote whose exact taxonomic position is unclear. The prevailing view, until recently, favored a protozoan classification because of its susceptibility to antiprotozoal agents. Recent studies analyzing ribosomal RNA have demonstrated that P. carinii is more closely related to fungi. Additionally, dihydrofolate reductase and thymidylate synthase, two major enzymes in P. carinii, have been shown not to be physically or genetically linked. On the other hand, in protozoa, these enzymes appear to be located on the same polypeptide chain. Finally, biochemical studies have demonstrated that the wall of P. carinii cysts contains large amounts of beta-glucan. A 1,3-β-glucanase (zymolyase) that has been useful in analyzing fungi has been shown to cleave the cell wall and surface antigens of P. carinii. Taken together, these findings suggest that P. carinii may well be a fungal organism rather than a protozoan.

EPIDEMIOLOGY

The epidemiologic characteristics of P. carinii are poorly understood. P. carinii is likely acquired by inhalation of an airborne particle at an early age. The fungal nature of P. carinii raises the possibility that unidentified stage(s) (spores) or environmental sources may be importantly involved in its epidemiologic background. Most children develop antibody to P. carinii by the age of 4 years. Persistent asymptomatic infection is difficult to document because P. carinii is not usually visualized in normal lungs at autopsy. The organism is believed to become a part of the resident microbial flora in the host and to propagate if and when the host's immune function becomes compromised.

Alternatively, P. carinii may result from exposure to an exogenous source. P. carinii might be spread through contact with infected persons or other environmental foci. These transmitted organisms could then be the source of a new infection or complicate a pre-existent latent infection in the immunocompromised host. The possibility of person-to-person spread of P. carinii is suggested by outbreaks of pneumocystis pneumonia among malnourished infants, in hospitals caring for immunosuppressed patients, and in elderly patients.

CLINICAL PRESENTATION

Certain patient populations are at high risk for the development of this disease. The major predisposing conditions are characterized by impaired cellular immunity and include acquired immunodeficiency syndrome (AIDS), primary immunodeficiency diseases, the use of intensive cytotoxic chemotherapeutic agents for malignant tumors, the use of corticosteroids, the use of immunosuppression in transplant recipients, protein malnutrition, prematurity, and patients with adult T-cell leukemia. The risk of P. carinii in patients with human immunodeficiency virus (HIV) infection correlates with the number of CD4 cells. P. carinii pneumonia occurs almost exclusively in patients whose CD4 counts are below 200 cells/mm^3 and particularly in those whose counts are less than 100 cells/mm^3. An HIV-infected individual with a CD4 count greater than 700 cells/mm^3 has only a 3.8% chance of developing P. carinii pneumonia within a 3-year period. A patient whose CD4 count is between 200 and 350 cells/mm^3 has a risk over this same period of 23%.

The presentation of pneumocystis pneumonia in HIV-infected patients is different from its presentation in those with other forms of immunodeficiency. In oncologic patients, its presentation is usually that of a rapidly progressive disease with fever, tachypnea, dyspnea with nonproductive or mildly productive cough, and crepitations (crackles). Severe hypoxemia usually develops within 5 to 10 days of initial manifestations. In HIV-infected patients, the onset of symptoms is usually more insidious, with nonspecific symptoms, such as a low-grade fever, mild cough, dyspnea on exertion, fatigue, and weight loss, being present for weeks to months before pulmonary symptoms become sufficiently bothersome to prompt medical intervention. Certain features have been shown to be of value in predicting the clinical course of AIDS-related P. carinii pneumonia. Duration of symptoms does not correlate with prognosis; however, a normal chest x-ray at the time of admission is a good prognostic sign. A wide alveolar-arterial gradient, a low PaO$_2$ (less than 50 or 60 mm Hg), and a respiratory rate equal to or greater than 30 have all been associated with a poor prognosis. If an initial PaO$_2$ is less than 50 or 60 mm Hg, the mortality rate approaches 50%. Mortality of untreated P. carinii pneumonia approaches 100%.

The diagnostic method(s) of choice for P. carinii pneumonia has undergone considerable evolution during the past decade. The examination of expectorated sputum in P. carinii pneumonia not associated with AIDS rarely yields the diagnosis, but detection of organisms in AIDS-associated P. carinii pneumonia may be more readily accomplished because of the larger numbers of organisms present. Examination of the sputum obtained by hypertonic saline nebulization yields a diagnostic sensitivity of 78%. The use of monoclonal antibodies can increase the sensitivity of the procedure to greater than 90%. Although a negative induced sputum is not sensitive enough to exclude the diagnosis, the patients with positive sputum are spared the need for bronchoscopic procedures. If sputum or nonbronchoscopic lavage is negative, fiberoptic bronchoscopy is the procedure of choice. Bronchoalveolar lavage (BAL) alone or with transbronchial biopsy can make the diagnosis rapidly in nearly all cases of HIV-associated P. carinii pneumonia. No cases of P. carinii pneumonia were missed in 373 patients when all diagnostic components of a bronchoscopy were performed (i.e. transbronchial biopsy with fixed tissue specimen and touch imprints, BAL, and brush biopsy). Open lung biopsy is only slightly more sensitive than BAL alone, and repeated bronchoscopic BAL and biopsy give an equivalent yield. Therefore, open lung biopsy is rarely necessary and is undertaken only if the possibility for other diagnoses is strong entertained (i.e. Kaposi's sarcoma, a lymphocytic interstitial pneumonitis).

TREATMENT

- Two antibiotic regimens are available, trimethoprim-sulfamethoxazole (TMP/SMX) and parenteral pentamidine isethionate. The efficacies of these two regimens in the therapy of AIDS-associated P. carinii pneumonia appear to be generally comparable, although TMP/SMX is preferable because of its lower incidence of severe side effects
- In moderate to severe disease, TMP/SMX should be given IV (in divided doses) at a total daily dose of 20 mg trimethoprim and 100 mg sulfamethoxazole/kg body weight. In mild cases, oral administration is preferable. Peak sulfamethoxazole levels should be monitored, especially when the drug is given orally, to assure adequate serum levels (100 to 150 μg/ml). Additionally, the frequency of adverse reaction is lessened if sulfamethoxazole levels are below 200 μg/ml
- The appropriate duration of treatment with either agent has not been established conclusively, but most clinicians prefer to treat episodes of AIDS-associated P. carinii pneumonia for 21 days

Response rates range from 60 to 80%. Ninety-day survival rates after P. carinii pneumonia are similar in patients with and without AIDS, but relapse is more frequent in the AIDS-related group, occurring in at least 20 to 40% of surviving patients. The incidence of side effects from either drug is quite high, in excess of 60% in most series.

- Dapsone is another antifolate that can be utilized for treatment of P. carinii. Dapsone alone is not as effective as conventional therapy or dapsone plus trimethoprim. Dapsone plus trimethoprim may be as ef-

fective, better tolerated, and associated with fewer side effects than conventional agents. Dapsone plus trimethoprim may, therefore, be an acceptable alternative to TMP/SMX or pentamidine in some patients
- Trimetrexate, an inhibitor of dihydrofolate reductase that is 1,000-fold more potent than trimethoprim, induces a response rate of 77 to 92% when administered by IV infusion. A major drawback of trimetrexate therapy thus far has been the high relapse rate (up to 60%) when this drug is used as a single agent. Combinations of this drug with other agents or prompt institution of prophylaxis after completion of acute therapy might reduce this high relapse rate
- P. carinii causes respiratory failure and death, especially in patients with moderate to severe hypoxemia at the time therapy is initiated. The prognosis for AIDS patients who have severe pulmonary dysfunction at the time of initial presentation or who are developing respiratory failure after initiation of specific therapy can be improved substantially by the use of adjunctive corticosteroid therapy. Deterioration in respiratory function, need for mechanical ventilation, and death can all be reduced significantly by the use of corticosteroids. Early adjunctive corticosteroid therapy should be utilized in individuals with an alveolar-arterial oxygen difference greater than 35 mm Hg or a PaO_2 less than 70 mm Hg on room air at the time therapy is initiated. Adjunctive corticosteroids should be started as early as possible and no later than within 72 hours of initiating specific antimicrobial therapy for P. carinii pneumonia. No data are available regarding the efficacy of adjunctive steroids for patients who fail to respond after more than 3 days of antimicrobial therapy, and accordingly, no recommendations regarding salvage therapy can be made. Although the optimal steroid regimen has not been determined, the regimen recommended is prednisone 40 mg bid (days 1 to 5), prednisone 20 mg bid (days 6 to 10), and prednisone 20 mg daily (days 11 to 21). Life-threatening adverse consequences of corticosteroid therapy have not been noted in any of the published studies, but standard surveillance should be employed. Clinical relapse may occur following abrupt, simultaneous discontinuation of corticosteroids and specific microbial therapy

Preferred Therapy

- Trimethoprim-sulfamethoxazole; trimethoprim, 20 mg/kg/d IV or PO in 3 or 4 doses for 21 days
- Prednisone, 40 mg PO bid, days 1 to 5
  Prednisone, 20 mg PO bid, days 6 to 10
  Prednisone, 20 mg PO daily, days 11 to 21
- Prednisone, for patients with $PaO_2 \leq 70$ mm Hg or A-a gradient ≥ 33 mm Hg

Alternate Therapy

- Pentamidine, 3 to 4 mg/kg, IV qd for 21 days
- Trimethoprim, 5 mg/kg PO q6h for 21 days + dapsone, 100 mg PO daily for 21 days

PROPHYLAXIS

Prophylactic therapy is required in patients with P. carinii pneumonia because approximately 60% of AIDS patients relapse within 1 year of their first episode of pneumonia. Additionally, primary prophylaxis markedly reduces the risk of pneumocystis pneumonia in pediatric patients with acute leukemia and other childhood malignant disorders. Both TMP/SMX and aerosolized pentamidine have been utilized for prophylactic therapy. CD4 cell counts constitute a reliable indicator of the relative risk of an HIV-infected individual acquiring P. carinii pneumonia, and accordingly, CD4 counts should be monitored every 3 to 6 months to determine when prophylaxis should begin. Prophylaxis with TMP/SMX or aerosolized pentamidine should begin when CD4 counts fall below 200 cells/mm^3. Secondary prophylaxis is recommended for all patients with a history of P. carinii pneumonia regardless of CD4 counts.

TMP/SMX prophylaxis involves administration of 1 double-strength tablet daily. Aerosol pentamidine (300 mg) is administered monthly via a Respirguard II nebulizer. Prior to beginning aerosolized pentamidine therapy, active tuberculosis should be ruled out to prevent spread of tuberculosis to both other patients and staff. Patterns of P. carinii pneumonia are changed following aerosol prophylaxis, with a predominance of upper lobe involvement and an increase in extrapulmonary P. carinii. Adverse effects include hypoglycemia (1%), airway irritation with cough (10 to 20%), and bronchospasm (1 to 2%).

Preliminary information regarding a clinical trial or TMP/SMX vs aerosolized pentamidine given in conjunction with zidovudine for prevention of recurrent P. carinii pneumonia in patients with AIDS suggests that 1 double-strength tablet of TMP/SMX was superior to aerosolized pentamidine, 300 mg every 4 weeks. In the 310 participants, 50 recurrences were reported during the study, 14 of which were among those assigned to TMP/SMX and 36 of which were among those assigned to aerosolized pentamidine. The risk of developing recurrent P. carinii pneumonia for participants randomized to aerosolized pentamidine was estimated to be 3 to 25 times that of participants randomized to TMP/SMX. No differences in hematologic or hepatic adverse effects were noted.

Preferred Therapy

- TMP/SMX, 1 double-strength tablet daily
- Prophylaxis when CD4 count < 200 cells/mm^3
- Secondary prophylaxis for all patients with a history of P. carinii pneumonia

Alternate Therapy

- Aerosolized pentamidine, 300 mg every 4 weeks using the Respirgard II nebulizer

SPECIFIC DRUGS

Trimethoprim-sulfamethoxazole (TMP/SMX)

TMP/SMX blocks folate metabolism at two sites. TMP inhibits dihydrofolate reductase and also inhibits dihydrofolic synthetase. TMP has at least a 2,000-fold greater affinity for microbial than mammalian dihydrofolate reductase. SMX interferes with dihydrofolic synthetase, an enzyme found only in microbes. TMP and SMZ have a broad spectrum of antimicrobial activity, are well absorbed after oral administration, and have similar peak concentrations and half-lives. Peak serum levels occur at 1 to 3 hours, and the serum half-life is 12 to 13 hours. Common adverse reactions that necessitate discontinuance of the drug include a rash with exfoliation or mucositus, severe neutropenia, thrombocytopenia, or hepatitis. Less severe adverse reactions include nausea, vomiting, and hyponatremia.

Pentamidine

Pentamidine is an aromatic diamidine whose mechanism of action is unknown. Pentamidine interferes with folate metabolism, oxidative phosphorylation, nucleic acid replication, and anaerobic glycolysis. Peak serum levels occur within 1 hour, and the half-life of the drug is between 6 and 10 hours. The tissue half-life of pentamidine may be as long as 30 days in the lung. Parenteral administration is necessary because gastrointestinal (GI) absorption is poor. The drug is best administered IV over a period of 60 to 90 minutes in 250 ml of 5% dextrose. Intramuscular (IM) administration should be avoided because of subcutaneous abscess formation at the injection site. Adverse reactions to pentamidine include hypoglycemia, azotemia, neutropenia, chemical hepatitis, nausea with vomiting, and cardiac arrhythmias. Pentamidine may induce damage to beta cells in the pancreas and may result in diabetes mellitus. Although cardiac arrhythmias are rare, they are difficult to manage because of the long tissue half-life of pentamidine.

Dapsone-Trimethoprim (DA/TMP)

DA/TMP is another antifolate combination that inhibits purine synthesis. Each drug in this combination interferes with the metabolism of the other; thus, an optimal dosage regimen is not known. Adverse effects include mild to severe nausea, vomiting, and a rash. Hyperkalemia, methemoglobinemia, elevated liver enzyme neutropenia, and thrombocytopenia also occur.

Trimetrexate

Trimetrexate is a potent inhibitor of mammalian and protozoal dihydrofolate reductase. This agent is lipid soluble and easily enters both mammalian cells and P. carinii. Folinic acid (leucovorin), which is not lipid soluble, is actively transported into mammalian cells but not into P. carinii.

Folinic acid must be administered to protect host tissues from toxic anti-folate effects.

FUNGAL DISEASE

ASPERGILLUS

EPIDEMIOLOGY

Aspergillus spp (A. fumigatus, A. flavus, A. niger) are ubiquitous in the environment, and infection with these septated fungi may occur via environmental exposures or via endogenous reactivation of latent spores in susceptible (immunocompromised) hosts. Host defenses against Aspergillus spp involve both granulocytes (PMNs) and mononuclear phagocytes; abrogation of both lines of defenses appears necessary to predispose to clinical disease. Thus, invasive aspergillosis occurs in patients with severe aberrations in *both* cellular immunity and granulocyte number or function. Infection most commonly occurs by endogenous spread in granulocytopenic patients previously colonized with Aspergillus spp; reinfection is common among previously infected leukemic patients (even after completion of antifungal therapy) when chemotherapy is continued. Nosocomial outbreaks of invasive aspergillosis in severely immunocompromised patients have also been described to result from inhalation of Aspergillus spores from contaminated air vents, operating rooms, and hospital wards. Clinical features of invasive aspergillar infections are protean. Aspergillus spp may affect virtually any organ, but have a distinct predilection for the lung and central nervous system. Pulmonary involvement occurs in more than 80% of patients; extrapulmonary dissemination (most commonly brain, GI tract, and skin) occurs in 20 to 30% of patients. Tissue invasion has been described following traumatic inoculation in devitalized tissue in nonimmunosuppressed hosts, but this occurrence is rare. More than 90% of cases of invasive aspergillosis occur in two settings: granulocytopenic patients with hematologic malignant conditions and organ transplant recipients on intensive immunosuppressive therapy. Multiple predisposing factors are usually present concomitantly and include prior corticosteroid or immunosuppressive therapy, recent antibiotic therapy, and severe (and sustained) granulocytopenia. Duration of granulocytopenia has been shown to be a critical determinant of risk of developing aspergillosis among patients with hematologic malignant conditions or bone marrow transplants. In this context, the risk of developing aspergillosis has been less than 1% when granulocytopenia resolves within 2 weeks; by contrast, infection rates of 4 to 15% have been noted when duration exceeds 24 to 30 days. Invasive aspergillosis may also complicate solid organ transplantation, even with normal granulocyte levels, because corticosteroids and immunosuppressive agents adversely affect granulocyte function. The frequency of invasive aspergillosis has been highly variable among institutions and varies considerably according to the transplanted organ. Aspergillosis occurs in only 1 to 5% of renal and hepatic transplant recipients, but is the most common fungal infection complicating heart, heart-lung, lung, and bone marrow transplants. At Stanford University, invasive aspergillosis occurred in 14% of 400 heart transplant recipients and 15% of the first 75 heart-lung transplant recipients; lower prevalence rates (ranging from 2 to 10%) have been noted in most other centers performing cardiac or lung transplantation. Bone marrow transplant recipients are most susceptible to invasive aspergillosis, with prevalence rates approaching 20% in some centers. The majority of cases occur within the first 40 days, thereby suggesting nosocomial acquisition. Aggressive prophylaxis with antifungal agents and the use of environmental control measures to reduce exposure to aspergillus spores may limit the development of clinical aspergillar infections in these patient populations. Aspergillar infections rarely complicate AIDS, which likely reflects the preservation of granulocyte number and function in this disorder. Only 3 cases of aspergillosis were described among the first 1,762 cases of AIDS reported to the Centers for Disease Control. In 1991, however, Denning and colleagues reported 13 cases of pulmonary aspergillosis among patients with AIDS seen at several medical centers within a 12-month period. Aspergillosis invariably developed late in the course of disease and followed multiple opportunistic infections (including Pneumocystis carinii pneumonitis in 10). Neutropenia was present in 6 patients; 4 had received prior treatment with corticosteroids. This finding suggests that pulmonary aspergillar infections may become more prevalent in patients with AIDS as survival is prolonged (with the use of zidovudine [AZT]) and with the increasing use of corticosteroids in AIDS (for *P. carinii* pneumonitis). With few exceptions, invasive aspergillosis develops only after *severe* and *sustained* impairment of host defenses and is confined to the few high-risk populations previously listed (e.g. granulocytopenic patients, organ transplant recipients, and patients late in the course of AIDS). Intensive corticosteroid and immunosuppressive/cytotoxic therapy may predispose to aspergillar infection in other populations as well (e.g. collagen vascular disorders and systemic vasculitis), but this outcome has been rare.

CLINICAL PRESENTATION

Invasive aspergillosis involves the lung (either primarily or in the context of widespread dissemination) in more than 80% of cases. Brain and GI involvement occur in 10 to 15% of cases. Prognosis with cerebral aspergillosis is grim, with a fatality rate of more than 95%. Aspergillosis involving the maxillary or ethmoidal sinuses may extend into the orbit or intracerebral vessels in neutropenic hosts. Ocular invasion may necessitate surgical enucleation in addition to medical therapy. GI involvement is rarely recognized ante mortem, but has been noted at necropsy in as many as 20% of series of invasive aspergillosis. Virtually all such cases have included concomitant pulmonary involvement. Primary cutaneous infection has been described in association with Hickman catheters in granulocytopenic patients with hematologic malignant conditions or in bone marrow transplant recipients. Rare sites of involvement include the ocular cavities and their adjacent cavities (endophthalmitis), liver, spleen, upper airway, bone, wounds, epidural space, urinary tract, pericardium, and endocardium (endocarditis).

BRONCHOPULMONARY INVOLVEMENT

Aspergillus spp may cause a wide spectrum of pulmonary disease, including allergic bronchopulmonary aspergillosis (ABPA), mycetoma (fungal ball), chronic necrotizing aspergillosis, and invasive aspergillosis. More recently, locally invasive aspergillosis involving the tracheobronchial tree in immunocompromised hosts has been described. ABPA represents a hypersensitivity response to aspergillus antigens in asthmatic patients, and is revealed by blood and tissue eosinophilia, wheezing, pulmonary infiltrates, high serum IgE, and positive immediate skin tests to aspergillus. Corticosteroids (to ablate the exaggerated antigenic response) are the mainstay of therapy. This syndrome does not result in systemic dissemination and does not require antifungal therapy. Aspergillus spp may also infect pre-existing pulmonary cavities in patients with chronic granulomatous or obstructive lung disease, thereby resulting in the formation of a distinct mass or fungal ball (i.e. aspergilloma or mycetoma). A crescent, with an intracavitary mass of hyphae, may be observed on chest x-rays or computed tomographic (CT) scans. Hemoptysis may result from erosion of the fungal hyphae into pulmonary vessels; specific antifungal therapy is of no value in this context. Surgical resection should be accomplished when feasible, although in many patients severe impairment in pulmonary function may contraindicate surgery. Chronic necrotizing aspergillosis is a rare condition, distinct from mycetoma, in which chronic aspergillar infection occurs within pre-existing cavitary disease (e.g. obstructive lung disease, destructive granulomatous disease) in otherwise immunologically normal hosts and extends or invades contiguous lung parenchyma. A distinct fungal ball is not observed, and extrapulmonary spread is rare. In contrast to invasive aspergillosis in immunocompromised hosts, which is often rapidly fulminant and lethal, the course of chronic necrotizing aspergillosis is indolent and rarely fatal. Amphotericin B is warranted, but data affirming its efficacy are limited. In contrast to the syndromes just reviewed, invasive aspergillosis represents tissue invasion with Aspergillus spp and is almost exclusively confined to individuals with serious deficits in immunity. The most common initial features of invasive pulmonary aspergillosis are new or persistent infiltrate(s) on the chest x-ray and fever. Radiographic features are variable; patchy bronchopneumonia, single or multiple nodular infiltrates, and cavitary lesions are characteristic. Lobar consolidation indistinguishable from bacterial pneumonia occurs in 5 to 15% of patients, however. Diffuse miliary or interstitial changes are unusual. Progressive parenchymal necrosis may lead to cavitation or even mycetoma (fungal ball). CT scans of the chest may be an invaluable adjunct; the demonstration of a "halo sign" on CT scan is characteristic of pulmonary aspergillosis. Pleuritic chest pain and hemoptysis are common associated symptoms and may reflect vascular invasion. Aspergillus spp have a propensity to invade the pulmonary vasculature; intravascular thrombosis, necrosis, and massive (sometimes exsanguinating) hemorrhage may result. The course of invasive aspergillosis, in the absence of therapy, is usually fulminant, with death within 2 to 4 weeks in most cases. More recently, aspergillus selectively invading the tracheobronchial tree has been described in patients with AIDS; in leukemic patients; and in heart-lung, lung, and bone marrow transplant recipients. Bronchoscopy may demonstrate necrotizing tracheitis, destruction of cartilage, ulcerations, or pseudomembranes overlying the bronchial mucosa; extension to lung parenchyma or widespread dissemination may also occur. Amphotericin B, combined with surgical debridement, is recommended.

DIAGNOSIS

The diagnosis of invasive pulmonary aspergillosis is difficult, as only 10 to 30% of sputum cultures are positive in this context. Further, isolation of Aspergillus spp from sputum or tracheobronchial secretions suggests, but does not *prove*, the presence of invasive disease. Isolation of Aspergillus spp from sputum or BAL has been associated with invasive disease in only 30 to 80% of patients at risk; in the remaining cases, positive cultures simply have represented asymptomatic colonization. Blood cultures are invariably negative. Serologic studies for aspergillar antigens using immunodiffusion and counterimmunoelectrophoretic (CIE) techniques are of no practical value. A *definitive* diagnosis of invasive aspergillosis requires demonstration of the typical septated hyphal forms within tissue. The fungal elements may be identified on hematoxylin-eosin stains, but silver-methenamine stains more clearly reveal the organisms. The histopathologic response to aspergillar infection is variable; either an acute suppurative response or a mixed mononuclear cell infiltrate (or both) may be observed. A frank granulomatous response rarely occurs. Necrosis is a hallmark; vascular invasion, with intra-arterial thrombosis, is common. Fiberoptic bronchoscopy, including transbronchial lung biopsy and BAL, has a diagnostic yield of 40 to 70% when invasive pulmonary aspergillosis is present; higher yields (exceeding 70%) have been reported with percutaneous needle aspiration (PNA), although PNA has usually been performed in the context of discrete nodular lesions. We believe that fiberoptic bronchoscopy is the initial invasive diagnostic procedure of choice when the disease is diffuse or involves an entire segment or lobe; however, PNA is superior for small, localized, nodular densities not accessible by bronchoscopic techniques. Open lung biopsy is rarely required. Unfortunately, delay in initiation of antimycotic therapy by even a few days may markedly reduce the chance for cure. Thus, empiric treatment of *suspected* cases should be considered in patients at high risk for invasive disease, even though the histopathologic diagnosis may not have been rigorously established. In granulocytopenic patients with fever or pulmonary infiltrates, isolation of aspergillus from nasal or tracheobronchial secretions warrants empiric treatment with amphotericin B while awaiting the results of ancillary studies; bronchoscopy or PNA may substantiate the diagnosis.

TREATMENT

Mortality from invasive pulmonary aspergillosis exceeds 50 to 80% in most series; cerebral involvement has been associated with greater than 95% mortality. The most important factors determining outcome are the status of the underlying disease and the ability to restore immune function. Even with aggressive antifungal therapy, prognosis has been poor among patients with hematologic malignant conditions in relapse or in bone marrow transplant recipients (>90% mortality). By contrast, mortality rates of less than 20% have been noted when aggressive antifungal therapy is initiated *early* (within 2 to 4 days of onset of symptoms) *and* remission of the underlying disease, resolution of granulocytopenia, or reduction of corticosteroid or immunosuppressive therapy has been achieved in a timely fashion. Resolution of granulocytopenia (when present) appears to be essential for recovery among patients with hematologic malignant conditions or among bone marrow transplant recipients. Similarly, among patients with persistent impairments in host defenses, mortality exceeds 80%. For example, 10 of 13 patients with AIDS and pulmonary aspergillosis reported by Denning and colleagues died at a median of 3 months after the diagnosis despite aggressive antifungal therapy with amphotericin B, itraconazole, or both in all but 2 patients. Randomized controlled studies regarding the treatment of invasive aspergillosis have not been performed.

- Amphotericin B remains the mainstay of therapy; high daily doses (1 to 1.5 mg/kg/day) and a prolonged course (1.5 to 3 g) are recommended for optimal cure rates. The advantage of high-dose amphotericin B over low-dose amphotericin B has not been critically analyzed; however, the low levels of amphotericin B achieved in bronchial secretions and the high minimal isorrheic concentration (MIC) for some strains of aspergillus suggest that the higher dose (1 to 1.5 mg/kg/day) may be preferable in neutropenic patients (i.e. those at highest risk for poor outcome) despite the potential for serious side effects. By contrast, lower doses of amphotericin B (0.5 mg/kg/day) may be adequate in transplant allograft recipients in whom the level of immunosuppression can be reduced. Unfortunately, the combination of amphotericin B and cyclosporine A often results in significant nephrotoxicity. Because of a high failure rate with amphotericin B alone, the combination of amphotericin B with alternative agents has been tried. In this context, 5-fluorocystosine (flucytosine, 5-FC) has been the most promising agent for *adjunctive* therapy. Flucytosine penetrates well into cerebrospinal fluid (CSF), bone, and vitreous (areas in which amphotericin B achieves low concentrations)
- Flucytosine *alone* exhibits weak activity against Aspergillus spp in vitro or in animal models; however, flucytosine may confer synergy (with amphotericin B) in some studies. This effect has not been consistent. In one recent review, Denning and Stevens culled a total of 63 patients treated with a combination of flucytosine and amphotericin B for invasive aspergillosis. Two thirds responded favorably, including 11 of 19 (58%) patients with acute leukemia, 14 of 16 (88%) nonimmunocom-

promised patients, and 9 of 11 (82%) renal transplant recipients. These data suggest that the combination of flucytosine and amphotericin B is superior to single-agent therapy

- The combination of flucytosine with other antifungals (ketoconazole or fluconazole) appears not to offer any advantage over single agent therapy; the combination of flucytosine and itraconazole is currently being investigated. Similarly, the combination of amphotericin B with ketoconazole may be antagonistic or indifferent; disparate results have been noted with combinations of amphotericin B and itraconazole. Although firm data supporting the clinical efficacy of combination therapy are not available, the combination of amphotericin B with flucytosine is advisable for serious aspergillar infections. Serum levels of flucytosine should be measured, aiming for peak levels between 30 to 90 µg/ml. Unfortunately, flucytosine has potential marrow toxicity and thus may not be suitable for patients with limited marrow reserve. Hematologic toxicity, however, has been rare in patients with persistently therapeutic serum concentrations. High-dose amphotericin B together with flucytosine has also been successfully used as prophylaxis against reactivation of infection among leukemic patients with previous invasive aspergillosis who are once again receiving chemotherapy
- Rifampin has also been used as adjunctive therapy (with amphotericin B) for invasive aspergillosis. Rifampin exhibits in vitro activity against Aspergillus spp, and observations in animal models in vivo and anecdotal clinical experience in humans suggest that the combination of rifampin and amphotericin B may be superior to amphotericin B alone; however, no firm evidence supports the superiority of combination therapy. Rifampin induces hepatic enzymes, and may markedly depress cyclosporine A levels; therefore, rifampin should be avoided in transplant recipients. Alternative delivery systems for amphotericin B involving lipids (liposomal amphotericin B or complexes of amphotericin B with lipids) exhibit activity in vitro and in animal models and may be less toxic than free amphotericin B. Preliminary data in humans suggest efficacy, but numbers are small and liposomal amphotericin B is not yet commercially available for humans
- Surgical resection, drainage, or debridement or devitalized, necrotic involved tissue may be critical as adjunctive therapy when the disease is localized (e.g. sinusitis, skin, bone, single pulmonary cavity). When localized cavitary pulmonary aspergillosis is identified, initial treatment with amphotericin B, followed by surgical resection, provides the greatest chance for cure
- The imidazole antifungal agents, miconazole and ketoconazole, have minimal activity against Aspergillus spp and have no clinical therapeutic role. Fluconazole, a newer azole, has excellent activity against Candida spp, penetrates well into lung, sputum, and CSF, and can be administered orally or intravenously. Fluconazole is more active than ketoconazole against Aspergillus spp in vitro, but is less effective than amphotericin B in vitro and in animal models of aspergillosis. Fluconazole has not been used in clinical aspergillar infections in man; thus, this agent cannot be recommended for aspergillosis in humans

- Itraconazole, a new oral triazole not yet released in the United States, has excellent activity against Aspergillus spp in vitro and in animal models and appears comparable (and possibly superior) to amphotericin B. Itraconazole achieves high tissue concentrations (including the lungs) and is well tolerated, with much lower toxicity than amphotericin B. Side effects of itraconazole are relatively minor and include nausea, vomiting, hypokalemia, gynecomastia, abnormalities in liver function tests, and hypertriglyceridemia; serious side effects warranting discontinuation of therapy occur in fewer than 5% of patients. Itraconazole has great promise as an antimycotic agent, but data in humans with invasive aspergillosis are limited. In uncontrolled trials in Europe, oral itraconazole (200 to 400 mg/day), alone or in combination with amphotericin B or flucytosine, has been curative in 50 to 80% of cases of chronic necrotizing aspergillosis or invasive aspergillosis. In the United States, itraconazole was administered to 189 patients with a variety of systemic mycoses as part of the Mycoses Study Group of the National Institutes of Allergic and Infectious Diseases from 1984 to 1989, but only 23 patients (12%) had aspergillosis. No direct comparison with amphotericin B or other antifungal agents was made. Denning and colleagues in the United States noted favorable responses to itraconazole in 12 of 15 evaluable patients with invasive aspergillosis, including 4 of 5 with pulmonary involvement. Only 10 of these patients, however, were immunocompromised. Further, concomitant surgical resection may have contributed to the response in 3 patients. Few neutropenic patients with invasive pulmonary aspergillosis have been treated with itraconazole alone. In a recent study from Stanford University, itraconazole was curative in 5 to 6 heart-lung or lung transplant recipients with locally invasive aspergillosis at the site of the transplant anastomotic site; 1 patient had fatal relapse. Itraconazole markedly depresses cyclosporine serum concentrations; consequently, adjustment of cyclosporine A dosage is usually required among organ transplant recipients receiving this agent. Itraconazole has also been effective as a prophylactic agent in two uncontrolled studies of granulocytopenic patients at high risk for aspergillar infections. While itraconazole is an attractive alternative to amphotericin B, this agent is not available in the United States except for compassionate use among patients in whom amphotericin B has failed or who suffered serious side effects from amphotericin B. A chronic course of therapy (minimum of 6 months) is recommended.

Preferred Therapy

- Amphotericin B (plus 5-fluorocytosine when possible)
- Restoration of immune function (or reverse underlying disease)
- Surgical resection or drainage may be required as *adjunctive* therapy
- Itraconazole (200 mg bid) promising but not yet available in the United States except in selected patients for compassionate use of amphotericin B or serious amphotericin B toxicity)

Note: Ketoconazole, miconazole, and fluconazole are not recommended.

BLASTOMYCOSIS

EPIDEMIOLOGY

Blastomycosis is produced by the soil-dwelling dimorphic fungus, Blastomyces dermatitidis. The endemic area of the fungus has been defined on the basis of reported cases. The western border of the endemic area extends from the Canadian province of Manitoba southward to east Texas and Louisiana. The endemic area extends eastward across the midwest and southern United States, overlapping the endemic area for histoplasmosis. The isolation of blastomycosis from soil is difficult, but the organism presumably grows in nitrogen-enriched soil.

PATHOGENESIS

Blastomycosis enters the host via the lung. After inhalation of the conidia, the yeast form of the fungus multiplies and induces a neutrophilic inflammatory response. The development of cell-mediated immunity activates macrophages. B. dermatitidis may disseminate to skin, bones, genitourinary tract, and meninges.

CLINICAL PRESENTATION

Most exposed individuals are believed to be asymptomatic. Symptomatic blastomycosis usually appears with cough with purulent sputum production, fever, chills, myalgias, and arthralgias. Chest roentgenographic abnormalities include lower lobe infiltrates, nodules, and pleural disease. Skin is the most frequent extrapulmonary site of involvement, and subcutaneous ulcerative nodules are commonly seen.

DIAGNOSIS

Identification of the organism by culture or histopathologic observation is the only reliable means of diagnosing blastomycosis. A doubly refractile yeast (8 to 20 μm) with a wide bud is a characteristic finding on 10% potassium hydroxide (KOH), digested sputum, or pus. The periodic acid-Schiff (PAS) or silver stain may be useful in aiding with identifying the organism.

TREATMENT

Ketoconazole is the treatment of choice for chronic pulmonary and non-meningeal disseminated blastomycosis. Ketoconazole cures 80% of pulmonary, skin, and bone infections. The usual dose is 400 mg/day for 6 months. A 2-g course of amphotericin B should be given if the patient is severely ill, or if improvement does not result with ketoconazole treatment. Fluconazole and itraconazole are active in animal models of blastomycosis, but neither agent is FDA approved for blastomycosis therapy.

Preferred Therapy

- Ketoconazole, 400 mg/day for 6 months
- If new foci develop in first month, increase dose to 600 to 800 mg/day

Alternate Therapy

- Amphotericin B, 0.4 mg/kg/day for 42 days, then 0.8 mg/kg/day for 28 doses. Total dose, 2 g.

COCCIDIOIDOMYCOSIS

Coccidioidomycosis is an illness caused by the pathogenic fungus, Coccidioides immitis. C. immitis is a dimorphic fungus that grows in the soil as a mold and in tissues as an endosporulating spherule. The endemic area for C. immitis includes the southwestern United States, including California, Nevada, Arizona, New Mexico, and Texas. The endemic area for C. immitis coincides closely with the climatic conditions that define the lower Sonoran Life Zone. Windy conditions and disruption of the soil lead to contaminated air. Outdoor recreational activities, excavation, and agriculture all contribute to aerosol formation.

PATHOGENESIS

Arthrospores enter the host via the lung, where they settle in alveoli and germinate to produce the giant spherule (50 to 100 μ). Spherules multiply by the formation of endospores. Spherules stimulate both a granulocytic and mononuclear inflammatory response and sensitize T cells. Cell-mediated immunity develops and successfully localizes most infection. Certain groups of patients are at high risk, including blacks, Philippinos, diabetic patients, immunosuppressed patients, transplant patients, and patients with AIDS.

CLINICAL PRESENTATION

Primary pulmonary coccidioidomycosis produces an influenza-like illness similar to that seen with other fungal diseases. Common symptoms include cough, fever, and chest pain. Headache and sore throat occur commonly. A rash is noted in approximately 50% of patients, whereas erythema nodosum and erythema multiforme occur less frequently. Most patients do not seek medical attention. When the infective dose is high, the patient may be toxic with high fever, and adult respiratory distress syndrome may develop. Coccidioidal pleural effusion is generally considered part of a primary infection. Pleural effusions may be a minor feature of the illness or may overshadow the pneumonia. The most common radiographic manifestation of primary coccidioidomycosis is patchy infiltrates, ranging in size from segmental to lobar infiltrates.

In most instances primary coccidioidomycosis resolves. But in some instances persistent primary coccidioidomycosis develops. This term is used to describe cases where signs and symptoms persist for 6 weeks or longer. X-rays may show a sizeable infiltrate or effusion that does not decrease, or extrapulmonary illness might ensue. Thin-walled cavities may develop, or pulmonary fibrosis and calcification may occur. Chronic progressive fibrocavitary disease, an illness that resembles chronic pulmonary tuberculosis, may develop. Symptoms of this illness include productive cough, hemoptysis, chest pain, and low-grade fever. Radiographically the disease involves primary upper zones of the lung and is slowly progressive.

Common sites of extrapulmonary spread include the skin and soft tissues, bones, and meninges. Meningitis is the most dreaded complication of coccidioidal infections. Spinal fluid examination is essential when central nervous system involvement is suspected. Complement fixation antibodies against coccidioidin can be identified in spinal fluid in 75% of patients.

AIDS

The exact frequency of coccidioidomycosis in association with AIDS is uncertain, but may be as high as 30% among patients in endemic areas. Progressive and disseminated infections are far more common in patients with AIDS than in nonimmunocompromised hosts. Common presentations among patients with AIDS include pneumonia and lymphadenopathy, meningoencephalitis, hepatosplenomegaly, osteomyelitis, arthritis, thyroid infection, and adrenal lesions. Prostatic involvement and subcutaneous abscesses have also been reported. Histopathologic evaluation typically reveals many more spherules than are seen in the tissues of comparable patients without AIDS.

DIAGNOSIS

The diagnosis of coccidioidomycosis depends on the identification of C. immitis within the body tissues or fluids. Histologic demonstration of spherules is acceptable in lieu of positive culture. Large quantities of CSF may be required for positive results. Serologic diagnosis may aid in indirectly identifying the infecting organism and may provide some assistance in determining the severity and extent of disease. The complement fixation (CF) test is the serologic gold standard. Titers of 1:8 to 1:16 are common in pulmonary infection, and a titer of 1:32 or greater or a rising titer suggests dissemination. If the CF test is used to guide treatment, the test must be performed in a reference laboratory and specimens must be tested together to ensure comparable results. Because the results of serologic tests in patients with AIDS may be falsely negative, biopsy or culture results are of primary importance in these patients.

TREATMENT

The usual primary pulmonary infection requires no treatment

- Treatment with ketoconazole, 400 mg/day, is advised for symptomatic immunosuppressed patients and other patients with high risks of dissemination (diabetic patients, blacks, Philippinos, and pregnant women). Additionally, ketoconazole is recommended for individuals with severe or persistent infection. Chronic pulmonary coccidioidomycosis and disseminated coccidioidomycosis require treatment. Ketoconazole, 400 mg/day, is the treatment of choice because the drug can be administered by mouth and produces side effects that are fewer and less severe than those caused by amphotericin B. Although most patients experience relief of signs and symptoms of the infection and radiographs usually improve, recurrence of disease after discontinuance of ketoconazole is seen in 25% of pulmonary and 30% of disseminated cases. Doses of up to 1,200 mg of ketoconazole per day have been administered, but marked increases in toxicity have limited this approach to therapy. An alternate choice of therapy for disseminated coccidioidomycosis is amphotericin B. An initial course of 2.5 g is provided, and if remission is not achieved, prolonged courses of 4 to 5 g may be administered

- Coccidioidal meningitis always requires IV and intrathecal amphotericin B. Prolonged therapy is required and cures are rare. Intrathecal amphotericin B (0.1 to 1 mg) is administered daily via an intraventricular reservoir (placed neurosurgically). In some instances treatment may be given 3 times per week. Treatment should be continued until the CSF count is normal and CF and titers are low or absent. The interval between doses then can be increased to once per week and continued for 1 to several years
- Standard treatment for progressive coccidioidomycosis in patients with AIDS involves the use of IV amphotericin B with added intrathecal amphotericin B if meningitis is present. Patients with AIDS are less likely to respond than are patients without AIDS, and the organism is eradicated in few, if any, instances. Itraconazole and fluconazole may be used for chronic suppressive therapy. Neither the optimal regimen nor the ultimate role for these two drugs has been established.

Preferred Therapy

- Primary coccidioidomycosis: No therapy
- Symptomatic primary coccidioidomycosis in immunosuppressed patients or patients at high risk (diabetic patients, blacks, Philippinos, pregnant women): Ketoconazole, 400 mg/day for 6 months
- Pulmonary and extrapulmonary: Ketoconazole, 400 mg/day for 6 months
- Coccidioidal meningitis: Amphotericin B IV 0.4 mg/kg/day for 42 days, then 0.8 mg/kg/day for 28 doses (total dose $\geq$2.5 g) plus amphotericin B intrathecally, 0.1 to 0.3 mg via an intraventricular reservoir until CSF is normal
- AIDS patients: Amphotericin B IV 0.4 mg/kg/day for 42 days, then 0.8 mg/kg/day for 28 doses (total dose $\geq$2.5 g)

CRYPTOCOCCOSIS

EPIDEMIOLOGY

Cryptococcosis is an invasive disease caused by Cryptococcus neoformans. C. neoformans is a ubiquitous encapsulated yeast with worldwide distribution. C. neoformans has been widely identified in nature, particularly in soil, in the excreta of birds, in animals, and on fruits.

PATHOGENESIS

C. neoformans is inhaled either as a small yeast (less than 10 μm) or a basidiospore. Under the influence of high carbon dioxide tensions in the lung, the organism forms a permanent polysaccharide capsule. The initial pulmonary host defenses against this organism involve complement, polymorphonuclear leukocytes, and macrophages. Cryptococci are found both within and outside phagocytic cells in the lung. C. neoformans is readily differentiated from other fungi by the presence of a polysaccharide capsule, which is likely important because of its antiphagocytic properties. The importance of cell-mediated immunity in this infection cannot be denied, and in fact, early recognition of its importance led to the mistaken assumption that cell-mediated immunity was the only protective immune response. Cell-mediated immunity develops over 2 to 4 weeks and involves both CD4 and CD8 lymphocytes. Following the development of cell-mediated immunity, macrophages are activated and intracellular and possibly extracellular killing of C. neoformans occurs. Antibody to cryptococcal polysaccharide neutralizes its protective effect, but cryptococcal polysaccharide is not strongly antigenic, and antibody may not be formed sufficiently early to provide protective effects.

Dissemination of the organism occurs frequently from the lungs in primary infections in animal models, but dissemination might possibly occur as a result of late breakdown of old foci. C. neoformans seems trophic for, and is certainly refractory to, host defenses in the central nervous system (CNS). Involvement of the CNS is the most serious and frequent clinical manifestation of cryptococcosis.

Direct human-to-human or animal-to-human infection is not known to occur. Certain factors that predispose to infection include AIDS, Hodgkin's disease, chronic lymphocytic leukemia, other lymphomas, organ transplantation, sarcoidosis, diabetes, treatment with corticosteroids, and cytotoxic chemotherapy. In approximately 50% of patients, no abnormality in host defenses or predisposing conditions are noted.

CLINICAL PRESENTATION

C. neoformans can induce a broad spectrum of pulmonary disease. Patients may present with chronic cough and fever. Chest pain is also a common symptom. Pulmonary involvement may be subacute or chronic, and in the extreme instances with severe immune depression, patients can develop the adult respiratory distress syndrome. The radiographic presentations of cryptococcal lung disease may be any type of infiltrate, a nodule, or a pleural effusion. The radiologic presentation of cryptococcal lung disease may mimic other mycoses, tuberculosis, bacterial infections, and infections with other opportunists, such as Pneumocystis carinii and Aspergillus.

Although the lung is the portal of entry, the usual clinical presentation is that of disseminated disease, particularly meningitis. Meningitis may be asymptomatic or may include some acute symptoms, such as low-grade fever, headache, meningismus, nausea, vomiting, and papilledema. CSF shows modest pleocytosis (10 to 30 cells/mm^3), and cellular reaction is characteristically lymphocytic.

Several dermatologic manifestations of cryptococcosis have been described, including subcutaneous swelling, nodules, and ulcers. Cryptococcal cellulitis and lesions resembling molluscum contagiosum (in patients with AIDS) have been described.

AIDS

Prior to the advent of AIDS, approximately 400 new cases of cryptococcosis were diagnosed yearly in the United States. With the advent of AIDS, the incidence of Cryptococcus neoformans has increased markedly. Approximately 8% of patients with AIDS developed C. neoformans infections between 1981 and 1987, and rates approaching 15% have been reported in patients with AIDS in the southeastern United States. In approximately 85% of C. neoformans infections in patients with AIDS, cryptococcosis has represented the initial opportunistic infection that defined AIDS.

Pulmonary lesions are frequently the initial presenting feature of cryptococcosis in AIDS. Fever, cough, dyspnea, and pleuritic chest pain occur. Chest x-rays reveal lymphadenopathy and pleural effusions with or without localized or diffuse pulmonary infiltrates. Pulmonary cryptococcosis may be accompanied by progressively severe shunting and hypoxemia and may be mistaken for infections caused by Pneumocystis carinii. Involvement of the CNS, revealed by meningoencephalitis, occurs in 82 to 90% of patients with cryptococcosis. Cryptococcus neoformans also disseminates to various other tissues, including lymph nodes, bone marrow, liver, spleen, kidneys, bones, joint, skin, eyes, pericardium, heart, thyroid, pancreas, adrenal, and ovaries. Certain cutaneous manifestations are seen largely in association with AIDS, including vesicular herpetiform lesions and molluscum contagiosum-like pigment papules.

DIAGNOSIS

Definitive diagnosis is made by visualizing the organism or culturing the organism from body fluid or body tissues. C. neoformans can usually be isolated from sputum, BAL fluid, or lung biopsy specimen in 4 to 7 days. Histopathologic study of tissue or cytologic examination of fluids demonstrates encapsulated yeasts with stains, such as methenamine silver, alcian blue, or mucicarmine. Normal individuals may harbor cryptococci as part of their normal respiratory tract flora. Accordingly, recovery of the organism does not define infection.

Serologic studies may help to document cryptococcal infection. Although no antibody test is commercially available, an excellent latex agglutination antigen test can reliably detect circulating cryptococcal polysaccharide antigen in serum or in CSF. Most patients with infection limited to the lung have no detectable polysaccharide antigens circulating in the serum. If antigen is found in the serum, one should seriously consider the possibility of a disseminated infection. A lumbar puncture should be performed on any patient, including asymptomatic patients and patients without underlying disease, from whose respiratory tract C. neoformans has been isolated. Diagnosis of cryptococcal meningitis depends on the demonstration of cryptococci in the CNS, antigen detection, or culture. The cryptococcal latex agglutination test has remarkable sensitivity and specificity and allows rapid detection of cryptococcal antigen when controlled for the presence of rheumatoid factor. A false-positive rate of as high as 9% may be seen in the presence of rheumatoid factor. The diagnosis of cryptococcal meningitis is sometimes difficult, and repeated lumbar punctures may be required to make the diagnosis. In patients with AIDS-associated cryptococcosis, abnormalities in CSF protein, glucose, and leukocyte count are frequently minimal or totally absent. In most instances, however, many organisms are easily identified on india ink smears. Titers of cryptococcal antigen in both CSF and serum obtained from patients with AIDS are enormously elevated. Titers as high as 1:2,000,000 have been reported in patients with AIDS.

TREATMENT

Unfortunately, few absolute guidelines exist for the treatment of cryptococcal pulmonary disease. A dilemma for the physician is created by the frequency of respiratory isolates that are harmless commensals, the fact that some lesions are discovered at surgical resection, and the toxicity of combination therapy with amphotericin B and flucytosine. In the absence of a clear-cut consensus, the following guidelines are suggested

- Pulmonary cryptococcal disease usually disseminates if the patient is immunosuppressed. Accordingly, patients with pulmonary disease and evidence of immune compromise either from chemotherapeutic agents or from an underlying disease, must receive antifungal treatment
- A lumbar puncture must be performed even in patients without CNS symptoms to ascertain whether the patient has cryptococcal meningitis, a condition that always requires treatment
- Treatment is recommended even in the apparently normal host who has C. neoformans isolated from the respiratory tract if radiographic evidence of parenchymal lung disease and pulmonary symptoms exist
- Treatment is not provided for patients who have only cryptococcal colonization without radiographic evidence of lung disease. Commonly, these patients have chronic obstructive pulmonary disease
- Patients who are apparently normal hosts with lung nodules or masses removed surgically are also not treated but followed with periodic visits

Immunosuppressed patients with cryptococcal pneumonia should be treated with a 2-g course of amphotericin B. Patients with cryptococcal meningitis should be treated with amphotericin B (0.3 to 0.5 mg/kg/day) and flucytosine (150 mg/kg/day divided in 4 equal doses). This highly effective, but toxic, regimen is continued for 6 weeks, if possible. The duration of therapy is arbitrary, with some patients requiring longer treatment and others not being able to tolerate this length of treatment. Flucytosine clearly can produce life-threatening bone marrow suppression and diarrhea. In patients who receive the drug for more than 2 weeks, or who have reduced renal function, flucytosine serum levels should be measured. A drug level between 30 and 100 μg/ml 2 hours after a dose is optimal; levels greater than 100 μg/ml should be avoided.

Patients with AIDS present a particular problem. Results of treatments of cryptococcosis in AIDS patients with combined amphotericin B and flucytosine for 6 weeks have been disappointing. Flucytosine is often not well tolerated because of leukopenia or GI side effects, and thus doses of this drug frequently must be reduced to less than 100 mg/day, if the drug can be administered at all. Amphotericin B, if used alone, requires prolonged treatment. The desire for effective oral therapy with a low toxicity profile has led to extensive trials of fluconazole. The proportion of responders to fluconazole (53%) was similar to that for amphotericin B (49%). Moreover, the mortality within each treatment group that adhered to the protocol was the same (23%). Culture conversion in the CSF was significantly slower in fluconazole treatment, and when all patients were analyzed, mortality rates were three-fold higher in patients treated with fluconazole than in those treated with amphotericin B. Moreover, smaller studies have suggested that aggressive therapy with amphotericin B and flucytosine produces better results than treatment with fluconazole or amphotericin B alone. Although fluconazole (400 mg/day, sometimes 800 mg/day) is the standard treatment for cryptococcosis in some parts of the world, amphotericin B plus flucytosine is still the recommended therapy. Future studies with fluconazole and itraconazole may change this recommendation.

Fluconazole, usually in doses of 200 to 400 mg/day, has been effective in the long-term prevention of relapse in most patients included in therapeutic trials. Accordingly, chronic suppressive therapy with fluconazole is recommended in patients with AIDS.

Preferred Therapy

- Pulmonary disease: Amphotericin B, 0.4 to 0.5 mg/kg/day for 6 weeks
- Pulmonary disease only, immunosuppressed patient: Amphotericin B, 0.4 mg/kg/day for 42 days, then 0.8 mg/kg/day for 28 doses (total dose, 2 g)
- Meningitis: Amphotericin B, 0.4 mg/kg/day for 42 days, then 0.8 mg/kg/day for 28 doses (total dose, 2.5 g) plus flucytosine, 25 to 37.5 mg/kg PO q6h for 6 weeks
- AIDS patients: Amphotericin B, 0.4 mg/kg/day for 42 days, then 0.8 mg/kg/day for 28 doses (total dose, 2.5 g) plus flucytosine, 25 to 37.5 mg/kg PO q6h for 6 weeks
- Chronic suppressive therapy for all patients with AIDS: Fluconazole, 200 mg PO daily indefinitely

Alternate Therapy

- Nonmeningeal cryptococcosis: Fluconazole, 400 mg on first day, then 200 mg/day for undetermined duration

HISTOPLASMOSIS

Histoplasmosis was originally described by Samuel Darling from autopsy specimens from a laborer who died of disseminated disease while working on the Panama Canal. Darling believed the organism was a protozoan and that it was encapsulated. Both of these assumptions were proved false. Histoplasmosis is a systemic disease caused by the dimorphic fungus, Histoplasma capsulatum, which exists in mycelial form in the soil and in yeast form at body temperature.

EPIDEMIOLOGY

The Mississippi and Ohio River areas are endemic areas of histoplasmosis. The organism exists in large quantities in soil that has been mixed with the excreta of chickens, starlings, and pigeons. Cleaning chicken houses and cutting or bulldozing trees in which birds have roosted often results in the inhalation of many spores that lead to human infections. The overall incidence of histoplasmin sensitivity in the United States is about 22%, but close to 100% of individuals under 18 years of age are positive in certain areas of the Mississippi and Ohio River Valleys.

PATHOGENESIS

Human infection with H. capsulatum almost always results from inhalation of microconidia of H. capsulatum into the alveoli of the lung, where germination leads to conversion into the yeast form. Multiplication of the organism occurs in the lung, and early fungemia spreads organisms to lymph nodes, liver, and spleen. The initial inflammatory response is an infiltration of polymorphonuclear leukocytes, which is followed by the appearance of mononuclear phagocytes. The fungus is ingested by mononuclear phagocytes, but is not destroyed. The fungus multiplies intracellularly for 2 to 3 weeks until cell-mediated immunity develops, thereby activating macrophages and enabling macrophages to kill the fungal organism.

CLINICAL PRESENTATION

H. capsulatum produces a wide spectrum of clinical syndromes. Acute primary histoplasmosis occurs in individuals previously unexposed to H. capsulatum and is asymptomatic or produces symptoms that are so minimal that medical attention is not sought. When present, symptoms are influenza-like with fever, malaise, headache, nonproductive cough, and roentgenographic infiltrates. Erythema nodosum and erythema multiforme are skin lesions that may occur during acute histoplasmosis. In most instances primary infections resolve completely, but in some patients, the infection becomes progressive. Chronic histoplasmosis most frequently occurs in patients with underlying chronic obstructive disease. Pulmonary infiltrates may wax and wane or cavitation may occur. In patients without cavitation, 80% resolve, but in those patients with cavitation only 20%

resolve spontaneously. Symptoms of chronic pulmonary histoplasmosis are chronic sputum production, fever, weight loss, and hemoptysis. Five-year mortality rates may approach 50% in untreated patients.

Disseminated histoplasmosis is a multisystem disease that may appear as a mild chronic disease or acute life-threatening disease. Acute life-threatening disease occurs in patients with deficiencies in cell-mediated immunity, whereas chronic disease is found in adults without previous identifiable deficiencies in whom cell-mediated immunity fails to develop or is inadequate. The clinical manifestations include fever, interstitial pneumonia, hepatosplenomegaly, adrenal involvement, oropharyngeal ulcers, and meningitis. Anemia, leukopenia, and thrombocytopenia may be found. Histoplasmomas and pulmonary nodules occur when concentric layers of necrosis and fibrosis surround an area of old histoplasmosis. These lesions calcify sequentially to form a target lesion and are of no physiologic significance. Histoplasmomas occasionally enlarge over time and thus appear as expanding pulmonary nodules that are difficult to differentiate from malignant tumors. Mediastinal granulomatosis and fibrosis are believed to be the result of a reaction to antigenic but nonviable organisms.

AIDS

Histoplasmosis is a formidable illness in patients with AIDS. Histoplasmosis may mimic sepsis in individuals with diffuse pneumonia and may present a picture similar to that of adult respiratory distress syndrome. Alternatively, progressive histoplasmosis may present with hepatosplenomegaly, lymphadenopathy, leukopenia, thrombocytopenia, anemia, chorioretinitis, meningoencephalitis, pancreatic or renal lesions, endocarditis, adrenal or thyroid lesions, prostatitis, testicular lesions, or as oral mucosal, cutaneous, or GI ulcerations. Fever of unknown origin in these patients may also be caused by H. capsulatum. Blood cultures are frequently positive, and organisms may be present in sufficient numbers to be visualized on smears of leukocyte buffy coats.

DIAGNOSIS

A definitive diagnosis of histoplasmosis can be made only by demonstrating the presence of H. capsulatum in tissue specimens or secretions either by culturing the organism or by visualizing the organism in histopathologic materials. Growth may occur after as early as a few days or may require up to 6 weeks. In patients with diffuse diseases, the blood or bone marrow should be cultured and the organism should be searched for with PAS or silver stains. A variety of quantitative serologic tests may be utilized in diagnosis. CF tests are positive 3 to 6 weeks after exposure and may remain positive for years. A fourfold rise in paired sera or a titer greater than 1:32 is suggestive of infection with H. capsulatum. CF titers are usually low in chronic histoplasmosis. CF tests of greater than 1:8 in CSF suggests H. capsulatum meningitis. Immunodiffusion studies measure precipitating antibodies to the M and H antigens. The H band is specific for active infection, but is present less often than the M band.

TREATMENT

- Acute primary histoplasmosis is usually self-limited and does not require treatment
- If symptoms persist for longer than 3 weeks, or if gas exchange abnormalities develop, amphotericin B is the treatment of choice. Treatment should be continued until the patient is asymptomatic or an accumulated dose of 500 mg has been reached
- Ketoconazole, 400 mg/day for 1 month, is an effective alternative mode of treatment
- Chronic cavitary histoplasmosis can be effectively treated with ketoconazole, 400 mg/day for 6 months. Alternatively, chronic cavitary histoplasmosis is also well treated with a 2-g course of amphotericin B. Although the response to amphotericin B is quicker, and fewer relapses occur, amphotericin B is a toxic regimen that requires prolonged IV therapy. Accordingly, amphotericin B should be reserved for patients with severe infections
- Progressive, disseminated histoplasmosis can also be treated with ketoconazole (400 mg/day for 6 months) in individuals who are immunocompetent and have subacute disease. In patients with severe disseminated disease, amphotericin B is probably superior. If disseminated histoplasmosis is suspected in patients with AIDS, therapy should be initiated before culture results are available
- Patients with AIDS should be treated with 2.5 to 3.5 g of amphotericin B. Relapse is frequent and, accordingly, ketoconazole, 400 mg once daily, should be administered following amphotericin B for an indefinite period of time

Preferred Therapy

- Acute histoplasmosis: Seldom requires treatment; ketoconazole, 400 mg/day for 1 month, if symptomatic
- Pulmonary disease, localized disease, disseminated disease in immunocompetent patients: Ketoconazole, 400 mg/day for 6 months
- All disease in immunocompromised patients, including patients with AIDS: amphotericin B, 0.4 mg/kg/day for 42 days, then 0.8 mg/kg/day for 28 doses (total dose, ≥2.5 g)
- Patients with AIDS: Should receive ketoconazole, 400 mg/day, indefinitely following amphotericin B

MUCORMYCOSIS (MUCORACEAE)

Mucormycosis refers to deep mycotic infection caused by nonseptated fungi belonging to the order Mucorales within the species Zygomycetes. Fourteen families are within the order Mucorales; most pathogens have been identified within the family Mucoraceae. Genera within Mucoraceae include Rhizopus, Absidia, Cunninghamella, and Mucor, and each of these fungi may cause clinical infections in immunocompromised individuals. Mucoraceous infections are among the rarest of fungal infections (fewer than 100 cases have been reported) and are exclusively confined to patients with severe impairments in immune function. Both cell-mediated immune mechanisms and granulocytes are important in host defense against these fungi. Alveolar macrophages and mononuclear phagocytes are important in engulfing inhaled spores, whereas neutrophils kill the organisms once the spores have germinated. Thus, derangements in *both* granulocyte and mononuclear phagocytic function are key elements predisposing to infection with Mucor spp. High-dose corticosteroid or immunosuppressive therapy, malignant hematologic disease, severe granulocytopenia, diabetes mellitus, metabolic acidosis, renal failure, and chronic dialysis have been identified as important risk factors for acquisition of mucormycosis. Mucormycosis rarely complicates AIDS, thus suggesting that defects in lymphocyte number or function or cell-mediated immunity are not sufficient to predispose to mucormycosis.

CLINICAL PRESENTATION

The major forms of mucoraceous infections include rhinocerebral, pulmonary, gastrointestinal, disseminated, and cutaneous. Rhinocerebral mucormycosis predominates among patients with diabetes mellitus and usually begins with infection of the nose, nasal septum, and paranasal sinuses. Extension through the ethmoids to involve the orbit, sphenoidal or cavernous sinuses, and brain may result in visual loss, cranial nerve palsies, and even death. Pulmonary or disseminated mucormycosis typically affects patients with malignant hematologic disorders, profound granulocytopenia, or global impairment in host defenses. These fungi (Phycomyces, Mucor) have a predilection to invade the vasculature; ischemia, infarction, and severe (even fatal) hemorrhage may occur in this context. Pulmonary mucormycosis may occur as a disease limited to the lung or in the context of widespread disseminated disease. Chest x-rays may demonstrate patchy bronchopneumonia, nodular infiltrates, consolidation, or cavities. Hyphae may penetrate bronchial walls and invade pulmonary blood vessels, thereby leading to thrombosis, distal hemorrhagic infarction, and (rarely) pseudoaneurysm formation. Massive, fatal hemoptysis may result from erosion of the mucoraceous process through a pulmonary artery. An aggressive surgical approach, in addition to therapy with amphotericin B, is recommended for mucormycosis involving pulmonary vessels. Mucormycosis involving large airways (trachea and bronchi) with pseudomembrane formation and extensive mucosal ulceration has also been described. Mortality with invasive pulmonary (or endobronchial) mucormycosis exceeds 80%; only 2 of 35 patients survived among 3 published series.

DIAGNOSIS

Diagnosis may be difficult. Several series have documented a low rate of diagnosis ante mortem; in three large series of pulmonary mucormycosis, the diagnosis was first made at necropsy in 29 of 35 patients. Sputum cultures are positive in only 10 to 40% of invasive infections; blood cultures are uniformly negative. No useful serologic or skin test exists. Thus, invasive techniques (e.g. bronchoscopy, percutaneous needle aspiration biopsy) are usually required to substantiate the diagnosis. A *definitive* diagnosis requires demonstration of the typical fungal hyphae in tissue specimens or on culture. Fungi of the order Mucorales are broad, nonseptated hyphae that branch at right angles; as with other fungi, Mucorales fungi may best be revealed by silver methenamine stains. Histologically, extensive parenchymal necrosis and hyphal invasion of blood vessels are typical. A neutrophilic suppurative response is characteristic; well-formed granulomata are not seen. Black necrotic pus or debris overlying sites of necrosis or ulceration may be a clue to the presence of Mucorales. Isolation of Mucoraceae by culture should be considered presumptive evidence for invasive disease, because false-positive results are rare. Fungal cultures have often been negative, even when histopathologic specimens reveal the characteristic fungal elements.

TREATMENT

- Optimal therapy for mucormycosis involves amphotericin B in addition to surgical resection or debridement of involved tissue (when possible). In view of the rarity of mucormycosis, no controlled therapeutic trials have been performed. Amphotericin B is the cornerstone of medical therapy, however; optimal dose and duration of therapy are not known, but a minimum total dose of 2 g of amphotericin B is recommended. Other antifungal agents (ketoconazole, miconazole, and fluconazole) have no significant activity against Mucoracea. Unfortunately, even with aggressive medical therapy, mortality with invasive pulmonary or disseminated mucormycosis exceeds 90% in patients with malignant hematologic disease in relapse; occasional cures have been noted in diabetic patients, organ transplant recipients, or immunocompromised hosts when control of the underlying disease or reduction in the level of immunosuppression has been achieved
- Surgical debridement or resection of involved tissue appears critical to improving outcome. This has been most evident in the management of rhinocerebral mucormycosis in diabetic patients; however, higher cure rates among patients with pulmonary cavitary mucormycosis who have undergone surgical resection plus amphotericin B therapy have been suggested. Therefore, most respirologists agree that surgical resection combined with amphotericin B offers the best chance for cure when the disease is localized and amenable to excision

Preferred Therapy

- Amphotericin B combined with surgical resection or debridement of involved tissue

SPECIFIC DRUGS

AMPHOTERICIN B

Amphotericin B is an antimycotic polyene antibiotic obtained from a strain of Streptomyces nodosus. The polyene group of antibiotics exists as a chemical and biologic subdivision of macrolides. The prime site of action of amphotericin B is the cell membrane where the polyene binds to sterols, chiefly ergosterol, to produce defects in membrane function. The binding is irreversible, and the membrane is made more permeable after specific attachment. The size of the defect induced in the membrane varies, depending on the molecular structure of the polyene. The alteration in cell permeability allows small molecules, notably potassium and glucose, to leak out. The polyene does not penetrate past the cell membrane and has no known effect on intermediary metabolism or DNA synthesis. Passage of intracellular molecules into the extracellular space is believed to arrest the growth of the organism or cause death of the cell. Yeast, animal cells, and artificial membranes appear to have a similar common pathway of injury. The involvement of amphotericin B with mammalian membranes may account for some side effects noted with this agent. Additionally, the defects in membrane permeability may permit entry of other antifungal agents, such as flucytosine, that might impede fungal growth by interfering with nucleic acid synthesis. Conversely, ketoconazole, which also interferes with ergosterol synthesis, reduces binding sites on the membrane and, therefore, interferes with and reduces activity of amphotericin B in experimental animals and in vitro.

Amphotericin B is associated with significant toxicity and, accordingly, requires careful monitoring. A test dose, 1 mg, in 500 ml of 5% dextrose and water should be infused over 3 to 4 hours, and the patient should be observed for the presence of an anaphylactic reaction. If the test dose is tolerated, the patient should then be infused with a daily dose of 10 mg, increasing the daily dose 10 mg each day until 50 mg/day is reached. A daily dose is continued until a clinical response is evident (often within 1 week). Subsequent doses then can be given on an every-other-day basis. Dosage should be adjusted to the requirements of each patient, because individual tolerance to amphotericin B varies. Amphotericin B should then be administered IV over 4 to 6 hours on an every-other-day basis. The use of this regimen would require approximately 18 weeks to complete a 2-g course of therapy.

Unpleasant reactions to amphotericin B are virtually universal. Fever, shaking chills, nausea, vomiting, anorexia, and headache are frequent complaints. Pretreatment with aspirin, diphenhydramine, or hydrocortisone (20 to 50 mg) may be helpful. Local phlebitis and thrombophlebitis may occur at the injection site. Heparin, 500 U, may decrease the phlebitis associated with IV delivery. Acute reactions tend to improve as the treatment course progresses.

The patient should be monitored carefully for adverse reactions, some of which are dangerous. Abnormal renal function, including azotemia, hypokalemia, hypomagnesemia, renal tubular acidosis, and nephrocalcinosis, are often observed. Normocytic, normochromic anemia may also result. Serum creatinine, blood urea nitrogen (BUN), electrolytes, magnesium, and a complete blood count (CBC) should be evaluated weekly during amphotericin B therapy. Serum creatinine rises in almost all subjects, and no adjustment in dose is required until the creatinine level reaches 2.5 mg/dl (221 µmol/l). Improvement in renal function usually occurs with interruption of therapy, but permanent impairment can occur with cumulative doses greater than 3 g. Other nephrotoxic antibiotics and chemotherapeutic agents should not be given concomitantly unless absolutely required.

In summary, amphotericin B is considered the gold standard of antifungal therapy, especially for systemic mycoses. Amphotericin B has several significant drawbacks, including

- The necessity of IV administration
- Poor penetration to cerebrospinal fluid
- Intolerance by many patients because of unpleasant side effects
- Significant toxicity to bone marrow and kidneys

AZOLE ANTIFUNGAL DRUGS

Several antifungal azoles are useful in therapy of fungal disease, including clotrimazole, miconazole, ketoconazole, and fluconazole. Two additional investigational drugs, itraconazole and SCH 39304, are also azole compounds. Antifungal azoles are composed of a 5-member azole ring that is attached by a carbon/nitrogen bond to other aromatic rings. Ketoconazole is an imidazole, thereby indicating the presence of two nitrogen atoms in the azole ring. Itraconazole, fluconazole, and SCH 39304 are triazoles, thereby indicating the presence of three nitrogen atoms in the azole ring. All antifungal azoles appear to exert their adverse effect on fungi primarily by impairing the synthesis of ergosterol, which is a vital component of fungal cell membranes. Synthesis is inhibited by inhibiting a demethylase enzyme that is involved in the demethylation of 14-alpha-methylsterols to form ergostol.

Ketoconazole

Ketoconazole is well adsorbed orally with peak serum levels occurring 1 to 6 hours after ingestion. Metabolism and excretion of ketoconazole occur by hepatobiliary mechanisms; little active drug is excreted in the urine. Ketoconazole requires gastric acidity for dissolution and absorption. The data on the effect of food on the absorption of ketoconazole are conflicting. Cimetidine and antacids that impair absorption should be withheld until 2 hours after the administration of a dose of ketoconazole. Many physicians prefer to administer the drug just prior to a meal. Oral ketoconazole possesses some undesirable properties

- A low, but real, potential for hepatotoxicity
- Dose-related inhibition of testoserone and adrenal corticosteroid synthesis

- Adverse interactions with other drugs, especially rifampin and cyclosporin

Symptomatic hepatic toxicity has been reported to occur in 1 in 10,000 to 12,000 treatment courses. Two deaths attributable to ketoconazole-induced hepatitis were reported in 1 series. A second series reported symptomatic, potentially serious hepatotoxicity in 1 in 15,000 patients. Decreases in serum testosterone have been reported in patients receiving 200 to 600 mg daily of ketoconazole. This suppression of testosterone may be accompanied by decreased sperm counts, decreased libido, impotence, and gynecomastia. These effects of ketoconazole are reversible when the drug is withdrawn. Ketoconazole also blunts the response to adrenocorticotropic hormone (ACTH) stimulation. This effect on steroid synthesis appears to be the result of P450 enzyme inhibition, thereby leading to decreased steroid synthesis. Additionally, ketoconazole has been shown to block glucocorticoid receptor sites by competitive binding. Hypoadrenalism is rare.

Concurrent administration of rifampin and ketoconazole has led to lower serum ketoconazole levels, probably caused by alteration in hepatic handling of the drug. Ketoconazole may enhance the anticoagulant effect of coumarin-like drugs. Keotconazole increases blood levels of cyclosporin A, and accordingly, blood levels of cyclosporin A should be monitored if the two drugs are given concomitantly. Concomitant administration of ketoconazole with phenytoin may alter the metabolism of one or both drugs. Both ketoconazole and phenytoin should be monitored if both drugs are given concurrently. Because severe hypoglycemia has been reported in patients concomitantly receiving oral miconazole and oral hypoglycemic agents, the potential interaction of ketoconazole and oral hypoglycemic agents should be monitored.

Fluconazole

Fluconazole is a water-soluble triazole whose mode of action is inhibition of the demethylase enzyme that is involved in the synthesis of ergosterol. Oral absorption is rapid and nearly complete within 2 hours. Oral absorption of fluconazole is more uniform than that of ketoconazole. Elimination of the drug is predominantly renal, and dose modification is required in moderate or severe renal insufficiency. Fluconazole has good penetration into CSF. Numerous studies have shown that CSF levels of fluconazole are 60 to 80% of simultaneous serum concentrations, even in the presence of uninflamed meninges. Because of its high level of penetration into CSF, high volume of distribution to body tissues, good absorption after oral dosing, and long half-life, fluconazole is an attractive alternative to IV amphotericin B for the treatment of fungal meningitis.

Oral fluconazole is generally well tolerated. Inhibition of testicular and adrenal steroidogenesis has not been seen at the doses studied. The frequency of GI complaints and hepatic toxicity is lower than that found with ketoconazole. Fluconazole interferes with phenytoin, cyclosporin, and warfarin. Drug levels of these agents should be monitored when given concomitantly with fluconazole. Interest in this new drug has been propelled by its favorable profile and by the paucity of effective antifungal agents for the treatment of fungal infections in AIDS. Although this drug has been approved for use in cryptococcosis and candidal infections, many important questions regarding the efficacy and optimal use of this drug await further studies.

Itraconazole

Itraconazole is the most water soluble of the azole drugs. Like fluconazole, it appears to be less toxic than ketoconazole. Despite relatively poor penetration of itraconazole into CSF, animal models and limited human data suggest that this drug will be more effective than ketoconazole for therapy of meningitis. Although this drug is not approved for use at present, several ongoing, noncomparative clinical trials suggest that itraconazole is at least as effective as oral ketoconazole for therapy of non–life-threatening forms of histoplasmosis, blastomycosis, and coccidioidomycosis. Studies of in vitro murine models and limited human studies suggest that itraconazole may be effective therapy for aspergillosis.

SCH 39304

SCH 39304 is an investigational drug that shares with fluconazole such pharmacologic features as good absorption after oral dosing and significant excretion of active drug in the urine. The half-life of SCH 39304 is 2.5 times longer than of fluconazole, and SCH 39304 has a plasma concentration time curve about 2 times that of fluconazole, thereby suggesting that single-day dosing yield persistently high steady-state concentrations in serum. Future studies of this azole are required.

FLUCYTOSINE

Flucytosine is a fluorinated pyrimidine analog that was initially synthesized as an antileukemic agent. Flucytosine has a narrow spectrum of activity and is never used alone because secondary resistance develops quickly. Flucytosine is water soluble and is rapidly and completely absorbed from the GI tract. Flucytosine is a small molecule that rapidly distributes to all tissues, including CSF. The kidneys secrete more than 90% of the drug unchanged. Flucytosine exerts its antifungal effect in fungi that possess cytosine deaminase. This enzyme metabolizes the drug to 5-fluorouracil, an antimetabolite that is incorporated into fungal RNA and interferes with protein synthesis. Antifungal activity might also be mediated by effects on DNA synthesis. Cytosine permease is required for entrance of flucytosine into the cell. Resistant fungi either lack the deaminase or have reduced cytosine permease activity.

Flucytosine is usually used in combination with amphotericin B. Amphotericin B, which causes changes in fungal cell wall permeability, may enhance the entrance of flucytosine into the cell. Alternatively, other authors have suggested that amphotericin B impedes entrance of flucytosine into the cell and that the two drugs interact in a sequential rather than a synergistic fusion.

Toxicity of flucytosine includes leukopenia and thrombocytopenia, which occur in as many as 5% of patients and may be life threatening. Cytopenias are most common in patients with impaired renal function and correlate with high serum concentrations, usually above 100 μg/ml. Flucytosine should be given in the usual single dose (37.5 mg/kg) twice daily if the creatinine clearance is between 20 to 40 ml/min and once daily if it is between 10 to 20 ml/min. Direct measurements of blood levels are necessary to prevent toxicity for all patients with decreased renal function at the beginning of treatment and for all patients receiving concomitant amphotericin B if their serum creatinine is increasing.

NOCARDIA SPECIES

EPIDEMIOLOGY

Nocardia spp are gram-positive filamentous branching rods within the genus Nocardia and the family Actinomycetaceae. Although originally misclassified as fungi, Nocardia spp are true bacteria. Nocardia spp are commonly found in soil, decaying organic matter, and environmental sources, but are not part of normal human flora. The three species of Nocardia capable of causing disease in humans are N. asteroides, N. brasiliensis, and N. caviae. The usual route of infection with N. asteroides is via inhalation into the lung, whereas cutaneous inoculation is the predominant mechanism implicated for N. brasiliensis. N. asteroides accounts for 80 to 95% of cases of nocardiosis; N. brasilienis accounts for 3 to 9% of cases; and N. caviae accounts for 1 to 3% of cases. Nocardial infections are rare; even large referral centers encounter only 1 to 3 new cases per year. Cell-mediated immune mechanisms (activated T-lymphocytes and macrophages) are of paramount importance in the clearance and killing of nocardial organisms; however, polymorphonuclear leukocytes and humoral antibodies also play contributory roles in host defenses against these organisms. Severe and sustained defects in both cellular immune and granulocyte function may provide a milieu for propagation of these relatively low virulence organisms. Of infections caused by Nocardia spp, 75 to 85% occur in patients with severe defects in immunity. Risk factors for acquisition of nocardial infections include high-dose corticosteroids or immunosuppressive therapy, organ transplantation, chronic granulomatous disease, and malignant hematologic disorder; however, 15 to 30% of cases occur in individuals without pre-existing immunologic deficits. Nocardiosis among organ transplant recipients has been virtually eliminated in programs using TMP/SMX as prophylaxis against Pneumocystis carinii infections, because TMP/SMX also inhibits Nocardia spp. Nocardiosis complicates AIDS in only 0.2 to 0.3% of cases; in a recent review, 6 cases of nocardiosis were diagnosed among 2,167 patients with AIDS at a New York Hospital between 1980 and 1989.

CLINICAL PRESENTATION

All species may disseminate, but the clinical expression of these various species differs. N. asteroides has a propensity to involve the lung, CNS, and skin; by contrast, more than half of all infections caused by N. brasiliensis are localized to skin or subcutaneous tissues. N. caviae is a rare pathogen, but may cause pulmonary or disseminated disease in immunocompromised individuals. Dissemination to bone, joints, heart, spleen, liver, kidney, or lymph nodes occurs in 1 to 4% of cases of nocardiosis (all species). Nocardial infections involve the lung in 56 to 85% of patients, and may appear as acute, subacute, or chronic pneumonitis. An acute, necrotizing pneumonia, with chills and rigors, has been described; however, a chronic, indolent course, with symptoms progressing over several weeks, is more characteristic. In this context, weight loss, anorexia, and constitutional symptoms are common concomitant features. Bronchopleural fistulae and empyema may rarely complicate chronic pulmonary nocardiosis. As many as one third of patients with pulmonary nocardiosis are asymptomatic, with incidental changes noted on chest x-ray. A myriad of changes in the chest x-ray have been described, e.g. cavitation, nodular infiltrates, bronchopneumonia, and lobar consolidation. Pleural effusions have been noted in 20 to 30% of patients, almost always in conjunction with parenchymal abnormalities. Extrapulmonary involvement occurs in 20 to 45% of patients. CNS involvement (by hematogenous spread) occurs in 15% of patients. Brain abscess is the most frequent CNS manifestation, but involvement of the spinal cord, epidural space, eyes, and meninges may occur. Skin or soft tissue involvement occurs in 10 to 20% of patients and may be the sole site of disease in infections caused by N. brasiliensis but usually reflects disseminated disease with other Nocardia spp. Cutaneous manifestations are protean, and include pustules, draining sinus tracts, subcutaneous or cutaneous nodules, mass lesions, and cellulitis. Direct inoculation of nocardial organisms into skin or soft tissue via abrasions or local trauma may result in localized infection; such an outcome is particularly characteristic of N. brasiliensis.

DIAGNOSIS

The diagnosis of nocardiosis is usually difficult. Smears and cultures of clinically involved sites (e.g., sputum, skin, pleural fluid, wound, and sinus tracts) are important, but are positive in a minority of cases. Sputum smears and cultures are positive in only 20 to 50% of cases of pulmonary nocardiosis, even when multiple samples are obtained. Blood cultures are invariably negative. On Gram's stain, Nocardia spp are gram-positive, coccobacillary rods that exhibit a filamentous or beaded appearance; these organisms are weakly positive by Kinyoun-modified Ziehl-Neelsen acid-fast stains. Oil immersion microscopy may better delineate the delicate nocardial filaments, which are only 0.5 to 1 μ in diameter. Nocardia spp have complex growth requirements in culture, and media may be overgrown by other organisms. Nocardia spp grow slowly, and identification may take 1 to 4 weeks. Because routine cultures are often discarded after

3 to 4 days of negative growth, the microbiologic laboratory must be specifically informed that Nocardia is a consideration. False-positive cultures for Nocardia spp are rare. Isolation of Nocardia spp from sputum has been reported in patients without serious immune impairments and without clinical evidence of disease and may reflect colonization. Isolation of Nocardia spp from any immunocompromised host, however, warrants treatment whether or not symptoms are present, because fatal dissemination may occur later. Nocardia spp are virtually never recovered as laboratory contaminants. Because delay in initiation of therapy may increase mortality, invasive techniques are usually required to substantiate the diagnosis. PNA biopsy is recommended for localized nodular lesions, with diagnostic yields of up to 80%. Fiberoptic bronchoscopy with transbronchial lung biopsy and BAL is the preferred procedure for diffuse disease or when the disease is segmental or lobar in distribution with consolidation. Histologically, a suppurative response, associated with significant necrosis, is characteristic; lymphocytic and mononuclear cellular infiltrates may also be observed. Well-formed granulomas are rare. Nocardia spp are not visible on hemotoxylin-eosin stains, but may be detected on silver methenamine stains or modified Ziehl-Neelsen stains. Sinus drainage may reveal sulfur granules from cutaneous, subcutaneous, or pleural lesions. The diagnosis of nocardiosis at extrapulmonary sites requires needle aspiration or biopsy of involved sites. In cases of CNS involvement, a careful search for Nocardia spp at other sites is appropriate and may obviate the need for invasive procedures of cerebral or intracranial lesions. CT imaging may be invaluable in the detection and staging of cerebral nocardiosis. In nocardial abscess, an area of decreased density in the center of the lesion, surrounded by a dense ring in the periphery of the abscess, is characteristic. IV contrast demonstrates ring enhancement in more than 80% of patients. Serial CT scans of the head may be helpful in following the course of cerebral nocardiosis. Serologic or skin tests for detection of nocardiosis are not commercially available.

TREATMENT

- Sulfonamides (sulfisoxazole, sulfadiazine, or sulfamethoxazole), alone or in combination with trimethoprim, have been associated with cure rates exceeding 80% and are the treatment of choice. Most treatment failures have occurred in immunocompromised patients with CNS involvement or widespread disease or when treatment is initiated late in the course of the illness. Mortality with isolated pulmonary nocardiosis has been less than 10%. Controlled studies have not been performed, but sulfisoxazole (4 to 12 g/day), sulfadiazine (6 to 8 g/day), or TMP/SMX (480 mg TMP and 2,400 mg SMX/day in divided doses) appear equally efficacious. The combination of TMP and SMX, however, may exhibit synergy against Nocardia spp in vitro, and the penetration of TMP into the CSF is superior to that of SMX. Thus, TMP/SMX is preferred to sulfonamides alone. Excellent serum levels are achieved with oral TMP/SMX. A chronic course of therapy (for 12 months) is recommended, because relapses may occur with short-course treatment. Surgical resection or debridement may be essential for cutaneous, soft tissue, or bone infections; its role in CNS disease is controversial. For pulmonary nocardiosis, medical therapy with sulfa-containing regimens is usually curative. Some strains of Nocardia are resistant to sulfonamides and TMP; in this context, minocycline may be an acceptable alternative

- Minocycline has excellent activity against Nocardia spp in vitro and in vivo and is preferred therapy for patients allergic to or unable to tolerate sulfonamides
- Cefuroxime, cefotaxime, cetriaxone, amikacin, ciprofloxacin, and imipenem/cilastin have good to excellent activity against Nocardia spp in vitro, but limited data are available in vivo. These agents, particularly imipenem, cefuroxime, and amikacin, have occasionally been beneficial as adjunctive therapy (with TMP/SMX) in patients with fulminant or widespread nocardiosis to confer synergistic killing
- Imipenem/cilastin displays exceptional activity against Nocardia spp in vitro and was more active than TMP/SMX in a murine model of cerebral nocardiosis. Owing to its expense, toxicity, and need for IV administration, imipenem is not recommended as primary therapy. A brief (10 to 14 days) course of imipenem with TMP/SMX is a reasonable option, however, in debilitated, immunocompromised patients with disseminated or cerebral nocardiosis. Penicillins, clindamycin, erythromycin, and first-generation cephalosporins are ineffective

Preferred Therapy

- TMP/SMX (480 to 640 mg/day TMP component in divided doses) (equivalent to 6 to 8 single-strength tablets daily)
- Surgical resection or debridement may be critical as adjunctive therapy (particularly for cutaneous or soft tissue infections)

Alternate Therapy

- Minocycline (300 mg orally bid for 6 to 12 months); not reliable for CNS infections.
- Imipenem, cefuroxime, amikacin, ciprofloxacin (reserve for treatment failure on TMP/SMX or minocycline)

TUBERCULOSIS

Many health care providers believe that tuberculosis no longer exists or, at most, is a minor problem. Unfortunately, both perceptions are incorrect. Although the number of cases of tuberculosis reported annually in the United States declined steadily from 1953 (84,304) to 1984 (22,255), this trend was dramatically reversed when the number of cases rose by 3% in 1986 and by 5% in 1989 (23,495). This resurgence of tuberculosis is largely related to the HIV epidemic.

MICROBIOLOGY

Mycobacteria are aerobic, nonmotile, curved or straight rods that are occasionally branched. Mycobacteria are free-living saprophytes that form part of the natural ecology of the soil. Mycobacterium tuberculosis is the major cause of human disease and depends on host transmission for its survival.

PATHOGENESIS

Transmission of infection with M. tuberculosis is primarily from person to person by aerosolization of microdroplets (1 to 5 μm) that usually contain 3 or fewer tubercle bacilli. Droplets of this size reach the alveoli, where macrophages ingest the organisms and process and present mycobacterial antigens to T-cells. In naive hosts, macrophages have a limited ability to kill the organism, which proliferates within and outside macrophages. Specific immune responses develop following presentation of antigens to T-cells. Sensitized T-lymphocytes secrete lymphokines, which activate macrophages, thereby greatly enhancing their capacity to ingest and kill mycobacteria. The time required for the generation of a specific immune response is unknown but probably requires approximately 6 weeks. During the interval between inhalation of the aerosol and the development of T-cell immunity, a clinically silent bacillemia, which seeds the lung as well as other organs in the host, usually occurs. With the development of cell-mediated immunity, the majority of organisms are killed throughout the body, although few dormant bacilli remain in most hosts. Clinically apparent tuberculosis develops in approximately 10% of infected patients either soon after infection (primary infection) or years later (reactivation tuberculosis). Both of these consequences are thought to be the result of defects in T-cell or macrophage function or both.

CLINICAL PRESENTATION

Primary Tuberculosis

Infection of the naive host usually produces a subclinical syndrome whose only manifestation is the development of a positive purified protein derivative (PPD). Occasionally fever, nonproductive cough, or shortness of breath may occur. Chest x-rays show an infiltrate in the apical or posterior segment of the upper lobes or in the middle or lower lobes. Alternatively, primary tuberculosis may present with a pleural effusion with pleurisy but no parenchymal infiltrate. The patient frequently complains of pleuritic chest pain, nonproductive cough, fever, chills, sweats, and dyspnea. The finding of a unilateral exudative pleural effusion in a patient with a positive PPD is highly suggestive of this diagnosis. When untreated, a high percentage of these patients develop active tuberculosis within 5 years.

Progressive Primary Tuberculosis

Progressive primary tuberculosis results from a failure to develop cell-mediated immunity. Its appearance is usually cryptic, with unexplained fever being common. Alternatively, a clinical syndrome of low-grade fever, night sweats, fatigability, loss of appetite, cough, hemoptysis, and the development of cavitary lung lesions may occur. This syndrome is differentiated from reactivation tuberculosis only by documentation of the natural history of the disease.

Reactivation Tuberculosis

Reactivation tuberculosis is the most common manifestation of infection with M. tuberculosis. Cavitary disease involving the posterior segments of the upper lobes or the apical segments of the lower lobes is common. Symptoms include night sweats, chills, fatigue, fever, and hemoptysis.

Extrapulmonary Tuberculosis

Approximately 15% of cases of tuberculosis are extrapulmonary. Lymphatic tuberculosis is the most common form of extrapulmonary tuberculosis. In patients over 12 years of age, 95% of lymphadenitis in the context of tuberculous infection is caused by M. tuberculosis. Genitourinary tuberculosis usually produces symptoms and signs of a urinary tract infection. Vertebral tuberculosis is a major source of morbidity because of resultant kyphosis and spinal cord abnormalities. The patient typically appears after weeks to months of back pain, fever, and weight loss. Tuberculous meningitis is a dreaded complication of tuberculosis. Fever, weight loss, and malaise predate CNS involvement in many patients, and most patients have CNS symptoms for less than 2 weeks. Other sites of extrapulmonary tuberculosis include tuberculous peritonitis, involvement of the distal ileum, and involvement of the skin.

DIAGNOSIS

The diagnosis of tuberculosis requires the isolation of M. tuberculosis from the infected host. A presumptive diagnosis may be made if acid-fast bacilli are noted in specimens or tissues obtained from patients. At least three samples of sputum obtained from the lower respiratory tract should be evaluated. Culture of M. tuberculosis requires 3 to 6 weeks for growth. If sputum cultures are negative, bronchoscopy with transbronchial biopsy can be performed. At present, evaluation of tissue or body fluids for mycobacterial RNA or DNA does not offer improved sensitivity. The role of polymerase chain reaction amplification of mycobacterial DNA is uncertain.

The tuberculin skin test is a useful diagnostic and epidemiologic tool. Concepts concerning the cutoff point for a positive test undergo continuous revision. The cut-off point of 5 mm has been proposed for HIV-infected patients, household contacts, or patients whose chest x-ray suggests prior tuberculosis. The cutoff point of 10 mm has been proposed for patients with recent skin test conversion and for patients with predisposing conditions. The cutoff point of 15 mm may be appropriate in otherwise healthy individuals with no known contact with an active case.

Patients with HIV Infection

The incidence of tuberculosis in patients with AIDS is almost 500 times the incidence in the general population. The risk of tuberculosis varies with the prevalence of infection with mycobacteria in the specific patient at risk. Foreign-born patients, IV drug abusers, and male homosexuals have the highest risk. Infection with tuberculosis usually precedes the diagnosis of AIDS. Extrapulmonary tuberculosis in patients with HIV infection has been an AIDS-defining condition since 1987. Among patients with relatively well-preserved immune function, findings on chest x-ray are similar to those of reactivation tuberculosis in immunocompetent patients and include cavitation and upper lobe infiltrates. In severely immunocompromised patients with HIV infection, findings on chest x-ray are typically those of primary tuberculosis and include hilar adenopathy, pleural effusions, and/or a miliary pattern. Lymphadenitis, meningitis, brain abscess, and bone, pericardial, peritoneal, and gastric involvement are the main outcomes of extrapulmonary tuberculosis. Blood cultures are positive in 50% of patients.

TREATMENT

Antituberculous chemotherapy is based on three basic principles

- Treatment should always include two drugs to which the organisms are susceptible
- The duration of treatment must continue for a sufficient period of time (at present, 6 months is the minimal duration)
- Promoting and monitoring compliance are central for treatment to be successful

Tuberculous chemotherapy can be successful only if the clinical and social management of patients and their contacts are considered.

Initial Treatment Regimen

The American Thoracic Society and Centers for Disease Control recommend a 6-month regimen consisting of a 2-month period of daily isoniazid (5 mg/kg, up to 300 mg), rifampin (10 mg/kg, up to 600 mg), and pyrazinamide (20 to 35 mg/kg, up to 2 g), followed by 4 months of twice weekly isoniazid (20 to 40 mg/kg, up to 90 mg) along with rifampin (10 mg/kg, up to 600 mg). Ethambutol should be included in the initial phase when isoniazid resistance is suspected. A 9-month regimen consisting of isoniazid and rifampin is also highly successful. When resistance to isoniazid is documented, rifampin and ethambutol, perhaps supplemented initially by pyrazinamide, should be given for a minimum of 12 months. Although little data exist regarding treatment for extrapulmonary tuberculosis, the above 9-month regimen is known to be effective. Regimens of 6 months are probably as effective in extrapulmonary disease as in pulmonary disease, but data are not presently available. Longer therapy may be necessary for lymphadenitis and bone and joint tuberculosis.

Patients treated for tuberculosis should have baseline measurements of hepatic enzymes, bilirubin, serum creatinine or BUN, serum uric acid, and a CBC. All patients should be monitored clinically at least monthly during therapy and should be specifically questioned regarding symptoms suggestive of drug toxicity. Symptoms of concern include nausea and vomiting, fatigue or weakness for more than 3 days' duration, dark urine, icterus, rash, paresthesias and/or fever for more than 3 days' duration, and right upper quadrant tenderness. Routine laboratory monitoring for subclinical drug toxicity is not necessary.

The response to antituberculous chemotherapy should be monitored and is best evaluated with examinations of sputum. Sputum should be cultured monthly until sputum conversion is documented, or at a minimum, sputum should be obtained after 3 months of therapy. After 3 months of therapy, more than 90% of patients should have converted to negative. If patients have not converted by the end of 3 months of therapy, serious consideration should be given to administering the treatment under direct observation. Patients whose sputum is negative after 3 months of treatment should have sputum smear and culture performed at the completion of therapy. Patients who have completed a 9-month course of isoniazid-rifampin and who have had a prompt bacteriologic response do not require further follow-up treatment. Patients who have completed a 6-month regimen should have follow-up evaluations 6 and 12 months after completion of therapy.

Patients whose sputum has not converted after 5 to 6 months of treatment are considered treatment failures. Susceptibility of the organism should be determined on the patient's current regimen. The regimen should be adjusted in accordance with the susceptibility tests, and treatment should be administered under direct observation. Patients whose organisms are susceptible to treatment at the outset of treatment and who relapse after the completion of an approved regimen usually relapse with organisms that remain susceptible to isoniazid and rifampin. Reinstitution of the isoniazid-rifampin previously used is recommended for these patients.

Preventive Therapy

Preventive therapy with isoniazid is useful in infected patients judged at high risk of progression to disease. Priorities for preventive therapy must compare the risk of developing tuberculosis to the risk of isoniazid toxicity. Preventive therapy is recommended for

- Household members and other close associates of persons with potentially infectious tuberculosis
- Newly infected persons

- Persons with past tuberculosis
- Persons with significant reaction to tuberculin skin tests and abnormal chest x-rays
- Persons with significant reactions to tuberculin skin tests who have special clinical conditions, such as silicosis, diabetes mellitus, prolonged therapy with adrenal corticosteroids, immunosuppressive therapy, such hematologic and reticuloendothelial disease as leukemia or Hodgkin's disease, AIDS, end-stage renal disease, and conditions associated with rapid weight loss and chronic undernutrition
- Persons with tuberculin skin test reactions who are younger than 35 years of age and have none of the previously mentioned risk factors

Isoniazid (300 mg/day for adults, 10 to 14 mg/kg/day for children not to exceed 300 mg/day) is used alone for preventive therapy. Isoniazid has been given for 12 months in most clinical trials, but good evidence suggests that 6 months of preventive therapy confers a nearly comparable degree of protection. Household contacts have a 2 to 4% risk of developing active disease in the first year. Young children and adolescents may have twice the adult risk. Accordingly, all persons in contact with a patient with tuberculin skin test of 5 mm or more should be treated with isoniazid. Preventive therapy for 3 months is prudent even if the skin test is negative. Initially, nonreactive household members should all undergo repeated skin testing after 3 months. If negative, isoniazid can be discontinued in children who have received 3 months of therapy. If positive, isoniazid should be continued. Patients receiving preventive therapy should be monitored in person or by phone at monthly intervals. The symptoms suggestive of toxic side effects mentioned earlier should be specifically sought.

Patients with HIV Infection

More prolonged treatment is recommended in patients with HIV infection because the efficacy of standard therapy in such patients is uncertain. Isoniazid, rifampin, and pyrazinamide are given daily for 2 months, followed by isoniazid and rifampin for 7 months, or for 6 months after cultures are negative, whichever is longer. If patients are intolerant to rifampin, several investigators suggest isoniazid, pyrazinamide, and ethambutol for 18 to 24 months, or for 12 months after cultures are negative, whichever is longer.

Of HIV-infected patients with positive tuberculin skin tests, 8% are diagnosed with tuberculosis each year. Accordingly, chemoprophylaxis for patients coinfected with HIV and M. tuberculosis is a critical public health priority. The initial evaluations of all patients with HIV infection should include the intradermal administration of 5 tuberculin units of PPD tuberculin and at least 2 companion antigens, such as candida, mumps, or tetanus toxoid. A 5-mm cutoff point is considered positive in patients with HIV infection because their delayed hypersensitivity response is reduced. Patients with a positive PPD should receive chemoprophylaxis regardless of age, unless a specific contraindication exists. Chemoprophylaxis should be administered to anergic HIV-seropositive patients with a documented history of a positive tuberculin skin test and who have not received treatment, to those with abnormalities on chest x-ray suggestive of previously untreated tuberculosis, and to those in close contact with patients with tuberculosis. Persons with skin test results of 5 mm or larger who refuse serologic testing for HIV but are suspected of having HIV infection should be considered candidates for preventive therapy regardless of age. The duration of chemoprophylaxis in confirmed or presumed HIV-infected patients is 12 months.

Preferred Therapy

Active Tuberculosis
Nonimmunocompromised hosts
- 6-month regimens are effective
- First 2 months: Isoniazid 5 mg/kg/day, maximum 300 mg/day; rifampin 10 mg/kg/day, maximum 600 mg/day; and pyrazinamide 25 mg/kg/day, maximum 2 g/day
- Final 4 months: Isoniazid daily (as above) or twice weekly, 15 mg/kg/day, maximum 900 mg/day; and rifampin daily (as above) or twice weekly, 10 mg/kg/day, maximum 600 mg/day
- Patients with positive sputum at 6 months are considered treatment failures

AIDS
- First 2 months: Isoniazid 5 mg/kg/day, maximum 300 mg/day; rifampin 10 mg/kg/day, maximum 600 mg/day; and pyrazinamide, 25 mg/kg/day, maximum 2 g/day
- Final 7 months: Isoniazid daily (as above) or twice weekly, 15 mg/kg/day, maximum 900 mg/day; and rifampin daily (as above) or twice weekly, 10 mg/kg/day, maximum 600 mg/day

Extrapulmonary
- 9-month and probably 6-month regimens are effective

Infection Without Disease (+PPD)
Nonimmunocompromised
- Isoniazid 5 mg/kg/day, maximum 300 mg/day for 6 to 12 months
- Results with 6 months (65%) nearly as good as with 12 months (75%) in reducing disease

AIDS
- Isoniazid 5 mg/kg/day, maximum 300 mg/day for 12 months
- All persons with PPD >5 mm should be treated regardless of age

SPECIFIC DRUGS

Isoniazid

Isoniazid is the most widely used of the antituberculosis agents. This bactericidal, nontoxic, easily administered, inexpensive agent is an ideal drug. Oral administration (3 to 5 mg/kg) produces a peak concentration of approximately 5 μg/ml 1 to 2 hours after administration. Most strains of M. tuberculosis are inhibited by concentrations of 0.05 to 0.20 μg/ml.

Hepatitis is the major toxic effect of isoniazid. The rate of hepatitis increases directly with increase in age to 65 years. Patients younger than 20 years of age had no hepatitis: Hepatitis occurred in 0.3% of patients 24–34 years of age, in 1.2% of patients 35 to 49 years of age, and in 2.3% of patients 50 to 64 years of age. Peripheral neuropathy caused by interference with metabolism of pyridoxine is also associated with isoniazid administration. In patients with diabetes, uremia, alcoholism, and malnutrition, pyridoxine, 10 to 25 mg/day, should be given with isoniazid. The interaction of isoniazid and phenytoin increased the serum concentration of both drugs, and accordingly, serum levels of phenytoin should be monitored.

Rifampin

Rifampin is bactericidal for M. tuberculosis. It is rapidly absorbed from the GI tract. Oral administration produces peak concentrations of 6 to 7 mg/ml 1 to 2 hours after ingestion. Most M. tuberculosis is inhibited in vitro by concentrations of 0.5 μg/ml. Rifampin is 75% protein bound but penetrates well into tissues and cells. Penetration through noninflamed meninges is poor, but therapeutic concentrations are achieved in CSF when the meninges are inflamed.

Adverse reactions to rifampin include hepatitis, GI upset, skin eruptions, and rarely thrombocytopenia. The rate of these reactions is variable, but hepatitis occurred in only 3.1% of the patients in a recent study of isoniazid-rifampin treatment administered for 6 months. Twice-weekly administration of higher doses of rifampin is associated with an influenza-like syndrome, hemolytic anemia, acute renal failure, and thrombocytopenia. Rifampin is excreted in urine, tears, sweat, and other body fluids and colors them orange. Patients should be advised of possible prominent discoloration of soft contact lenses. Rifampin may accelerate clearance of methadone, coumadin derivatives, glucocorticoids, estrogens, oral hypoglycemic agents, digitalis, anticonvulsants, ketoconazole, and cyclosporin. Rifampin may interfere with the effectiveness of oral contraceptives.

Pyrazinamide

Pyrazinamide is bactericidal for M. tuberculosis in an acid environment. The drug is particularly active against organisms in macrophages, presumably because of the acid environment within the cell. Administration of the drug in doses of 20 to 25 mg/kg results in serum concentrations of 30 to 50 μg/ml 2 hours after ingestion. At a pH of 5.5, the minimal inhibitory concentration of pyrazinamide for M. tuberculosis is 20 μg/ml. Penetration of the drug into cells and tissues seems to be good, although data are limited. The most important adverse reaction to pyrazinamide is liver injury, but apparently a significant increase in hepatotoxicity does not occur when pyrazinamide is added to a regimen of isoniazid and rifampin during the initial 2 months of therapy. Hyperuricemia also occurs, but clinical gout is uncommon. Diffuse arthralgias, apparently not related to hyperuricemia, occur frequently.

Ethambutol

Ethambutol in usual doses has a bacteriostatic effect on M. tuberculosis. Following administration of 15 mg/kg, peak concentrations of 4 μg/ml are noted 2 to 4 hours after ingestion. Inhibitory concentrations for this drug range from 1 to 5 μg/ml. CSF concentrations are low even in the presence of meningeal inflammation.

Retrobulbar neuritis is the most frequent and serious adverse effect of ethambutol. This complication occurs in less than 1% of patients at a daily dose of 15 mg/kg. Symptoms include central scotomata, blurred vision, and red-green color blindness. The frequency of ocular complications is increased in patients with renal failure.

Streptomycin

Streptomycin is bactericidal in an alkaline environment. Streptomycin must be given parenterally. Following administration of 15 mg/kg, the peak concentration in serum is 40 μg/ml 1 hour after an intramuscular dose. The drug should be used in reduced dosage and with extreme caution in patients with renal insufficiency. Streptomycin enters the CSF only in the presence of meningeal inflammation.

The most common adverse effect of streptomycin is ototoxicity. Vertigo is more common, but hearing loss may also occur. Nephrotoxicity occasionally occurs, and patients with pre-existing renal insufficiency or who are simultaneously using other nephrotoxic drugs are at increased risk. A total dose of more than 120 g should not be given. Ototoxicity and nephrotoxicity are more common in persons older than 60 years of age, and streptomycin should be avoided, if possible, in this group.

Second-Line Drugs

The five second-line antituberculous agents are para-aminosalicyclic acid, ethionamide, cycloserine, kanamycin, and capreomycin. Amikacin is also active against M. tuberculosis and may be useful in some circumstances.

VIRAL INFECTIONS

Infections with DNA viruses (cytomegalovirus, herpes simplex, varicella zoster, adenovirus) occur with increased frequency in immunocompromised hosts, and may give rise to serious pneumonias in this context.

CYTOMEGALOVIRUS

Cytomegalovirus (CMV) is the most important cause of severe viral infections in immunocompromised patients. CMV rarely causes clinical infections in normal hosts; however, serum antibodies are present in 45 to 80%

of normal adults, thus suggesting that asymptomatic infection occurs commonly. Serious CMV infections are almost exclusively confined to severely immunocompromised hosts (typically patients with AIDS or organ transplant recipients); other groups at risk include patients on high-dose corticosteroid or immunosuppressive therapy or patients with malignant hematologic disease receiving intensive chemotherapy. CMV is the most common pathogen complicating both bone marrow and solid organ transplantation. The incidence of CMV infection in allogeneic bone marrow transplant recipients ranges from 50 to 70%; approximately one third of infected patients develop CMV pneumonitis, which has been associated with a mortality of 60 to 90%. Clinical CMV infections among solid organ transplant recipients range from 40 to 80%, but only 10 to 20% develop clinical pneumonitis. Higher rates of serious pneumonia have been noted among heart-lung and lung transplant recipients. Predisposing factors for CMV infections among organ transplant recipients include receipt of organs or blood products from CMV-infected donors or previous seropositivity (i.e. latent CMV infection) in the recipient. Primary infections (i.e. arising from donor organ or blood products) typically are far more severe than secondary (reactivation) infections in previous seropositive recipients.

CLINICAL PRESENTATION

The manifestations of CMV infections are diverse. Asymptomatic viral shedding (viruria, viremia) is frequent among organ transplant recipients; however, disseminated disease or fulminant CMV pneumonitis may be fatal. The most common manifestation of CMV infection in immunocompromised patients is an atypical mononucleosis syndrome with fever, circulating atypical lymphocytes in peripheral blood, anemia, leukopenia, and abnormal liver function tests. Pneumonia occurs in 10 to 20% of infected patients, but higher rates (exceeding 50%) have been noted in lung transplant recipients receiving positive donor organs. Diffuse interstitial or alveolar infiltrates on chest x-ray are characteristic of CMV pneumonitis; however, focal infiltrates mimicking bacterial pneumonia may be observed. A miliary pattern on chest x-ray reflects hematogeneous spread, and is often associated with a more fulminant course. Large nodular infiltrates or cavities, which are virtually never seen with primary CMV pneumonitis, suggest alternative diagnoses. More than 80% of patients with CMV pneumonitis are viremic, which usually antedates the development of pulmonary infection by 7 to 14 days. CMV infections are confined to a relatively well-defined time period post organ transplantation. Virtually all infections occur from 30 to 120 days post transplantation, with a mean of 40 to 55 days. Infections before day 21 or after 6 months are rare. The mortality associated with CMV pneumonitis has been high in some patient populations (exceeding 80% in bone marrow transplant recipients), whereas the contribution of CMV pneumonitis to mortality among patients with AIDS is doubtful. Secondary complications may occur, however. Infection with CMV interferes with cell-mediated immunity and has been associated with a high rate of bacterial, fungal, and protozoan opportunistic superinfections; these secondary infections may markedly contribute to mortality. In addition, CMV may upregulate class II HLA antigen expression and may potentiate allograft dysfunction and rejection. Among lung transplant recipients, CMV pneumonitis may be associated with a higher rate of allograft rejection and increased mortality.

DIAGNOSIS

The diagnosis of CMV pneumonitis can be established by demonstrating the typical large CMV-infected cells containing intranuclear inclusions (an "owl's eye" appearance) and multiple smaller cytoplasmic inclusion bodies in lung tissue or cytologic specimens. These basophilic intranuclear inclusions can be demonstrated readily by hematoxylin-eosin, Wright's, Giemsa, or Papanicolaou's stains. Conventional viral cultures are positive in 70 to 90% of confirmed cases, but may take 2 to 6 weeks to grow. More recently, several new techniques have been employed to substantiate the diagnosis in a more timely fashion. Immunofluorescent (IF) studies using monoclonal antibodies against CMV antigens (shell vial cultures) enable a rapid diagnosis (within 24 hours) of CMV-infected cells in BAL fluid, blood, urine, or tissue, with diagnostic accuracy comparable to or exceeding that of conventional cytologic and cultural techniques. Other techniques using in situ hybridization with specific cDNA probes against CMV-viral DNA appear comparable to IF techniques, but are cumbersome to perform and require 2 to 3 days to complete. Surveillance cultures of buffy coat cells, urine, and throat washings have been positive for CMV antigen in more than 80% of patients with clinical CMV pneumonitis and typically antedate the development of pneumonia by 1 to 3 weeks. Isolation of CMV from buffy coat blood cultures has been associated with an increased risk of developing CMV pneumonitis; by contrast, isolation of CMV from urine has no predictive value.

TREATMENT

Ganciclovir [9-(1-3-dihydroxy-2-propoxymethyl)guanine] (also known as DHPG) is the treatment of choice for serious CMV infections. Early studies performed prior to the availability of ganciclovir and employing other antiviral agents for CMV were disappointing. Adenine arabinoside (vidarabine), alpha-interferon (alpha-IFN), or combinations of vidarabine and alpha-IFN failed to benefit clinical CMV infections and were associated with significant toxicity. Acyclovir, a guanosine analog that selectively inhibits herpesvirus DNA polymerase and inhibits herpes and CMV virus replication, may be efficacious as prophylaxis against CMV infections (when administered in high doses of 3,200 mg/day) but does not influence mortality in established CMV pneumonitis or serious CMV infections. Ganciclovir is 10 to 100 times more active than acyclovir against CMV, and favorable responses have been achieved in 20 to 80% of patients. Initial studies in patients with AIDS confirmed that ganciclovir resulted in clinical and virologic improvement in CMV retinitis and suppressed excretion of CMV from respiratory secretions; however, survival was not prolonged among AIDS patients with CMV pneumonitis. More favorable results have been reported among organ transplant recipients, with 60 to 80% success rates achieved when treatment is initiated early. The propensity for relapse upon discontinuation of therapy has led to more prolonged therapy among patients at risk. Foscarnet (trisodium phosphonoformate), a potent inhibitor of herpesvirus DNA polymerase, also has modest activity against CMV. Favorable responses to foscarnet have been reported in 50% of cases of CMV pneumonitis in organ transplant recipients in Europe, but this agent is not currently available in the United States. A recent trial in AIDS patients indicated that foscarnet slowed the progression of CMV retinitis, reduced serum levels of HIV-1 (p24) antigen, and more effectively cleared CMV viremia when compared to placebo. Marrow toxicity of foscarnet is less than that of ganciclovir. Foscarnet can usually be used in conjunction with zidovudine, whereas ganciclovir may be problematic in this context. Foscarnet, however, has considerable toxicity, including nausea, electrolyte disturbances (hypomagnesemia and hypocalcemia), nephrotoxicity, and the potential for seizures. Ganciclovir and foscarnet appear comparable in activity and in therapeutic efficacy against CMV, but no trials have directly compared these agents. At present, ganciclovir is the only antiviral agent with proven efficacy against CMV available for clinical use in the United States.

Preferred Therapy

- Ganciclovir (DHPG) initial dose of 10 mg/kg/day in 2 divided doses for 21 days, followed by 5 mg/kg/day for period of risk (as long as 90 to 120 days for organ transplant recipients)
- High-dose (3,200 mg/day) acyclovir may substitute for 5 mg/kg/day ganciclovir for long-term prophylaxis among patients who have received initial induction therapy with 10 mg/kg/day ganciclovir for 21 days

Alternate Therapy

- Foscarnet sodium (60 mg/kg q8h for 21 days, followed by maintenance); not yet available in the United States

PROPHYLAXIS

Prophylactic strategies against CMV infections have been applied primarily among organ transplant recipients and continue to evolve. Because of the greater severity of disease among previously seronegative recipients who receive seropositive donor organs or blood products, "passive" prevention strategies have included use of seronegative blood products when both the donor and the recipient are seronegative for CMV and avoiding use of seropositive donor organs in seronegative recipients. Such avoidance may not be practical, however, given the current shortage of donor organs. Thus, prophylactic therapy with antiviral agents among patients at high risk for CMV infection (i.e. recipient seropositive for CMV or donor organ positive for CMV) has also been tried. Passive immunization with high-titer anti-CMV immunoglobulin ("hyperimmune") globulin before and after transplantation was ineffective in two trials in seropositive bone marrow recipients, but appears to confer protection among renal transplant recipients; results with seropositive liver and heart transplant recipients have yielded conflicting results. The combination of hyperimmune globulin with acyclovir reduced serious "primary" CMV infections among hepatic transplant recipients at risk. The first-generation antiviral agents (vidarabine, cytarabine, alpha-interferon) did not prevent CMV reactivation in several early prophylactic trials in high-risk organ transplant recipients; however, high-dose acyclovir reduced the incidence and severity of CMV infections in seropositive bone marrow transplant and seropositive renal transplant recipients in separate studies. Early "pre-emptive" therapy with ganciclovir among asymptomatic seropositive bone marrow transplant recipients at high risk for developing CMV pneumonitis may reduce morbidity and mortality from CMV pneumonitis. In a recent study, Schmidt and colleagues randomly administered either IV ganciclovir (administered for 14 days at 10 mg/kg/day, followed by 5 mg/kg/day 5 days weekly until day 120) or placebo to allogenic bone marrow transplant recipients with normal chest x-rays and no pulmonary symptoms but with evidence for CMV respiratory tract infection/colonization (by shell vial cultures on surveillance bronchoscopy performed on day 35 post transplantation). A marked reduction in clinical CMV pneumonitis was observed among patients receiving ganciclovir. In a recent double-blind, controlled study, Goodrich and associates randomly administered either ganciclovir (5 mg/kg bid for 1 week, then 5 mg/kg/day for the first 100 days post transplantation) or placebo to 72 allogeneic bone marrow recipients who were excreting CMV in clinical specimens (blood, urine, BAL, or throat swabs) but had no clinical evidence for CMV disease. By day 100 following transplantation, CMV disease developed in 15 of 35 (43%) patients receiving placebo but in only 1 of 37 (3%) patients receiving ganciclovir. Excretion of CMV virus was reduced substantially in patients treated with ganciclovir, as compared to those treated with placebo. More importantly, mortality at 100 and 180 days was lower in the ganciclovir group. Similar prophylactic strategies are currently being investigated in lung allograft recipients at high risk for CMV infections. CMV pneumonitis has been a major cause of morbidity among lung allograft recipients, and may contribute to allograft rejection and mortality.

The incidence of clinical CMV pneumonitis among CMV-negative recipients receiving CMV-positive donor organs has been exceedingly high, ranging from 70 to 100%, with mortality rates approaching 40%. Secondary infections among seropositive recipients tend to be less severe than primary infections in previously seronegative recipients acquiring CMV infection from donor organs or blood products. Thus, aggressive prophylaxis is mandated in this latter context. Initial studies employing prophylactic low-dose acyclovir (800 to 2,400 mg/day) for 3 months or ganciclovir for 21 days (beginning on day 7 post transplant) without subsequent additional antiviral prophylaxis in patients at high risk for CMV infections have been associated with an unacceptably high rate of clinical infections. Hyperimmune globulin prophylaxis did not prevent clinical CMV infection among seronegative recipients receiving CMV-positive lung allografts in a study from Toronto. Several centers have adopted prophylactic regimens employing IV ganciclovir (beginning on day 7 post transplantation and continuing for 14 to 21 days) followed by low-dose ganciclovir (5 mg/kg/ day) up to 90 days. Alternative regimens employing initial therapy with ganciclovir (for 14 to 21 days) followed by high-dose acyclovir (3,200 mg daily) for 90 to 120 days are currently in progress. These strategies have not been validated in large prospective trials. All these regimens are expensive, logistically difficult, and have potential toxicity; thus, additional studies are required to affirm their efficacy.

HERPES SIMPLEX VIRUS (HSV)

Primary herpes simplex pneumonitis may rarely accompany serious mucocutaneous herpes simplex infections in immunocompromised hosts; in more than 80 to 90% of patients, herpetic lesions involving the lip or oropharynx precede or occur simultaneously with the pulmonary lesion. Individuals at greatest risk are children with acute leukemia and organ transplant recipients. Herpetic infections involving the lower respiratory tract have been associated with a wide gamut of clinical manifestations. Mild extension of HSV from the oropharynx may result in a mild tracheobronchitis; more fulminant hemorrhagic pneumonitis has also been described, but is rare. In severe cases, bronchoscopy may demonstrate punctate ulcerations of tracheal or bronchial mucosa, edema, and thick pseudomembranes within the tracheobronchial tree. With fulminant HSV penumonitis, pulmonary edema and hemorrhage may ensue. Radiographic findings are diverse; both focal pneumonia and diffuse interstitial infiltrates have been described. Cavitation does not occur. Bacterial or fungal superinfection complicates HSV pneumonitis in as many as 50% of patients and may contribute to mortality.

DIAGNOSIS

Herpes simplex may be demonstrated by cytologic methods or cultures of BAL fluid or lung biopsies; eosinophilic intranuclear inclusions and multinucleated (syncytial) giant cells may be detected in infected tissue. Distinction of colonization from clinical HSV pneumonitis is difficult, however. In many patients, HSV colonizes the lower respiratory tract as a saphrophyte while other pathogens are present concomitantly. In documented HSV pneumonitis, mortality may exceed 80% in severely ill, immunocompromised patients; however, concomitant infections and host factors may contribute to this observed high mortality.

TREATMENT

Acyclovir has been efficacious in mucocutaneous and disseminated HSV infections and is effective prophylaxis against HSV infections in organ transplant recipients. Limited data are available regarding acyclovir as therapy for HSV pneumonitis. IV acyclovir is recommended, however. Outcome largely depends on the immune status of the host and the presence or absence of complicating superinfections rather than on antiviral therapy.

Preferred Therapy

- IV acyclovir 250 mg/m² q8h for 7 to 10 days (reduce level of immuno-suppression when possible)

VARICELLA ZOSTER (VZ)

As with HSV, varicella zoster (VZ, "chickenpox") has the potential to cause a rapidly progressive hemorrhagic pneumonia in susceptible hosts. Life-threatening VZ infections or pneumonia are rare, however, even with disseminated zoster. The cutaneous exanthem of zoster, with grouped vesicles on an erythematous base ("shingles"), precedes pulmonary manifestations by 1 to 7 days. Chest x-rays typically demonstrate interstitial infiltrates, with a peribronchiolar distribution; lobar pneumonia has been described, but is rare. Histologic and cytologic features of VZ pneumonia are identical to those of HSV pneumonitis. Acyclovir, alpha-interferon, and vidarabine reduce viral shedding and accelerate healing of cutaneous zoster in immunocompromised patients; however, IV acyclovir is the treatment of choice for VZ pneumonia. Mortality of VZ pneumonia in the absence of therapy in immunocompromised patients ranges from 15 to 25%; with acyclovir, mortality is less than 10%. Reduction of level of immunosuppressive/corticosteroid therapy may accelerate healing and prevent dissemination.

Preferred Therapy

- IV acyclovir for 7 to 10 days
- Reduce level of immunosuppression (when possible)

ADENOVIRUS

Adenovirus may give rise to lower or upper respiratory tract infections in both normal and compromised hosts; fatal, hemorrhagic pneumonia may occur. Adenovirus is a rare opportunist, but has been associated with frequent pulmonary and hepatic involvement, and a high mortality, in immunocompromised hosts. Adenovirus was isolated from 5% of 1,050 bone marrow transplant recipients in 1 series, and was responsible for 15 clinical infections (including 12 pneumonias) during an 11-year period at UCLA. Pneumonia caused by adenovirus is characterized histologically by interstitial infiltrates and necrosis, sloughing of bronchial mucosa, pulmonary edema, and alveolar hemorrhage. Chest x-rays typically demonstrate diffuse interstitial or alveolar infiltrates; unilateral involvement has also been described. CNS involvement with diffuse meningoencephalitis and progressive hepatic necrosis is a rare complication. Unfortunately, no specific therapy is available.

REFERENCES

PNEUMOCYSTIS CARINII

General

1. Davey RT, Masur H: Recent advances in the diagnosis, treatment, and prevention of Pneumocystis carinii pneumonia. Antimicrob Agents Chemother, 34:499, 1990.
2. Glatt AE, Chirgwin K: Pneumocystis carinii pneumonia in human immunodeficiency virus-infected patients. Arch Intern Med, 150:271, 1990.

Microbiology

3. De Stefano JA, Cushion MT, Puvanesarajah V, Walzer PD: Analysis of Pneumocystis carinii cyst wall. II. Sugar composition. Protozool 1990; 37:436–41.
4. Edman JC, Kovacs JA, Masur H, et al: Ribosomal RNA sequence shows Pneumocystis carinii to be a member of the fungi. Nature, 334:519, 1988.
5. Edman U, Edman JC, Lundgren B, Santi DV: Isolation and expression of the Pneumocystis carinii thymidylate synthase gene. Proc Natl Acad Sci USA, 86:6503, 1989.
6. Jacobs JL, Libby DM, Winters RA, et al: A cluster of Pneumocystis carinii pneumonia in adults without predisposing illnesses. N Engl J Med, 324:246, 1991.
7. Stringer SL, Stringer JR, Blase MA, et al: Pneumocystis carinii: sequence from ribosomal RNA implies a close relationship with fungi. Exp Parasitol, 86:6503, 1989.

Clinical

8. Bigby TD, Margolskee D, Curtis JL, et al: The usefulness of induced sputum in the diagnosis of Pneumocystis carinii pneumonia in patients with the acquired immunodeficiency syndrome. Am Rev Respir Dis, 133:515, 1986.
9. Brenner M, Ognibene FP, Lack EE, et al: Prognostic factors and life expectancy of patients with acquired immunodeficiency syndrome and Pneumocystis carinii pneumonia. Am Rev Respir Dis, 136:1199, 1987.
10. Efferen LS, Nadarajad D, Palat DS: Survival following mechanical ventilation for Pneumocystis carinii pneumonia in patients with the acquired immunodeficiency syndrome: a different perspective. Am J Med, 87:401, 1989.
11. Garay SM, Greene J: Prognostic indicators in the initial presentation of Pneumocystis carinii pneumonia. Chest, 95:769, 1989.
12. Golden JA, Holander H, Stulbarg MS, Gamsu G: Bronchoalveolar lavage as the exclusive diagnostic modality for Pneumocystis carinii pneumonia. A prospective study among patients with acquired immunodeficiency syndrome. Chest, 90:18, 1986.
13. Haron E, Bodey GP, Luna MA, et al: Has the incidence of Pneumocystis carinii pneumonia in cancer patients increased with the AIDS epidemic? Lancet, 2:904, 1988.
14. Hopewell PC: Pneumocystis carinii pneumonia: diagnosis. J Infect Dis, 157:1115, 1988.
15. Jacobs JL, Libby DM, Winters RA, et al: A cluster of Pneumocystis carinii pneumonia in adults without predisposing illnesses. N Engl J Med, 324:246, 1991.
16. Jacobson MA, Mills J, Rush J, et al: Morbidity and mortality of patients with AIDS and first-episode Pneumocystis carinii pneumonia unaffected by concomitant pulmonary cytomegalovirus infection. Am Rev Respir Dis, 114:6, 1991.
17. Julyes-Elysee KM, Stover DE, Zaman MB, et al: Aerosolized pentamidine: effect on diagnosis and presentation of Pneumocystis carinii pneumonia. Ann Intern Med, 112:750, 1990.

18. Kovacs JA, Hiemenz JW, Macker AM, et al: Pneumocystis carinii pneumonia: a comparison between patients with the acquired immunodeficiency syndrome and patients with other immunodeficiencies. Ann Intern Med, 100:663, 1984.

19. Kovacs JA, Ng VL, Masur H, et al: Diagnosis of Pneumocystis carinii pneumonia: improved detection in sputum with use of monoclonal antibodies. N Engl J Med, 318:589, 1988.

20. Levine SJ, Masur H, Gill VJ, et al: Effect of aerosolized pentamidine prophylaxis on the diagnosis of Pneumocystis carinii pneumonia by induced sputum examination in patients infected with the human immunodeficiency virus. Am Rev Respir Dis, 144:760, 1991.

21. Masur H, Ognibene FP, Yarchoan R, et al: CD4 counts as predictors of opportunistic pneumonias in human immunodeficiency virus (HIV) infection. Ann Intern Med, 111: 223, 1989.

22. Nesone GS, Ward DJ, Pierce PF: Spontaneous pneumothorax in patients with acquired immunodeficiency syndrome treated with prophylactic aerosolized pentamidine. Arch Intern Med, 150:2167, 1990.

23. Raviglione MC: Extrapulmonary pneumocystosis: the first 50 cases. Rev Infect Dis, 12: 1127, 1990.

24. Zaman MK, White DA: Serum lactate dehydrogenase levels and Pneumocystis carinii pneumonia: diagnostic and prognostic significance. Am Rev Respir Dis, 137:796, 1988.

Therapy

25. Allegra CJ, Chabner BA, Tuazone CV, et al: Trimetrexate for the treatment of Pneumocystis carinii pneumonia in patients with the acquired immunodeficiency syndrome. N Engl J Med, 317:978, 1987.

26. Bozzette SA, Sattler FR, Chiu J, et al: A controlled trial of early adjunctive treatment with corticosteroids for Pneumocystis carinii pneumonia in the acquired immunodeficiency syndrome. N Engl J Med, 323:1451, 1990.

27. Centers for Disease Control: Guidelines for prophylaxis against Pneumocystis carinii pneumonia for persons infected with human immunodeficiency virus. MMWR, 38(S5): 1, 1989.

28. Conte JE, Hollander H, Golden JA: Inhaled or reduced-dose intravenous pentamidine for Pneumocystis carinii pneumonia. A pilot study. Ann Intern Med, 107:495, 1987.

29. Davey RT, Masur H: Recent advances in the diagnosis, treatment and prevention of Pneumocystis carinii pneumonia. Antimicrob Agents Chemother, 34:499, 1990.

30. Fischl MA, Dickinson GM, LaVoie L: Safety and efficacy of sulfamethoxazole and trimethoprim chemoprophylaxis for Pneumocystis carinii pneumonia in AIDS. JAMA, 259: 1185, 1988.

31. Gagnon S, Boota AM, Fischl MA, et al: Corticosteroids as adjunctive therapy for severe Pneumocystis carinii pneumonia in the acquired immunodeficiency syndrome. A double-blind, placebo-controlled trial. N Engl J Med, 323:1444, 1990.

32. Godrin FM, Simon GL, Wofsy CB, Mills JB: Adverse reactions to trimethoprim-sulfamethoxazole in patients with the acquired immunodeficiency syndrome. Ann Intern Med, 100:49, 1984.

33. Hirschel B, Lazzari A, Chopard P, et al: A controlled study of inhaled pentamidine for primary prevention of Pneumocystis carinii pneumonia. N Engl J Med, 324:1079, 1991.

34. Hughes WT, Rivera GK, Schell MJ, et al: Successful intermittent chemoprophylaxis for Pneumocystis carinii pneumonitis. N Engl J Med, 316:1627, 1987.

35. Kemper CA, Tucker RM, Lang OS, et al: Low-dose dapsone prophylaxis of Pneumocystis carinii pneumonia in AIDS and AIDS-related complex. AIDS, 4:1145, 1990.

36. Leoung GS, Feigal DW, Montgomery AB, et al: Aerosolized pentamidine for prophylaxis against Pneumocystis carinii pneumonia. N Engl J Med, 323:769, 1990.

37. Leoung GS, Mills J, Hopewell PC, et al: Dapsone-trimethoprim for Pneumocystis carinii pneumonia in the acquired immunodeficiency syndrome. Ann Intern Med, 105:45, 1986.

38. Masur H: Prevention of Pneumocystis carinii pneumonia. Rev Infect Dis, 11(*Suppl 7*): S1664, 1989.

39. Medine I, Mills J, Leoung G, et al: Oral therapy for Pneumocystis carinii pneumonia in the acquired immunodeficiency syndrome. N Engl J Med, 323:776, 1990.

40. Mills J, Leoung G, Media I, et al: Dapsone treatment of Pneumocystis carinii pneumonia in the acquired immunodeficiency syndrome. Antimicrob Agents Chemother, 32:1057, 1988.

41. Montaner JSC, Lawson LM, Levitt N, et al: Corticosteroids prevent early deterioration in patients with moderately severe Pneumocystis carinii pneumonia and the acquired immunodeficiency syndrome. Ann Intern Med, 113:14, 1990.

42. Montgomery AB, Debs RJ, Luce JM, et al: Aerosolized pentamidine as a sole therapy for Pneumocystis carinii pneumonia in patients with the acquired immunodeficiency syndrome. Lancet, 2:480, 1987.

43. Murphy RL, Lavelle JP, Allan JD, et al: Aerosol pentamidine prophylaxis following Pneumocystis carinii pneumonia in AIDS patients: results of a blinded dose comparison study using an ultrasonic nebulizer. Am J Med, 90:418, 1991.

44. National Institute of Allergy and Infectious Disease, National Institutes of Health: Important therapeutic information on prevention of recurrent Pneumocystis carinii pneumonia in persons with AIDS. Executive Summary, October 11, 1991.

45. Sands M, Kron MA, Brown RB: Pentamidine: a review. Rev Infect Dis, 7:625, 1985.

46. Sattler FR, Cowan R, Nielsen DM, Ruskin J: Trimethoprim-sulfamethoxazole compared with pentamidine for treatment of Pneumocystis carinii pneumonia in patients with the acquired immunodeficiency syndrome. Ann Intern Med, 109:280, 1988.

47. Wharton JM, Coleman DL, Wofsy CB, et al: Trimethoprim-sulfamethoxazole or pentamadine for Pneumocystis carinii pneumonia in the acquired immunodeficiency syndrome. A prospective, randomized trial. Ann Intern Med, 105:73, 1986.

48. Wolsy CB: Use of trimethoprim-sulfamethoxazole in the treatment of Pneumocystis carinii pneumonitis in patients with acquired immunodeficiency syndrome. Rev Infect Dis, 9:S184, 1987.

FUNGAL DISEASE

Fungal Pneumonias

49. Cairns MR, Durack DT: Fungal pneumonia in the immunocompromised host. Semin Respir Infect, 1:166, 1986.

50. Robertson MJ, Larson RA: Recurrent fungal pneumonias in patients with acute nonlymphocytic leukemia undergoing multiple courses of intensive chemotherapy. Am J Med, 84:233, 1988.

51. Zeluff BJ: Fungal pneumonia in transplant recipients. Semin Respir Infect, 5:80, 1990.

Aspergillus

52. Binder RE, Faling LJ, Pugatch RD, et al: Chronic necrotizing pulmonary aspergillosis: a discrete clinical entity. Medicine, 61:109, 1982.

53. Burch PA, Karp JE, Merz WG, et al: Favorable outcome of invasive aspergillosis in patients with acute leukemia. J Clin Oncol, 5:1985, 1987.

54. Clarke A, Skelton J, Fraser RS: Fungal tracheobronchitis: report of 9 cases and review of the literature. Medicine, 70:1, 1991.

55. Denning DW, Follansbee S, Scolaro M, et al: Pulmonary aspergillosis in AIDS. Predisposing factors, clinical features, and therapeutic outcome. N Engl J Med, 324:654, 1991.

56. Denning DW, Stevens DA: Antifungal and surgical treatment of invasive aspergillosis: review of 2,121 published cases. Rev Infect Dis, 12:1147, 1990.

57. Gerson SL, Talbot GH, Hurwitz S, et al: Prolonged granulocytopenia: the major risk factor for invasive pulmonary aspergillosis in patients with leukemia. Ann Intern Med, 100:345, 1984.
58. Gustafson TL, Schaffner W, Lavely GB, et al: Invasive aspergillosis in rental transplant recipients: correlation with corticosteroid use. J Infect Dis, 148:230, 1983.
59. Kramer MR, Denning DW, Marshall SE, et al: Ulcerative tracheobronchitis after lung transplantation. A new form of invasive aspergillosis. Am Rev Respir Dis, 144:552, 1991.
60. Rinaldi MG: Invasive aspergillosis. Rev Infect Dis, 5:1061, 1983.
61. Yu VL, Muder RR, Poorsattar A: Significance of isolation of aspergillus from the respiratory tract in diagnosis of invasive pulmonary aspergillosis: Results from a three-year prospective study. Am J Med, 81:249, 1986.

Blastomycosis

62. Brown LR, Swensen SJ, Van Scoy RE, et al: Roentgenologic features of pulmonary blastomycosis. Mayo Clin Proc, 66:29, 1991.
63. Dismukes WE, Cloud G, Bowles C, et al: Treatment of blastomycosis and histoplasmosis with ketoconazole: results of a prospective randomized trial. Ann Intern Med, 103:861, 1985.
64. Recht LD, Davies SF, Eckman MR, Serosi GA: Blastomycosis in immunosuppressed patients. Am Rev Respir Dis, 125:359, 1982.
65. Serosi GA, Davies SF: Blastomycosis. Am Rev Respir Dis, 120:911, 1979.

Coccidioidomycosis

66. Ampel NM, Wieden MA, Galgiani JN: Coccidioidomycosis: clinical update. Rev Infect Dis, 11:897, 1989.
67. Bayer AS: Fungal pneumonias: pulmonary coccidioidal syndromes. Chest, 79:686, 1981.
68. Bronnimann DA, Adam RD, Galgiani JN, et al: Coccidioidomycosis in the acquired immunodeficiency syndrome. Ann Intern Med, 106:372, 1987.
69. Graybill JR, Lundberg D, Donovon W, et al: Treatment of coccidioidomycosis with ketoconazole: clinical and laboratory studies of 18 patients. Rev Infect Dis, 2(4):661, 1980.

Cryptococcosis

70. Bennett JE, Dismukes WE, Duma RJ, et al: A comparison of amphotericin B alone and combined with flucytosine in the treatment of cryptococcal meningitis. N Engl J Med, 301:126, 1979.
71. Campbell DG: Primary pulmonary cryptococcosis. Am Rev Respir Dis, 94:236, 1966.
72. Chuck LS, Sande MA: Infections with Cryptococcus neoformans in the acquired immunodeficiency syndrome. N Engl J Med, 321:794, 1989.
73. Dismukes WE, Cloud G, Gallis HA, et al: Treatment of cryptococcal meningitis with combination amphotericin B and flucytosine for four as compared with six weeks. N Engl J Med, 317:334, 1987.
74. Duperval R, Hermans PE, Brewer NS, et al: Cryptococcosis with emphasis on the significance of isolation of Cryptococcus neoformans from the respiratory tract. Chest, 72: 13, 1977.
75. Hammerman KJ, Powell KE, Christianson CS, et al: Pulmonary cryptococcosis: clinical forms and treatment. Am Rev Respir Dis, 108:1116, 1973.
76. Kerkering TM, Duma RJ, Shadomy S: The evolution of pulmonary cryptococcosis. Ann Intern Med, 94:611, 1981.
77. Kovacs JA, Kovacs AA, Polis M, et al: Cryptococcosis in the acquired immunodeficiency syndrome. Ann Intern Med, 103:533, 1985.

78. Sugar AM, Sanders C: Oral fluconazole as suppressive therapy of disseminated cryptococcosis in patients with acquired immunodeficiency syndrome. Am J Med, 85:481, 1988.
79. Sugar AM, Stern JJ, Dupont B: Overview treatment of cryptococcal meningitis. Rev Infect Dis, 12:S338, 1991.
80. Tynes B, Mason KN, Jennings AE, et al: Variant forms of pulmonary cryptococcosis. Ann Intern Med, 69:1117, 1968.
81. Warr W, Bates JH, Stove A: The spectrum of pulmonary cryptococcosis. Ann Intern Med, 69:1109, 1968.
82. Wasser L, Talavera W: Pulmonary cryptococcosis in AIDS. Chest, 92:692, 1987.
83. Zuger A, Schuster M, Simberkoff MS, et al: Maintenance amphotericin B for cryptococcal meningitis in the acquired immunodeficiency syndrome. Ann Intern Med, 109:592, 1988.

Histoplasmosis

84. Graybill JR: Histoplasmosis and AIDS. J Infect Dis, 158:623, 1988.
85. Mody CH, Toews GB: Histoplasmosis. *In* Current Therapy of Respiratory Disease. Edited by RM Chemiak. Ontario, B. C. Decker, 1989.
86. Wheat LJ, Slama TJ, Zeckel ML: Histoplasmosis in acquired immune deficiency syndrome. Am J Med, 78:203, 1985.

Mucormycosis

87. Lehrer RI, Howard DH, Sypherd PS, et al: Mucormycosis. Ann Intern Med, 93:93, 1980.
88. Parfey NA: Improved diagnosis and prognosis of mucormycosis: a clinicopathological study of 33 cases. Medicine (Baltimore), 1:166, 1986.
89. Rangel-Guerra R, Martinez HR, Saenz C: Mucormycosis: report of 11 cases. Arch Neurol, 42:578, 1985.
90. Rinaldi MG: Zygomycosis. Infect Dis Clin North Am, 2:19, 1989.

Antifungal Drugs

91. EORTC International Antimicrobial Therapy Cooperative Group: Empirical antifungal therapy in febrile granulocytopenic patients. Am J Med, 86:668, 1989.
92. Walsh TJ, Lee J, Lecciones J, et al: Empiric therapy with amphotericin B in febrile granulocytopenic patients. Rev Infect Dis, 13:496, 1991.

Amphotericin B

93. Bates JH: Amphotericin B, amphotericin B methylester and other polyenes. *In* Fungal Diseases of the Lung. Edited by GA Sarosi and SF Davies. New York, Grune & Stratton, 1986.
94. Christiansen KJ, Bernard EM, Gold JWM, Armstrong D: Distribution and activity of amphotericin B in humans. J Infect Dis, 152:1037, 1985.
95. Kennedy MS, Deeg HJ, Siegel M, et al: Acute renal toxicity with combined use of amphotericin B and cyclosporine after marrow transplantation. Transplantation, 35:211, 1983.
96. Lopez-Berestein G, Bodey GP, Fainstein V, et al: Treatment of systemic fungal infections with liposomal amphotericin B. Arch Intern Med, 149:2533, 1989.
97. Perfect JR, Pickard WW, Hunt DL, et al: The use of amphotericin B in nosocomial fungal infection. Rev Infect Dis, 13:474, 1991.

Azoles

98. Dismukes WE: Azole antifungal agents: old and new. Ann Intern Med, 109:177, 1988.
99. Saag MS, Dismukes WE: Azole antifungal agents: emphasis on new triazoles. Antimicrob Agents Chemother, 32:1, 1988.

KETOCONAZOLE

100. Brass C, Galgiani JN, Blashke TF, et al: Disposition of ketoconazole, an oral antifungal, in humans. Antimicrob Agents Chemother, 21:151, 1982.
101. Brass C, Galgiani JN, Campbell SC, Stevens DA: Therapy of disseminated or pulmonary coccidioidomycosis with ketoconazole. Rev Infect Dis, 2(4):656, 1980.
102. Catanzara A, Einstein H, Levine B, et al: Ketoconazole for treatment of disseminated coccidioidomycosis. Ann Intern Med, 96:436, 1982.
103. Craven PC, Graybill JR, Jorgensen JH, et al: High dose ketoconazole for treatment of fungal infection of the central nervous system. Ann Intern Med, 98:160, 1983.
104. Fainstein V, Bodey GP, Elting L, et al: Amphotericin B or ketoconazole therapy of fungal infections in neutropenic cancer patients. Antimicrob Agents Chemother, 31:11, 1987.
105. Graybill JR, Craven PC, Donovon W, Matthew EB: Ketoconazole therapy for systemic fungal infections. Inadequacy of standard dosage regimens. Am Rev Respir Dis, 126:171, 1982.
106. National Institute of Allergy and Infectious Diseases Mycoses Study Group: Treatment of blastomycosis and histoplasmosis with ketoconazole. Results of a prospective randomized clinical trial. Ann Intern Med, 103:861, 1985.
107. Slama TG: Treatment of disseminated and progressive cavitary histoplasmosis with ketoconazole. Am J Med, 74 (suppl 1b):70, 1983.
108. Sugar AM, Alsip SG, Galgiani JN, et al: Pharmacology and toxicity of high-dose ketoconazole. Antimicrob Agents Chemother, 31:1874, 1987.

FLUCONAZOLE

109. Bozette SA, Larsen RA, Chiu J, et al: A placebo-controlled trial of maintenance therapy with fluconazole after treatment of cryptococcal meningitis in the acquired immunodeficiency syndrome. N Engl J Med, 324:580, 1991.
110. Classen DC, Burke JP, Smith CB: Treatment of coccidioidal meningitis with fluconazole. J Infect Dis, 158:903, 1988.
111. Galgiani JN: Fluconazole, a new antifungal agent. Ann Intern Med, 113:177, 1990.
112. Ikemoto H: A clinical study of fluconazole for the treatment of deep mycoses. Diagn Microbiol Infect Dis, 12:239S, 1989.
113. Larsen RA, Leal ME, Chan LS: Fluconazole compared with amphotericin B plus flucytosine for cryptococcal meningitis in AIDS. Ann Intern Med, 113:138, 1990.
114. Lazar JD, Wilner KD: Drug interactions with fluconazole. Rev Infect Dis, 12:S327, 1990.
115. Robinson PA, Knirsch AK, Joseph JA: Fluconazole for life-threatening fungal infections in patients who cannot be treated with conventional antifungal agents. Rev Infect Dis, 12:S349, 1990.
116. Stern JJ, Hartman BJ, Sharkey P, et al: Oral fluconazole therapy for patients with acquired immunodeficiency syndrome and cryptococcosis: experience with 22 patients. Am J Med, 85:477, 1988.
117. Tucker RM, Galgiani JN, Denning DW: Treatment of coccidioidal meningitis with fluconazole. Rev Infect Dis, 12:S380, 1990.
118. Van't Wout JW, Mattie H, van Furth R: A prospective study of the efficacy of fluconazole (UK-49,858) against deep-seated fungal infections. J Antimicrob Chemother, 1:665, 1988.

ITRACONAZOLE

119. Denning DW, Tucker RM, Hanson LH, et al: Iraconazole therapy of cryptococcal meningitis and cryptococcosis. Arch Intern Med, 149:2301, 1989.
120. Denning DW, Tucker RM, Hanson LH, Stevens DA: Treatment of invasive aspergillosis with itraconazole. Am J Med, 86:791, 1989.
121. Dupont B: Itraconazole therapy in aspergillosis: study in 49 patients. J Am Acad Dermatol, 23:607, 1990.
122. Faggian G, Livi U, Bortolotti U, et al: Itraconazole therapy for acute invasive pulmonary aspergillosis. Transplant Proc, 21:2506, 1989.
123. Grant SM, Clissold SP: Itraconazole: a review of its pharmacodynamic and pharmacokinetic properties, and therapeutic use in superficial and systemic mycoses. Drugs, 18: 310, 1989.
124. Kramer MR, Marshall SE, Denning DW, et al: Interaction between cyclosporine and itraconazole in heart and lung transplant recipients. Ann Intern Med, 113:327, 1990.
125. Tucker RM, Denning DW, Dupont B, Steven DA: Itraconazole therapy for chronic coccidioidal meningitis. Ann Intern Med, 112:108, 1990.
126. Tucker RM, Haq Y, Denning DW, Stevens DA: Adverse events associated with itraconazole in 189 patients on chronic therapy. J Antimicrob Chemother, 26:561, 1990.
127. Tucker RM, Williams PL, Stevens DA: Treatment of mycosis with itraconazole. Ann NY Acad Sci, 544:451, 1988.
128. Viviani MA, Tortorano AM, Langer M, et al: Experience with itraconazole in cryptococcosis and aspergillosis. J Infect, 18:151, 1989.

Flucytosine

129. Bennett JE: Flucytosine. Ann Intern Med, 86:319, 1977.
130. Stamm AM, Diasio RB, Dismukes WE, et al: Toxicity of amphotericin B plus flucytosine in 194 patients with cryptococcal meningitis. Am J Med, 83:236, 1987.

NOCARDIA

131. Berkey P, Bodey G: Nocardial infection in patients with neoplastic disease. Rev Infect Dis, 2(3):407, 1989.
132. Chapman SW, Wilson JP: Nocardiosis in transplant recipients. Semin Respir Infect, 5: 74, 1990.
133. Dewsnup DH, Wright DN: In vitro susceptibility of Nocardia asteroides to 25 antimicrobial agents. Antimicrobob Agents Chemother, 25:165, 1984.
134. Goldstein FW, Hautefort B, Acar F: Amikacin-containing regimens for treatment of nocardiosis in immunocompromised patients. Eur J Clin Microbiol, 6:198, 1987.
135. Gombert ME: Susceptibility of Nocardia asteroides to various antibiotics including newer beta-lactams, trimethoprim-sulfamethoxazole, amikacin, and N-formimidoyl thienamycin. Antimicrob Agents Chemother, 21:1011, 1982.
136. Gombert ME, Aulicino TM: Synergism of imipenem and amikacin in combination with other antibiotics against Nocardia asteroides. Antimicrob Agents Chemother, 24:810, 1983.
137. Gombert ME, Aulicino TM, du Bouchet L, Berkowitz LR: Susceptibility of Nocardia asteroides to new quinolones and beta-lactams. Antimicrob Agents Chemother, 31:2013, 1987.
138. Gombert ME, Aulicino TM, du Bouchet L, et al: Therapy of experimental cerebral nocardiosis with imipenem, amikacin, trimethoprim-sulfamethoxazole, and minocycline. Antimicrob Agents Chemother, 30:270, 1986.
139. Kim J, Minamoto GY, Grieco MH: Nocardial infection as a complication of AIDS: Report of six cases and review. Rev Infect Dis, 13:624, 1991.

140. Rolfe M, Strieter RM, Lynch JP III: Nocardiosis. Semin Respir Med 1992 13(3):216, 1992.
141. Simpson GL, Stinson EG, Egger MJ, Remington JS. Nocardial infections in the immunocompromised host: a detailed study in a defined patient population. Rev Infect Dis, 3:492, 1981.
142. Smego RA, Gallis HA: The clinical spectrum of Nocardia brasiliensis infection in the United States. Rev Infect Dis, 6:164, 1984.
143. Wallace RJ, Septimus EJ, Williams TW, et al: Use of trimethoprim-sulfamethoxazole for treatment of infections due to Nocardia. Rev Infect Dis, 4:315, 1982.
144. Wilson JP, Turner HR, Kirchner KA, Chapman SW: Nocardial infections in renal transplant recipients. Medicine, 68:38, 1989.

TUBERCULOSIS

Clinical

145. Barnes PF, Bloch AB, Davidson PT, Snider DE Jr: Tuberculosis in patients with human immunodeficiency virus infection. N Engl J Med, 324:1644, 1991.
146. Baughman RP, Dohn MN, Loudon RG, Frame PT: Bronchoscopy with bronchoalveolar lavage in tuberculosis and fungal infections. Chest, 99:92, 1991.
147. Bloch AB, Rieder HL, Kelly GD, et al: The epidemiology of tuberculosis in the United States. Semin Respir Infect, 4:157, 1989.
148. Brudney K, Dobkin J: Resurgent tuberculosis in New York City: human immunodeficiency virus, homelessness, and the decline of tuberculosis control programs. Am Rev Respir Dis, 144:745, 1991.
149. Chaisson RE, Schecter GF, Theuer CP, et al: Tuberculosis in patients with the acquired immunodeficiency syndrome: clinical features, response to therapy, and survival. Am Rev Respir Dis, 136:570, 1987.
150. Comstock GW, Daniel TM, Snider DE Jr, et al: The tuberculin skin test. Statement of American Thoracic Society. Am Rev Respir Dis, 124:356, 1981.
151. Dannenberg AM Jr: Pathogenesis of pulmonary tuberculosis. Am Rev Respir Dis, 125: 24, 1982.
152. DeGracia J, Curull V, Vidal R, et al: Diagnostic value of bronchoalveolar lavage in the suspected pulmonary tuberculosis. Chest, 93:329, 1988.
153. Ellner JJ, Barnes PF, Wallis RS, Modlin RL: The immunology of tuberculous pleurisy. Semin Respir Infect, 3:335, 1988.
154. Johnson JL, Ellner JJ: Tuberculosis meningitis. In Prognosis in Neurological Disease. Edited by RW Evans, DS Baskins, FM Yatsu. New York, Oxford University Press, 1990.
155. Khan MA, Kovanat DM, Bachus B, et al: Clinical and roentgenographic spectrum of pulmonary tuberculosis in the adult. Am J Med, 62:31, 1977.
156. Kim JH, Langston AA, Gallis HA: Miliary tuberculosis: epidemiology, clinical manifestations, diagnosis, and outcome. Rev Infect Dis, 12:583, 1990.
157. Kramer F, Modilevsky T, Waliany AR, et al: Delayed diagnosis of tuberculosis in patients with human immunodeficiency virus infection. Am J Med, 89:451, 1990.
158. McAdam JM, Brickner PW, Scharer LL, et al: The spectrum of tuberculosis in a New York City men's shelter clinic (1982–1988). Chest, 97:798, 1990.
159. Pitchenik AE, Rubinson HA: The radiographic appearance of tuberculosis in patients with the acquired immune deficiency syndrome (AIDS) and pre-AIDS. Am Rev Respir Dis, 131:393, 1985.
160. Reider HL, Cauthen GM, Kelly GD, et al: Tuberculosis in the United States. JAMA, 262: 385, 1989.
161. Shafer RW, Goldberg R, Sierra M, Glatt AE: Frequency of Mycobacterium tuberculosis bacteremia in patients with tuberculosis in an area edemic for AIDS. Am Rev Respir Dis, 140:1611, 1989.

162. Stead WW: Tuberculosis among elderly persons: an outbreak in a nursing home. Ann Intern Med, 94:606, 1981.
163. Stead WW, Dutt AK: Tuberculosis in the elderly. Semin Respir Infect, 4:189, 1989.
164. Stead WW et al: Tuberculosis as an endemic and nosocomial infection among the elderly of nursing homes. N Engl J Med, 312:1483, 1985.
165. Update: tuberculosis elimination—United States. MMWR, 39:153, 1990.

Therapy

166. American Thoracic Society: Treatment of tuberculosis and tuberculosis infection in adults and children. Am Rev Respir Dis, 134:355, 1986.
167. Chaisson RE, Hopewell P: Survival after active tuberculosis in patients with HIV infection. Am Rev Respir Dis, 142:259, 1990.
168. Cohn DL, Catlin BJ, Peterson KL, et al: A 62-dose, 6-month therapy for pulmonary and extrapulmonary tuberculosis. Ann Intern Med, 112:407, 1990.
169. Combs DL, O'Brien RJ, Geiter LJ: USPHS tuberculosis short-course chemotherapy trial 21: effectiveness, toxicity, and acceptability. Ann Intern Med, 112:397, 1990.
170. Davidson PT: Drug resistance and the selection of therapy for tuberculosis. Am Rev Respir Dis, 136:255, 1987.
171. Guidelines for preventing the transmission of tuberculosis in health-care settings, with special focus on HIV-related issues. MMWR, 39:RR-17:1, 1990.
172. Hong Kong Chest Service/British Medical Research Council: Controlled trial of 2, 4, and 6 months of pyrazinamide in 6-month, three-times-weekly regimens for smear-positive pulmonary tuberculosis, including an assessment of a combined preparation of isoniazid, rifampin, and pyrazinamide: results at 30 months. Am Rev Respir Dis, 143:700, 1991.
173. O'Brien RJ: Present chemotherapy of tuberculosis. Semin Respir Infect, 4:216, 1989.
174. Singapore Tuberculosis Service/British Medical Research Council: Assessment of a daily combined preparation of isoniazid, rifampin, and pyrazinamide in a controlled trial of three 6-month regimens for smear-positive pulmonary tuberculosis. Am Rev Respir Dis, 143:707, 1991.
175. Small PM, Schecter GF, Goodman PC, et al: Treatment of tuberculosis in patients with advanced human immunodeficiency virus infection. N Engl J Med, 324:289, 1991.

VIRAL INFECTIONS

176. Glezen WP: Serious morbidity and mortality associated with influenza epidemics. Epidemiol Rev, 4:25, 1982.
177. Glezen WP, Decker M, Joseph S, et al: Acute respiratory diseases associated with influenza epidemics in Houston, 1981–1983. J Infect Dis, 155:1119, 1987.

Adenovirus

178. Zahradnik JM: Adenovirus pneumonia. Semin Respir Infect, 2:104, 1987.

Cytomegalovirus

Epidemiology and Clinical Features

179. Burke CM, Glanville AR, Macoviak JA, et al: The spectrum of cytomegalovirus infection following human heart-lung transplantation. J Heart Transplant, 5:267, 1986.
180. Duncan AJ, Dummer JS, Paradis IL, et al: Cytomegalovirus infection and survival in lung transplant recipients. J Heart Lung Transplant, 10:638, 1991.
181. Grundy JE, Shanley JD, Griffiths PD: Is cytomegalovirus interstitial pneumonitis an transplant recipients an immunopathological condition? Lancet, 2:996, 1987.

182. Klotman ME, Hamilton JD: Cytomegalovirus pneumonia. Semin Respir Infect, 2:95, 1987.
183. Maurer JR, Tullis E, Scavuzzo M, Patterson GA: Cytomegalovirus infection in isolated lung transplantations. J Heart Lung Transplant, 10:647, 1991.
184. Miles PR, Baughman RP, Linnemann CC: Cytomegalovirus in the bronchoalveolar lavage fluid of patients with AIDS. Chest, 97:1072, 1990.
185. Millar AB, Patou G, Miller RF, et al: Cytomegalovirus in the lungs of patients with AIDS: respiratory pathogen or passenger? Am Rev Respir Dis, 141:1474, 1990.
186. Wreghitt TG, Hakim M, Gray JJ, et al: Cytomegalovirus infection in heart and heart-lung transplant recipients. J Clin Pathol, 41:660, 1988.

Therapy

GANCICLOVIR

187. Buhles WC Jr, Mastre BJ, Tinker AJ, et al: Ganciclovir treatment of life- or sight-threatening cytomegalovirus infection: experience in 314 immunocompromised patients. Rev Infect Dis, 10 (Suppl 3):S495, 1988.
188. Collaborative DHPG Treatment Study Group: Treatment of serious cytomegalovirus infections with 9-(1,3-dihydroxy-2-propoxymethyl) guanine in patients with AIDS and other immunodeficiencies. N Engl J Med, 314:801, 1986.
189. Faulds D, Heel RC: Ganciclovir: a review of its antiviral activity, pharmacokinetic properties and therapeutic efficacy in cytomegalovirus infections. Drugs, 39:597, 1990.
190. Goodrich JM, Mori M, Gleaves, CA, et al: Early treatment with ganciclovir to prevent cytomegalovirus disease after allogeneic bone marrow transplantation. N Engl J Med, 325:1601, 1991.
191. Keay S, Petersen E, Icenogle T, et al: Ganciclovir treatment of serious cytomegalovirus infection in heart and heart-lung transplant recipients. Rev Infect Dis, 10:S563, 1988.
192. Reed EC, Bowden RA, Bandliker PS, et al: Treatment of cytomegalovirus pneumonia with ganciclovir and intravenous cytomegalovirus immunoglobulin in patients with bone marrow transplants. Ann Intern Med, 109:783, 1988.

FORSCARNET

193. Deray G, Martinez F, Katlama C, et al: Forscarnet nephrotoxicity: mechanism, incidence, and prevention. Am J Nephrol, 9:316, 1989.
194. Jacobson MA, Crowe S, Levy J, et al: Effect of foscarnet therapy on infection with human immunodeficiency virus in patients with AIDS. J Infect Dis, 158:862, 1988.
195. Oberg B: Antiviral effects of phosphonoformate (PFA, forscarnet). Pharmacol Ther, 19: 387, 1989.
196. Palestine AG, Polis MA, de Smet MD, et al: Forscarnet in the treatment of cytomegalovirus retinitis in patients with AIDS. Ann Intern Med, 115:665, 1991.

Prophylactic Strategies

197. Balfour HH, Chace BA, Stapleton JT, et al: A randomized, placebo-controlled trial of oral acyclovir for the prevention of cytomegalovirus disease in recipients of renal allografts. N Engl J Med, 320:1381, 1989.
198. Bowden RA, Meyers JD: Prophylaxis of cytomegalovirus infection. Semin Hematol, 27: 17, 1990.
199. Schmidt GM, Horak DA, Hiland JC, et al: A randomized, controlled trial of prophylactic ganciclovir for cytomegalovirus pulmonary infection in recipients of allogeneic bone marrow transplants. N Engl J Med, 324:1005, 1991.

200. Snydman DR, Werner BG, Heinze-Lacey B, et al: Use of cytomegalovirus immune globulin to prevent cytomegalovirus disease in renal transplant recipients. N Engl J Med, 317:1049, 1987.
201. Snydman DR, Werner BG, Tilney NL, et al: Final analysis of primary cytomegalovirus disease prevention in renal transplant recipients with a cytomegalovirus-immune globulin: comparison of the randomized and open-label trials. Transplant Proc, 23:1357, 1991.
202. Stratta RJ, Shaefer MS, Cushing KA, et al: Successful prophylaxis of cytomegalovirus disease after primary CMV exposure in liver transplant recipients. Transplantation, 51: 90, 1991.

Herpes Simplex/Varicella Zoster Viruses

203. Corey L, Spear PG: Infections with herpes simplex viruses. N Engl J Med, 314:686, 749, 1986.
204. Feldman S, Stokes DC: Varicella zoster and herpes simplex virus pneumonias. Semin Respir Infect, 2:84, 1987.
205. Graham BS, Snell JD: Herpes simplex virus infection of the adult lower respiratory tract. Medicine (Baltimore), 62:384, 1983.
206. Ramsey PG, Fife KH, Hackman RC, et al: Herpes simplex virus pneumonia. Clinical, virologic, and pathologic features in 20 patients. Ann Intern Med, 97:813, 1982.
207. Shepp DH, Dandliker PS, Meyers JD: Treatment of varicella-zoster virus infection in severely immunocompromised patients. A randomized comparison of acyclovir and vidarabine. N Engl J Med, 314:208, 1986.

26

PLEURAL DISEASES, PLEURAL EFFUSIONS

Richard W. Light

Approximately 1 million patients in the United States develop a pleural effusion each year. Anytime a patient with an abnormal chest x-ray is evaluated, the possibility of a pleural effusion should be considered. Increased densities on the chest x-ray are frequently attributed to parenchymal infiltrates, although they actually represent pleural fluid. The earliest radiologic sign of a pleural effusion is blunting of the posterior costophrenic sulcus on lateral x-ray. If this angle is blunted, bilateral decubitus chest x-rays should be obtained to ascertain whether free pleural fluid is present. The presence of pleural fluid can be documented by one of the following

- Bilateral decubitus x-rays of the chest
- Computerized tomographic (CT) scan of the chest
- Ultrasonic examination of the chest

PHYSIOLOGY OF PLEURAL FLUID FORMATION

Fluid can enter the pleural space from

- Capillaries in the parietal pleura
- Capillaries in the visceral pleura
- Interstitial spaces of the lung

Pleural fluid accumulates when the rate of fluid formation exceeds the rate of fluid absorption. This situation can be caused by either an increased rate of formation or a decreased rate of absorption. Rate of formation is normally 0.01 ml/kg/hr, whereas capacity for absorption is 0.20 ml/kg/hr

- Absorption is almost exclusively via the lymphatics in the parietal pleura
- Lymphatics in the visceral pleura do not communicate with the pleural space
- Little fluid exits the pleural space via capillaries

Fluid entry into the pleural space from the capillaries follows Starling's equation. The following factors increase the rate of pleural fluid formation from the capillaries

- Increased hydrostatic pressure in the capillaries in either the visceral or the parietal pleura
- Decreased pressure in the pleural space
- Decreased oncotic pressure in the blood
- Increased oncotic pressure in the pleural fluid

The rate of fluid entry into the pleural space from the interstitial spaces of the lungs increases when

- Interstitial fluid is increased
- The lymphatics that normally drain the lung become disrupted, such as occurs with lung transplantation

CLINICAL MANIFESTATIONS

SYMPTOMS OF PLEURAL EFFUSION

- Dyspnea on exertion
- Chest tightness
- Pleuritic chest pain

SIGNS OF PLEURAL EFFUSION

- Dullness to percussion over fluid
- Absent tactile fremitus over effusion
- Decreased breath sounds over effusion

APPROACH TO PATIENTS WITH PLEURAL EFFUSION

Pleural effusions can occur as complications of many different diseases (Table 26–1). The vigor with which various diagnoses are pursued depends on the likelihood that the individual has that particular disease. Rough estimates as to the incidence of the most common causes of pleural effusions are provided in Table 26–2.

When a patient has a pleural effusion that measures more than 10 mm on the decubitus x-ray, a diagnostic thoracentesis usually should be performed. If the patient has obvious congestive heart failure, consideration can be given to postponing the thoracentesis until the heart failure is treated. The characteristics of pleural fluid change little with diuresis over several days. If, however, such a patient is febrile or has pleuritic chest pain, or if the effusions are not of comparable size on both sides, a thoracentesis should be performed without delay.

PERFORMING A DIAGNOSTIC THORACENTESIS

This procedure is usually performed while the patient sits upright. A table should be available for the patient to rest his arms upon. The patient's back should remain relatively vertical, for if the patient leans forward too

TABLE 26–1. DIFFERENTIAL DIAGNOSES OF PLEURAL EFFUSIONS

I. TRANSUDATIVE PLEURAL EFFUSIONS
   A. Congestive heart failure
   B. Cirrhosis
   C. Peritoneal dialysis
   D. Nephrotic syndrome
   E. Superior vena cava obstruction
   F. Fontan procedure
   G. Urinothorax
   H. Myxedema
   I. Pulmonary emboli
II. EXUDATIVE PLEURAL EFFUSIONS
   A. Neoplastic diseases
      1. Metastatic disease
      2. Mesothelioma
   B. Infectious diseases
      1. Bacterial infections
      2. Tuberculosis
      3. Fungal infections
      4. Viral infections
      5. Parasitic infections
   C. Pulmonary embolization
   D. Gastrointestinal disease
      1. Acute pancreatitis
      2. Chronic pancreatic pleural effusion
      3. Esophageal perforation
      4. Intra-abdominal abscesses
      5. Diaphragmatic hernia
      6. Postabdominal surgery
      7. Endoscopic variceal sclerotherapy
   E. Collagen vascular diseases
      1. Rheumatoid pleuritis
      2. Lupus erythematosus
      3. Churg-Strauss syndrome
      4. Familial mediterranean fever
      5. Immunoblastic lymphadenopathy
   F. Drug-induced pleural disease
      1. Nitrofurantoin
      2. Dantrolene
      3. Methysergide
      4. Bromocriptine
      5. Procarbazine
      6. Amiodarone
   G. Asbestos exposure
   H. Postcardiac injury syndrome
   I. Pericardial disease
   J. Postcoronary artery bypass surgery
   K. Uremia
   L. Yellow nail syndrome
   M. Sarcoidosis
   N. Trapped lung
   O. Meigs' syndrome

TABLE 26–2. APPROXIMATE ANNUAL INCIDENCE OF VARIOUS TYPES OF PLEURAL EFFUSIONS IN THE UNITED STATES

CAUSES	INCIDENCE (REPORTED CASES)
Congestive heart failure	500,000
Pneumonia (bacterial)	300,000
Malignant disease	200,000
Lung	60,000
Breast	50,000
Lymphoma	40,000
Other	50,000
Pulmonary embolization	150,000
Viral disease	100,000
Cirrhosis with ascites	50,000
Gastrointestinal disease	25,000
Collagen vascular disease	6,000
Asbestos exposure	2,000
Mesothelioma	1,500
Tuberculosis	1,000

far, the lowest part of the hemithorax may move anteriorly and no fluid will remain posteriorly.

The site for insertion of the needle should be determined with care

- Insert the needle posteriorly where the ribs are easily palpable and where the fluid gravitates
- Make the first attempt one interspace below the level where the tactile fremitus is lost
- Most unsuccessful thoracentesis procedures result from attempting to perform the thoracentesis at a level that is too low
- Insertion of the needle at a low level is dangerous because the spleen or liver may be lacerated
- Evaluate with ultrasound if fluid is not obtained after two or three attempts

The actual performance of the procedure is as follows

- Thoroughly cleanse the skin over the site
- Anesthetize the skin with lidocaine using a short 25-gauge needle
- Anesthetize the periosteum of the underlying rib and the parietal pleura by performing the following steps with a 22-gauge needle 1.5 inches long. Move the needle up and over the rib with frequent injections of small amounts (about 0.1 ml) of lidocaine. Once superior to the rib, slowly advance the needle toward the pleural space, with aspiration followed by the injection of 0.1 to 0.2 ml lidocaine every 1 to 2 mm. Once pleural fluid is obtained through the anesthetizing needle, withdraw the needle.
- Withdraw the fluid by using a second 22-gauge needle attached to a 50- to 60-ml syringe that contains 0.5 to 1.0 ml heparin. Slowly insert the

needle along the same tract with constant aspiration until pleural fluid is obtained. Continue aspiration until the syringe is filled
- Withdraw the needle

If more than 60 ml of pleural fluid is to be removed, a plastic catheter rather than a sharp needle should be utilized.
Complications of thoracentesis include

- Pneumothorax, which occurs in 10% of patients; 20% of these patients require a chest tube
- Infection of the pleural space
- Hemothorax from laceration of an intercostal artery or vein, the spleen, or the liver
- Seeding of the needle tract with tumor cells
- Vasovagal reaction with bradycardia and hypotension

SEPARATING TRANSUDATIVE FROM EXUDATIVE PLEURAL EFFUSIONS

The first question to be answered with a diagnostic thoracentesis is whether the patient has a transudative or an exudative pleural effusion. An exudative effusion results from disease of the pleural surfaces, whereas a transudative effusion results from alterations in the systemic factors that influence the formation and reabsorption of pleural fluid.

This differentiation can be made by simultaneous analysis of the protein and lactic acid dehydrogenase (LDH) levels in the pleural fluid and in the serum. Exudative pleural effusions meet at least one of the following criteria, whereas transudative pleural effusions meet none:

- Ratio of pleural fluid to serum protein >0.5
- Ratio of pleural fluid to serum LDH >0.6
- Absolute level of pleural fluid LDH $>\frac{2}{3}$ upper normal limit for serum

If none of the above criteria is met, the patient has a transudative pleural effusion, and the pleura itself can be ignored while the congestive heart failure, cirrhosis, or nephrosis is treated. Remember, however, that transudative pleural effusion can result from pulmonary embolization.

If a transudative pleural effusion is probable, the most cost effective use of the laboratory is initially to measure only the pleural fluid protein and LDH levels. Other diagnostic tests, such as cytology, cell count, and differential, amylase, glucose, and cultures, are obtained only if the patient is proved to have an exudative pleural effusion.

TRANSUDATIVE PLEURAL EFFUSIONS

CONGESTIVE HEART FAILURE

Congestive heart failure is the disease most responsible for pleural effusions.

PATHOPHYSIOLOGY

The accumulation of pleural fluid in patients with congestive heart failure appears to be related more to left ventricular than to right ventricular failure

- Left ventricular failure leads to increased interstitial fluid, which then traverses the visceral pleura to enter the pleural space. In animal experiments, approximately 25% of pulmonary edema fluid moves directly from the lung into the pleural space

CLINICAL MANIFESTATIONS

Patients with pleural effusions secondary to congestive heart failure usually have other signs and symptoms

- Increasing dyspnea on exertion
- Increasing peripheral edema and orthopnea or paroxysmal nocturnal dyspnea
- Auscultation may reveal an S_3 gallop and crepitations (crackles), as well as signs of the pleural effusions (see Chapter 5)
- The chest x-ray may reveal cardiomegaly (see Chapter 5)
- Pleural effusions are usually bilateral and roughly equivalent in size
- The pleural fluid is a transudate

DIAGNOSIS AND TREATMENT

The diagnosis is usually suggested by the clinical picture of congestive heart failure

- Perform thoracentesis to demonstrate that fluid is a transudate when the patient does not respond to therapy, when effusions are not roughly the same size, and when patient is febrile or has pleuritic chest pain
- Treatment consists of digitalis, diuretics, and afterload reduction
- A rare patient has dyspnea from a large persistent pleural effusion despite optimal medical therapy. If dyspnea is relieved by a therapeutic thoracentesis, consideration can be given to attempting a pleurodesis with a sclerosing agent

HEPATIC HYDROTHORAX

Pleural effusions sometimes develop in patients with cirrhosis, particularly if ascites is present. The incidence of pleural effusion is approximately 6% in patients with cirrhosis and ascites, but is less than 1% in patients with cirrhosis with hypoalbuminemia but without ascites.

PATHOPHYSIOLOGY

The predominant mechanism is the movement of the ascitic fluid directly from the peritoneal cavity through the diaphragm into the pleural space

- Small pores in diaphragm have been demonstrated

CLINICAL MANIFESTATIONS

The pleural effusion with hepatic hydrothorax tends to be large because of the large reservoir of fluid in the peritoneal cavity that can flow directly into the pleural space with its lower pressure

- Usually tense ascites is present, but occasionally the ascites is subclinical
- A large effusion may produce severe dyspnea
- The pleural effusions are usually right-sided (67%), but may be left-sided (16%) or bilateral (17%)

DIAGNOSIS AND TREATMENT

In a patient with cirrhosis, tense ascites, and a pleural effusion, the diagnosis is easy

- Both a paracentesis and a thoracentesis should be performed to ascertain that both fluids are transudates. The pleural fluid protein level, although usually slightly higher than the ascitic fluid protein level, is still <3.0 g/dl
- Patients with hepatic hydrothoraces are prone to develop bacterial infections of the pleural space
- Primary treatment is geared toward treatment of the ascites because the hydrothorax is an extension of the peritoneal fluid. A low-salt diet is recommended and diuretics should be administered judiciously. Serial therapeutic thoracenteses are not indicated because the pleural fluid rapidly reaccumulates and the thoracenteses deplete the patient of body protein

If the pleural effusion persists despite optimal therapy directed toward the ascites, three therapeutic options, none of which is ideal, are available

- Tube thoracostomy followed by the injection of a sclerosing agent; however, electrolyte depletion can lead to death
- Implantation of a peritoneal-to-venous shunt; however, these shunts frequently do not control the effusion
- Thoracotomy with surgical repair of the diaphragmatic leak; however, thoracotomy is a major surgical procedure

OTHER TRANSUDATIVE PLEURAL EFFUSIONS

Although congestive heart failure and hepatic hydrothorax account for most transudative pleural effusions, the following conditions also cause transudative pleural effusions.

PERITONEAL DIALYSIS

Large pleural effusions occasionally complicate peritoneal dialysis

- Dialysate appears to move directly through the diaphragm
- Incidence is 10% in those on continuous ambulatory peritoneal dialysis

- The effusion is almost always on the right side
- The pleural fluid has biochemical characteristics between those of the dialysate and of the serum
- Treat with chemical pleurodesis combined with a short period of small-volume, intermittent peritoneal dialysis

NEPHROTIC SYNDROME

Pleural effusion occurs in approximately 20% of patients with the nephrotic syndrome

- Effusions are usually bilateral transudates because of the low oncotic pressure in the serum
- Pulmonary embolus must be ruled out in this situation because emboli are common in patients with the nephrotic syndrome
- Primary treatment is aimed at treating the nephrotic syndrome, but chemical pleurodesis occasionally may be performed

SUPERIOR VENA CAVAL SYNDROME

Pleural effusions are not present in most patients with superior vena caval obstruction

- Pleural effusions do occur in neonates with superior vena caval thrombosis, however

FONTAN PROCEDURE

This procedure is used to treat infants and children with hypoplastic right ventricles

- The right ventricle is bypassed with an anastomosis between the superior vena cava, the right atrium, or the inferior vena cava and the pulmonary artery
- Almost all patients develop postoperative bilateral pleural effusions, which are frequently large and clinically significant
- With refractory effusions, consider chemical pleurodesis or a pleuro-peritoneal shunt

URINOTHORAX

Pleural fluid can accumulate in the presence of retroperitoneal urinary leakage secondary to urinary obstruction, trauma, or retroperitoneal inflammatory or malignant processes

- Effusion develops within hours of the precipitating event
- Pleural fluid looks and smells like urine
- Diagnosis is confirmed by demonstrating a higher creatinine level in the pleural fluid than in the serum
- Effusion resolves once urinary tract obstruction is relieved

MYXEDEMA

Pleural effusions occasionally occur as a complication of myxedema

- Incidence is probably <5%
- Pleural fluid may have biochemical characteristics of either a transudate or an exudate

MISCELLANEOUS CAUSES OF TRANSUDATIVE PLEURAL EFFUSIONS

- About 20% of the pleural effusions secondary to pulmonary embolism are transudative
- Although pleural effusions secondary to Meigs' syndrome and sarcoidosis have been described as transudative, this is probably not the case

EXUDATIVE PLEURAL EFFUSIONS

Once a patient is known to have an exudative pleural effusion, one should attempt to determine which of the diseases listed in Table 26-1 is responsible. Pneumonia, malignant disorders, and pulmonary embolization account for most exudative pleural effusions. The following tests should be performed on the pleural fluid from a patient with an exudative pleural effusion of unknown origin: glucose level, amylase level, LDH level, differential cell count, microbiologic studies, and cytology. In selected patients, other tests on the pleural fluid, such as the pH, antinuclear antibody level, adenosine deaminase level, rheumatoid factor level, and lipid analysis, may be of value.

TESTS ON PLEURAL FLUID

APPEARANCE

The gross appearance of the pleural fluid should always be described and its odor noted

- Bloody fluid: Obtain hematocrit. If hematocrit is more than 50% that of peripheral blood, hemothorax is present and tube thoracostomy should be considered
- Cloudy fluid: Centrifuge fluid. If supernatant is clear, the initial cloudiness was caused by cells or debris. If supernatant is cloudy, the initial cloudiness was caused by high lipid levels and the patient has chylothorax or pseudochylothorax
- Putrid odor indicates bacterial infection (probably anaerobic) of the pleural space
- Urine-like odor strongly suggests urinothorax

GLUCOSE

Measurements of the pleural fluid glucose level are indicated, because a reduced level (<60 mg/dl) narrows the diagnostic possibilities to the following 7 conditions

- Parapneumonic effusion
- Malignant effusion
- Tuberculous effusion
- Rheumatoid effusion
- Hemothorax
- Churg-Strauss syndrome
- Paragonimiasis

AMYLASE

Measurement of the pleural fluid amylase level is indicated, because an elevated level (above the upper normal limit of serum) indicates that the patient has one of the following three diseases

- Esophageal perforation. Important to establish diagnosis early because mortality is high if not properly treated
- Pancreatic disease. Patients with chronic pancreatic pleural effusions often appear to have cancer
- Pleural malignancy. Salivary type amylase in this situation

LDH

The pleural fluid LDH level is not used in the differential diagnosis of exudative pleural effusion. Nevertheless, a pleural fluid LDH level should be measured every time a diagnostic thoracentesis is performed because it is a good indicator of the degree of inflammation in the pleural space. Increasing levels with serial thoracenteses indicate that the degree of inflammation is worsening and one should pursue the diagnosis more aggressively.

WHITE BLOOD CELL COUNT AND DIFFERENTIAL CELL COUNT

The absolute pleural fluid white blood cell count has limited utility

- Counts >10,000/mm^3 are most common with parapneumonic effusions, but are also seen with pancreatitis, pulmonary embolism, collagen vascular disease, malignant disorders, and tuberculosis
- The differential cell count on the pleural fluid is of more utility than is the absolute cell count
- Presence of predominantly polymorphonuclear leukocytes indicates an acute disease process, such as pneumonia, pulmonary embolization, pancreatitis, intra-abdominal abscess, or early tuberculosis
- Presence of predominantly mononuclear cells indicates a chronic disease process, such as malignant disease, tuberculosis, or a resolving acute process
- Presence of predominantly small lymphocytes indicates that the patient probably has tuberculosis or a malignant disease
- Presence of >10% eosinophils usually indicates that the patient has had either blood or air in the pleural space. If neither air nor blood is present

in the pleural space, several unusual diagnoses should be considered: benign asbestos pleural effusions, pleural effusions caused by drug reactions, paragonimiasis, or the Churg-Strauss syndrome. Diagnosis is never determined for approximately 20% of exudative pleural effusions, and interestingly, pleural fluid eosinophilia is found in approximately 40% of these effusions

- The presence of >5% mesothelial cells in the pleural fluid basically rules out a diagnosis of pleural tuberculosis

CYTOLOGY

Pleural fluid cytology is quite useful in establishing the diagnosis of malignant pleural effusion

- Cytologic results are positive in 40 to 90% of malignant pleural effusions and depend on the type of tumor (difficult with lymphomas), the amount of fluid submitted (more fluid, higher yield), and the skill of the cytologist
- Immunohistochemical tests using monoclonal antibodies are complementary to cytology
- Flow cytometry can demonstrate abnormal numbers of chromosomes in approximately two thirds of patients with malignant pleural effusions. The number of chromosomes is normal in benign cells
- Diagnosis of malignancy can be facilitated via electron microscopy

CULTURE AND BACTERIOLOGIC STAINS

The following pleural fluid cultures should be obtained on patients with undiagnosed exudative pleural effusions

- Aerobic and anaerobic bacterial cultures plus a Gram's stain
- Mycobacterial cultures
- Fungal cultures and fungi

pH

The pleural fluid pH is most useful in determining whether chest tubes should be inserted in patients with parapneumonic effusions

- If the pleural fluid pH is <7.00, tube thoracostomy should be instituted
- If the pleural fluid pH is >7.20, the patient probably does not require tube thoracostomy

The reduction of pleural fluid pH to <7.20 can occur with nine other conditions

- Systemic acidosis (pleural fluid pH approximates blood pH normally)
- Esophageal rupture caused by concurrent infection
- Rheumatoid pleuritis
- Tuberculous pleuritis

- Malignant pleural disease (if tumor burden is large)
- Hemothorax
- Paragonimiasis
- The Churg-Strauss syndrome (the patient also has asthma)
- Urinothorax (protein and LDH levels may be low)

When the pleural fluid pH is used as a diagnostic test, the pleural fluid must be measured with the same care as arterial pH

- The fluid should be collected anaerobically in a heparinized syringe
- The fluid should be placed in ice between collection and analysis
- The analysis should be performed with a blood gas machine

IMMUNOLOGIC STUDIES

Patients with systemic lupus erythematosus (SLE) or rheumatoid arthritis may have a pleural effusion during the course of their disease

- The best screening test for lupus pleuritis is the pleural fluid antinuclear antibody (ANA) titer. With lupus pleuritis, the pleural fluid ANA titer is greater than or equal to 1:160 or greater than or equal to the serum titer. The test is both sensitive and specific
- Only patients with rheumatoid pleuritis have a pleural fluid rheumatoid factor titer greater than or equal to 1:320 or greater than or equal to the serum titer

OTHER DIAGNOSTIC TESTS

Several other tests are useful at times in the differential diagnosis of pleural effusions

- Pleural fluid adenosine deaminase (ADA) levels. Levels >70 U/L are virtually diagnostic of tuberculous pleuritis, whereas levels <40 U/L virtually rule out this diagnosis
- Pleural fluid lipid analysis: A pleural fluid triglyceride level >110 mg/dl is diagnostic of chylothorax. With pseudochylothorax, the pleural fluid cholesterol level is elevated.
- Perform lipoprotein analysis of the pleural fluid in confusing cases. The demonstration of chylomicrons in the pleural fluid establishes the diagnosis of chylothorax
- Measurements that have not been unequivocally demonstrated to be of value in the differential diagnosis of pleural effusions are carcinoembryonic antigen, hyaluronic acid, lysozyme, alkaline, and acid phosphatase.

INVASIVE TESTS FOR UNDIAGNOSED EXUDATIVE PLEURAL EFFUSIONS

In most patients, the cause of the pleural effusion is apparent after the initial clinical assessment and a diagnostic thoracentesis. If the diagnosis is not apparent, the following invasive tests might be considered: needle biopsy of the pleura, pleuroscopy, bronchoscopy, and open biopsy of the pleura. Because pulmonary embolism is one of the leading causes of pleural effusion, this diagnosis should be considered in all patients with an undiagnosed pleural effusion

- Perfusion lung scan is the best screening test
- Pulmonary angiography is often necessary (see Chapter 30)

A diagnosis is never established for approximately 20% of the exudative pleural effusions that resolve spontaneously leaving no residua. Three factors should influence the vigor with which one pursues the diagnosis in patients with undiagnosed exudative effusions

- The symptoms and clinical course of the patient: If the symptoms are minimal or improving, a less aggressive approach is indicated
- The trend of the pleural fluid LDH level: If the pleural fluid LDH tends to increase with serial thoracenteses, a more aggressive approach is indicated because the process is getting worse
- The attitude of the patient: If the patient is desperate to know why a pleural effusion has developed, an aggressive approach should be taken

NEEDLE BIOPSY

With special needles, small specimens of the parietal pleura can be obtained relatively noninvasively

- Useful mainly to establish the diagnosis of malignant or tuberculous pleural effusion
- The initial biopsy is positive for granulomas in 50 to 80% of patients with pleural tuberculosis. The demonstration of granulomas on the pleural biopsy is virtually diagnostic of tuberculous pleuritis. Culture of a portion of the pleural biopsy specimen for mycobacteria increases the diagnostic yield
- The initial biopsy is positive in about 40% of patients with malignant pleural disease
- Overall, the yield from pleural fluid cytology is higher than that obtained by needle biopsy
- When malignant disease is strongly suspected, pleural biopsy should be performed only if initial cytology is nondiagnostic

PLEUROSCOPY

With this procedure, also called thoracoscopy, a rigid scope or a fiberoptic scope is introduced through the chest wall into the pleural space after a pneumothorax has been induced on the side of the pleural effusion

- Excellent results are obtained when the procedure is done by experienced personnel
- In this country, only a few physicians are well trained in pleuroscopy
- This procedure is nearly as invasive as open pleural biopsy
- Diagnoses of benign disease are rarely made

- The open biopsy procedure is generally preferable unless personnel experienced in pleuroscopy are available

BRONCHOSCOPY

Bronchoscopy is at times useful in the evaluation of patients with an undiagnosed exudative pleural effusion. The procedure is recommended for undiagnosed pleural effusions in following situations

- Parenchymal infiltrate is apparent on chest x-ray or CT scan
- Presence of hemoptysis
- Diagnostic yield should exceed 70% in these 2 situations

OPEN BIOPSY

Thoracotomy with direct biopsy of the pleura is the most invasive procedure used to diagnose pleural effusion

- Open biopsy provides the best visualization of the pleura and the best biopsy specimens
- The procedure does not provide a definitive diagnosis in a substantial percentage of patients
- Open biopsy should be done in conjunction with pleural abrasion to prevent recurrence

MALIGNANT PLEURAL EFFUSIONS

The annual incidence of malignant pleural effusions is approximately 200,000 in this country. The 3 tumors that cause approximately 75% of all malignant pleural effusions are lung carcinoma (30%), breast carcinoma (25%), and tumors of the lymphoma group (20%).

PATHOGENESIS

The initial step in the development of pleural metastases is the embolization of the tumor to the lung and/or visceral pleura

- Parietal pleura is involved via secondary seeding from the visceral pleura or the pleural fluid

Direct mechanisms

- Pleural metastases can increase the permeability of the pleural surfaces so more fluid is formed
- Lymphatic involvement can lead to decreased pleural fluid clearance
- The thoracic duct can be interrupted, thereby leading to a chylothorax
- Bronchial obstruction can lead to markedly decreased pleural pressure and a pleural effusion
- Pericardial involvement with a malignant tumor is frequently associated with the accumulation of pleural fluid

Indirect mechanisms

- Hypoproteinemia can decrease the serum oncotic pressure and lead to pleural effusion
- Patients with a malignant disorder have a higher incidence of pulmonary embolism, which may cause a pleural effusion
- The postobstructive pneumonia secondary to bronchogenic carcinoma may cause a parapneumonic effusion
- The therapy for the tumor (radiation or chemotherapy) may itself cause the effusion

CLINICAL MANIFESTATIONS

The most common symptom reported by patients with malignant pleural effusions is dyspnea, which occurs in about 50% of patients

- Only about 25% of patients with malignant pleural effusions have chest pain. The pain is usually dull and aching rather than pleuritic in nature
- Symptoms attributable to the tumor itself are frequent, e.g., weight loss in 32%, malaise in 21%, and anorexia in 14%
- The pleural fluid is an exudate
- The ratio of pleural fluid to serum protein level is <0.5 in about 20% of patients with pleural malignancy, but the LDH ratio >0.60, or the absolute pleural fluid LDH meets exudative criteria in this 20%
- The fluid may be serous or bloody
- The predominant cells can be lymphocytes, other mononuclear cells, or polymorphonuclear leukocytes
- Pleural fluid eosinophilia is uncommon
- The pleural fluid glucose level is reduced to <60 mg/dl in 15 to 20% of malignant pleural effusions, thereby indicating that the patient has a high tumor burden. Mean survival is less than 2 months. (The pleural fluid pH is also reduced in most patients with a low glucose malignant pleural effusion)

DIAGNOSIS

The diagnosis of a malignant pleural effusion is established by demonstrating malignant cells in the pleural fluid or in the pleura itself

- Diagnosis is most commonly established with pleural fluid cytology, which is positive in approximately 60% of patients
- Needle biopsy of pleura is positive in 40% of patients
- Immunohistochemical tests using monoclonal antibodies directed against various antigens are useful in differentiating malignant from benign pleural effusions and adenocarcinomas from mesotheliomas
- Chromosomal abnormalities demonstrated by flow cytometry are highly suggestive of malignant disease
- Pleuroscopy effectively establishes the diagnosis, as does open biopsy

TREATMENT

The initial step is to identify the location of the primary tumor

- The clinician must determine whether the tumor is of a type that is responsive to chemotherapy. Small-cell lung carcinoma, lymphomas, leukemias, and rarely germ-cell tumors may have an associated pleural effusion and respond to chemotherapy
- Obliteration of the pleural space via a pleurodesis or removal of fluid via a pleuroperitoneal shunt should be considered if the patient is symptomatic (dyspnea at rest or during exercise) from the presence of the pleural fluid and the dyspnea is relieved with a therapeutic thoracentesis
- Pleurodesis should not be attempted if the mediastinum is shifted toward the side of the effusion
- Tetracycline, the most commonly used sclerosing agent for the past decade, is no longer available. The following five agents are reasonable alternatives—minocycline 300 mg intrapleurally; doxycycline 500 mg intrapleurally; bleomycin 60 IU intrapleurally (cost exceeds $700); Mitoxantrone hydrochloride (Novantrone) 30 mg intrapleurally (cost exceeds $600); and talc (an excellent sclerosing agent but must be used in conjunction with pleuroscopy or open biopsy)
- The goal of a chemical pleurodesis is obliteration of the pleural space so that room is not available for the pleural fluid to reaccumulate
- Intense inflammatory response results in fusion of the visceral and parietal pleurae and obliteration of the intervening space
- A chest tube should be inserted
- Systemic sedation and local anesthesia (4 mg/kg lidocaine) should be given because the procedure at times is painful
- The sclerosing agent should be injected only if the underlying lung has expanded
- After injection, the patient is repositioned frequently and the chest tube is clamped for 1 to 2 hours
- Suction is maintained for at least 48 hours and until the pleural drainage is <150 ml/day

Pleurodesis effectively controls the pleural effusions in 80 to 90% of properly selected patients. Most failures occur because of poor patient selection; either the mediastinum is shifted toward the side of the pleural effusion or the lung does not expand after the chest tube is inserted.

An alternative to pleurodesis is a pleuroperitoneal shunt

- This device consists of two catheters connected with a valved pump chamber. The two one-way valves in the pump chamber are positioned so that fluid can flow only from the pleural space to the pump chamber to the peritoneal cavity. The pumping chamber must be used to move fluid from the pleural cavity to the peritoneal cavity because the pleural pressure is lower than the peritoneal pressure
- Advantages of the shunt are that total hospitalization time is less than that required for chemical pleurodesis; the amount of pain is less than that caused by tetracycline pleurodesis; the procedure can be done on

an outpatient basis; and the procedure can be effective even if the underlying lung does not completely reexpand
- The disadvantages of the shunt are that the shunt becomes obstructed in some patients; insertion of the pump frequently requires general anesthesia; and the patient must use the pump daily

MALIGNANT MESOTHELIOMA

These highly malignant tumors are thought to arise from the mesothelial cells that line the pleural cavities

- Malignant mesothelioma is much more common in individuals with a history of asbestos exposure. The current incidence is 2,000 cases per year
- The usual presentation is the insidious onset of chest pain or shortness of breath. Pain is usually nonpleuritic and is frequently referred to the upper abdomen or shoulder
- The chest x-ray almost always reveals a pleural effusion, and frequently the effusion is large, occupying 50% or more of the hemithorax. The CT scan is suggestive of the diagnosis
- The fluid is exudative and has lower mean glucose and pH levels than does the fluid from metastatic carcinoma
- The diagnosis of malignant mesothelioma is difficult and usually requires either thoracoscopy or an open pleural biopsy
- Malignant mesothelioma has no effective treatment. Patients are best managed symptomatically; oxygen is administered for dyspnea and opiates are given to help to relieve chest pain

PARAPNEUMONIC EFFUSIONS AND BACTERIAL INFECTIONS OF THE PLEURAL SPACE

A parapneumonic effusion is any pleural effusion associated with bacterial pneumonia, lung abscess, or bronchiectasis. Parapneumonic effusions are probably the most common exudative pleural effusions in the United States. Approximately 40% of the 1.2 million individuals who develop a bacterial pneumonia in the United States each year have a pleural effusion.
The subcategories of parapneumonic effusions are

- Complicated parapneumonic effusions, which require tube thoracostomy for their resolution
- An empyema, which is an exudative effusion on which the Gram's stain of the pleural fluid is positive

PATHOGENESIS

The evolution of a parapneumonic effusion can be divided into three stages that represent a continuous spectrum

- The exudative stage is the first stage and is characterized by the collection of sterile fluid in the pleural space. The pleural fluid in this stage is an

exudate with primarily polymorphonuclear leukocytes, a normal glucose level, and a normal pH level. Appropriate antibiotic therapy effects resolution of both the pneumonic process and the pleural disease
- The fibropurulent stage is the next stage and is characterized by infection with the offending bacteria of the previously sterile pleural fluid. The pH and glucose levels of the pleural fluid become progressively lower while the LDH level of the pleural fluid becomes progressively higher. As this stage progresses, the pleural space becomes loculated as the result of the formation of fibrin membranes
- The organization stage is the final stage and is characterized by fibroblasts growing into the exudate from both the visceral and the parietal pleural surfaces to produce an inelastic membrane called the pleural peel. This peel encases the lung and renders it nearly functionless

BACTERIOLOGY

Prior to the antibiotic era, Streptococcus pneumoniae or hemolytic streptococci were responsible for most empyemas

- At present, anaerobic organisms, aerobic organisms, and mixed infections with aerobes and anaerobes each account for about one third of culture-positive parapneumonic effusions

CLINICAL MANIFESTATIONS

The clinical picture depends on whether organisms are aerobic or anaerobic

- If aerobic, an acute febrile illness with chest pain, sputum production, and leukocytosis ensues
- If anaerobic, a subacute illness with weight loss, anemia, and leukocytosis ensues. Most patients also have a history of an episode of unconsciousness or some other factor that predisposes them to aspiration and anaerobic pneumonia

DIAGNOSIS

The possibility of a parapneumonic effusion should be considered whenever a patient with a bacterial pneumonia is initially evaluated

- Obtain bilateral decubitus chest x-rays if either of the posterior costophrenic angles is blunted on the lateral chest x-ray or if either diaphragm is not visible throughout its length
- Semiquantitate the amount of pleural fluid by measuring the distance between the inside of the chest wall and the outside of the lung. If the thickness of the fluid is <10 mm, the effusion is not clinically significant and a thoracentesis is not indicated. If the thickness of the fluid is >10 mm, a diagnostic thoracentesis should be performed immediately

TREATMENT

One can identify a complicated parapneumonic effusion only by examining the pleural fluid. A diagnostic thoracentesis should be performed as soon as the presence of a significant amount of pleural fluid is demonstrated

- Aliquots of the pleural fluid should be sent for measurement of the pleural fluid glucose, LDH, amylase and protein levels, pH, a differential and total white blood cell count, Gram's stain, and aerobic and anaerobic bacterial cultures
- Usually the fluid also is submitted for mycobacterial and fungal smears and cultures, as well as for cytologic studies

At the time of the initial evaluation, the pleural effusion of some patients with parapneumonic effusions is already loculated

- Ultrasonic examinations of the pleural space are quite effective in distinguishing loculated fluid from pneumonic infiltrates
- Perform thoracentesis with ultrasonic guidance
- Loculated fluid by itself is not an indication for tube thoracostomy

When a patient with pneumonia and pleural effusion is initially evaluated, the decision whether to initiate tube drainage of the pleural space must be made and an appropriate antibiotic must be selected

- Individuals who require tube thoracostomy must be identified immediately. A delay of even 24 hours increases morbidity and mortality
- Indications for chest tube insertion are the presence of gross pus in the pleural space; organisms on the pleural fluid Gram's stain; pleural fluid glucose <60 mg/dl; and pleural fluid pH <7.00

Even when none of these criteria is met, tube thoracostomy should still be considered if the pleural fluid pH is <7.20 or if the pleural fluid LDH is >1,000 IU/L

- In borderline cases, serial thoracenteses at 12- to 24-hour intervals are quite useful in deciding whether to place chest tubes. If the pleural fluid LDH tends to decrease and the pleural fluid pH and glucose levels tend to increase with serial thoracenteses, the patient is improving and tube thoracostomy is not indicated. Alternatively, if the LDH is increasing and the pH and glucose levels are decreasing, tube thoracostomy should be performed without delay

A relatively large chest tube should be utilized (small tubes are likely to become obstructed with fibrin and debris)

- Position tube in the most dependent part of the effusion
- Leave tube in place until the volume of the pleural drainage is <50 ml/ 24 hr and until the draining fluid becomes clear yellow
- If no clinical and radiologic improvement occur within 24 hours, either the pleural drainage is unsatisfactory or the patient is receiving the wrong antibiotic
- Review culture results

- If drainage is inadequate, check position of chest tube and consider facilitating drainage with intrapleural streptokinase or urokinase

Certain factors can help to predict whether closed tube drainage will be sufficient therapy for a complicated parapneumonic effusion. In general, when a patient has a purulent empyema that is loculated, chest tubes alone usually are not sufficient therapy. The following scheme is a useful classification of complicated parapneumonic effusions

- Class I, low pH pleural effusion: Pleural fluid pH is <7.20, but pleural fluid cultures are negative. Tube thoracostomy by itself is usually successful
- Class II, classic empyema: Pleural fluid cultures are positive, but no loculations. Patient may need thrombolytic therapy in addition to chest tubes
- Class III, complicated empyema: Multiple loculations on chest x-ray, initially or subsequently, or trapped lung. Almost all patients require thrombolytic therapy and many require decortication or open drainage procedure

TUBERCULOUS PLEURAL EFFUSIONS

In many parts of the world, the most common cause of an exudative pleural effusion is tuberculosis. Such pleural effusions, however, are relatively rare in the United States with an annual incidence of 1,000 cases.

Tuberculous pleural effusions are thought to result when a subpleural caseous focus in the lung ruptures into the pleural space

- Delayed hypersensitivity is responsible for pleural effusion
- Tuberculous pleuritis can appear as an acute or a chronic illness. The acute presentation is characterized by cough and chest pain; the chronic presentation is characterized by low-grade fever, weakness, and weight loss
- The effusion is almost always unilateral and is usually small to moderate in size, although at times it may be massive. One third of patients have concurrent parenchymal infiltrates
- When untreated, the effusion resolves, but most patients subsequently develop tuberculosis
- Pleural fluid is an exudate with predominantly small lymphocytes
- The diagnosis is established by needle biopsy of the pleura demonstrating granuloma or positive mycobacterial cultures of the pleural fluid or pleural biopsy specimen. Elevated levels of ADA or gamma interferon in the pleural fluid are suggestive of the diagnosis
- Appropriate therapy is the administration of 2 antituberculous drugs for 9 months. All patients with an undiagnosed exudative pleural effusion and a positive purified protein derivative (PPD) should be treated

PLEURAL EFFUSIONS IN PATIENTS WITH AIDS

- Pleural effusions are uncommon in patients with AIDS
- The most common cause is Kaposi's sarcoma (KS). Diagnosis is difficult, and open biopsy usually is required

- Parapneumonic effusions are the second most common cause, followed by tuberculosis, cryptococcosis, and lymphoma
- Effusions are unusual with Pneumocystis carinii infection
- Patients with AIDS and pleural effusion should undergo diagnostic thoracentesis. If no diagnosis, a needle biopsy of pleura is performed if fluid is exudative. If still no diagnosis, one should consider treatment for tuberculosis. If the patient is symptomatic, a pleuroperitoneal shunt should be implanted or chemical pleurodesis should be attempted

PLEURAL EFFUSIONS CAUSED BY PULMONARY EMBOLIZATION

Although pulmonary embolism is one of the most common causes of pleural effusion (Table 26-2), it is frequently not considered in the differential diagnosis of pleural effusion

- Effusion may be either a transudate or an exudate with any cell type. Pleural fluid may or may not be bloody
- Patients have usual symptoms of pulmonary embolization
- Parenchymal infiltrate is also apparent in 50% of patients
- The initial diagnostic study is usually a perfusion lung scan. If the perfusion scan is abnormal, a ventilation lung scan should be obtained. If doubt still exists after these tests, a pulmonary arteriogram should be performed (see Chapter 30)
- The treatment is the same as that for any patient with a pulmonary embolus. If effusion enlarges during treatment, thoracentesis should be repeated to rule out infection or hemothorax

PLEURAL EFFUSIONS CAUSED BY DISEASES OF THE GI TRACT

Several different gastrointestinal diseases may have an associated pleural effusion.

ACUTE PANCREATITIS

Approximately 20% of patients with acute pancreatitis have an exudative pleural effusion

- The effusion probably results from diaphragmatic inflammation
- Occasionally chest symptoms dominate the clinical picture
- The pleural fluid is an exudate with predominantly polymorphonuclear leukocytes and an elevated amylase
- The effusion does not alter the treatment plan for a patient with acute pancreatitis

CHRONIC PANCREATIC PLEURAL EFFUSION

The possibility of a chronic pancreatic pleural effusion should be considered in all patients who seem to have a malignant pleural effusion but in whom the pleural fluid cytologic results are negative

- Results from a sinus tract leading from the pancreas through the aortic or esophageal hiatus into the mediastinum
- Clinical picture is dominated by chest symptoms such as dyspnea, cough and chest pain
- Effusion is usually very large and recurs rapidly after a therapeutic thoracentesis
- Markedly elevated pleural fluid amylase level is key to the diagnosis
- Usually therapy requires abdominal exploration with ligation or excision of the sinus tract and drainage or partial resection of the pancreas

ESOPHAGEAL PERFORATION

This diagnosis should be considered in all acutely ill patients with exudative pleural effusions, because if this condition is not treated rapidly and appropriately, the mortality approaches 100%

- Usually follows instrumentation of esophagus, but may occur spontaneously
- Severe symptoms result from intense infection of the mediastinum
- Pleural fluid amylase level is a good screening test. The amylase level is markedly elevated because saliva, with its high amylase content, enters the mediastinum through a hole in the esophagus. The diagnosis is confirmed with contrast studies of the esophagus
- The treatment of choice for esophageal perforation is exploration of the mediastinum with primary repair of the esophageal tear and drainage of the pleural space and mediastinum

INTRA-ABDOMINAL ABSCESS

Approximately 80% of subphrenic abscesses, 40% of pancreatic abscesses, 30% of splenic abscesses, and 20% of intrahepatic abscesses have an accompanying pleural effusion

- Effusion results from diaphragmatic irritation
- The possibility of an abscess should be considered strongly in any patient with an undiagnosed exudative pleural effusion containing predominantly polymorphonuclear leukocytes when pulmonary parenchymal infiltrates are absent
- The diagnosis of intra-abdominal abscess is best established with abdominal CT scanning
- Treatment consists of drainage of the abscess

PLEURAL DISEASE CAUSED BY COLLAGEN VASCULAR DISEASES

RHEUMATOID PLEURITIS

Approximately 5% of patients with rheumatoid arthritis develop a pleural effusion in the course of their disease

- The pleural effusion usually develops only after the arthritis has been present for several years

- Most patients are male, older than 35 years, and have subcutaneous nodules
- The pleural fluid is characterized by a glucose level <30 mg/dl, a LDH level >700 IU/L, a pH <7.20, and a rheumatoid factor titer > 1:320
- No treatment has proved effective for rheumatoid pleuritis

LUPUS PLEURITIS

The incidence of pleural effusion with either systemic or drug-induced lupus erythematosus is about 40%

- Arthritis or arthralgias are usually present before effusion develops
- Almost all patients with lupus pleuritis have pleuritic chest pain and most are also febrile
- Many different drugs have been incriminated for producing drug-induced lupus erythematosus. Hydralazine, procainamide, isoniazid, phenytoin, and chlorpromazine are most commonly indicted. The presenting signs, symptoms, and radiographic abnormalities are similar to those of spontaneous lupus
- The pleural fluid is an exudate that may have predominantly polymorphonuclear leukocytes or lymphocytes. The pleural fluid glucose level is usually >60 mg/dl, the LDH level is <500 IU/L, and the pH is >7.20
- Measurement of the level of antinuclear antibody (ANA) in the pleural fluid is the best test for lupus pleuritis. With lupus, the ANA titer is ≥1:160 or the pleural fluid to serum ANA ratio is ≥1
- Oral corticosteroids are effective therapy for lupus pleuritis

PLEURAL EFFUSIONS CAUSED BY DRUG REACTIONS

Administration of the following drugs has been associated with the development of a pleural effusion

- Nitrofurantoin, the urinary antiseptic
- Dantrolene, the muscle relaxant
- Methysergide, the antimigraine drug
- Bromocriptine, the antiParkinson's drug
- Procarbazine, the antineoplastic drug
- Amiodarone, the antiarrhythmic drug

Individuals with drug-induced pleural effusions may appear with acute, subacute, or chronic illnesses

- Concomitant pulmonary infiltrates are sometimes present
- Characteristics of fluid are poorly described, but it is frequently eosinophilic

BIBLIOGRAPHY

Albertine KH, Wiener-Kronish JP, Staub NC: The structure of the parietal pleura and its relationship to pleural liquid dynamics in sheep. Anat Rec, *208*:401, 1984.
Broaddus VC, Wiener-Kronish JP, Berthiaume Y, Staub NC: Removal of pleural liquid and protein by lymphatics in awake sheep. J Appl Physiol, *64*:384, 1988.

Light RW: Pleural Diseases. Philadelphia, Lea & Febiger, 1991.

Little AG, Kadowaki MH, Ferguson MK, et al: Pleuro-peritoneal shunting. Alternative therapy for pleural effusions. Ann Surg, *208*:443, 1988.

Shinto RA, Light RW: The effects of diuresis upon the characteristics of pleural fluid in patients with congestive heart failure. Am J Med, *88*:230, 1990.

Van Way C III, Narrod J, Hopeman A: The role of early limited thoracotomy in the treatment of empyema. J Thorac Cardiovasc Surg, *96*:433, 1988.

27

ACID-BASE DISORDERS

Paul L. Marino
David Nierman

The interpretation and management of acid-base disorders is an essential skill in patient care, but physician performance in acid-base disturbances has been far from skilled. In one study of physician attitudes about computerized acid-base interpretations, 70% of the physicians surveyed claimed they were competent in acid-base interpretations and did not need computer assistance.[1] However, this same group of physicians correctly identified only 39% of the acid-base disorders from a sample of arterial blood gas measurements. Another report from a university-affiliated hospital shows a diagnostic accuracy of only 17% for physician interpretation of combined acid-base disorders.[2] Finally, an audit of physician performance in life-threatening situations at a university-affiliated hospital revealed that 33% of the therapeutic decisions made by physicians in response to life-threatening blood gas abnormalities were inappropriate or untimely.[3] These reports show a disturbing lack of knowledge in acid-base balance, and they are mentioned here to emphasize the need for clinicians to maintain a working knowledge of the information in this chapter.

RULE-BASED ACID-BASE INTERPRETATIONS

Acid-base regulation is a well-defined process that allows for a highly organized approach to identifying acid-base disorders. A "rule-based" method is used in the acid-base interpretations in this chapter. This method creates predictions based on the observed behavior of acid-base regulation, and these predictions are used as statements or instructions (rules) that will identify acid-base abnormalities. Rules create rigid guidelines that reduce uncertainty and simplify the problem-solving process; these attributes can improve the accuracy of acid-base interpretations.

ACID-BASE RELATIONSHIPS

The principal features of acid-base regulation are defined by the chemical relationship between pH, carbon dioxide, and bicarbonate ions in the extracellular fluid. This relationship is expressed below, using the partial

794

TABLE 27–1. EXPECTED COMPENSATORY RESPONSES	
PRIMARY DISORDER	**EXPECTED RESPONSE**
Metabolic Acidosis	Expected PCO_2 = 1.5 × HCO_3^- + 0.8 (+2)
Metabolic Alkalosis	Expected PCO_2 = 0.7 × HCO_3^- + 20 (+1.5)
Respiratory Acidosis	$\Delta pH/\Delta PCO_2$ = $\dfrac{0.008 \text{ (Acute)}}{0.003 \text{ (Chronic)}}$
Respiratory Alkalosis	$\Delta pH/\Delta PCO_2$ = $\dfrac{0.008 \text{ (Acute)}}{0.017 \text{ (Chronic)}}$

pressure of carbon dioxide (PCO_2) and the concentration of bicarbonate ions [HCO_3] and hydrogen ions [H^+] in circulating blood.

$$(\text{mEq/l}) \quad [H^+] = 24 \times (PCO_2/[HCO_3])$$

This relationship defines the PCO_2/HCO_3 ratio as the principal factor in determining the acid-base properties of extracellular fluid. As such, the PCO_2/HCO_3 ratio can be used to describe the different types of acid-base disorders (see Table 27–1). The "primary" acid-base disorders are defined by the component of the PCO_2/HCO_3 ratio that is initially altered or is altered by the greatest magnitude; i.e., the "respiratory" acid-base disorders indicate a primary change in PCO_2, and the "metabolic" acid-base disorders identify HCO_3 as the primary abnormality. "Secondary" or compensatory adjustments are identified as a decrease in the magnitude of change in PCO_2/HCO_3 produced by the primary acid-base disorder.

COMPENSATORY CHANGES

The goal of acid-base regulation is to reduce or eliminate the change in pH (i.e., change in PCO_2/HCO_3 ratio) produced by an acid-base disturbance. This is accomplished by compensatory adjustments to primary acid-base changes, and these adjustments are aimed at reducing the change in the PCO_2/HCO_3 ratio produced by the primary disturbance. For example, an increase in PCO_2 (primary respiratory acidosis) must be accompanied by an increase in HCO_3 (compensatory metabolic alkalosis) to limit the change in the PCO_2/HCO_3 ratio caused by the change in PCO_2. In other words, compensatory responses to primary respiratory acid-base disorders will involve changes in serum bicarbonate levels in the same direction as the PCO_2 changes. These adjustments in serum bicarbonate are produced in the kidneys and represent changes in urinary bicarbonate excretion. These renal adjustments require 3 to 5 days for completion, thus creating a period of "partial compensation." Table 27–1 shows the changes in pH associated with partial and full compensation. Note that the compensatory changes are not enough to maintain constant pH; i.e., compensation differs from correction.

Compensation for primary metabolic acid-base disorders involves a change in ventilation that changes the arterial PCO_2 in the same direction as the original change in serum bicarbonate level. These responses are mediated by chemoreceptors that respond to changes in pH and modulate the activity of the respiratory centers in the lower brainstem. Metabolic acidosis produces an increase in ventilation and a decrease in PCO_2, while metabolic alkalosis depresses ventilation and raises the PCO_2. Table 27–1 shows the expected changes in PCO_2 in each type of metabolic acid-base disorder. Note that there is no period of partial compensation; i.e., the respiratory response is fully developed at onset.

RULES FOR ACID-BASE DISORDERS

The equations in Table 27–1 define the changes expected in the different types of acid-base disorders. These relationships have been used to generate the following rules.

Rule 1. A primary metabolic disorder is present if:

A. The pH and PCO_2 change in the same direction, or
B. The pH is abnormal but the PCO_2 is normal.

Rule 2. In primary metabolic disorders, a secondary disturbance is identified by a difference between the PCO_2 expected from respiratory compensation and the PCO_2 measured in arterial blood.

A. For Primary Metabolic Acidosis, Expected PCO_2 = $1.5(HCO_3)$ + $8(\pm 2)$
*B. For Primary Metabolic Alkalosis, Expected PCO_2 = $0.7(HCO_3)$ + $20(\pm 1.5)$

Measured PCO_2 > Expected PCO_2 = Associated Respiratory Acidosis
Measured PCO_2 < Expected PCO_2 = Associated Respiratory Alkalosis

* The respiratory response to metabolic alkalosis can be variable and unpredictable, creating some concern about the validity of the expected PCO_2 in metabolic alkalosis. Several equations are available for predicting the PCO_2 in metabolic alkalosis; this one was selected because it is currently the most popular. The accuracy of this relationship when the HCO_3 exceeds 40 mEq/l is not known.

Rule 3. A primary respiratory disorder is present if the pH and PCO_2 change in opposite directions.

Rule 4. In primary respiratory disorders, the relative changes in pH and PCO_2 will determine the extent of compensation and identify secondary metabolic disturbances, using the following guidelines:

A. For Respiratory Acidosis:

pH/PCO$_2$	Disorder
>0.008	Associated metabolic acidosis
0.008	Acute uncompensated acidosis
0.003–0.008	Partially compensated acidosis
<0.003	Associated metabolic alkalosis

B. For Respiratory Alkalosis:

pH/PCO$_2$	Disorder
>0.008	Associated metabolic alkalosis
0.008	Acute uncompensated alkalosis
0.002–0.008	Partially compensated acidosis
<0.002	Associated metabolic acidosis

Rule 5. A mixed metabolic–respiratory disorder is present if the pH is normal and the PCO$_2$ is abnormal.

ACID-BASE INTERPRETATIONS

The rules in the previous section are now applied to acid-base interpretations, and the flow diagrams for this approach are shown in Figure 27–1 and Figure 27–2. These interpretations are based on the relationships between pH and PCO$_2$, and are organized according to the change in pH. The normal ranges for acid-base parameters in arterial blood are as follows: pH = 7.36 to 7.44; PCO$_2$ = 36 to 44 mmHg; HCO$_3$ = 22 to 26 mEq/l.

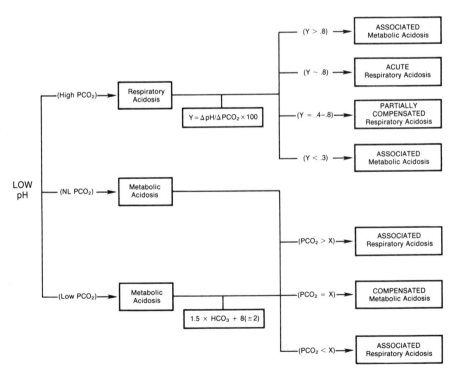

FIG. 27–1. Flow diagram for acid-base interpretation when arterial pH is below normal. (See text for explanation.) From: Marino PL: The ICU Book. Philadelphia, Lea & Febiger, 1991.

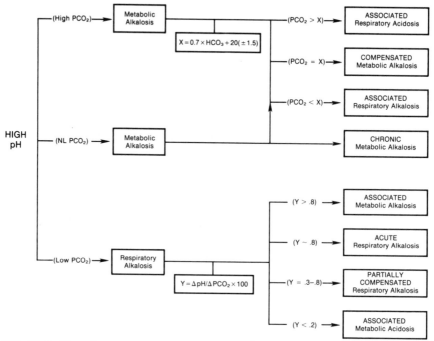

FIG. 27–2. Flow diagram for acid-base interpretation when arterial pH is above normal. (See text for explanation.) From: Marino PL: The ICU Book. Philadelphia, Lea & Febiger, 1991.

If pH is LOW:

A. A low or normal PCO_2 indicates a primary metabolic acidosis (See Rules 1A and 1B).

   1. The equation in Rule A $[PCO_2 = 1.5(HCO_3) + 8(\pm2)]$ is then used to identify an associated respiratory disorder.

B. A high PCO_2 indicates a primary respiratory acidosis (See Rule 3).

   1. The change in the pH/PCO_2 ratio is then used to determine the degree of compensation and to identify an associated metabolic disorder (See Rule 4).

If pH is HIGH:

A. A high or normal PCO_2 indicates a primary metabolic acidosis (See Rules 1A and 1B).

   1. The equation $[PCO_2 = 0.9(HCO_3) + 9]$ in Rule 4B is then used to identify an associated respiratory disorder.

B. A low PCO_2 indicates a primary respiratory alkalosis (See Rule 3).

   1. The pH/PCO_2 ratio is then used to determine the degree of compensation and to identify an associated metabolic disorder (See Rule 4B).

If pH is NORMAL:

A. A high PCO_2 indicates a mixed respiratory acidosis–metabolic alkalosis (See Rule 5).
B. A low PCO_2 indicates a mixed respiratory alkalosis–metabolic acidosis (See Rule 5).
C. A normal PCO_2 may indicate normal acid-base status but does not rule out combined metabolic acidosis–metabolic alkalosis. In this situation, the anion gap can prove to be valuable.

RESPIRATORY ACIDOSIS

Respiratory acidosis, defined as an increased PCO_2, results from alveolar hypoventilation. Physiologically, there will be either decreased total minute ventilation V_E (e.g., narcotic overdose or neuromuscular weakness) or increased physiologic dead space (e.g., increased V_D/V_T ratio as in COPD) (Table 27–2). Distinguishing the underlying physiology becomes important when deciding upon diagnosis and treatment. To differentiate these two physiologic causes, the Arterial-alveolar (A-a) gradient can be calculated on room air ($FIO_2 = 0.21$) using the shortened alveolar gas equation:

$$PAO_2 = 150 - PCO_2/0.8$$

$$\text{A-a gradient} = PAO_2 - PaO_2$$

If the increased PCO_2 is from a decreased minute ventilation, the A-a gradient will be normal. However, if it is from ventilation–perfusion abnormalities, the A-a gradient should be increased.

RESPIRATORY ALKALOSIS

Respiratory alkalosis, defined as a decreased PCO_2, occurs as a result of increased alveolar ventilation from hyperventilation (Table 27–3).

METABOLIC ACIDOSIS

Metabolic acidosis is defined as a primary decrease in plasma bicarbonate[4] and is caused either by the accumulation of fixed exogenous inorganic or endogenous organic acids or loss of HCO_3^- buffer, as in diarrhea. Aci-

---

TABLE 27–2. RESPIRATORY ACIDOSIS

Central nervous system depression:
  Narcotics, sedatives, head trauma, CNS infections, CVAs, cerebral ischemia, obesity-hypoventilation syndrome
Spinal cord and peripheral nerve disease:
  Guillain-Barre syndrome, myasthenia gravis, botulism
Musculoskeletal disorders:
  Kyphoscoliosis, flail chest, bilateral phrenic nerve damage, polymyositis
Pleural disease:
  Massive pleural effusion, pneumothorax
Intrinsic lung disease:
  COPD, advanced ARDS, large pulmonary emboli, severe pneumonia, severe pulmonary edema, stage IV asthma

TABLE 27–3. RESPIRATORY ALKALOSIS

Central nervous system disease or stimulants:
   Anxiety (voluntary hyperventilation), fever, pain, third trimester pregnancy, salicylates, progesterone, sepsis, liver cirrhosis, brain trauma, infection, CVAs, tumors
Thoracic disease:
   Small to moderate pleural effusion, pneumothorax
Intrinsic lung disease:
   Interstitial fibrosis, pneumonia, mild pulmonary edema, stages I + II asthma

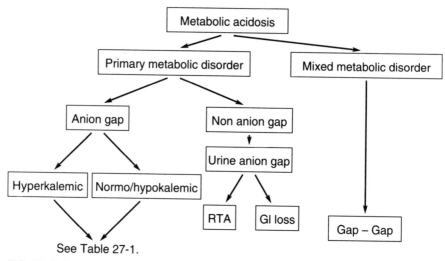

See Table 27-1.

FIG. 27–3. Diagnostic evaluation of metabolic acidosis.

demia refers to a plasma pH that is decreased. Interpretation of a metabolic acidosis follows a straightforward algorithm (Fig. 27–3).

ANION GAP

First, decide whether there is a normal or increased anion gap (Fig. 27–4). The anion gap, calculated by $[Na^+ - (Cl^- + HCO_3^-)]$, is normally 12 ± 4 mEq (mmol)/l and is composed of negatively charged proteins (largely albumin), phosphate, sulfate, and other organic anions. When a fixed acid donates a proton (H^+) to the serum, the bicarbonate should decrease 1 mEq/l for every 1 mEq/l of H^+ added. Therefore, the anion gap should increase by the same amount, and an increase in the anion gap almost always indicates acid accumulation.[4] In contrast, if bicarbonate is lost in the urine or stool, the kidneys will hold on to chloride to compensate, thereby maintaining the total negative equivalency and keeping the calculated anion gap normal.

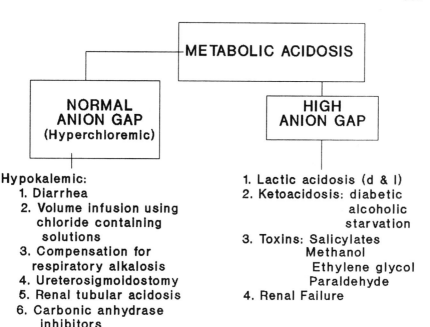

FIG. 27–4. Classification of metabolic acidosis.

Recently, the sensitivity of the anion gap in stratifying metabolic acidoses has been questioned.[5,6] The main problem is which value to choose as the upper limit of normal. Most laboratories currently use ion-selective electrodes to measure Na^+, K^+, and Cl^-. This technology frequently gives higher Cl^- levels and lower Na^+ levels than older photometric or colorimetric assays, yielding a consistently smaller normal anion gap. Using this new technology, the upper limit of normal for the anion gap is often ≤6 mmol/l and practically always ≤11 mmol/l.[6] However, even when using 11 as the upper limit of normal, 29% of surgical ICU patients with elevated lactate levels were not identified.[5] The anion gap was least sensitive for patients with mildly elevated lactate levels between 2.5 and 4.9 mmol/l.

HYPOALBUMINEMIA

The serum albumin contributes about half (11 mEq/l out of a total of 23 mEq/l) of the total unmeasured anion pool. Assuming normal serum electrolytes, a 50% reduction in serum albumin will reduce the calculated anion gap by 5 to 6 mEq/l; this should be added to the calculated number when deciding in which category to place the acidosis.[7,8] Since hypoalbuminemia is very common in ICU patients, this correction should be kept in mind whenever the calculation is made, as this may help recategorize a previously unsuspected elevated anion gap acidosis.

HYPONATREMIA

For unclear reasons, hyponatremia may also decrease the calculated anion gap. Since most causes of hyponatremia occur from net increases in free water, one would expect that the serum chloride would drop as much as the sodium, yielding a normal calculated anion gap. However, the chloride often does not drop equally. It may be that other unmeasurable anion concentrations such as albumin also decrease.

URINARY ANION GAP

The next step in interpretation is to further subcategorize these two broad groups. Normal anion gap acidoses are subdivided into hypokalemic and hyperkalemic groups (Fig. 27–4). In patients with a normal anion gap and hypokalemic hyperchloremic acidosis, the urinary anion gap can help differentiate a renal tubular acidosis from gastrointestinal bicarbonate loss (Fig. 27–4). The major unmeasured cation in the urine is ammonium, which is the excretable form of titratable acid. When urine acidification is deranged and the kidneys are unable to excrete acid, the urine anion gap becomes more positive. Measuring the urinary anion gap requires a spot urine for Na^+, K^+, Cl^-, and pH.[7]

$$\text{Urinary Anion Gap:} \quad \text{Total Anions} = \text{Total Cations}$$

$$UA + Cl^- = Na^+ + K^+ + UC$$

$$\text{Anion gap:} \quad UA - UC = (Na^+ + K^+) - Cl^-$$

Urine anion gap	Urine pH	Diagnosis
Negative	<5.5	Normal
Positive	>5.5	RTA
Negative	>5.5	Diarrhea

RATIO OF ANION GAP EXCESS TO DECREASE IN SERUM BICARBONATE

The final step in analysis is to look at the ratio of anion gap excess to the decrease in serum bicarbonate,[7] referred to as the "gap–gap" ratio (Fig. 27–5).

"Gap–gap ratio": AG Excess/HCO_3 Deficit = $[AG - 12/24 - HCO_3]$. This ratio has the following three uses

- To determine whether there is a mixed metabolic acidosis, which is a common occurrence in the ICU. When an organic acid such as lactic acid is added to blood, there will be an equal drop in HCO_3 for every mEq acid added to the anion gap, and the gap–gap ratio will remain 1. When

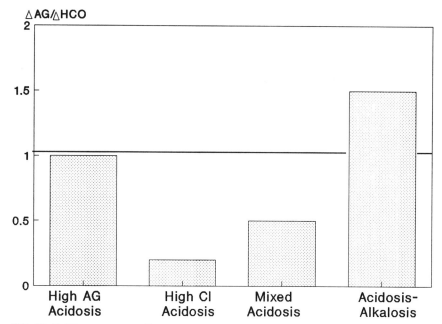

FIG. 27–5. The gap–gap ratio.

there is a hyperchloremic acidosis from loss of HCO_3, the numerator remains low as the denominator increases and the ratio will approach zero. When there is a mixed metabolic acidosis, the ratio will fall between 0 and 1

- To follow responses to treatment in diabetic ketoacidosis. Prior to treatment, when serum ketones are elevated and serum bicarbonate is low, the gap–gap ratio will be high. Once treatment has begun with fluids and insulin, the ketone level drops, but the serum HCO_3 may remain low because of the dilutional effect of intravenous fluids. Although this low HCO_3 may be incorrectly interpreted as an inadequate response to treatment, the drop in gap–gap ratio actually indicates that the ketones are being cleared and that the acidosis is changing from a high gap acidosis to a low one
- To evaluate the presence of a mixed metabolic acidosis and alkalosis. In the presence of a high anion gap acidosis, adding alkali will make the gap–gap ratio greater than 1

LACTIC ACIDOSIS

Lactic acidosis is a common cause of acute metabolic acidosis in critically ill patients and usually results from inadequate tissue oxygenation.

Lactate is produced within all cells in the body by the conversion of pyruvate to lactate, a reaction catalyzed by the enzyme lactate dehydrogenase (LDH). Cellular levels of lactate are mainly determined by mitochondrial function; therefore, states of impaired mitochondrial function (such as cellular hypoxia) will cause cellular levels of lactate to increase, which will then be added to the circulation. Hyperlactatemia is not synonymous with lactic acidosis. In situations such as beriberi or Reye's syndrome, lactate accumulation without an acidosis can occur (formerly referred to as Type B1 Lactic Acidosis).[9] Although all cells except red blood cells are capable of extracting lactate from the circulation, most is removed by the liver and kidneys and converted back to pyruvate via LDH for either gluconeogenesis or energy production. A normal liver is capable of increasing lactate clearance to 10 times the baseline.[10]

Normal serum lactate levels are 2 mEq/l or less (normal arterial blood is less than 1.5 mmol/l, and normal venous blood is less than 2.0 mM/l). Increased production by the tissues and/or decreased clearance of lactate by the liver will result in increased serum levels.

Cardiogenic shock and septic shock are common states in which the oxygen supply may be inadequate to meet the needs of the tissues. Although there may not be frank hypotension (a common criterion used to indicate systemic shock), elevated lactate levels with acidosis in these settings still imply shock at a cellular level. In any case of clinical shock, an elevated lactate level carries a poor prognosis.[9]

When discussing inadequate oxygen supply–demand ratios, it is worthwhile to review the determinants of oxygen delivery:

$$DO_2 = (Cardiac\ output) \times [(Hb)(saturation)(1.34) + (pO_2)(0.003)].$$

Lack of adequate cardiac output resulting in a peripheral low flow state is the most important contributor to the development of lactic acidosis. Although hypoxemia (a low PO_2) is commonly listed as a cause of lactic acidosis, patients with respiratory insufficiency have been shown to tolerate an arterial PO_2 as low as 22 mmHg without developing an acidosis. Although anemia is also listed as a cause of lactic acidosis, there are many patients (for example, Jehovah's Witnesses) who are able to tolerate hemoglobins as low as 3.0 g/dl without this happening, as long as the cardiac output can increase to compensate. If the cardiac output in an anemic patient cannot appropriately increase to compensate for the drop in delivery, a lactic acidosis may appear.[7]

THIAMINE DEFICIENCY

Another cause of lactic acidosis that is being increasingly recognized in ICU patients is thiamine deficiency. Thiamine causes increased lactates by reducing the mitochondrial oxidation of pyruvate. Pyruvate, instead of being converted to acetyl CoA, is diverted into the production of lactate. In patients with elevated lactate levels out of proportion with the degree of clinical hemodynamic instability, serum thiamine levels should be checked while empiric thiamine is given.[9]

D-LACTIC ACIDOSIS

A diagnostic entity that physicians must be aware of is d-lactic acidosis. Lactate is a stereoisomer and exists in l and d forms. Anaerobic human cells produce the l-isomer, a molecule that is readily metabolized by l-lactate dehydrogenase. Anaerobic bacteria, such as Bacteroides fragilis, Eubacterium, Lactobacillus, and Bifidobacterium, and some enteric aerobes, such as E. coli, produce both l and d isomers. Some patients who have undergone extensive bowel surgery, when exposed to high carbohydrate enteral diets, can develop a syndrome of "d-lactate-associated encephalopathy." In this setting, large amounts of d-lactate are produced by these enteric bacteria, which are then absorbed into the bloodstream and distributed across the extracellular fluid compartment, including the cerebrospinal fluid. Since mammalian cells lack d-lactate dehydrogenase and d-lactate is very slowly metabolized through unclear enzymatic pathways, d-lactate accumulates.

Patients with this syndrome present with slurred speech, confusion, lethargy, ataxia, and changed mental status and are frequently thought to be drunk or intoxicated. Laboratory tests show an increased anion gap acidosis with normal l-lactate levels. When suspected, special d-lactate levels may be measured by the laboratory, either by enzymatic means using an in vitro kit with d-lactate dehydrogenase or by nuclear magnetic resonance spectrophotometry. Treatment is effective and consists of oral nonabsorbable antibiotics and a carbohydrate-restricted diet.

Since human cells are unable to produce d-lactate, an intriguing area of investigation is the possible use of d-lactate levels in blood or urine of patients as a marker for bacterial infection.[11] After experimentally produced Klebsiella peritonitis, rats have been shown to develop detectable blood levels of d-lactate. This remains a future area of research.

LACTIC ALKALOSIS

Severe alkalosis (pH > 7.6) can cause increased lactate production by red blood cells, probably by enhancing certain pH-dependent enzymes in the glycolytic pathway. In normal flow states, the liver is usually able to handle the increased lactate production. However, in low flow states where hepatic clearance is reduced, serum lactate levels may climb, particularly with exogenous alkali therapy.[7]

DIAGNOSIS

Intensivists should have a low threshold for obtaining serum lactate levels. Although the patient with a high anion gap acidosis in circulatory shock will clearly have an elevated lactate level, so might the patient with a relatively normal anion gap and only mildly lowered bicarbonate.[5,9] There are no distinctive clinically significant features that suggest l-lactic acidosis, and levels elevated only slightly to 2.5 mmol/l already have a marked increase in mortality.[9] In any patient suspected of having inadequate tissue oxygen supply, lactate levels are essential for diagnosis and management.

Arterial blood will reflect both production and clearance of lactate, whereas blood drawn from a peripheral vein will only reflect regional production. Excellent correlation has been shown between arterial blood and either superior vena cava or pulmonary artery blood (mixed venous), and these sites can be used. The blood sample should either be placed immediately on ice or drawn into a vacuum tube containing a glycolytic inhibitor such as sodium fluoride to limit further lactate production by the red blood cells.

KETOACIDOSIS

Ketoacidosis is characterized by the metabolism of free fatty acids by the liver with the generation of acetoacetate, Beta-hydroxybutyric acid, and acetone. In order for ketoacidosis to occur, there are two requirements. First, there must be increased delivery of free fatty acids from the peripheral adipose tissue to the liver, a process primarily induced by relative or absolute insulin deficiency. Next, the liver must channel these fatty acids into ketone bodies rather than through the normal pathway of triglyceride synthesis, a process apparently induced by a rise in the ratio of glucagon to insulin in portal blood.

There are three ketoacidoses

- *Diabetic ketoacidosis:* The result of either an absolute or relative insulinopenia. Concentrations of free fatty acids may reach two to four times that of a normal fasting state, which drives ketone production and results in a metabolic acidosis. Treatment of diabetic ketoacidosis consists of two simultaneous goals—the correction of the ketoacidosis by adequate exogenous insulin and the correction of fluid and electrolyte deficits
- *Alcoholic ketoacidosis:* Usually arises in alcoholics who abstain from alcohol 1 or more days prior to presentation[2] and requires three simultaneous factors to occur. First, low caloric intake leads to reduced liver glycogen stores and decreased insulin. Next, dehydration decreases renal clearance of ketone bodies. Finally, oxidation of ethanol impairs hepatic gluconeogenesis and increases the NADH:NAD ratio, which results in the conversion of acetoacetate to beta-hydroxybutyrate. Alcoholic ketoacidosis usually resolves within 24 hours with infusion of saline and glucose and does not require additional insulin
- *Starvation ketoacidosis:* Occurs from the mobilization of fatty acids from peripheral tissues and is usually mild. In prolonged fasting, serum insulin levels, although low, are present and are enough to prevent free fatty acid levels in plasma from continuing to increase

DIAGNOSIS

Diagnosis of a ketoacidosis is made by a positive nitroprusside test. This colorimetric reaction, in which either a nitroprusside tablet or stick turns purple, only measures serum acetoacetate at levels over 3 mEq/l but not beta-hydroxybutyric acid. Acetoacetate and beta-hydroxybutyric acid exist in equilibrium with each other, with their interconversion catalyzed by the enzyme beta-hydroxybutyrate dehydrogenase.

$$Acetoacetate + NADH + H^+ \xrightarrow{BHBDH} \beta\text{-Hydroxybutyrate} + NAD^+$$

Tissue hypoxia can lead to decreased availability of intracellular NADH. This will increase the ratio of $NADH/NAD^+$, which drives the above reaction to the right. Since the nitroprusside reaction does not occur with beta-hydroxybutyrate, it is possible to have a severe ketoacidosis and hypoxia yet a negative or trace positive nitroprusside test.[4]

TREATMENT

Should a metabolic acidosis be treated?

Metabolic acidosis has established detrimental effects, especially on cardiovascular function. In vivo, myocardial dysfunction, a reduced threshold for ventricular fibrillation, direct arterial vasodilation, indirect sympathetic-mediated vasoconstriction, and direct venous vasoconstriction can occur.[12] In addition, metabolic acidosis can cause marked increases in pulmonary vascular resistance resulting in increased right heart afterload. Finally, although mild acidosis causes tachycardia secondary to catecholamine release, as the acidosis worsens, bradycardia occurs. Despite all this, it is not clear if these are clinically applicable. Acidemia causes catecholamine release and the vasodilation may counteract the drop in cardiac output. Additionally, patients with diabetic ketoacidosis can tolerate pH levels as low as 7.0 without cardiovascular compromise.

There are data that suggest that elevated blood lactate can have harmful negative inotropic effects independent of pH.[10] Increased intracellular lactate suppresses the activity of glyceraldehyde 3-phosphate dehydrogenase, thereby inhibiting glycolysis and limiting myofibril ATP production.[10]

Although avoiding the detrimental effects of a severe acidosis may be desirable, there is no clear consensus concerning when or how to treat. Any treatment decision must be made firmly in the context of what is causing the acidosis, whether the accumulation is of inorganic or organic acids and whether it is a primary process as with poisonings or a reflection of other pathology, as in lactic acidosis or ketoacidosis. Appearance of a lactic acidosis in a critically ill patient usually indicates inadequate oxygen delivery to meet the metabolic oxygen demand of the tissues. Therefore, the focus of treatment should not be on exogenous bicarbonate replacement but on aggressively correcting VO_2/DO_2 imbalances.

Is bicarbonate beneficial?

A debate has raged for years over the use of sodium bicarbonate to correct lactic acidosis. Bicarbonate therapy can produce a number of harmful effects, including hyperosmolarity, hypercapnea, and aggravation of intracellular acidosis, hypotension, and ionized hypocalcemia. In hypoxic dogs, bicarbonate therapy has been shown to worsen lactic acidosis.[9] Most importantly, the use of bicarbonate has never been shown to either improve hemodynamics in critically ill patients with lactic acidosis or to improve their outcome.[13]

When lactic acid is buffered by sodium bicarbonate, PCO_2 is generated by the following process:

$$\text{Lactate-} H^+ + NaHCO_3 \rightarrow Na^+\text{lactate-} + H_2O + CO_2.$$

In shock situations where microvasculature circulation is decreased or in other settings where ventilation is fixed (e.g., the patient has been de-

TABLE 27–4. ALKALI SOLUTIONS		
	CARBICARB	**NaHCO₃**
Na⁺	1,000	1,000 (mmol/L)
HCO₃	333	1,000
CO₃²⁻	333	0
PCO₂	3	over 200 (mm Hg)
pH 25 C°	9.6	8.0
Osmolality	1,667	2,000 (mOsm/kg)

From: Sun JH, Filley GF, Hord K: Carbicarb: An effective substitute for NaHCO₃ for the treatment of acidosis. Surgery, *102*:835, 1987.

liberately paralyzed), PCO_2 will accumulate in the tissues, rapidly pass into cells, and cause an intracellular acidosis, with harmful effects. A clear example of this has been shown in cardiac arrest. Closed cardiac massage can, at most, generate 20 to 25% of the normal cardiac output. Arterial blood drawn at this time will reveal a normal to low $PaCO_2$ (depending on the effectiveness of ventilation). Mixed venous blood drawn simultaneously will show a markedly elevated $PaCO_2$, reflecting tissue respiratory acidosis. Giving exogenous bicarbonate, which both contains PCO_2 and is converted to PCO_2 in the tissues, will only add to this venous acidosis and worsen the situation.[10]

Other alkalinizing agents have been developed that do not cause this undesirable CO_2 production

- *Carbicarb:* (Table 27–4) Carbicarb, which consists of ⅓ M Na_2CO_3 and ⅓ M $NaHCO_3$ and has the same alkalinity as bicarbonate, has been found to raise blood pH without raising PCO_2. Clinical experience with carbicarb is limited at present, but the preliminary results are encouraging[14]
- *Dichloroacetate:* Sodium dichloroacetate stimulates pyruvate dehydrogenase and diverts pyruvate away from lactate production toward mitochondrial oxygenation. Although DCA has been shown to decrease serum lactate levels, this has not translated into improved clinical outcome[15]

If bicarbonate is to be used, the standard recommendation is to keep the serum pH above 7.2. To calculate the approximate amount to give, the space of distribution is approximately 0.5% of body weight, but this may be twice as large with severe acidosis. With a normal PCO_2, a goal of a serum bicarbonate of 15 mEq/l should be sufficient.

$$HCO_3 \text{ deficit} = 0.5 \times \text{wt (kg)} \times (\text{desired } HCO_3 - \text{serum } HCO_3)$$

One half of the calculated deficit is given IV bolus and the rest is added to hyponatremic solution and run over 4 to 6 hours. Periodic determinations of acid-base balance are necessary to titrate therapy.

The treatment for lactic acidosis resulting from cellular hypoxia is correction of the cellular hypoxia. There should be aggressive attempts to increase flow to the tissues, using invasive hemodynamic monitoring. The

VO_2, the DO_2, and the extraction ratio are closely followed. A lower than normal extraction ratio in the setting of lactic acidosis implies that the peripheral tissues are unable to remove the required oxygen from the circulation, probably because of an endothelial defect. This is a poor sign. If the extraction ratio is normal or high, with a decreased DO_2, the next step is to increase delivery. First, volume load with colloid or crystalloid and follow the above parameters. If the DO_2 remains low despite volume loading, add inotropic agents. If possible, avoid using PRBCs because of concerns about increasing viscosity and sludging at the microvascular level.

The use of exogenous alkalinizing agents for a lactic acidosis is a temporizing measure and is doomed to failure unless the cause of the acidosis is resolved.

METABOLIC ALKALOSIS

Metabolic alkalosis is the most common acid-base disorder in hospitalized patients.[4] The hallmark of a metabolic alkalosis is a serum bicarbonate that is greater than expected for the patient's PCO_2. While a drop of pH to between 7.0 and 7.2 may be tolerated by many patients without adverse effects, a pH above 7.55 has an associated mortality of 40% in the critically ill.[4] Overall, the most common causes of metabolic alkalosis in the ICU are loss of gastric juice protons and chloride through either NG suction or vomiting and renal retention of bicarbonate secondary to hypovolemia and chloride depletion.

Metabolic alkalosis can be categorized into three broad groups for both diagnosis and treatment strategies. Differentiating these two groups requires a spot urinary chloride (Fig. 27–6)

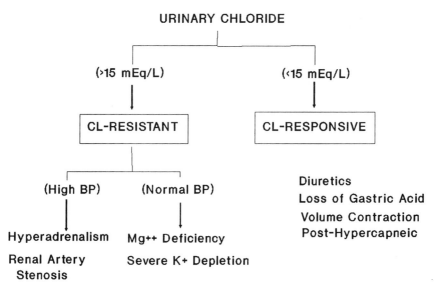

FIG. 27–6. Classification of metabolic alkalosis.

- Chloride-responsive: Urinary chloride < 15 mEq/l. Chloride is the only nonbicarbonate anion that contributes to ECF volume. Therefore, in conditions where chloride is depleted, the kidney holds on to bicarbonate as compensation to maintain the total anion equivalency.
  (a) Gastric acid loss: Will cause depletion of both H^+ and Cl^- ions
  (b) Diuretics: Cause loss of K^+, Mg^{++}, and most importantly, Cl^-. By contributing to an increase in renal acid excretion, diuretics lead to a disproportionate loss of fluid rich in Cl^- and a transcellular shift of hydrogen ions. Some of this can be prevented by either using or adding potassium-sparing diuretics such as triamterene or spironolactone
  (c) Extracellular volume contraction
  (d) Post hypercapneic
- Chloride-resistant: Urinary chloride > 15 mEq/l. The chloride-resistant alkaloses are usually mild and hypervolemic, and treatment is directed toward the underlying disorder. These alkaloses are generated and maintained by the kidneys and result from either a chloride-reabsorptive defect (i.e., Bartter's syndrome) or from a hypermineralocorticoid state (i.e., Hyperaldosteronism, Cushing's syndrome)
- Alkali administration: Exogenous bicarbonate administration rarely causes a metabolic alkalosis, secondary to the kidneys' tremendous ability to excrete excess bicarbonate[8]

COMPLICATIONS

- Hypoventilation: The ventilatory response to a metabolic alkalosis is variable and may be absent. The following equation shows that there must be a relatively severe metabolic alkalosis to cause significant CO_2 retention; e.g., a HCO_3 of 40 only results in a PCO_2 of 49.

$$\text{Expected } PCO_2 = 0.7 \times HCO_3 + 20 \ (\pm 1.5)$$

A more important respiratory consequence of a metabolic alkalosis is shift of the oxyhemoglobin dissociation curve to the left, therefore making less oxygen available to the peripheral tissues[7]
- Neuromuscular: When the pH is greater than 7.55, neuromuscular irritability may occur, ranging from a positive Chvostek or Trousseau sign, to muscle cramping and spasms, to frank tetany (at a pH > 7.55 to 7.6), and finally to lethargy, stupor, and coma. The central nervous system manifestations are more common in patients with low ionized Ca^{2+} levels, prior seizures, or cerebrovascular disease.
- Myocardial irritability: Includes increased digitalis toxicity.
- Decreased ionized Ca^{2+}: Although the total calcium may remain normal, alkalosis causes increased binding of the ionized fraction to plasma proteins. It is not clear whether this is clinically significant. Once a metabolic alkalosis is established, a vicious cycle may ensue. The combination of extracellular fluid contraction, hypokalemia and chloride depletion results in a secondary hyperaldosteronism, which leads to more alkalosis. This self-perpetuating cycle may be the most important aspect of this acid-base disorder, with treatment required to break the cycle[8]

TREATMENT

FLUID THERAPY

Most of the metabolic alkalosis encountered in the intensive care unit, and practically all of the serious alkaloses ($HCO_3 > 40$) belong in the hypovolemic chloride-responsive group. Therefore, initial treatment strategies first involve chloride replacement using either NaCl, KCl, HCl, or combinations of these three

- NaCl: Patients who are volume depleted generally respond well to treatment with 0.9% NaCl. The chloride deficit is calculated by the following equation:

$$Cl\ Deficit\ (mEq) = 0.27 \times Wt\ (kg) \times (100 - Present\ Cl)$$

Since a liter of normal saline contains 154 mEq of Cl^-, the volume of NaCl needed is:

$$Normal\ Saline\ Replacement\ (mEqs) = Cl\ Deficit/154$$

- KCl: Because of the prohibitive amount of K^+ that would be needed, KCl alone is not adequate to provide adequate chloride replacement. If hypokalemia is present, however, it must be corrected, because hypokalemia will sustain the metabolic alkalosis even after the calculated Cl^- deficit has been replaced. Correction of hypokalemia has a crucial important role in the treatment of metabolic alkalosis
- HCl: In severe alkalosis, dilute hydrochloric acid may be necessary. Hydrochloric acid must be administered through a central line to avoid its sclerosing actions, glass bottles must be used, and the IV tubing must be changed frequently. The solution that is used is 0.1 N HCl, which contains 100 mEq H^+/l. To calculate the amount needed, the following equations are used:

$$H^+\ Deficit\ (mEq) = 0.5 \times Wt\ (kg) \times (Present\ HCO_3 - Desired\ HCO_3)$$

$$Volume\ (L)\ pf\ 0.1N\ HCl = H^+\ Deficit/100$$

$$Infusion\ Rate = 0.2\ mEq/kg/hr$$

Arginine HCl, lysine HCl, and NH_4Cl are solutions that were previously used but are no longer commercially available

DRUG THERAPY

Drug therapy has a role when there is a chloride-responsive metabolic alkalosis in normovolemic or hypervolemic patients.[16] Neither Diamox nor H_2 blockers will correct a preexisting alkalosis

- Acetazolamide: Diamox (250 to 1,000 mg/day divided doses), a carbonic anhydrase inhibitor, blocks bicarbonate resorption in the proximal tubule and may be useful when extracellular volume is high. Unfortunately, Diamox may also cause additional K^+ and volume depletion, which as mentioned above, can perpetuate an alkalosis.

- H₂ Blockers: Can be used to prevent H^+ loss with loss of gastric juice and may have a particular role in normovolemic chronic renal failure patients.[16] It is important to first check the gastric secretions to identify the presence of acid. The treatment goal is to keep the pH greater than 5.[7] Because of concerns about gastric superinfection, aspiration, and translocation of bacteria through the gut, the use of H₂ blockers in the ICU should be avoided.

DIALYSIS

A final option for a severe metabolic alkalosis in patients with renal failure is hemodialysis with a high chloride, low acetate bath. If the patient has a high volume status, another alternative is to use CAVH with simultaneous IV chloride replacement.

REFERENCES

1. Hingston DM: A computerized interpretation of arterial pH and the blood gas data: Do physicians need it? Respir Care, *27*:809–815, 1982.
2. Schreck DM, Zacharias D, Grunau CFV: Diagnosis of complex acid-base disorders: Physician performance vs. the microcomputer. Ann Emerg Med, *15*:164–170, 1986.
3. Broughton JO, Kennedy TC: Interpretation of arterial blood gases by computer. Chest, *85*:148–149, 1984.
4. Riley LJ, Ilson BE, Narins RG: Acute metabolic acid-base disorders. Crit Care Clin, *5*:699–746, 1987.
5. Iberti TJ, Leibowitz AB, Papadakos PJ, Fischer EP: Low sensitivity of the anion gap as a screen to detect hyperlactatemia in critically ill patients. Crit Care Med, *18*:275–277, 1990.
6. Winter SD, Pearson JR, Gabow PA, et al.: The fall of the serum anion gap. Arch Intern Med, *150*:311, 1990.
7. Marino PL: The ICU Book. Philadelphia, Lea & Febiger, 1991.
8. Kokko JP, Tannen RL (Eds.): Fluids and electrolytes. Philadelphia, W.B. Saunders Company, 1990, pp. 27–53.
9. Kruse JA, Carlson RW: Lactate metabolism. Crit Care Clin, *5*(4):725–726, 1987.
10. Hindman BJ: Sodium bicarbonate in the treatment of subtypes of acute lactic acidosis: physiologic considerations. Anesthesiology, *72*:1064–76, 1990.
11. Smith SM, Eng RHK, Buccini F: Use of d-lactic acid measurements in the diagnosis of bacterial infections. J Infect Dis, *154*(4):658–64, 1986.
12. McLaughlin ML, Kassirer JP: Rational treatment of acid-base disorders. Drugs, *39*:841–855, 1990.
13. Cooper DJ, Walley KR, Wiggs BR, Russell JA: Bicarbonate does not improve hemodynamics in critically ill patients who have lactic acidosis. Ann Intern Med, *112*:492–498, 1990.
14. Kucera RR, Shapiro JI, Whalen MA, et al.: Brain pH effects of NaHCO₃ and Carbicarb in lactic acidosis. Crit Care Med, *17*:1320–1323, 1989.
15. Stacpoole PW, Lorenz AC, Thomas RG, Harman EM: Dichloroacetate in the treatment of lactic acidosis. Ann Intern Med, *108*:58–63, 1988.
16. Quintanilla A, Singer I: Metabolic alkalosis in the patient with uremia. Am J Kidney Dis, *XVII*(5):591–95, 1991.

28

ACUTE RESPIRATORY FAILURE AND ADULT RESPIRATORY DISTRESS SYNDROME

Amy O'Brien-Ladner
Susan K. Pingleton

ACUTE RESPIRATORY FAILURE

Acute respiratory failure is defined not as a disease but as an abnormality of the normally well balanced homeostasis of the lung gas exchange function. As a result of disturbance in the exchange of oxygen or carbon dioxide between the alveolus and the pulmonary capillaries, respiratory failure occurs. This definition is complicated by the fact that acute respiratory failure can develop despite normal lungs. Thus, the classification of acute respiratory failure is based on the underlying mechanism precipitating the disturbance in gas exchange.

DIAGNOSIS OF ACUTE RESPIRATORY FAILURE

Acute respiratory failure is diagnosed by abnormalities in arterial blood gases. Clinically, it can be obvious in a patient who is apneic secondary to drug overdose or head trauma; however, in other instances during early phases of respiratory failure, a high level of clinical suspicion is necessary in the diagnosis of acute respiratory failure. Measuring arterial gas tensions (P_aO_2, P_aCO_2) and pH is most useful in evaluating the severity of respiratory dysfunction and failure. These measurements provide an indication of the status of integrated cardiorespiratory function and acid base balance. Essentially, two types of abnormalities are found when arterial blood gases are evaluated.

HYPOXIA

Hypoxia is defined as a reduction of arterial oxygen tension (P_aO_2)

- $P_aO_2 < 50$ mm Hg on room air or FiO_2 0.21

The most common mechanisms by which reductions in P_aO_2 are produced include

- Alveolar hypoventilation ($P_aCO_2 > 40$ mm Hg)
- Ventilation–perfusion mismatching
- Right to left intrapulmonary or intracardiac shunting of blood

It is important to determine which of these mechanisms is operative in the hypoxemic patient. Hypoxemia, which is caused primarily by hypoventilation, suggests that the lung is normal and that the only necessary therapeutic goal is to increase ventilation. This type of hypoxemia is characterized by normal alveolar to arterial difference ($P_AO_2 - P_aO_2$), which is determined using the alveolar gas equation. Alveolar oxygen tension (P_AO_2) is calculated by a simple equation

- P_AO_2 = [(barometric pressure – water vapor pressure)(FiO$_2$)] – ($P_aCO_2/0.8$)
- 770 mm Hg = barometric pressure at sea level
- 47 mm Hg = water vapor pressure
- FiO$_2$ = oxygen concentration
- 0.8 = respiratory quotient

- $P_AO_2 - P_aO_2 = (770 - 47)\text{FiO}_2 - \dfrac{P_aCO_2}{0.8} - P_aO_2$

Arterial oxygen tension (P_aO_2) is determined from actual arterial blood gas samples. This value is subtracted from the calculation of P_AO_2 value. For example, on room air with a normal P_aO_2 of 90 Hg and P_aCO_2 of 40 mm Hg, the $P_AO_2 - P_aO_2$ difference can be determined by inserting the values.

$$= (770 - 47)0.21 - \left(90 + \frac{40}{0.8}\right)$$
$$= 10 \text{ (normal)}$$

Another example of acute respiratory failure secondary to hypoventilation is exemplified by a P_aO_2 of 60 mm Hg and a P_aCO_2 of 70 mm Hg. Calculated P_AO_2 is 68 mm Hg; P_aO_2 gradient difference is 8 mm Hg, a normal value. In this instance of acute respiratory failure, the normal A–a gradient suggests that the mechanism of hypoxia is hypoventilation and not abnormal lung structure. Hypoventilation can cause increased alveolar arterial oxygen gradients when severe.

Acute respiratory failure often occurs with an increased A–a gradient. For example, in a patient with pneumonia, a P_aO_2 of 55 mm Hg and a P_aCO_2 of 35 mm Hg would result in an A–a gradient greater than 60 mm Hg, suggesting significant lung dysfunction. Mechanisms of hypoxemia with a widened $P_AO_2 - P_aO_2$ gradient include ventilation–perfusion mismatch and shunting. Shunted blood is blood that traverses the capillary beds and never "sees" alveolar air. When hypoxemia resulting from ventilation–perfusion mismatch occurs, ventilation is inappropriate to the level of alveolar capillary perfusion or vice versa. The distinction between ventilation–perfusion mismatch and shunting can be made by measuring the response of the hypoxic patient to the administration of 100% oxygen. Normal arterial oxygenation will increase to values of nearly 600 mm Hg if the hypoxemia is due purely to ventilation–perfusion mismatching. With shunt, however, arterial oxygen tension is markedly reduced in relation to the magnitude of shunt flow. This is because shunted blood has no capacity to be oxygenated, despite high levels of inspired oxygen tension. Figure 28–1 shows the relationship between P_aO_2 and FiO_2 with different shunt fractions. Figure 28–2 demonstrates the effect of increasing amounts of mismatch of ventilation to perfusion on P_aO_2 with different FiO_2 values.

It is important to determine the mechanism of hypoxemia in acute respiratory failure because the approach to treatment varies considerably depending on which mechanism has caused the hypoxemia. Small amounts of supplemental oxygen can increase the P_aO_2 with ventilation–perfusion mismatching. However, when shunting is the mechanism of hypoxemia, high levels of inspired oxygen and even mechanical ventilation are required.

HYPERCAPNIA

Hypercapnia is defined as elevation of carbon dioxide tension

- $P_aCO_2 > 50$ mm Hg on room air

Hypercapnia is caused by alveolar hypoventilation. It can occur secondary to

- Increase in production of CO_2
- Decrease in ventilation
- Increase in wasted ventilation or dead space

Most commonly, hypercapnia results from decreased ventilation caused by the lung, either from disease (e.g., chronic obstructive pulmonary disease) or suppressed ventilatory drive. The calculation of dead space requires knowledge of the P_aCO_2 tension and the partial pressure of carbon dioxide in mixed expired air. Dead space is commonly expressed as a fraction of tidal volume; normal values for the V_D/V_T ratio are 0.3 to 0.35.

Acute hypercapnic respiratory failure can result in respiratory acidosis, which is characterized by an increase in P_aCO_2. The relationship between P_aCO_2 and plasma bicarbonate concentrations determines the arterial pH. However, the relationship between P_aCO_2 and arterial pH varies while the P_aCO_2 becomes elevated. The acuity or chronicity of carbon dioxide elevation can be inferred by examining the relationship between P_aCO_2, arterial pH, and serum HCO_3^-

- Acute increases in P_aCO_2 are accompanied by small increases in bicarbonate, and arterial pH changes in a nearly linear fashion. For every 1 mm Hg change in P_aCO_2, there is approximately a 0.008 pH unit change in the opposite direction. For example, an acute rise in P_aCO_2 from 40 to 60 mm Hg would be expected to cause a decrease in arterial pH to 7.25

In addition to respiratory acidosis, metabolic acidosis and alkalosis, caused by metabolic or respiratory problems, can be threatening to a patient with severe respiratory dysfunction. A serious case of metabolic acidosis resulting from imbalance between oxygen delivery and oxygen consumption may lead to anaerobic metabolism and lactic acid production. Patients

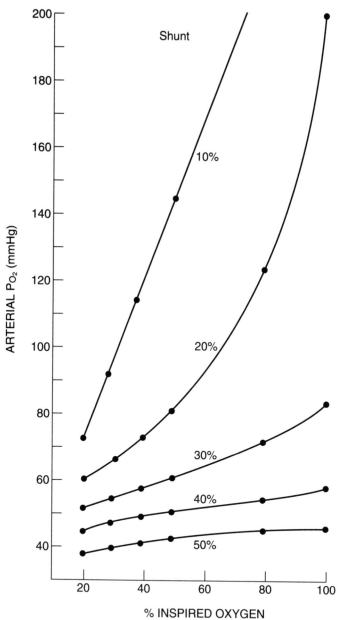

FIG. 28–1. The relationship between inspired oxygen concentration and arterial PO_2 for lungs with varying degrees of shunt. The increase in PO_2 is small for lungs with large shunts. Reproduced with permission from: Dantzker DR: Gas exchange in the adult respiratory distress syndrome. Clin Chest Med, *3*:57, 1982.

VENTILATION/PERFUSION MISMATCH

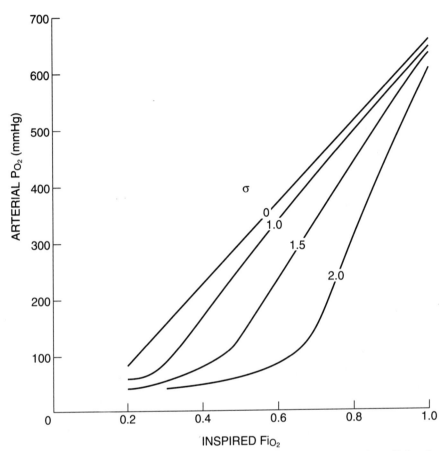

FIG. 28–2. The relationship of P_aO_2 to FiO_2 with increasing amounts of ventilation to perfusion mismatching (0 = standard deviation of log normal distribution of ventilation and perfusion). Note that even with marked mismatching, the P_aO_2 increases to nearly normal values with a very high FiO_2. From: West JR: Pulmonary Pathophysiology: The Essentials. Baltimore, Williams & Wilkins, 1977.

in acute respiratory failure may not be able to lower P_aCO_2 to compensate for decreased pH, and the resulting metabolic acidosis can be quite severe.

Metabolic alkalosis, often secondary to volume contraction, may actually cause increased hypoventilation in efforts to compensate for the elevated serum bicarbonate. Alkalosis predisposes arrhythmia, decreases cardiac output, and reduces the threshold for seizures. Hypocapnia, with or without alkalosis, reduces cerebral blood flow and may depress the level of consciousness.

CLINICAL EVALUATION

In most instances, the symptomatic hallmark of respiratory failure is dyspnea. In dyspnea, the patient must be aware of the sensation and be able to convey that awareness. This sensation is related to the increased work of breathing and not to hypoxia directly. For example, the patient who hypoventilates after narcotic administration may not be dyspneic in the presence of marked gas exchange abnormalities. Dyspnea is more intense when it develops rapidly. In respiratory failure that develops slowly, dyspnea appears first only with exertion, but the process may become more severe and the dyspnea constant, even at rest. As acute respiratory failure progresses, hypoxemia and hypercarbia both blunt the sensation of dyspnea and occasionally result in misleading symptomatic assessment. Unfortunately, although dyspnea is frequent in respiratory failure, it is impossible to quantitate and it correlates very poorly with the severity of respiratory failure.

The clinical signs of hypoxia include confusion, restlessness, impaired coordination, coma, and death. Physiologic parameters suggesting hypoxia include tachycardia, hypertension, and tachypnea. During progressive hypoxemia, physiologic parameters may change to include bradycardia, hypotension, cardiac arrhythmias, vasoconstriction, and cyanosis. Cyanosis requires 5 g/dl of reduced hemoglobin in the circulation. Thus, for the severely anemic patient, cyanosis is usually not apparent in acute respiratory failure. In a nonanemic patient, cyanosis is usually obvious with a P_aO_2 of approximately 40 mm Hg oxygen ($S_aO_2 < 75\%$), but at this stage the patient's life is threatened.

The signs and symptoms of hypercapnia are dependent on the time during which the P_aCO_2 becomes elevated. When the P_aCO_2 rises rapidly, clinical symptoms include primarily central nervous system (CNS) disturbances such as apprehension, confusion, sedation, and coma. Physiologic parameters during acute hypercarbia include vasodilatation causing headache, engorged retinal vessels, encephalopathy, asterixis, and perspiration. Tachycardia and hypertension secondary to increased catecholamine levels may also be present. If carbon dioxide retention progresses over several days to weeks, the kidneys allow for compensation by the retention of bicarbonate. In this instance, even with P_aCO_2 greater than 80, the clinical and physiologic parameters may be nonapparent or very mild and the patient usually maintains a near normal pH.

The general assessment of the severity of the patient's illness from the physical appearance, including the degree of respiratory distress as determined by the respiratory rate, to the mental status, provides important information. The respiratory rate, although influenced by a number of factors, may serve as an indicator of the severity of respiratory distress and can be used to monitor response to therapy. Severely tachypneic patients will be able to speak only a few words at a time. Retraction of the sternum and the supraclavicular, supersternal, and intercostal spaces indicates an increased work of breathing. In obstructive lung disease, these findings correlate with the severity of airway obstruction. In asthma, the decrease in arterial systolic blood pressure that occurs with inspiration (pulsus paradoxus) also correlates with the severity of airway obstruction.

Unfortunately, examination of the lung does not always provide specific information concerning the severity of respiratory dysfunction. The following is notable

- Although wheezing is a characteristic feature of severe airway obstruction, the absence of wheezing may be more important. In severe airway obstruction, airflow may be reduced and inadequate to produce flow rates required for wheezing. Secondly, asymmetry of breath sounds is important in the evaluation of respiratory distress. The absence of sounds on one side may suggest pneumothorax, which is especially important to mechanically ventilated patients because of the greater likelihood of a tension pneumothorax

CATEGORIES OF ACUTE RESPIRATORY FAILURE

The treatment of acute respiratory failure depends on the underlying mechanism causing respiratory failure. Therefore, it is essential to identify the etiology of the process. Appropriate treatment for one type of acute respiratory failure may be entirely inappropriate for another. Thus, acute respiratory failure is grouped into the following etiologic categories

- Acute respiratory failure with normal lung function
- Acute respiratory failure with abnormal lung function
- Acute respiratory failure with hypoxia and normocapnia or hypocapnia

ACUTE RESPIRATORY FAILURE WITH NORMAL LUNG FUNCTION

Hypoventilation

Hypoventilation, a decreased amount of air entering the lungs and reaching the alveoli, is manifest by excess amounts of arterial carbon dioxide, as reflected by an elevated P_aCO_2 tension in arterial blood gases. In normal lungs, the ability to oxygenate blood is not as dependent on alveolar ventilation as on the removal of CO_2. Thus, hypoxia does not manifest itself unless the degree of hypoventilation is extreme. In this type of acute respiratory failure, lung structure and function may be normal. What is abnormal is the function of the respiratory muscles, thoracic cage, or respiratory center, which is responsible for the respiratory drive. The causes of acute respiratory failure in normal lungs would include

- Thoracic cage abnormalities such as flail chest or kyphoscoliosis
- Upper airway obstruction such as laryngeal edema or epiglottitis
- Diseases of the brain stem, cerebral vascular accident, trauma
- Respiratory center depression (narcotics or general anesthesia)
- Neurologic disease (polio, amyotrophic lateral sclerosis)
- Hypoventilation of obesity (Pickwickian Syndrome)
- Diseases of muscles (muscular dystrophy, polymyositis)
- Sleep apnea

- Sudden infant death syndrome
- Botulism
- Heavy metal intoxication
- Organic phosphate poisoning
- Aminoglycoside antibiotics (rarely)
- Severe electrolyte disorders such as hypokalemia and hypophosphatemia

Characteristically, patients who develop acute respiratory failure because of neurologic compromise have a forced vital capacity (FVC) less than 4 to 5 ml/kg body weight, a progressive inability to handle oral secretions, and a cough. An FVC of less than 1 liter in this situation indicates the need for consideration of mechanical ventilation. This leaves the patient at risk for lobar atelectasis and pneumonia, which may result in hypoxia and elevated A–a gradient.

ACUTE RESPIRATORY FAILURE WITH ABNORMAL LUNG FUNCTION

Acute respiratory failure is most frequently caused by abnormal lung function. Two types of acute respiratory failure occur, either hypoxemic and hypercapnic respiratory failure or simple hypoxemic respiratory failure without aberrancy in CO_2 elimination.

Chronic Obstructive Pulmonary Disease

The primary diagnosis of patients with hypoxemic hypercapnic respiratory failure is usually chronic obstructive lung disease (COPD). COPD, a common disorder, is approximately the fifth leading cause of death in the United States. Patients with hypercapnic respiratory failure often have a combination of chronic bronchitis and emphysema, which is linked to tobacco use and is usually apparent between age 50 and 70.

Respiratory failure develops when acute exacerbations of COPD occur. Patients exhibit severe pulmonary impairment as a baseline characteristic, and additional minor insults precipitate respiratory failure, requiring hospital admission and intensive therapy. It is important to identify and correct reversible factors before progression to respiratory muscle fatigue and failure. The pathophysiology of respiratory failure is at least partly due to respiratory muscle fatigue. High work loads placed on the respiratory muscles secondary to abnormal lung mechanics of the chronically obstructed airway cause early respiratory muscle fatigue. Since the primary gas exchange problem is hypoventilation (assuming pneumonia and/or pulmonary edema are not present), hypoxemia responds well to supplemental oxygen administration. However, because ventilatory drive in severe COPD may be dependent on a low oxygen level, increasing hypoventilation can occur with the removal of hypoxemia by aggressive supplemental oxygen use. Adequate oxygenation is a primary goal and the concern of increasing hypercapnia should not inhibit the use of oxygen, but careful observation of the arterial blood gases is necessary.

Conditions that can precipitate acute respiratory failure in the patient with COPD are multiple

- Infection, either upper or lower airway (acute bronchitis, pneumonia)
- Cardiac arrhythmia
- Heart failure
- Pulmonary embolus
- Pneumothorax
- Pleural effusion
- Rib fracture
- Metabolic derangement such as hypophosphatemia, hypocalcemia, hypokalemia, and metabolic alkalosis
- Medicine noncompliance
- Medicine toxicity such as theophylline
- Sedative agents such as benzodiazepenes or barbiturates

Interventional considerations in the COPD patient with hypercapnic respiratory failure should include several modalities

- Management within a critical care or hospital unit with close observation
- Supplemental oxygen with a P_aO_2 goal of approximately 60 mm Hg
- Bronchodilators (beta agonists, aerosolized anticholinergics, oral or intravenous aminophylline)
- Intravenous steroids

As in all cases of acute respiratory failure consideration of intervention with general diagnostic tests and support is important

- Antibiotics for possible upper or lower respiratory infections
- Capacity for the institution of mechanical ventilation
- Analysis of electrolytes and blood count
- X-ray analysis to rule out pneumothorax or large pleural effusion
- ECG to rule out cardiac arrhythmias such as atrial fibrillation and multifocal atrial tachycardia
- Consideration of congestive heart failure and the use of diuretics for preload reduction and vasodilators for afterload reduction (see Chapter 19)

Asthma

The hallmark of respiratory failure in asthma is the marked obstruction to airflow. The initial event is contraction of bronchial smooth muscle as a result of an immunologically mediated process, direct stimulation of irritant receptors within the airways, or both. The increased resistance to airflow occurs primarily during expiration, which leads to air trapping and hyperinflation as in the patient with COPD. Because the airflow obstruction is not uniform, the distribution of inspired air is uneven, causing mismatching of ventilation–perfusion and hypoxemia. Hyperinflation forces the intercostal, accessory, and diaphragmatic muscles to work at a mechanical disadvantage. The combination of airway obstruction, diaphragmatic muscle fatigue, and wasted ventilation results in CO_2 retention.

Assessment of severity during an asthmatic episode involves a careful history. Severe asthma is more common in patients with a history of serious attacks. The duration of the current attack is important because the mechanism of airway obstruction changes as the attack persists. Early, the mechanism is mainly bronchial smooth muscle spasm, while later airway obstruction is due to mucous plugging and mucosal edema. Spasm can resolve within minutes, but days may be required to improve the obstruction that is caused by edema and plugging. Important factors signifying severe asthma and possible pending respiratory failure have been identified

- History of prior hospitalization or mechanical ventilation for asthma
- History of chronic corticosteroid therapy
- Failure to respond to usual bronchodilator therapy
- Length of attack
- Silent chest (absence of wheezing secondary to insufficiency of airflow)
- Disturbance in mental status
- Hypertension or tachycardia
- Cardiac arrhythmia
- Cyanosis
- Prominent accessory muscle use
- Pulsus paradoxus greater than 10 mm Hg is significant, greater than 18 mm Hg is usually life threatening
- Pneumothorax or mediastinal air
- FEV_1 less than 1 liter or 20% of predicted normal
- Normal P_aCO_2 in the setting of tachypnea or severe respiratory distress
- Acute respiratory acidosis or severe hypoxemia

The causes of exacerbations in asthma are similar to those in COPD, including the following

- Infection of the upper or lower airway
- Medicine noncompliance
- Recent steroid taper
- Pneumothorax
- Stress
- Exposure to known airway irritants
- A significant number of exacerbations involve no known insult

Supportive care of patients with asthma and impending respiratory failure involve considerations similar to those in COPD

- Supplemental oxygen, but at high concentrations, as opposed to controlled low flow in COPD
- Bronchodilators (inhaled beta$_2$ agonists, inhaled anticholinergic therapy)
- IV corticosteroid therapy is crucial
- IV theophylline
- Consideration of the use of antibiotics
- Consideration and capacity for mechanical ventilation
- IV hydration to restore normovolemia
- Careful analysis of a chest x-ray

Death from asthma is uncommon, however, and is increasing in incidence (see Chapter 21).

ACUTE RESPIRATORY FAILURE IN PATIENTS WITH HYPOXEMIA AND NORMOCAPNIA OR HYPOCAPNIA

The causes of acute respiratory failure in patients with primarily hypoxic respiratory failure are those processes involving the pulmonary vascular bed, the lung interstition, or the alveoli of the lung. These disorders are primarily manifest by a decrease in diffusion and not alveolar hypoventilation. Thus, hypercapnia is rarely found. However, any process involving the lung parenchyma, given enough time and severity, may result in an elevated P_aCO_2.

Causes of acute respiratory failure involving the parenchyma of the lung include

- Pneumonia (bacterial, viral, or fungal)
- Adult Respiratory Distress Syndrome (ARDS) or noncardiogenic pulmonary edema
- Cardiogenic pulmonary edema
- Interstitial lung diseases
- Autoimmune lung diseases (idiopathic pulmonary fibrosis, systemic lupus erythematosus, scleroderma, rheumatoid arthritis, Wegener's granulomatosis, Goodpasture's disease)
- Pulmonary emboli

DIAGNOSTIC TESTS

CHEST X-RAY

The chest x-ray is very important in the diagnosis of acute respiratory failure. However, on occasion, the x-ray will only verify what the physical exam has suggested, such as alveolar infiltrate in an area in which crackles were auscultated. However, the x-ray may also reveal a concomitant disorder, such as pleural effusion, pneumothorax, bilateral infiltrates, and/or atelectasis, that was not evident on physical examination. Identification of these disorders by x-ray allows for earlier intervention and improvement in the course of the patient with acute respiratory failure. The chest x-ray is also important in following the course of a patient with respiratory failure. Entities evident radiographically that complicate the diagnosis and course of acute respiratory failure include

- Atelectasis
- Pneumothorax
- Nosocomial pneumonia
- Pleural effusion
- Enlarging cardiac silhouette
- Pulmonary artery catheters, central lines, and feeding tubes

ELECTROCARDIOGRAM

The electrocardiogram (ECG), while not diagnostic of any specific etiology of acute respiratory failure, may assist in evaluation of the heart and its tolerance of acute respiratory failure. In chronic lung disease, the ECG may demonstrate abnormalities such as P pulmonale, right heart hypertrophy, and rightward axis. Acute changes on the ECG, signifying right heart strain or shift in axis, may also be helpful in the diagnosis of massive pulmonary emboli. The myocardium is vulnerable to hypoxia in the face of increased work, resulting in ECG changes of ischemia or infarction during respiratory dysfunction. In this setting, more aggressive management of the respiratory failure and interventions such as hospital admission, oxygen supplementation, and even earlier support with mechanical ventilation may be required. Acute myocardial infarction in the setting of acute respiratory failure has an ominous prognosis.

PULMONARY FUNCTION STUDIES

Pulmonary function studies may be helpful in early acute respiratory failure, especially in the face of asthma or COPD. In this setting, spirometry may indicate decreased forced expiratory volumes at one second (FEV_1) and decreased forced vital capacity (FVC). The ratio of these two values should be less than 75% if airway obstruction is present. In patients with COPD, the comparison of baseline spirometry with that during an acute exacerbation can be helpful in determining the severity of the episode. However, in the setting of acute respiratory failure with airway obstruction, the patient's ability to cooperate and, thus, the validity of pulmonary function studies is quite marginal. Serial measurement of the vital capacity is required in patients with normal lungs and pulmonary function impairment secondary to neuromuscular disease. Monitoring the patient's vital capacity serially is a sensitive indicator of the progression of acute respiratory failure in these patients. A vital capacity of greater than one liter is considered adequate pulmonary function. However, if the patient's weakness progresses, such that the vital capacity is less than one liter, ventilatory support should be strongly considered. Pulmonary function tests should be obtained after a bout of acute respiratory failure if there is a possibility of significant lung injury. Residual pulmonary function abnormalities may potentially limit the rehabilitation of the patient. Lung volumes and diffusion capacity can be especially helpful in this situation.

PULMONARY ARTERY CATHETER

Bedside pulmonary artery catheterization is quite helpful in determining whether the left heart plays a role in acute respiratory failure. The measurement of the pulmonary capillary wedge pressure (PCWP) or pulmonary artery occlusion pressure (PAOP) estimates the left ventricular end diastolic filling pressure if placed and inflated properly. The catheter may be inserted via the subclavian, internal jugular, femoral, or antecubital vein. Careful calibration, taking into account the effects of respiration on pressure measurements, is very important for the acquisition of reliable data. Accurate measurements of pulmonary artery pressure can be particularly difficult in patients with acute severe airway obstruction. In order to overcome the high airway resistance, positive intrathoracic pressure is generated throughout expiration. This leads to elevated pulmonary artery pressures and/or elevated wedge pressures as detected by the catheter balloon. The measurement of PCWP also assists in distinguishing cardiogenic pulmonary edema from noncardiogenic pulmonary edema or ARDS. ARDS will be discussed more thoroughly in the next section.

Systemic Arterial Catheterization

Monitoring systemic arterial blood pressure is useful in patients who are hemodynamically unstable by placement of an arterial catheter. In addition, blood can be withdrawn from the catheter, thus avoiding repeated percutaneous venous and arterial sticks. In the patient with severe COPD in exacerbation who may not tolerate increasing concentration of oxygen, an arterial cathether can be quite helpful in acquiring the frequent arterial blood gas samples required for serial arterial gas analysis. Careful attention must be paid to percutaneous insertion with aseptic technique and assessment of collateral circulation by the Allen test, which determines adequacy of collateral arterial flow. Arterial catheters are well tolerated. Complications involve distal embolization, which may require thrombectomy when distal ischemia is present. Infection and careful maintenance of equipment attachments also require special considerations.

SUPPORTIVE CARE FOR ACUTE RESPIRATORY FAILURE

The treatment and support of the patient in acute respiratory failure are dependent on the underlying mechanisms by which the process has been caused. The first priority in treating a patient with acute respiratory failure is adequate oxygenation.

SUPPLEMENTAL OXYGEN

Oxygen supplementation is required in the treatment and support of acute respiratory failure. Hypoxic damage of end organ systems (renal, cardiovascular) can complicate the course and worsen the prognosis of patients with acute respiratory failure. Thus, the patient's need for oxygen should not be underestimated. The decision to use mechanical ventilation with endotracheal intubation or an external oxygen delivery depends on three factors

- The amount of oxygen needed
- The level of patient cooperation
- The potential consequence of failure to provide oxygen if the external device is malpositioned

A variety of external oxygen delivery systems are available; nasal prongs are the simplest and most comfortable. However, the FiO_2 provided cannot be quantitated reliably and humidification is poor. Open face masks or tents provide a high flow of well humidified gas with a moderately reliable FiO_2 set by a Venturi device. Tight-fitting masks with a non-rebreathing valve and reservoir bag can be used to provide even higher concentrations of oxygen, perhaps an FiO_2 of 0.7 to 0.8 for short periods. These masks can be quite uncomfortable and require a high level of patient cooperation. Another version of oxygen delivery involves the constant positive airway pressure (CPAP), in which a constant pressure is delivered throughout inspiration and expiration. The use of this device in acute respiratory failure is unpredictable in patients who are experiencing airway obstruction and elevated P_aCO_2. Investigations now demonstrate some early success with CPAP during exacerbation of COPD. Mechanical ventilation delivered by face mask has been reported and is usually reserved for the patient with chronic respiratory failure in decline as an alternative to endotracheal intubation.

Ventilatory Assist Devices and Mechanical Ventilation

Indications for endotracheal intubation are difficult to define. Certainly, the level of hypoxemia and hypercapnia are taken into account. However, other objective criteria such as patient awareness, ability to cooperate, level of fatigue, as well as course over a period of several hours may be as important in the decision to intubate. Regardless of the situation, intubation should be performed on a semi-elective basis rather than emergently; close patient monitoring is required to assess the effect of therapy in a patient course. Endotracheal tubes may be passed through the nose or the mouth. The mouth allows for a larger diameter tube, which is not as comfortable for the patient. Oral intubation requires more sedation, while the spontaneously ventilating awake patient may be nasally intubated.

Immediately after the tube is placed, either by direct laryngoscopy or blindly nasally, the lungs should be auscultated to determine if air is entering both lungs. Because of the anatomical advantage at the main carina, the endotracheal tube will often enter the right main stem bronchus. Position should be confirmed by chest x-ray or bronchoscope. The tube should be secured by taping or another measure to avoid malposition and extubation. All endotracheal tubes should be fitted with a low pressure cuff to avoid tracheal mucosal injury. Overinflation of the cuff should be avoided, since this may cause pressure necrosis of adjacent tracheal mucosa.

There is no absolute time limit for endotracheal intubation beyond which tracheostomy is indicated. The institution of tracheostomy depends on the prognosis of the patient, previous failure to wean from mechanical ventilation, patient comfort, and rehabilitation. It is not unreasonable to consider tracheostomy after 14 to 21 days of mechanical ventilation.

AIRWAY MAINTENANCE

Airway maintenance in the nonintubated and intubated patient with reactive airways generally requires aerosolized beta agonists, anticholinergics, and possibly IV corticosteroids. In mechanically ventilated patients, the use of aerosolized bronchodilators is routine. Careful attention to suctioning of secretions is also a high priority in the mechanically ventilated patient. This is especially true during the period of weaning.

INFECTION

Infection is a common cause of acute respiratory failure in patients with chronic lung disease. Cultures of sputum, blood, and urine should be routinely acquired. Careful identification of infection risks, especially factors leading to an immunocompromised state (e.g., diabetes, renal failure), must also be entertained and a broader spectrum of antibiotics used in this patient group. In the immunocompromised patient, bronchoscopy for acquisition of alveolar samples by bronchial alveolar lavage and protected specimen brush (PSB) can be helpful in identifying causative agents of uncommon processes.

Nosocomial pneumonia is a common complication of patients treated in an intensive care unit (ICU). The patient with mechanical ventilated needs is more susceptible. Unfortunately, current clinical parameters for diagnosis of pneumonia in the ICU are inadequate. Radiographic infiltrates, transient fevers, and elevated white blood counts are not specific indicators of pneumonia in the ICU. Thus, different mechanisms for acquiring cultures have been developed. Bronchoscopy via an endotracheal tube is a low risk procedure in the intubated patient. Samples from alveolar spaces can be taken via protective specimen brush in areas involved in infiltrates. Significant growth in culture of an agent suggests pneumonia; quantitative cultures are necessary if results are to be useful. These methods of diagnosing pneumonia in the ICU are necessary not only to adequately treat pneumonia but also to avoid the consequences of prolonged broad spectrum antibiotic use in the ICU. These consequences include infection with more virulent strains of bacteria as well as increased mortality (see Chapter 24).

NUTRITION

Nutritional support in the ICU has made great gains over the past decade. It is generally accepted that the involvement of the gut in feeding is more advantageous than total parenteral nutrition (TPN) in the ICU patient. Patients in acute respiratory failure are often unable to maintain adequate caloric intake secondary to respiratory distress, anorexia, endotracheal intubation, and/or higher caloric needs. Nutritional needs should be defined and adequate total calories, protein, carbohydrates, and fats should be prescribed. The goal of nutritional support in a patient with acute respiratory failure is maintenance of total body mass, the avoidance of protein catabolism, and loss of muscle mass, especially regarding to muscle strength.

PROPHYLAXIS FOR GASTROINTESTINAL BLEEDING

The use of H_2 blockers and antacids has been routine in the ICUs. The rationale has included the protection of the gastric mucosa during a period of nonfeeding and a subsequent decrease in gastric stress ulceration and GI bleeding. This has come under some scrutiny in the last few years, and there is evidence that the use of antacids may be associated with increased nosocomial pneumonia due to gastric colonization with gram-negative bacilli. There is no clear evidence that H_2 blockade alone or sucralfate has been associated with an increased incidence of nosocomial pneumonia. Further studies with H_2 blockers are needed.

OPEN LUNG BIOPSY

The acquisition of lung tissue is indicated in the setting of acute respiratory failure when x-ray infiltrates are present, but the etiology for the parenchymal process cannot be identified by nonsurgical techniques including bronchoalveolar lavage and transbronchial biopsy, cultures, VQ scans or associated systemic processes. Open lung biopsy can be obtained with relatively low risk and supplies invaluable information regarding the etiology and prognosis in acute respiratory failure.

Each case of acute respiratory failure must be individualized and a different course must be taken depending on the underlying cause. After the first round of investigation, which involves arterial blood gas, ECG, physical examination, review of past history, as well as laboratory examination of serum electrolytes, blood counts, and baseline renal and liver studies, decisions must be made involving diagnostic and therapeutic considerations. Diagnostic considerations include ventilation–perfusion scans, cultures of sputum, blood, and urine, as well as the consideration of the need for tissue examination by either transbronchial biopsy or open lung biopsy. Therapeutic decisions depend on the specific etiology of acute respiratory failure. In the past three decades, gains in the support of the patient in respiratory failure have been immense. However, this cannot replace the high level of knowledge and expertise required by the clinician for the diagnosis and therapeutic intervention of acute respiratory failure.

ADULT RESPIRATORY DISTRESS SYNDROME

Adult respiratory distress syndrome (ARDS) or noncardiogenic pulmonary edema is a form of acute respiratory failure occurring in a wide variety of medical, surgical, obstetric and gynecologic, and trauma patients. A complex inflammatory cascade follows a severe systemic or pulmonary injury and results in a constellation of findings, including severe hypoxemia, diffuse infiltrates on chest x-ray, and decreased respiratory compliance. Petty and Ashbaugh originally characterized the clinical syndrome of acute lung injury in 1967. The ARDS associated mortality rate approached 90% at that time; however, over the last decade it has dropped to 60%.

In general, several diagnostic characteristics of ARDS can be identified

- Acute lung injury as evidenced by diffuse alveolar damage, including interstitial and alveolar edema and hyaline membranes
- The lack of elevated left heart filling pressures by pulmonary artery catheter measurement, which account for noncardiogenic pulmonary edema
- Association with previously identified clinical disorders or inciting factors
- Association with progressive multiple organ systems dysfunction or failure

LUNG INJURY IN ARDS

Murray and Matthay recommend evaluation of four parameters of lung injury to define ARDS: the chest x-ray, the hypoxemia score, compliance, and the need for positive end expiratory pressure (PEEP)

- The chest x-ray: Radiographically, ARDS can be a patchy process; however, it often progresses to include all five lobes of the lungs. Usually, the chest x-ray in ARDS demonstrates a diffuse five-lobe alveolar infiltrate. The chest x-ray is important in the diagnosis of ARDS as well as to identify potential reversible processes that may be remedied by simple therapy. These include pleural effusions, cardiogenic pulmonary edema, and pneumothorax. The chest x-ray also is important to monitor during a course of ARDS. Many complications of the ARDS treatment with mechanical ventilation and associated high peak inspiratory pressures may be apparent by chest x-ray: interstitial air, pneumothorax, pneumomediastinum, subcutaneous emphysema. Other processes that occur with lung parenchyma after significant injury can also be reflected in the chest x-ray: cavitation, consolidation, atelectasis, pneumatocele formation
- Hypoxemia score = P_aO_2/FiO_2: The hypoxemia score is defined as the ratio of arterial oxygen tension divided by the inspired oxygen concentration. It is a reflection of the severity of the disease process and, therefore, the difficulty in oxygenating the patient. The information gained from the $P_AO_2 - P_aO_2$ difference equation is similar, in that it reflects the severity of gas exchange dysfunction; however, the hypoxemia score is simpler to calculate and does not take CO_2 into account. An example: a patient with P_aO_2 of 67 mm Hg on a ventilator delivering an FiO_2 of 0.6 has a P_aO_2/FiO_2 ratio of 112. A range of <100 (severe injury) to >300 (minimal to no injury) is observed
- Compliance: This is defined as the ratio of tidal volume delivered by the pressure required to deliver that volume. In a ventilated patient, it is calculated by dividing the tidal volume over the plateau airway pressure minus the PEEP. Compliance reflects the "flexibility" of the interstitium. Initially in ARDS, a compliance can be near normal, but with progression of disease, compliance decreases and the classic "stiff" lung results. The progression of a decline in compliance prognostically is an ominous factor. An example: A 65-kg patient is delivered a 750-ml tidal volume (V_T) breath by mechanical ventilation. The pressure after the breath is delivered and airflow has stopped is 50 cm H_2O; PEEP is 5 cm H_2O. The compliance of this patient would be 750 ml/50 to 5 ml of H_2O = 17 ml/cm H_2O. Normal compliance is greater than 40 ml/cm H_2O
- Positive end expiratory pressure (PEEP): PEEP is end expiratory pressure that is positive instead of the normal negative end expiratory pressure. PEEP is begun in patients requiring mechanical ventilation who have failed to oxygenate adequately with conventional ventilation. Thus, the addition of added pressure support at the end expiratory phase is made to recruit distal alveoli that have been lost secondary to collapse and/or filling with an inflammatory exudate. PEEP can be a very helpful mo-

dality in improving oxygenation; however, its association with pulmonary barotrauma such as pneumothorax can be a serious problem

CLINICAL DISORDERS ASSOCIATED WITH ARDS

ARDS is characteristically associated with a wide variety of clinical disorders that result in lung insult and subsequent acute lung injury. Unfortunately, the associated entities are often multiple, and the risk of ARDS increases with the number of clinical disorders that occur in each patient.

Despite the heterogeneity of associated clinical disorders, the time course from any insult to the development of ARDS is less than 24 hours in most patients and often less than 12 hours in patients with sepsis-related ARDS. The importance of the earliest hours of ARDS is the clarification and possible intervention of whichever mechanism is responsible for the development of the lung injury. Common clinical disorders associated with acute lung injury of ARDS have been identified

- Sepsis is the most common disorder associated with the development of ARDS. It is difficult to establish the true incidence of sepsis in associated ARDS since there has been a lack of consensus on the definition of sepsis. In general, definitions now cover a range of disease severity
- Bacteremia indicates positive blood cultures for bacteria, pathogenic virus, fungi, rickettsia, or mycobacteria
- Sepsis suggests clinical evidence of infection and signs of a systemic response to the infection such as tachypnea, tachycardia, and hyperthermia or hypothermia. Blood cultures demonstrating bacteremia are not required
- Sepsis syndrome includes parameters of sepsis plus evidence of altered organ perfusion. For example: P_aO_2/FiO_2 no higher than 280, lactate level at the upper limit of normal, oliguria, and altered mental status
- Early septic shock includes the above description plus hypotension (systolic blood pressure <90 mm Hg) for less than 1 hour, which responds to fluids or pharmacologic intervention
- Refractory septic shock includes hypotension for more than 1 hour despite adequate volume and vasopressors (dopamine >6 ug/kg/minute administered for 1 hour)

Fully developed ARDS occurs in about 25% of patients with sepsis; however, another 35% demonstrate transient derangements in gas exchange suggestive of mild to moderate lung injury. ARDS is probably a manifestation of a systemic disease, and its occurrence is related to the degree of injury at the capillary endothelium outside the pulmonary parenchyma. A marker of endothelial injury, the von Willebrand factor, is markedly elevated in septic patients who develop ARDS. These preliminary data suggest that the von Willebrand factor antigen may be a marker of the risk for the development of ARDS after sepsis. However, this is still at an investigational stage.

Despite the presence of clinical sepsis, the site of infection is not always clear. In clinical sepsis, associated with ARDS, postmortem examination has shown that if the site of infection is unclear and the blood cultures are positive, the source is often the abdomen. If blood cultures are negative but septic physiology has been present, the source is most commonly the lung.

Infection is the most common cause of ARDS in nonsurvivors. Adequate antibiotic treatment does not favorably influence survival in this patient group. Overall, survival in ARDS associated with sepsis is estimated to be approximately 20 to 40%. Sepsis is also the most common cause of early and late deaths in patients with ARDS

- Aspiration of gastric contents is another important cause of ARDS. Prognosis depends on the degree of injury. In witnessed episodes of aspiration, prognosis is correlated with the oxygen requirements of the patient at 1 hour
- Major trauma such as that secondary to motor vehicle accidents and crush injuries may develop ARDS on a multifactorial basis. Examples include lung contusion, hypotension, transfusion, sepsis, and fat emboli (long bone fractures)
- Overdose of various pharmacological agents is associated with ARDS. Common agents include aspirin, narcotics, tricyclic antidepressants, and barbiturates. Often, the exact disorders causing the ARDS is not clear because these patients may also be hypotensive, aspirate, and/or have direct lung injury caused by the ingested drug
- Cardiopulmonary bypass is another important clinical condition associated with acute lung injury and ARDS. This procedure, commonly used for coronary artery bypass surgery or open heart surgery, has the best prognosis of any entities associated with ARDS. The survival rate approaches 100%
- In contrast, ARDS associated with bone marrow transplantation or hepatic failure has an approximately 0% survival rate
- Early death in ARDS secondary to the respiratory tract occurs in approximately 10% of patients. Only 20% of patients surviving 1 week of ARDS will die secondary to respiratory failure. The clinical disorders associated with ARDS clearly affect survival and must be identified for a realistic assessment of prognosis and appropriate intervention

PATHOPHYSIOLOGY

The pathologic features of the lung in ARDS derive from severe injury to the alveolar capillary unit. Because of the injury, the capillary "leaks" with extravasation of intravascular fluid into the alveolus, thus the term "permeability pulmonary edema." This process is at least partly responsible for the resultant hypoxia. The histologic appearance of this damage can be divided into three phases

- Exudative phase of edema and hemorrhage
- Proliferative phase of organization and repair
- Fibrotic phase of end-stage fibrosis

The source of injury to the alveolus may enter from its vascular bed, as in sepsis, and fat emboli or from within the lung as in aspiration and pneumonia. It must be emphasized that the course and prognosis of ARDS are dependent on the mechanism by which it occurred.

The mediation of inflammation has recently been proposed to involve the circulating and tissue macrophages because of their ability to produce and release the newly described class of peptide mediators termed "cytokines." Because ARDS involves intense inflammation in the lung, no review of this is now possible without a brief discussion of cytokines, which refers to cell-derived peptide molecules that cause a target cell to alter one or more of its functional activities. Multiple cytokines have been implicated in the pathogenesis of ARDS, including the following

- Tumor necrosis factor (TNF) is produced by the alveolar macrophage and circulating monocyte. TNF can cause fever, neutrophil sequestration in the lung, and hemorrhage and edema of many organs, including the kidney, gut, and lung. Antibodies to TNF attenuate its effects during ARDS and sepsis in animal models
- Interleukin-1 (IL-1) is a cytokine produced by the alveolar macrophage and circulating monocyte. It has many characteristics clinically similar to TNF. Injected into animal models, it can reproduce the septic physiology in end organ changes

The most important modification of the ARDS concept in recent years is the recognition that there are significant extrapulmonary components to this syndrome. Dysfunction and failure of the renal, hepatic, cardiovascular, gastrointestinal, and central nervous systems can also occur.

Systemic physiologic derangements occur in ARDS. For reasons that are not entirely clear, the uptake of oxygen at the cellular level is dependent on delivery of oxygen to tissues at nearly all levels of oxygen uptake in patients with ARDS. Normally, oxygen uptake is independent of oxygen delivery as long as a certain threshold is reached. Two basic changes in physiology allow for this derangement in oxygen delivery and uptake

- Altered blood flow distribution: Oxygenated blood bypasses nutrient capillary beds, often redistributing portions of the cardiac output to lower oxygen extraction tissues
- Endothelial and/or parenchymal cell injury: Edema with increased diffusion distances and/or decrease in capillary surface area may account for the inability of oxygen to leave the circulation. When injured, the endothelium and other cells within the parenchyma are potent inflammatory mediators that may impair basic protective responses of normal physiology such as the maintenance of blood pressures or shunting of blood to vital organs

These may account for at least part of the multisystem injury in ARDS. In simple terms, the scenario may occur in three phases

- Initially, multisystemic interactions between neutrophils and endothelial cells occur. This results in microvascular injury and involves endothelium throughout the vascular bed. The lung has more dramatic consequences, because the intact permeability barrier is a unique prerequisite for respiratory "success." At this point, only clinical signs of ARDS may be present

- Secondly, recurrent or sustained injury, possibly by endotoxemia, is probably necessary for endothelial dysfunction to progress to extrapulmonary organ dysfunction
- In the terminal phase, overt multisystem failure occurs

It is recognized that the high likelihood of association of nonpulmonary organ failure and death in ARDS occurs after secondary multi-organ failure, and not necessarily respiratory failure.

MULTI-ORGAN DYSFUNCTION

The discussion of ARDS would not be complete without the consideration of nonpulmonary organ failure. A similar process by which ARDS develops is involved systemically and may involve a variety of organ systems. Unfortunately, no uniform definitions of each organ dysfunction have been established. The incidence of organ involvement with ARDS has been estimated

- Renal: 40 to 55%
- Hepatic: 12 to 95%
- CNS: 7 to 30%
- GI: 7 to 30%
- Hematologic: 0 to 26%
- Cardiac: 0 to 23%

Renal manifestations such as oliguria or advancing azotemia are criteria for involvement of that system with ARDS.

- Creatinine >2 mg/dl (200 μmol/l)
- Urine output <600 ml over 24 hours

The etiology of impairment may be based on the systemic injury seen in many cases of ARDS but cannot be distinguished from the injury resulting from hypotension and nephrotoxic drugs. Nonoliguric renal failure caused by nephrotoxic drugs appears to have the best prognosis.

Available estimates indicate that 7 to 30% of patients with ARDS have a significant gastrointestinal disturbance such as an ileus, malabsorption, hemorrhage, or perforation. Gastrointestinal hemorrhage and perforation are important examples of injury at the bowel level. However, the gut's role in host defense may be the most bothersome dysfunction. When injured, the gastrointestinal tract may permit the systemic translocation of resident bowel organisms into the systemic circulation. Translocation of enteric organisms results in sustained delivery of endotoxin to hepatic macrophages and hepatic export of cytokines and other mediators active in the amplification of inflammation.

Fulminant hepatic failure is uncommon in ARDS. Less than 10% of patients with ARDS develop hepatic failure; however, transient elevation of serum transaminases, bilirubin, or clotting parameters is common. Significant hepatic dysfunction includes a variety of parameters

- Bilirubin >4 to 5 mg/dl (68 to 85 μmol/l)

- PT >1.5 × control
- Albumin <2.0 g/dl (20 g/l)

The liver is an important source in host defense, although this difficult to quantify. The proximity of the pulmonary vascular bed to the liver is important if the liver is unable to produce or clear toxic substances, including endotoxin, bloodborne from the gut. The pulmonary endothelium is first in line for injury after hepatic dysfunction.

Cardiovascular parameters suggesting significant cardiovascular dysfunction include

- Cardiac index <2 liters/min per m²
- Reversible ventricular fibrillation or asystole
- Mean arterial pressure <60 mm Hg

The alterations in cardiac function most often associated with sepsis are decreased left and right heart function, reflected in decreased ejection fractions. Ventricular end systolic and end diastolic volumes are increased; stroke volume is decreased. Serum from patients with septic shock depresses myocardial cell contractility in vitro, suggesting a bloodborne myocardial depressed factor. TNF, a potent mediator of inflammation, has been implicated in this ability to depress myocardial function.

Hematologic dysfunction in the critically ill patient with ARDS is difficult to define; however, generally accepted parameters to assess the status of the hematologic system in ARDS patients include

- Platelet count <50,000 cu mm (50 × 10⁹/l)
- Fibrinogen <100 mg/dl (1 g/l)
- White blood cell <1,000 cu mm (1.0 × 10⁹/l)

By this evaluation criteria, approximately 26% of critically ill patients develop hematologic dysfunction. The Central Nervous System (CNS) is probably the least investigated system in ARDS. The Glasgow coma scale can be used to evaluate even intubated patients on a verbal, motor, and visual response basis (best score: 15; worst score: 3). The CNS is significantly involved if confusion, seizures, and coma occur. Unlike other organ systems, a uniform approach is available to measure CNS dysfunction.

PREVENTION AND TREATMENT OF ARDS

As sepsis is the most common cause of ARDS, prevention tactics are geared toward blunting the inflammatory response. Unfortunately, although current strategies are promising, they are in the preliminary stages of therapeutic application

- Antiendotoxin therapy is aimed at removing or inactivating lipopolysaccharide (LPS). This toxic bacterial component of the gram-negative bacterial cell wall is a potent inducer of systemic cytokine release, including TNF and IL-1. Ziegler and associates demonstrated a significant advantage in the outcome of patients with gram-negative sepsis by using polyclonal antibody to the cell wall of J5 strain *Escherichia coli*. Preliminary reports using monoclonal antiendotoxin antibodies have demon-

strated decreased mortality from the septic syndrome if overt shock had not developed by the time therapy was initiated. Unfortunately, antiendotoxin therapy would be effective only in gram-negative sepsis.
- Anti-inflammatory is aimed at a variety of pathways throughout the immune cascade. Corticosteroid treatment in sepsis has been disappointing in that it has no benefit in prevention of ARDS or multisystem dysfunction. In fact, steroids may increase the mortality by increasing the incidence of serious secondary infections. Prostaglandin E1 has anti-inflammatory properties, and initial reports in trauma patients demonstrated that it may improve survival in patients with ARDS. However, follow-up reports now suggest no effect in the outcome of ARDS patients. Nonsteroidal anti-inflammatory drugs such as ibuprofen may benefit hemodynamics and ventilation. However, the assessment of its role in attenuation of ARDS and multisystem dysfunction is incomplete
- Antibodies to various cytokines or their receptors are in early stages of investigation. Blocking or neutralizing the TNF response may have therapeutic potential. However, a brief half-life in the circulation may narrow the window of opportunity. The advantage of cytokine blockade is that it would be effective in both gram-positive and gram-negative sepsis. For example, levels of TNF are as high in patients with gram-positive sepsis as in those with gram-negative sepsis. However, the potential of dysfunctional inflammatory response is of concern and there are no clear data suggesting the routine use of anti-TNF antibodies
- Support efforts have improved the ARDS mortality rate of 95% when the entity was first described in 1967 to a current mortality rate between 40 and 60%. This is probably attributable to the improvement of ventilatory and hemodynamic support as well as the improvement of antibiotics and nutritional awareness.

MECHANICAL VENTILATION

A few points concerning the mechanical ventilation of patients with ARDS should be made. This topic is discussed thoroughly in Chapter 29.

- Of all forms of acute respiratory failure, ARDS often requires mechanical ventilation because support with high tidal volumes re-expands atelectatic and partially fluid-filled alveoli. PEEP is especially helpful in recruiting alveoli for ventilation. This aids in reducing the fraction of inspired oxygen required and may avoid oxygen toxicity
- One of the most difficult problems in managing patients with ARDS is determining the optimal level of PEEP. While PEEP is used to improve oxygenation and avoid toxic levels of oxygen, it may also decrease cardiac output and tissue oxygen delivery. While evaluating the level of PEEP that improves oxygenation but does not compromise cardiac output significantly, the use of the pulmonary artery catheter is quite helpful
- Data suggest that oxygen concentrations in the range of 50 to 60% or less are unlikely to contribute in a major way to progressive, acute lung injury. Thus, a reasonable goal is to adjust the level of PEEP to achieve an FiO_2 of around 60%

- Patients with ARDS may not tolerate the addition of PEEP secondary to the relative reduction in preload that is caused by increased thoracic pressures. Volume expansion may improve the tolerance of PEEP
- Patients requiring mechanical ventilation and high levels of PEEP often require muscle paralysis. Paralysis alleviates added resistance to ventilation that may be manifest by muscle tone in the thoracic cage. If the patient is paralyzed, a sedative and/or anxiolytic agent must be used as well

Other modalities involving mechanical ventilation such as inverse ratio ventilation, jet ventilation, and high frequency ventilation have been used in patients with ARDS with varying success. No modality has proven predictably superior to conventional ventilation with PEEP. Extracorporeal membrane oxygenation for patients with severe ARDS also has not improved mortality. Currently, several centers are experimenting with extracorporeal CO_2 removal, although the preliminary data is not promising.

HEMODYNAMIC MONITORING

In the early phases of ARDS, hemodynamic monitoring of pulmonary vascular pressures may be helpful

- Measurement of pulmonary artery wedge pressures can help confirm the cause of pulmonary edema as noncardiogenic
- It has been shown that some patients with primary acute lung injury have coexistent modest elevations of pulmonary artery wedge pressures. The use of diuretics may be particularly helpful in these patients, although recently there has been some concern that patients who are at risk for multisystem dysfunction may actually benefit from full-volume expansion and even supernormal cardiac output. Because the patient with ARDS often has associated systemic hypotension, a pulmonary artery catheter can be quite helpful in guiding IV fluid, transfusion, and plasma expander therapy

NUTRITION

Malnutrition or inadequate nutritional support has adverse effects on thoracoabdominal function, including decreased respiratory muscle strength, diminished ventilatory drive, and altered lung defense mechanisms. Clinical sequelae of these adverse effects can result in increased infection, especially pneumonia; the added difficulty in weaning from mechanical ventilation due to decreased strength. All ARDS patients who are malnourished or unable to maintain adequate oral intake should receive nutritional supplementation. Routes of nutritional support are either enteral via nasogastric or nasoduodenal tubes or parenterally with total parenteral nutrition (TPN). The enteral route is the first choice of nutritional support because it is less invasive, less expensive, and more physiologic than TPN. Additionally, recent data suggest that enteral nutrition may decrease the frequency of bacterial translocation from the bowel to systemic circulation.

Decreased inflammatory mediators or cytokine release is seen with enteral nutrition as compared to TPN.

NOSOCOMIAL PNEUMONIA

As many as 20 to 40% of mechanically ventilated ARDS patients develop nosocomial pneumonia, i.e., pneumonia occurring after the onset of ARDS. The pathophysiologic mechanism where by ARDS patients develop nosocomial pneumonia is aspiration of colonized tracheobronchial, oropharyngeal, or gastric secretions. Nosocomial pneumonia only rarely develops from hematemegous dissemination or inhalation of organisms from contaminated respiratory therapy devices. Colonization of the nasopharynx and stomach is directly related to the severity of the illness. Critically ill patients, such as those with ARDS, have a high likelihood of developing gram-negative nasopharyngeal or gastric colonization. Aspiration of a small amount of colonized secretions may result in pneumonia.

Diagnosis of nosocomial pneumonia in a ventilated ARDS patient with infiltrate is difficult. Clinical criteria of pneumonia (fever, leukocytosis, radiographic infiltrate, and purulent sputum) raise the clinical suspicion for pneumonia but are inadequate for a diagnosis in the clinical setting. Recently, quantitative culture of the lower airway by a protected specimen brush or bronchoalveolar lavage with or without bronchoscopy have been shown to be more sensitive and specific than routine tracheal aspirate cultures.

Therapy of nosocomial pneumonia requires identification of a potential pathology (usually gram-negative organism) and administration of appropriate antibiotics. Mortality is high in nosocomial pneumonia in ARDS, even with the appropriate antibiotics, suggesting that the basic disease process may be more important in ultimate outcome than choosing the right antibiotic.

Efforts to avoid gastric and/or nasopharyngeal colonization have included aerosolized antibiotics and selective gut decontamination, as well as preformed antibody. However, these studies are in investigational stages and are not currently recommended.

Other considerations include

- The use of subcutaneous heparin therapy in the ICU for prophylaxis against pulmonary emboli is generally accepted. The patient requiring mechanical ventilation of ARDS is often paralyzed. The opportunity for venous stasis in deeper thigh and pelvic veins with embolization to the pulmonary artery is a concern
- Dopamine is particularly useful as an agent to increase renal bloodflow if the patient is at risk for multi-organ system dysfunction. However, dopamine may cause a mild increase in PCWP. For the patient who has difficulty oxygenating, an alternative is required. Dobutamine is the preferred agent, especially in the setting of lower limit cardiac indices (see Chapter 16).

The course of ARDS can often be long and complicated, necessitating intense patient and family support. This dimension of patient care should not be lost in the confusion of the complicated therapy required for these patients.

SEQUELAE

Early information suggests that most survivors of ARDS recovered nearly normal lung function within 12 months. However, recent data do not support this

- Some degree of pulmonary impairment as defined by pulmonary function testing is apparent in approximately 60% of patients tested at 1 year. The diffusion was found to be the best test for detecting impairment both early and late after ARDS. This is probably related to the injury at the capillary level with thickened alveolar capillary interfaces. Surprisingly, the study has shown no association between symptoms and the laboratory evidence of impairment. Several risks for pulmonary function impairment have been identified
- Extremes of age, either early or late
- Physiologic indices of severity of ARDS, such as compliance, peak pulmonary pressures, and maximal PEEP requirements, were also found to correlate with the presence of impairment at 1 year after ARDS
- Other studies have found an association with FiO_2 requirements greater than 50 or 60% and a relationship of time ventilated

BIBLIOGRAPHY

Ashbaugh DG, Bigelow DB, Petty TL, et al.: Acute respiratory distress in adults. Lancet, 2: 319, 1967.

Bergofsky EH. Respiratory failure in disorders of the thoracic cage. Am Rev Respir Dis, *119*: 643, 1979.

Baum GL, Wolinsky E: Textbook of pulmonary diseases. Boston, Little Brown and Company, 1989.

Bernard GR, Luce JM, Sprung CL, et al.: High-dose corticosteroids in patients with the adult respiratory distress syndrome. N Engl J Med, *317*:1565, 1987.

Bone RC, Fisher CJ, Clemmer TP, et al.: A controlled clinical trial of high-dose methylprednisolone in the treatment of severe sepsis and septic shock. N Engl J Med, *317*:653, 1987.

Bone RC: Review: pathogenesis of sepsis. Annals Int Med, *115*:457, 1991.

Chastre J, Fagon JY, Soler P, et al.: Diagnosis of nosocomial bacterial pneumonia in intubated patients undergoing ventilation: Comparison of the usefulness of bronchoalveolar lavage and the protected specimen brush. Am J Med, *85*:499, 1988.

Chernow B (ed.): New insights into the science of critical care medicine. Chest, 100(Suppl.): 1535, 1991.

Danek SJ, Lynch JP, Weg JG, et al.: The dependence of oxygen uptake on oxygen delivery in the adult respiratory distress syndrome. Am Rev Respir Dis, *122*:387, 1980.

Dorinsky PM, Gadek JE: Multiple organ failure. Clin Chest Med, *11*:581, 1990.

Fukuda Y, Ishizake M, Masuda Y, et al.: The role of intra-alveolar fibrosis: The process of pulmonary structural remodeling in patients with diffuse alveolar damage. Am J Pathol, *126*:171, 1987.

Hollenberg SM, Cunnion RE, Lawrence M, et al.: Tumor necrosis factor depresses myocardial cell function: Results using an in vitro assay of myocyte performance. Clin Res, *37*:528A, 1989.

Jacobs RF, Tabor DR, Burke AW, et al.: Elevated interleukin release by human alveolar macrophages during ARDS. Am Rev Respir Dis, *140*:1686, 1989.

Marini JJ: Obtaining meaningful data from the Swan-Ganz catheter. Respir Care, *30*:572, 1985.

Mohsenifar Z, Goldbach P, Tashkin DP, et al.: The relationship between O_2 delivery and O_2 consumption in the adult respiratory distress syndrome. Chest, *84*:267, 1893.

Matuschak GM, Rinaldo JE: Organ interactions in the adult respiratory distress syndrome during sepsis: Role of liver in host defense. Chest, *94*:400, 1988.

Mollow WD, Dobson K, Girling L, et al.: Effects of dopamine on cardiopulmonary function and left ventricular volumes in patients with acute respiratory failure. Am Rev Respir Dis, *130(3)*:396, 1984.

Murray JF, Matthay MA, Luce JM, et al.: An expanded definition of the adult respiratory distress syndrome. Am Rev Respir Dis, *138*:720, 1988.

Pingleton SK, Bone RC, Ruth WE, Pingleton WW: Efficacy of low dose heparin in prevention of pulmonary emboli in a respiratory intensive care unit. Chest, *79*:647, 1981.

Pingleton SK, Harmon G: Nutritional management of acute respiratory failure. JAMA, *257*: 3094, 1987.

Pingleton SK: Complications of acute respiratory failure—State of the art review. Am Rev Respir Dis, *137*:1463, 1987.

Pingleton SK, Hinthorn D, Lui C: Enteral nutrition of patients receiving mechanical ventilation—multiple sources of tracheal colonization include the stomach. Am J Med, *80*:827, 1986.

Shoemaker WC, Appel PL, Kram HB, et al.: Prospective trial of supranormal values of survivors as therapeutic goals in high-risk surgical patients. Chest, *94*:1176, 1988.

Rubin DB, Matthay MA, Weinberg PF, et al.: Factor VIII antigen: Possible plasma marker of progressive acute lung injury in patients with sepsis. Am Rev Respir Dis, *131*:A142, 1985.

Schumacher PT, Samsel RW: Oxygen delivery and uptake by peripheral tissues: Physiology and pathophysiology. Critical Care Clinics, *5*:255, 1989.

Simmons RS, Berdine GG, Seidentfeld JJ, et al.: Fluid balance and the adult respiratory distress syndrome. Am Rev Respir Dis, *135*:924, 1987.

Stauffer JL, Silverstri RE: Complications of endotracheal intubation tracheostomy and artificial airways. Respir Care, *27*:417, 1982.

Suchyta MR, Clemmen TP, et al.: The adult respiratory distress syndrome: A report of survival and modifying factors. Chest, *101*:1074, 1992.

Weinberg PF, Matthay MA, Webster RO, et al.: Biologically active products of complement and acute lung injury in patients with sepsis syndrome. Am Rev Respir Dis, *130*:791, 1984.

Weisman IM, Rinaldo JE, Rogers RM: Positive end-expiratory pressure in adult respiratory failure. N Engl J Med, *307*:1381, 1982.

Westerman DE, Benatar SR, Potgieter PD, et al.: Identification of the high risk asthmatic patient. Am J Med, *66*:565, 1979.

Ziegler EJ, McCutchan L, Fierer J, et al.: Treatment of gram negative bacteremia and shock with human antiserum to a mutant Escherichia coli. N Engl J Med, *307*:1225, 1982.

29

MECHANICAL VENTILATION: PRINCIPLES AND MANAGEMENT

Paul L. Marino

CONVENTIONAL MECHANICAL VENTILATION

Conventional mechanical ventilation involves the use of positive-pressure devices that inflate the lungs by pushing gas into the upper airways, which is referred to as intermittent positive-pressure ventilation (IPPV). There are two principal methods of delivering IPPV in adults: pressure-cycled ventilation and volume-cycled ventilation.[1]

PRESSURE-CYCLED VENTILATION

Pressure-cycled ventilators inflate the lungs until a preset pressure is reached; the lung inflation is then terminated and exhalation is begun. The major drawback of this type of ventilation is the tendency for the inflation volume to vary with changes in the mechanical properties of the lungs (e.g., inflation volume will decrease if resistance in the airways increases or if the lungs become less distensible). For this reason, pressure-cycled ventilation is not recommended for patients with abnormal or unstable pulmonary function.

INDICATIONS

- Short-term ventilation of patients with normal lung function (e.g., postoperative awakening or respiratory failure due to neuromuscular disease)

Periodic inflations with pressure-cycled ventilators have been used to deliver nebulized bronchodilators and to reduce the risk for atelectasis in postoperative patients. However, these applications have been replaced by more effective and less expensive methods and are no longer recommended as routine practices.

CONTRAINDICATIONS

- Longterm ventilation of patients with underlying pulmonary disease
- Patients who are at risk for developing pulmonary complications during mechanical ventilation

840

Since most patients who require longterm mechanical ventilation either have underlying pulmonary disease or are at risk for developing pulmonary complications, pressure-cycled ventilation is not a common method of mechanical ventilation.

VOLUME-CYCLED VENTILATION

Volume-cycled ventilators are designed to inflate the lungs until a preset volume is reached, thereby ensuring a constant inflation volume even with changes in the mechanical properties of the lungs.

INDICATIONS

- The standard technique for patients with pulmonary disease, also recommended for ventilator-dependent patients at risk for developing pulmonary complications

AIRWAY PRESSURES

The waveforms produced by volume-cycled ventilators are shown in Figure 29–1. As shown in the upper graphs, the inspiratory flow rate ($\dot{V}$) is constant, producing a linear increase in lung volume (V). The pressure in the proximal airways (Pprox) shows a sharp initial deflection, produced by resistance in the larger airways, whereas the pressure in the distal airspaces (Palv) shows only a gradual rise throughout lung inflation. When airway resistance increases, the initial rise in proximal airway pressure is exaggerated, while the alveolar pressure is unchanged. When the compliance (distensibility) of the lungs diminishes, the rate of pressure increase is exaggerated in both the proximal and distal airways. These patterns illustrate two notable features of conventional mechanical ventilation

- When airway resistance is high (e.g., obstructive lung disease), the proximal airway pressure is not an accurate reflection of alveolar pressure
- When the lungs are stiff (e.g., pulmonary edema), the inflation pressure is easily transmitted to distal airspaces, increasing the risk for alveolar rupture and compression of the pulmonary microvessels

Thus, the proximal airway pressure, which is commonly displayed on the front panel of mechanical ventilators, must be interpreted according to the presence and type of underlying lung disease in each individual patient. An increase in proximal airway pressure will have different consequences in a patient with obstructive lung disease and a patient with pulmonary edema; this is an important consideration when excessive proximal airway pressures exist (see later discussion).

CARDIOVASCULAR INTERACTIONS

The influence of IPPV on the cardiovascular system is complex and is determined by the type of pulmonary disease (which determines the transmissibility of pressure to the distal airspaces) and by the balance between intravascular and intrathoracic pressures

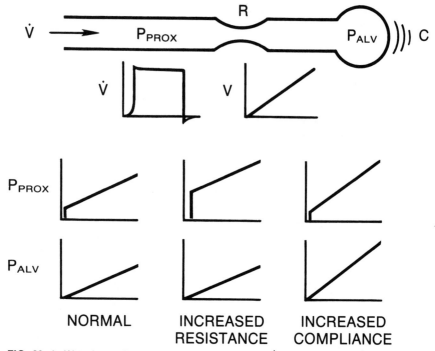

FIG. 29–1. Waveforms for volume-cycled ventilation. $\dot{V}$ = inspiratory flow rate; V = inflation volume; R = airway resistance; Pprox = proximal airway pressure; Palv = alveolar pressure. Lower series of graphs illustrate the effects of lung mechanics on airway pressures.

- Positive intrathoracic pressure can increase the cardiac output when the blood volume is normal.[2] This is the result of a decrease in left ventricular afterload; i.e., afterload is defined as the peak transmural pressure across the wall of the ventricle, and positive pressure around the heart will decrease this transmural pressure

- Positive intrathoracic pressure will decrease cardiac output when intravascular volume is reduced.[2,3] This is the result of a decrease in venous return and a drop in ventricular end-diastolic volume

The ability of positive intrathoracic pressure to augment cardiac output in normovolemic subjects has been proposed as the underlying mechanism for the ability of closed chest compressions to promote cardiac output during cardiopulmonary resuscitation.[4] This mechanism is called the "thoracic pump," while the traditional view of squeezing the heart between the sternum and bony spine during CPR is called the "cardiac pump" mechanism. This highlights the potential value of positive intrathoracic pressure in assisting cardiac function and stresses the value of preventing hypovolemia during mechanical ventilation.

INDICATIONS FOR MECHANICAL VENTILATION

INDICATIONS FOR ASSISTED VENTILATION

- The inability to maintain adequate arterial oxygenation (i.e., arterial PO_2 > 60 mmHg or oxyhemoglobin saturation > 90%) during spontaneous ventilation, despite supplemental oxygen inhalation
- When toxic levels of inspired oxygen (i.e., fractional concentration of oxygen in inspired gas above 50%) required to maintain adequate arterial oxygenation
- Acute respiratory acidosis
- Respiratory distress with high minute ventilation (i.e., above 10 L/min) without an acute respiratory alkalosis. Stated another way, the inability of hyperventilation to eliminate CO_2. This state indicates a high degree of "dead space" ventilation, where alveolar gas does not equilibrate fully with pulmonary capillary blood

INDICATIONS FOR ENDOTRACHEAL INTUBATION

The following indications for endotracheal intubation do not necessarily mandate the need for mechanical ventilation

- Depressed mental status, with risk for aspiration and/or inability to clear secretions
- Trauma to the head-and-neck region

There is a tendency to delay intubation and mechanical ventilation as long as possible, in the hopes that it will not be necessary, and this can be dangerous. If the patient's condition is severe enough to warrant consideration of intubation and mechanical ventilation, then it is wise to proceed with this course of action without delay. In other words, "whenever in doubt, intubate and ventilate." Once the airway is controlled and the patient's ventilation is supported, the subsequent evaluation and initiation of therapy can be carried out more safely.

INITIATING MECHANICAL VENTILATION

Some recommendations for initial ventilator settings are listed in Table 29–1, and each is briefly discussed below.

MODE OF VENTILATION

The initial mode of ventilation that is most commonly selected is the assist/control mode, in which the patient can initiate the mechanical breath by generating a small negative intrathoracic pressure (assisted ventilation) or the ventilator will automatically deliver lung inflations at a preset rate if the patient has no spontaneous efforts (controlled ventilations). Patients with excessive respiratory rates may pose a problem during assisted ventilation because of the tendency to create auto-PEEP (described later in this

TABLE 29–1 RECOMMENDATIONS FOR INITIAL VENTILATOR SETTINGS*

Ventilatory Mode:	Assist–Control Ventilation
Tidal Volume (Vt):	10–15 ml/kg (ideal body weight)
	If peak inflation pressure > 30 cmH$_2$O, consider 5–6 ml/kg
Respiratory Rate:	12–14 breaths/minute
	or
	RR × Vt = 80–90 ml/kg
Inspiratory–Expiratory Time Ratio:	1:3
Inspired Oxygen (FIO$_2$):	100%, then decrease to lowest FIO$_2$ for SaO$_2$ > 90% by pulse oximetry

* From Ponte J: Indications for mechanical ventilation. Thorax, 45:885, 1990.

chapter). In this situation, the options are to sedate the patient or select a mode of ventilation that is designed to augment spontaneous ventilation, such as intermittent mandatory ventilation (IMV) or pressure-support ventilation (PSV), which are described later in this chapter.

INFLATION VOLUME

Mechanical ventilators are commonly set to deliver inflation volumes of 10 to 15 ml/kg ideal body weight; these volumes are considerably larger than the normal tidal volumes of 5 to 6 ml/kg recorded in healthy adults.[5–7] The high inflation volumes were adopted in the early days of positive pressure ventilation, when the inability to deliver periodic "sighs" created the fear of promoting progressive atelectasis during prolonged periods of mechanical ventilation. However, the addition of mechanical sighs (1.5 times the inflation volume, delivered at a rate of 10 to 20 per hour, in pairs) has not been shown to produce a sustained improvement in lung function.[8] In addition, the introduction of mechanical sighs to conventional mechanical ventilation does not prompt a decrease in the recommended inflation volumes. The results of these excessive inflation volumes are a common tendency for overventilation with respiratory alkalosis during mechanical ventilation[9] and the risk of barotrauma, with disruption of alveolar and capillary integrity.[10] The latter risk has gained much attention in recent years and has led to recommendations to use inflation volumes of 5 or 6 ml/kg when the conventional inflation volumes cause excessively high proximal airway pressures.[6,11] When delivering mechanical ventilation to patients with lung resection, the inflation volume should be adjusted to keep the peak inflation pressure below 20 cmH$_2$O.[6]

Also important is the influence of the connector tubing between the patient and the ventilator on the inflation volume that reaches the patient. This tubing will expand in response to positive pressure, and the volume of gas taken up by this expansion is lost from the inflation volume that reaches the patient. As such, this volume must be subtracted from the original inflation volume to determine the actual volume that enters the patient's lungs. The volume of gas lost in this process is a function of the peak inflation pressure (Ppk) and the compliance (or distensibility) of the specific tubes being used. The usual compliance of ventilator tubing is 3 to 4 ml/cm H_2O, which means that 3 to 4 ml of inflation volume is lost for every 1 cm H_2O of positive inflation pressure exerted on the walls of the tubing. Thus, at high inflation pressure, a considerable volume can be lost in the tubing. This is illustrated in the following example.

For a tidal volume (Vt) of 700 ml and tube compliance of 4 ml/cm H_2O

- If Ppk = 20 cm H_2O, actual Vt = 620 ml
- If Ppk = 40 cm H_2O, actual Vt = 540 ml
- If Ppk = 80 cm H_2O, actual Vt = 380 ml

At the highest Ppk, over half of the original inflation volume is lost in the tubing and never reaches the patient; this can produce inadequate alveolar ventilation and can aggravate the underlying respiratory failure. This complication occurs primarily in patients with very stiff lungs (e.g., pulmonary edema) and necessitates an increase in machine inflation volume to help compensate for the lost volume. Newer ventilators can adjust for the lost volume to ensure that the patient is receiving the desired volume.

RESPIRATORY RATE

The rate of lung inflation is commonly set between 12 and 16 breaths/minute, but patients who are able to trigger the ventilator will breathe at their intrinsic respiratory rate. Therefore, the respiratory rate set on the ventilator is not necessarily the respiratory rate experienced by the patient. The rate of lung inflation should be kept under 20 breaths/minute to minimize the risk of air trapping in distal airspaces due to inadequate time for exhalation.

INSPIRATORY–EXPIRATORY TIME RATIO

The combination of high inflation volumes and increased resistance in the airways creates a tendency for air trapping in the distal airspaces; thus, it is important to allow sufficient time for exhalation. This is performed by adjusting the rate of gas flow during lung inflation so that the inflation time is one-half to one-third of the exhalation time, an Inhalation:Exhalation time ratio (I:E ratio) of 1:2 or 1:3. The ratio is displayed continuously on the front panel of the ventilator and can easily be monitored while adjusting the inspiratory gas flow until the desired ratio is achieved. This is usually performed by the respiratory therapists, but physicians should keep track of this ratio when making "ventilator rounds." A recently introduced method of ventilation that features a reversal of the I:E ratio (i.e., inflation time greater than exhalation time) has generated some interest in patients who are refractory to conventional ventilation (see later discussion in this chapter).

INSPIRED OXYGEN

The fractional concentration of inspired oxygen (FIO_2) should be high initially to prevent undesirable hypoxemia in the time period that preceeds the first blood gas analysis. If pulse oximetry is being used, the FIO_2 can be decreased rapidly, as long as the arterial O_2 saturation is above 90%. The goal is to achieve the lowest possible FIO_2 needed to maintain adequate arterial oxygenation (see later discussion of O_2 inhalation and O_2 toxicity).

SPECIAL MODES OF VENTILATION

A variety of specialized patterns of ventilation are available on modern mechanical ventilators, each with specific benefits as well as drawbacks. There is a tendency to view these special modes of ventilation as a form of therapy, but it is unlikely that turning a knob on a ventilator will arrest or reverse a pathologic process in the patient, and there is no clear evidence that any of these ventilatory patterns will hasten recovery. Five of the more common modes of mechanical ventilation are described in this section.

INTERMITTENT MANDATORY VENTILATION

• Designed to augment spontaneous minute ventilation
• Used primarily for patients with respiratory alkalosis from assist/control ventilation and for weaning patients from mechanical ventilation
• Benefits over conventional mechanical ventilation are unproven

Intermittent mandatory ventilation (IMV) intersperses positive-pressure lung inflations with the patient's spontaneous breaths, using a circuit like the one shown in Figure 29–2. The patient is connected to the source of inhaled gas through two parallel circuits, one containing the ventilator and one containing a reservoir bag with the inhaled gas mixture. A unidirectional valve in the circuit allows the patient to breathe spontaneously from the reservoir bag when a ventilator breath is not being delivered. The pattern of ventilation that results is illustrated in Figure 29–3. The upper panel shows the pattern obtained with the early IMV systems. Note that the mechanical breath (solid line) is delivered at the height of the spontaneous inspiration (dashed line). This random style of delivery was poorly tolerated by patients; the system was modified so that machine breaths were delivered only when the patient first started to inhale. The modified IMV system produces a breathing pattern like the one shown in the middle

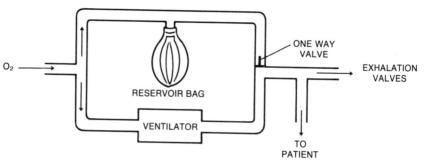

FIG. 29–2. Schematic diagram of the circuit for intermittent mandatory ventilation (IMV). FIO_2 is the fractional concentration of inspired oxygen.

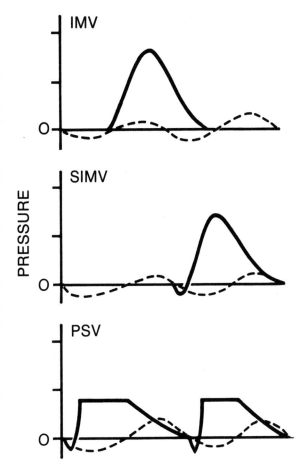

FIG. 29–3. Proximal airway pressure profiles for three methods used to augment spontaneous ventilation. IMV: intermittent mandatory ventilation; SIMV: synchronized IMV; PSV: pressure support ventilation (PSV). Augmented breaths shown as solid lines; spontaneous breaths shown as dashed lines. Proximal airway pressure on vertical axis.

panel of Figure 29–3. This is referred to as synchronized IMV (S-IMV) and is standard on most ventilators. IMV and S-IMV will be used interchangeably in this chapter.

USE AND MISUSE

Shortly after its introduction, IMV was proposed as an alternative method for weaning adults from mechanical ventilation[12] and, despite any evidence that it is superior to conventional methods of weaning,[13] IMV has become the most popular method of weaning patients from mechanical ventilation in this country. However, the focus in this section will be the utility of IMV as a mode of ventilation rather than a mode of weaning (see later discussion for a description of IMV in weaning).

TABLE 29-2 INTERMITTENT MANDATORY VENTILATION (IMV) VERSUS CONVENTIONAL MECHANICAL VENTILATION (CMV)		
ADVANTAGES OF IMV VERSUS CMV	PROVEN	UNPROVEN
Less respiratory alkalosis	X	
Improves cardiac output		X
Prevents respiratory muscle atrophy		X
DISADVANTAGES OF IMV VERSUS CMV		
Increases work of breathing	X	
Promotes respiratory muscle fatigue		X
Unresponsive to patient's ventilatory needs	X	

A brief list of the advantages and disadvantages of IMV relative to conventional mechanical ventilation (CMV) is shown in Table 29-2. Few of the proposed advantages of IMV have been validated or tested in clinical studies,[13] and the following is a brief summary of current knowledge.

OVERVENTILATION

Overventilation with respiratory alkalosis is a common occurrence during mechanical ventilation with the conventional assist/control mode of ventilation[9] and is particularly prevalent in patients with rapid breathing. Although IMV reduces the tendency for respiratory alkalosis during mechanical ventilation, the higher arterial PCO_2 during IMV compared to CMV is caused by an increase in the rate of CO_2 production rather than a decrease in alveolar ventilation.[14] This indicates that the effect of IMV on arterial PCO_2 is due to an increased work of breathing, which is not desirable.

CARDIAC OUTPUT

The ability of CMV to reduce cardiac output by reducing venous return to the heart (described earlier) is one of the principal reasons for the popularity of IMV,[15] since the ability for negative-pressure breathing with IMV should pose less of a risk for reducing venous return. However, the available evidence indicates that cardiac output does not increase when IMV is substituted for CMV and can actually decrease when IMV is imposed on patients with left ventricular dysfunction.[16,17]

DIAPHRAGM STRENGTH

Although the diaphragm is not a voluntary muscle, there is a popular belief that the diaphragm becomes weak from disuse atrophy during mechanical ventilation. If this were the case, the ability to breathe spontaneously during IMV could be beneficial by permitting continued contraction of the diaphragm. However, there is no evidence that diaphragm strength is greater with IMV than with CMV.[13]

PRESSURE SUPPORT VENTILATION

- Designed to augment tidal volume during spontaneous breathing
- Used primarily to aid in weaning from mechanical ventilation
- Benefits over conventional methods of weaning are unproven

Pressure support ventilation (PSV) is, like IMV, a method for augmenting a patient's spontaneous ventilation, but while IMV augments minute ventilation, PSV augments tidal volume.[18] The airway pressure profile from PSV is illustrated in Figure 29–3 (lower panel). At the onset of each spontaneous breath, the negative pressure generated by the patient opens a valve that delivers the inspired gas at the desired pressure (usually 5 to 10 cm H_2O). This increases the tidal volume while reducing the work of breathing.[18]

The level of pressure selected during PSV can be taken as either maximum inspiratory pressure (PImax) generated during spontaneous breathing or the difference between peak airway pressure and plateau pressure during mechanical ventilation.[19]

$$Pressure = PImax/3 \text{ or } Ppk - Ppl$$

The use of PImax assumes that a patient will not be able to generate three times the PImax without developing fatigue. The proximal airway pressure method uses the notion that the difference $Ppk - Ppl$ is the pressure needed to overcome resistance in the larger airways and the endotracheal tube, and that PSV could reduce the work of breathing by overcoming this resistance.

INDICATIONS

PSV has become a popular method for weaning patients from mechanical ventilation. However, there is no evidence that PSV is superior to conventional methods of weaning.[10] The benefits of PSV are unproven.

POSITIVE END-EXPIRATORY PRESSURE

- Designed to prevent alveolar collapse in conditions that reduce lung distensibility
- Primarily indicated for decreasing inhaled oxygen to nontoxic levels in patients with the adult respiratory distress syndrome.[20,21] It does not reduce lung water (i.e., it is not therapeutic) and can actually increase edema formation if excessive[22–24]
- Can be harmful if used in localized lung disease (e.g., pneumonia)[20,21]
- Tends to decrease cardiac output, which can offset any improvement in arterial oxygenation.[20,21,25–28] Therefore, monitoring arterial oxygenation alone can be misleading for determining the influence of positive end-expiratory pressure (PEEP) on systemic oxygen delivery in individual patients

PEEP ventilation maintains a positive pressure in the distal airspaces through the ventilatory cycle, thereby reducing the tendency for collapse

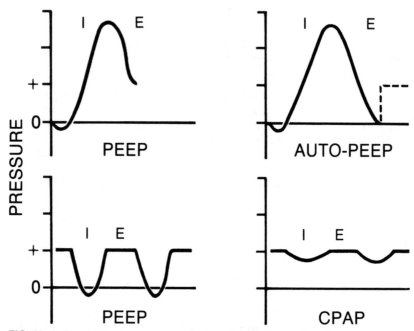

FIG. 29–4. Proximal airway pressure profiles for positive end-expiratory pressure (PEEP) and continuous positive airway pressure (CPAP). Upper panels show profiles from mechanical ventilation; lower panels are spontaneous breaths. I denotes inhalation, E denotes exhalation.

of the distal airspaces. The airway pressure profile with PEEP ventilation is shown in Figure 29–4. A pressure-limiting valve in the expiratory tubing does not allow the pressure in the airways to return to atmospheric (zero) pressure at the end of expiration. The positive pressure in the alveoli at end-expiration helps maintain the functional residual capacity (resting lung volume) and thereby preserves the gas exchange between alveoli and pulmonary capillaries. When applied to patients with noncardiogenic pulmonary edema or adult respiratory distress syndrome (ARDS), PEEP increases lung distensibility and decreases intrapulmonary shunting, thereby improving arterial oxygenation and allowing a decrease in the level of inspired oxygen (FIO_2). This is particularly valuable when the levels of inhaled oxygen are in the toxic range (i.e., $FIO_2 > 50\%$).

CARDIOVASCULAR EFFECTS

The cardiac effects of PEEP are identical to the cardiac effects of positive-pressure ventilation described earlier. Cardiac output can be augmented when airway pressures are not excessive and the lungs are normal; when airway pressures are high and the lungs are stiff, PEEP often produces a decrease in cardiac output.[20,25–28] The latter effect is primarily due to a decrease in ventricular filling, but systolic function can also be de-

TABLE 29–3 SPECTRUM OF PEEP EFFECTS ON OXYGEN TRANSPORT			
ARTERIAL O$_2$ SAT	**CARDIAC OUTPUT**	**O$_2$ DELIVERY**	**INTERPRETATION**
A. ↑	→	↑	Benefit
B. ↑	↓	→	No help
C. ↑	↓ ↓	↓	Harmful

pressed.[20,28] The mechanism for the negative inotropic effects of PEEP includes a reduction in coronary blood flow[27] and the release of a negative inotropic substance from the lungs.[28]

OXYGEN DELIVERY

The rate of oxygen delivery in arterial blood is determined by the cardiac output (Q), the arterial hemoglobin concentration (Hb), and the percent saturation of hemoglobin with oxygen (SaO$_2$).

$$O_2 \text{ Delivery} = Q \times Hb \times SaO_2 \text{ (ml/min)}$$

The influence of PEEP on oxygen delivery depends on the net balance between the changes in SaO$_2$ and cardiac output. This is demonstrated in Table 29–3. The three situations in this table represent equivalent increases in SaO$_2$. In situation A, there is an increase in oxygen delivery because the cardiac output does not decrease. In situation B, the increase in SaO$_2$ is offset by a decrease in cardiac output and O$_2$ delivery is unchanged. In situation C, the decrease in cardiac output exceeds the increase in SaO$_2$ and O$_2$ delivery is diminished. This illustrates the lack of correlation between arterial oxygenation and systemic oxygen delivery during ventilation with PEEP. In other words, the arterial PO$_2$ can be misleading during ventilation with PEEP, and it is advisable to monitor oxygen delivery to determine the effects of PEEP.

APPLICATIONS

- The major indication for PEEP is in patients with pulmonary edema (or any diffuse lung process that decreases FRC) when toxic levels of inspired oxygen (FIO$_2$ > 50%) are required to maintain adequate arterial oxygenation (SaO$_2$ > 90%)

When the pathologic process is confined to a portion of the lung (e.g., lobar pneumonia), PEEP can worsen the hypoxemia by overdistending the normal lung and directing flow to the diseased segment.[19] When lung disease is localized, hypoxic vasoconstriction in the diseased area directs blood flow away from that area and toward normal areas of lung, which helps preserve gas exchange. When PEEP is applied in this situation, it is distributed unevenly because it is applied more to normal lung areas. This overdistends the normal alveoli and redirects blood back to the diseased segments, counteracting the inherent tendencies to maintain ventilation–

perfusion balance. Therefore, PEEP is not recommended for localized lung disease unless it is selectively applied to the diseased lung using differential lung inflation techniques

- Prophylactic PEEP has been recommended in patients at risk for developing the adult respiratory distress syndrome (ARDS). However, the routine use of PEEP does not reduce the incidence of ARDS in susceptible patients[29]

There is a tendency to apply low levels of PEEP to all patients who are intubated because of the widespread belief that low levels of PEEP are created in normal individuals by glottic closure at the end of expiration. However, end-expiratory glottic closure (or physiologic PEEP) has been demonstrated only in neonates with respiratory distress, and the routine application of PEEP in adults has no proven benefit[30]

- PEEP is commonly applied following thoracotomy to prevent or control mediastinal bleeding. However, there is no convincing evidence that PEEP reduces the risk of postoperative mediastinal bleeding[31] or that it reduces the severity of bleeding once it starts[32]

The application of PEEP for intrathoracic hemorrhages has little basis in the physiology of intrathoracic pressure transmission. That is, PEEP will be transmitted, at least in part, into the lumen of intrathoracic blood vessels, so the transmural pressure will not change appreciably. Since transmural pressure is the pressure governing the tendency for bleeding, this should not be reduced by the application of PEEP.

COMPLICATIONS

In addition to the decrease in cardiac output, PEEP can cause any one of the following complications

- Barotrauma (e.g., pneumothorax)
- Fluid retention
- Increased intracranial pressure

Barotrauma from PEEP is controversial. Some studies report a higher incidence of pneumothorax with PEEP,[33] while others observed no correlation between PEEP and barotrauma.[34] The variable correlation between PEEP and barotrauma is not surprising since peak inspiratory pressure may be the more important factor in determining the risk of barotrauma.[24] The other important factor is the type of lung disease. Pulmonary barotrauma is discussed in more detail later in this chapter.

Fluid retention is common with positive-pressure ventilation and with PEEP.[34] Several mechanisms have been proposed, including depression of atrial natriuretic factor (ANF) and stimulation of antidiuretic hormone (ADH). Compression of the atria from hyperinflated lungs is the proposed mechanism for the decrease in ANF and the increase in ADH.[35] Stimulation of the sympathetic nervous system may also be responsible for a redistribution of renal blood flow favoring perfusion of sodium-conserving nephrons.[34] The purpose of the fluid retention may be to promote cardiac output in the face of high intrathoracic pressures, but the disadvantages of fluid overload are not to be overlooked.

Intracranial hypertension is a variable finding when PEEP is administered to head-injured patients.[36] The mechanism is probably the increase in pressure in the superior vena cava associated with PEEP, and the effect is more prominent in patients with reduced cerebral compliance. The variability of the response may be due to the lack of monitoring peak and mean intrathoracic pressures in the available studies. Intracranial pressure monitoring is advised when high intrathoracic pressures are present in head injury patients who are prone to increased intracranial pressure.

CONTINUOUS POSITIVE AIRWAY PRESSURE

Continuous positive airway pressure (CPAP) is defined as "a pressure above atmospheric maintained at the airway opening throughout the respiratory cycle during spontaneous breathing."[37] The breathing pattern produced by CPAP is shown in Figure 29–4, along with the pattern produced by PEEP during spontaneous breathing (lower left panel). Note that the end-expiratory pressure is the same with CPAP and PEEP, but the pressure excursion during inspiration is much greater with PEEP. The larger excursion with PEEP increases the work of breathing, which is the fundamental difference between spontaneous PEEP and CPAP.

The difference in inspiratory pressure excursion between CPAP and PEEP is due to differences in the pressure across a one-way valve in the circuits (see Figure 29–5). The valve in both circuits requires a pressure gradient of 2 cm H_2O to open. The valve in the PEEP circuit has atmospheric pressure on the side opposite the patient, so the patient must generate a pressure equal to the PEEP plus 2 cm H_2O. The CPAP circuit uses an anesthesia bag to apply a positive pressure to the side of the valve opposite the patient so that the pressure generated by the patient to open the valve is reduced by the amount of positive pressure applied. This is how CPAP reduces the work of breathing.

INDICATIONS

- The major use of CPAP is to postpone or prevent intubation in patients with ARDS and refractory hypoxemia

CPAP is delivered via specially designed masks equipped with pressure-limiting valves. These masks must be tightly fitted and cannot be removed to allow patients to eat. Because of poor patient tolerance, these masks are used as temporary measures only. CPAP can also be applied through artificial airways and was once popular for weaning patients from mechanical ventilation. However, CPAP weaning has largely been abandoned.

INVERSE-RATIO VENTILATION

- Characterized by an I:E ratio = 2:1 to 4:1
- Used in cases of refractory hypoxemia to prevent pulmonary oxygen toxicity

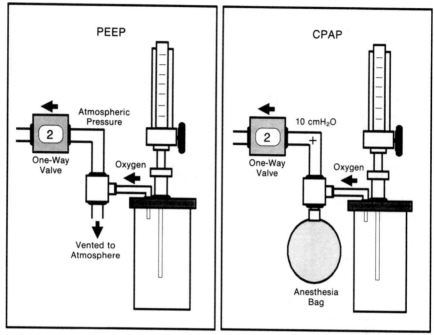

FIG. 29–5. Diagrams of the inhalation circuits for CPAP (right side) and "spontaneous PEEP." Unidirectional valve in each circuit opens when pressure differential reaches 2 cmH$_2$O. See text for explanation.

Inverse-ratio ventilation (IRV) is characterized by an increase in inspiratory time to at least twice the expiratory time, thereby reversing the inspiratory–expiratory time from a normal I:E ratio of 1:2 to 1:4 (see Table 29–1) to an I:E ratio of 2:1 to 4:1.[38] This is meant to recruit alveolar units that have collapsed, thereby improving gas exchange from alveoli to pulmonary capillaries and improving arterial oxygenation. Pressure-cycled ventilation is recommended during IRV because the inspiratory flow rate decreases exponentially during inflation in pressure-cycled ventilation, which should help minimize the risk of overinflation and alveolar rupture during IRV.[39] Although clinical experience with IRV is limited, the available reports show that IRV is associated with dramatic improvements in arterial oxygenation without adverse effects on cardiac output.[39] More experience is needed with IRV before this mode of ventilation is recommended for routine clinical use.

MONITORING LUNG FUNCTION DURING MECHANICAL VENTILATION

Despite the fact that severe pulmonary dysfunction is the most common cause for prolonged mechanical ventilation, there are few methods for accurately assessing pulmonary functions at the bedside in ventilator-dependent patients. The proximal airway pressure has been used to assess the mechanical properties of the lungs at the bedside;[40] the following paragraphs will describe this method and its applications in the intensive care unit.

INTERPRETATION OF AIRWAY PRESSURES

The pressure in the proximal airways is monitored continuously during mechanical ventilation and displayed on the front panel of the ventilator. Figure 29–6 illustrates how this pressure can be used to assess the mechanical properties of the lungs. At a given inflation volume, the Ppk varies directly with the resistance (R) in the airways and inversely with the compliance (C) or distensibility of the lung parenchyma (i.e., Ppl $\propto$ R + 1/C). An increase in Ppk can signal either an increase in airway resistance, a decrease in lung compliance, or both. The two components of lung me-

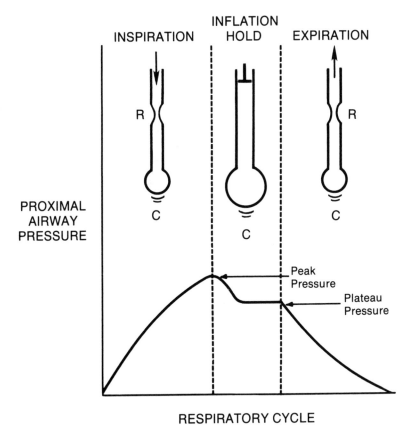

FIG. 29–6. Proximal airway pressure during an "inflation hold" maneuver. See text for explanation.

chanics can be separated by occluding the expiratory tubing at the end of inspiration to hold the inflation volume in the lungs (see Figure 29–6). This removes airflow, which will remove the influence of airway resistance on Ppk. The pressure obtained in the absence of airflow, called the plateau pressure (Ppl), represents the elastic recoil pressure of the lungs and the chest wall structures. Since compliance is the reciprocal of elastance, then Ppl is inversely related to compliance (Ppl $\propto$ 1/C). Thus, as the lungs become stiffer (less compliant), the plateau pressure will increase and vice versa. Finally, the difference between Ppk and Ppl is the pressure needed to overcome airflow resistance and is proportional to the resistance in the airways. These relationships are summarized below:

$$Ppk \propto 1/C$$

$$Ppk - Ppl \propto R$$

It is important to emphasize that the proximal airway pressure is measured as a transthoracic pressure (i.e., measured relative to atmospheric pressure) and not a transpulmonary pressure (i.e., measured relative to intraplural pressure). Therefore, it can be influenced by the chest wall structures as well as the lungs. For this reason, it is imperative to ensure that the patient is completely at rest when measuring this pressure, to eliminate any contribution from contraction of the chest wall muscles.

COMPLIANCE

The "compliance" of a structure is a measure of its distensibility or deformability and is the reciprocal of elastance. The compliance of a container like the thorax is expressed as the ratio of change in volume to change in pressure in the container. The static compliance (Cstat) of the thorax can then be derived by determining the Ppl associated with a specific inflation volume, as shown in the example below:

When Vt $= 800$ ml and Ppl $= 10$ cm H_2O:

$$Cstat = Vt/Ppl = 800/10$$

$$= 80 \text{ ml/cm } H_2O$$

Since compliance is actually a measure of the change in volume and pressure, the correct method for determining compliance is to measure Ppl at more than one tidal volume and generate a pressure–volume curve like the one shown in Figure 29–7. The slope of this curve varies directly with Cstat (i.e., a decrease in slope indicates a decrease in compliance) and vice versa.

The Cstat in normal subjects during spontaneous breathing is >0.09 L/cm H_2O,[41] while the value in intubated patients without lung disease is reported at 0.05 to 0.07 L/cm H_2O.[42] Most of the lung diseases that are responsible for acute respiratory failure cause a decrease in lung compliance (e.g., pulmonary edema, pneumonia), while resolution of the disease will result in a return of the compliance to normal or baseline levels.

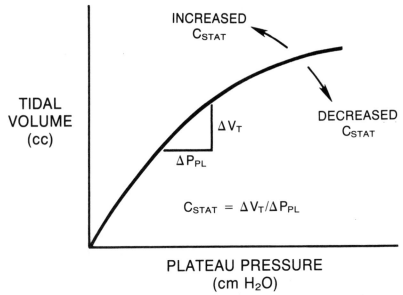

TIDAL VOLUME (cc)

INCREASED C_{STAT}

DECREASED C_{STAT}

ΔV_T

ΔP_{PL}

$C_{STAT} = \Delta V_T / \Delta P_{PL}$

PLATEAU PRESSURE
(cm H_2O)

FIG. 29–7. Static pressure–volume curve. C_{stat} = static compliance of the lungs and chest wall; P_{pl} = plateau pressure; V_t = tidal (inflation) volume.

AIRWAY RESISTANCE

The resistance to airflow during inspiration (R) can be estimated by determining the pressure needed to overcome airflow resistance (i.e., Ppk − Ppl) and dividing this by the inspiratory flow rate (Vinsp). An example of this calculation is shown below:

When Ppk = 22 cm H_2O, Ppl = 10 cm H_2O, and Vinsp = 40 L/sec,

$$R = Ppk - Ppl/Vinsp$$
$$= 22 - 10/40$$
$$= 0.3 \text{ cm } H_2O/L/sec$$

This resistance represents the summed resistance of the connector tubing, the tracheal tube, and the airways. However, changes in R should represent changes in airway resistance as long as the inspiratory flow rate and the size of the tracheal tube and connector tubing are constant. In intubated patients without lung disease, Rinsp is 4 to 6 cm $H_2O/L/sec$.[42,44]

The major limitation in the resistance measurement may be the sensitivity of inspiratory resistance as an indication of resistance in the small airways. That is, airflow obstruction in the small airways is usually measured during expiration (particularly forced expiration), and the distending pressures delivered by the ventilator during inspiration may keep the small airways open. If this is the case, measurement of airflow resistance during inspiration may not be a sensitive measure of changes in small airway resistance.[45] However, measurement of airflow resistance during expiration cannot be performed routinely in a clinical setting, therefore, the inspiratory resistance measurement is the only index of airway resistance routinely available at the bedside.

PRACTICAL APPLICATIONS

The pressures in the proximal airways may be valuable in the following clinical situations:

Troubleshooting

When a ventilator-dependent patient develops sudden onset of respiratory distress or worsening blood gases, the proximal airway pressures can provide a simple, rapid method to identify the problem at the bedside. This approach is outlined in Figure 29–8

- If the peak pressure is increased but the plateau pressure is unchanged, the problem is an increase in airways resistance. The major concerns are: 1) obstruction of the tracheal tube, 2) secretions, and 3) bronchospasm
- If the peak and plateau pressures are increased, the problem is a decrease in compliance of the lungs and/or chest wall (or the presence of auto-PEEP, which is described later in this chapter). The major concerns are: 1) pneumothorax, 2) lobar atelectasis, and 3) pulmonary edema
- If the peak pressure is decreased, the problem may be an air leak in the system. The major concerns are: 1) an air leak around the endotracheal tube cuff, 2) the patient is not connected to the ventilator circuit, 3) hyperventilation; i.e., the patient is generating enough negative intrathoracic pressure to pull air into the lungs

The sensitivity of the proximal airway pressures in detecting changes in the mechanical properties of the lungs is not known, but the method is probably not sensitive to changes in pulmonary function. Therefore, the absence of a change in proximal airway pressures should not be used as evidence for the absence of a change in lung function.

Monitoring Clinical Course

In patients with decreased lung compliance from pulmonary edema, diffuse pneumonia, etc., routine monitoring of plateau pressures may help in following the clinical course of the disease. The tidal volume must be constant when interpreting changes in plateau pressure.

In patients with airway disease from asthma, COPD, etc., the difference between peak and plateau pressures can be used to follow the resistance in the airways. Once again, the tidal volume should be constant when interpreting changes in these pressures.

Assessing Response to Bronchodilators

The routine administration of bronchodilators is a common practice in patients requiring mechanical ventilation, but there is no clear documentation that this is beneficial for all patients. In any patient, the response

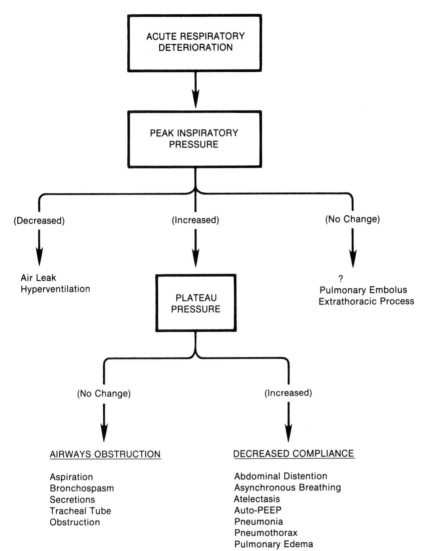

FIG. 29–8. Flow diagram for interpreting changes in proximal airway pressures. See text for explanation.

to inhaled bronchodilators can be evaluated using the peak inspiratory pressure. Inhaled beta agonists decrease airway resistance and increase lung compliance,[46] and either of these effects should decrease peak inspiratory pressures. Therefore, to determine whether a nebulized bronchodilator is effective, the peak pressure should be monitored just before giving the agent and again 30 to 60 minutes later. A decrease in peak pressure can then be used as evidence that the bronchodilator is having an effect.

Evaluating PEEP. The application of PEEP should keep alveoli open and, thus, PEEP should decrease lung compliance. The plateau pressure should provide a means of assessing the effects of PEEP on lung function at the bedside; i.e., the plateau pressure should decrease after the application of PEEP. It is important to remember to subtract the amount of PEEP from the plateau pressure when interpreting changes in Ppl.

AUTO-PEEP

Overinflation is common in ventilator-dependent patients due to the prevalence of obstructive airway disease and the tendency for rapid breathing in these patients, coupled with the high inflation volumes used in conventional mechanical ventilation. These combine to produce incomplete exhalation and positive alveolar pressure at the end of exhalation. Figure 29–9 illustrates the principle involved in this phenomenon.

Pathogenesis

In the normal lung, there is no airflow at the end of expiration, and the pressure in the alveoli is the same as the pressure in the most proximal airways (i.e., atmospheric pressure). However, when exhalation is incom-

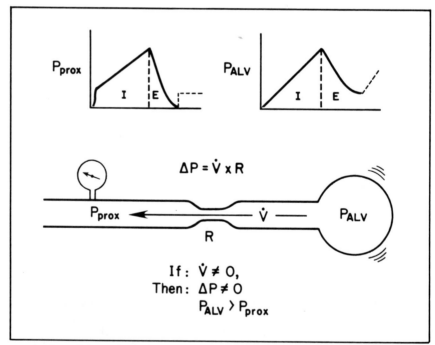

FIG. 29–9. The principle of auto-PEEP. Q = airflow; R = resistance to flow in airways; P_{ALV} = alveolar pressure; Pprox = proximal airway pressure; I = inhalation; E = exhalation. Graph in upper left shows proximal airways after tube occlusion at end-expiration. Graph in upper right shows the proximal pressure profile with externally added PEEP.

plete and there is airflow at the end of expiration, there will be a pressure difference between the alveoli and the proximal airways, creating a positive alveolar pressure at end-expiration. This PEEP is commonly called intrinsic PEEP or auto-PEEP[47] and has the same physiologic effects described earlier for PEEP that is externally applied. Auto-PEEP is common (and may be universal) in patients with obstructive lung disease who are receiving mechanical ventilation, and it is particularly troublesome in patients with status asthmaticus.[48]

Diagnosis

Auto-PEEP is often overlooked because the proximal airway pressure (monitored on the front panel of the ventilator) often returns to zero at end-expiration, despite the presence of positive pressure in the distal airspaces. However, when the expiratory tubing is occluded at the end of expiration to eliminate airflow and thereby eliminate the pressure drop along the airways, the presence of auto-PEEP will be signaled by a sudden increase in the proximal airway pressure (see upper left panel in Figure 29–9). The magnitude of auto-PEEP is difficult to determine precisely, because manual occlusion cannot be timed to the very end of expiration.

Routine Monitoring

Routine monitoring for auto-PEEP is recommended for ventilation-dependent patients because

- Auto-PEEP is prevalent in ventilator-dependent patients, particularly those with underlying obstructive lung disease[34]
- Auto-PEEP has the same adverse consequences as externally applied PEEP (e.g., a decrease in cardiac output)
- Auto-PEEP increases the proximal airway pressures (peak and plateau pressure) and can falsely lower the estimated lung compliance
- Auto-PEEP can be transmitted into the intrathoracic blood vessels, producing false elevations in the central venous pressure and the pulmonary capillary wedge pressure
- The response to bronchodilators can be assessed by monitoring changes in auto-PEEP

When auto-PEEP is present, the peak and plateau airway pressures will be increased by the same amount as the auto-PEEP, and this can lead to a spuriously low compliance determination.[1] The following relationship is applicable for compliance determinations in the presence of auto-PEEP:

$$Cstat = Vt \times (Ppl - PEEP)L/cm\ H_2O$$

Auto-PEEP can also be transmitted into the pulmonary circulation and can falsely elevate the ventricular filling pressures, which will lead to errors in interpretation and unnecessary therapeutic maneuvers. For example, a patient who suddenly becomes tachypneic and displays an increase in the pulmonary capillary wedge pressure is commonly felt to have heart failure. However, the problem could be auto-PEEP from rapid breathing, which would produce a spurious increase in the wedge pressure without heart failure. This demonstrates the importance for routine monitoring of auto-PEEP.

Management

When auto-PEEP is detected, it is important to minimize the factors that create overinflation. The following maneuvers should help to reduce the tendency for overinflation

- Decrease the inflation volume
- Increase exhalation time by decreasing the respiratory rate and increasing the rate of lung inflation
- Add external PEEP

The last maneuver in this list seems contradictory, but it could be beneficial for two reasons. First, the external peep could provide a stent to keep airways open at the end of expiration, thereby promoting more complete exhalation. Second, external PEEP will reduce the work of breathing during auto-PEEP by reducing the pressure excursion needed to trigger the ventilator,[49] i.e., the alveolar pressure needs only to drop below the PEEP level instead of below the zero level to initiate lung inflation. The clinical impact of this is not clear.

COMPLICATIONS OF MECHANICAL VENTILATION

Several complications are possible during mechanical ventilation, but this section will present only those directly related to mechanical ventilation; i.e., the complications of artificial airways and pulmonary barotrauma. Other complications, such as pneumonia, can be a result of the patient's underlying clinical condition, and these complications are not included here. A comprehensive review of the spectrum of complications encountered in ventilator-dependent patients (including over 400 citations) is included in the bibliography at the end of this chapter (see reference no. 34).

ARTIFICIAL AIRWAYS

The risks of tracheal intubation are determined, in part, by the route of entry, which is either translaryngeal (endotracheal) or transtracheal (tracheostomy).[50,51] Translaryngeal intubation is achieved by inserting endotracheal tubes through either the nose or mouth. The nasal route is often preferred because the insertion technique is less involved and there is no risk for dental trauma. The oral route is usually reserved for comatose patients or for immediate intubation (e.g., cardiac arrest). Some comparative risks of the insertion routes are listed below.[50,52]

Risk Factor	Nasotracheal	Orotracheal
Intubation	Epistaxis	Dental trauma
	Esophageal intubation	Aspiration
Tube in place	Sinusitis	Tube occlusion
	Retained secretions	Laryngeal damage

The major problem with longterm nasal intubation is the risk of sinusitis. The major problem with oral intubation is the risk of laryngeal damage (due to greater mobility of orotracheal tubes) and tube occlusion (anxious or confused patients who bite down on the tubes).

SELECTIVE INTUBATION

As many as 15% of intubations will result in accidental entry of one lung, most commonly the right lung, and tension pneumothorax develops in 15% of unilateral lung intubations.[9] Recent evidence confirms that auscultation of the lungs is inadequate for detecting unilateral lung intubation,[53] and routine chest X-rays are necessary to reduce the incidence of missed diagnoses.[54]

SINUSITIS

Nasal tubes can obstruct the sinus ostia and produce a purulent sinusitis that can be life-threatening. Paranasal sinusitis has been demonstrated in as many as 40% of patients with indwelling nasotracheal tubes,[55] and sinusitis has been reported as the cause of at least 5% of unexplained fevers in intubated patients.[56] The maxillary sinus is almost always involved.[55,57] Computed tomographic scans are considered the procedure of choice for identifying sinusitis, but portable chest X-rays are often revealing.[58] The appearance of acute purulent sinusitis on an anteroposterior view (Water's view) taken at the bedside is shown in Figure 29–10. Since portable films like this are less expensive and do not impose the risks and inconvenience of moving the patient out of the ICU, single view (Water's view) portable sinus films have been recommended as a screening procedure for patients with suspected sinusitis.[58] However, the appearance of abnormal radiographic findings does not secure the diagnosis of infection, and aspiration of the involved sinus for gram stain and culture is necessary to confirm the presence of infection.[55,57]

LARYNGEAL DAMAGE

Damage to the larynx is the most common and most feared complication of endotracheal intubation. However, this is not clinically evident until after the endotracheal tube is removed. The risk for laryngeal injury is the rationale for tracheostomy if prolonged intubation is anticipated. The risk factors for laryngeal injury include the route of intubation (orotracheal tubes are believed to cause more damage to the larynx than nasotracheal tubes), the ease of intubation, tube diameter, the duration and number of intubations, and self-extubation with the cuff inflated.

Evidence of laryngeal injury is almost always present visually when endotracheal tubes are removed, but the incidence of serious complications is low.[59–61] Laryngeal edema may be evident immediately after extubation or it can become evident in the first few hours after extubation. In the latter situation, the lateral wall pressure exerted by the endotracheal tube in place prevents edema formation, and the edema begins to form only when the

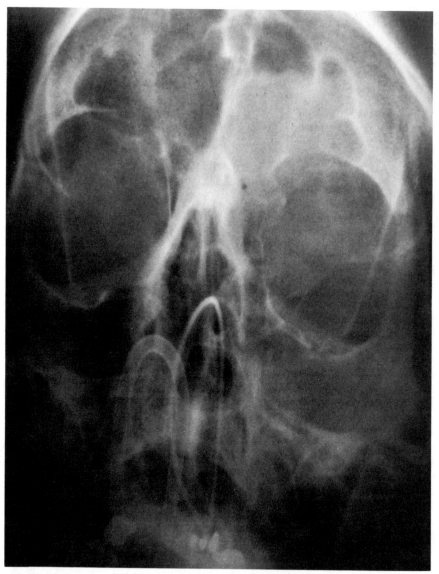

FIG. 29–10. Bedside anteroposterior view of the paranasal sinuses in a patient with documented purulent sinusitis. Note the complete opacification of the left maxillary sinus, and the air-fluid level in the left frontal sinus. Note also bilateral nasal intubation with nasotracheal and nasogastric tubes.

tube is removed. Respiratory distress following extubation almost always indicates laryngeal obstruction and should prompt immediate reintubation. Inspiratory stridor is not a sensitive sign of laryngeal obstruction, particularly at low airflows, and the absence of stridor should not be interpreted as the absence of laryngeal obstruction.

The proper therapy for laryngeal edema from endotracheal tubes includes tracheostomy and removal of the endotracheal tube. Steroid administration has no proven value in reducing the extent of edema[62] and is not recommended as a substitute for tracheostomy in this setting.

CUFF-RELATED COMPLICATIONS

All tracheal tubes for adults are equipped with an inflatable cuff at the distal end that seals the trachea and prevents air from escaping through the larynx. The major complications associated with these cuffs are aspiration, air leaks, and mucosal damage.

Aspiration

Although there is a tendency to believe that cuff inflation ensures against aspiration of mouth secretions into the lower airways, this is not the case. The soft, pliable cuffs that have become popular because they reduce the risk of pressure necrosis of the tracheal wall are quite capable of allowing secretions to pass. Aspiration of dye placed in the mouth has been documented in 20% of patients with endotracheal tubes[63] and 40% of patients with tracheostomy tubes[64] despite cuff inflation. The risk of aspiration decreases if cuff pressure is increased to 25 cm H_2O,[64] but this is the highest cuff pressure allowed to limit tracheal damage. The only defense against aspiration of mouth secretions is frequent suctioning and the patient's own defense mechanisms (cough, etc.).

Cuff Leaks

A leak is defined as air passing around the cuff and escaping through the larynx. Cuff leaks are usually detected by a sound during lung inflation that represents air passing over the vocal cords. The exhaled volume registered on the ventilator will be diminished and can be used to quantitate the volume of the leak.

The most common cause of a cuff leak is nonuniform contact between the cuff and the trachea. Another common source is the one-way valve on the pilot balloon. These valves can become faulty, allowing air to escape from the cuff. Cuff leaks are rarely due to disruption of the cuff itself.

When a leak is detected, the patient must be separated from the ventilator and the lungs must be manually inflated with an anesthesia bag to determine if the origin of the leak is at the cuff site. If a cuff leak is present, the cuff is inflated with a few ml of air until the sound disappears. If the cuff pressure exceeds 25 cm H_2O, the tracheal tube is replaced. If the cuff pressure is acceptable, the tube is observed for return of the leak. If the leak returns quickly, the problem is likely to be in the pilot balloon valve and the tube should be changed. If the valve is faulty, the inflation tube can be clamped to keep the cuff inflated until the tube is replaced.

Tracheal Injury

Pressure necrosis of the trachea from cuff inflation has decreased significantly since high compliance cuffs were developed in the early 1970s. The newer cuffs are larger and more elliptic, so the pressure is dispersed over a larger surface area. The systolic pressure in the mucosal vessels of the trachea is 20 to 25 mmHg,[51,64] and the cuff pressure is kept below 25 cm H_2O (18.4 mmHg) to prevent pressure necrosis of the tracheal mucosa. A preferential cuff design is a foam rubber cuff that is normally inflated and must be deflated with syringe suction to insert the tube into the trachea. The main advantage of this types of cuff is that it seals the trachea at zero (atmospheric) intracuff pressure, thereby minimizing the risk for pressure-induced injury to the tracheal mucosa. This tube (called the Fome-Cuff®) should be available in most hospitals and is worth considering for prolonged intubations.

TRACHEOSTOMY

Tracheostomy is preferred in patients who require prolonged mechanical ventilation. The advantages of tracheostomy over endotracheal intubation include patient comfort, more effective clearing of secretions, and absence of laryngeal injury.[51] Selected patients can take food orally and can speak with the aid of special tracheostomy tubes. The complications of tracheostomy are related to three factors: the surgical procedure, the tracheal stoma, and the patient population.

SURGICAL COMPLICATIONS

Tracheostomy is associated with serious complications in 5% of cases[51] and has a reported mortality of 2 to 3%.[50] Immediate postoperative complications include pneumothorax (5%), stomal hemorrhage (5%), and accidental decannulation.[50,51]

Accidental decannulation in the first few days after surgery can be a serious problem because the tracheostomy tract closes quickly. Attempts to reinsert tubes can create false tracts. If a tracheostomy tube has to be replaced in the first week after surgery, a suction catheter (12 French) should be used as a guidewire to reduce the risk of a traumatic or unsuccessful reintubation.

TRACHEAL STENOSIS

Tracheal stenosis usually occurs at the stoma site and not at the site where the cuff seals the trachea.[50–52,59] Tracheal stenosis is the most feared complication of tracheostomy but is a late complication and appears after the patient leaves the ICU.

GENERAL COMPLICATIONS

The complications from tracheostomy are more frequent than the complications from endotracheal intubation[52] but this may be due largely to the characteristics of the patients. That is, patients who require tracheostomy are usually more ill than patients who are intubated, they have been in the hospital for a longer period of time, and they have been intubated prior to the tracheostomy. These factors must be weighed when considering complications like pneumonia, which is reported in 50% of patients with a tracheostomy.[51]

TIMING

The optimal time for changing from endotracheal tube to tracheostomy is a time-honored controversy. The central issue in this decision involves the relative advantages and disadvantages of each method. These are summarized below[51,52,61]

- The proponents of early tracheostomy (3 to 7 days after intubation) maintain that tracheostomy is more comfortable, provides less resistance to airflow, allows for more effective care of the airways, and permits oral feeding
- The advocates of prolonged endotracheal intubation (3 weeks or longer) maintain that tracheostomy is a costly surgical procedure with a high morbidity and an associated mortality rate. Moreover, the duration of intubation does not seem to determine the incidence or severity of complications (for at least 3 weeks)[52]
- A popular approach to this issue is to allow 1 week of endotracheal intubation and if extubation seems unlikely in the next week, tracheostomy should be initiated

PULMONARY BAROTRAUMA

Pulmonary barotrauma occurs in 1 to 20% of patients receiving mechanical ventilation, and the consequences can be devastating.[66,67]

PATHOGENESIS

Although the term barotrauma indicates pressure-induced injury, the culprit in mechanical ventilation is overinflation (i.e., volume). When the airspaces rupture, air can dissect along tissue planes (interstitial emphysema) or can travel along the bronchovascular bundles into the mediastinum (pneumomediastinum) and up into the neck (subcutaneous emphysema). The air can also rupture through the visceral pleura (pneumothorax) or can enter the peritoneal cavity (pneumoperitoneum).

Predisposing factors include excessive inflation volume and high intrathoracic pressures. In one study, the incidence of barotrauma was 43% if the peak inflation pressure exceeded 70 cm H_2O, while no patient experienced barotrauma if the inflation pressure remained below 40 cm H_2O.[68]

Also important is the tendency of the lung to rupture; predisposing illnesses include asthma, necrotizing pneumonia, and gastric acid aspiration. Asymmetric lung disease is not mentioned enough in pathogenesis.[66] In this situation, normal lung regions receive excessive volumes and pressures from the ventilator because the inflation volume from ventilators will preferentially travel to areas of least resistance and greater distensibility. All pulmonary disorders are nonuniform to some degree, and this mechanism is operative in all cases of barotrauma.

DIAGNOSIS

Vigilance and early recognition are the hallmarks of the approach to pneumothorax, as emphasized by the following observation

- Delays in diagnosis can prove fatal in one of every three ventilator-dependent patients who develop a pneumothorax[66]

Clinical signs can be absent and, when present, are usually nonspecific. Common signs of pneumothorax in ventilator-dependent patients include tachycardia and sudden hypotension.[14] Breath sounds are notoriously unreliable in ventilator-dependent patients, and sounds transmitted from the ventilator tubing can be mistaken for airway sounds,[53] thereby leading to missed diagnoses for pneumothorax.

SUBCUTANEOUS AIR

The presence of subcutaneous air in the neck or upper thorax is pathognomonic of pulmonary barotrauma. In one study, subcutaneous air was palpable in all 74 patients who developed a pneumothorax during mechanical ventilation.[69] This indicates that palpation for subcutaneous air in the neck and upper thorax may be the most valuable bedside test for the early diagnosis of pulmonary barotrauma in ventilator-dependent patients.

CHEST RADIOGRAPHS

Pulmonary barotrauma is often detected on routine chest films before the clinical diagnosis is evident. The following are some radiographic features of barotrauma that are useful in the ICU patient population

- One of the early signs of barotrauma is pulmonary interstitial emphysema (PIE), which appears as small parenchymal cysts or linear streaks projecting toward the hilum. This represents air that is dissecting along the pulmonary interstitium

In one study, five of 13 patients with radiographic evidence of PIE developed pneumothorax within the next 12 hours.[70] This indicates that PIE can be a harbinger of pneumothorax

- In the supine position, pleural air collects in the anterior costophrenic sulcus at the base of the hemithorax, and searching for air at the apex of the hemithorax can be misleading[71]

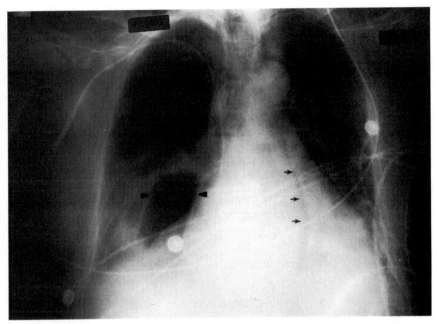

FIG. 29–11. Portable chest x-ray showing air collection in anteromedial recess on the left (lower arrows). Upper arrow indicates subcutaneous emphysema. Sharp line delineating the descending thoracic aorta is air behind the inferior pulmonary ligament.

Some of the atypical patterns of pleural air collection in supine patients are shown in the radiograph in Figure 29–11. The hyperlucency outlined at the right lung base represents air in the anterior costophrenic recess. The sharp line outlining the descending aorta is produced by air trapped behind the inferior pulmonary ligament. Note the subcutaneous air at the base of the neck (upper arrow).

GOALS OF MANAGEMENT

The management of patients with acute respiratory failure who require mechanical ventilation involves specific goals, regardless of the underlying cardiopulmonary problem. The goals are listed below and are illustrated in the schematic diagram in Figure 29–12.

- Prevent fluid accumulation in the lungs
- Maintain systemic oxygen transport
- Limit inhaled oxygen to the minimally acceptable concentration
- Monitor for nosocomial diseases (e.g., pneumonia)

FLUID ACCUMULATION

As mentioned earlier, there is a tendency for fluid accumulation during positive pressure mechanical ventilation,[34,35] and this will increase capillary hydrostatic pressures (Pc). In addition, the increase in total body water

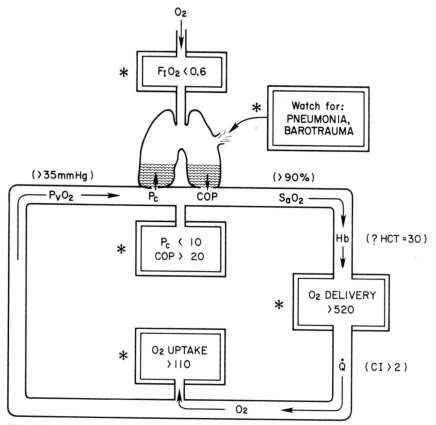

FIG. 29–12. Goals of management for patients who require prolonged mechanical ventilation. See text explanation. Systemic oxygen delivery (DO_2), oxygen uptake (VO_2), and cardiac output (Q) are expressed in ml/min/m². Arterial PO_2 (PaO_2) and colloid osmotic pressure (COP) of plasma are measured in mmHg. Hematocrit (%) expressed as fractional volume of blood taken up by erythrocytes. See text for explanation.

will dilute serum proteins, leading to a decrease in the colloid osmotic pressure (COP) of blood. According to the Starling relationships governing fluid movement across capillaries, an increase in Pc above the COP of plasma will favor the net movement of fluid into the interstitium. Therefore, as indicated in Figure 29–12, the goal of fluid management during mechanical ventilation is to keep the Pc in the pulmonary microcirculation below the plasma COP. Diuretics should be ideal for achieving this goal because diuresis will decrease vascular volume (decrease Pc) while also concentrating plasma proteins (increasing plasma COP). Albumin infusion has also been utilized as a means of limiting lung water accumulation by increasing the plasma COP.

- Neither aggressive diuretic therapy nor infusion of albumin solutions has proven effective in reducing fluid accumulation in the lungs in ventilator-dependent patients[72,73]

- Intravenous furosemide can reduce cardiac output,[74] and aggressive therapy with furosemide can be detrimental in patients with pulmonary hypertension[75]

Despite these observations, routine administration of diuretics remains a common practice in the care of ventilator-dependent patients. In the absence of invasive hemodynamic monitoring, this practice is to be discouraged. The value of invasive hemodynamic monitoring in ventilator-dependent patients is presented in the following section on systemic oxygen transport.

The practice of infusing albumin to limit extravascular fluid accumulation is not supported by the physiology of albumin distribution in the human body. That is, over 50% of the total body albumin is located outside the vascular space and, thus, albumin infusion should not be expected to increase preferentially the vascular volume. Infusion of colloid solutions like 5% albumin is, however, superior to crystalloid (saline) fluid infusion for increasing vascular volume and promoting cardiac output in critically ill patients,[76] and colloid administration is not to be discouraged as a means of volume support in the intensive care unit.

SYSTEMIC OXYGEN TRANSPORT

The ultimate goal in managing any patient with respiratory failure is to maintain the delivery of oxygen to the vital organs. The common practice of monitoring arterial blood gases provides little information about the transport of oxygen to the vital organs, and this practice is no longer considered adequate for monitoring seriously ill patients who require mechanical ventilation. The clinical parameters that are used to assess systemic oxygen transport are shown in Table 29–4.[77] The two principal measures of systemic oxygen transport are the oxygen delivery rate in arterial blood (DO_2) and the rate of oxygen uptake from the systemic microcirculation (VO_2). Both parameters require the measurement of cardiac output and thus require indwelling pulmonary artery catheters equipped with thermistors (to measure cardiac output by thermodilution). Note that the partial pressure of oxygen in arterial blood (PaO_2) is not included in the determination of either DO_2 or VO_2, demonstrating why arterial blood gases provide little information about systemic oxygen transport.

The flow diagram in Figure 29–13 provides a stepwise approach to maintaining adequate tissue oxygenation in patients with acute respiratory failure. The salient features of this approach are listed below

TABLE 29–4 THE OXYGEN TRANSPORT VARIABLES		
PARAMETER	**DEFINITION**	**UNITS**
Oxygen content	$1.3 \times Hb \times SaO_2$	ml/100 ml
Oxygen delivery	$Q \times 13 \times Hb \times SaO_2$	ml/min/m^2
Oxygen uptake	$Q \times 13 \times Hb \times (SaO_2 - SvO_2)$	ml/min/m^2

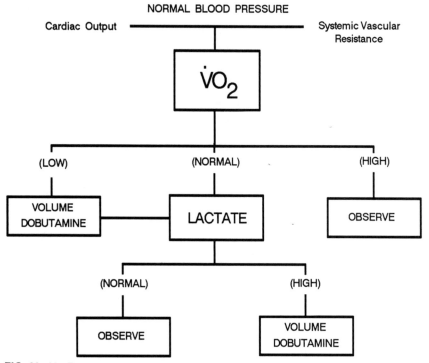

FIG. 29-13. Flow diagram for assessing and maintaining tissue oxygenation in patients with acute respiratory failure. See text for explanation.

- The initial goal of management is to achieve a DO_2 of at least 520 ml/min/m^2 and a VO_2 of at least 110 ml/min/m^2 (i.e., the lower limits of normal for systemic oxygen transport)
- If the oxygen transport variables are abnormally low, cardiac output with volume and/or inotropic therapy should be promoted, and anemia should be corrected, if severe (see later discussion for more details on these maneuvers)
- When oxygen transport is normal, check the serum lactate level; if the lactate is greater than 2 mEq/l, then continue to increase cardiac output or correct anemia to achieve a serum lactate level less than 2 mEq/l

The lactate level in "mixed venous" (pulmonary artery) blood is used to assess the balance between oxygen availability and the oxygen utilized by aerobic metabolism in the vital organs.[78] When the rate of oxygen utilization exceeds the rate oxygen uptake from the microcirculation, the venous lactate levels should begin to rise, so that an elevated serum lactate level is used as evidence for inadequate oxygen transport in individual patients. Although the sensitivity of the serum lactate for detecting inadequate tissue oxygenation is unknown (and is probably insensitive), the serum lactate is the only clinical test of bioenergetic failure that is currently available and an elevated lactate level with associated metabolic acidosis, as distinguished from hyperlactatemia without metabolic acidosis,[79] carries a poor prognosis and warrants immediate attention.

CARDIAC OUTPUT

The principal means of supporting systemic oxygen transport is to support the cardiac output

- The goal is a cardiac output > 2 l/min/m^2 (indexed to body surface area) and a serum lactate < 2 mEq/l
- If support is necessary, infuse volume first to achieve a left ventricular end-diastolic pressure (pulmonary capillary wedge pressure) $= 18$ to 20 mmHg
- Once ventricular filling is adequate, further support of cardiac output can be achieved with dobutamine (initial dose $= 5$ μg/kg/min, usual dose range $= 5$ to 15 μg/kg/min)
- Intravenous amrinone (initial dose $= 0.75$ mg/kg as bolus, then 2 μg/kg/min, usual dose range $= 2$ to 10 μg/kg/min) can be used as an adjunct to dobutamine therapy,[80] but this agent is more a vasodilator than a positive inotropic agent,[81] and it is not recommended as a single agent for inotropic support
- Dopamine should be avoided whenever possible because of the tendency for this agent to constrict pulmonary veins,[72,82] which can increase pulmonary capillary hydrostatic pressure and aggravate lung fluid accumulation. Furthermore, dobutamine is more effective than dopamine in augmenting cardiac output in patients with respiratory failure.[82]
- Vasodilator therapy is not recommended routinely in patients with respiratory failure because of the tendency for vasodilator agents to increase intrapulmonary shunting and thereby aggravate the underlying abnormality in gas exchange.[83]

ERYTHROCYTE TRANSFUSIONS

Transfusion of erythrocyte concentrates (i.e., packed red cells) is a common practice in seriously ill patients with serum hemoglobin levels below 10 g/dl. However, this practice has no proven benefit[84] and can be detrimental.[85] The influence of blood transfusion on systemic oxygen uptake in postoperative patients with respiratory failure is shown in Figure 29–14. In a majority of the 20 patients included in this study, the increase in serum hemoglobin (mean increase $= 21.6\%$) was not associated with an increase in systemic oxygen uptake. The absence of a consistent improvement in tissue oxygen uptake following erythrocyte transfusions illustrates the need for monitoring systemic oxygen transport to identify the few patients in the ICU who will benefit from blood transfusion therapy.

OXYHEMOGLOBIN SATURATION

Virtually all the oxygen that is transported in blood is bound to hemoglobin. Therefore, the oxyhemoglobin saturation (expressed as a fraction of the total hemoglobin in blood) is an important determinant of systemic oxygen transport

CELL DAMAGE

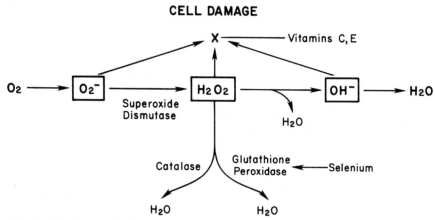

FIG. 29–14. The metabolic pathway for the reduction of molecular oxygen to water, including the endogenous antioxidant defense system. See text for details.

- The consensus is to maintain an arterial oxyhemoglobin saturation (SaO_2) above 90%.[86]

The flat portion of the oxyhemoglobin dissociation curve begins at an SaO_2 of around 90% in healthy individuals. The maintenance of an SaO_2 above 90% reduces the risk of sharp declines in SaO_2 when the PaO_2 declines from baseline. Because of the toxic potential of inhaled oxygen (see following section), it is wise to keep the SaO_2 just above 95%, thereby maintaining the level of inhaled oxygen at the lowest acceptable level.

REDUCING RISK OF OXYGEN TOXICITY

Animal studies reveal that inhalation of oxygen can be fatal within days when the fractional concentration of inhaled oxygen (FIO_2) exceeds 60%.[87] The culprit is an acute lung injury similar to the adult respiratory distress syndrome.[87,88] Although the effects of breathing high FIO_2 mixtures have not been studied in humans, the observations from animal studies have led to the consensus recommendation that the FIO_2 not exceed 60% in patients with acute respiratory failure. However, as shown in the following paragraphs, the use of a universal threshold for oxygen toxicity in all patients does not take into account the endogenous antioxidant system and the potential for this system to become depleted in seriously ill patients.[89,90] A safer practice would be to maintain the FIO_2 at the lowest possible level required to maintain adequate arterial oxygenation (i.e., SaO_2 just above 90%).

PATHOGENESIS

The conversion of molecular oxygen to water by cytochrome oxidase is accomplished in a series of single electron reductions, creating molecular intermediates that have an unpaired electron in their outer orbitals (free radicals) and are thereby rendered highly reactive.[87,91,92] The metabolic pathway for oxygen is shown in Figure 29–14; the reactive intermediates identified are the superoxide anion (O_2), hydrogen peroxide (H_2O_2), and the hydroxyl radical (OH·). These compounds (particularly OH·) oxidize polyunsaturated fatty acids in cell membranes (lipid peroxidation) and are capable of widespread and self-sustaining damage to all cell membranes.

Toxic oxygen intermediates are produced by all cells endowed with aerobic metabolism, but the toxicity of these intermediates is limited by endogenous mechanisms.[87,89] The principal protection against oxidant injury in man is the glutathione redox pathway,[93] which facilitates the reduction of hydrogen peroxide directly to water, thereby bypassing the formation of the highly destructive hydroxyl radical. Glutathione peroxidase is the catalytic enzyme in this system, and the enzyme in humans requires selenium as a cofactor.[87] A second line of defense against oxidant injury is provided by substances that can donate a hydrogen ion to reduce and detoxify the hydroxyl radical. Two of the major scavengers that function in this capacity are alpha tocopherol (vitamin E) and ascorbic acid (vitamin C). Vitamin E is situated in cell membranes, where it can break the chain of lipid peroxidation, while vitamin C is considered to act primarily as an extracellular antioxidant.

ANTIOXIDANT STRATEGIES

The endogenous antioxidant defenses can become overwhelmed and depleted from persistent hyperoxia or serious illness.[87–90] In fact, the lack of attention given to supporting the antioxidant systems in serious illness or prolonged hyperoxia would seem to favor the depletion of antioxidants in these conditions. Although there are currently no general guidelines for monitoring or maintaining antioxidant defenses, a few considerations are worth mentioning.

Selenium deficiency may be common in critically ill patients,[15] and it is not unwise to monitor selenium status in patients at risk for oxygen toxicity. This can be accomplished by measuring the serum selenium concentration or by measuring the activity of glutathione peroxidase in erythrocytes (both tests are available in clinical laboratories).[94,95] The recommended daily allowance for selenium is 10 µg,[95] with the maximum safe dose set at 200 µg/day.[96] Selenium can be administered intravenously, and the higher doses may be given in four divided doses.

Vitamin E deficiency is also common in hospitalized patients; one study reported low levels of vitamin E in 37% of random plasma samples from hospitalized patients.[96] The recommended daily allowance for vitamin E is 10 mg,[95] and vitamin E supplements are given via the enteral route.

Thiamine plays an important role in the pentose-phosphate pathway, which generates the NADPH necessary for proper functioning of the glutathione redox pathway. The body stores of thiamine are limited, and depletion occurs after 18 days of a thiamine-free diet in healthy adults.[98] In hypermetabolic patients, thiamine depletion may occur more rapidly; one study of trauma victims reported that all patients showed evidence of thiamine deficiency after one week.[99] Thiamine status is assessed by either the serum thiamine level (normal = 3.5 − 5 μg/100 ml) or by the activity of a transketolase enzyme in red blood cells. Either test should be available in most clinical laboratories; the erythrocyte transketolase activity test is the most sensitive of the two for thiamine deficiency.[99] The recommended daily allowance for thiamine is 1 to 1.5 mg in adults,[95] and replacement therapy can be given intravenously.

WEANING FROM MECHANICAL VENTILATION

Removing the patient from prolongèd mechanical ventilation is a practice that is common but has a few consensus guidelines. Two points are relevant at the outset

- The diaphragm is not a voluntary muscle and is not expected to develop disuse atrophy during mechanical ventilation; i.e., the situation is not the same as having a limb immobilized in a cast
- The primary focus on weaning should be to successfully treat the underlying cardiopulmonary problem

BEDSIDE CRITERIA

The common bedside criteria for weaning are listed in Table 29–5.[100,108] These criteria will be unreliable as predictors of weanability in at least one-third of patients and are not to be applied as absolute rules for weaning. Before applying these criteria, it is mandatory that gas exchange is adequate, with a nontoxic level of inhaled oxygen and no PEEP.

OXYGEN COST OF BREATHING

In the normal adult, the act of quiet breathing consumes only 5% of the total oxygen consumption (VO_2). When breathing is labored or minute ventilation is excessive, the relative proportion of oxygen consumed by the respiratory muscles will increase (see Fig. 29–15). As the minute ventilation increases above 10 liters per minute, the VO_2 begins to increase geometrically. This increase in VO_2 is called the oxygen cost of breathing and represents the oxygen consumed by the respiratory muscles in performing the work of breathing.[107,108] This is a measure of the efficiency of breathing

TABLE 29–5 BEDSIDE WEANING CRITERIA	
PARAMETER	**DESIRED VALUE**
PaO_2/FIO_2	>100
Tidal volume	5 ml/kg
Vital capacity	10 ml/kg
Minute ventilation	<10 L/min
Maximum inspiratory pressure (PImax)	> −30 cmH$_2$O
Oxygen cost of spontaneous breathing	Spontaneous VO_2 < 20% higher than ventilator VO_2

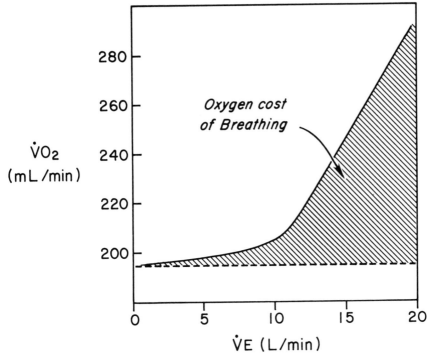

FIG. 29–15. The relationship between oxygen consumption (VO_2) and the minute ventilation. See text for explanation.

or the relationship between the work performed and the energy needed to perform the work. At a given workload, an efficient engine consumes less energy than an inefficient engine.

This principle has been applied to the evaluation of patients for weaning. The VO_2 is measured at the bedside using a metabolic cart or the pulmonary artery catheter. The measurement is obtained while the patient is resting on the ventilator and again shortly after removal from the ventilator. The difference in VO_2 in the two conditions is the O_2 cost of breathing. If the VO_2 increases less than 10% after removal from the ventilator, the patient should wean successfully. If the VO_2 increases more than 20% after removal, the wean is likely to be unsuccessful.[108]

METHODS OF WEANING

There are two methods of weaning, and each is analogous to an electrical switch: one is abrupt like an on–off toggle switch, while the other is gradual like a variable-resistance rheostat. The abrupt method is called the "T-piece" method because of the shape of the tubing in the circuit. The gradual method uses the IMV mode of ventilation described earlier in this chapter. A survey of ICU directors conducted in 1987 indicated IMV as the most popular method of weaning in the United States,[109] but as presented below, there it little evidence to justify this preference.

The T-Piece

The circuit design in Figure 29-16 has an adaptor that is shaped like the letter "T," hence it is commonly called a "T-piece" circuit. Oxygen-rich gas is delivered at constant flow from the inlet 3 arm of the apparatus and flows past the patient to exit the circuit at the other end. When the patient takes a breath, the gas is drawn into the lungs from the inlet side only. The high flow of gas along the upper arms of the circuit prevents the patient from entraining room air. When the patient exhales, this high gas flow also carries the exhaled gas out of the circuit so the patient cannot rebreathe the exhaled gas.

The original T-piece circuit was not connected to the ventilator, which made it difficult to monitor tidal volume and respiratory rate during the wean. The newer ventilators are equipped with circuits that allow a T-piece wean while monitoring tidal volume and rate on the ventilator. This is done by using the CPAP mode of ventilation. When no pressure (CPAP) is applied in this mode, the patient will receive the inspired O_2 concentration from the ventilator at constant flow. The only drawback to the CPAP circuit is that a valve must be opened by the patient to receive the inhaled

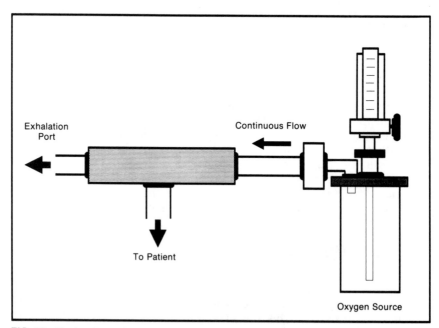

FIG. 29-16. A schematic representation of the T-shaped circuit used for weaning. A continuous flow of gas passes along the horizontal arm of the T-circuit to prevent the patient from entraining room air or rebreathing exhaled gas.

gas and the pressure required to open the valve can increase the work of breathing. For normal subjects, this increase in work would not be deleterious. However, in a patient with borderline respiratory function, the added workload can be enough to eventually fatigue the patient and prevent extubation. Therefore, when a difficult wean is anticipated, the stand-alone circuit is preferred.

When a T-piece wean trial is started, the patient is allowed to stay off the ventilator as long as tolerated. If it is not possible for the patient to wean at this point, a wean schedule can be started using trials of shorter duration (to prevent any further muscle fatigue) alternating with periods of total ventilatory support.

Intermittent Mandatory Ventilation

The IMV method provides a backup level of ventilation for the patient while allowing the patient to breathe spontaneously between ventilator breaths. The backup rate is usually started at 8 to 10 breaths/minute and is gradually reduced in increments of 1 to 2 breaths/minute until there is no input from the ventilator. The period of time over which the IMV rate is tapered is extremely variable and is determined by the condition of the patient.

There is a tendency to view IMV as safer than the T-piece method because IMV provides a ventilator backup. This produces a false sense of security with IMV weaning, which can be dangerous. The ventilator backup is misleading because the IMV circuit is not a closed-loop feedback system. That is, the ventilator is unable to sense changes in the patient's ventilatory demands and adjust the backup rate. If the patient's minute ventilation decreases, the ventilator will not increase ventilatory input to keep overall minute ventilation constant. Therefore, the patient can get into trouble with IMV despite the presence of backup ventilator breaths. This can be dangerous because patients weaned with IMV tend to be unattended more than those weaned with the T-piece method.

T-Piece Versus IMV Weaning

Neither the T-piece nor the IMV method of weaning has proven to be superior,[110,111] so the method selected is largely one of personal preference. T-piece trials are preferred for the following reasons

- IMV can prolong weaning in patients who could be easily weaned and extubated (e.g., postoperative patients). Since IMV ends up as a T-piece trial, the time needed to taper the IMV rate is wasted time for patients who would wean easily
- The T-piece method forces the physician to watch the patient more closely during the wean, which is a safer environment for weaning
- T-piece is superior to IMV for increasing muscle strength in patients with respiratory muscle weakness. The traditional method of strengthening skeletal muscle groups is to alternate periods of exercise and periods of rest (similar to the T-piece trials) and not to continually use the

fatigued muscles, which is what IMV does. This concept is very simplified, particularly since the diaphragm is continually in use in either method of weaning. However, the concept of rest for a fatiguing muscle is valid, and at least the accessory muscle will rest periodically using the T-piece method of weaning

Finally, it is important to stress that the choice of weaning method is not the primary issue in the ability to wean from mechanical ventilation; i.e., weaning is not a therapy for the removal of mechanical ventilation. The ability to wean is dependent on the severity of the underlying problem and not on the method of weaning. When the underlying problem is corrected, the patient will wean regardless of the method used.

TROUBLESHOOTING

The following problems can appear during a difficult wean and often pose the problem of whether to continue the wean or resume mechanical ventilation.

Tachypnea

The most common scenario in a difficult wean is the appearance of agitation and tachypnea, and the task is to distinguish anxiety from a cardiopulmonary problem. When tachypnea appears during a wean, the spontaneous tidal volume can be a valuable measure (see Fig. 29–16). Failure to wean is often associated with a diminishing tidal volume,[112] but not invariably.[15] The interpretation of the tidal volume in the setting of tachypnea is shown in Figure 29–17. An increase in the tidal volume suggests hyperventilation from anxiety, while a drop in tidal volume suggests muscle weakness or a cardiopulmonary problem.

The alveolar–arterial PO_2 (A-a PO_2) gradient might help to differentiate anxiety from a cardiopulmonary problem; i.e., an increase in A-a PO_2 gradient indicates a ventilation–perfusion imbalance or a reduced venous PO_2 while a normal or unchanged A-a PO_2 gradient indicates anxiety or muscle weakness. Unfortunately, an increase in A-a PO_2 gradient might not always rule out anxiety as a cause of hypoxemia. There are two mechanisms whereby anxiety could elevate the A-a PO_2 gradient. First, the anxiety-induced tachypnea could produce auto-PEEP and thereby create a ventilation–perfusion mismatch. Second, increased work of breathing from anxiety could increase oxygen consumption and reduce mixed venous PO_2. Both processes would increase A-a PO_2 gradient.

To summarize the above

- In the setting of tachypnea, measure the tidal volume. If the tidal volume is reduced, resume full mechanical ventilation. If the tidal volume is unchanged, obtain an arterial blood sample, and determine the A-a PO_2 gradient. If the A-a PO_2 has increased, then resume mechanical ventilation. If the A-a PO_2 is unchanged, then the problem may be nonpulmonary anxiety; continuing the wean and sedating the patient should be considered.

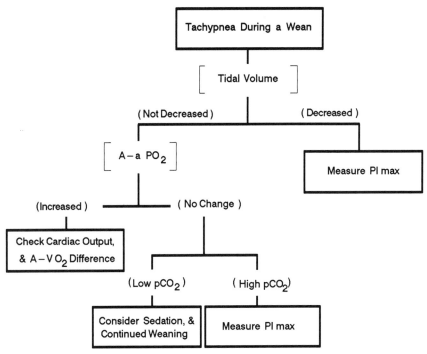

FIG. 29–17. The bedside approach to tachypnea during a wean. See text for explanation.

Hypercapnia

The appearance of hypercapnia during a wean is an ominous sign and usually indicates immediate return to mechanical ventilation. The bedside approach to hypercapnia is outlined in Figure 29–18.[113] The end-tidal PCO_2 ($ETCO_2$) should be monitored during a difficult wean because the gradient between $ETCO_2$ and arterial PCO_2 ($PaCO_2$) can help to identify the problem.

- An increase in the $PaCO_2–ECTO_2$ gradient indicates an increase in dead space ventilation while a constant gradient suggests an extrapulmonary etiology

Extrapulmonary Causes

- Respiratory muscle weakness
- Increased CO_2 production

The strength of the inspiratory muscles can be monitored during the wean by measuring the PImax at regular intervals. A decrease in PImax to below 25 to 30 cm H_2O is taken as evidence for muscle weakness. Hypercapnia alone can depress the contractile strength of the diaphragm[3] and this will confuse the interpretation of a decrease in PImax during a wean.

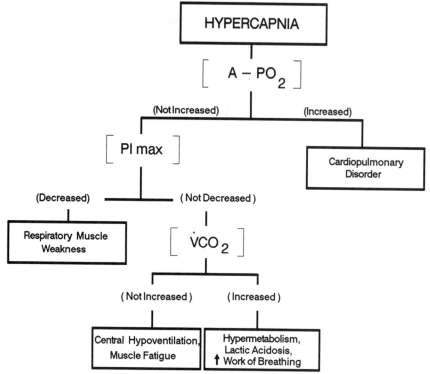

FIG. 29–18. The bedside approach to hypercapnia during a wean. See text for explanation.

Dead space ventilation

- Low cardiac output from negative pressure breathing
- Auto-PEEP from high respiratory rates

The cardiac output can be monitored at regular intervals during a difficult wean, but auto-PEEP can be monitored only during mechanical ventilation. However, the combination of tachypnea and an increase in dead space ventilation suggests auto-PEEP. In this situation, the judicious use of sedation is not unreasonable if the CO_2 retention is acute and the degree of elevation is mild.

Aminophylline

The observation that aminophylline increases the contractility of the diaphragm has led to the recommendation that aminophylline be used to facilitate a difficult wean.[114] There are two problems with this recommendation. First, it assumes that respiratory muscle weakness is a major factor in the inability to wean. This may not be the case, at least for the diaphragm.[115] Secondly, the usual approach to skeletal muscle weakness is to rest the muscle rather than stimulate it continuously. Constant stimulation of a weak muscle (in this case, with aminophylline) will deplete the high energy phosphate stores in the muscle and add to the problem. For these reasons, there is no evidence to justify the use of aminophylline in patients who are difficult to wean.

REFERENCES

CONVENTIONAL MECHANICAL VENTILATION

1. Grum CM, Chauncey JB: Conventional mechanical ventilation. Clin Chest Med, *9*:37, 1988.
2. Biondi JW, Schulman DS, Mattahy RA: Effects of mechanical ventilation on right and left ventricular function. Clin Chest Med, *9*:55, 1988.
3. Abel JG, Salerno TA, Panos A, et al.: Cardiovascular effects of positive-pressure ventilation in humans. Ann Thorac Surg *43*:198, 1987.
4. Weil MH, Gazmuri RJ, Rackow EC: The clinical rationale of cardiac resuscitaiton. Disease-a-Month, *36*:423, 1990.
5. Grum CM, Morganroth ML: Initiating mechanical ventilation. Intensive Care Med, *3*:6, 1988.
6. Ponte J: Indications for mechanical ventilation. Thorax, *45*:885, 1990.
7. Kacmarek RM, Venegas J: Mechanical ventilatory rates and tidal volumes. Respiratory Care, *32*:466, 1987.
8. Novak RA, Shumaker L, Snyder JV, Pinsky MR: Do periodic hyperinflations improve gas exchange in patients with hypoxemic respiratory failure. Crit Care Med, *15*:108, 1987.
9. Zwillich CW, Pierson DJ, Creagh CE, et al.: Complications of assisted ventilation. Am J Med, *57*:161, 1974.
10. Tsuno K, Prato P, Kolobow T: Acute lung injury from mechanical ventilation at moderately high airway pressures. J Appl Physiol, *69*:956, 1990.
11. Lee PC, Helsmoortel CM, Cohn CM, Fink MP: Are low tidal volumes safe? Chest, *97*: 425, 1990.

SPECIAL MODES OF VENTILATION

12. Downs JB, Klein EF, Desautels D, et al.: IMV: A new approach to weaning patients from mechanical ventilators. Chest, *64*:331, 1973.
13. Weisman IM, Rinaldo JE, Rogers RM, Sanders MH: Intermittent mandatory ventilation. Amer Rev Respir Dis, *127*:641, 1983.
14. Hudson LD: Does intermittent mandatory ventilation correct respiratory alkalosis in patients receiving assisted mechanical ventilation? Am Rev Respir Dis, *132*:1071, 1985.
15. Robotham JL, Scharf SM: Effects of positive and negative pressure ventilation on cardiac performance. Clin Chest Med, *4*:161, 1983.
16. Mathru M, et al.: Hemodynamic response to changes in ventilatory patterns in patients with normal and poor left ventricular reserve. Crit Care Med, *10*:423, 1982.
17. Hastings PR, et al.: Cardiorespiratory dynamics during weaning with IMV versus spontaneous ventilation in good-risk cardiac surgery patients. Anesthesiology, *53*:429, 1980.
18. MacIntyre NR: Pressure-support ventilation. *In* Mechanical Ventilation and Assisted Respiration. Contemporary Management in Critical Care. Edited by A. Grenvik, J. Downs, J. Rasanen, R. Smith. New York, Churchill Livingstone, 1991, pp. 51–62.
19. Hughes CW, Popovich J Jr.: Uses and abuses of pressure support ventilation. J Crit Illness, *4*:25, 1989.
20. Petty TL: The use, abuse and mystique of positive end-expiratory pressure. Am Rev Respir Dis, *138*:475, 1988.

21. Shaprio BA, Cane RD, Harrison RA: Positive end-expiratory pressure therapy in adults with special reference to acute lung injury: A review of the literature and suggested clinical correlations. Crit Care Med, *12*:127, 1984.

22. Saul GM, Feeley TW, Mihm FG: Effect of graded administration of PEEP on lung water in noncardiogenic pulmonary edema. Crit Care Med *10*:667, 1982.

23. Helbert C, Paskanik A, Bredenberg CE: Effect of positive end-expiratory pressure on lung water in pulmonary edema caused by increased membrane permeability. Ann Thorac Surg, *36*:42, 1983.

24. Kanarek DJ, Shannon DC: Adverse effect of positive end-expiratory pressure on pulmonary perfusion and arterial oxygenation. Am Rev Respir Dis, *112*:457, 1975.

25. Guyton RA, Chiavarelli M, Padgett CA, et al.: The influence of positive end-expiratory pressure on intrapericardial pressure and cardiac function after coronary artery bypass surgery. J Cardiothorac Anesth, *1*:98, 1987.

26. Martin C, Saux P, Albanese J, et al.: Right ventricular function during positive end-expiratory pressure. Chest, *92*:999, 1987.

27. Tittley JG, Fremes SE, Weisel RD, et al.: Hemodynamic and myocardial metabolic consequences of PEEP. Chest, *88*:496, 1985.

28. Pick RA, Handler JB, Friedman AS: The cardiovascular effects of positive end-expiratory pressure. Chest, *82*:345, 1982.

29. Pepe PE, Hudson LD, Carrico CJ: Early application of positive end-expiratory pressure to patients at risk for the adult respiratory distress syndrome. N Engl J Med, *311*:281, 1984.

30. Good JT, Wolz JF, Anderson JT, et al.: The routine use of positive end-expiratory pressure after open heart surgery. Chest, *76*:397, 1979.

31. Banasik JL, Tyler ML: The effect of prophylactic positive end-expiratory pressure on mediastinal bleeding after coronary revascularization surgery. Heart & Lung, *15*:43, 1986.

32. Zurick AM, Urzua J, Ghattas M, et al.: Failure of positive end-expiratory pressure to decrease postoperative bleeding after cardiac surgery. Ann Thorac Surg, *34*:608, 1982.

33. Peterson GW, Baier H: Incidence of pulmonary barotrauma in a medical ICU. Crit Care Med, *11*:67, 1983.

34. Pingleton SK: Complications of acute respiratory failure. Am Rev Respir Dis, *137*:1463, 1988.

35. Leithner C, Frass M, Pacher R, et al.: Mechanical ventilation with positive end-expiratory pressure decreases release of alpha atrial natriuretic peptide. Crit Care Med, *15*:484, 1987.

36. Shapiro HM, Marshall LF: Intracranial pressure responses to PEEP in head-injured patients. J Trauma, *18*:254, 1978.

37. Kirby RR, Taylor RW: PEEP and CPAP for respiratory failure. When, where and why. J Crit Illness, *2*:42, 1987.

38. Marcey TW, Marini JJ: Inverse ratio ventilation. Rationale and implementaiton. Chest, *100*:494, 1991.

39. Papadakos PJ, Halloran W, Hessney JI, et al.: The use of pressure-controlled inverse ratio ventilation in the surgical intensive care unit. J Trauma, *31*:1211, 1991.

MONITORING LUNG FUNCTION

40. Tobin MJ: Respiratory monitoring in the intensive care unit. Amer Rev Resp Dis, *138*:1625, 1988.

41. Berger R, Burki NK: The effects of posture on total respiratory compliance. Am Rev Respir Dis, *125*:262, 1982.

42. Bergman NA: Measurement of respiratory resistance in anesthetized subjects. J Appl Physiol, *21*:1913, 1966.

43. Katz JA, Zinn SE, Ozanne GM, Fairley BB: Pulmonary, chest wall and lung-throax elastances in acute respiratory failure. Chest, *80*:304, 1981.

44. Gomez-Rubi JA, SanMartin A, Gonzalez Diaz G, et al.: Assessment of total pulmonary airways resistance during mechanical ventilation. Crit Care Med, *11*:633, 1980.
45. Marino PL, Barkin P, Shaw D, et al.: Bronchodilator effects on inspiratory and expiratory airflow resistance during mechanical ventilation. Am Rev Respir Dis, *127*:263, 1983.
46. DeTroyer A, Yernault JC, Rodenstein D: Influence of beta-2 agonist aerosols on pressure-volume characteristics of the lungs. Am Rev Respir Dis, *118*:987, 1978.

AUTO-PEEP

47. Pepe PE, Marini JJ: Occult positive end-expiratory pressure in mechanically ventilated patients with airflow obstruction. Amer Rev Respir Dis, *126*:166, 1982.
48. Qvist J, Pemberton M, Bennike KA: High-level PEEP in severe asthma. N Engl J Med, *307*:1347, 1982.
49. Tobin M, Lodato RF: PEEP, auto-PEEP, and waterfalls. Chest, *96*:449, 1989.

ARTIFICIAL AIRWAYS

50. Consensus conference on artificial airways in patients receiving mechanical ventilation. Chest, *96*:178, 1989.
51. Heffner JE, Miller S, Sahn SA: Tracheostomy in the intensive care unit. Parts 1 and 2. Chest, *90*:269, 1986.
52. Stauffer JL, Olson DE, Petty TL: Complications and consequences of endotracheal intubation and tracheostomy. Am J Med, *70*:65, 1981.
53. Brunel W, Coleman DL, Schwartz DE, et al.: Assessment of routine chest roentgenograms and the physical examination to confirm endotracheal tube position. Chest, *96*: 1043, 1989.
54. Caplan RA, Posner KL, Ward RJ, Cheney FW: Adverse respiratory events in anesthesia: A closed claims analysis. Anesthesiology, *72*:828, 1990.
55. Salord F, Gaussorgues P, Marti-Flich J, et al.: Nosocomial maxillary sinusitis during mechanical ventilation: A prospective comparison of orotracheal versus nasotracheal route for intubation. Intensive Care Med, *16*:390, 1990.
56. Knodel AR, Beekman JF: Unexplained fevers in patients with nasotracheal intubation. JAMA, *248*:868, 1982.
57. Gridlinger GA, Niehoff J, Hughes L, et al.: Acute paranasal sinusitis related to nasotracheal intubation of head-injured patients. Crit Care Med, *15*:214, 1987.
58. Williams JW Jr., Roberts L, Distell B, Simel DL: Diagnosing sinusitis by X-ray: Comparing a single Water's view to 4:view paranasal sinus radiographs. Clin Sci, *38*:937 A, 1990.
59. Whited RE: A prospective study of laryngotracheal sequelae in long-term intubation. Laryngoscope, *94*:367, 1984.
60. Dunham CM, LaMonica C: Prolonged tracheal intubation in the trauma patient. J Trauma, *24*:120, 1984.
61. Colice G, Stukel T, Dain B: Laryngeal complications of prolonged intubation. Chest, *96*: 877, 1989.
62. Gaussorgues P, Boyer F, Piperno D, et al.: Do corticosteroids prevent postintubation laryngeal edema? A prospective study of 276 adults. Crit Care Med, *16*:649, 1988.
63. Spray SB, Zuidema GD, Cameron JL: Aspiration pneumonia. Am J Surg, *131*:701, 1976.
64. Bernhard WN, Cottrell JE, Sivakumaran C, et al.: Adjustment of intracuff pressure to prevent aspiration. Anesthesiology, *50*:363, 1979.
65. Shapiro M, Wilson RK, Cesar G, et al.: Work of breathing through different sized endotracheal tubes. Crit Care Med, *14*:1028, 1986.

PULMONARY BAROTRAUMA

66. Haake R, Schlichtig R, Ulstad DR, et al.: Barotrauma. Pathophysiology, risk factors and prevention. Chest, *91*:608, 1987.
67. Powner DJ: Pulmonary barotrauma in the intensive care unit. Intensive Care Med, *3*: 224, 1988.

68. Petersen GW, Baier H: Incidence of pulmonary barotrauma in a medical ICU. Crit Care Med, *11*:67, 1983.
69. Steir M, Ching N, Roberts EB, Nealon TF: Pneumothorax complicating continuous ventilatory support. J Thorac Cardiovasc Surg, *67*:17, 1974.
70. Woodring JH: Pulmonary interstitial emphysema in the adult respiratory distress syndrome. Crit Care Med, *13*:786, 1985.
71. Chiles C, Ravin CE: Radiographic appearance of pneumothorax in the intensive care unit. Crit Care Med, *14*:677, 1986.

MANAGEMENT

72. Broaddus VC, Berthiaume Y, Biondi JW, et al.: Hemodynamic management of the adult respiratory distress syndrome. Intensive Care Med, *2*:190, 1987.
73. Jing DL, Kohler JP, Rice CL, et al.: Albumin therapy in permeability pulmonary edema. J Surg Res, *33*:482, 1982.
74. Francis GS, Siegel RM, Goldsmith SR, et al.: Acute vasoconstrictor response to intravenous furosemide in patients with chronic congestive heart failure. Ann Intern Med, *103*:1, 1986.
75. Mathur PN, Pugsley SO, Powles P, et al.: Effects of diuretics on cardiopulmonary performance in severe chronic airflow obstruction. Arch Intern Med, *144*:2154, 1984.
76. Rackow EC, Falk JL, Fein IA, et al.: Fluid resuscitation in circulatory shock: A comparison of the cardiorespiratory effects of albumin, hetastarch, and saline solutions in patients with hypovolemic and septic shock. Crit Care Med, *11*:839, 1983.
77. Shoemaker WC: Relationship of oxygen transport patterns to the pathophysiology and therapy of shock states. Intensive Care Med, *13*:230, 1987.
78. Kruse JA, Haupt MT, Puri V, Carlson RW: Lactate levels as predictors of the relationship between oxygen delivery and oxygen consumption in ARDS. Chest, *98*:959, 1990.
79. Mizock B: Controversies in lactic acidosis. JAMA, *258*:497, 1987.
80. Uretsky BF, Lawless CE, Verbalis JG, et al.: Combined therapy with dobutamine and amrinone in severe heart failure. Chest, *92*:657, 1987.
81. Franciosa JA: Intravenous amrinone: An advance or a wrong step? Ann Intern Med, *102*:399, 1985.
82. Malloy DW, Ducas J, Dobson K, et al.: Hemodynamic management in clinical acute hypoxemic respiratory failure: dopamine vs dobutamine. Chest, *89(5)*:636, 1986.
83. Hales CA, Westphal D: Hypoxemia following the administration of sublingual nitroglycerin. Am J Med, *65*:911, 1978.
84. Kahn RC, Zaroulis C, Goetz W, Howland WS: Hemodynamic and oxygen transport and 2,3-diphosphoglycerate changes after transfusion of patients in acute respiratory failure. Intensive Care Med, *12*:22, 1986.
85. Brinson ME, Alexander JW: Mechanisms of transfusion-induced immunosuppression. Transfusion, *30*:651, 1990.
86. ACCP-NHLBI National Conference on Oxygen Therapy. Chest, *86*:234, 1984.
87. Jenkinson SG: Oxygen toxicity. Intensive Care Med, *3*:137, 1988.
88. Brigham KL: Role of free radicals in lung injury. Chest, *89*:850, 1986.
89. Heffner JE, Repine JE: Pulmonary strategies of antioxidant defense. Am Rev Respir Dis, *140*:531, 1989.
90. Sugino K, Dohi K, Yamada K, Kawasaki T: Changes in the levels of endogenous antioxidants in the liver of mice with experimental endotoxemia and the protective effects of the antioxidants. Surgery, *105*:200, 1989.
91. Chance B, Sies H, Boveris A: Hydroperoxide metabolism in mammalian organs. Physiol Rev, *59*:527, 1979.
92. Southorn PA, Powis G: Free radicals in medicine. II. Involvement in human disease. Mayo Clin Proc. *63*:390, 1988.

93. Suttorp N, Toepfer W, Roka L: Antioxidant defense mechanisms of endothelial cells: Glutathione redox cycle versus catalase. Am J Physiol, *20*:C671, 1986.
94. Hesselvik F, Carlsson C, von Schenck H, Sorbo B: Low selenium plasma levels in surgical intensive care patients: Relation to infection. Clin Nutrition, *6*:279, 1987.
95. Food and Nutrition Board, National Academy of Sciences—National Research Council. Recommended Dietary Allowances, 1989.
96. Stead NW, Leonard S, Carroll R: Effect of selenium supplementation on selenium balance in the dependent elderly. Am J Med Sci, *290*:228, 1985.
97. Dempsey DT, Mullen JL, Rombeau JL, et al.: Treatment effects of parenteral vitamins in total parenteral nutrition patients. J Parent Ent Nutrit, *11*:229, 1987.
98. Winslet MC, Donovan IA, Aitchison F: Wernicke's Encephalopathy in association with complicated acute pancreatitis and morbid obesity. Br J Clin Pract, *44*:771, 1990.
99. McConachie I, Hasken A: Thiamine status after major trauma. Intensive Care Med, *14*: 628, 1988.

WEANING

100. Karpel JP, Aldrich TK: Respiratory failure and mechanical ventilation: Pathophysiology and methods to promote weaning. Lung, *164*:309, 1986.
101. Sporn PHS, Morganroth ML: Discontinuation of mechanical ventilation. Clin Chest Med, *9*:113, 1988.
102. Morganroth ML, et al.: Criteria for weaning from prolonged mechanical ventilation. Arch Intern Med, *144*:1012, 1984.
103. Benedixen HH, et al.: Respiratory Care. St. Louis, C.V. Mosby Co., 1965, pp. 137–156.
104. Stetson JB: Introductory essay in prolonged tracheal intubation. Int Anesthesiol Clin, *8*: 774, 1970.
105. Pontoppidan H, Laver MA, Geffin B: Acute respiratory failure in the surgical patient. Adv Surg, *4*:163, 1970.
106. Sahn SA, Lakshminarayan S: Bedside criteria for discontinuation of mechanical ventilation. Chest, *63*:1002, 1973.
107. Harpin RP, Baker JP, Downer JP, et al.: Correlation of the oxygen cost of breathing and length of weaning from mechanical ventilation. Crit Care Med, *15*:807, 1987.
108. Nashimura M, Taenaka N, Takezawa J, et al.: Oxygen cost of breathing and inspiratory work of ventilator as weaning monitor in critically ill. Crit Care Med, *12*:258, 1984.
109. Venus B, Smith RA, Mathru M: National survey of methods and criteria used for weaning from mechanical ventilation. Crit Care Med, *15*:530, 1987.
110. Ashutosh K: Gradual vs. abrupt weaning from respiratory support in acute respiratory failure and advanced chronic obstructive lung disease. South Med J, *76*:1244, 1983.
111. Prakash O, Meij MS, Van Der Borden B: Spontaneous ventilation test vs. intermittent mandatory ventilation. Chest, *81*:403, 1982.
112. Tobin MJ, Perez W, Guenther SM, et al.: The pattern of breathing during successful and unsuccessful trials of weaning from mechanical ventilation. Amer Rev Respir Dis, *134*: 1111, 1986.
113. Weinberger SE, Schwartzstein RM, Weiss JW: Hypercapnia. N Engl J Med, *321*:1223, 1989.
114. Aubier M, DeTroyer A, Sampson M, et al.: Aminophylline improves diaphragm contractility. N Engl J Med, *305*:249, 1981.
115. Swartz M, Marino PL: Diaphragm strength during weaning from mechanical ventilation. Chest, *88*:736, 1985.

30

Pulmonary Embolism

Lucy B. Palmer
M. Gabriel Khan

In the United States, the incidence of pulmonary embolism has been estimated to exceed 600,000 cases per year. A common and difficult clinical problem, pulmonary embolism is the third most frequent cause of death in the United States. Approximately 10% of patients with pulmonary embolism will die in the first hour, and another 20% will die later in the course of the illness. When a timely diagnosis is made, over 90% of patients will survive; however, when pulmonary embolism is overlooked, 30% of cases will result in death. Prevention, early diagnosis, and treatment of this serious disease are vital.

PATHOGENESIS

Pulmonary emboli arise from a number of sites, but the primary sources are the deep iliofemoral and thigh veins. Other sites include the pelvic veins and, less commonly, the right atrium and ventricle. The calf veins do not give rise to significant emboli but may extend upward in about 15% of cases.

Risk factors include any processes that increase venous stasis, damage the intima of the venous system, or cause a hypercoagulable state. Certain clinical conditions present particularly high risk for pulmonary embolism. Patients with these conditions must be considered for prophylactic measures and a diagnostic workup must be initiated promptly if there are any symptoms of pulmonary embolism. High-risk clinical conditions include the following

- History of thromboembolic disease
- Prolonged anesthesia associated with surgery
- Surgery or injury to the lower extremities or pelvis
- Bed rest
- Pregnancy (particularly postpartum) or use of estrogen-containing compounds
- Congestive heart failure
- Malignancy

- Obesity
- Hypercoagulable diathesis (protein C, S, or antithrombin III deficiency). This condition comprises < 15% of cases of deep venous thrombosis (DVT)

PATHOPHYSIOLOGY

The effects of pulmonary emboli on gas exchange are multifold

- Increase in dead space
- Bronchoconstriction in the area of the embolus
- Hyperventilation
- Hypoxemia

Hypoxemia has been attributed to multiple causes, including increased shunt (both intrapulmonary and intracardiac, in cases of patent foramen ovale), widening of the arteriovenous O_2 difference caused by acute changes in cardiac output secondary to right heart failure, increased perfusion to low V/Q units secondary to elevated pulmonary pressures, and atelectasis associated with the loss of surfactant.

Hemodynamic effects of pulmonary emboli depend not only on the size of the embolus but on the patient's baseline cardiopulmonary status. Normal individuals can tolerate an embolic event of substantial size without significant changes in pulmonary artery pressures. Pulmonary hypertension may occur when 30% or more of the vascular bed is obstructed. But in patients with significant underlying pulmonary vascular disease, smaller emboli can result in cor pulmonale if acute elevations of the mean pulmonary arterial pressure exceed 40 mm Hg. Pulmonary hypertension appears to be due not only to decreased cross-sectional area of the vascular bed but to pulmonary artery constriction, which may result from hypoxemia and neural and humoral factors. In a patient with no preexisting cardiopulmonary disease, shock is caused by obstruction of more than 50% of the pulmonary circulation.

PROGNOSIS

The prognosis for patients with pulmonary embolism is usually excellent if they survive the first hour and the diagnosis is made. The degree and rate of resolution are most abnormal in patients with underlying cardiopulmonary disease. Recurrent thromboembolism is uncommon in patients with an acute presentation of pulmonary embolism if treated appropriately. The rate of resolution has been examined using hemodynamic, angiographic, and scan abnormalities

- Hemodynamic improvement may be minimal the first week after a large embolus
- Most scans and angiograms will show significant improvement in 3 weeks
- Complete angiographic resolution can occasionally occur as soon as 7 days after the embolic event

- There will be minimal further resolution after 2 to 3 months
- With underlying cardiopulmonary disease, complete resolution may never occur

CLINICAL HALLMARKS

The diagnosis of pulmonary embolism should be strongly considered in patients who manifest one or more of the following clinical patterns.

ACUTE UNEXPLAINED DYSPNEA

- Patients present with tachypnea and possibly tachycardia
- The chest x-ray and ECG are usually normal
- Patients frequently have sustained a large embolus or have underlying cardiopulmonary disease

PULMONARY HEMORRHAGE AND/OR INFARCTION

- Patients usually have sustained, submassive embolus.
- Most will have pleuritic chest pain, dyspnea, hemoptysis, and chest x-ray infiltrate. At least three out of four of these findings are usually present

Other common findings, including fever, occasional friction rub, mild wheeze, and/or crepitations may be detected on auscultation. Leukocytosis may also occur, but there is a conspicuous absence of band cells that are virtually always present in patients with a bacterial pneumonia, which is frequently the main differential diagnosis.

A small pleural effusion with blunting of the costophrenic-angle and pleural-based consolidation are frequent. Large effusions with bronchial breathing, which may persist for some weeks, occasionally occur. The effusion is often blood-tinged or frankly hemorrhagic and has the qualities of an exudate; however, up to 20% of cases yield a transudative pattern. When an exudative effusion is present, a pH less than 7.2 suggests infection. When requesting pH of the pleural aspirate, it is crucial to use the same technique for collecting and transporting the pleural aspirate as is used for arterial blood gas analysis (see Chapter 26).

As lung parenchyma is oxygenated by the airways as well as by the pulmonary and bronchial circulation, infarction usually occurs when there is damage to two of the three supplies. Therefore, pulmonary infarction occurs more commonly in patients with underlying cardiopulmonary disease. After an infarct, the necrosis of intra-alveolar septae with dense hemorrhage undergoes slow resolution with fibrosis and scar formation, as opposed to complete resolution in patients with no underlying disease.

ACUTE COR PULMONALE AND CARDIOGENIC SHOCK

Massive emboli cause obstruction or large filling defects in two or more lobar arteries. If greater than 70% of the pulmonary vascular cross-sectional area is obstructed, this results in acute pulmonary hypertension exceeding

40 to 45 mm Hg. Acute right ventricular dilation and failure supervene, but blood pressure may be temporarily preserved because of an increase in systemic vascular resistance caused by adrenergic reflexes. Over one-half of deaths due to thromboembolic disease result from massive pulmonary embolism, which is responsible for the majority of deaths that occur within the first hour after the onset of symptoms. The mortality rate of patients with massive pulmonary embolism and shock is approximately 33%. Symptoms and signs include the following

- Presyncope or syncope
- Abrupt unexplained severe dyspnea and signs that may simulate an acute exacerbation of chronic obstructive lung disease
- Oppressive central chest pain (usually nonpleuritic)
- Marked apprehension
- Clouding of consciousness
- Cold, clammy skin
- Signs of cardiogenic shock (see Chapter 16)
- Intensified pulmonic component of the second heart sound, accompanied by wide physiologic splitting of the second heart sound due to prolonged right ventricular ejection

CHRONIC COR PULMONALE IN PATIENTS WITH RECURRENT PULMONARY EMBOLISM OR AN UNDETERMINED CAUSE

While must pulmonary emboli resolve over weeks, residual obstruction persists in a small group of patients resulting in pulmonary hypertension and cor pulmonale. This may be secondary to persistent major vessel obstruction or to recurrent small emboli or possible in situ thrombosis. In patients with major vessel obstruction, the diagnosis is often not made at the time of the initial embolic event. Clinical features include the following

- Patients present with increasing dyspnea and fatigue, as well as signs of right ventricular failure. These symptoms appear to be due to pulmonary hypertension, which causes further vessel damage
- The perfusion scan may reveal large bilateral perfusion defects without ventilation abnormality
- Right heart catheterization and pulmonary angiography are required for diagnosis

APPROACH TO DIAGNOSIS

Certain symptoms and signs, while nonspecific, are quite sensitive and, when combined with significant risk factors (see Tables 30–1, 30–2, and 30–3), increase the likelihood of pulmonary embolism. Tables 30–1 and 30–2 show the most commonly demonstrated signs and symptoms in the National Heart Lung Blood Institute Prospective Investigation of Pulmonary Embolism Diagnosis (PIOPED), a large multicenter study examining the accuracy of lung scans compared to pulmonary angiography

- Dyspnea and pleuritic pain are the most common symptoms

TABLE 30–1. SYMPTOMS: NO PREEXISTING CARDIAC OR PULMONARY DISEASE

	PULMONARY EMBOLISM N = 117 NUMBER (%)	NO PULMONARY EMBOLISM N = 248 NUMBER (%)
Dyspnea	85 (73)	178 (72)
Pleuritic pain	77 (66)	146 (59)
Cough	43 (37)	89 (36)
Leg swelling	33 (28)	55 (22)
Leg pain	30 (26)	60 (24)
Hemoptysis	15 (13)	20 (8)
Palpitations	12 (10)	44 (18)
Wheezing	10 (9)	28 (11)
Angina-like pain	5 (4)	15 (6)

No significant differences were seen.
Reproduced with permission from Stein PD, Terrin ML, Hales CA, et al.: Clinical, laboratory, roentgenographic and electrocardiographic findings in patients with acute pulmonary embolism and no pre-existing cardiac or pulmonary disease. Chest, *100*:600, 1991.

TABLE 30–2. SIGNS OF ACUTE PULMONARY EMBOLISM: NO PREEXISTING CARDIAC OR PULMONARY DISEASE

	PULMONARY EMBOLISM N = 117 NUMBER (%)	NO PULMONARY EMBOLISM N = 248 NUMBER (%)
Tachypnea (20/min)	82 (70)	169 (68)
Crackles	60 (51)	98 (40)*
Tachycardia (> 100 min)	35 (30)	59 (24)
Fourth heart sound	28 (24)	34 (14)*
Increased P_2	27 (23)	33 (13)*
Deep venous thrombosis	13 (11)	27 (11)
Diaphoresis	13 (11)	20 (8)
Temperature > 38.5	8 (7)	29 (12)
Wheezes	6 (5)	21 (8)
Homan's sign	5 (4)	6 (2)
Right ventricular lift	5 (4)	6 (2)
Pleural friction rub	3 (3)	6 (2)
Third heart sound	3 (3)	11 (4)
Cyanosis	1 (1)	5 (2)

* $p < 0.05$
Reproduced with permission from Stein PD, Terrin ML, Hales CA, et al.: Clinical, laboratory, roentgenographic and electrocardiographic findings in patients with acute pulmonary embolism and no pre-existing cardiac or pulmonary disease. Chest, *100*:600, 1991.

TABLE 30–3. RISK GROUPS FOR THROMBOEMBOLISM		
RISK GROUP	**INCIDENCE OF VENOUS THROMBOSIS (%)**	**INCIDENCE OF FATAL PE (%)**
Medical patients	15	1
General and gynecologic surgery	15–20	1
Neurologic surgery	15–20	1
Urologic surgery	15–20	5
Total knee replacement	40–70	5
Hip replacement	40–70	1–2
Hip fracture	40–70	1–5

Data from Hyers T, Hull R, Weg J: 2nd American College of Chest Physicians Conference on Antithrombotic Therapy, Antithrombotic Therapy for Venous Thromboembolic Disease. Chest, *95*:37S, 1989 (with permission).

- Tachypnea and crepitations are the most common findings on physical examination

Combining the results of clinical diagnosis and lung scanning can greatly increase the accuracy of diagnosis in certain settings and help direct decision-making as soon as the result of the lung scan is available (see Figure 30–1). This was demonstrated in PIOPED. When a clinical impression of high probability of pulmonary embolism was combined with a high probability scan, the condition was present in 96% of the cases. Conversely, if both scan and clinical impression were low probability for embolism, the diagnosis was correctly excluded in 96% of the cases. For example, if a patient presents with sudden pleuritic pain and becomes hypoxemic on the fifth postoperative day and the chest x-ray shows a small area of atelectasis, the diagnosis of pulmonary embolism is likely. If the scan is high probability, it is not necessary for the workup to proceed. This is a logical approach, but unfortunately, it does not embrace many scenarios that may be encountered and the assignment of high probability and low probability to clinical assessment is still quite subjective. In PIOPED, the majority of assessments were intermediate, with 20 to 79% likelihood of pulmonary embolism.

STANDARD LABORATORY TESTS

Complete blood count and blood chemistries are nonspecific. As mentioned above, leukocytosis may be present. Lactate dehydrogenase may be elevated in approximately 80% of cases; however, it may be a nonspecific and delayed finding.

CHEST X-RAY

Numerous radiographic abnormalities have been described. None of them, however, are specific or sensitive

- Atelectasis
- Pleural effusion

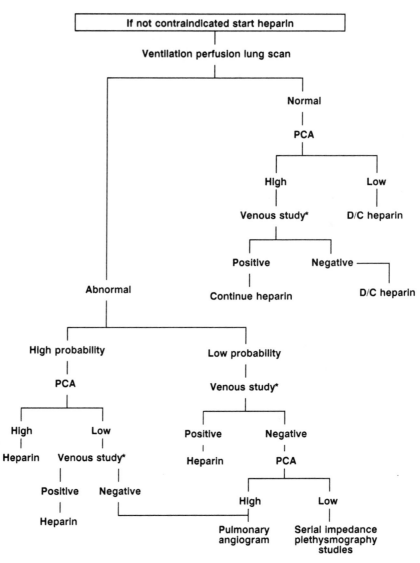

PCA = Probability from clinical assessment
D/C = Discontinue
* Venous study = Impedance plethysmography, venogram, or Duplex scanning

FIG. 30–1. Algorithm for the management of suspected pulmonary embolism.

- Elevated hemidiaphragm
- Pleural-based consolidation (Hampton's hump)
- Pulmonary artery enlargement
- Abrupt vessel cutoff (knuckle sign)
- Area of hyperlucency: Oligemia (Westermark's sign)

- Dilation of azygos vein
- Enlargement of any chamber of the heart

ARTERIAL BLOOD GAS (ABG)

The most common abnormalities of the arterial blood gas include

- Hypoxemia: P_aO_2 less than 80 mm or less than age predicted is present in over 70% of cases but is nonspecific. Importantly, more than 30% of patients with proven pulmonary embolism have a P_aO_2 greater than 80 mm Hg, on room air, especially if the blood sample is drawn several hours after the event. The alveolar–arterial (A–a) gradient exceeds 20 mm Hg in up to 86% of patients with proven pulmonary embolism, but as with hypoxemia this is nondiagnostic
- Respiratory alkalosis: This is a common finding and usually will be present even in patients with chronic obstructive pulmonary disease and CO_2 retention. CO_2 retention from pulmonary emboli is seen only in the setting of massive emboli

SWAN-GANZ CATHETER

Many patients who present with severe hypoxemia while in the intensive care unit setting may have a Swan-Ganz catheter in place. Elevated pulmonary artery pressures and the inability to obtain a good wedge tracing may suggest a massive embolus. If the embolus is massive and sufficient to cause right ventricular failure and decreased cardiac output, pulmonary artery pressures may be only moderately elevated.

ELECTROCARDIOGRAM

- Sinus tachycardia is common but too nonspecific to assist in diagnosis
- A pattern of acute cor pulmonale: S1 Q3 T3 (T wave inversion in 3) with lead 2 following the pattern in lead 1 rather than lead 3; a finding that is unlike inferior infarction
- S1 S2 S3
- Right axis deviation
- Right ventricular strain pattern: Inverted T waves V1 to V3 with more prominent S waves in V5, V6 due to right ventricular dilation
- Transient right bundle branch block
- Nonspecific ST segment or T wave inversion (in up to 33% of patients)
- ST segment depression V4 to V6 (may be due to poor coronary perfusion in patients with ischemic heart disease)

These findings are uncommon and nonspecific but may occur suddenly; their transient appearance increases the likelihood of pulmonary embolism. Patterns of acute right heart strain should raise the concern of a large embolic event.

LUNG SCAN

The first-line investigation for patients with suspected pulmonary embolism is a ventilation/perfusion scan, except for patients with acute cor pulmonale pattern and/or cardiogenic shock, in whom emergency pulmonary

---

TABLE 30–4. PIOPED CENTRAL SCAN INTERPRETATION CATEGORIES AND CRITERIA

HIGH PROBABILITY

≥ Two large (>75% of a segment) segmental perfusion defects without corresponding ventilation or x-ray abnormalities.

≥ Two moderate segmental (≥25% and ≤75% of a segment) perfusion defects without matching ventilation or chest x-ray abnormalities and one large mismatched segmental defect.

≥ For moderate segmental perfusion defects without ventilation or chest x-ray abnormalities.

INTERMEDIATE PROBABILITY (INDETERMINATE)

Not falling into normal, very low, low, or high probability categories.

Borderline high or borderline low.

Difficult to categorize as low or high.

LOW PROBABILITY

Nonsegmental perfusion defects (e.g., very small effusion causing blunting of the costophrenic angle, cardiomegaly, enlarged aorta, hila and mediastinum, and elevated diaphragm).

Single moderate mismatched segmental perfusion defect with normal chest x-ray.

Any perfusion defect with a substantially larger chest x-ray abnormality.

Large or moderate segmental perfusion defects involving no more than four segments in one lung and no more than three segments in one lung region with matching ventilation defects either equal to or larger in size and chest x-ray either normal or with abnormalities substantially smaller than perfusion defects.

> Three small segmental perfusion defects (< 25% of a segment) with a normal chest x-ray.

VERY LOW PROBABILITY

≤ Three small segmental perfusion defects with a normal chest x-ray.

NORMAL

No perfusion defects present.

Perfusion outlines exactly the shape of the lungs as seen on the chest x-ray (hilar and aortic impressions may be seen, chest x-ray and/or ventilation study may be abnormal).

Reproduced from: The PIOPED Investigators: Value of the ventilation/perfusion scan in acute pulmonary embolism. JAMA, *263*: 2755, 1990.

angiography is essential. It must be emphasized that the lung scan may not be useful in many patients with underlying cardiopulmonary disease who will have an indeterminate scan. The PIOPED study did reveal, however, that the specificity of a high probability scan in patients with prior cardiopulmonary disease was similar to patients with no underlying disease (97% versus 98%). Many radiologists request a scan prior to angiographic study to guide their injection and permit a selective study if appropriate. The perfusion scan should be performed first because a normal scan will usually negate the need for further workup. The following rules govern the properly interpreted lung scan report. (See Table 30–4 for definition of scans in PIOPED study.)

NORMAL SCANS

A normal scan associated with a normal chest x-ray usually indicates the absence of pulmonary embolism. Although some investigations have revealed a 2 to 4% incidence of positive pulmonary angiograms, it has been shown that patients with normal scans who have negative studies of their lower extremities for venous thrombosis have an excellent prognosis without anticoagulation. In this setting, it is likely that a clot undetected by a scan is not clinically significant.

NONDIAGNOSTIC LUNG SCANS

Recent data from large multicenter studies suggest that nondiagnostic lung scans should include all scans other than normal and high probability scans. Previously, scans have been rated in compartments of likelihood of pulmonary embolus. With the exception of high probability and normal scans, these terms are frequently misleading and may be dangerous because of the high frequency of low probability scans in patients with angiographic pulmonary embolism. Both PIOPED and a large series by Hull have shown that pulmonary emboli may be present in 25 to 40% of patients with low probability scans (see Table 30–5).

HIGH PROBABILITY SCANS

These scans reveal multiple segmental perfusion defects with ventilation mismatch. These scans are specific but lack sensitivity, which can be as low as 40%. In the PIOPED study, sensitivity of these scans was 97%, but only 102 of 251 patients (41%) with positive angiograms had high probability scans. Similarly, in an investigation by Hull, only 52 of 98 (41%) with pulmonary embolism by angiogram had high probability scans.

FEMORAL VENOGRAPHY AND IMPEDANCE PLETHYSMOGRAPHY

Above-the-knee deep venous thrombosis is present in 70 to 90% of patients with angiographic pulmonary embolism. Thus, evaluation of the lower extremities is often warranted in decision making in patients suspected of having pulmonary embolism. Femoral venography remains the gold standard against which other methods are measured, but there are sufficient

TABLE 30–5. LUNG SCAN AND THE INCIDENCE OF PULMONARY EMBOLUS

LUNG SCAN REPORT	PULMONARY EMBOLISM PRESENT*	
	Ref. 5	Ref. 11
Normal	2%	4%
High probability	57%	88%
Nondiagnostic	42%	16–33%

* Differences between these two large clinical studies are most likely due to different definitions of subgroups of scans.

Ref. 5—Hull RD, Raskob GE: Low probability lung scan findings: A need for change. Ann Int Med, *174*:142, 1991.

Ref. 11—Pioped Investigators: Value of the ventilation-perfusion scan in acute pulmonary embolism. JAMA, *263*:2753, 1990.

data to support the use of impedance plethysmography for the diagnosis of acute venous thrombosis of less than 7 days' duration, as it will detect 95% of clots involving the popliteal vein or above. Recent data also support the use of Duplex scanning as a sensitive and specific technique for DVT. DVT and its management is discussed in Chapter 11.

PULMONARY ANGIOGRAPHY

Pulmonary angiography is the final step necessary in properly selected patients.

INDICATIONS

Pulmonary angiography is performed to confirm or exclude the diagnosis of pulmonary embolism in the following situations

- Nondiagnostic lung scan with a negative femoral venogram or impedance plethysmography and remaining suspicion of pulmonary embolism
- As an emergency procedure for diagnostic confirmation prior to embolectomy in patients with acute cor pulmonale pattern and/or cardiogenic shock. In this setting, lung scan is not indicated
- High probability scan in a patient with a history of pulmonary emboli (these scans have less specificity in this group)
- High probability scan with a high risk of bleeding

RISKS

- Allergic reaction to contrast material. The procedure can be carried out, if strongly warranted, using premedication with corticosteroids and antihistamine with epinephrine standby
- Cardiac perforation (occurs in up to 0.3%, but is virtually nonexistent in experienced hands)
- Arrhythmias (usually easily controlled)
- Depression of myocardial contractility may precipitate heart failure within minutes to 1 hour of the procedure in patients with left ventricular dysfunction. Also, a large volume of contrast material is required and imposes an osmotic load; thus, intravenous (IV) furosemide may be required
- Pulmonary hypertension may be exacerbated by the procedure, but selective injections are often possible and are well tolerated
- The morbidity rate is 2 to 4%; the mortality rate is less than 0.2%

THERAPY

HEPARIN

Heparin (5,000 to 10,000 units) is given as an IV bolus if there is no contraindication to anticoagulant therapy. The bolus is followed immediately by an infusion of heparin 1,000 units/hour. Partial thromboplastin time

(PTT) is done 6 hours later and the infusion adjusted to maintain the PTT 1.5 to 2 times the patient control level. Heparin is usually continued for 7 to 10 days, and coumadin is started between the first and fifth day. See Chapter 11 for instructions on heparin and coumadin therapy. For submassive pulmonary embolism however, coumadin can be commenced on on the first or second night and heparin is discontinued when the prothrombin time is in the therapeutic range of 1.3 to 1.5 times the control or International Normalized Ratio (INR). This approximately 5-day course of IV heparin can result in considerable savings for patients and hospitals. Coumadin is continued for 3 to 6 months. In some patients with ongoing risk factors, prolonged therapy may be required.

THROMBOLYTIC AGENTS

Thrombolytic therapy is of value to restore circulation in patients with hemodynamic compromise in the setting of massive emboli or shock. Streptokinase, urokinase, and tissue plasminogen activator (tPA) are the three agents currently available. Despite their ability to accelerate the early rate of resolution, there has been no proven benefit in long-term morbidity or mortality compared to heparin therapy alone. The unknown benefits must be weighed against the significant bleeding risks associated with the use of these agents. Despite early speculation that tPA might be associated with less bleeding, early investigations have not shown this to be true (see Chapter 3).

The current indication for thrombolytic agent use is massive pulmonary embolism and hemodynamic compromise.

Dosage: The two most commonly used agents are streptokinase and urokinase.

- Streptokinase: 250,000 units/30 minutes IV, then infusion of 100,000 units for 12 to 24 hours followed by IV heparin
- Urokinase: 4,400 IU/kg for 12 hours followed by IV heparin

After 3 hours of treatment with either agent, testing should be done to ensure a "lytic state." This can be monitored with a number of tests, including *euglobulin* lysis time, fibrinogen level, fibrinogen degradation products, PT or PTT. This testing is not used to adjust dosing but to determine whether systemic fibrinolysis has been achieved. If it has not, then the patient may need to be rebolused. See Chapter 3 for contraindications and further discussion of thrombolytic agents.

PULMONARY EMBOLECTOMY

This is a controversial treatment reserved for patients with massive embolism and hypotension who have not responded to conventional therapy. The mortality is approximately 50%, which most likely reflects the severity of the process being treated (frequently these patients have already arrested and are requiring cardiopulmonary resuscitation). This option is a viable one in only a few institutions. When pulmonary embolectomy is performed, the patient must also have placement of a vena caval filter.

INFERIOR VENA CAVA BARRIER

This useful intervention prevents the migration of large clots. Currently, the ideal method is transvenous insertion of a filter device that permits blood flow to prevent occlusion and longterm complications. There are a variety of types and sizes of devices available, and these vary from institution to institution.

INDICATIONS

- Patients recovering from life-threatening pulmonary embolism to prevent further massive embolism
- Contraindication for anticoagulants
- Recurrent emboli during adequate anticoagulation
- Patients undergoing pulmonary embolectomy

PREVENTION IN PATIENTS AT RISK

Patient populations have been stratified into risk categories for deep venous thrombosis and pulmonary emboli. Methods of prevention are modified for the individual clinical groups and their risk of bleeding

- For patients at low to moderate risk, low-dose heparin should be given (5,000 units subcutaneously every 8 to 12 hours starting at the time of risk)
- Neurosurgical procedures, major knee surgery, and urologic surgery should be treated with intermittent pneumatic compression
- Patients undergoing hip surgery should be treated with adjusted-dose heparin to keep PTT in upper half of normal range or with warfarin to prolong PT to 1.3 to 1.5 times control (INR 2 to 3 times control)
- Hip fracture patients should receive prophylactic therapy to prolong the PT to 1.3 to 1.5 times control (INR 2 to 3)
- In some high-risk patients, there may be a role for combined modalities, e.g., pneumatic compression and anticoagulation

BIBLIOGRAPHY

Bell WR, Simon GL, DeMets DL: The clinical features of submassive and massive pulmonary emboli. Am J Med, *62*:35, 1977.

Caracci BF, Rumbolo PM, Mainini S, et al.: How accurate are ventilation-perfusion scans for pulmonary embolism? Am J Surg, *156*:477, 1988.

Dalen JE, Alpert JS: Natural history of pulmonary embolism. Prog Cardiovasc Dis, *42*:259, 1975.

Dantzker PR, Bower JS: Clinical significance of pulmonary function tests: alterations in gas exchange following pulmonary thromboembolism. Chest, *81*:495, 1982.

Hull RD, Raskob GE: Low-probability lung scan findings: A need for change. Ann Intern Med, *174*:142, 1991.

Hull RD, Hirsh J, Carter CJ, et al.: Pulmonary angiography, ventilation lung scanning and venography for clinically suspected pulmonary embolism with abnormal perfusion lung scan. Ann Intern Med, *98*:891, 1983.

Hyers JM, Hull RD, Weg JE: Antithrombotic therapy for venous thromboembolic disease. Chest, *95*:375, 1989.

McBride K, LaMorte WW, Menzoian JO: Can ventilation-perfusion scans accurately diagnose pulmonary embolism. Arch Surg, *121*:754, 1986.

Meyer G, Sors H, Charbonnier B, et al.: Effects of intravenous urokinase versus alteplase on total pulmonary resistance in acute massive pulmonary embolism: A European multicenter double-blind trial. J Am Coll Cardiol, *19*:239, 1992.

Moser KM: Venous thromboembolism. Am Rev Respir Dis, *141*:235, 1990.

Moser KM, Spragg RG, Utley J, et al.: Chronic thrombolic obstruction of major pulmonary arteries. Ann Intern Med, *99*:299, 1983.

PIOPED Investigators: Value of the ventilation-perfusion scan in acute pulmonary embolism. JAMA, *263*:2753, 1990.

Stein PD, Athanasoulis C, Alavi A, et al.: Complications and validity of pulmonary angiography in acute pulmonary embolism. Circuation, *85*:462, 1992.

Stein PD, Coleman RE, Gottschalk A, et al.: Diagnostic utility of ventilation/perfusion lung scans in acute pulmonary embolism is not diminished by pre-existing cardiac or pulmonry disease. Chest, *100*:604, 1991.

Stein PP, Terrin ML, Hales CA, et al.: Clinical laboratory, roentgenographic and electrocardiographic findings in patients with acute pulmonary embolism and no pre-existing cardiac or pulmonary disease. Chest, *100*:598, 1991.

31

LUNG CANCER AND THE SOLITARY PULMONARY NODULE

Thomas W. Shields

LUNG CANCER

Lung cancers may be divided into three major categories: non-small cell carcinomas, small cell carcinomas, and carcinoids (Table 31–1). Other malignant tumors are infrequently encountered and are of less clinical importance. Some clinicians have combined small cell tumors and carcinoids into the category of neuroendocrine (NE) tumors (Table 31–2) because of similar embryologic derivation, pathologic features, and observed functional activities (expression of amine precursor uptake and decarboxylation cell properties). Nonetheless, because the investigation, staging, and therapeutic management of these two tumor types are so different, they should be considered as separate entities rather than as NE tumors.

DIAGNOSTIC INVESTIGATION

RADIOGRAPHIC STUDIES

Radiographic Features on Standard Radiographs

The radiographic findings caused by carcinoma of the lung result from the tumor itself, changes in the pulmonary parenchyma distal to an obstructed bronchus (atelectasis, infection, or both), and spread of the tumor to extrapulmonary, intrathoracic sites (hilar and mediastinal lymph nodes, pleura, chest wall, and other mediastinal structures). The findings vary with the location, the cell type, and the length of time that the tumor has been present.

The chest x-ray is abnormal in 97 to 98% of all patients with lung cancer. The abnormality is most suggestive of tumor in more than 80% of all these patients.

Early Radiographic Features

The early radiographic signs of lung tumors are listed in Table 31–3. The incidence of these early features in a screening program revealed a peripheral nodule or mass in 33%, a peripheral "infiltrate" in 25%, and a

TABLE 31–1. HISTOLOGIC CLASSIFICATION OF LUNG CARCINOMA

Squamous Cell—Epidermoid—Carcinoma
  Spindle cell (squamous) variant
Adenocarcinoma
  Acinar adenocarcinoma
  Papillary adenocarcinoma
  Bronchioloalveolar carcinoma
  Solid carcinoma with mucous formation
Large Cell Undifferentiated Carcinoma
  Giant cell variant
  Clear cell variant
Undifferentiated Small Cell Carcinoma
  Oat cell—typical small cell—carcinoma
  Intermediate—polygonal, fusiform—cell type
  Combined—mixed—cell type
Adenosquamous Carcinoma
Carcinoid Tumor
  Typical
  Atypical
Other Tumors

TABLE 31–2. NEUROENDOCRINE CARCINOMAS OF THE LUNG

Carcinoid tumors—"typical" carcinoids
Well-differentiated cell type—"atypical" carcinoids
Intermediate cell type—polygonal or fusiform small cells
Small cell type—"typical" or oat cells

TABLE 31–3. EARLY RADIOLOGIC FINDINGS IN LUNG CANCER

Homogeneous parenchymal density
  Nodular or linear-shaped
Nonhomogenous parenchymal density
Cavitation within a solid mass
Local infiltration along a blood vessel
Segmental consolidation or atelectasis
Enlargement of the hilar area
Pleural effusion
Obstructive emphysema

TABLE 31-4. RADIOLOGIC ABNORMALITIES ASSOCIATED WITH LUNG CANCER

REGION	TYPE OF INVOLVEMENT
Hilus	Hilar enlargement without discrete mass Hilar mass Perihilar mass
Parenchyma	Small peripheral mass 3 cm or less, distinct or indistinct border Large peripheral mass greater than 3 cm Bronchial obstruction Atelectasis, consolidation, or obstructive pneumonitis (loss of lung volume) Lung abscess with thick irregular wall Localized obstructive emphysema
Intrathoracic extrapulmonary structures	Mediastinal mass or widening Chest wall invasion with bony destruction Pleural effusion Paralyzed, elevated hemidiaphragm

TABLE 31-5. RADIOGRAPHIC FINDINGS IN 200 PATIENTS WITH LUNG CANCER

Tumor in the periphery of the lung	39.5%
Hilar tumor	19.5%
Atelectasis	13.5%
Pleural effusion	7.0%
Hilar invasion	5.0%
Normal	4.0%
Infiltrative shadow in the periphery	3.0%
Other	8.5%

Adapted with permission from Amemiya R, Oho K: X-ray diagnosis of lung cancer. *In* Lung Cancer Diagnosis. Edited by Y Hayata. New York, Igaku-Shoin, 1982.

hilar enlargement in 28% of the patients. Atelectasis or a pleural effusion each occurred in 3% of patients, and obstructive emphysema was seen in only 1%.

Usual Radiographic Manifestations

The radiographic features are classified as hilar, pulmonary parenchymal, and intrathoracic extrapulmonary (Table 31-4). The incidences of the initial presenting radiographic findings are presented in Table 31-5.

Special Radiographic Studies

In addition to the standard x-rays of the chest taken with the patient in the posteroanterior and lateral positions, other x-rays can be obtained with the patient in the right or left anterior oblique, the lordotic, or other special positions to delineate further any suspected lesion. Other radiographic studies, such as standard tomography, 55° oblique tomography, bronchography, contrast study of the esophagus, angiography, azygography, and pneumomediastinography, are rarely indicated.

Conventional Tomography

Conventional tomography is indicated only to evaluate a solitary pulmonary nodule. The study is not included in the routine evaluation of the patient with lung cancer.

Computed Tomography

Computed tomography (CT) is almost routinely performed in patients suspected of having lung cancer.

Advantages

- Permits evaluation of the size of the superior mediastinal lymph nodes (Table 31–6, Fig. 31–1)
- Better than 55° oblique tomography for evaluation of hilar lymph nodes
- Good for demonstrating vertebral body invasion, less effective for rib cage
- May reveal presence of small, undetected pleural effusion
- May suggest encirclement of vital structures by the tumor

Lymph nodes in the superior mediastinum normally measure less than 1 cm in the short axis of the node. In the subcarinal area, normal lymph nodes may measure as large as 1.5 cm. The threshold size for nodal enlargement in the various stations is shown in Table 31–7.

Disadvantages

- Cannot differentiate between inflammatory tissue and tumor
- Of little or no value in the identification of the inferior mediastinal lymph nodes (paraesophageal and pulmonary ligament stations)
- Evaluation of parietal, mediastinal, or diaphragmatic pleural invasion is difficult
- Invasion of mediastinal structures is difficult to determine

When obvious invasion or encirclement of a mediastinal structure is absent and the tumor mass only abuts the structure the CT must be considered indeterminate, even in the absence of a fat plane. When the contact with the mediastinum is 3 cm or less, when contact with the aorta is less than 90°, or when mediastinal fat is present between the mass and the mediastinal structure, resection of the tumor can be done. In 75% of such patients, mediastinal invasion is absent, and in the remaining 25%, only limited focal invasion is present.

A CT scan of the thorax should include the upper abdomen, even in asymptomatic patients, because a small incidence of occult metastasis to either the liver or the adrenals may be suggested.

TABLE 31–6. PROPOSED DEFINITIONS OF REGIONAL NODAL STATIONS FOR PRETHORACOTOMY STAGING

X	Supraclavicular nodes.
2R	Right upper paratracheal (suprainnominate) nodes: Nodes to the right of the midline of the trachea, between the intersection of the caudal margin of the innominate artery with the trachea, and the apex of the lung. (Includes highest R mediastinal node.) (Radiologists may use the same caudal margin as in 2L.)
2L	Left upper paratracheal (supra-aortic) nodes: Nodes to the left of the midline of the trachea between the top of the aortic arch and the apex of the lung. (Includes highest L mediastinal node.)
4R	Right lower paratracheal nodes: Nodes to the right of the midline of the trachea between the cephalic border of the azygos vein and the intersection of the caudal margin of the brachiocephalic artery with the right side of the trachea. (Includes some pretracheal and paracaval nodes.) (Radiologists may use the same cephalic margin as in 4L).
4L	Left lower paratracheal nodes: Nodes to the left of the midline of the trachea between the top of the aortic arch and the level of the carina, medial to the ligamentum arteriosum. (Includes some pretracheal nodes.)
5	Aortopulmonary nodes: Subaortic and para-aortic nodes, lateral to the ligamentum arteriosum or the aorta or left pulmonary artery, proximal to the first branch of the LPA.
6	Anterior mediastinal nodes: Nodes anterior to the ascending aorta or the innominate artery. (Includes some pretracheal and preaortic nodes.)
7	Subcarinal nodes: Nodes rising caudal to the carina of the trachea but not associated with the lower lobe bronchi or arteries within the lung.
8	Paraesophageal nodes: Nodes dorsal to the posterior wall of the trachea and to the right or left of the midline of the esophagus. (Includes retrotracheal, but not subcarinal, nodes.)
9	Right or left pulmonary ligament nodes: Nodes within the right or left pulmonary ligament.
10R	Right tracheobronchial nodes: Nodes to the right of the midline of the trachea from the level of the cephalic border of the azygos vein to the origin of the right upper lobe bronchus.
10L	Left peribronchial nodes: Nodes to the left of the midline of the trachea between the carina and the left upper lobe bronchus, medial to the ligamentum arteriosum.
11	Intrapulmonary nodes: Nodes removed in the right or left lung specimen plus those distal to the main stem bronchi or secondary carina. (Includes interlobar, lobar, and segmental nodes.)*

* Post-thoracotomy staging: Nodes could be divided into stations 11, 12, 13 according to the AJC classification.

With permission of American Thoracic Society: Tisi GM, Fiedman PJ, Peters RM, et al.: Clinical staging of primary lung cancer. Am Rev Respir Dis, *127*:659, 1983.

Magnetic Resonance Imaging

The role of magnetic resonance imaging (MRI) in evaluating the patient with lung cancer has yet to be determined.

Advantages

- Requires no contrast material
- May be obtained in sagittal and coronal planes
- More accurate than CT in showing chest wall invasion and extrathoracic spread

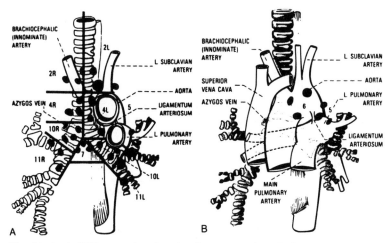

Fig. 31–1. *A*, ATS map of regional pulmonary nodes. *B*, Separation of nodal stations 5 and 6 requires anterior thoracostomy. Reproduced with permission of the American Thoracic Society: Tisi GM, Fiedman PJ, Peters RM, et al.: Clinical staging of primary lung cancer. Am Rev Respir Dis, *127*:659, 1983.

TABLE 31–7. THRESHOLD SIZES FOR NODAL ENLARGEMENT	
REGION	**SHORT-AXIS MEASUREMENT ABOVE WHICH NODE IS CONSIDERED ENLARGED (MM)**
2R	7
2L	7
4R	10
4L	10
5	9
6	8
7	11
8R	10
8L	7
10R	10
10L	7

From Glazer GM, Gross BH, Quint LE, et al.: Normal mediastinal lymph nodes: number and size according to American Thoracic Society mapping. AJR, *144*: 261, 1985.

- May be more valuable than CT in demonstrating invasion of mediastinal structures

Disadvantages

- Poor spatial resolution
- Longer scan times

- Thicker image slices
- Inability to detect calcium

As with CT scanning, controversy persists as to the value of MRI in the determination of metastatic involvement of mediastinal lymph nodes. Some authors have suggested that T_1 relaxation values may differentiate benign and malignant lymph node tissue, but such postulation has not gained universal acceptance. Most clinicians believe that relaxation time measurements of mediastinal lymph nodes will prove to have limited value in assessing the presence of mediastinal lymph node metastatic disease.

SPUTUM CYTOLOGY

With appropriate cytologic study of several sputum specimens, tumor cells are found in 45% to as many as 90% of patients. Cell type agrees with the final histologic diagnosis in approximately 85% of patients. The accuracy of such testing is approximately 90 to 100% for small cell carcinoma, 92 to 96% for squamous cell carcinoma, and 87 to 97% for adenocarcinoma. The undifferentiated carcinomas, the poorly differentiated epidermoid carcinomas, and combined carcinomas are more difficult to type correctly.

Cytologic studies are most often positive in patients with large tumors that involve a major bronchus. Peripheral lesions frequently do not communicate with a bronchus, and thus, the diagnostic results are less rewarding. Bronchial brushing or biopsy may be carried out to improve the yield.

A few patients with carcinoma of the lung without a pulmonary lesion revealed on the chest x-rays are identified because of an incidental finding of tumor cells in the sputum during a screening examination. At least 75% of these findings are from squamous cell lesions. These occult lung carcinomas may represent a readily identifiable lesion of the bronchus on bronchoscopic examination, but in approximately 25% of patients, the primary lung tumor is not initially identified by bronchoscopy and biopsy of a visualized lesion. Complete examination of the oropharynx and esophagus is required to rule out other orodigestive tumors; repeated bronchoscopy with brushing of individual lobes then is necessary. Approximately 50% of this subset of patients requires 2 to 5 examinations before localization is obtained. The examinations should be spaced at 8- to 12-week intervals.

TUMOR MARKERS

Tumor markers have little clinical value in the diagnosis of lung cancer (Table 31–8). They are of some value in determining the possible response to therapy and the prognosis of small cell lung carcinoma.

RADIONUCLIDE STUDIES

Radionuclide scanning of the lung is satisfactory for identifying the primary tumor but is not diagnostic. Scanning with ^{67}Ga may identify metastatic tumor deposits in the mediastinal lymph nodes as well as at distant sites.

TABLE 31–8. TUMOR MARKERS IN LUNG CANCER

	FREQUENCY OF OCCURRENCE IN		
SUBSTANCE	Non-small cell	Small cell	Carcinoid
Polypeptide hormones			
ACTH[a]	+	+ +	+
ADH (arginine vasopressin)[ab]	±	+ +	±
neurophysins			
Calcitonin[b]	+	+ + +	+
Bombesin (gastrin-releasing	+	+ + +	+
peptides)			
Human chorionic gonadotropin	+	+	
Parathyroid hormone	+	−	
Enzymes			
Dopa decarboxylase	−	+ +	
Neuron-specific enolase	−	+ +	+
Histaminase	−	+ +	
Creatine kinase	−	+ +	
Synaptophysin	−	+ +	+
Biogenic amines			
Serotonin	−	+ +	+
5-Hydroxytryptophan	−	+	
Histamine	−	+	
Tumor-associated antigens			
Carcinoembryonic antigen[b]	+ +	+ +	
Morphologic markers			
Electron-dense granules	±	+ +	+
Specific chromosome	−	+	
abnormality			

[a] Clinical syndrome associated with elevated marker level
[b] Clinically useful for monitoring therapy

The use of ^{67}Ga scans for detection of possible mediastinal lymph node involvement has been supplanted by CT evaluation of the mediastinum. Other scans also are more efficient for detecting distant metastases.

The use of radionuclide-labeled monoclonal antibodies for identifying primary lung tumors, regional metastases, and tumor recurrences is under active investigation. Immunoscintigraphy may detect 75% of the primary lung tumors and may identify tumor spread that CT imaging has failed to identify.

Ventilation and perfusion scans are useful in evaluating preoperative and predicting postoperative pulmonary function in poor-risk candidates for surgical resection. A predicted postoperative forced expiratory volume in one second (FEV_1) of 40% is the lowest allowable limit for pneumonectomy.

BRONCHOSCOPY AND TRANSBRONCHIAL NEEDLE ASPIRATION

The tracheobronchial tree in all patients suspected of having a tumor of the lung should be examined with either the rigid or the flexible fiberoptic bronchoscope

- Permits direct visualization or positive biopsy findings in 25 to 50% of patients
- Positive biopsy more frequent in squamous and large cell undifferentiated tumors than in adenocarcinomas. Small cell tumors readily identified. Centrally located suspected carcinoid tumors should be biopsied
- Length of normal bronchus proximal to the tumor should be noted
- Rigidity or loss of mobility of either the main stem bronchus or the bronchus intermediates suggests metastatic lymph node disease

Transbronchial fine-needle aspiration is indicated when rigidity is present and when enlarged mediastinal lymph nodes are identified by CT examination, even though endobronchial abnormality is not present. The sensitivity of fine-needle aspiration of enlarged lymph nodes in patients with non-small cell carcinoma may be as high as 82%. A positive aspiration obviates the more invasive diagnostic procedure of mediastinal exploration.

PERCUTANEOUS TRANSTHORACIC NEEDLE ASPIRATION

Needle aspiration of a suspected carcinoma of the lung is often performed without indication.

Indications

- In the patient with an undiagnosed but clinically nonresectable tumor
- In a patient who is not a medical candidate or who refuses resection of an otherwise resectable tumor and in whom a tissue diagnosis cannot be obtained by other means

Complications

- A postaspiration pneumothorax is seen in 25% of patients
- Of these patients, approximately 25% (6% of all patients) require a closed tube thoracostomy
- Hemoptysis occurs infrequently

Contraindications

- A hemorrhagic diathesis
- Pulmonary hypertension
- Severe emphysema with multiple bullae

Needle biopsy of the pleura (usually with a cutting needle) in the presence of pleural effusion is positive for tumor in 60 to 75% of patients with proven bronchial carcinoma.

THORACOSCOPY

Thoracoscopic examination of the pleural space rarely is indicated in patients with suspected bronchial carcinoma. A cytologically undiagnosed pleural effusion is the most frequent indication. On occasion, direct visualization of the lung and directed biopsy of an indeterminate mass by use of thoracoscopy may be of value, especially in the patient in whom a standard thoracotomy is contraindicated. It has been suggested that video-assisted thoracoscopic visualization of the pleural space be done immediately prior to thoracotomy. Previously undetected pleural seeding or locally nonresectable extension of the tumor beyond the lung would contraindicate the planned thoracotomy. The efficacy of this procedure is undetermined since such findings are identified in less than 5% of patients believed to have resectable disease at the completion of appropriate preoperative evaluation.

SUPRACLAVICULAR LYMPH NODE BIOPSY

Any palpable cervical lymph nodes should be excised or aspirated for histologic study; most of these are involved by tumor. Biopsy of nonpalpable lymph nodes in the scalene area is not indicated.

MEDIASTINAL LYMPH NODE BIOPSY

The most valuable invasive diagnostic procedure other than a thoracotomy is a prethoracotomy mediastinal exploration. The choice of a standard mediastinoscopy, an extended cervical mediastinoscopy, an anterior mediastinotomy, or a combination of these procedures depends on the location of the enlarged mediastinal lymph node(s) as demonstrated on the CT scan.

Indications

- Mediastinal lymph nods 1 cm or greater in size in patients with known non-small cell carcinoma
- Multiple lymph nodes of normal size in patients with adenocarcinoma
- In patients with potentially resectable central tumors in whom a tissue diagnosis has not been established
- All potential surgical candidates with known small cell carcinoma

Results

- 60 to 85% of enlarged lymph nodes in patients with non-small cell carcinoma contain metastatic tumor
- 15 to 40% of enlarged lymph nodes in non small-cell carcinoma are only inflammatory or hyperplasic without tumor

Routine mediastinal exploration has a positive yield of metastatic disease of 34%. Only 7% of lymph nodes of normal size (in the absence of associated enlarged lymph nodes with tumor) contain "occult" metastasis. Metastatic involvement of lymph nodes of normal size is more common in adenocarcinoma than in squamous carcinoma; the incidence in small cell tumors is highest.

The policy of foregoing a mediastinal exploration based on clinical (bronchoscopic and radiologic) findings without CT examination is inappropriate except in patients with a small peripheral tumor with normal hilar and mediastinal shadows. The incidence of mediastinal node involvement is approximately 5% in these patients. In over 90%, a complete resection can be done. In most other patients who are believed to have no nodal involvement or at most only lobar or hilar disease but whom mediastinal node disease is discovered at thoracotomy a complete resection can be accomplished in only 50%. Similarly, in patients with enlarged mediastinal nodes identified by CT scan but no prethoracotomy exploration and in whom metastatic disease is identified at thoracotomy, only a 50% complete resection rate can be obtained. In either of these two situations, an excessively high incidence of inappropriate thoracotomies has therefore been done. Thus, with the exception noted, all patients with a potentially resectable carcinoma should undergo a CT scan and all those in whom enlarged mediastinal nodes are identified should be evaluated by a preoperative mediastinal exploration.

INVESTIGATION FOR DISTANT METASTASES

CT scans of the brain and upper abdomen and radionuclide bone scans are the preferred diagnostic procedures for determining the presence of extrathoracic metastatic disease.

Indications

- Presence of symptoms or physical or laboratory findings (elevated alkaline phosphatase or LDH levels) suggestive of metastatic disease in any extrathoracic organ system in patients with non-small cell tumors or carcinoids
- In all patients, symptomatic and asymptomatic, with small cell tumors

Routine "metastatic" evaluation is not indicated in asymptomatic patients with non-small cell tumors. Yield of useful information from a routine brain CT scan is less than 1%, from an upper abdominal CT scan 1 to 3%, and from a bone CT scan less than 4%.

STAGING

Once the diagnosis has been established and the extent of the disease determined, the disease should be staged by one of two morphologic classifications. In addition the functional status should be determined, usually by the Karnofsky and Burchenal's classification (Table 31–9). A Clinical-Severity Staging, which takes into consideration the clinical features presented by the patient, has been suggested. This staging system may give a better guide to the individual patient's prognosis, especially those with advanced disease.

NON-SMALL CELL LUNG CARCINOMA

The morphologic staging system is most appropriate in determining the treatment options and the prognosis of patients with non-small cell lung cancer. The extent of tumor is codified by the descriptor T, the presence of lymph node metastases by the descriptor N, and the status of distant metastasis by the descriptor M (Table 31–10). The combinations of the TNM

TABLE 31–9. KARNOFSKY SCALE OF PERFORMANCE STATUS

CONDITION	PERCENTAGE	COMMENTS
A: Able to carry on normal activity and to work. No special care is needed.	100	Normal, no complaints, no evidence of disease
	90	Able to carry on normal activity, minor signs or symptoms of disease
	80	Normal activity with effort, some signs or symptoms of disease
B: Unable to work. Able to live at home, care for most personal needs. A varying degree of assistance is needed.	70	Cares for self, unable to carry on normal activity or to do active work
	60	Requires occasional assistance, but is able to care for most needs
	50	Requires considerable assistance and frequent medical care
C: Unable to care for self. Requires equivalent of institutional or hospital care. Disease may be progressing rapidly.	40	Disabled, requires special care and assistance
	30	Severely disabled, hospitalization indicated although death not imminent
	20	Hospitalization necessary, very sick, active supportive treatment necessary
	10	Moribund, fatal processes progressing rapidly
	0	Dead

designations are separated into four stage categories to denote the extent of the disease process (Table 31–11). These categories can be determined at the completion of the diagnostic evaluation (clinical), at time of thoracotomy (surgical), or by examination of the resected specimen (pathologic).

Problems with Present Classification

- Classification of N2 disease as stage IIIA
- How to classify tumors with satellite tumor nodules
- How to classify patients with two primary synchronous tumors
- Classification of patients without evident pleural involvement but positive cytologic pleural lavage at thoracotomy

Most patients with N2 disease have nonsurgical disease. Only a 2% long-term salvage rate is reported in patients with N2 disease confirmed prior

---

TABLE 31–10. NEW INTERNATIONAL STAGING SYSTEM: TNM CLASSIFICATION

Primary Tumor (T)

TX   Tumor proven by the presence of malignant cells in bronchopulmonary secretions but not visualized roentgenographically or bronchoscopically, or any tumor that cannot be assessed as in a retreatment staging.

T0   No evidence of primary tumor.

Tis   Carcinoma in situ.

T1   A tumor that is 3.0 cm or less in greatest diameter, surrounded by lung or visceral pleura, and without evidence of invasion proximal to a lobar bronchus at bronchoscopy.*

T2   A tumor more than 3.0 cm in greatest diameter, or a tumor of any size that either invades the visceral pleura or has associated atelectasis or obstructive pneumonitis extending to the hilar region. At bronchoscopy, the proximal extent of demonstrable tumor must be within a lobar bronchus or at least 2.0 cm distal to the carina. Any associated atelectasis or obstructive pneumonitis must involve less than an entire lung.

T3   A tumor of any size with direct extension into the chest wall (including superior sulcus tumors), diaphragm, or the mediastinal pleura or pericardium without involving the heart, great vessels, trachea, esophagus, or vertebral body, or a tumor in the main bronchus within 2.0 cm of the carina without involving the carina.

T4   A tumor of any size with invasion of the mediastinum or involving heart, great vessels, trachea, esophagus, vertebral body, or carina, or presence of malignant pleural effusion.†

Nodal Involvement (N)

N0   No demonstrable metastasis to regional lymph nodes.

N1   Metastasis to lymph nodes in the peribronchial or the ipsilateral hilar region, or both, including direct extension.

N2   Metastasis to ipsilateral mediastinal lymph nodes and subcarinal lymph nodes.

N3   Metastasis to contralateral mediastinal lymph nodes, contralateral hilar lymph nodes, and ipsilateral or contralateral scalene or supraclavicular lymph nodes.

Distant Metastasis (M)

N0   No (known) distant metastasis.

M1   Distant metastatis present. Specify site(s).

---

* The uncommon superficial tumor of any size with its invasive component limited to the bronchial wall, which may extend proximal to the major bronchus, is classified as T1.

† Most pleural effusions associated with lung cancer result from tumor. Cytopathologic examination of pleural fluid (on more than one specimen) in a few patients is negative for tumor, however, and the fluid is nonbloody and is not an exudate. When these elements and clinical judgment dictate that the effusion is not related to the tumor, the patient should be staged as T1, T2, or T3, excluding effusion as a staging element.

From Mountain CF: A new international staging system for lung cancer. Chest(Suppl), *89*:225S, 1986.

to thoracotomy. "Occult" N2 disease discovered at thoracotomy may be resected, resulting in long-term salvage rates of 30 to 45%. The overall salvage rate in patients with N2 disease is no greater than 5 to 8%; patients with evident N2 disease should be classified as having stage IIIB disease.

Patients with satellite nodules, synchronous tumors, or positive pleural lavage have salvage rates of 18 to 22%. All these manifestations should be classified as stage IIIA disease.

TABLE 31–11. NEW INTERNATIONAL STAGING SYSTEM STAGE GROUPING	
TX N0 M0	An occult carcinoma with bronchopulmonary secretions containing malignant cells, but without other evidence of the primary tumor or evidence of metastasis to the regional lymph nodes or distant metastasis.
Stage 0 Tis N0 M0	Carcinoma in situ.
Stage I T1 N0 M0 T2 N0 M0	A tumor that can be classified T1 or T2 without any metastasis to nodes or distant metastasis.
Stage II T1 N1 M0 T2 N1 M0	Any tumor classified as T1 or T2 with metastasis to the lymph nodes in the peribronchial or ipsilateral hilar region only.
Stage IIIA T3 N0 M0 T3 N1 M0 T1 N2 M0 T2 N2 M0 T3 N2 M0	A tumor that can be classified as T3 without nodal metastasis or with metastasis limited to the peribronchial, ipsilateral hilar, and ipsilateral mediastinal lymph nodes. T1 and T2 tumors that have metastasized to the level of the ipsilateral mediastinal lymph nodes only are also included.
Stage IIIB Any T, N3 M0 T, any N, M0	Any tumor more extensive than T3 or any tumor with supraclavicular or contralateral mediastinal lymph node involvement or any tumor with a malignant pleural effusion, but without evidence of distant metastasis.
Stage IV Any T, any N, M1	Any tumor with distant metastatic spread.

From Mountain CF: A new international staging system for lung cancer. Chest(Suppl), *89*:225S, 1986.

SMALL CELL LUNG CARCINOMA

The morphologic staging of small cell lung cancer is less detailed. It is generally only categorized as limited or extensive disease. Limited disease is defined as disease confined to the ipsilateral hemithorax with or without contralateral hilar or ipsilateral supraclavicular lymph node involvement. Extensive disease is any disease that extends beyond these limits.

Patients with limited disease that is clinically a potential surgical lesion should be further staged as to their T and N status.

CARCINOID TUMORS

No evidence suggests that carcinoid tumors should be staged by the International Staging System. No extensive preoperative staging procedures are indicated. A CT scan of the chest is necessary only when radiographic evidence suggests mediastinal lymph node enlargement. The tumors are classified postoperatively as typical or atypical, with or without lymph node metastasis.

FUNCTIONAL STATUS

The performance status of most surgical candidates is less important than the morphologic stage because almost all have a Karnofsky score of 80 or higher. In patients with stage IIIB or IV non-small cell tumors or in patients with small cell carcinomas, functional status is important relative to the patient's response to therapy and prognosis. The lower the Karnofsky score, the poorer the outcome for each.

TREATMENT

Treatment options consist of surgical resection, radiation therapy, chemotherapy, supportive medical care, or a combination of these options. Surgical resection should be considered in all patients when it can completely remove all tumor and is curative in intent. A palliative (more rightly called "incomplete") resection confers no benefit in the outcome of the disease and must be avoided. Radiation therapy and chemotherapy may be used with either intent, but most often are palliative in result.

The selection of the appropriate therapeutic approach depends on the cell type of the tumor, the stage of the disease, the medical condition of the patient, and at times the presence or absence of symptoms.

SURGICAL THERAPY

Non-Small Cell Lung Carcinoma

Surgical resection is the most effective therapy for non-small cell carcinoma of the lung even though it is applicable to fewer than one fourth of all new patients seen. Surgical candidates are primarily most of the patients with stage I or II disease and a few patients with stage IIIA disease. Patients with stage IIIB or IV disease are considered as potential surgical patients only in exceptional situations.

Contraindications to Definitive Surgical Resection

Based on the Extent and Location of the Tumor

- Extensive N2 disease
- N3 or T4 disease
- M1 disease

Controversy persists regarding whether resection should be carried out for some patients with N2 disease discovered by a prethoracotomy mediastinal exploration. N2 disease in 1 nodal station (low superior mediastinal [stations 3, 4, or 5] or subcarinal [station 7], preferably in only 1 lymph node and without capsular invasion or fixation) may be considered as potential surgical disease.

Tumors involving a main stem bronchus within 2 cm of the tracheal carina (T3) or involving the tracheal carina or encroaching upon the tracheal wall (T4) are generally nonresectable. Rarely, a small tumor without lymph node involvement can be removed by a main stem bronchoplastic procedure or a tracheal sleeve pneumonectomy.

On rare occasion, solitary brain metastasis identified in a patient with a resectable lung carcinoma may be excised, followed by whole-brain irradiation. Resection of the lung tumor then may be considered. The primary disease should preferably be stage I, but certainly no more advanced than stage II.

Based on Medical Status of Patient

- FEV_1 reduced to ≤ 1 L
- Predicted postoperative FEV_1 <30%
- Postoperative carbon monoxide diffusion capacity (DL_{CO}) <40%
- Decrease in oxygen saturation during maximal exercise $\geq 2\%$
- Presence of hypoxia at rest or after mild exercise
- Presence of hypercapnia, CO_2 >45 mm Hg
- Recent myocardial infarction (within 3 months)
- Uncontrolled heart failure
- Uncontrollable arrhythmia

The patient history and electrocardiogram (ECG) are sufficient to evaluate the patient's cardiac status when both are normal. When the ECG is abnormal, when an arrhythmia is present, or when the patient has a history of angina, of a previous myocardial infarct, or of controlled failure, a stress test should be performed. When the stress test is normal, other studies need not be done. If the stress test is not completed or is equivocal, a ^{201}Tl scan to evaluate myocardial perfusion should be done. When either the stress test or the ^{201}Tl scan is abnormal, a coronary angiogram should be obtained. When a patient is a candidate for myocardial revascularization or other cardiac procedures and has a resectable lung cancer, both procedures should be done at the same time when possible.

Advanced age alone does not preclude surgical resection. Acceptable mortality rates and satisfactory long-term survival have been obtain in patients 80 years of age and older.

Based on Thoracotomy Findings

- Metastatic seeding of the parietal pleura
- Undetected T4 disease (direct involvement of vertebral body, vena cava, aorta, heart)
- Extensive N2 disease with extracapsular growth and/or fixation to surrounding structures
- Inability to safely control the blood supply to the lung
- Required resection greater than can be tolerated by the patient

The percentage of patients in whom one or more of these local contraindications are found varies with the preoperative selection of the patients and the aggressiveness of the individual surgeon in the operative management. A nonresection rate should be no higher than 5 to 10%.

Definitive Surgical Resection

The goal of a definitive surgical resection is the complete removal of all gross and microscopic tumor within the involved hemithorax. Anything less must be regarded as an incomplete resection and should be avoided.

TABLE 31–12. OPERATIVE PROCEDURES IN NON-SMALL CELL CARCINOMA OF THE LUNG		
OPERATIONS	**APPROXIMATE FREQUENCY (%)**	**OPERATIVE MORTALITY (%)**
Lobectomy	62	3
Bilobecotomy	6	4
Sleeve Lobectomy	1	5
Pneumonectomy	25	6
Segmentectomy	3	2
Lesser Resection	3	<1

Lung tissue preservation without compromising the adequacy of the tumor removal is recommended. Lobectomy and pneumonectomy and their modifications (bilobectomy, sleeve resection) are the standard procedures. A properly selected segmentectomy is appropriate, but lesser resections (wedge resection or even a more limited local resection) should be considered as a compromise necessitated by the patient's pulmonary or cardiac status. Any of these operations may be combined with the en bloc resection of an involved adjacent nonvital structure.

A lobectomy is the most common operative procedure (Table 31–12). Radiographic occult tumors that have been localized only by bronchial brushing or by biopsy of a suspicious mucosal lesion generally require a lobectomy, but some occult tumors necessitate a bilobectomy or pneumonectomy because of their location.

All procedures should be accompanied by sampling of the ipsilateral mediastinal and subcarinal lymphatic stations or by a standard, systematic mediastinal lymph node dissection.

The advantages of a lobectomy are that it permits conservation of lung parenchyma and is better tolerated in the long term than is a pneumonectomy. The 30-day postoperative mortality is approximately 3%. In patients older than 70 years of age, the mortality may be increased. A sleeve lobectomy for excision of a tumor involving the upper lobe orifice may be done to negate the necessity of a pneumonectomy.

A standard pneumonectomy is required when a lobectomy or one of its modifications is not sufficient to remove the local disease or its metastases to the lobar or hilar lymph nodes. In properly selected patients, the mortality rate is approximately 6%. The late development of pulmonary hypertension and subsequent ventilatory disability, however, are additional disadvantages of the procedure, particularly in older patients.

In patients with small peripheral tumors without lymph node involvement (T1N0), segmentectomy has been advocated to preserve more functional lung tissue in older patients and in those with major defects in pulmonary function. The mortality rate is low, 2 to 5%. A wedge resection or even a local cautery or laser excision of a small lesion without lymph node involvement can be done as a compromise procedure. The local recurrence rate after segmentectomy or lesser procedure is greater than that observed after a lobectomy. Video-assisted thoracoscopic surgical resection of small (<2 cm) peripherally located carcinomas has been reported. This may be an option in the management of a poor risk patient but should not be considered as standard practice. No longterm survival data are available, and the incidence of local recurrence is not known.

Extended resections to excise T3 lesions extending into the parietal pleura, chest wall, diaphragm, or pericardium are indicated when all the disease can be removed by the procedure. Mediastinal lymph node involvement decreases markedly the value of any extended procedure. Resection of the vena cava or other greater vessels in the chest is rarely indicated.

When the tumor involves the apex of the chest and adjacent structures (superior sulcus tumor) and no vertebral body invasion or Horner's syndrome is present, an en block resection may be carried out. Preoperative irradiation is used initially. Radiation therapy in the range of 35 to 45 Gy should be given preoperatively. If no evidence of distant spread occurs 1 month after completion of this therapy, resection is undertaken. When lymph nodes are positive or when extensive vertebral bony involvement is present, resection is contraindicated. In such instances, additional irradiation is given after thoracotomy.

Results of Surgical Treatment

The overall 5-year salvage rates after surgical resection vary from as low as 7.5% to as high as 45%; the average figures are usually between 20 and 35%. The prognosis after resection primarily depends on the postsurgical TNM classification of the tumor (Table 31–13).

Adjuvant Therapy

Depending on the stage of the disease at the time of resection, 28 to more than 75% of patients with lung carcinoma die from metastases or local recurrence of the carcinoma. Some form of adjuvant therapy would appear

TABLE 31–13. SURVIVAL RELATIVE TO TNM CLASSIFICATION

TNM SUBSET	CLINICAL		Surgical	
	No.	% Surviving	No.	% Surviving
T1N0M0	591	61.9	429	68.5
T2N0M0	1,012	35.8	436	59.0
T1N1M0	19	33.6	67	54.1
T2N1M0	176	22.7	250	40.0
T3N0M0	221	7.6	57	44.2
T3N1M0	71	7.7	29	17.6
Any N2M0	497	4.9	168	28.8
Any M1	1,166	1.7	—	—
Total	3,753		1,436	

Reproduced with permission from Mountain CE: A new international staging system for lung cancer. Chest(Suppl), *89*:225S, 1986.

to be indicated in most patients. Unfortunately, with few exceptions, the use of irradiation, chemotherapy, or immunotherapy has not been successful to date.

Preoperative Irradiation

- No benefit relative to survival
- Some patients may be harmed by its use
- Absence of tumor after irradiation has no effect on survival
- Routine use contraindicated

Postoperative Irradiation in Stage II and Stage III

- Reduction of local recurrence observed
- No survival benefit
- Timing of irradiation, immediate versus delayed, is undetermined

Chemotherapy

- Prolongation of disease-free interval in Stage II and Stage IIIA adenocarcinoma
- Consensus is that routine use not indicated

Immunotherapy

- No indication for its use at present

Neoadjuvant Therapy. Recent interest has grown in the use of preoperative chemotherapy with or without radiation therapy in marginally resectable or nonresectable stage IIIA disease, particularly in those with known N2 involvement, in an attempt to convert the local disease into a resectable lesion. The more common regimens have used cisplatin and fluorouracil infusion with 30 to 40 Gy of irradiation. A critical analysis of the present status of neoadjuvant therapy for stage IIIA non-small cell lung cancer reveals response rates to cisplatin-based chemotherapy to be approximately 50% regardless of the actual regimen used. The addition of radiation therapy does not appear to be of any major benefit and may complicate the technical aspects of the operative procedure. The addition of irradiation may increase the toxocity to doxorubicin and mitomycin C. Serious toxicity consisting of profound neutropenia, mitomycin lung toxicity, and esophagitis is observed. A 3.2% mortality rate from the adjuvant therapy is reported. Several complete local responses have been reported (no tumor present in the resected specimen), and in other patients, tumors initially thought to be unresectable could be removed. The relationship of this local control to longterm survival remains unknown, however.

Small Cell Lung Carcinoma

Surgical resection is applicable to only 5 to 8% of all patients with small cell lung cancer. The surgical candidates are those with stage I, selected stage IIIA non-N2 patients, and possibly stage II disease. Chemotherapy

TABLE 31–14. SURVIVAL IN SURGICALLY RESECTED SMALL CELL LUNG CANCER		
STAGE	TORONTO STUDY* (%)	INTERNATIONAL SOCIETY OF CHEMOTHERAPY LUNG STUDY** (%)
I	71	60
II	38	36
IIIA	18	33
Total	36	47

* 5-year survival—Initial chemotherapy followed by surgical resection
** 4-year survival—Initial resection followed by chemotherapy

is an integral part of the multimodality approach and may be given either pre- or postoperatively. Local irradiation to the chest in patients with positive lymph nodes may be indicated postoperatively. The efficacy of postoperative prophylactic cranial irradiation is under question because of observed neurologic defects in the longterm survivors. Because the rate of brain relapse is only 15% in stage I disease, some authors negate its routine use. Longterm survival in surgically treated patients with small cell cancer is seen in Table 31–14.

Carcinoid Tumors

Typical carcinoid tumors are managed with the most conservative surgical resection possible. Lymph nodes should be removed when grossly abnormal. Bronchoscopic resection is contraindicated except as a palliative measure. Atypical carcinoids, although of greater malignant potential, are managed in the same manner. The long-term survival rate for patients with typical carcinoids is over 90%, and for those with atypical tumors, the rate is 50%.

ENDOBRONCHIAL MANAGEMENT OF LUNG CANCER

Recurrent tumor obstructing the lower trachea or main stem bronchi may be coagulated endoscopically to prevent death from strangulation. The development of laser technique has made the endoscopic approach more satisfactory.

Both carbon dioxide (CO_2) and neodymium-YAG lasers can be used to remove obstructing cancerous tissue. Phototherapy with hematoporphyrin derivative has also been evaluated experimentally.

Laser Therapy

Laser therapy is more suitable than phototherapy. YAG laser is better than CO_2 laser because it can be used with the flexible fiberscope, its light wavelength is not absorbed appreciably by either water or blood, and its energy can penetrate several millimeters. The CO_2 laser requires rigid-tube endoscopy, its depth of penetration is less than 1 mm, and its efficacy relies on an absolutely dry field.

The YAG laser produces a thermal necrosis that debulks the tumor, and it controls any superficial bleeding. The technique is not without danger. Bleeding from perforation of a large vessel may occur, as may late hemorrhage from tumor necrosis.

Indications for YAG Laser Therapy

- The airway obstruction is unresponsive to other reasonable therapy
- The lesion protrudes into the bronchial lumen without obvious extension beyond the cartilage
- The axial length of the endobronchial component of the tumor is <4 cm
- The bronchoscopist can see the bronchial lumen
- Functioning lung tissue exists beyond the obstruction

Satisfactory palliation of severe obstruction or hemoptysis may occur in 79% of patients with advanced malignant tumors involving the trachea or main stem bronchi by the use of the YAG laser.

Bronchoscopic Phototherapy with Hematoporphyrin Derivative (HpD-PT)

This method can be used to manage advanced, previously treated tumor causing significant airway obstruction. HpD-PT has not been as successful as either CO_2 or neodymium-YAG lasers. Clinical trials are being carried out to define its usefulness and to improve its technique.

In a small subset of patients with radiographic occult lesions, bronchoscopic phototherapy has been successfully used as the primary treatment method. The lesion must be confined to the mucosa or be an in situ carcinoma less than 3 cm^2 in surface area.

Endoscopic Management of Carcinoid Tumors

Most of the growth of an endobronchial carcinoid occurs outside the involved bronchial lumen. Endoscopic removal results in an incomplete excision in almost all patients. This technique is recommended only in patients in whom surgical resection of the tumor is contraindicated.

RADIATION THERAPY

Non-Small Cell Lung Carcinoma

The role of radiation therapy as a curative treatment method for patients with lung cancer is minor. In potentially operable good-risk candidates who do not undergo resection, a reported 22.5% 5-year survival rate was obtained following a radiation dose of 40 to 55 Gy. In poor-risk patients (elderly patients with poor pulmonary or cardiac function), a survival rate of only 6% was reported. In patients with nonresectable extensive stage

TABLE 31–15. PALLIATION OF SYMPTOMS IN PATIENTS FOLLOWING RADIATION THERAPY

SYMPTOM	PERCENTAGE*
Hemoptysis	84 to 95
Chest pain	61 to 72
Dyspnea	60
Atelectasis	
SCLC	57
Non-SCLC	15

* Percentage of patients experiencing palliation.
SCLC = small cell lung cancer.
Non-SCLC = non-small cell lung cancer.
From Weisenburger TH: Non-small cell lung cancer: definitive radiotherapy and combined modality therapy. In Thoracic Oncology. Edited by JA Roth, JC Ruckdeschel, TH Weisenburger. Philadelphia, WB Saunders, 1989.

IIIA and IIIB disease, the longterm survival rate is reduced to 3%. Although greater survival rates have been published (10 to 16%), irradiation clearly has little to offer as a curative treatment. A selective approach to its use should be practiced. The use of radiation therapy as the sole therapeutic method in superior sulcus tumors, however, has been suggested to be efficacious, with a projected 5-year survival rate of 23%.

As a palliative method to decrease symptoms or to relieve the patient of symptoms (Table 31–15), irradiation produces results better than those afforded by any other palliative therapeutic intervention. Radiation therapy is the mainstay of treatment for the patient with nonresectable symptomatic non-small cell carcinoma.

Small Cell Lung Carcinoma

Thoracic irradiation is considered by most clinicians to have a valuable role in the multimodality management of localized small cell lung carcinoma. The best regimen for its use with intensive chemotherapy remains unresolved. In patients with extensive disease, radiation therapy is primarily used as a palliative measure to control persistent or recurrent symptoms.

Bronchial Carcinoid Tumors

These tumors are resistant to irradiation. Its use is rarely indicated for recurrent or metastatic disease.

CHEMOTHERAPY

Non-Small Cell Lung Carcinoma

Chemotherapy, other than possibly neoadjuvant therapy, has no role as a curative treatment method. Its use as a palliative method in nonresectable disease is controversial. Randomized trials of multidrug therapy, particularly cisplatin-based regimens, have shown some superiority over supportive care alone. The aggregate median survival is approximately 2 months greater in the chemotherapy-treated groups. The qualitative impact on survival is undetermined, but the toxic effects as well as costs of the chemotherapy are well known. Its use, other than in clinical trials, should be discouraged except in the few symptomatic, advanced-stage patients with a good initial performance status who cannot be enrolled in an appropriate clinical trial.

Small Cell Lung Carcinoma

Multidrug chemotherapy, with or without local irradiation, is the treatment of choice in all but the few patients with very localized disease. It is most effective in patients with limited-stage disease and in those with disseminated disease who still have a good performance status.

Limited-Stage Disease

Frequently used chemotherapy combinations are listed in Table 31–16. No best combination is as yet known. The response rates are 70 to 90%. The value of late intensification therapy, the use of alternating non–cross-resistant drugs, and the duration of therapy continue to be under investigation. Whereas, in the past, treatment for 12 to 24 months was standard, with maintenance therapy considered essential, now 6 courses of chemotherapy with adjuvant thoracic irradiation appear to be as satisfactory as prolonged treatment regimens. The timing and radiation dosage are under intensive investigation. Prophylactic cranial irradiation is usually recommended for the complete responders. This therapeutic intervention decreases the number of brain relapses but does not prolong survival. Neurologic toxicities in patients with longterm survival are forcing a reevaluation of the use of radiation and of the manner in which it is given.

TABLE 31–16. FREQUENTLY USED CHEMOTHERAPY COMBINATIONS FOR SMALL CELL LUNG CANCER

CHEMOTHERAPY COMBINATION	ABBREVIATION
Cyclophosphamide, Adriamycin (doxorubicin), vincristine	CAV
Cyclophosphamide, methotrexate, lomustine (CCNU)	CMC$_N$
Etoposide (VP-16), cisplatin	VpP
Cyclophosphamide, Adriamycin (doxorubicin), etoposide (VP-16)	CAVp
Cyclophosphamide, Adriamycin (doxorubicin), etoposide (VP-16), cisplatin	CAVpP
Etoposide (VP-16), carboplatin	VpCP

From Feld R, Ginsberg RJ, Payne DG: Treatment of small cell lung cancer. *In* Thoracic Oncology. Edited by JA Roth, JC Ruckdeschel, TH Weisenburger. Philadelphia, WB Saunders, 1989.

Extensive Disease

Similar chemotherapeutic regimens are used in the management of patients with extensive disease. Response rates of 50 to 75% are achieved. Local thoracic and prophylactic cranial irradiation is not used routinely. Either may be used in patients who have obtained a complete response to the chemotherapy. Radiation therapy in patients with extensive disease is most often used as a palliative measure for the management of uncontrolled or recurrent symptoms.

Treatment Results

In patients with localized disease, survival equal to or greater than 2 years is reported to be between 15% to as high as 43%. Five-year survival rates have varied between 5 to 20%. Significant favorable independent variables for prolonged survival are listed in Table 31–17.

In patients with extensive disease, survival times of 1 year or greater are reported to be between 21 and 42%. Survivals of 2 years or more are 3 to 19%; 5-year survival is rarely observed in this group (<1%). Similar favorable prognostic factors as recorded for patients with limited disease appear to be applicable to patients with extensive disease. Prognostic factors with a negative effect on survival are listed in Table 31–18.

TABLE 31–17. FAVORABLE FACTORS FOR SURVIVAL IN LIMITED SMALL CELL LUNG CANCER

Good performance status
Female sex
70 years of age or younger
No pleural effusion
Tumor confined to lung
Normal LDH value
"Classic" growth pattern (vs "variant") in culture

TABLE 31–18. NEGATIVE PROGNOSTIC FACTORS FOR SURVIVAL OF PATIENTS WITH SMALL CELL LUNG CANCER WITH EXTENSIVE DISEASE

Poor performance status
Weight loss
More than one site of distant metastasis
Liver or brain metastasis
Local extension beyond the lung
Increase CEA, LDH, neuron-specific enolase
Variant growth pattern in culture

Carcinoid Tumors

The use of chemotherapy in patients with local recurrent or metastatic disease is experimental. Because of the neuroendocrine similarities among the atypical carcinoid tumors and the small cell tumors, similar treatment regimens may be attempted in these patients.

IMMUNOTHERAPY

At present, immunotherapy appears to have no place in the therapeutic management of patients with lung cancer.

THE SOLITARY PULMONARY NODULE

A solitary pulmonary nodule (SPN) is most often an incidental finding on a routine radiographic examination of the chest in an asymptomatic patient. It may be identified in either the posteroanterior or the lateral view and is frequently identified in only one of these views. Lordotic, oblique, and stereoscopic views may be profitably used to define an indistinct or questionable lesion.

RADIOGRAPHIC LIMITS OF VISIBILITY

The lower limit of radiographic visibility is between 6 and 7 mm. Such small lesions frequently are identified only when located in an intercostal space at a distance from the chest wall, diaphragm, or mediastinum. Lesions as small as 3 mm may be identified, but such SPNs are recognized only in retrospect.

Experimentally 3-mm discs with sharp borders may be visualized but once the borders become rounded or ill-defined, this low limit of visibility is lost. Because most pulmonary nodules are spherical, the presence of an SPN usually is not appreciated until it is 1 cm in size.

DEFINITION

The definition of an SPN is controversial.

TYPICAL FEATURES

- Spherical or ovoid in shape and relatively well demarcated
- May be associated with other pulmonary disorder but should be distinct from it
- Surrounded by air-containing lung, but may be located just beneath the visceral pleura
- Margins may be sharply demarcated to ill defined
- Margins may be smooth, umbilicated, nodular, or spiculated
- Some clinicians inappropriately exclude nodules that contain readily recognizable calcifications on the standard radiologic views

- Cavitation may be present, but a thin-walled lesion containing air or an air fluid level is best considered a pulmonary cavitary
- May be associated with small satellite nodules
- Invasion into the chest wall, diaphragm, or mediastinum should be absent
- Grossly discernible mediastinal lymphadenopathy should not be present

The most controversial feature is the size of the lesion. Many series have included any lesion as large as 6 or even 8 cm in diameter, but more recent reports consider only lesions 4 cm or less in size as SPNs. A suggested cutoff of 3 cm would conform to the size of a T1 lesion in the various classifications of carcinoma of the lung. SPNs larger than 3 cm in size in most reported surgical series are usually malignant with the exceptions of a large noncalcified granuloma or a hamartoma.

ETIOLOGY

An SPN is an important finding because it may represent an early carcinoma of the lung. The percentage these primary lung tumors represent in a series of SPNs varies with the population pool from which the series is derived. The percentage may be as low as 5% in a routine radiographic survey of all adults in a geographic catchment area to as high as 75% in a highly selected surgically resected group. The other causes of an SPN are other tumors (benign or metastatic), granulomas, other inflammatory processes, vascular lesions, and miscellaneous lesions (Table 31–19). A typical distribution of the major causes is seen in Table 31–20.

TABLE 31–19. CAUSES OF SOLITARY PULMONARY NODULE

Neoplasms	Inflammatory Lesions	Malformations
Primary carcinoma	Tuberculoma and	Arteriovenous
Solitary metastasis	tuberculous lesions	malformations
Hamartoma	Histoplasmosis	Vascular endothelioma
Primary sarcoma	Coccidioidomycosis	Sequestrated segment
Bronchial carcinoid	Cryptococcus	
Reticuloses	Nonspecific	Traumatic Lesions
Fibroma	granuloma	Hematoma
Myxoma	Chronic lung abscess	
Neurogenic tumor	Lipoid pneumonia	Hernias
Lipoma	Massive fibrosis	
Myoblastoma	Rheumatoid	Cysts
Hibernoma	granuloma	Bronchogenic
Solitary fibrous tumor	Gumma	Pericardial
of the pleura	Mycetoma	Dermoid
Leiomyoma		Teratoma
Plasmocytoma	Parasitic Lesions	
Sclerosing	Echinococcus	Pulmonary Infarct
hemangioma	granulosus	Rounded Atelectasis
Thymoma	Ascaris lumbricoides	
Endometriosis	Dirofilaria immitis	
Sugar tumor		

Adapted with permission from Bateson EM: Analysis of 155 solitary lung lesions illustrating the differential diagnosis of mixed tumors of the lung. *Clin Radiol*, *16*:60, 1965.

TABLE 31–20. INCIDENCE OF COMMON TYPES OF SOLITARY PULMONARY NODULES	
Malignant	(%)
Primary carcinoma of the lung	28
Carcinoid tumor	2
Metastatic tumor	10
Benign	
Infectious granuloma	50
Noninfectious granuloma	2
Benign tumors	2
Miscellaneous	6

From Lillington GA: Pulmonary nodules: solitary and multiple. Clin Chest Med, *3*:361, 1982.

MALIGNANT SOLITARY PERIPHERAL NODULES

Primary Lung Tumors

Most solitary peripheral malignant primary lung tumors are either adenocarcinomas, including the bronchioloalveolar subtype, or squamous cell tumors. Large cell and small cell undifferentiated tumors are less frequently observed. Bronchial carcinoids, both typical and atypical cell types, are less commonly present.

Solitary Metastatic Nodule in Lung

Of all SPNs, 10% are metastatic tumors. Only 1 to 2% of metastatic tumors to the lung, however, occur as solitary nodules. The incidence is 2% for adenocarcinoma of the colon and 1.2% for breast carcinoma.

A patient with a previous or concurrent (unless uncontrolled) squamous cell primary extrapulmonary tumor rarely has a solitary metastasis to the lung. A new SPN in such patients, except for a small incidence of a granulomatous or other benign lesion, is usually a second primary tumor in the lung, regardless of the cell type of the lung tumor.

In patients with an extrapulmonary primary adenocarcinoma, the possibility that the new SPN is a metastatic lesion is approximately 50%; a few benign lesions have been observed.

In patients in whom the original extrapulmonary tumor was a sarcoma or a melanoma, the new SPN is almost always a metastatic lesion; infrequently it may be a benign lesion and rarely a new primary lung carcinoma.

Other Malignant Lung Tumors

Primary malignant lung tumors, such as soft tissue sarcomas (fibrosarcoma, leiomyosarcoma, and other mesenchymal-derived tumors) and pulmonary blastomas (embryoma), may occur as an SPN.

BENIGN PULMONARY LESIONS

Granulomas

Infectious granulomas comprise the largest percentage of SPNs, approximately 50% or more. The cause of the infectious granulomas varies with geographic area of the population under review.

In the catchment area of the Mississippi River Valley and its tributaries, histoplasmosis is the common cause; in the Southwest, coccidioidomycosis is the more common cause. In Europe, tuberculosis is the most common cause of the SPN. Cryptococcosis may be encountered, but has no specific geographic distribution.

Parasitic lesions rarely are causes of pulmonary granulomas, but lesions caused by Echinococcus granulosus, Ascaris lumbricoides, and Dirofilaria immitis have been reported.

Noninfectious granulomas, such as lipoid pneumonia, rheumatoid granuloma, resolving hematoma, and pulmonary infarct, have appeared as an SPN.

Benign Lung Tumors

Hamartomas are the most common benign tumors that occur as SPNs (2 to 5%). They comprise 77% of all benign lung tumors. Slow growth of these tumors may be observed. Occasionally, benign mesenchymal tumors of the lung, such as fibromas, lipomas, and leiomyomas, occur as SPNs. Rarely, a neurogenic tumor or a clear cell tumor (a sugar tumor) may occur in this manner.

Vascular Lesions

A solitary pulmonary arteriovenous fistula is one of the vascular lesions that should be considered in the differential diagnosis of an SPN. Other lesions to be considered are a sclerosing hemangioma, an endothelioma, and a pulmonary infarct.

BENIGNANCY VERSUS MALIGNANCY

CRITERIA OF MALIGNANCY

No single criterion identifies a malignant SPN.

Suggestive Features

- A patient older than 40 years (the risk increases with advancing age)
- A history of smoking
- A history of a previous malignancy elsewhere
- The absence of calcification
- An ill-defined, umbilicated, or spiculed ("corona radiata") margin
- A large size

Only 4 to 15% of T1 carcinomas are smaller than 1 cm in diameter, whereas more than 53% are larger than 2 cm.

CRITERIA OF BENIGNANCY

As with malignancy of an SPN, no one criterion establishes benignancy with absolute certainty.

Suggestive Features

- Very rapid or slow or no rate of growth
- Specific types of calcification
- Density of the SPN
- A fatty density within the nodule
- Characteristic shape of a scar on tomographic examination

Rate of Growth of SPN

The absence of growth over a 2-year period as established by retrospective review of previous available chest x-rays may be considered as almost an absolute criterion of benignancy. Rare examples of a primary adenocarcinoma behaving in this manner have been noted.

With the availability of previous chest x-rays, the rate of growth (the "doubling time") can be estimated. A 25% increase in the diameter of the SPN represents approximately a doubling of the volume of the mass. A 3- to 5-mm increase in the diameter of an SPN represents about 1 doubling time of an initial 1-cm to 2-cm SPN, respectively. A rapid doubling time (less than 36 days) or a slow doubling time (more than 465 days) can be accepted as representative of a benign process. Doubling times between 36 to 465 days can occur in either a benign or a malignant SPN.

Presence of Calcification

The presence of a central nidus, laminar layers, diffuse homogeneous distribution, or "popcorn" distribution (observed in some hamartomas) of calcification on radiologic examination (including conventional or computed tomography) can be accepted as denoting benignancy. Eccentric or dystrophic calcification regardless of its size cannot be considered as signifying a benign lesion. Either type of calcification can occur in a primary lung tumor. Calcification may occur in a bronchial carcinoid (30% on CT) and in some metastatic lesions (osteogenic sarcoma, chondrosarcoma, mucinous adenocarcinomas of the endometrium, as well as rarely some lesions from the gastrointestinal tract).

Density of Nodule

Many benign granulomas that appear to be noncalcified by conventional radiographic studies contain microcalcifications, which increase the density of an SPN. Malignant lesions do not contain microcalcifications and their density is less. The density can be evaluated by computed tomographic densitometry, which is measured in Hounsfield units (HU)

• Density is estimated by averaging density numbers within the nodule and deriving a representative CT number expressed in HU
• A mean CT number greater than 164 HU is presumed to represent a granulomatous lesion
• Of all indeterminate (noncalcified) nodules eventually proved to be benign, 60% had CT numbers of this magnitude
• CT densitometry most effective in SPNs measuring less than 3 cm in diameter with smooth or lobulated borders

Initially these results could not be confirmed by other workers because of differences in the technique, the equipment used, and the variations that could be attributed to the size of the patient and the location of the nodule. The development of a reference phantom that could reduce the sources of densometric error and provide a standard independent of scanner variations has overcome this problem. In a multicenter study, CT densitometry could be generalized in any scanner once standardization was achieved. In 2 studies, 30 to 35% of the noncalcified, indeterminate SPNs were found to be more attenuating (higher density) than the phantom. Benignancy was confirmed in these SPNs by long-term follow-up examination.

Fat Within a Nodule

CT examination may reveal tissue consistent with the density of fat. This finding may be seen in one third of hamartomas and in the rare lipoid pneumonias. Fatty tissue is not found in malignant lesions. Some authors have suggested that the SPN can be considered a benign lesion when fatty tissue is identified on CT.

Shape and Size

A well-demarcated, smoothly marginated SPN or an SPN with a bosselated margin, especially of less than 1 cm in size, frequently is a benign lesion, but malignancy cannot be ruled out. Some authors have suggested, however, that if the SPN is linear in shape, consistent with scarring, the lesion can be considered benign. This determination is best made by conventional tomography. There should be no nodularity or irregularities. The SPN may be angular in shape, with smooth tapering margins ending in points. Another variation is an SPN consisting of a conglomeration of multiple tiny nodules. In 1 study, all 38 uncalcified SPNs characterized by these features were proved to be benign. Further corroboration of this observation is necessary.

The finding of vascular connections to an SPN suggests the possibility of an arteriovenous fistula or an embolus; contrast enhancement CT or angiographic studies can confirm the vascular nature of the SPN.

EVALUATION OF THE PATIENT WITH A SOLITARY PULMONARY NODULE

HISTORY

- Age of the patient is most important. Only 1 to 3% of SPNs are malignant in patients 35 years of age or younger. In patients over the age of 50 years, approximately 50% of SPNs are malignant, and the incidence increases with advancing age
- A history of smoking markedly increases the possibility that the SPN is malignant
- Acute respiratory symptoms may suggest the presence of an inflammatory process
- A granuloma is more common in an immunocompromised host
- Symptoms or other findings related to another organ system suggest the possibility of a primary tumor in a site other than the lung
- Hemoptysis is unusual with an SPN and suggests the possibility of a radiographically unidentified endobronchial lesion
- A history of a previous malignancy raises the possibility that the SPN is a solitary metastasis or a new primary lung tumor
- An SPN in an asymptomatic patient negates an extensive search for an occult primary tumor. The incidence of an SPN representing a metastasis from a truly occult tumor is less than 0.5%

PHYSICAL EXAMINATION

Examination of the thorax should be complete to rule out the possibility that the observed radiographic mass is a skin or readily palpated bone or soft tissue tumor. The supraclavicular fossa should be evaluated for the presence of cervical lymphadenopathy. The thyroid, breasts, prostate, and testes should be examined for the presence of an asymptomatic mass.

SPUTUM CYTOLOGY AND SKIN TESTS

Sputum cytology may be obtained but is only infrequently positive for tumor (<5%) in a malignant SPN. When positive, the cytologic cell type may agree with the final histologic diagnosis in 85 to 90% of cases.

Skin tests for tuberculous or fungal infections are of little or no value in evaluating an SPN. At best, if negative, they render the diagnosis of a specific granuloma unlikely. A positive skin test has no relevant value in the management of the patient.

RADIOGRAPHIC STUDIES

Standard Radiographic Studies

If the SPN possibly could represent a nipple shadow, nipple markers with repeat radiographs should be obtained. When the SPN is indistinct, radiographs in other positions (lordotic, oblique views) may be helpful. The

SPN should be examined for features highly suggestive of malignancy or benignancy, and any chest x-rays taken should be compared with available previous chest x-rays. When the nature of the SPN can be determined with reasonable certainty at this point, a therapeutic decision can be made. The indeterminate nodule requires further evaluation.

The pulmonary hilar and mediastinal shadows should be critically examined. If both these areas are normal, CT evaluation of the mediastinum for the presence of enlarged nodes is unnecessary.

Conventional Tomography

The indeterminate SPNs should be evaluated by conventional tomography guided by appropriate location by low kV fluoroscopy. If characteristic benign calcification or a linear shape (scar) is present, the SPN may be considered benign. If neither of these features is present, the SPN remains indeterminate.

Computed Tomography

The remaining indeterminate SPNs should be evaluated by standard CT (8- to 10-mm sections), high resolution tomography (2- to 5-mm sections), or by CT densitometry.

Standard Computed Tomography

Standard CT is recommended for

- Patients with an extrathoracic primary tumor
- Presence of abnormal or obscured hilar or mediastinal shadows
- Indeterminate SPNs larger than 2 cm in size

Patients with a previous history of a metachronous primary tumor or a synchronous primary tumor outside the chest should be evaluated to determine the presence of multiple lesions. Multiple lesions are identified by CT in 45% of such patients; 80% of these are metastatic nodules (the others are small benign granulomas or small intrapulmonary lymph nodes).

In patients with an associated abnormal or obscured hilar or mediastinal shadows, CT permits investigation of the mediastinum for the presence of enlarged lymph nodes as further examination of the nodule.

High-Resolution CT and Densitometry

- Permits identification of unsuspected calcification within a benign SPN that may have been undetected by previous examinations
- Calcification must be distributed in what has been described as a benign pattern
- Particular caution is necessary in interpreting the calcifications in a lesion in a patient with a known extrathoracic malignant tumor because some of these may be calcified

- When calcification is not visually evident, the density of the lesion should be compared with a reference densitometry phantom

Despite these radiographic studies, some SPNs will remain indeterminate. Additional diagnostic studies should be used in a selective manner to resolve the nature of the lesion. Thoracotomy may be the final diagnostic procedure.

BRONCHOSCOPIC EXAMINATION

Bronchoscopic evaluation with transbronchoscopic biopsy or aspiration of an SPN of the size defined ($\leq$ 3 cm) is not indicated as a separate procedure. Results are positive in fewer than 20% of the patients with malignant nodules. This evaluation may be considered in larger lesions (>3 cm), but otherwise the bronchoscopic examination of the tracheobronchial tree need be done only at the time of operation if one is indicated.

TRANSTHORACIC FINE-NEEDLE ASPIRATION BIOPSY

Routine Fine-Needle Aspiration

Routine fine-needle aspiration of an SPN is not needed to prove a preoperative diagnosis in nodules believed to be malignant. The argument that the SPN may represent a small cell carcinoma and that this procedure would rule out a resection is not valid. Recent reports from North America, Europe, and Japan have shown that excellent results can be obtained by primary resection of stage I small cell tumors followed by aggressive chemotherapy; projected 62 to 73% 5-year survival rates have been reported. The rare occurrence of development of tumor in the needle tract after a fine-needle aspiration of a malignant SPN has been recorded, thus further negating the unnecessary routine use of the procedure.

Aspiration performed to attempt to establish a benign diagnosis in the indeterminate SPN is controversial. Although some authors report that benignancy can be established in 85% of truly benign lesions, several reports have emphasized a false-negative yield (the lesion subsequently proved to be malignant) in as many as 30 to 35% of indeterminate SPNs diagnosed as not being malignant.

Selective Fine-Needle Aspiration

A fine-needle biopsy may be justified in a few clinical settings.

Indications

- Patient's refusal of a recommendation for operation: Patient refuses resection of an SPN unless a preoperative diagnosis of tumor is established or desires some other therapeutic (radiation therapy) management
- Medical condition precludes operative intervention: The presence of insufficient pulmonary function, noncorrectable cardiac contraindications, or a recent myocardial infarction carry a prohibitive operative risk. When

a diagnosis of malignancy is obtained, other therapy may be recommended

- Suspected hamartoma: Indicated if the appearance is suggestive of a hamartoma but neither calcification nor fatty tissue is identified on high-resolution computed tomography. Although often attended with an increased risk of postoperative pneumothorax, conformation of diagnosis negates an unnecessary thoracotomy
- Immunocompromised patient: Indicated when attempting to identify a specific opportunistic inflammatory process, such as cryptococcus or an atypical mycobacterial or fungal infection
- Patient with a previous malignant melanoma: Rules out the remote possibility of a secondary primary lung tumor that should be resected. If a benign lesion is identified, the resection is not indicated because its removal has little or no influence on the subsequent longevity of the patient. Removal of a metastatic melanoma is controversial

METASTATIC EVALUATION

A "metastatic" evaluation (brain, upper abdominal, and bone scans) is contraindicated in the asymptomatic patient with an SPN. The rate of discovery of an occult metastasis is too small (1 to 3%) to justify the "metastatic" evaluation.

VIDEO-ASSISTED THORACOSCOPIC REMOVAL

The video-assisted surgical resection of a peripherally located small (<2 cm) indeterminate SPN has become the procedure of choice for diagnosis. Although techniques have been described for the resection of more centrally located SPN deep within the lung substance, such lesions are best resected by an open thoracotomy.

THORACOTOMY

The ultimate diagnostic procedure is thoracotomy with resection of the indeterminate SPN. With the appropriate preoperative evaluation, no more than 25 to 35% of the resected SPNs should be benign; the other SPNs are malignant tumors.

OTHER DIAGNOSTIC OPTIONS

Artificial Intelligence

Computer-aided diagnosis of an SPN by discriminant analyses or based on the use of the Bayesian theorem has been reported to be useful. The data in these studies, however, are unique to the given institutional study pattern and are not applicable to all situations. Refinement of such analyses may result in wide applicability for all patients in the future.

Period of "Watchful Waiting"

The periodic observation of an indeterminate SPN by serial chest x-rays to determine whether the nodule is growing at a malignant rate is unacceptable in most situations. The exceptions are an SPN in patients under the age of 35 years who have never smoked cigarettes, SPNs discovered in association with an acute lower respiratory infection, and SPNs less than 1 cm in size (with a well-defined, smooth border) in nonsmokers who are high operative risks because of concurrent cardiac, pulmonary, or other life-threatening comorbid conditions.

RECOMMENDED PLAN OF MANAGEMENT

Several optional courses can be taken in the management of the patient with an asymptomatic SPN. The selection of one over another depends on the age of the patient, the availability of previous chest x-rays, the radiographic characteristics of the nodule, and a history or the presence of a primary extrathoracic malignancy.

AGE OF PATIENT

In patients under the age of 35 years, a period of observation is justified unless the radiographic characteristics strongly support a presumptive diagnosis of tumor (large size, spiculated or markedly ill-defined borders, and the absence of calcification or fatty tissue). Radiographs should be obtained at 3-month intervals for a least 2 years. If growth is observed, transthoracic fine-needle biopsy may be justified to establish a diagnosis. If tumor is present or the diagnosis remains in doubt, video-assisted surgical resection or thoracotomy is indicated.

AVAILABILITY OF PREVIOUS CHEST X-RAYS OR DOUBLING TIME

If previous chest x-rays reveal no growth over a 2-year period or if more recent films show a rapid doubling time (<30 days) or slow growth (>465 days), the lesion may be considered benign and should be observed at periodic intervals. If the doubling time falls between these two extremes, further radiographic evaluation of the SPN is indicated.

NONAVAILABILITY OF PREVIOUS CHEST X-RAYS OR INDETERMINATE DOUBLING TIME

If the SPN is noncalcified on the standard radiographic views, fluoroscopic evaluation and conventional tomography should be done to identify any typically benign pattern of calcification within the nodule. A linear benign shape of the mass may also be discerned by this examination. If neither is demonstrated, standard or high-resolution CT should be carried out to identify any "typical" calcification pattern or the presence of fatty tissue within the mass. A pulmonary arteriovenous malformation may be identified by its vascular connections, as well as by their pattern of enhancement on dynamic CT imaging. If none of these features is present, CT densitometry should be obtained. If the lesion can be presumed to be benign by any of these studies, periodic radiographic re-evaluation of the mass can be recommended. If the nodule remains "indeterminate," thoracotomy and resection should be carried out.

SYNCHRONOUS OR METACHRONOUS PRIMARY EXTRATHORACIC MALIGNANCY

The approach to a patient with an SPN who has a history of a previous extrathoracic neoplasm or in whom the SPN was discovered at the time of evaluation should be tailored to the type and site of the extrathoracic primary tumor and to the clinical situation existing at the time of the discovery of the SPN.

Clinical Status of Patient

The extrathoracic tumor must be controlled or controllable locally, and no evidence of metastases to other sites should be present or detectable. The potential sites of other metastatic involvement vary with the type of original primary tumor and must be appropriately evaluated. For example, a patient with breast or prostatic cancer should have a radionuclide bone scan, and a patient with colon carcinoma should have an abdominal CT study to evaluate the liver and the local site of resection to rule out recurrence. If available, tumor markers (alpha-fetoprotein and human chorionic gonadotropin levels for patients with nonseminomatous testicular tumors, acid phosphatase in a patient with prostatic cancer) should be obtained. Radioactive iodine uptake study should be done in a patient with a previous thyroid carcinoma. If any of these studies is positive, resection is best delayed, and the patient should be managed with chemotherapy, hormonal therapy, or irradiation (radioactive I^{131}) as indicated.

Radiographic Evaluation

All potential surgical patients should undergo conventional CT of the chest for evaluation of the presence of multiple nodules. When multiple nodules are present, the lesions can be assumed to be metastatic. The management of multiple pulmonary metastases is not germane to this presentation.

If the nodule is solitary, high-resolution CT for the possible establishment of benignancy of the nodule is indicated. If a criterion for benignancy is not met, prompt resection is indicated.

Cell Type of Original Primary Tumor

All potential solitary metastases, with the exceptions previously noted, should be resected. Some authors have questioned the efficacy of this procedure in actually improving the patient's ultimate prognosis. This question is unanswerable. The most compelling reason for resecting an SPN in patients with a previous squamous cell primary tumor is that the SPN most often represents a new primary lung cancer; in patients with a previous adenocarcinoma, the possibility is 50%. In patients with a previous sarcoma, on the other hand, the SPN rarely represents a primary lung cancer.

PROGNOSIS

RADIOGRAPHIC OBSERVATION

Solitary nodules that have met the radiographic or at times the cytologic criteria of benignancy should be observed periodically over a period of time because these lesions rarely eventually prove to be malignant. The prognosis is near 100% for long-term survival in these patients.

Prospective observation for growth of small lesions is to be condemned except in nonsmoking patients under the age of 35 years or in those whose clinical condition or personal beliefs negate resection. Watchful waiting, which may permit the growth of a lung cancer, increases the likelihood of locoregional and distant metastasis. An increased size of a malignant SPN also has an unfavorable effect on the patient's prognosis.

SURGICAL RESECTION

Benign Nodule

The prognosis after resection is excellent.

Primary Lung Tumor

The resection of a primary malignant SPN of the lung results in an overall 60 to 70% 5-year survival. The smaller the lesion, the better the prognosis. Nodules smaller than 1 cm have an 80% long-term survival rate, those between 1 and 2 cm have a 74% rate, and those larger than 2 cm have a 51% survival rate.

Metastatic Malignant Solitary Pulmonary Nodule

The resection of a solitary pulmonary metastasis results in overall long-term survival rates of 20 to 30%.

BIBLIOGRAPHY

Aberg T, Malmberg KA, Nilsson B, Nou E: The effect of metastasectomy: fact or fiction? Ann Thorac Surg, *30*:378, 1980.

Albain KS, Crowley JJ, Livingston RB: Long-term survival and toxicity in small cell lung cancer. Chest, *99*:1425, 1991.

Albertucci M, DeMeester TR, Rothberg M, et al: Surgery and the management of peripheral lung tumor adherent to the parietal pleura. J Thorac Cardiovasc Surg, *103*:8–13, 1992.

Armstrong JG, Minski, BD: Radiation therapy for medically inoperable stage I and II non-small cell lung cancer. Cancer Treat Rev, *16*:247, 1989.

Arroliga AC, Buzaid AC, Matthay RA: Which patients can safely undergo lung resection. J Respir Dis, *12*:1080–1086, 1991.

Backer CL, Shields TW, Lockhart CG, et al: Selective preoperative evaluation for possible N2 disease in carcinoma of the lung. J Thorac Cardiovasc Surg, 93:337, 1987.

Black WC, Armstrong P, Daniel TM: Cost effectiveness of chest CT in T1N0M0 lung cancer. Radiology, 167:373, 1988.

Bleyer WA: Hobson's choice in CNS radioprophylaxis of small cell lung cancer (editorial). Int J Radiat Oncol Biol Phys, 15:783, 1988.

Bourguet P, Dazord L, Desrues B, et al: Immunoscintigraphy of human lung squamous cell carcinoma using an iodine-131 labelled monoclonal antibody (P066). Br J Cancer, 61:230, 1990.

Buhr J, Berghauser KH, Moor H, et al.: Tumor cells in intraoperative pleural lavage. An indicator for the poor prognosis of bronchogenic carcinoma. Cancer, 65:1801, 1990.

Burt M, Wronski M, Arbit E, et al: Resection of brain metastases from non-small cell lung carcinoma. Results of therapy. J Thorac Cardiovasc Surg, 103:399–441, 1992.

Calhoun P, Feldman PS, Armstrong P, et al: The clinical outcome of needle aspiration of the lung when cancer is not diagnosed. Ann Thorac Surg, 41:592, 1986.

Casey JJ, Stempel BG, Scanlon EF, Fry WA: The solitary pulmonary nodule in the patient with breast cancer. Surgery, 96:801, 1984.

Caskey CL, Templeton PA, Zerhouni EA: Current evaluation of the solitary pulmonary nodule. Radiol Clin North Am, 28:511, 1990.

Chang AE, Schaner EG, Conkle DM, et al: Evaluation of computed tomography in the detection of pulmonary metastases. Cancer, 43:913, 1979.

Cooper JD, Pearson FG, Todd TRJ, et al: Radiotherapy alone for patients with operable carcinoma of the lung. Chest, 87:289, 1985.

Coppage L, Shaw C, Curtis AM: Metastatic disease to the chest in patients with extrathoracic malignancy. J Thorac Imaging, 2:24, 1987.

Cortese DA: Endobronchial management of lung cancer. Chest, 89:234S, 1986.

Cummings SR, Lillington GA, Richard RJ: Estimating the probability of malignancy in solitary pulmonary nodules: A Bayesian approach. Am Rev Respir Dis, 134:449, 1986.

Cummings, SR, Lillington GA, Richard RJ: Managing solitary pulmonary nodules. The choice of strategy is a "close call." Am Rev Respir Dis, 134:453, 1986.

Curran WJ Jr, Stafford PM: Lack of apparent difference in outcome between clinically staged IIIA and IIIB non-small cell lung cancer treated with radiation therapy. J Clin Oncol, 8:409, 1990.

Dales RE, Stark RM, Raman S: Computed tomography to stage lung cancer. Approaching a controversy using meta-analysis. Am Rev Respir Dis, 141:1096, 1990.

Deschamps C, Pairolero PC, Trastek VF, et al: Multiple primary lung cancers: results of surgical treatment. J Thorac Cardiovasc Surg, 99:769, 1990.

Deslauriers J, Brisson J, Cartier R, et al: Carcinoma of the lung: evaluation of satellite nodules as a factor in influencing prognosis after resection. J Thorac Cardiovasc Surg, 97:504, 1989.

Diggs CH, Engler JE, Prendergast EJ, Kramer K: Small cell carcinoma of the lung. Treatment in the community. Cancer, 69:2075–2083, 1992.

Eagan RT, Rund C, Lee RE, et al: Pilot study of induction therapy with cyclophosphamide, doxorubicin, and cisplatin (CAP) and chest irradiation prior to thoracotomy in initially inoperable stage III MO non-small cell lung cancer. Cancer Treat Rep, 71:895, 1987.

Edell ES, Cortese DA: Bronchoscopic phototherapy with hematoporphyrin derivative for treatment of localized bronchogenic carcinoma: a 5-year experience. Mayo Clin Proc, 62:8, 1987.

Edwards FH, Schaefer PS, Cohen AJ, et al: Use of artificial intelligence for preoperative diagnosis of pulmonary lesions. Ann Thorac Surg, 48:556, 1989.

Feinstein AR, Wells CK: A clinical-severity staging system for patients with lung cancer. Medicine (Baltimore), 69:1, 1990.

Feld R, Ginsberg RJ, Payne DG: Treatment of small cell lung cancer. *In* Thoracic Oncology. Edited by JA Roth, JC Ruckdeschel, TH Weisenburger. Philadelphia, WB Saunders, 1989.

Glazer HS, Kaiser LR, Anderson DJ, et al: Indeterminate mediastinal invasion in bronchogenic carcinoma: CT evaluation. Radiology, 173:37, 1989.

Goldstein MS, Rush M, Johnson P, Sprung CL: A calcified adenocarcinoma of the lung with very high CT numbers. Radiology, *150*:785, 1984.

Goldstraw P: The practice of cardiothracic surgeons in the perioperative staging of non-small cell lung cancer. Thorax, *47*:1–2, 1992.

Gross DH, Glazer GM, Orringer MB, et al: Bronchogenic carcinoma metastatic to normal-sized lymph nodes: frequency and significance. Radiology, *166*:71, 1988.

Harpole DH Jr, Johnson CM, Wolf WG, et al: Analysis of 945 cases of pulmonary metastatic melanoma. J Thorac Cardiovasc Surg, *103*:743–750, 1992.

Harrow EM, Oldenburg FA, Lingenfelter MS, Smith AM Jr: Transbronchial needle aspiration in clinical practice. A five-year experience. Chest, *96*:1268, 1989.

Heavey LR, Glazer GM, Gross BH, et al: The role of CT in staging radiographic T1N0M0 lung cancer. AJR, *146*:285, 1986.

Huston J III, Muhm JR: Solitary pulmonary nodule evaluation with a CT reference phantom. Radiology, *163*:481, 1987.

Huston J III, Muhm JR: Solitary pulmonary nodule evaluation with a CT reference phantom. Radiology, *170*:653, 1989.

Ichinose Y, Hara N, Ohta M, et al: Preoperative examination to detect metastasis is not advocated for asymptomatic patients with stages I and II non-small cell lung cancer. Preoperative examination for lung cancer. Chest, *96*:1104, 1989.

Ichinose Y, Hara N, Ohta M, et al: Brain metastases in patients with limited small cell lung cancer achieving complete remission. Correlation with TNM staging. Chest, *96*:1332, 1989.

Ishida T, Yokoyama H, Kaneko S, et al: Long-term results of operation for non-small cell lung cancer in the elderly. Ann Thorac Surg, *50*:919, 1990.

Israel RH, Poe RH: The solitary pulmonary nodule: What to do, and why. J Respir Dis 13: 308–318, 1992.

Johnson BE, Becker B, Goff WB III, et al: Neurologic, neuropsychologic, and computed cranial tomography scan abnormalities in 2- to 10-year survivors of small cell lung cancer. J Clin Oncol, *3*:1659, 1985.

Johnson DH, Einhorn LH, Bartolucci A, et al: Thoracic radiotherapy does not prolong survival in patients with locally advanced, unresectable non-small cell lung cancer. Ann Intern Med, *113*:33, 1990.

Karnofsky DA, Burchenal JH: The clinical evaluation of chemotherapeutic agents in cancer. *In* Evaluation of Chemotherapeutic Agents. Edited by CM McLeod. New York, Columbia University Press, 1949.

Karrer K, Shields TW, Denk H, et al: The importance of surgical and multimodality treatment for small cell bronchial carcinoma. J Thorac Cardiovasc Surg, *97*:168, 1989.

Kerrigan DC, Spence PA, Crittenden MC, Tripp MD: Methylene blue guidance for simplified resection of a lung lesion. Ann Thorac Surg, *53*:163–164, 1992.

Khouri NF, Meziane MA, Zerhouni EA, et al: The solitary pulmonary nodule. Assessment, diagnosis, and management. Chest, *91*:128, 1987.

Klastersky J, Feld R, Kleisbauer JP, Rocmans P: Treatment of N2 non-small cell lung cancer (NSCLC). Chest, *96*(Suppl):835, 1989.

Klein JS, Webb WR: The radiologic staging of lung cancer. J Thorac Imag, *7*:29–47, 1991.

Kormas P, Bradshaw JR, Jeyasingham K: Preoperative computed tomography of the brain in non-small cell bronchial carcinoma. Thorax, *47*:106–108, 1992.

Kreisman H, Wolkove N, Quoix E: Small cell lung cancer presenting as a solitary pulmonary nodule. Chest, *101*:225–231, 1992.

Kuhlman JE, Fishman EK, Kuhajda FP, et al: Solitary bronchioloalveolar carcinoma: CT criteria. Radiology, *167*:379, 1988.

Lad T, Rubinstein L, Sadeghi A: The benefit of adjuvant treatment for resected locally advanced non-small cell lung cancer. J Clin Oncol, *6*:9, 1988.

Landreneau RJ, Hazelring SR, Ferson PF, et al: Thoracoscopic resection of 52 pulmonary lesions. Presented at the 28th Annual Meeting of the Society of Thoracic Surgeons, Orlando FL, February 4, 1992. (To be published in Ann Thorac Surg)

Landreneau RJ, Herlan DB, Johnson JA, et al: Thoracoscopic neodymium: yittrium-aluminum garnet laser-assisted pulmonary resection. Ann Thorac Surg, 52:1176–1178, 1991.

Lauer RC, Fleck JF, Antony A, Einhorn LH: Is prophylactic cranial irradiation indicated in small cell lung cancer? *In* Proceedings of the American Society of Clinical Oncology (New Orleans). Vol. 7. Philadelphia, WB Saunders, 1988.

Lewis RJ, Caccavale RJ, Sisler GE: Video assisted thoracic surgical resection of malignant lung tumors. Presented at 72nd Annual Meeting of the American Association for Thoracic Surgery, Los Angeles CA, April 27, 1992. (To be published in J Thorac Cardiovasc Surg)

Little AG, Stitik FP: Clinical staging of patients with non-small cell lung cancer. Chest, 97: 1431, 1990.

Mack MJ, Gordon MJ, Postma TW, et al: Percutaneous localization of pulmonary nodule for thoracoscopic lung resection. Ann Thorac Surg, 53:1123–1124, 1992.

Magilligan DJ Jr, Duvernoy BS, Malik G, et al: Surgical approach to lung cancer with solitary cerebral metastasis: twenty-five years' experience. Ann Thorac Surg, 42:360, 1986.

Mathisen DJ, Grillo HC: Carinal resection for lung cancer. (To be published in J Thorac Cardiovasc Surg).

Miller JD, Gorenstein LA, Patterson A: Staging: The key to rational management of lung cancer. Ann Thorac Surg, 53:170–178, 1992.

Mills SE, Cooper PH, Walker AN, Kron IL: Atypical carcinoid of the lung: a clincopathologic study of 17 cases. Am J Surg Pathol, 6:643, 1982.

Mountain CF: A new international staging system for lung cancer. Chest, 89(Suppl):225S, 1986.

Murren JR, Buzaid AC, Hait EH: Critical analysis of neoadjuvant therapy for stage IIIA non-small cell lung cancer. Am Rev Respir Dis, 143:889, 1991.

Nathan MH, Collins VP, Adams RA: Differentiation of benign and malignant nodules by growth rate. Radiology, 79:321, 1962.

Naunheim KS, Kesler KA, D'Orazio SA: Thoracotomy in the octogenarian. Ann Thorac Surg 51:547–551, 1991.

Neff TA: The science and humanity of the solitary pulmonary nodule. Am Rev Respir Dis, 134:433, 1986.

Okumura M, Ohshima S, Kotake Y, et al: Intraoperative pleural lavage cytology in lung cancer patients. Ann Thorac Surg, 51:599, 1991.

Payne WS, Bernatz, PE, Pairolera PE, et al: Localization and treatment of radiographically occult lung cancer. *In* Lung Cancer. Edited by NC Delarue, H Eschapasse. Philadelphia, WB Saunders, 1985.

Penketh AR, Robinson AA, Barber V, Flower CD: Use of percutaneous needle biopsy in the investigation of solitary pulmonary nodules. Thorax, 42:967, 1987.

Pogrebniak HW, Strovroff M, Roth JA, Pass HI: Resection of pulmonary metastasis from malignant melanoma: Results of a 16 year experience. Ann Thorac Surg, 46:20, 1988.

Read RC, Schaefer RF, North W, Walls R: Diameter, cell type and survival in stage I primary non-small cell lung cancer. Arch Surg, 123:446, 1988.

Reed JG, Rubin SA, Schnodig VJ: Interventional procedures used for diagnosing and treating lung cancer. J Thorac Imag, 7:48–56, 1991.

Rosengart TK, Martini N, Ghosn P, Burt M: Multiple primary lung carcinomas: prognosis and treatment. Ann Thorac Surg, 52:772–779, 1991.

Rotte KH, Meiske W: Results of computer-aided diagnosis of peripheral bronchial carcinoma. Radiology, 125:583, 1977.

Schenk DA, Strollo PI, Pichard JS, et al: Utility of the Wang 18-gauge transbronchial histology needle in the staging of bronchogenic carcinoma. Chest, 96:272, 1989.

Schulten M, Heiskell CA, Shields TW: The incidence of solitary pulmonary metastasis from carcinoma of the large bowel. Surg Gynecol Obstet, 143:727, 1976.

Seyfer AE, Walsh DS, Graeber GM, et al: Chest wall implantation of lung cancer after thin-needle aspiration biopsy. Ann Thorac Surg, 48:284, 1989.

Shepherd FA, Evans WK, Feld R, et al: Adjuvant chemotherapy following surgical resection for small-cell carcinoma of the lung. J Clin Oncol, 6:832, 1988.

Shepherd FA, Ginsberg RJ, Patterson A, et al: A prospective study of adjuvant surgery after chemotherapy for limited small cell lung cancer. A University of Toronto Lung Oncology Group Study. J Thorac Cardiovasc Surg, 97:177, 1989.

Shepherd FA, Laskey J, Evans WK, et al: Cushing's syndrome associated with ectopic corticotropin production and small cell lung cancer. J Clin Oncol, 10:21–27, 1992.

Shields TW: The use of mediastinoscopy in lung cancer: the dilemma of mediastinal lymph nodes. *In* Current Controversies in Thoracic Surgery. Edited by CF Kittle. Philadelphia, WB Saunders, 1986.

Shields TW: The "incomplete" resection. Ann Thorac Surg, 47:487, 1989.

Shields TW: Behavior of small bronchial carcinomas. Ann Thorac Surg, 50:691, 1990.

Shields TW: The significance of ipsilateral mediastinal lymph node metastasis (N2 disease) in non-small cell carcinoma of the lung. A commentary. J Thorac Cardiovasc Surg, 99:48, 1990.

Shields TW: Mediastinal Surgery. Philadelphia, Lea & Febiger, 1991.

Shirakusa T, Tsutsui M, Iriki N, et al: Results of resection for bronchogenic carcinoma in patients over the age of 80. Thorax, 44:189, 1989.

Siegelman SS, Khouri NF, Scott WW Jr, et al: Pulmonary hamartoma: CT findings. Radiology, 160:313, 1986.

Siegelman SS, Zerhouni EA, Leo FP, et al: CT of the solitary pulmonary nodule. AJR, 135:1, 1980.

Stewart JG, MacMahon H, Vyborny CJ, Pollak ER: Dystrophic calcification in carcinoma of the lung: demonstration by CT. AJR, 148:29, 1987.

Sugio K, Ishida T, Kaneko S, et al: Surgically resected lung cancer in young adults. Ann Thorac Surg, 53:127–131, 1992.

Talton B, Constable W, Kersh C: Curative radiotherapy in non-small cell carcinoma of the lung. Int J Radiol Oncol Biol Phys, 19:15–21, 1990.

Van Houtte P, Rocmans P, Smets P, et al: Postoperative radiation therapy in lung cancer: a controlled trial after resection of curative design. Int J Radiat Oncol Biol Phys, 6:983, 1980.

Vokes EE, Bitran JD, Vogelzang NJ: Chemotherapy for non-small cell lung cancer. The continuing challenge. (Editorial). Chest, 99:1326, 1991.

Warren WH, Faber LP, Gould VE: Neuroendocrine neoplasms of the lung. A clinicopathologic update. J Thorac Cardiovasc Surg, 98:321, 1989.

Webb WR: The role of magnetic resonance imaging in the assessment of patients with lung cancer: a comparison with computed tomography. J Thorac Imaging, 4:65, 1989.

Wilkins EW, Grillo HC, Moncure AC, Scannel JG: Changing times and surgical management of bronchopulmonary carcinoid tumors. Ann Thorac Surg, 38:339, 1984.

Winning AJ, McIvor J, Seed WA, et al: Interpretation of negative results in fine needle aspiration of discrete pulmonary lesions. Thorax, 41:875, 1986.

Wolfe WG, Sabiston DC Jr: Management of benign and malignant lesions of the trachea and bronchi with the neodymium-yttrium-aluminum-garnet laser. J Thorac Cardiovasc Surg, 91:40, 1986.

Yashar J, Weitberg AB, Glicksman AS, et al: Preoperative chemotherapy and radiation therapy for Stage IIIa non-small cell carcinoma of the lung. Ann Thorac Surg, 53:440–444, 1992.

Zerhouni EA, Boukadoum M, Siddiky MA, et al: Standard phantom for quantitative CT analysis of pulmonary nodules. Radiology, 194:767, 1983.

Zrhouni EA, Stitik FP, Siegelman SS, et al: Computed tomography of the pulmonary nodule: A national cooperative study. Radiology, 160:319, 1986.

Zhang H, Yin W, Zhang L, et al: Curative radiotherapy of early operable non-small cell lung cancer. Radiother Oncol, 14:89–94, 1989.

INDEX

Page numbers in *italics* indicate illustrations; numbers followed by "t" indicate tables.

943